The New Our Bodies, Ourselves

A BOOK BY AND FOR WOMEN

Preface by Byllye Avery, Helen Rodriguez-Trias and Gloria Steinem

The Boston Women's Health Book Collective

A TOUCHSTONE BOOK
Published by Simon & Schuster
New York London Toronto Sydney Tokyo Singapore

TOUCHSTONE
Rockefeller Center
1230 Avenue of the Americas
New York, NY 10020

Designed by Barbara Marks

Manufactured in the United States of America

10 9 8 7 6 5 4 3 2

Library of Congress Cataloging in Publication Data

The New our bodies, ourselves : a book by and for women / Boston
    Women's Health Book Collective.
        p. cm.
    "A Touchstone book."
    Includes bibliographical references and index.
    1. Women—Health and hygiene. 2. Women—Diseases. 3. Women—
Psychology. I. Boston Women's Health Book Collective.
RA778.N67 1992
613'.04244—dc20   92-1627
                              CIP
ISBN: 0-684-82352-7

Special Acknowledgments

1992 Update coordinated by Amy Alpern, Leah Diskin and Judy Norsigian, with Rachel Lanzerotti, Wendy Sanford, Norma Swenson, Laura Weil and Laurie Williams.

1992 Library Staff: Jamie Penney, Brenda Reeb, Sally Whelan.

Other Staff: Judy Norsigian, Susan Quass, Esther Rome, Norma Swenson, Laurie Williams.

1984 Edition:

Editors and Midwives:
Jane Pincus and Wendy Sanford worked with each writer to help give the book shape, clarity and unity. In the editing process, they shortened and wrote and/or rewrote parts of every chapter.

Project Coordinators:
Nancy Hawley and Wendy Sanford kept in their minds all the people, tasks and stages of this project in the three years from the initial negotiations to the final production of the book.

Resource Coordinators:
Pamela Morgan and Judy Norsigian fielded every possible question, sending us to the appropriate resources in order to make the new book as informative and accurate as possible.

Special thanks to:
Ann Godoff, our editor, whose persistence, patience and tactful advocacy pulled us through the last stages of this labor;

Ruth Hubbard, who, red pencil in hand, clarified the language of nearly every chapter in the book;

Jo Polk-Matthews, who relayed many of the chapters to thoughtful outside readers and made sure we got the comments and criticisms we needed;

Gina Prenowitz, who cast her careful eye on the language and politics of important sections of the book;

Nancy Schlick, whose copyediting was respectful, attentive and wonderfully intelligent;

Catherine Shaw, who was an eager, enthusiastic and patient reader of the sprawling first manuscript;

Irv Zola, who had the pleasure of reading and carefully criticizing all our most problematic chapters, and whose advice never failed to be right on the mark;

Our families, lovers and housemates, who lived with us, fed us, complained and loved us anyway and soundly rejoiced when the project was complete.

Sue Ade	Agnes Norsigian
Davida Andelman	Kyra Zola Norsigian
Polly Attwood	Roy Norsigian
Alan Berger	Julia Perez
Laurel Berger	Ben Pincus
Noah Berger	Ed Pincus
Belle Brett	Sami Pincus
Abraham Brown	Minrose Quinn
Ethel Brown	Judah Rome
Robert S. Cohen	Micah Rome
Trudy Cox	Nathan Rome
Aaron Diskin	Alan Rosen
Leah Diskin	Megan Crowe-Rothstein
Martin Diskin	Natalie Rothstein
Bruce Ditzion	Peter Rothstein
Robbie Ditzion	Daniel Salk
Sammy Ditzion	Nikki Salk
Benjamin Doress	Stephen Salk
Hannah Doress	Toni Sandmaier
Caitlin Fisher	Matthew Sanford
Dan Fisher	Cheryl Schaffer
Philip Hart	Jeremy Schwartz
Gina Hawley	Dan Sipe
Josh Hawley	John Swenson
Vilma Hunt	Sarah Swenson
Kathryn Jewell	David Wegman
Patrice Keegan	Jesse Wegman
Cheryl Kennedy	Marya Wegman
Philip Kraft	Alexi Wolf
Nancy Lessin	Lea Wolf
Jeffrey McIntyre	Tom Wolf
Noah McIntyre	Allen Worters
Halford Meras	Amanda Zola
Nellie Meras	Warren Zola

General Acknowledgments

Many thanks to the following people for their help:

Bonnie Acker
Lois Alix
Carol Altobelli
Majeeda Amadadeen
Vicky Anderson
Beth Andrews
George Annas
Naomi Armon
Hilde Armour
Harriet Arnoldi
Connie Arsenault
Arthritis and Health
  Resource Center
Gisela Ashley
Diane Austras
Byllye Avery
Tricia Axsom
Diane Balser
Kim Bancroft
David Banta
Faith Nobuko Barcus
Phoebe Barnes
Kathleen Barry
Pauline Bart
Margaret Belbin
Ruth Bell
Riva Berkovitz
Davi Birnbaum
Alice Bonis
Bea Bookchin
Shafia Bossman
Ursula Bowring-Trenn
Pam Boyle
Almont Bracy
Etta Breit
Jan Brin
Linda Brion-Meisels
Steven Brion-Meisels
Kathy Brownback

Agnes Butcher
Norma Canner
Barbara Carmen
Casa Myrna Vasquez
Robin Casarjian
Mary Rae Cate
Susie Chancey
Wendy Chavkin
Donna Cherniac
Cindy Chin
Aram Chobanian
Ann Chronis
Peggy Clark
Savitri Clarke
Yarrow Anne Cleaves
Connie Clement
Cindy Cohen
Deborah Catherine
  Cohen
Nancy Cohen
Robert S. Cohen
Tom Conry
Liz Coolidge
Betty Corpt
Maria Corsaro
Mary Costanza
Terry Courtney
Olivia Cousins
Belita Cowan
Frannye Crocker
Emily Culpepper
John Cutler
Lynne Dahlberg
William Darrow
Martha Davis-Perry
Caro Dellenbaugh
Catherine DeLorey
Debby DeVaughn
Andrew Dibner

Annette Dickinson
Loretta Dixson
Rose Dobosz
Jan Dodds
Karen Dorman
Barbara Dow
Hugh Drummond
Kim Ducharme
Buffy Dunker
Wendy Dunning
Jane Dwinell
Sally Edwards
Susan Eisenberg
Helen Eisenstein
Carol Englander
Judy English
Carol Epple
Samuel S. Epstein
Wendy Roberts Epstein
Kitty Ernst
Tish Fabens
Martha Farrar
Lee Farris
Carolyn Fawcett
Richard Feinbloom
Geri Ferber
Fertility Consciousness
  Group
Cynthia Fertman
Ron Fichtner
JoAnne Fischer
Alice Fisher
Maureen Flammer
Mary Flinders
Becky Fowler
Cary Fowler
Dorothy Frauenhofer
Nancy Friedman
Stella Friml

Rose Frisch
Dana Gallagher
Paula Garbarino
Jean Gardelia
Linda Gardner
Linda Gaynor
Carole Geddis-Dlugasch
Tobin Gerhardt
Lois Gibbs
Paige Gidney
Cheryl Giles
Betty Gittes
Evelyn Gladu of Omega,
  Somerville, Mass.
Leonard Glantz
Pat Gold
Meg Goldman
Arnold A. Goldstein
Sharon Golub
Mary Moore Goodlett
Jennifer Gordon
Jocelyn Gordon
Ruth Gore and the
  Goldennaires, Freedom
  House, Roxbury, Mass.
Benina Gould
Gray Panthers
Meryl Green
Tova Green
Miriam Greenspan
Betsy Grob
Ione Gunnerson
Joan Gussow
Cynthia Hales
Diana Long Hall
Eleanor Hamilton
Jalna Hanmer
Sandie Harris
Michelle Harrison

GENERAL ACKNOWLEDGMENTS

Pat Haseltine
Robert Hatcher
Marie Hayes
Lester Hazell
Muriel Heiberger
Lori Heise
Ingeborg Helling
Susan Helmrich
Judy Herman
Curdina Hill
Ruth Hill, Black
  Women's Oral History
  Project, Radcliffe
  Institute
Hella Hoffman
Kate Hoffman
Beryl-Elise Hoffstein
Joanne Holt
Barbara Homan
Barbara Horgan
Mary Howell
Jeanne Hubbuch
Maile Hulihan
Suzanne Ingrao
Rick Ingrasci
Jeanne Jackson
Sandy Jaffe
Mary Jane Jarrett
Pat Jerabek
Gail Johnson
Leila Joseph
Myla Kabat-Zinn
Alexandra Kaplan
Peg Kapron
Amy Kasanjian
Linda Katzman
Augusta Kaufman
David Kaufman
Jay Kaufman
Peggy Hershenson
  Kaufman
Lorrie Kendler
Jamie Keshet
Edith Kessler
Nina Kimche
Joanne Klys
Jenny Knaus
Joan Knight
Thurmond Knight
Pat Kraepelian-Bartels
Helen Kramer
Mark Kramer
Karen Kruskal
Ruth Kundsin
Ann LaCasse
Eben LaCasse
Kirsten LaCasse
Marianne LaLuz
Hildegarde Lambrom
Nan Lassin
Nancy Lastoff
Tesair Lauve
Stephen Lester
Maggie Lettvin
Debbie LeVan

Jane Levin
Mitch Levine
Myrna Lewis
Heidi Lewitt
Rinchen Lhamo
Frederick Li
Ricky Lieberman
Bonnie Liebman
Dottie Limont
Lee Lindbert
Liz Linderman
Jessica Lipnak
Judy Lipshutz
Mary Logan
Dylan Loman
Carin Layne Lomon
Susan Love
Barbara Low
Ruth Lubic
Brinton Lykes
Peggy Lynch
Ana Machado de Oliveira
P'nina Macher
Howie Machtinger
Catherine MacKinnon
Una MacLean
Brian MacMahon
Elizabeth MacMahon
Carol Mamber
Elizabeth Markson
Lisa Marlin
Irene Marotta
Caroline Marvin
Eliot Masters
Raquel Matas
Lourdes Mattei
Elizabeth Matz
Charlotte Mayerson
Art Mazer
Katie Mazer
William M. Mazer
Renee Mazon
Maggie McCarthy-Herzig
Bill McCormack
Patty McLean
Martha P. Megee
Jeanne Melvin
Mary Beth Menaker
Barbara Menning
Irma Meridy
Donald Miller
Jean Baker Miller
Miriam Miller
William Minniciello
Denise Minter
Nora Mitchell
Ramona Monteverde
Montreal Health Press
Helen Boulware Moore
Susanne Morgan
Beth Morrison
Marilyn Morrissey
Sonia Muchnick
Charlotte Muller
J. B. Mulligan

Multinational Monitor
  Staff
Sister Angela Murdaugh
Maryann Napoli
Ruth Nelson
Network of Women in
  Trade and Technical
  Jobs
Holly Newman
Marjorie Newman
Louise Newton
Nancy Nichols
Steve Nickerson
Nine-to-Five Health and
  Safety Committee
Barbara Norfleet
Abigail November
Older Women's League
Oral History Project of
  the Cambridge Arts
  Council
Pat O'Reilly
Julie Snow Osherson
Patricia Papernow
Jane Patterson
Cynthia Pearson
Donald Pedicini
Jamie Penney
Jackie Petrillo
Robbie Pfeufer
Connie Phillips
Beatrice Pitcher
Jackie Pitullo
Sara Poli
Jane Porcino
Ruth Porham
Clare Potter
Terri Powell
Abraham Press
Helane Press
Janet Press
Rosellen Primrose
Susan Quass
Kathleen Quinlan
Pat Rackowski
Jill Rakusen
Carolyn Ramsey
Eloise Rathbone-McCuan
Brenda Reeb
Elsie Reethof
Mira Reicher
Margaret Reid
C. J. Reilly
Erica Reitmayer
Susan Rennie
Ulrike Rettig
Susan Reverby
Naomi Ribner
Marcie Richardson
Claudia Richter
Pat Ricker
Virginia Robison
Lisa Rofel
Eva Rooks
Lynn Rosenberg

Anita Rossien
Alice Rothchild
Donna Roux
Alice Ryerson
Alma Sabatini
Pat Sacry
Carol Sakala
Jackie Samson
Linda Sanford
Frank Santora
Miriam Schocken
Cyprienne Schroeppel
Allyson Schwartz
Janet Schwartz
Helen Scott
Mary Scully
Barbara Seaman
Eli Shapiro
Rene Shaw
Susan Shaw
Beth Shearer
Helen Sheingold
Karen Sheingold
Sayre Sheldon
Laurie Shields
Andrea Siani
Sergio Siani
Ben Siegel
Jane Siegel
Diane Siegelman
Sandra Signor
Marge Silver
Phyllis Silverman
Yehudit Silverman
Jane Simmons-Nashinoff
Barbara Sindriglis
Joan Sing
Susan Siroty
Peggy Sloane
Seymour Small
Annette Smith
Barbara Smith
Lee Smith
Mary Smith
Leni Sollinger
Tish Sommers
Ethel Sondik
Heidi Spoerle
Selma Squires
Karen Stamm
Cecilia Stanley
Karen Starr
Judith Stein
Susan Steiner
Sheila Stillman
John Stoeckle
Carol A. Stollar
Sheera Strick
Suzanne Stuart
Jana Suchankova
Edith Bjornson Sunley
Carol Sussman
Judy Sutphen
Kate Swan
Chris Sweeney

GENERAL ACKNOWLEDGMENTS

Cheryl Tabb
Linda Tate
Claire Taylor
Rosemary Taylor
Marsha Tennis
Bernice Thomas
Winnie Thomas
Helen Thornton
Peggy Thurston
Jean Tock
Sally Tom
Barbara Tomaskovic-
  Devey
Donald Tomaskovic-
  Devey
Melinda Tuhus
Trude Turnquist

Kathy Ullman
Stephanie Urdang
Carol Doyle Van
  Valkenburgh
Martha H. Verbrugge
Gretchen Von Mering
Margo Wallach
Lila Wallis
Susan Wanger
Gail Washor-Liebhaver
Barbara Waxman
Michelle Weiner
Joan Caplan Weizer
Phoebe Wells
Laura Wexler
Sally Whelan
Beatrice Whiting

Lillian Whitney
Paul Wiesner
Valerie Wilk
Diane Willow Williams
Fran Wiltsie
Susan Winick
Ann Withorn
Glorianne Wittes
Simon Wittes
Will Wittington
Karen Wolf
Alice Wolfson
Jean Wolhandler
Women of the Boston-
  Area Socialist-Feminist
  Group

WOOSH (Women Organ-
  izing for Occupational
  Safety and Health)
Lisa Yost
Geraldine Zetzel
Jane Sprague Zones

Coordinator of
  photographs:
  Nancy Hawley

1992 Update:
  Laurie Williams

Coordinator of graphics:
  Esther Rome

Contents

Preface to the 25th Anniversary Edition

One of my introductions to the women's health movement came in 1971, from two women—Carol Downer and Lorraine Rothman—in Gainesville, Florida. They came to talk to us about claiming our bodies. After much sharing, we learned for the first time about the demystification of medicine and why it's important for women to understand and be in control of their own bodies. We were intrigued and excited by the thought of taking charge of our reproduction, of having the power to change our lives. We were told that women all over the country were beginning to question their medical care and that people were starting to develop women-specific health information. The Boston Women's Health Book Collective was just such a group, and with their first publication of *Our Bodies, Ourselves*, they showed us an example of women taking health care into their own hands.

This meeting occurred at a turning point in my life. My husband, at age thirty-three, had just suffered a massive heart attack and died. The trauma of this event made me question everything, particularly the medical system and how health information was disseminated. In the early seventies, an awareness of the dangers of high blood pressure was not common knowledge. Although my husband and I were both educated, I with a master's degree and Wesley just four months away from his doctorate, in the end it didn't matter how much education we had. If you don't know how to take care of yourself, you are basically ignorant. I also realized that health information had to be shared within the context of one's life in order for it to produce lifestyle changes.

It was easy for me to be receptive to the words of these women as they talked about the *right* to have medical information and the importance, or even necessity, of active patient participation. Their words were so inspiring that five of us (Judy Levy, Margaret Parrish, Joan Edelson, Betsy Randall-David and I) opened the doors of the Gainesville Women's Health Center (GWHC) in May 1974. This center provided first-trimester abortions and well-woman gynecological services.

The political climate of the seventies encouraged the continual growth of the women's health movement. And at the heart of this activism was the Boston Women's Health Book Collective, which convened the historic conference of 1975 in Boston, with five of us from the GWHC attending. The impact of that conference still resonates today in the hearts and souls of many of us, as it taught us to question the status quo and create a sensitive health care delivery system. In fact, it confirmed my commitment to the women's health movement. In 1978, I cofounded an alternative birthing center, Birthplace, and founded the National Black Women's Health Project in 1981.

Our Bodies, Ourselves is the bible for women's health. Countless women have told me that they consult it before physician visits and after diagnosis and are always comforted by its straightforward, honest approach. I have given away hundreds of copies to all kinds of women, those who can read it openly as well as those who are embarrassed and need to read it privately.

Our Bodies, Ourselves modeled for us the importance of talking about health problems with other women. Most of us participated in the conspiracy of silence. We felt ashamed about our illnesses, and this isolation contributed to further ill health. The truth of the matter is, *Our illness is our business.* Over the years, many of us have learned that we don't need to suffer in silence anymore. We now know that sharing helps us make knowledgeable decisions about our health and our lives.

The women's health movement started health care reform in the seventies. Women spoke out about the lack of health information given, the abuse of medical procedures and the unavailability of safe contraceptives. They said no to the disease approach to natural female processes such as birth and menopause and established the rationale for outpatient surgical procedures. Over the years, we have seen many of the demands of the women's health movement incorporated into standard health care procedure. Since the United States sees itself as the best health care system in the world, we are justified in making sure it lives up to its reputation.

Our Bodies, Ourselves has served as a way for women, across ethnic, racial, religious and geographical boundaries, to start examining their health from a perspective that will bring about change. The change begins with the individual, who then brings about effective community change. The struggle continues. *La lucha continua.*

Byllye Avery

In 1970, a young woman training to become a pediatrician gave me a copy of a book by women and about women, printed on newspaper stock and cheaply bound. I was forty-one and just beginning to heal from a traumatic few years of a disastrous marriage. I had just arrived from Puerto Rico and was struggling to find my identity as a Puerto Rican professional and a single mother in New York City. When I read that first edition, titled *Women and Their Bodies*, I felt a surge of joy. The authors spoke to me as if I had been part of their discussion group.

This incredibly talented group of women, initially meeting about their frustration with doctors, had decided to empower themselves. They learned about their bodies, discussed their feelings and shared their knowledge with other women. Their individual and collective strength shone from the pages, giving me strength to grow as well. Their book validated my own nascent perceptions of our need for a different kind of medicine, one that respected and valued people's wisdom and autonomy. The courage and clarity of the women in valuing themselves and one another, in drawing the political lessons from their personal experiences, helped me start what became my lifelong work. I joined other advocates for our right to health. I joined the women's health movement. I became a charter member of the National Women's Health Network, a strong voice for women on health issues.

In the early seventies, my staff at Lincoln Hospital, a beleaguered city hospital in the South Bronx, included a group of pediatricians-in-training who were activists striving to change social inequities. As part of a group of doctors, nurses and other hospital workers known as the Lincoln Collective, they were not always in harmony with hospital rules and regulations or other staff. The Lincoln Collective's goal was to improve health care for disfranchised communities. As a result, our library copies of the various editions of *Our Bodies, Ourselves* were dogeared and worn. Their contents were used for classes, discussions and teaching materials for community groups.

I believe those readings, discussions and organizing efforts that the Book Collective sparked sensitized doctors and nurses to listen to and respect women as partners in seeking health. I hope it also led them to question accepted health care practices for women that women were questioning. I know that women who used the book challenged the young professionals into new ways of communicating with their patients.

Through the years, the Book Collective has undertaken difficult revisions, additions and expansions. New knowledge and changing needs, political realities and points of view compelled the authors to renew each edition. What has made each generation of women rejoice in discovering themselves in *Our Bodies, Ourselves* is that it still emanates from women's experiences as faithfully as ever. The idea that women's self-knowledge is the source of our knowledge of health, health promotion and health care is as valid now as it was twenty-five years ago.

Women now constitute an unprecedentedly high proportion of health care professionals and administrators. Although underrepresented in the higher ranks of pay and power, they exert a growing influence on the way women are treated by the health care system. But health care is undergoing radical changes, from a system controlled by doctors to large corporate entities controlled by managers far removed from patients and doctors. This calls for greater vigilance. In the world of "managed care," cost control rules, not quality or quantity of care.

Now, more than ever, we women must empower ourselves and our communities to participate knowingly in mounting health efforts. Promotion of health and prevention of illness must become paramount on our agenda. Women must lead the struggles to reverse the trend toward denying health care access to growing numbers of women—women of low income, of color, immigrant, with disabilities or who are aging are particularly vulnerable. The majority of the over 40 million people without health care coverage in this country are women and children—a national disgrace.

The New Our Bodies, Ourselves speaks to us, helping us understand and take better care of ourselves, and of one another. As the Book Collective has done for a quarter of a century, it challenges us and equips us to organize and fight for our rights to health. The women of the Collective make it clear that we cannot achieve a healthier us without achieving a healthier, more equitable health care system and ultimately a more equitable society.

Helen Rodriguez-Trias

When the group that was to become the Boston Women's Health Book Collective first met in 1969, I was working as a political columnist for *New York* magazine. I was also white and thirty-five years old and had become middle-class courtesy of going to college. In other words, I was part of that small demographic slice of people most likely to get the best health care information. As a journalist, I was even in a position to research what I didn't know.

Yet what "best" meant in those largely prefeminist days was whatever limited information the medical establishment considered appropriate— for patients in general and for women in particular. As a result, I assumed that my body needed attention only when it didn't work, and that the large portions of animal fat, refined sugar, hormones and chemicals in our recommended diets couldn't be too dangerous or they wouldn't be there. Like the third or so of American women who had abortions even when they were illegal, I believed that if I needed an abortion, I had no choice but to risk my life and safety in a criminal underworld. After having one abortion and to avoid taking this risk a second time, I followed the "best" medical advice and took the high-dose contraceptive pill for a decade. In addition to such self-destructive acts, I had many habits based on unchallenged beliefs: for instance, that binging on sugar was okay as long as my weight was normal, that only heart attack–prone men had to worry about cholesterol or cardiovascular fitness, and that male violence was inevitable and could only be avoided by female caution.

All these conditions of life seemed to be the price for being female. So did submitting our female bodies to doctors who were over 90 percent male (though childbearing meant that women used the health care system about 30 percent more than men did), and lying feet up like a dying bug in the common gynecological position (a horizontal pose so uniform that even women giving birth were forced to do so against gravity).

I often tell these personal observations because trusting, comparing and compiling our own experience is the revolutionary act taught to us by the Boston Women's Health Book Collective—as it is by feminism in all areas of life. Only remembering a prefeminist time of even greater disempowerment will allow us to see how revolutionary and prescient the message of twenty-five years ago really was. If women with the most resources had to endure ignorance, humiliation and a lack of empathy for female bodies (plus such special punishments as the mysteriously high rate of hysterectomies among women who could afford them), then those with fewer resources risked punishments that were far more lethal (for instance, higher mortality rates for breast cancer due to late discovery among poor women).

Much has changed in this past quarter century of a forceful and populist women's health movement, from increased mental health and life expectancy among women to the increased confidence and influence of women health consumers. Though there are still unacceptable differentials by race, class, age, sexuality and ability, the lives of the female half of America have been touched in a way that shows us how lifesaving a raised consciousness and collective activism can be. Indeed, the lives of men, too, have been improved and perhaps lengthened by such female-led reforms as labeling drugs with information about side effects (a cause advanced by protests against the contraceptive pill) and counselors who accompany a patient through procedures (an innovation pioneered by abortion clinics).

Nonetheless, there are still life-threatening reasons to keep learning from one another's experience, and to increase our activism. A medical and sexual double standard still tries to convince us that males, whether as doctors or lovers, know more about women's bodies than women do. Everyone from profiteering polluters to the beauty police still sends us to the medical establishment for unnecessary fixing. Drug companies still have more profit motive and government support for discovering expensive "cures" than for instituting already known, inexpensive preventions. The few still get better health care than the many.

But we now know that we can topple hierarchies by starting with our bodies. After all, male-dominant, racist and other unjust systems must control female bodies as the most basic means of production, the means of reproduction, in order to "own" children through systems of legitimacy, to decide how many workers and soldiers the nation needs, and to maintain the degree of race (and class) "purity" that keeps hierarchical systems going. Whether we are insisting on good nutrition when we are pregnant or safe abortions when we choose not to be pregnant, whether we're exposing male violence as a major health danger or exposing household chemicals as carcinogens, whether we're exercising our sexual rights or using our health consumer rights, we are taking control of our own bodies—and freedom.

Any and all of these acts make us part of the women's health movement. It is worldwide—as is *Our Bodies, Ourselves*. From its heretical beginnings, this book has been adapted and adopted by women in many different countries and cultures. It is now available in more than fourteen languages—and still growing.

Within these pages, you will find the voice of a women's health movement that is based on shared experience. Listen to it—and add your own.

Gloria Steinem

Preface to the 1992 Edition

With this updated edition we have eliminated any outdated information and replaced it with more current material. We have included many additional items as resources, although we retained some of the classics. In addition, we have added new topics such as AIDS, new birth control methods and special disorders that affect primarily women—subjects we did not cover in the 1984 edition.

The basic organization and format of the book remain the same, as this is an update and not a complete revision. We have changed a few diagrams and charts, and substituted some of the photographs. As always, we welcome your ideas, opinions, knowledge and experiences for future revisions.

Our organization has changed in many ways over the past decade. However, we still operate a Women's Health Information Center, now located in Somerville, MA. You can write to us at P.O. Box 192, West Somerville, MA 02144.

Preface/Introduction* to 1984 Edition

BY JANE PINCUS AND
JOAN DITZION

Earlier Prefaces: I by Vilunya
Diskin and Wendy Sanford;
II by Wendy Sanford.

In 1969, there was practically no women's health information easily available, and every fact we learned was a revelation. Our first publication of *Our Bodies, Ourselves* helped spark many women to explore the health issues most important to them. Since then, women throughout this country and the world have generated such a wealth of information and resources—research papers, books, health groups and centers, newsletters and journals—that this time around we turned to *them* for help in rewriting the book.

Rewriting has been a challenging, remarkable experience. Every writer (and consultant) ended up working on the book much longer than she ever expected to, with immense goodwill and patience, for very little pay. A typical chapter went through at least three drafts, each commented on and criticized by most Collective members and a wide range of outside readers. Several chapters were themselves written by small groups. Sometimes one person's insight would cause a whole chapter to be rethought. The end result of all this work is an almost totally new *Our Bodies, Ourselves*.

This rewrite reflects our Collective's longtime commitment to keeping the book up-to-date. Health and medical information changes quickly;

new health problems come to the fore; legal and political realities shift, changing people's access to information and care. Equally important, our own political awareness keeps changing: the more we learn, the less we believe that the medical system as it is structured today can or will alter to meet our needs. So in this book, less medically oriented than previous editions, we emphasize what we as women can do for ourselves and for one another, and we often discuss nonmedical perspectives and remedies as well as medical ones. The thousands of women who contact us in person, in letters and by phone have opened up whole new subjects and issues for revisions: "I looked in your book for a discussion of *in vitro* fertilization and couldn't find it." "You've got to include the experiences of differently abled [disabled] women next time." "This is what happened to me when I got PID [pelvic inflammatory disease]; tell other women about it so they will be forewarned and know how to get the right kind of treatment." "Could you please say more about lesbians and medical care?" Such comments in the past have led to the book's becoming denser and longer each time. This edition is no exception. It was difficult to decide what to cut, especially when every chap-

Some of the many women who wrote chapters and sections of this book.
Phyllis Ewen

*The following chapters were included in prior editions but are not in this current edition: "Our Changing Sense of Selves," by Joan Ditzion; "Considering Parenthood," by Joan Ditzion.

ter turned out to be twice as long as we had room for. To include and condense so much information has meant oversimplifying some subjects and shortchanging others. (Many authors have written long, annotated bibliographies, available from our office upon request.)

We expanded some of the original sections, such as Women in Motion and Violence Against Women, into chapters in their own right. Some entirely new chapters are "Health and Healing: Alternatives to Medical Care"; "Alcohol, Mood-Altering Drugs and Smoking"; "Environmental and Occupational Health"; "New Reproductive Technologies." After noting that in previous editions our discussions of the life cycle always ended with menopause, older women vehemently told us that indeed there *is* life after menopause. Together with them we wrote an all-new chapter on growing older. The chapter on international issues grew out of our correspondence and conversations with women whom some of us met in Asia, Latin America and Europe, and who visit our office to tell us about the health situations of women in their own countries as they collect information to bring back home. While this continues to be a book written primarily by white women, it includes experiences and information gathered by women of color.

Not all of us in the Collective agree with the content and style of every chapter and section. For instance, we had a long debate about psychotherapy—are women more helped than hurt by it? After many difficult discussions and rewrites we reached a compromise that we could live with.

Though we labored over several pages about pornography intended for the "Violence Against Women" chapter, we ended up leaving it out because we couldn't agree about the topic ourselves and could not do the controversies justice in such limited space. As of this writing, some of us still don't agree with the decision to leave this discussion out of the book.

Our Collective consists of the same core group who worked on the 1973 edition of *Our Bodies, Ourselves* (minus one). One of us now lives in California, another in Vermont. We have been meeting once a week for twelve years and have become a kind of family to one another. We have written together in twos and threes, looked after each other's children, had family picnics and celebrations, played music together and met for meals, given workshops with each other around New England and throughout the country and spent hours in long conversations. Four new babies were born in the past two years, making twenty-one children in all. We have seen one another through four divorces and three marriages, one case of hot flashes and some long, dramatic affairs with men and women. Three children have gone off to college and nine are in the midst of adolescence. We have comforted each other the best we could through four parents' deaths and the illnesses of several others. Most of us have other work in addition to working for the Collective. Now that revisions are over, we plan to do more public speaking nationwide about many of the issues in this book. Most important, we will be raising funds to keep our health information center going and vital. It is located in a large, bright room in the basement of a church in Watertown, Massachusetts, filled wall to wall with all forms of women's health information. Community groups often meet there; women are welcome to come and use our files. The center is staffed by a few Collective members and several terrific women who have worked closely with us over the past years.

It is clear that the same forces which created the need for *Our Bodies, Ourselves* twelve years ago exist today as strongly as ever. The medical system is a vast business, now tied more closely than ever to other businesses in this profit-oriented economy. Rich and poor receive very different types of health and medical care. Not only is preventive health care a low national priority, but reimbursement policies actually discourage prevention. Industries continue to pollute the environment. Misogynist archconservative mentality, money and policy drive women out of the workforce, deprive women of needed prenatal, abortion and birth control services and cut down access to health information. Drug companies continue to make huge profits by selling products often harmful to women, "dumping" into other countries

Some staff of the Boston Women's Health Book Collective.
Ellen Shub

Cambridge Women's Quilting Project.   Bonnie Burt

Staff and residents of a homeless women's shelter.

Ellen Shub

those drugs judged to be too old or unsafe here. So now, more than ever before, we hold to our original goals:

- To fit as much information on women's health between the covers of this book as we can.
- To let women's different voices and experiences speak out in its pages.
- To reach as many women as possible with the tools that will enable them to take greater charge of their own health care and their lives, deal with the existing medical system and fight whenever possible for improvements and changes.
- To support those women and men working for change both within and outside the existing system of health and medical care.
- To work to create a more just society in which good health is a right, not a luxury, a society that does not perpetuate unequal relationships between the sexes.

Above all, we want to encourge women to get together—to meet, talk and listen to each other. Most of us in the Collective grew up in the decades after World War II, when girls' lives centered around finding a man and women's lives around husband and children. Before we began working on this book fourteen years ago, most of us had moved away from our home communities. In 1968–1969, we became active in the early women's movement because of the political ferment of those years, and as a way out of the isolation we were experiencing. As we talked in small groups about our lives, we reclaimed an important part of our heritage, for women in traditional families and small communities have always exchanged experiences and wisdom with one another. In learning to support each other in our daily lives, we were not only continuing a tradition but doing something different too. With only a few exceptions, our own grandmothers and great-grandmothers had not dared speak openly about their

feelings and experiences—about sexual feelings, for example, or abortions, which so many of them had had. Religious and cultural taboos had kept too many of them locked in ignorance and silence. Most of them had not felt entitled to protest and resist the circumstances of their lives or had found no context in which to do so. But we began to distinguish between the habits, roles and traditions that nurtured us and gave us strength and those that limited and repressed us. We realized that sexism restricted our options and opportunities. We encouraged each other to change unsatisfactory or painful life situations. We saw the tremendous political strength we gained by identifying common problems and standing in unity with one another. In becoming aware of our own and other women's passions and potentialities, we discovered that we belonged to a family of women, a family larger than we had ever dreamed of.

We are increasingly proud of our dependence upon one another in a culture that so prizes independence. Yet our efforts (along with so many others') to form a community of women are still evolving and, despite their strengths, are quite fragile. A competitive society like ours makes it difficult to work collectively, to be open, to trust one another. It is more difficult to be a feminist these days than it was in the optimistic climate of the early seventies. And when the many women with backgrounds and experiences different from our own speak up and tell the truth about their lives, they make it clear just how diverse this huge community is. Sometimes the great differences between us—race, class, ethnicity, sexual preference, values and strategies—turn us against one another. Keeping in mind our common ground as women must be one of our main tasks. Acknowledging the past and present hurts, the inner fears of difference and the external realities which separate us can enable us to learn to hear each and every woman's voice clearly, to nurture each and every woman's life.

*Remember the dignity
of your womanhood.
Do not appeal,
do not beg,
do not grovel.
Take courage,
join hands,
stand beside us,
Fight with us . . .*

CHRISTABEL PANKHURST
English suffragist,
1858–1928

From

Norma	Nancy	Vilunya	Wendy
Pam	Paula	Esther	Joan
Judy	Ruth	Jane	

While the information contained in *Our Bodies, Ourselves* will hopefully empower you and give you useful tools and ideas, this book is not intended to replace professional health and medical care.

OUR FACES BELONG TO OUR BODIES

*Our faces belong to our bodies.
Our faces belong to our lives.*

*Our faces are blunted.
Our bodies are stunted.
We cover our anger with smiles.*

*Our faces belong to our bodies.
Our faces belong to our lives.*

*Our anger is changing our faces, our bodies.
Our anger is changing our lives.*

*Women who scrub have strong faces
Women who type have strong faces
Women with children have strong faces
Women who love have strong faces*

*Women who laugh have strong faces
Women who fight have strong faces
Women who cry have strong faces
Women who die have strong faces.*

*Our love is changing our faces, our bodies.
Our love is changing our lives.*

*Our sisters are changing our faces, our bodies.
Our sisters are changing our lives.*

*Our anger is changing our faces, our bodies.
Our anger is changing our lives.*

*Our power is changing our faces, our bodies.
Our power is changing our lives.*

*Our struggle is changing our faces, our bodies.
Our struggle is changing our lives.*

Boston Women's Health Book Collective in 1982.

Elizabeth Cole

The Boston Women's Health Book Collective is a nonprofit organization devoted to education about women and health. Our many projects and services include a Women's Health Information Center, open to the public; extensive distribution of free materials to women and organizations in the United States and other countries; several midwifery and reproductive health projects; and a speakers bureau. Royalties income from the sale of *Our Bodies, Ourselves* is not sufficient to support our work. Therefore, the Collective continually needs additional funding from contributions and grants. Tax-deductible donations (made payable to BWHBC) are welcome. Send to Box 192, West Somerville, MA 02144. Thank you.

PART I

Taking Care of Ourselves

Introduction

BY WENDY SANFORD

With special thanks to Nancy P.
Hawley and Jane Pincus.

The following chapters offer some of the basic information we as women need to take care of our health—at home and in the workplace. Though medical care sometimes helps us when we are sick, it does not keep us healthy. To a great extent what makes us healthy or unhealthy is how we are able to live our daily lives—what we eat, how we exercise, how much rest we get, how much stress we live with, how much we use alcohol, cigarettes or drugs, how safe or hazardous our workplaces are, whether we experience the threat or reality of sexual violence. Some of these things are under our control as individuals. Many, however, are not; we can influence them only by working with others to bring changes: pressuring an employer to remove hazards, forming a co-op for cheaper high-quality food, protesting the pollution from a nearby chemical plant, starting a "safelight" network for women alone on the streets at night. Many of these daily health factors are dependent on how much money we have: in an unjust society some people can afford to take better care of their health than others. It is a major aim of the feminist movement to make the crucial tools for health and survival available to everyone.

All through this book we emphasize wherever possible *what women can do*—for ourselves, for each other—in staying healthy, healing ourselves and working for change. Women have a long and proud history as healers (see p. 689.) Our friends and women's groups are sources of comfort, insight, courage and healing. We *do* need professional help with health problems, even when medical approaches are not always the best, with their excessive emphasis on drugs, surgery and crisis intervention. So we have included a number of nonmedical alternatives in Chapter 5. We have also included a brief discussion of psychotherapy, because so many women use it as a tool for taking care of themselves in a society that presents many barriers to true emotional health.

HEALTHISM

Healthism, simply put, is an overemphasis on keeping healthy. Social critic Robert Crawford believes that many persons today (particularly, he notes, the more affluent) are *too* focused on staying healthy.* He suggests that people have become preoccupied with controlling the more manageable health factors like smoking or diet because they feel powerless to change major factors like

---

*See Robert J. Crawford, "Healthism and the Medicalization of Everyday Life," *International Journal of Health Services*, Vol. 10, No. 3 (1980).

financial uncertainty or potential nuclear disaster. When we are overly focused on healthiness or a "healthy lifestyle" as goals to strive for (or as the measure of a "healthy" society), we deflect attention from the more important goals of social justice and peace.

Crawford also points out that even though prevention is crucial, and dangerously glossed over by conventional medicine, it, too, can be overemphasized. In expanding the concept of prevention ever further, we risk defining more and more aspects of life in terms of health and illness—that is, according to a medical model. We may end up seeing exercise, eating, meditation, fresh air, dance, for example—all pleasures in their own right—simply as measures of our potential health or nonhealth. In this way, ironically, we further medicalize our lives.

Keeping healthy can also become a moral issue. Individuals are made to feel guilty for getting sick. People shake their heads disapprovingly over those who "don't take care of themselves." In many cases this amounts to blaming the victim; it shows a failure to recognize the social and economic influences on health habits and illness. With personal habits, too, a certain judgmentalness creeps in: "She *should* have more control over her smoking" or "She *should* get more exercise, stop eating so much sugar." Even when these are matters of personal choice, a moralistic healthism is inappropriate. And it doesn't help people change, even when they may want to.

STRESS

Common to most of the chapters in this unit is a new understanding of stress as a major health factor. Humans, like all animals, have innate stress-alarm systems originally designed to help us fight or run away when faced with danger. In earlier, simpler times this fight-or-flight response was appropriate. In today's world, however, the dangers are no longer so obvious or so simple. We experience multiple, prolonged, often ambiguous stresses (see box) for which immediate action is often impossible. We squelch the fight-or-flight response over and over again in the course of a single

---

CAUSES AND SYMPTOMS OF STRESS

Some Causes of Stress

- Financial insecurity.
- Job loss.
- Death of somebody we love and/or need.
- Ending or beginning of a relationship.
- Job changes; a new job.
- Having a baby.
- Moving.
- Being discriminated against because of race, class, age, looks, sexual preference or physical disability.
- An illness for which we can find no appropriate care.
- A diet low in fresh foods and high in sugar, white flour, caffeine, additives and salt.
- Environmental pollution.
- The threat of nuclear war.

Stresses Specific to Women

- A majority of women now combine outside jobs with full responsibility for home and children. In addition, we may feel—from others, from ourselves—the pressure to be "perfect" at each of these.
- Most jobs pay women little and don't allow us to use our abilities.
- Many women are single parents; many are poor.
- Some of us are at home all day with small children.
- We face sexual harassment and abuse on the street, in workplaces, at home.

Symptoms of Excessive Stress

- Headaches.
- Neck, back and shoulder pains.
- Nervous twitches, "tics."
- Insomnia.
- Skin rashes.
- Greater susceptibility to colds, influenza or other illnesses.
- Worsening of existing conditions or illnesses.
- Depression, anxiety, irritability, nervousness, despair.
- Jaw pains and toothaches (from grinding teeth).
- Cankers, cold sores.
- Stomachaches, diarrhea, loss of or increase in appetite.
- Increased frequency of herpes episodes.

day. One commonly expressed theory is that years of failing to discharge the body's stress response can damage the body's immune (disease-fighting) system and result in many different kinds of ill health. Possible long-term consequences of living with too much stress are ulcers, high blood pressure, higher risk of coronary heart disease, rheumatoid arthritis and cancer.

We can minimize the effects of stress in various ways such as exercise, better food, meditation, foot rubs, long hot baths, time to ourselves. It helps to complain when we need to, ask our friends for encouragement, laugh. But it is important, too, to try to identify the *causes* of negative or excessive stress in our lives, and to change as many as we can.* This isn't always easy or possible, especially by ourselves. The following chapters seek to distinguish carefully between what we can do as individuals and the social factors which we must change by working together.

---

*Many businesses have introduced "stress reduction" programs for employees. These programs, however, emphasize only what *individuals* can do and rarely address the *sources* of stress in the workplace, because to do so would mean expensive changes such as reducing the workload or eliminating safety hazards.

1

Body Image

By WENDY SANFORD

With special thanks to the women of Boston Self-Help, including Frances Deloatch, Mary Fitzgerald, Jean Gillespie, Oce, Rosemarie Ouilette, Marsha Saxton and Janna Zwerner; and to Joan Lastovica, Judith Stein, Nancy Hawley, Esther Rome, Jane Pincus and Jill Wolhandler.

1992 Update by Demetria Iazzetto.

Imagine yourself naked in front of a mirror. Turn around slowly. Do you like what you see? Stroke your body's contours. Do you like what you feel? Try saying something appreciative to each part of yourself. It may be difficult at first. Almost every woman judges some part of her body—sometimes all of it—as "not right," tries to hide it from view, feels ashamed of it even with friends or lovers.

We often feel negative about our physical selves. Our hair is too straight or too curly, nose too small or too large, breasts too big or too small, stomach or thighs too fat, frame too bony. We don't like our body hair or odors. Our genitals—well, we just try to ignore them; after all, they really "belong" to lovers or doctors, not to us. We often compare ourselves to others; we're never okay the way we are. We feel ugly, inadequate. If others say we are beautiful, we don't/can't believe it, or we worry about losing our beauty. We spend precious time and money trying to change our looks. We may also subject ourselves to health hazards: cosmetics and vaginal deodorants that contain dangerous chemicals, low-calorie diets that deprive us of needed nutrients, hair dyes with cancer-causing ingredients, clothes and shoes that severely hamper our freedom of movement, and questionable surgery like liposuction or a face-lift. Looks are too often a matter of survival: many employers require that we look a particular way in order to get or keep our jobs. It's hard not to judge ourselves—and each other—on the "acceptability" of our bodies.

Talking with other women about body image helps us see that we can come to think differently about our bodies and come to accept ourselves more fully. It's a process which we can begin at any point in our lives and continue as long as we live.

One freeing step is to take a critical look at the pressures on us to look a certain way. Growing up, we are taught to think of our bodies mainly in terms of *how we look*. Early on we get the message: you've got to look good in order to be acceptable, to please men.

My husband gave me a full-length mirror for my thirtieth birthday to remind me I'd better keep an eye on my looks.

Every society throughout history has had standards of beauty, but at no time has there been such an intense media blitz telling us what we *should* look like. Magazine covers, films, TV shows, billboards surround us with images which fail to reflect the tremendous diversity among us. Never before have there been hundreds of businesses that profit by convincing us we don't look good enough.

Whole industries depend on selling us products through slick ads depicting "beautiful" women, playing on our insecurities and fears of imperfection.

We naturally want to look and feel good, to wear colors and materials that are beautiful to us, to feel attractive and appreciated. The trouble is that the media defines "looking good" so narrowly that few of us ever feel we have made it. Picture for yourself the "ideal" woman in the dominant culture of America today. She is thin, shapely or muscular, white, able-bodied, smooth-skinned, young and glamorous. She may change from decade to decade (big breasts are out this year, little breasts are in), yet we always have to measure up to some image.* Media images encourage us to strive to achieve that body/beauty ideal.

If we are passably close to the current media image of beauty we may not be aware of the intense pressures working on us. But if we are more obviously "different"—fat, old, women of color or with a disability, for instance—we encounter the pressures more openly and every day. Women who don't "fit" the image experience painfully the negative judgments, fears and hatreds which in subtle or unsubtle ways make it hard for nearly every woman in our society to love and accept herself as she is. If friends and family like us as we are, media images can have less impact on us.

---

*Those of us who are feminists and/or lesbians may not worry so much about pleasing men. Yet we may replace one ideal with another, substituting muscular for shapely, for instance, or Amazon for covergirl, so that there is still an image we feel we have to live up to. Those of us who are nonwhite or non-Anglo Saxon often feel torn between the dominant culture's standards and those of our own community.

PHYSICAL DISABILITY AND THE PRESSURE TO BE PHYSICALLY "PERFECT"

Author's note: Several women from Boston Self-Help (a self-help organization for people with physical disabilities) were generous with their time in talking with us, suggesting books and articles and reading over what we'd written here. Many of us in the Collective didn't know we knew women with physical disabilities; our meetings with the Boston Self-Help group began to change both how we see disabled women and how we see ourselves. We have chosen to use the pronouns "we" and "us" in this section because both groups discovered at those meetings that many of the issues we face as women are similar, because the women in the group said that to use the third-person "they" would be too distancing, and because it is important to them that able-bodied women be conscious that they are only "temporarily" able-bodied. By remembering that this state could change at any time through accident or illness, we are more likely to see women with disabilities as more similar than different.

Several million women in this country walk with a limp, move in a wheelchair or with crutches, have impaired sight, speech or hearing, have lost a limb to fire or accident or disease, need special assistance with simple bodily functions or wear the scars of some damaging event. Many of these millions of women are silent and invisible— many of us choose to hide in order to avoid the pain of being stared at and objectified, and the public, in fear, does not acknowledge and accept us.

With a body that doesn't "measure up," we learn pretty quickly what our culture really wants from women.

Having a disability made me very aware at an early age of the messages I was receiving from the larger society about how I was supposed to look and how you're supposed to be. Also, as the doctors poked and studied me endlessly, I learned more quickly than some nondisabled women that I'm seen as an object.

My family's thing was that girls dated in order to find a prospective mate. Since I had cerebral palsy, they assumed I was never going to marry. So why should I date? And I've only just begun to wear a dress this year, because I was always encouraged to wear pants. There was no reason for me to dress like

This woman is postpolio and has no use of her arms and hands. She takes care of her daughter using her teeth and toes and love.
                                                    Jean Gillespie

a woman because I wasn't one. That wasn't part of my identity.

The more we vary from "the norm," the less families, friends, physicians expect or allow us to be sexual (see Sex and Physical Disabilities, p. 223). If we can't have children, we are pitied for not being "real" women. If we we aren't "pleasing" to look at, we are expected to compensate, and we come to expect it of ourselves: we learn to smile a lot and be sweet, or clown around, so people won't feel so uncomfortable around us. Or, believing in our own unworthiness, we fall into the background.

Other "female" stereotypes surface quickly—we are weak, less intelligent, need protection. If we can't control our movements or bodily functions people think we are mentally incompetent. ("My family thinks of epilepsy as a mental illness." "People see my body and don't expect me to be smart.") Like many women, only more so, we are treated like children far into our adult lives. ("People will pinch me on the cheek and use words that you would use to a first- or second-grader." "The doctors still talk to my parents or to the person with me instead of directly to me, as though I'm a child, and I'm sick of it.") As women with physical disabilities, it is difficult but important to assert our adulthood, our power, our individuality and intelligence. This process is crucial for *all* women.

Severe job discrimination penalizes us for having "unacceptable" bodies and creates strong economic incentive for "fitting in" and minimizing differences. This pressure to keep a low profile if we are disabled makes us feel isolated and less free to get the help we need and deserve both physically and emotionally. Inaccessible buildings and public accommodations also make it difficult for us to participate fully in society. As one woman said, "We are not disabled; it is society that disables us by being so unsupportive."

Sooner or later, if we're lucky, we realize how angry we are at always having had to hide our true feelings and the realities of our lives.

After I got my braces removed at age twelve, I did everything I could to hide my skinny, scarred legs, including wearing knee socks or long pants in the hottest weather. Slowly my anger grew at the restrictions I was accepting. Partly with the help of other disabled women, I came to see my underlying feeling that if people saw my legs they'd not only reject me for being ugly, but they'd somehow see the years in the hospital or how dependent and scared I'd been. I began to reevaluate these experiences as simply things that had happened, not who I am. I wear shorts when I want to now, and I like my legs the way they are.

If coming to love and accept our bodies is a difficult process for every woman in this society, it is especially hard with a disability.

Finally I like my body, and because of my disability that statement has added significance. There is something "WRONG" with my body, so how can I possibly feel good about it or enjoy life in it? Simple answers are: I have no choice *and* I want to. *The more complex answer is that* there is nothing wrong with my body. *It falls within the wide range of human experience and is therefore both natural and normal. I've been in this body all my life, I was born with it and I'll die with it. It's part of who I am, and I'd be someone else without this body just the way it is.*

Dialogue between disabled and nondisabled women reveals that we have much in common. A woman with a brittle bone condition wrote:

I can't quite pinpoint when I began to listen to the experiences of able-bodied women and relate them to my own. It may have been when someone said that she couldn't go out of the house because her skin was so spotty, or when a beautiful black woman told me how all her life she had wanted to be white and blotchy like her friend at school, or it could have been when a friend of mine who had always been my envy for being followed around by drooling men said that she was so lonely because people only reacted to her stunning body and never to the person inside it. It may have been when my family began to talk about one of its female members who had put on weight and had, in their eyes, become not only unattractive but somehow outrageously undutiful in her role as an ornament. It may have been none of this that made the turning point for me, but instead it could have been the way some of the women put their arms around me and called me their beautiful sister that made me begin to see that we are not so

Bonnie Burt

different after all. We are all made to feel that our role is firstly to be beautiful in a highly stereotyped way, secondly to be interesting and amusing company to men and thirdly, good servants. My experience of finding that I was not necessarily any of those things is the experience of most women sooner or later. I have been lucky enough to discover that I am still a whole and worthwhile person and feel that all those dark years linked me profoundly to other women.[1]

BODY IMAGE AND WEIGHT*

In most cultures and historical periods women have been proud to be large—being fat was a sign of fertility, of prosperity, of the ability to survive. Yet fear of fat and bigness reigns in most sectors of American culture today. The reducing, medical and advertising industries all insist that thin is beautiful and that fatness is a dangerous problem in need of correction. Fat women encounter daily hostility and discrimination.

No wonder so many of us worry about our weight no matter what we weigh, spend precious hours counting calories, feel guilty when we "splurge."

I don't like myself heavy, I want to feel thin, stream-lined and spare, and not like a toad. I have taken antifat thinking into myself so deeply that I hate myself when I am even ten pounds "overweight," whatever that means.

Low-calorie dieting has become a national obsession. Fat activists suggest that making women afraid to be fat is a form of social control. Fear of fat keeps women preoccupied, robs us of our pride and energy, keeps us from *taking up space*. Says activist Vivian Mayer, "Mass starvation of women is the modern American culture's equivalent of foot-binding, lip-stretching and other forms of female mutilation."[2]

Recent research indicates that the "ideal" body weight for each woman is at least ten pounds higher than that stated by medical charts and that no one at this point *knows* a given woman's ideal weight.† The Metropolitan Life Insurance Company recently revised its optimum-weight charts upward by several pounds. Many health problems blamed on overweight turn out to have a more complex relationship to weight than doctors once assumed. Studies suggest that dieting is usually not successful in the long run, and that repeated low-calorie dieting is in fact a major cause of ill health.

These developments offer women a chance to become more relaxed about weight:

- By experimenting with what weight feels *comfortable* to us rather than trying primarily to be thin.
- By being more accepting of weight variations through the life cycle.
- By developing a clearer understanding of which health problems are truly associated with weight—some (e.g., diabetes and overly high blood pressure) may be, but not others; we must learn to distinguish what facts exist among the many, often damaging fictions.
- By exercising and eating nutritious food to feel healthy, and letting our body weight set itself accordingly.
- If we do diet, by choosing a program that emphasizes exercise and helps us change eating patterns but doesn't starve us.

WORKING TOGETHER FOR CHANGE

In moving toward a more positive self-image, we are stronger if we can talk with other women. We need each other's help to change the deeply entrenched attitudes that make us dislike our bodies. Here are some things groups of women can do together:

- Look at ads and criticize how they demean women and limit our ideas of beauty. Find ways to make your protest known to the companies advertised* and to let the media know you want to see more varied and realistic images of women.
- Learn more about how our bodies work, through self-help sessions and/or discussion (see Chapter 25, "The Politics of Women and Medical Care").
- Plan together how to challenge men who judge, choose and discard women on the basis of appearance.
- Form or join a group or organization that promotes self-acceptance and self-love for all our sizes and in all our diversity.
- Work together on tackling the fears and stereotypes which make us all discriminate against people who are "different."

If we can begin to eliminate the hatred and ridicule levied against women who don't fit the

---

*For more on this topic, especially on health issues and low-calorie dieting, see Chapter 2, "Food."
†Unpublished manuscript by Judith Stein and others.

*See Today and Tomorrow in Chapter 8, "Violence against Women," for an example. See also mailings from a group called Women Against Violence in Pornography and Media, P.O. Box 14635, San Francisco, CA 94114.

BEING FAT IN AN ANTIFAT SOCIETY*

Being fat in the United States means that we walk down the street to comments like "fat bitch" or "pig." We are expected to laugh at fat jokes. People laugh at us when we try to be physically active or if we show an interest in sex. Friends and family try to get us to diet instead of helping us love ourselves. At public events the seats are too small and uncomfortable. We search for days to find clothes that fit and have a harder time than thin women finding a job or getting into college. Like many other minorities, we never see *our* image on TV or in the movies except as comic or pathetic characters. We often hear that our fatness is the cause of everything that goes wrong in our lives. We are judged as weak-willed or morally lax because we "indulge" ourselves. We live for long stretches in a state of starvation (called "being on a diet") because our appearance touches people's fear of their own appetites.

If we are fat, health practitioners often attribute our health problems to "obesity," postpone treatment until we lose weight, accuse us of cheating if we don't, make us so ashamed of our size that we don't go for help and make all kinds of assumptions about our emotional and psychological state ("She must have emotional problems to be so fat"). In fact, much of our ill health as fat women results from the *stress* of living with fat-hatred—social ridicule and hostility, isolation, financial pressures resulting from job discrimination, lack of exercise due to harassment and, perhaps most important, the hazards of repeated dieting.

Recently there has been an increase in support groups and positive resources for fat women. Women in one Fat Liberation group suggest:†

No matter what anyone says to you (or what you fear they are saying about you), you have the right to go anywhere and do anything you like: to eat whatever you want in restaurants, to go dancing, to enjoy life. If someone or some place makes you feel uncomfortable (by rude remarks, aisles too narrow or chairs too small) it is up to them to change, not you.

You have the right to respond angrily to the nasty things people say to you or about you. Practice a few good withering glances or comebacks.

Take up all of the space your body occupies—no more hunching or slumping to try to look smaller. Stand up tall and relax. Practice being big. Or pretend you're a lion afraid of nothing and very, very strong. Move around your house remembering to breathe deeply, keeping your shoulders and back straight. Be loose and big in your movements. Work to create the feeling that you are entitled to go wherever you want and the world should make room for your wonderful presence. Whatever the size of your stomach (thighs, rear end), stop sucking in your stomach muscles. Insist on the right to be comfortable all the way out to your skin. Try to buy clothes that fit easily. Pleated pants or ones with elastic in the waist are less likely to bind your stomach in. Tight clothes don't make us look thinner—but they do make it harder to get out and move around.

*See in particular, William Bennett and Joel Gurin's book *The Dieter's Dilemma*, New York: Basic Books, 1983.
†Thanks especially to Judith Stein and Rea Rea Sears of Boston Area Fat Liberation.

"norm," we can lessen the stress of "not fitting in" and, with it, a lot of stress-related illness. We also open the possibility of building a social-change movement of many different kinds of women. Working together to change the attitudes and conditions that restrict us, we feel proud and more able to take control of our lives.

A better self-image doesn't pay the rent or cook supper or prevent nuclear war. Feeling better about ourselves doesn't change the world by itself, but it can give us more energy to do what we want and can to work for change.

NOTES

1. Jo Campling, ed. "Micheline," *Images of Ourselves: Women with Disabilities Talking*. London: Routledge and Kegan Paul, 1981, pp. 26–27.
2. Vivian Mayer Aldebaran. "Uptight and Hungry: The Contradiction in Psychology of Fat." *The Radical Therapist: Journal of Radical Therapy*, p. 6.

RESOURCES

Books

Brown, S., et al., eds. *With the Power of Each Breath: A Disabled Women's Anthology*. San Francisco: Cleis

Members of Wallflower Order Dance Collective—now performing as the Dance Brigade.   Ellen Shub

Press, 1985. Excellent collection of stories, essays and poetry by women with disabilities.

Campling, Jo, ed. *Images of Ourselves: Women with Disabilities Talking*. London: Routledge and Kegan Paul, 1981. In this excellent book, twenty or more women with varied disabilities write informatively and movingly about their lives.

Chapkis, Wendy. *Beauty Secrets: Women and the Politics of Appearance*. Boston: South End Press, 1986. Insightful analysis of the roles of sexism, racism and classism in shaping images of beauty for women.

Chernin, Kim. *The Obsession: Reflections on the Tyranny of Slenderness*. New York: Harper & Row, 1981. Perceptive analysis of our culture's obsession with weight, how it affects every woman's life, and the eating disorders that result.

Corbette, K., A. Cupolo and V. Lewis. *No More Stares: A Role Model Book for Disabled Teenage Girls*. Disability Rights Education Defense Fund, 2032 San Pablo Ave., Berkeley, CA 94702, 1982.

Duffy, Yvonne. *All Things Are Possible*. A. J. Garvin and Associates, P.O. Box 7525, Ann Arbor, MI 48107, 1981.

Fine, Michelle, and Adrienne Asch, eds. *Women with Disabilities: Essays in Psychology, Culture and Politics*. Philadelphia: Temple University Press, 1988.

Freedman, Rita. *Bodylove: Learning to Like Our Looks—and Ourselves*. New York: Harper & Row, 1989.

Hutchinson, Marcia G. *Transforming Body Image*. New York: Crossing, 1985.

Kano, Susan. *Making Peace with Food*. New York: Harper & Row, 1989.

Lyons, Pat, and Debby Burgard. *Great Shape: The First Fitness Guide for Large Women*. Palo Alto, CA: Bull Publishing Co., 1990.

Martin, Emily. *The Woman in the Body: A Cultural Analysis of Reproduction*. Boston: Beacon Press, 1987.

Orbach, Susie. *Fat Is a Feminist Issue*. New York: Berkeley Publishing Corp., 1978. This book has some helpful material about accepting your own body weight.

It suffers, however, from the underlying assumptions that fat people eat compulsively, that it's better to be thin than fat and that if you're healthy you must be thin.

Roth, Geneen. *Feeding the Hungry Heart: The Experience of Compulsive Eating*. New York: Penguin/Signet, 1982.

Saxton, Marsha, and Florence Howe, eds. *With Wings: An Anthology of Literature by and about Women with Disabilities*. New York: Feminist Press, 1987.

Schoenfielder, Lisa, and Barb Wieser, eds. *Shadow on a Tightrope: Writings by Women About Fat Oppression*. Aunt Lute Book Co., P.O. Box 410687, San Francisco, CA, 94141. Anthology of all the best articles about fat liberation.

Walker, Alice. "Beauty: When the Other Dancer Is the Self," in *The Black Woman's Health Book*. Seattle, WA: Seal Press, 1990.

Woman of Power. Women's Bodies. Issue 18. Fall 1990. Available from Woman of Power, Inc. P.O. Box 2785, Orleans, MA 02653.

Articles

Brown, Laura. "Women, Weight and Power: Feminist Theoretical and Therapeutic Issues," *Women and Therapy*, Vol. 1 (1985), pp. 61–71.

Dworkin, Sari H. "Lesbians and the Cultural Oppression of Body Image," *Women and Therapy*, Vol. 8 (1988), pp. 27–38.

Thomas, V. G., and M. D. James. "Body Image, Dieting Tendencies and Sex Role Traits in Urban Black Women," *Sex Roles*, Vol. 18, Nos. 9/10 (1988), pp. 523–529.

Thompson, Becky. "Feeding Our Hunger, Feeding Ourselves," *Woman of Power*, Vol. 11 (1988), pp. 78–85.

Periodicals

Radiance: A Publication for Large Women
  P.O. Box 31703
  Oakland, CA 94604
  (510) 482-0680
  A magazine that celebrates large women. Good articles on body acceptance, health and well-being.

Audiovisual Materials

Killing Us Softly, a 16-mm, 30-minute film based on a lecture/slide show by Jean Kilbourne. Powerful and provocative presentation of the advertising industry's objectification of women's bodies. An excellent film for colleges, schools, church groups, women's centers. Highly recommended. Available from Cambridge Documentary Films, P.O. Box 385, Cambridge, MA 02139.

Lambert, S., and S. Gibson. *Size 10*, a 20-minute 1978 film. Available from Women Make Movies, 225 Lafayette St., Ste. 207, New York, NY, 10012, (212) 925-0606. Australian-made film shows how women's body image has been formed and deformed by advertising and sexism.

Throwing Our Weight Around, a 0.5-inch 60-minute VHS video produced by Sandy Dwyer, c. 1989, Roundabout Productions. Fat women talk about the prejudice and discrimination they've encountered, especially how their skills have been discounted or ignored. Some basic facts mixed into conversation. Good to stimulate discussion. Available from Boston Area Fat Liberation, PO Box 1836, Jamaica Plain, MA 02130.

Organization

Project on Women and Disability
  One Ashburton Place, Room 1305
  Boston, MA 02108
  (617) 727-7440
  (800) 322-2020 Voice and TDD
  Offers consultation and training on the issues of women and disability.

2

Food

BY ESTHER ROME

With special thanks to Marsha
Butman and Vivian Mayer.

*This chapter in previous editions was
called "Nutrition and the Food We
Eat" and was written by Judy
Norsigian.*

*1992 Update by Esther Rome with
help from Bonnie Liebman, Demetria
Iazzetto, Ruth Palumbo, Tricia
Copeland, Christine Rugen and other
staff members of ATTRA.*

Food touches practically every aspect of our lives and affects how we feel physically and emotionally. By eating well we take care of ourselves on the most basic level. Eating has enormous emotional importance for women because we are still usually the ones who have the responsibility for budgeting, planning and cooking for others in our households. Food often takes on magical powers of nurturance.

I like baked chicken, mashed potatoes, jellied cranberry sauce, salad, milk—they make me feel cared for. When I cook it for myself I become both my mother and me as a child.

Because we don't control food production, food can be a source of problems as well as joy. It's hard to get practical, reliable information about what is best to eat, and often hard to find what we need. Even when we know how to make good choices we may not have enough money to eat well.

I know I should buy fresh fruits and vegetables, but I can't afford them since I lost my job. We eat canned goods since they are cheaper and don't spoil.

About 80 percent of the poor in this country are women and children. Budget cutbacks increase the dependency of women and children on food subsidy programs like food stamps, school breakfast and lunch programs, meals for the elderly, and so on. These programs, even when most heavily funded, have never been adequate.*

Many of us want to share the responsibility for choosing, buying and preparing food in our households. This may mean changing our eating and cooking patterns, encouraging a husband or partner to learn to shop and cook, getting teenage children to cook once a week and sharing meals with friends.

When my husband and I first decided to take turns cooking it was very hard for me to let him take the responsibility. I would suggest recipes and look over his shoulder while he cooked, giving him helpful hints. Since he was unsure of himself, that only encouraged him to ask me how to do something every few minutes. When I realized that I might as well have been cooking myself, I decided to make sure I

---

*The Women, Infant and Children supplement program (WIC) at its height covered only 39 percent of the people eligible for it. (One study estimated that for every dollar spent on this program, three dollars was later saved in reduced medical costs.) Food stamps cover about half the cost of an adequate meal for healthy people and make no provision if special diets are needed.

stayed in a different room and answered most questions with "Why don't you experiment?" Now he's just as good a cook as I am. We have the added benefit of more variety since he makes different kinds of things than I do.

EATING WELL

Our Changing Diet*

With the abundance and variety of food in this country, you might be surprised that many nutritionists think we eat more poorly now than at the turn of the century. Even today, many middle-class Americans, who have enough money to buy whatever food they want, choose their food poorly. We eat too much fat, salt and sugar. We used to eat more whole foods, such as whole-wheat rather than white flour. Food generally was minimally processed; that is, changed little from its original state. This change usually involved the kind of cooking or preserving that could be done in a home kitchen. Now we have technology to refine and process food; that is, to change it radically in ways we never could before, by splitting it into its components and sometimes transforming, rearranging and adding to these parts. We also used to eat more complex carbohydrates, food with a lot of starch and/or natural sugars and fiber. Now we eat fewer carbohydrates (starches and sugars) and more is refined, like cane sugar.

Diet and Illness

Because of dietary changes previously mentioned we may be making ourselves more suscep-

*For an analysis of the development of "food science," see Naomi Aaronson, "Fuel for the Human Machine: The Industrialization of Eating in America" (Dissertation, Brandeis University, Waltham, MA 02154, 1978). Also excerpted in Jane Rachel Kaplan, ed., *A Woman's Conflict*, Englewood Cliffs, NJ: Prentice-Hall, 1980.

James R. Holland/Stock Boston

tible to various diseases; current research suggests many links. Many of us have found this research compelling enough to change what we eat. Others of us who have had health problems have found that changing what we eat improves our health. Few doctors have any special expertise about the effects of diet on illness. Only one-third of medical schools require any nutrition education and often it is cursory.

Government Guidelines for Good Eating

Nutrient Guidelines

We still do not know what an optimum diet is but the government is making some attempt to determine this. The U.S. Recommended *Daily* Allowances (U.S. RDAs) set by the U.S. Food and Drug Administration (FDA) that you see on food packages under "Nutritional Information per Serving" are based on the Recommended *Dietary* Allowances (RDAs) determined by a board of respected scientists, the Food and Nutrition Board

Disease	Possible Causes from Eating Patterns
Italics indicates research strongly supports connection. *Exercise and hereditary predisposition are other important factors for many of these problems.*	
Heart disease	Too many *saturated fats, cholesterol* and sugar; lack of fiber
Some cancers	Too many *fats*; lack of *fiber*
High blood pressure	Too much *salt*, alcohol, saturated fats; too little calcium, potassium
Diabetes	Lack of fiber
Osteoporosis	Lack of *calcium* and vitamin D
Cavities	Too much *sugar*
Gallstones	Lack of fiber
Diverticulitis and other intestinal disorders	Lack of *fiber*

of the National Academy of Sciences. The U.S. RDAs are not fixed; the numbers of nutrients and amounts recommended change from time to time with new information. The U.S. RDAs can be valuable for comparing the nutritional value of foods. However, those foods which are enriched or fortified look deceptively nutritious since the manufacturer is required to report only a handful of vitamins and minerals.

Many people take the U.S. RDAs too literally, thinking that if they follow them, they are protected. The U.S. RDAs are set generously for an "average" adult. They are not intended to assess individual needs, which may vary widely. But they are even less complete than the RDAs. We know that over twenty-eight vitamins and minerals are essential in some way; most labels list only seven. For some we don't know how much we need. Researchers think others are essential but haven't turned up final proof, and no doubt there are some yet to be discovered.

General Eating Guidelines

Because our changed eating habits have been linked to various diseases, the government has developed suggestions for eating in USDA and USDHHS's "Nutrition and Your Health: Dietary Guidelines for Americans" (1990). The authors of this book feel that the government's recommendations are more conservative than necessary and believe that research supports the following guidelines.*

1. Increase the level of complex carbohydrates we eat from 45 to 60 percent of our total calories. These foods include grains, legumes,† fruits and vegetables.

2. Decrease refined sugar intake to no more than 10 percent of our calories. It is now twice that.

3. Decrease fats to 20 percent from about 40 percent. Reduce saturated fats from 20 percent to 7 or 8 percent of calories. Saturated fats are fats which are solid at room temperature (about 70 degrees Fahrenheit): animal fats, hydrogenated (hardened) fats and two vegetable fats, coconut and palm oil. Most of our saturated fats come from red meats, cheese, ice cream, whole and 2 percent milk. Unsaturated fats are those which are liquid (oils), like corn, safflower or sesame. Those which are monounsaturated are liquid at room temperature but solidify easily in the refrigerator, like peanut, canola (rapeseed) or olive oil.

4. Reduce cholesterol in foods to 300 milli-

---

*See Resources and your local library and bookstore for specialized cookbooks to help you eat better. Some give a lot of information about the nutrient content of foods.
†Legumes are peas and beans like peanuts, split peas, lima beans, chick-peas or garbanzos, kidney beans, lentils, cowpeas, navy beans and pea beans.

NUTRIENTS LOST IN MAKING WHOLE WHEAT INTO WHITE FLOUR

Nutrients Lost	Nutrients Replaced by Enrichment
88% of cobalt	Iron
86% of vitamin E	Niacin
85% of magnesium	Riboflavin
85% of manganese	Thiamine
80% of riboflavin	
78% of sodium	
78% of zinc	
77% of potassium	
75% of iron	
71% of phosphorus	
70% of vitamin B_6	
68% of copper	
66% of folic acid	
60% of calcium	
50% of pantothenic acid	
48% of molybdenum	
40% of chromium	
16% of selenium	
Biotin (amount unknown)	
Fiber (amount unknown)	
Inositol (amount unknown)	
Niacin (amount unknown)	
para-Aminobenzoic acid (amount unknown)	
Thiamine (amount unknown)	

grams per day, about half of what it is now. Cholesterol is found only in animal products, mostly in egg yolks (one yolk fills the day's limit) and organ meats (liver, brain, etc.).

5. Reduce salt (actually sodium) to 2,400 milligrams per day.

6. Cut proteins in half to 10 to 12 percent of the calories you eat, unless you have specific needs. (See Chapter 19, "Pregnancy.")

7. Avoid excess caffeine, especially if you are pregnant. It is found in coffee, chocolate, black tea,

---

Putting good food into your mouth is only one part of nourishing yourself. You need to be active to help your blood and lymph fluids better deliver the nutrients to your cells where they are used. Exercise probably* plays a crucial role in regulating your metabolism.

*We say "probably" because most of the studies linking exercise with increased metabolism are done on men. Most studies on weight reduction are done on women.

some herb teas such as matte and many soft drinks, especially cola drinks, as well as in others with caffeine listed as an ingredient.

8. If you drink alcohol at all, reduce your intake to no more than one drink a day. This is one five-ounce glass of wine, a twelve-ounce bottle of beer or one and one-half ounces of hard liquor. (See section on alcoholism in Chapter 3.)

Making Changes

Would you like to see whether you can feel healthier and more energetic by eating differently? First of all, assess why you like the foods that you do and what factors influence your food choices. Do you use lots of sweet, salty and fatty foods as rewards? Do you eat when you're not hungry? Do you always eat certain foods when you are depressed, angry or upset? Are you nostalgic for certain foods you associate with childhood, special holidays or childhood rewards?

Sweets, especially ice cream, were always a treat and a comfort food in my family. I had changed my diet in all kinds of other ways, like eliminating white flour, but I didn't seriously consider cutting out sweets, even though I knew they weren't good for me. I figured I'd always have a sweet tooth. When my asthma acted up, one person suggested I eliminate dairy products and sugar from my diet. I felt so sick I was willing to try anything at that point. It was hard to do, so I took it one day at a time at first.

Now I have stopped craving sweets most of the time. I stopped eating ice cream, which I never thought I could.

Tips to Make the Guidelines Work for You

1. Introduce changes slowly, as they aren't always easy to make. Experiment with one thing at a time so you won't feel overwhelmed. This will help overcome resistance if you are cooking for others and will give your digestive tract a chance to adjust. And if you change too fast, you might find yourself craving what you are used to.

2. Look at what you eat as a whole. One day of high-fat high-sugar foods won't hurt you. (The exception to this is if you have trouble regulating your blood sugar, as with diabetes or hypoglycemia.) Think about what you eat over a one- or two-week period. Don't judge yourself for "indulging" in less-healthy foods. Given time, you will find a balance that's right for you.

3. Try new things when you aren't rushed.

4. Increase the whole foods in your diet. Generally, whole, minimally processed foods have a higher nutrient density than refined, highly processed foods. This means that for every calorie of food you eat you are getting more vitamins, minerals and other important goodies than in a low-nutrient-density food. Vegetables tend to have very high nutrient densities and foods high in fats and/or refined sugar are often low.

5. Change the snacks you keep around the house. Try fruits, vegetables or whole-wheat or rice crackers. Popcorn can be made either plain or with seasonings like chili powder. Use nuts, seeds and dried fruit in moderation. (They contain important nutrients but also a lot of fat or sugar.)

6. Gradually reduce the amount of processed foods you buy. These often are "convenience" foods. They tend to be high in salt, sugar and fats, often saturated. They also are more likely to have artificial colors, flavors and other questionable ingredients. You generally get less per dollar for the nutrients in heavily processed foods than in whole foods.

7. Bring your own food as often as possible rather than relying on fast-food restaurants, vending machines and food trucks, for the same reasons as given in number 6. If you eat from them regularly, you won't get enough fresh vegetables, fruits or whole grains.

8. Get together with your friends and help each other figure out how to eat healthily away from home.

9. If you eat in restaurants, you can request and often get foods prepared just for you. You can also ask about the method of preparation and the ingredients.

10. Next time you watch TV notice what kinds of foods are advertised and consider how they help or hurt your body. This can be fun to do with children.

11. Sometimes eat food that is just plain delicious whether or not it is nutritious.

Increasing Unrefined Carbohydrates

1. Make sure the bread label says "100 percent whole wheat" or "whole grain" and not just "wheat." Caramel and molasses may be added to make white bread look like whole wheat when it isn't. Use whole-wheat pastas instead of white-flour ones.

2. Try eating more kinds of legumes (peas and beans).

3. Eat at least three servings of vegetables and two servings of fruit every day. Seven servings total is even better. A serving is one-half cup cooked or one cup raw vegetables or one piece of fruit. Orange, yellow and dark-green vegetables and fruits are especially nutritious.

4. In baking, substitute pastry or all-purpose whole-wheat flour for white flour. Whole-wheat pastry flour* is not as widely available as all-

---

*It has less gluten, the wheat protein, than bread or all-purpose whole-wheat flour. Note that unbleached flour is white flour.

READING LABELS*

Elizabeth Cole

1. The ingredients are listed in order of amount by weight used in preparation; there's most of the first ingredient and least of the last. If you don't see any ingredients listed it's because the product conforms to minimal ingredients standards set up by the FDA. For example, peanut butter need only contain 90 percent peanut butter. A food labeled "imitation" is like the food it substitutes for, but doesn't meet the standard. For example, mayonnaise must contain a certain percent of fat; imitation mayonnaise usually has less.†

2. "Enriched" means that *some* of the nutrients removed during processing have been replaced by synthetic nutrients (sometimes used by your body the same as naturally occurring ones and sometimes not) to approximately the same levels found in the original food. If flour does not say "enriched" or "whole" or "whole grain," it is the poorest kind of flour you can get. Many bakeries and restaurants still use this. Ask!

3. "Fortified" means that nutrients have been added to foods. These nutrients may not normally be found in the food, as iodine in salt. They may be added in amounts greater than what naturally occurs, such as large amounts of vitamins added to breakfast cereals and to candy bars.

4. Labels must be truthful but may also be literal. For instance, "Beef with Noodles" will have more beef than "Noodles with Beef." The percentage of the named ingredients in the product determines how it is labeled. Or a product may boast that it has "more iron than milk" without also saying that milk is a poor source of iron.

5. Although the labeling must be truthful, a product's advertising can be misleading. "Cholesterol free" on a label may disguise that it is still high in saturated fat. Products advertised as "light" or "100 percent natural" may still contain high amounts of saturated fat and sugar. This *may* change.

6. On cans, look at how weight is listed. "Net weight" includes any liquid used for packing. "Drained" or "filled" weight tells you what the actual food weighs.

7. Check to see if there is a date listed. This can tell you how fresh the food is.

8. If you need more information about a packaged food, write to the manufacturer or distributor. The name and address must be on the label.

---

*The FDA has proposed stricter and more truthful labeling requirements to take effect in 1993, but the Administration may allow the food industry to force the FDA to back down. The FDA or a nutritionist can advise you of the changes.
†If you want to know the ingredients, labeling or grading requirements for any food, call or write to your local U.S. FDA office located in the nearest major city. Some helpful grading standards are regulated by the U.S. Department of Agriculture (USDA).

purpose whole-wheat flour, but will make lighter-colored and -textured baked goods.

5. Try using some whole grains like brown rice, buckwheat (kasha) or bulgur (a form of cracked wheat). They may take about twice as long to cook (forty minutes for brown rice, compared to twenty for converted white rice), but this is mainly a matter of remembering to start cooking them as soon as you begin to prepare the meal. You can use a pressure cooker to reduce preparation time.

6. For long-cooking foods, make twice as much and either freeze the leftovers or make them into something else the next day. You can buy many beans precooked in cans. Rinse to reduce added salt.

Decreasing Refined and Added Sugars
1. Check the sugar content of processed foods, which often have many types of sugar in them, though legally "sugar" means sucrose. The follow-

ing are all names for different forms of sugar: HFCS (high-fructose corn syrup), invert sugar, molasses, honey (refined by bees), corn sweetener, caramel, corn syrup, sucrose, lactose, maltose, dextrose, levulose, fructose, maple syrup, brown sugar, turbinado, rawkleen sugar, jam, jelly.

2. Drink more water or real fruit juice instead of soda or juice drinks. If you still want something fizzy, add seltzer to real fruit juices.

3. Drink 100 percent juice and not "juice drinks," which have only 35 to 69 percent real juice. "Fruit drinks" have 10 to 34 percent and "fruit flavored" drinks have zero to 10 percent. The rest is water and sugar. "No sugar added" means just that. Orange and grapefruit juice are more nutritious than apple and grape juice.

4. Some people find honey, molasses or malt syrup much sweeter than sugar and so use less of these than they would sugar. *Blackstrap* molassses has some good nutrients, like iron, but is still a highly concentrated sugar. Contrary to popular opinion, honey has no measurable benefits over sugar.*

5. Substitute sweet whole foods or real fruit juices for sugar in recipes. Try mashed cooked sweet potatoes; raisins soaked or boiled in water, then pureed in a blender; or very ripe mashed bananas instead of sugar where they can be substituted. That way you get other vitamins, minerals and fiber with sweetness.

6. If you use cold cereals, choose less sugary ones. Check the labeling on the side of the box for the number of grams of sucrose and other sugars per ounce of cereal. These cereals are moderately processed. Hot cereals, such as regular or quick (not instant) oatmeal, cracked wheat, cornmeal and buckwheat (kasha), take no more than fifteen to twenty minutes to prepare. Wheatena and Maltex are even quicker. They are minimally processed and contain no sugar unless added by you.

7. Use sweet spices and flavorings like cinnamon, ginger, cloves, allspice and vanilla to replace some of the sugar in the food you prepare.

8. Don't use sweets as a reward for kids (or adults!). They fill you up so you don't have room for nutritious foods. Ask relatives and friends to bring love, good stories and fruit for the children. If they persist, suggest they pick up the tab on dental bills.

Decreasing Fats and Changing the Ratio of Fats in Our Diets
1. Check the fats in the foods you buy. Avoid

ingredients listed as animal fat, shortening,* tallow, lard, hydrogenated, coconut oil, palm oil or palm kernel oil.

2. Increase your use of fresh fish.

3. When eating poultry, remove the skin. That's where 25 percent of the fat is.

4. Try some vegetarian main dishes one or more times a week. Use those that rely primarily on grains and beans (see Vegetarianism, p. 36).

5. Substitute 1 percent low-fat or nonfat milk or buttermilk and nonfat or low-fat yogurt for some or all of the whole milk you drink.

6. Cut back on red meat, since it is high in saturated fats even if none is visible. About a third of the fat in American diets comes from meat. If your meals don't feel as substantial, remember it's the fat, not the protein, that makes you feel so full after a meat meal.

7. Avoid processed meats like bacon, sausage and cold cuts, which are even higher in fat than fresh or frozen meat. About 80 percent of their calories are from fat.

8. Cut back on the use of hard and processed cheeses if you eat a lot of them.

9. If you fry foods, use small amounts of unsaturated or monounsaturated oil. Keep the oil below smoking temperatures and don't reuse it if it has darkened at all. Try boiling, baking, stewing or stir-frying instead.

10. Cut back on the butter, margarine, mayonnaise, cream and salad dressing you add to foods.

11. Reduce the amount of fatty pastries and fried foods you eat. These include pies, doughnuts, Danish, layer cakes, cheesecakes, chocolate bars, potato chips and french fries.

Reducing Salt
1. Reduce or avoid foods cured in salt, most condiments, hard and processed cheeses, salty snack foods including nuts, soy sauce, monosodium glutamate (MSG), ingredients with the word *salt* or *sodium*, bouillon and many canned soups, vegetables and meats. (Look at ingredients in over-the-counter medications also.) "Instant" and processed foods can be high in sodium.

2. Don't add salt to food before tasting it.

3. Some people use less salt when adding it during cooking. Others use less if they cook without salt and add some if necessary at the table. You can see which works better for you. Keep track of how much salt you buy.

4. Don't add softeners to drinking and cooking water because they add sodium to the water.

---

*Honey, however, can be produced locally, aiding diversification in farming and making possible a more ecological agricultural system.

*When just the word *shortening* appears, it is animal shortening and should be avoided. Vegetable shortenings are specified as such on the label.

5. Check the sodium level of your tapwater. If you are part of a municipal system, the water department will know what it is. If you have a well, you can get the water tested.

6. Substitute plain herbs, spices, onions and garlic for salt. Use oil and vinegar or lemon or other fruit juice to flavor salad and other vegetables.

7. Check food labels for sodium content.*

VEGETARIANISM

Many of us today are becoming interested in vegetarianism and are eating less meat or none at all. We may do this to reduce our exposure to saturated fats and/or cholesterol, which may reduce our risk of heart disease and certain cancers; to decrease the amount of pesticides or other contaminants we eat, especially if we breastfeed;† to eat more cheaply; to stop killing other living beings; and for other religious reasons.

It is absolutely possible to live a healthy life and never eat any animals.

As a child, I never liked to eat meat and followed mostly a vegetarian diet with occasional eggs and some dairy. This was before the time when people understood this diet well. I knew that it was right for me and quickly became labeled stubborn, a fussy eater, etc. But when the household came down with seasonal colds and flus, I was running around quite happy and healthy with an excellent resistance.

Most vegetarians eat both eggs ("ovo") and dairy ("lacto") products. Some eat only one or the other or none ("vegans"). If you are a vegan, it is much more difficult to get protein and certain essential vitamins than if you eat eggs or dairy products. Most children, pregnant women and nursing mothers should be especially careful to get enough protein, calcium, zinc and iron and perhaps enough calories to stay healthy. If you eat soy products and certain fermented foods like tempeh or miso or a supplement to get vitamin B_{12}, an essential nutrient, you may not need to eat any animal products. Consult a nutritionist familiar with a vegan diet.

In order to stay healthy, vegans, but not ovolacto vegetarians must know how the body uses plant proteins. Proteins are made up of amino

---

*"Sodium free" means less than 5 mg per serving. "Very low sodium" means 35 mg or less per serving. "Low sodium" means 140 mg or less per serving. "Reduced sodium" means processed to reduce the usual level of sodium by 75 percent. "Unsalted" means processed without salt when the food normally is processed with salt.
†This may not actually be the case. See the section on residues, p. 47.

SHOPPING IN A SUPERMARKET

1. Go with a list. Think about *whether you really need* items not on the list. Are they fulfilling a nutritional need or some other need?

2. Don't go when you are hungry or with someone else who is hungry, especially children.

3. Shop the outside aisles first. Most of the less processed foods are there. The specialty or international section may have more whole grains and legumes.

4. If the food is highly processed, read the label so you'll know what you are getting. If you use a lot of processed food, read one new label each time you shop.

5. If your supermarket doesn't carry a food you want, call up the manager and ask for it. Try to get other people to call, too. You can also contact people who shop at other stores that have the foods you want and go with them or ask them to buy food for you. Use mail order catalogs. Consider starting a food co-op.

6. If you have unit pricing (price per pound) in your area of the country, use it to compare brands and to see if a larger size is really cheaper. Check the total price on the unit price label to see if it is up-to-date. If you don't have unit pricing, try and organize some friends to pressure your food store to start using it. Failing that, use a calculator to determine the unit price.

7. End-of-aisle display items are not necessarily cheaper than similar items in their regular places. Compare before buying.

---

acids. Some your body cannot make and these must be eaten. You must also eat them in the right proportions to make use of them. Single sources of plant proteins, like most beans, grains and nuts, have the wrong proportions of amino acids for people. It is easy, though, to combine different types of plant foods so that you can get the right balance. These do not necessarily have to be combined in the same meal but should be eaten within three to four hours of each other. For a more complete description of how to combine vegetable proteins and lots of recipes, see Frances Moore Lappe's *Diet for a Small Planet* (New York: Ballantine Books, 1982) and Laurel Robertson et al., *Laurel's Kitchen* (Berkeley, CA: Ten Speed Press, 1986).

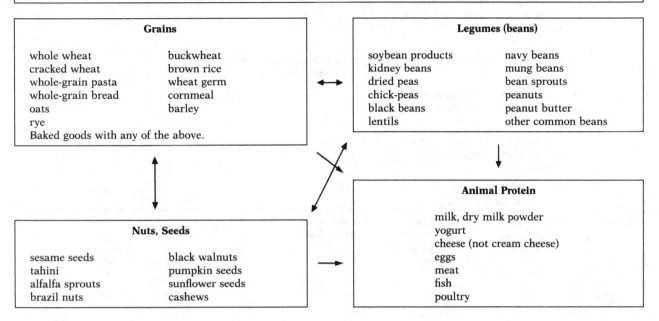

Protein Combination Chart*

To turn nonanimal foods into high-quality protein it is best to combine them with one of the foods pointed to. No arrows point out from the animal foods because they can stand alone but will enhance other groups.

Grains

whole wheat	buckwheat
cracked wheat	brown rice
whole-grain pasta	wheat germ
whole-grain bread	cornmeal
oats	barley
rye	

Baked goods with any of the above.

Legumes (beans)

soybean products	navy beans
kidney beans	mung beans
dried peas	bean sprouts
chick-peas	peanuts
black beans	peanut butter
lentils	other common beans

Nuts, Seeds

sesame seeds	black walnuts
tahini	pumpkin seeds
alfalfa sprouts	sunflower seeds
brazil nuts	cashews

Animal Protein

milk, dry milk powder
yogurt
cheese (not cream cheese)
eggs
meat
fish
poultry

*From Nikki Goldbeck, *As You Eat So Your Baby Grows*. Woodstock, NY: Ceres Press, 1977.

SHOULD YOU TAKE SUPPLEMENTS?

The most honest answer is that unless you have an obvious vitamin or mineral deficiency disease, no one really knows. People vary in their ability to absorb and use nutrients. At particular times you are likely to need specific extra vitamins and minerals—from birth through adolescence; when you take birth control pills; when you are pregnant and nursing; and after menopause, when you slowly become less efficient at absorbing nutrients. Some supplements may be particularly important for women. The average woman is 300 milligrams a day shy of the RDA for calcium, which is 800 milligrams a day. Postmenopausal women who live in the northern parts of the country get too little sunlight for their bodies to make vitamin D from October through May. Taking 400 international units (IU) a day during that time, along with enough calcium, can reduce bone loss. Women who are trying to get pregnant should take 400 micrograms a day of folic acid to reduce the risk of having a child with neural tube disorders, such as spina bifida. It's best to start before you are pregnant because the greatest benefit occurs in the first month of pregnancy. The amounts of vitamins mentioned are usually found in an ordinary multivitamin supplement.

Growing, but not yet conclusive, evidence suggests that some supplements, known as antioxi-dants, may reduce the risk of cancer, heart disease, cataracts and another age-related eye disorder called macular degeneration. These antioxidants are beta-carotene, which the body turns into vitamin A, and vitamins C and E. Unlike vitamin A, beta-carotene is not dangerous at high doses. It's too early to say that antioxidants can protect your health, but because they are safe in *moderate* doses and inexpensive some may want to take them.

In the United States today one-fourth of what we eat is often made up of foods which provide calories and not much else, like soda and sugary snacks and alcohol.[1] These "empty calorie" foods, combined with foods stripped of nutrients through processing or for other reasons, may mean we are not getting enough of all the nutrients we need. Your specific needs are based on a combination of your unique biochemical inheritance, which currently is difficult to assess; the environmental stresses in your life; and how well you eat.

You may be able to find out if you have a deficiency by experimenting with dietary changes or with nutritional supplements.* *If you feel better*

---

*Multivitamins sometimes contain more of the cheaper nutrients and less of the expensive ones. To choose a balanced supplement, check to see what percent of the U.S. RDA of each nutrient is contained in the product. (*Laurel's Kitchen* gives you guideline amounts to take so you don't overdose yourself.) Be especially careful with vitamins A and D. B vitamins must be balanced.

A PARTIAL LIST OF IMPORTANT NUTRIENTS

Nutrient	Chief Functions	Important Sources	Comments
Proteins	Provide nitrogen and amino acids for body proteins (in skin tissues, muscles, brain, hair, etc.), for hormones (substances that control body processes), for antibodies (which fight infections), and for enzymes (which control the rates of chemical reactions in our bodies)	Milk, cheese, yogurt, eggs, fish, poultry, meat, beans, tofu, certain vegetable combinations	
Fats	Provide concentrated sources of energy Carry fat-soluble vitamins (notably A, D and E) and essential fatty acids Provide insulation and protection for important organs and body structures Store calories to provide for pregnancy and nursing needs	Whole milk, most cheeses, butter, margarine, oils, nuts, meats	
Carbohydrates	Keep proteins from being used for energy needs, so they can be used primarily for body-building functions; also necessary for protein and fat utilization Provide our main source of energy Provide the glucose vital for certain brain functions	Grains and cereals, bread, vegetables, beans, fruits	
Vitamin A (fat soluble)	Helps prevent infection Helps eyes adjust to changes from bright to dim light (prevents night blindness) Needed for healthy skin and mucosal tissues, such as the inside of the mouth and lungs, bones and teeth	Fish liver oil, liver, whole milk, fortified margarine, butter, whole-milk cheeses, egg yolks, dark green, yellow and orange vegetables and fruits	Toxic in large doses
Vitamin D (fat soluble)	Regulates calcium and phosphorus absorption necessary for strong bones and teeth	Sunlight on bare skin, fortified milk, fish liver oil; small amounts in sardines, tuna, salmon, egg yolks	Toxic in large doses
Vitamin E (fat soluble)	Helps preserve some vitamins and unsaturated fatty acids (acts as an antioxidant) Helps stabilize biological membranes	Vegetable oils (wheat germ, corn and soybean), wheat and rice germ, egg yolks, legumes, corn, almonds	Destroyed by freezing
B vitamins (water soluble) including thiamine (B_1), riboflavin (B_2), niacin, pyridoxine, folic acid, cobalamin (B_{12}), choline, etc.	Needed for steady nerves, alertness, good digestion, energy production, healthy skin and eyes, maintenance of blood, disease resistance Needed for protein, fat and carbohydrate metabolism	Whole-grain breads and cereals, liver, wheat germ, nutritional yeast, green vegetables, lean meats, milk, cheese, molasses, peanuts, dried peas and beans, nuts and seeds, eggs, poultry, potatoes, fish	Heat, air and sometimes light destroy B and C vitamins; most water-soluble vitamins are *not* stored for long periods, so you need some every day

A PARTIAL LIST OF IMPORTANT NUTRIENTS

Nutrient	Chief Functions	Important Sources	Comments
Vitamin C (ascorbic acid) (water soluble)	Needed for healthy collagen (a protein that holds cells together), tendons and bones Helps wounds to heal; needed for iron absorption Spares or protects vitamins A and E and several B vitamins	Citrus fruits, sweet peppers, leafy greens, broccoli, cauliflower, tomatoes, fresh potatoes, berries, melons, bean sprouts	If you are taking large doses and want to stop, taper off gradually to avoid scurvy
Calcium	Needed for building bones and teeth, for blood clotting, for regulating nerve and muscle activity	Milk and milk products, leafy greens (except as noted), broccoli, artichokes, blackstrap molasses, ground sesame seeds, canned fish containing bones, tofu made with calcium lactate, soups made from bones plus a little vinegar or lemon juice	Too much phosphorus and leafy vegetables that contain oxalic acid (chard, spinach, beet greens) reduce calcium absorption
Phosphorus	Needed to metabolize fats and carbohydrates into energy in the body Makes up part of all the body's cells Needed with calcium for building bones and teeth	Milk, cheeses, lean meats, eggs, fish, nuts and seeds, poultry, legumes, whole grains, soft drinks	
Magnesium	Required for carbohydrate metabolism Helps regulate body temperature, nerve impulses and muscle contractions	Whole grains, leafy greens, beans, seafood, nuts	Large amounts lost in food processing
Potassium Sodium	Needed for healthy nerves and muscles Regulate fluid in cells Balance between these important	Potassium: fresh ripe fruits and vegetables (bananas, potatoes, dark leafy greens), legumes (limas, peanut butter), blackstrap molasses, fish, poultry, meat, milk Sodium: table salt, condiments (see tips on reducing salt, p. 35)	
Iron	Makes up an important part of hemoglobin, the compound in blood that carries oxygen from the lungs to the body cells	Lean meat, liver, egg yolks, leafy greens (dandelions and kale), nutritional yeast, wheat germ, whole-grain and enriched breads and cereals, blackstrap molasses, legumes, oysters, turkey, dried fruit	Daily intake is important
Water	Not really a nutrient, but an essential part of all tissues Often supplies important minerals such as calcium and fluorine	Tapwater, tea, coffee, juice, soups, fruit, vegetables	Most people need 6 to 7 glasses of fluid a day to keep good water balance in the body
Fiber	Also not a nutrient, but important for stimulating the intestinal muscles, encouraging the growth of certain intestinal bacteria and regulating absorption of nutrients	Fruits, vegetables, whole-grain bread and cereals, legumes	There are two kinds: insoluble, like cellulose; and soluble, like gums and pectins; both are important

the changes are probably what you needed. We need to pay attention to and trust our bodies to help us find out what our special needs are.

There are particular nutritional stresses that you may be putting yourself under. If you smoke, you need about 120 milligrams of vitamin C a day, about twice the usual amount. You can get this amount from two oranges. Many drugs affect vitamin and mineral use. Aspirin affects folic acid absorption and depletes tissues of vitamin C.

Even though supplements are fast and easy to take and you know exactly what you are getting, they cannot substitute for fresh whole food because we don't yet know all of the nutrients necessary for our health. You can't get some things easily from pills, like fiber. Also, many nutrients are useless or are less effective if taken by themselves.

HELPING KIDS EAT WELL

Mothers often have a lot of conflicts when feeding their kids. Even strangers may condemn us if our kids are "too" fat or skinny, though how we feed them may have little to do with how they look. Since most mothers work outside the home today, we may not be able to supervise our children's eating as much as we'd like. With young children we may have to make sure that the caretaker does not undermine our rules about good foods. Once children are in school, the task of changing the quality of cafeteria food may be bigger than we feel able to take on alone. Changing the food in the school vending machines from sweets to fruit, nuts and yogurt may seem overwhelming when the school football uniforms come out of the money collected and the coach doesn't believe that healthier foods will sell. Our children are under a lot of peer pressure to eat the foods advertised on television or to get a candy bar on the way home

from school even though they know you may disapprove of those choices.

One way to interest kids in eating better is to set an example by eating well ourselves. Children do remember what they eat at home and can learn to make good choices, especially if you explain the reasons for the choices. (This may not seem true if you have teenagers!)

I tell my four-year-old that some foods help him grow better than others, and he wants to grow as fast as he can.

Kids of all ages eat a significant portion of their food in the form of snacks, just like adults. This is fine if the snacks are nutritious. Older kids, especially teenagers, just need a lot of food. Cookies can have wheat germ, whole grains, dried fruit and nuts. Milkshakes can be made from yogurt, banana, crushed ice and vanilla. Stock up on fruits, vegetables, peanut butter and/or wedges of hard cheese. When kids are hungry they'll eat what's there, so make the snacks worth eating and enjoyable.

It's important to let kids decide when they are hungry and when they are full. They eat different amounts at different times depending on how fast they are growing and whether or not they are sick. Helping them to trust themselves in this way teaches them an important lesson they can use in regulating their eating all through life.

Involve children in growing, buying and preparing foods. Have them read product labels for you in the supermarket. Try to find a small space, even if you are in the city, to grow something. Have older kids take their turns at cooking meals. Younger kids usually will be eager helpers. Even a three-year-old can chop soft vegetables for a salad with a table knife, spread nut butters, help mix batters or add ingredients to almost any recipe.

PROBLEMS ASSOCIATED WITH EATING PATTERNS*

Fear of Fat

Low-Calorie Dieting

Do you find yourself worrying about your weight or thinking all the time about how everything you eat is fattening? Could it be because your lover says you are getting middle-age spread, because you don't look like the fashion models, be-

Esther Rome

*See the chart on p 31; check index to find diseases not covered in this chapter.

cause the supermarket magazines feature a new diet every month? Everywhere we look we see ads for foods, devices and diet support groups to help us lose weight. We spend over 10 billion dollars a year in the hopes of becoming slimmer. Most of us in the United States have been on at least one diet to lose weight and many of us go on several a year. ("Dieting" in this section means low-calorie dieting.) Dieting is medically endorsed as a cure for "obesity" and the diseases doctors think fatness contributes to. (For more on the social consequences of fatness, see Chapter 1, "Body Image.")

But dieting doesn't "cure" fatness.

Over a five-year period 98 to 99 percent of the women who diet regain their weight.[2] In fact, 90 percent regain more than they lost.[3] Dieting can make you fatter.

Studies show that diets don't work in the long run and that regaining weight is *not* a personal failure but a physiological adaptation to stress that our bodies have made to help us survive. After repeated dieting, many of us begin to feel we can never control our eating.

Dieting is debilitating, a form of self-starvation. The World Health Organization defines starvation as a calorie intake of less than 1,000 calories a day; reducing diets in this country commonly restrict calories to 700 to 1,000 a day. The average woman under fifty needs 2,200 calories and older women need 1,900 calories, though actual requirements vary with size and physical activity. At calorie levels below this you can easily be lacking necessary nutrients, especially if you consume a quarter or more of your calories from alcoholic beverages, sweets and other low-nutrient snacks. When you don't eat enough, your body reacts in specific ways to help you survive. It doesn't matter if you deliberately choose to eat less or if you can't get enough food. Starvation is starvation. The fewer calories you eat, the longer you do it for and the greater the number of times you do it, the more likely you are to permanently damage your body.*

Let's assume you are dieting and getting too few calories. (For some women the common 1,200-calorie diet is too few.) After a few days you are likely to feel physically listless. You may become

___
*Although rats on very low-calorie or protein diets live longer than those on regular laboratory rat rations, according to some experiments, these rats must have nutritional supplements, because their food does not provide sufficient nutrients for good health. The weight of these rats does not fluctuate as it does with people who diet repeatedly. Human studies do not always corroborate these rat studies. Also, these experiments do not try to assess the role of other kinds of stress or exercise in longevity.

apathetic, especially if you are on a low-carbohydrate diet. When fat from your body stores is broken down for energy, it doesn't provide any glucose, the fuel the brain normally uses. Your body must break down proteins from food and lean body tissues (muscles and organs, such as your heart) to provide this glucose. Processing the extra nitrogen from the proteins puts a strain on your kidneys. Fat metabolism without adequate carbohydrates leaves waste products called *ketones* in the blood. If the amount of ketones is too great, the critical acid-base balance of the blood can be upset. Extra blood ketones usually make you feel headachy, lethargic, dizzy, high or possibly lightheaded. After a couple of weeks the brain can adjust to using some of the ketones for fuel as a stopgap measure. You may feel irritable, partly because it is harder for you to control your blood sugar levels without adequate food. You may also find yourself becoming depressed and less interested in sex. You may become preoccupied with thoughts of food and obsessed with "quick energy" foods, especially sweets, and devour them uncontrollably as a way of replacing missing calories and glucose for the brain, the most immediate deficits. This carbohydrate craving may be especially severe if more than 10 percent of the diet is from protein. "High protein diets may actually generate cravings for carbohydrates and doom the dieter to periodic calorie-laden binges."[4] One woman describes how she stopped bingeing (and didn't try to be thin).

I worked at ignoring the rules and eating whatever I wanted. In the first month of "liberated eating" I craved only sweets. In effect, I was still bingeing. However, I chose not to berate myself for eating so much sugar. I reminded myself of all the sweets I'd been denied, and let feelings of nausea and hunger, rather than guilt, determine when I should eat again and what I should eat. At that point nausea and hunger were just about all I could be sure of. A month later, meat and dark green vegetables appealed to me very strongly. I chose a diet very high in protein and vitamins for a while. I think that during this period I was recovering from tissue damage due to previous years of dieting and bingeing. In the year that followed my cravings became more subtle and diverse. I ate smaller portions and greater varieties of food in one day.[5]

If you try to follow the often-cited rule that you'll lose one pound of body fat for every 3,500 calories you don't eat, you'll probably be disappointed. First of all, this calculation gives only average weight loss. For each month you continue eating the same low number of calories, your rate of weight loss is usually cut in half.[6] As a way of adjusting to a lower calorie intake, your body becomes more efficient at using and storing calories. Your basal metabolism (the calories you burn to keep your basic body functions going) can slow down by as much as 30 percent.[7] When you stop starving yourself you will probably replace or even exceed your original weight quickly, and mostly in the form of fat.[8] Your body is more efficient now, burning off fewer calories immediately and storing more fat for later use.

Fat often replaces the lean tissue lost from muscles and organs, and you may have done permanent damage. You may have as much as 40 percent more body fat than before you started.[9] On a total fast as much as two-thirds of the weight lost is a result of losing lean body tissue.[10] But usually muscle tissue can be developed again through vigorous exercise. If you continue dieting or adopt a pattern of repeat dieting, you risk amenorrhea, anemia, liver impairment, kidney stones, vitamin and mineral imbalances, gout and elevated blood fats.[11] If you have diverticulitis, tuberculosis, gout, Addison's disease, ulcerative colitis or regional ileitis, weight loss will make you sicker.[12]

Furthermore, a 1992 National Institutes of Health panel examining the safety and effectiveness of weight control techniques found a link between weight loss and increased death rates.

Most fat women believe that they eat more than their thin friends. However, careful studies show that, on the average, fat people do not eat more than thin people.[13]

Your general body shape probably resembles your relatives', due perhaps to heredity or to learned eating patterns. If one of your parents was fat, you have a 40 percent chance of being fat; if both were fat, you have an 80 percent chance.[14] We don't really know why people are different shapes and sizes. We do know that people's basal metabolism rates are different and that vigorous exercise may increase the rate. We don't know if fat people's cells (even when the person looks thin after weight loss) act differently from thin people's. Researchers have come up with many theories to account for different body types, from totally psychological to totally physical, but so far none is satisfactory.

Obesity (Fatness)

Ironically, the medical world considers fatness a disease. It is associated with and sometimes said to cause heart disease, high blood pressure, gall-

stones, diabetes and arthritis. Since doctors assume fat people are eating large amounts of food, a common method of treating many of these diseases is to recommend a severe reducing diet or fast. However, most studies in this country relating disease to fatness are done on people who are chronic dieters. Sudden and repeated weight loss may well be responsible for many of the diseases associated with fatness, but researchers don't consider this when drawing conclusions from their studies.* We have not been able to find any studies to show that over the *long* run thinned-down fat people avoid or are cured of diseases associated with fatness.† Slimming can improve high blood pressure and diabetes, but repeated or "yo-yo" dieting may make them worse.‡

Even worse than dieting are the various types of surgery medicine offers women labeled obese. They include liposuction, jaw-wiring and various ways to make the stomach and intestines smaller, decreasing a person's ability to eat and thereby absorb nutrients. These operations are performed almost entirely on women, may have a death rate as high as 10 percent and are only moderately effective in achieving the stated goal of weight loss. Doctors performing them really believe they are improving the woman's health, but they actually impair her ability to nourish herself properly. After intestinal tract operations a woman often gets severe diarrhea for several months and is at higher risk for getting gallstones and arthritis, two problems supposedly "cured" by weight loss.[15]

If You Choose to Diet

The authors of this book recommend against low-calorie dieting for weight loss. We include the following suggestions, however, because we are aware that many women will continue to diet even after learning about dieting's long-term ineffectiveness and its possible adverse consequences.

1. Become much more physically active. This may be the single most important change you can make in your life. It will increase your strength

---

*Fat Liberation was probably the first group to speak about this. See Resources.
†William Bennett and Joel Gurin, *The Dieter's Dilemma*, New York: Basic Books, 1983, Chapter 5, includes a summary of literature on fatness and disease.
‡A few studies have shown *no* strong correlation between fatness and several diseases usually associated with it. See *The Dieter's Dilemma* as well as two of several studies of heart attacks in Roseto, PA: C. Stout et al., "Unusually Low Incidence of Death from Myocardial Infarction: Study of an Italian Community in Pennsylvania," *Journal of the American Medical Association*, Vol. 188 (June 8, 1964), pp. 845–49; and S. Wolf et al., "Roseto Revisited: Further Data on the Incidence of Myocardial Infarction in Roseto and Neighboring Pennsylvania Communities," *Transactions of the American Clinical and Climatological Association*, Vol. 85 (1973), pp. 100–107.

and suppleness and probably your self-confidence as well as lifting depression. It may even lead to weight loss without dieting.[16] Be aware, however, if exercise becomes another obsession for you.

2. Eat a wide variety of foods and make every bit count nutritionally. Cut out the junk foods, including high-fat foods. Follow the general eating guidelines previously listed.

3. You are more likely to be successful if you lose weight slowly and if you set your goal within twenty pounds of your present weight.* Do not restrict your calorie intake more than 500 calories a day under what you eat when not on a diet. Even with careful eating, it is virtually impossible to get your major nutrients from food on less than 1,200 calories. You need more to get all your trace elements.

4. There are no magic foods or pills to help you lose weight. Most over-the-counter weight-loss pills contain phenylpropanolamine (PPA), which is a relative of amphetamine (speed) and may increase blood pressure or produce agitation and dizziness; it may even set off a stroke or bring on psychosis.[17]

5. Trust yourself and your body signals. Eat when you begin to get hungry. Don't wait until you are starved. If you feel ill, check what and when you are eating. You definitely should not have any severe symptoms, such as hair loss, shakiness, abnormally dry skin and so on.

6. Don't weigh yourself more than once every one or two weeks. Body water fluctuates daily.

7. Join with other women to discuss dieting, feelings about yourself and your body and societal issues, such as the way ideal body images, both sexual and medical, divert your attention from control over your life and from more productive work.†

Other Eating Problems

Most of us at one time or another have used food to numb or deny our feelings, to comfort ourselves or to put some order into our lives. Who among us hasn't at one time either binged or felt nauseous when scared, angry, depressed, lonely or sad? However, when we let food become the *major* outlet for expressing our feelings, we risk damaging our physical and emotional health. Eating this way is a common strategy many women have used to cope with a variety of abusive situations.

"Figure control is one of the few forms of control that women have been allowed to exercise."[18]

One problem is *anorexia nervosa,* a form of severe and deliberate self-starvation, sometimes leading to death. Another syndrome is *bulimia nervosa,* which is bingeing and then purging with vomiting or laxatives. Women can seriously injure their intestines or esophagus, develop severe tooth decay from regurgitated stomach acid and seriously upset their electrolyte balance, which can be life-threatening. A third is *compulsive* or *binge eating.** Women with these problems often seem to be acting out the ultimate stereotype of the female role: extreme self-denial, repression of anger and conflict, the desire to remain childlike and conformity to the idea that a woman must be thin. These problems reflect graphically how little control women feel they have over their lives.

My body was my ultimate and, to me, only weapon in my bid for autonomy. It was the only thing I owned, the only thing which could not be taken away from me. . . . I had discovered an area of my life over which others had no control. . . . What was going on in my body was as unreal, as devoid of meaning, as were the events in the outside world. The two were part of one whole, a whole of which "I" was no part. "I" had shrunk to a nugget of pure and isolated will whose sole purpose was to triumph over the wills of others and over the chaos ensuing from their conflicting demands.[19]

Some women who were sexually abused as children report that binge eating initially gave them a way to become bigger and gain a sense of control over their bodies. Over time, however, their eating large amounts of food became less a solution and more of a problem.

Because eating problems and sexual abuse are both body issues, I see them as connected. Both are acted out on my body, and the numbing—emotionally and psychologically—I did when I was sexually abused is not all that different from the numbing out of unpleasant feelings I used food for.

Learning other ways to express feelings of anger, frustration and powerlessness can eliminate our need to use food to express what we feel.

One woman who has successfully helped many others out of this pattern has found that building

---

*People tend to maintain a fairly stable long-term weight if they do not attempt to modify it by changing caloric intake. However, common short-term weight changes range over 10 kilograms (22 pounds).
†Fat Liberation is one such group. (See Resources and Chapter 1, "Body Image.") This group works to help people with diverse bodies gain physical, psychological, emotional and economic access to the wider world.

---

*If you have any of these problems or know someone who does, contact the American Anorexia Nervosa Association, Inc., 418 E. 76 Street, New York, NY 10021, (212) 734-1114, or Anorexia Nervosa and Related Eating Disorders, Inc., P.O. Box 5102, Eugene, OR 97405, (503) 344-1144, for the support and information group closest to you.

self-esteem, developing a sense of control over one's life and receiving support from others are key factors for recovery.[20]

Tooth and Gum Decay

Many of us forget that good teeth and gums are a significant part of good health. Without them we cannot eat many foods which provide important nutrients. Teeth are alive. Your saliva nourishes them through tiny passageways in the tooth. Poor nutrition can cause dental disease just as it causes other diseases of the body. Vitamins A and D, calcium, phosphorus and fluoride are important for tooth development. Reducing sugar in your diet is another way to keep your teeth healthy. Teeth are especially prone to decay in the six-month period after they come through the gums, before they are fully hardened.

Foods containing sugar cause tooth and gum decay in the following way. Certain types of bacteria found in saliva use sugar to make themselves a protective coating. This helps them cling to our teeth as a sticky substance called *dental plaque*, which saliva cannot wash away. These bacteria, tiny organisms known as *streptococci*, multiply rapidly and produce large amounts of acids, which dissolve the enamel and irritate the gums, causing disease. To remove the plaque and prevent this decay, it's important to brush and floss our teeth daily.

The least cavity-causing way to eat sweets is to have them with meals and not between. The number of times you eat sweets rather than the total amount determines how much acid the bacteria produces. But the amount of sweets influences the quality of your saliva. Avoid, if you can, sticky sweets that stay in your mouth a long time. Also try to brush and floss your teeth after eating sugary foods. Even rinsing your mouth with water is effective. Whenever possible, eat foods with fiber that scrape off plaque, acting as a toothbrush (raw carrot sticks, apples, celery sticks, whole grains, etc.).

Intestinal Problems

Adding fiber-rich foods, such as whole grains; pinto, black and other beans; peas; fruits and vegetables to the diet seems to help the intestinal tract. Appendicitis and diverticulitis are practically nonexistent in cultures that eat no refined foods. Different kinds of fiber help with diarrhea and constipation. Soluble fiber like pectin, found in many fruits, absorbs water, thickening the stool, and insoluble fiber like bran from whole grains softens the stool. Some researchers think that by decreasing the time it takes for food to go through the digestive system from one end to the other, fiber indirectly acts to hurry toxins through the system as well as diluting them so that there is less likelihood of developing bowel cancer.

Allergies and Other Reactions

Sometimes it's hard to figure out if you have a food allergy, since it can show up so many different ways. Your symptoms could be caused by many other problems. You may have rashes, hives, joint pains mimicking arthritis, headaches, irritability or depression.

The most common food allergies are to milk, eggs, seafood, wheat, nuts, seeds, chocolate, oranges and tomatoes. Many of these allergies will not develop if these foods are not fed to an infant until her/his intestines mature at around seven months. Breast milk also tends to be protective.

Migraines can be set off by foods containing tryamine, phenathylamine, monosodium glutamate or sodium nitrate. Common foods which contain these are chocolate, aged cheeses, sour cream, red wine, pickled herring, chicken livers, avocados, ripe bananas, cured meats, many Asian and prepared foods (read the labels!). Some people have been successful in treating their migraines with supplements of B vitamins, particularly B_6 and niacin. (High doses of vitamin B_6, 200 milligrams or more, can cause nerve damage, which is reversible.)

Children who are hyperactive may benefit from eliminating food additives, especially colorings, and foods high in salicylates from their diets. A few of these are almonds, green peppers, peaches, tea, grapes. This is the diet made popular by Benjamin Feingold.* Other researchers have had mixed results when testing the diet's effectiveness.

Cancer

See also Chapters 7 and 24.

A high-fat diet, all too common in this country, is linked with cancers of the breast and colon and probably of the ovary, pancreas and prostate gland. It's not clear whether the total fat content of your diet or the type of fat you eat is responsible. Saturated fats, especially from red meat, seem to increase the risk of colon cancer.

Some nutrients and foods seem to protect against cancer, though research on this is not conclusive. Foods high in vitamins C and E protect against several types of cancers. Beta-carotene, a precursor of vitamin A found in yellow and dark green vegetables and used as a food coloring, protects against lung cancer. Vegetables in the cabbage family as well as spinach, celery, citrus fruit,

---

*He has written several books that you can read if you want to explore this further. Many areas have Feingold Associations. Check your phone book.

General Foods plant, Woburn, Massachusetts.   Elizabeth Cole

beans and seeds help the body produce an anti-cancer enzyme.[21]

Certain food substances are likely to *increase* our chances of developing cancer. They may be natural constituents of our food, have been added to our foods purposefully by the food industry, or they may be contaminants in our diets. Sodium nitrite is used to cure and preserve meat and fish and to give the food a pinkish color. It doesn't have to be added at all because now there are other less harmful ways to preserve food, such as freezing. The nitrites combine with amines, found in the food or even in our saliva, to form nitrosamines, which are carcinogenic substances. Smoked foods are an additional source of nitrosamines. Saccharin and many artificial colors derived from coal tar have been linked to cancer or organ damage in animal studies but are still certified for use by our government because of food industry pressure.

Naturally occurring carcinogenic contaminants also exist. Aflatoxin is produced by a mold that thrives in damp weather. It most commonly occurs on peanuts but can also be found on corn, figs, grain sorghum, cottonseed and certain tree nuts. It sometimes gets into cows' milk from the grains the cows eat. Some aflatoxin reaches the marketplace and we eat it, although proper drying and storing of food can minimize it. Cutbacks in FDA funding result in contaminants like these being less closely monitored.

WHY EATING WELL DOESN'T COME EASILY

The agriculture and food businesses (agribusiness) are based on making a profit. This is a problem because many of the most immediately profitable methods of producing food deplete the growing ability of the soil and produce less nutritious and more expensive food.

Current planting practices may leave fields bare for periods of time, allowing precious topsoil to wash or blow away, or use herbicides to clear them. Widespread use of pesticides, herbicides and inorganic fertilizers destroys the organisms that control the structure of the soil and the balance and availability of nutrients to the plants, creates poisoning hazards for agricultural workers and contaminates groundwater. Irrigation practices may leave salts poisonous to plants in the soil or use up groundwater faster than it can be replaced.

As consumers, we also contribute to poor agricultural practices by demanding blemish-free produce, which makes pesticides a necessary component of commercial agriculture. However, an increasing number of farmers are interested in agricultural practices that conserve water, soil and wildlife. Consumers can support this trend by buying organically grown produce when possible, as well as encouraging Congress to increase the small amount of money for research on sustainable agriculture.

Business considers the most desirable foods to be those that are as uniform as possible and can withstand the abuse of mechanical harvesting and long-term shipping and storage. The land-grant colleges, supported by tax dollars and run by the states, have for years been responding to agribusiness influence by researching ways to develop complementary foods and labor-saving machines for large farms* while paying little attention to the nutritive qualities of the foods they develop or

---

*For more information on the intimate relationship between agribusiness and research at land-grant colleges, see Jim Hightower, *Hard Tomatoes, Hard Times*, Cambridge, MA: Schenkman Publishing Co., 1978.

the needs of the small farmer or consumer. Agricultural research has been partly responsible for the extraordinary decrease in the numbers of types of crops and varieties of seeds grown in the United States and elsewhere. Half the wheat acreage is planted in a handful of varieties out of 20,000 named varieties in the world. If a blight strikes, it strikes across the country, since all the varieties are so similar.*

One product of this system—the mechanically harvested tomato—took twenty-five years to develop. It is designed to be tough and is reputed to withstand a thirteen miles per hour impact without splitting. Normally picked completely green before its full nutritive value has developed, it is then conveniently "degreened" with gas as stores put in orders for "red" tomatoes. ("Vine ripened" means that it started to show color before being picked. Then it is either allowed to color up on its own or gassed to hasten the process.) Unfortunately, flavor didn't occur on the same gene with durability. We have a whole generation now that doesn't know what a real tomato tastes like! New gene-splicing techniques transform plants faster than previously possible. Already tomatoes can be made herbicide resistant, leading to an increased use of herbicides. Fuel-guzzling machines† now harvest these tomatoes, compacting the soil so plant roots have difficulty pushing through it and displacing farmworkers who were never retrained for other jobs.

Our food supply has become more and more centralized. In the last fifty years 5 million farms have gone out of business. Farmers grow most food in very few places in the country and ship it far. California produces 25 percent of the dollar value of the nation's food and 42 percent of the dollar value of the domestic fruits and vegetables. New England imports 85 percent of its food. There is a small revival going on in regional agriculture, but it still is hard to say how successful it will be.

Travel time from one part of the country to another can be substantial (an average of five to seven days; up to two weeks for fruits and vegetables to get to New York from California). In that time vegetables lose nutrients: in two days, 34 percent of the vitamin C in refrigerated broccoli is lost.

The length of time food is stored after arrival and how it is kept during that time are also important. Canned juice loses as much as 70 percent of its total vitamin C when stored in a hot warehouse, while juice stored at 45 degrees Fahrenheit keeps most of its vitamin C.

The Proliferation of Processed Foods

One effective way for agribusiness to multiply profits is to process food as much as possible, which results in the marketing of frozen peas in butter sauce rather than fresh peas; or to synthesize entirely new foods, like nondairy imitation whipped cream. Slight differences from one product to the next also help increase profits. Wheaties are sprayed with two cents' worth of vitamins and sold as Total for a substantial price increase. The food industry adds many substances to processed foods to ease manufacture and transportation, reduce manufacturing costs, replace costlier ingredients, improve appearance and texture and increase shelf life (how long the product is good after picking, processing, etc.). Yellow coloring gives bread the appearance of having eggs in it. Cheaper nonnutritive thickeners like modified foodstarch replace nutritive ones, perhaps eggs, because the parts don't separate as quickly, giving the illusion of a fresher product. Preservatives do the same thing by increasing shelf life, sometimes indefinitely.* We no longer can observe the original color, smell and texture of many foods to help us judge if they are good for us.

Even minimal processing of foods usually involves some nutrient losses. Frozen vegetables have to be blanched first and thereby lose B and C vitamins. Vitamin E is reduced by freezing. Sulfur dioxide on dried fruits destroys vitamin B_1 but reduces losses of vitamins A and C. Minerals, unless physically removed from food as in flour refining, usually are not lost. Canning generally is the least nutritious way to keep vegetables, because they are heated long enough to destroy many nutrients.

More Is Less

Advertisements suggest that the large number of processed foods available represents a wide variety of food choices. In reality, our nutritional choices are severely limited. We see a small num-

---

*Because we export hybrid seeds along with many industrialized agricultural practices to developing countries, local varieties of foods perfectly suited to the local conditions are being lost forever, so the base of our food supply is really shrinking. (See Cary Fowler and Pat Mooney, *Shattering: Food, Politics and the Loss of Genetic Diversity*, Tucson, AZ: University of Arizona Press, 1990.)
†In 1975, it took ten calories of energy to produce each calorie of food energy; in 1910 it was one for one. In 1980, the equivalent of ninety-five gallons of gasoline was used per *acre* of corn grown. This highly mechanized crop is our largest one.

---

*Preservatives can perform a positive function by making more of the food grown available to us, since about one-fifth of the food grown in the world goes bad or is eaten by other animals. They become counterproductive when there is no way to tell if food is a week old or five years old. Generally, the older food gets, the less nourishing it is. Also, some preservatives like salt and sugar are themselves problematic. Another, BHT, has been poorly tested and is known to sometimes cause allergic reactions yet protects vitamins A and D.

NUTRIENT PROFILE OF TANG AND ORANGE JUICE
% US RDA IN 6 OUNCES OF JUICE OR TANG

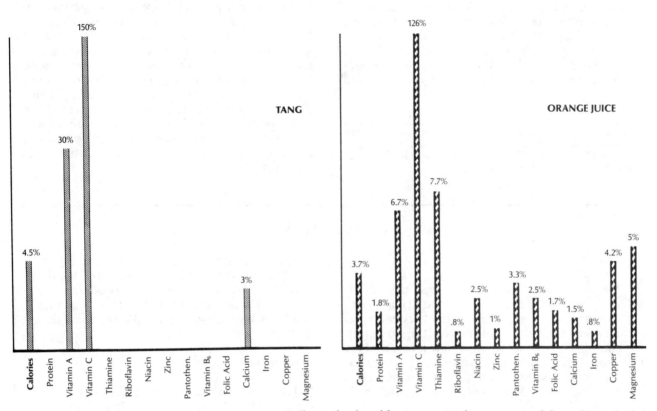

Charts developed by Annette Dickinson, artwork by Robbie Pfeufer

ber of basic foods transformed into many different forms, none of which are nutritionally equivalent to the original foods. A raw or baked-in-its-skin potato that would make a little under a cup's worth in volume contains 50 percent of the U.S. RDA for vitamin C. Prepared potato flakes or frozen-mashed-reheated potatoes have 20 percent or less of the original amount. Synthetic potato chips like Pringles, which have been freeze-dried, reconstituted, molded, fried in oil, salted, flavored and packed in a fancy box, contain 10 percent of the U.S. RDA for vitamin C in a serving. In addition, a pound of Pringles costs twenty to twenty-five times more than whole potatoes (1992 prices).

Residues

During food preparation, processors sometimes add chemicals that they don't intend the food to contain when it is eaten. Vegetable oils are usually chemically dissolved out of the plants that they come from by solvents, such as gasoline or carbon tetrachloride. Although the solvent is then boiled off before the oil is bleached chemically and deodorized by heat, chemical traces remain.

Some of the pesticides and herbicides applied in the fields remain on the food at harvest time.* Manufacturers ship abroad chemicals our government bans for agricultural use in this country, and farmers and farmworkers who do not know of their hazardous nature use them freely. Imported foods, including vegetables available in winter and tropical fruits, can contain residues. One examination of coffee beans showed that almost half had pesticide levels higher than U.S. law allows. Antibiotics that farmers use in animal feed to promote growth are a factor in the increasing resistance of microbes to antibiotics. These contaminants are in our foods because the large food corporations' desires strongly influence the regulation of our food supply.

The FDA and USDA

Consumers think the FDA and USDA protect us from contaminated and adulterated food, but they

---

*To remove some of the pesticide, wash food with dilute dish detergent or soak five minutes in dilute vinegar, then rinse; plain water is often ineffective.

are not nearly as effective as we think they are or wish they would be. The food industry influences how they are run in several ways. There are over eighty-five industry groups that maintain lobbyists in Washington to keep track of and influence pertinent legislation and regulations. Industry proposes most of the regulations and supplies test results when needed for the approval of new substances.* People often take jobs at the regulated industries after a stint at FDA or USDA. The people developing and implementing regulations have the industry viewpoint strongly in mind because if they promote regulations or rulings favorable to industry, they may have a good chance of being hired by industry with a far higher salary than the government pays. Their contacts inside government give the corporations information on where key links exist in the regulatory organizations to help bend them to their purposes. Partly because the industry wants it this way, Congress doesn't allot enough money in the federal budget for the FDA and USDA to be able to do very much independent testing and to enforce their own regulations very efficiently.

---

*Companies that do testing for the drug and food industry sometimes falsify or ignore detrimental results. See Douglas Foster and Mark Dowie, "The Illusion of Safety, Part 1," *Mother Jones*, Vol. 7, No. 5 (June 1982).

ARTIFICIAL FOODS

Fake Fats

Responding to America's obsession with dieting and the Surgeon General advising people to reduce the amount of fat that they eat, agribusiness multinationals are waiting to lap up the consumer's dollar with new fabricated fat substitutes, such as Simplesse and Olestra. The increased use of fat substitutes, however, may increase deficiencies of the fat-soluble vitamins A and E.

Fat substitutes are made by transforming foods lower in calories than fats into globules that slide over each other to give the feeling of fat in the mouth. There are two categories of fat substitutes that manufacturers are developing. One is made from starches—often from byproducts of the processing of other foods—like cornstarch, cellulose gel from wood pulp, whey or oatbran. A combination of heating, filtering and high-speed mixing forms it into rounded particles. Companies claim that the body metabolizes these substances just like any other starch, but of course they are pretty much stripped of the vitamins and minerals that usually accompany minimally processed starches.

The other type of fat substitute combines proteins, sugars and edible fatty acids from egg whites and whey to make molecules so big that they pass through the digestive system unchanged. Manufacturers claim there are no adverse effects. As of 1992, the Food and Drug Administration was still pondering the truth of this claim, and so had not yet allowed products with this type of fat substitute for commercial sale. The government treats starched-based fat substitutes as ordinary food.

The safest course is to gradually reduce the amount of fat you eat and use in cooking and to start to incorporate dishes from cuisines generally using less fat, as many of the Asian diets do.

Aspartame

Although approved for use, aspartame, marketed as NutraSweet or Equal, is still under a cloud of suspicion. Studies the manufacturer, Searle, submitted to the FDA never clearly proved its short-term safety. Brain tumors in rats resulting from aspartame ingestion have never been satisfactorily explained. Virtually nothing is known about its long-term safety. The FDA has received a long list of complaints that consumers believe result from consuming both high and low levels of aspartame. These include allergic reactions such as hives and rashes; behavioral disturbances, such as depression, hyperactivity or sleep problems; seizures; loss of vision; headaches; diarrhea; severe abdominal pain; menstrual irregularities; intense thirst; loss of control of diabetes and severe joint pain. As much as 10 percent of the population cannot digest the components that aspartame breaks into during metabolism: aspartic acid, phenylalanine and methyl alcohol. High levels of phenylalanine in the blood of a pregnant woman can lead to retardation of the baby. Because it may break down from heat or long storage, aspartame is frequently combined with saccharin, a known animal carcinogen. Nothing is known about the safety of this combination.

Advertising and Market Share

Through advertising, food companies influence us to buy certain foods, especially the most highly processed, least nutritious foods, because they are the most profitable. Advertising appeals not to our desire for a healthy or reasonably priced meal so much as to our desire for status, reward, popularity, satisfaction, increased fun, increased sexual potency or an illusion of superior quality. One advertising consultant complains that "the greater insistence on truth and accuracy in commercials also makes selling more difficult."[22] The most pernicious ads are aimed at kids and emphasize the fun of eating nonnutritious snacks between meals. Some large companies use children by linking sales of a certain brand to some cause that parents usually favor. For instance, large conglomerates—like Campbell—offer a school sports or play equipment if students collect a certain number of labels. If we tally actual costs, usually it's more expensive to buy the national brand than the store brand plus the cost of the equipment.

Corporations use advertising to get a larger market share. "To grow dramatically you have to introduce new products,"[23] says a General Foods executive. Proliferating new products, 80 percent of which fail, requires the company to advertise and to create needs for nonessential products. Food companies also capitalize on trends. An executive of a large food company points out that "people are consuming fewer calories as they watch their weight and that translates to less food tonnage."[24] To keep profits up, companies respond by making food with fewer calories so that people will eat more of it. They add water and air to whipped products and use artificial sweeteners and other nonnutritive additives.

In order to be able to charge more, companies are now putting brand names on basic produce that otherwise has a low profit margin. Advertising tries to convince the consumer that a brand-name product is superior to unbranded ones. Pioneers in this field are Chiquita and Cabana (Dole bananas), Sun Giant (Tenneco), Bud Antle (Castle and Cook) and Perdue chickens.

In advertising wars, conglomerates force out local companies since they have more resources. Particular strategies include coupon saturation and price cutting.

Large corporations don't limit sales and advertising to this country. Pepsi and Coke are known worldwide and are considered status drinks, even among very poor people. Infant formula is another example (see p. 717). In Indonesia processed foods account for 15 to 20 percent of the family food budget, even of the very poor.

Food Costs

Concentration in the Food Industry

Increasingly fewer corporations control food production, processing and distribution. Once a small group of companies controls 40 percent or more of the market (called an *oligopoly*), companies set prices beyond their costs according to what they think they can get for a product. In 1972 the Federal Trade Commission estimated that consumers paid more than $660 million annually because of concentration in the food industry. In another case the FTC said that ready-to-eat cereal manufacturers charge an extra fifteen cents on every dollar spent for cereal products.

Conglomerates buy up companies involved in every link of the food chain, from seed to supermarket shelf. For many commodities the people who plow the fields no longer control farming. To gain more control over raw materials, large corporations own and manage their own farms or hire farmers and specify how and what they grow and for what price, while the farmers assume the risks of financing and growing the crop. Farmers are not getting a share of the increased prices paid in the supermarket. Only 6 percent of the rise in food prices in the past twenty years has gone to the farmer. While we're taught to believe that in farming "bigger is better," the most efficient farms in terms of food produced per acre are family farms big enough to be able to use technology but small enough to run without outside help. But deliberate government policies have encouraged farmers to "get big or get out."

Other Factors Affecting Cost

Some of the other factors in the supermarket price of food include such things as financing, labor, taxes, the world export market, government price supports for some commodities, maintaining the corporate bureaucracy, lobbyists in Washington, and the price of crude oil, which affects fertilizers, pesticides, fuel and transportation costs.

Out of the sixty-one cents you might pay per pound of iceberg lettuce, 8.7 cents goes to the grower, 7.3 cents for packing, 5.8 cents to trans-

Power to control and profits from food production in this country are more concentrated than ever. Sixty years ago 40 percent of the population were farmers. Today 1 percent of the population are farmers.

port it to a city warehouse, 4.7 cents for the wholesaler, and 34.6 cents to the retailer.

Packaging increases price, with cans and glass bottles the most expensive containers. In 1979 the can and label on a ten-and-a-half-ounce can of vegetable soup was 27.4 percent of its retail price.

Advertising is expensive, and you pay for it in the price of the item. Companies employ television, magazines, newspapers, coupon promotions, sample giveaways and other gimmicks to get you to use a product.

WOMEN WORKERS IN THE FOOD SYSTEM[25]

On family farms in the past, women generally were equal partners in decision making as well as work. As farms become larger and are increasingly mechanized, men are trained to run the machinery and women are pushed out of farmwork. Women are often forced to supplement the farm income with low-paying nonfarm jobs like waitressing or factory work. In food factories, it's women who do the repetitive low-paying jobs, such as disemboweling and dressing turkeys in the assembly line, where it is cold, smelly, noisy and wet. Mechanization will most likely eliminate even these jobs. While more women are attending agricultural school today to go into large-scale farming, it remains to be seen whether we'll get the jobs we want.

Of those who are agricultural workers, migrant

Boston Urban Gardeners/Read D. Brugg

women are the hardest hit. Low wages make it difficult to buy sufficient food and other necessities. Most fields do not have toilets or provisions for water, making the women, particularly, more susceptible to many infections. Pesticide and herbicide exposure, harmful to all adults and children, is even more so to pregnant women. When nitrogen from fertilizers leaches into wellwater or reservoirs, it can poison infants who drink formula or other foods prepared with that water. Maternal and infant mortality is more than 100 percent higher among migrants than the national average. At the end of a long, grueling day in the fields, the women are expected to cook and clean and raise their children under the usually squalid circumstances found in migrant labor camps over which they rarely have control. U.S. agribusiness affects women in developing countries as well (see p. 715).

CHANGES

Starting on a personal level, each of us can intentionally work to make our diets more nutritious. Many cities have urban gardening programs through which you can get a plot of land to garden or get help with gardening in your yard or rooftop or porch (see National Gardening Association in Resources). If you have no gardening experience at all, try to find someone who has gardened before to help or who is at least willing to look at what you are doing and give advice. Often you can raise all your own vegetables and sometimes fruit in season this way. Not only is it cheaper, but it is also fresher.*

Sometimes a group will have organized a farmers' market near you, or there may be farm stands if you live in a rural area. When you buy at these places, you support local agriculture, benefiting farmers, the land and yourself. Consider preserving some of the foods through freezing, canning or drying.† It is surprisingly quick for some foods.

The next level of activity involves forming or joining a group. On the local level, look for a food co-op or form your own. Find other concerned parents who want to improve the school breakfast and lunch program or to try to get rid of junk food from the vending machines. Introduce nutritional education in the classroom or workplace. If you are at college, you can work with other students

---

*Beware of problems with heavy metals, such as lead, in the soil. See the Farallones Institute, *Integral Urban House* (San Francisco: Sierra Club Books, 1979).
†See Ruth Hertzberg, Beatrice Vaughn and Janet Greene, *Putting Food By*, New York: Viking Penguin, 1982. See also many standard cookbooks like *The Joy of Cooking* by Irma S. Rombauer and Marion Rombauer Becker (Indianapolis/New York: Bobbs-Merrill, 1975).

or co-workers to improve the quality and choice in the cafeteria. If you get your foods from vending machines or a truck at work, you can do the same. Work with or support one of many groups advocating and helping small farmers. There are many organic farming and gardening associations. Other groups have set up food banks to collect surplus foods and to distribute them to the poor.

Then there are political advocacy and information groups, some local or regional and some national. They try to inform the public about what is going on in big business and government, give expert testimony before Congress and sometimes institute lawsuits in the public interest. Groups like these have done important work around such issues as land-use policy, water rights, working conditions of farmworkers or food-processing plantworkers, the effects of tax law on land ownership, ways co-ops help or hinder cooperative behavior, energy use in agriculture and getting food to the hungry.

The food industry is powerful. The only way to challenge it is to work together so that we become powerful.

NOTES

1. Jane Brody. "Deficiencies of Vitamins," *The New York Times Magazine* (March 29, 1981); "Diets Won't Cure Teenage Obesity," *CNI Weekly Report*, Vol. 10, No. 33 (August 14, 1980), p. 4.
2. Alvan Feinstein. "How Do We Measure Accomplishment in Weight Reduction?" in Louis Lasagna, ed., *Obesity: Causes, Consequences and Treatment*, New York: Medcom Press, 1974, p. 86. Researchers have known for a while that dieting doesn't work for most women.
3. Llewellyn Louderback. *Fat Power*. New York: Hawthorn Books, Inc., 1970, p. 143, quoting Norman G. Jolliffe, M.D., of the New York City Department of Health: "At least 90 percent of all the people who lose weight on a diet gain back more than they have lost." This phenomenon is corroborated by the testimony of many dieters and a 1992 National Institutes of Health panel.
4. Judith Wurtman, quoted in Jane Brody, "Can Craving for Carbohydrates Be Controlled? Chemical Studies of Brain Point to New Approach," *The New York Times* (September 29, 1981).
5. Vivian Mayer. "Why Liberated Eating?" (ca. 1979), pp. 14–15. Available through Fat Liberator Publications (see Resources).
6. S. C. Wooley, O. A. Wooley and S. Dyrenforth. "Theoretical, Practical and Social Issues in Behavior Treatment of Obesity," *Journal of Applied Behavior Analysis*, Vol. 12, No. 1 (Spring 1979), p. 9.
7. H. J. Roberts. "Overlooked Dangers of Weight Reduction," *Medical Counterpoint* (September 1970), p. 15.

J. S. Garrow. *Energy Balance and Obesity in Man*, 2nd ed. New York/Amsterdam: Elsevier/North-Holland Biomedical Press, 1978, pp. 89–90 (see S. C. Wooley, et al., "Theoretical, Practical and Social Issues," p. 9).
8. See Jane Rachel Kaplan, ed., *A Woman's Conflict: The Special Relationship Between Women and Food*. Englewood Cliffs, NJ: Prentice-Hall, 1980, p. 50.
9. Jane Rachel Kaplan, ed. *A Woman's Conflict*, p. 50.
10. H. J. Roberts. "Overlooked Dangers of Weight Reduction," p. 15.
11. *Consumer Reports*, Vol. 43, No. 2 (February 1978), pp. 92–5.
12. H. J. Roberts. "Overlooked Dangers of Weight Reduction," p. 17. J. S. Garrow. *Energy Balance and Obesity in Man*, pp. 161, 163. See Louderback, *Fat Power*, p. 171.
13. J. S. Garrow, *Energy Balance and Obesity in Man*, p. 48, and studies listed in Kaplan, p. 45. This is common knowledge among researchers working in the weight-loss field, although lay people rarely believe it.
14. S. C. Wooley and O. W. Wooley. "Obesity and Women—I. A Closer Look at the Facts," *Women's Studies Int. Quart.*, Vol. 2 (1979), pp. 69–79.
15. J. S. Garrow. *Energy Balance and Obesity in Man*, p. 180; and Teis Andersen, Erik Juhl and Flemming Quaade. "Jejunoileal Bypass for Obesity: What Can You Learn from a Literature Study?" in *American Journal of Clinical Nutrition*, Vol. 33 (special supplement on weight-loss surgery) (February 1980), pp. 440–5.
16. William Bennett and Joel Gurin. *The Dieter's Dilemma: Eating Less and Weighing More*. New York: Basic Books, 1983, p. 224.
17. Douglas Foster and Mark Dowie. "The Illusion of Safety, Part 1," *Mother Jones*, Vol. 7, No. 5 (June 1982), p. 47. William Bennett and Joel Gurin. *The Dieter's Dilemma*, p. 224.
18. Vivian Mayer. "The Fat Illusion," *Hagborn*, Vol. 1, No. 4 (Winter 1980), pp. 3 ff. Also available through Fat Liberator Publications (see Resources).
19. Sheila MacLeod. *The Art of Starvation: A Story of Anorexia and Survival*. New York: Schocken Books, 1981, pp. 56, 66, 98. A perceptive autobiography and analysis of anorexia.
20. Marlene Boskind-White and William White have been working with bulimarexics for many years and have written *The People Pleasers: Women Who Binge and Purge*. New York: W. W. Norton, 1983.
21. Jane Brody. *Jane Brody's Nutrition Book*. New York: W. W. Norton, 1981, p. 442.
22. Fred A. Lemont, quoted in "Trouble for Packaged Goods," *The New York Times* (June 8, 1981).
23. Peter Rosow, general manager of General Foods dessert division, quoted in "Introducing a New Product," *The New York Times* (July 14, 1981).
24. William D. Smithburg, chief executive officer of Quaker Oats Co., quoted in "Quaker Oats Names New Chief Officer," *The New York Times* (July 10, 1981).
25. For more, see Sally Hacker, "Farming Out the Home: Women and Agribusiness," in Jane Rachel Kaplan, ed., *A Woman's Conflict*. This article also appeared in *The Second Wave: A Magazine of the New Feminism*, Vol. 5, No. 1 (Spring/Summer 1977), pp. 38–49; and *Science for the People* (March/April 1978).

RESOURCES

Nutritional Information

Authors' note: Most of these books assume that thin is better than fat, and that a reasonable way to achieve thinness is through low-calorie dieting.

Brody, Jane. *Jane Brody's Nutrition Book.* New York: Bantam Books, 1987. Many practical suggestions.

National Academy of Sciences. "Recommended Dietary Allowances," 10th ed., 1989. Available from the Office of Publications, National Academy of Sciences, 2101 Constitution Avenue N.W., Washington, DC 20418. The most complete summary of what we know about human nutrient needs at this time.

National Research Council. *Diet and Health: Implications for Reducing Chronic Disease Risk.* Washington, DC: National Academy Press, 1989.

U.S. Department of Agriculture. "Nutritive Value of Foods," Home and Garden Bulletin No. 72. Washington, DC: USDA. Available from U.S. Government Printing Office, Washington, DC 20402.

U.S. Department of Agriculture and U.S. Department of Health and Human Services. "Nutrition and Your Health: Dietary Guidelines for Americans," Publication No. 232. Washington, DC: USDA and USDHHS, 1990. Available from U.S. Government Printing Office, Washington, DC 20402.

U.S. Department of Health and Human Services. "The Surgeon General's Report on Nutrition and Health: Summary and Recommendations," Publication No. 88-50211. Washington, DC: DHHS, 1988. Available from U.S. Government Printing Office, Washington DC 20402.

U.S. Senate Select Committee on Nutrition and Human Needs. *Eating in America: Dietary Goals for the United States.* Cambridge, MA: The MIT Press, 1977. "First comprehensive statement by any branch of the federal government on risk factors in the American diet" (p. 1). The USDA then issued Dietary Guidelines based on these goals.

Vegetarianism

Adams, Carol. "The Inedible Complex: The Political Implications of Vegetarianism," *The Second Voice,* Vol. 4, No. 4 (Summer/Fall 1976). Weaves together vegetarianism and feminism.

Akers, Keith. *A Vegetarian Source Book.* Denver, CO: Vegetarian Press, 1989. Available from Vegetarian Press, P.O. Box 61273, Denver, CO 80206. Lists regional vegetarian societies.

Lappe, Frances Moore. *Diet for a Small Planet.* New York: Ballantine Books, 1982. The popular vegetarian cookbook that explains protein complementarity.

Robertson, Laurel, Carol Flenders and Bronwen Godfrey. *The New Laurel's Kitchen.* Berkeley, CA: Ten Speed Press, 1986. A wealth of nutritional information (especially on how to get specific nutrients) as well as recipes. Less reliance on eggs and dairy products than *Diet for a Small Planet.*

Untema, Sharon. *Vegetarian Baby: A Sensible Guide for Parents.* Ithaca, NY: McBooks Press, 1980. Available from McBooks Press, 106 N. Aurora Street, Ithaca, NY 14850. An informed guide for feeding child from pregnancy through two years. Includes information on a vegan diet. Recipes.

The Vegetarian Resource Group, P.O. Box 1463, Baltimore, MD 21203.

Women and Food

Heresies Collective. "Food Is a Feminist Issue," *Heresies,* No. 21 (1987). Special issue contains essays, articles, stories, poems, photos, drawings and cartoons examining women's involvement with food and the complexity of the relationship between women and their bodies.

ISIS, *Women in Development.* Philadelphia, PA: New Society Publishers, 1984. Available from NSP, 4527 Springfield Avenue, Philadelphia, PA 19143. Feminist. Additional resources listed.

Jensen, Joan M., ed. *With These Hands: Women Working on the Land.* Old Westbury, NY: The Feminist Press; New York, 1981. A chronological anthology of short excerpts of conversations with farming women in the United States from the days before European settlers arrived to the present. Good introductions for each section.

———. *Promise to the Land: Essays on Rural Women.* Albuquerque: University of New Mexico Press, 1991.

Fatness/Dieting and Other Eating Problems

Ample Opportunity, 5370 NW Roanoke, Portland, OR 97229, (503) 645-0497. Focuses on health and happiness rather than weight loss. Publishes newsletter *Ample Opportunity.*

Bennett, William, and Joel Gurin. *The Dieter's Dilemma: Eating Less and Weighing More.* New York: Basic Books, 1983. Shows role of exercise in weight reduction may be more important than how much you eat, but still out to get you thin. Draws on many of same scientific sources as Fat Liberation.

Bulimia and the Road to Recovery, a 27-minute 1988 color video. Available from Women Make Movies, 225 Lafayette Street, Suite 207, New York, NY 10012. Interviews with health professionals and women working through their problems of food, body image and sociocultural pressures. Excellent for college audiences.

Chernin, Kim. *The Obsession: Reflections on the Tyranny of Slenderness.* New York: Harper & Row, 1981. Recommended.

———. *The Hungry Self: Women, Eating, and Identity.* New York: Times Books, 1985. A provocative look at the meanings attached to women's bodies, their relationships to food and their struggles for self-identity in a culture in crisis over changing female roles.

Diet/Weight Liberation Project, CRESP, Anabel Taylor Hall, Cornell University, Ithaca, NY 14853. Nonprofit support and education group. Membership fee includes subscription to newsletter *Grace-Full Eating.*

Ernsberger, Paul, and P. Haskew. *Rethinking Obesity: An Alternative View of Its Health Implications.* New York: Human Sciences Press, 1987. Excellent, extensive review of the literature on fatness, in which the authors argue that fatness does not equal bad health.

Fat Liberator Publications (Judith Stein, P.O. Box 308, Kendall Square, Cambridge, MA 02142). An extensive list of well-researched publications.

I Don't Have to Hide: A Film About Anorexia and Bulemia, 20-minute 16-mm 1983 color film. Available from Fanlight Productions, 47 Halifax Street, Jamaica Plain, MA 02130. Good for use in high school and college settings.

Kano, Susan. *Making Peace with Food.* New York: HarperCollins, 1989. Excellent analysis and workbook to help women free ourselves from food obsession.

Kaplan, Jane Rachel, ed. *A Woman's Conflict: The Special Relationship Between Women and Food.* Englewood Cliffs, NJ: Prentice-Hall, 1980. An excellent anthology of issues vital to women. Good section on fatness.

Lambert-Lagace, Louise. *The Nutrition Challenge for Women: Now You Don't Have to Diet to Stay Healthy and Fit.* Palo Alto, CA: Bull Publishing Co., 1990.

Millman, Marcia. *Such a Pretty Face: Being Fat in America.* New York: Berkley Books, 1980. Explores both social and personal aspects.

National Association to Advance Fat Acceptance, Department GS, P.O. Box 188620, Sacramento, CA 95818, (916) 443-0303. Focuses on size acceptance through education, support and civil rights. Publishes newsletter. Many local chapters in the United States and Canada.

Nothing to Lose, a 30-minute color video. Available from Fat Lip Reader's Theatre, P.O. Box 7717, Berkeley, CA 94707, (415) 465-4688. Based on their funny, poignant theatrical production.

Polivy, Janet, and C. P. Herman. *Breaking the Diet Habit: The Natural Weight Alternative.* New York: Basic Books, 1983. Practical advice on how to stop dieting and eat/live normally.

Radiance: The Magazine for Large Women, P.O. Box 31703, Oakland, CA 96404, (510) 482-0680. Affirming of accepting yourself no matter what size. A good place to find other resources.

Roth, Geneen. *Breaking Free from Compulsive Eating.* Indianapolis, IN: Bobbs-Merrill, 1984. How to stop eating and exercising compulsively are effectively presented in this sensitive book.

Roundabout Productions. *Throwing Our Weight Around,* a 60-minute 1989 color video. Available from BAFL, P.O. Box 1836, Jamaica Plain, MA 02130. Fat women talk about prejudices they encounter and how they have come to accept their large bodies.

Schoenfielder, Lisa, and Barb Wieser, eds. *Shadow on a Tightrope: Writings on Fat Oppression.* Iowa City, IA: Aunt Lute, 1983.

Wooley, Susan C., and Wayne O. Wooley. "Woman and Weight Obsession: Redefining the Problem," in P. A. Treichler, C. Kramarae and B. Stafford, eds., *For Alma Mater: Theory and Practice in Feminist Scholarship.* Chicago: University of Illinois Press, 1985, pp. 350–72. A review of research that challenges the popular myths about fatness and dieting and a discussion that fat is more an ethical and political problem than a medical, psychiatric or behavioral problem.

Agribusiness and Related Issues

Berry, Wendell. *The Unsettling of America: Culture and Agriculture.* Pasadena, CA: Sierra Club Books, 1986. An important exploration of the impact society and agriculture have on each other.

Burbach, Roger, and Patricia Flynn. *Agribusiness in the Americas.* New York: 1980. Available from North American Congress on Latin America, 475 Riverside Drive, Room 454, New York, NY 10115. Analyzes the workings and impact of agribusiness on an international scale.

Financial pages of any major newspaper, for example, *The New York Times, The Wall Street Journal,* keep you current on the workings of agribusiness.

Fowler, Cary, and Pat Mooney. *Shattering: Food, Politics, and the Loss of Genetic Diversity.* Tucson: University of Arizona Press, 1990.

George, Susan, and Nigel Paige. *Food for Beginners.* New York: Writers and Readers Publishing, 1982. Food production facts and myths.

Gussow, Joan. *Chicken Little, Tomato Sauce, and Agriculture: Who Will Produce Tomorrow's Food.* New York: Bootstrap Press. Available from ITDGNA, 777 United Nations Plaza, New York, NY 10017. How agribusiness is pushing food production off the land and into the laboratory.

Gussow, Joan, and Paul Thomas. *The Nutrition Debate.* Palo Alto, CA: Bull Publishing Co., 1986.

Krebs, A. V. *The Corporate Reapers: The Books of Agribusiness.* Washington, DC: Central Books, 1992. Available from Central Books, P.O. Box 19405, Washington, DC 20036.

Lappe, Frances Moore, and Joseph Collins. *Food First: Beyond the Myth of Scarcity.* New York: Ballantine Books, 1981. How food for profit keeps the world hungry. Well documented.

Rodefeld, Richard D., Jan Flora, Donald Voth, Isao Fujimoto and Jim Converse, eds. *Changes in Rural America: Causes, Consequences and Alternatives.* St. Louis: C. V. Mosby Co., 1978. An anthology with good introductions to each section.

Resources for Change

Americans for Safe Food, a project of Center for Science in the Public Interest. See CSPI listing for address. Promotes sustainable agriculture through coalitions and education for changing policy and legislation on the state level. Encourages locally grown, organic food.

Appropriate Technology Transfer for Rural Areas, P.O. Box 3657, Fayetteville, AR 72702, (501) 442-9824 or (800) 346-9140. Works with commercial growers to encourage sustainable techniques and promote local marketing of produce.

Center for Science in the Public Interest, 1875 Connecticut Avenue, N.W., Suite 300, Washington, DC 20009-5728. Publishes *Nutrition Action* magazine and a long list of valuable books and posters. Does research and prods government. Send for publications list.

Farallones Institute. *The Integral Urban House.* San Francisco: Sierra Club Books, 1979. Section on food raising (plants and animals) contains much useful information for urban gardeners. Includes information on lead.

Harty, Sheila. *Hucksters in the Classroom: A Review of Industry Propaganda in Schools.* Washington, DC: Center for Study of Responsive Law, 1979. Available from Center for Study of Responsive Law, P.O. Box 19367, Washington, DC 20036. Excellent section on the food industry.

Hertzberg, Ruth, Beatrice Vaughn and Janet Greene. *Putting Food By.* New York: Viking Penguin, 1982. Comprehensive. Covers all methods of preservation that can be done at home.

Institute for Food and Development Policy, 145 Ninth Street, San Francisco, CA 94103. Publishes written and audiovisual material about the politics of food distribution and hunger.

National Center for Agricultural Law, Research and Information, School of Law, University of Arkansas, Fayetteville, AR 72701, (501) 575-7646. Free information on agricultural legal issues, from pesticide drift to commodities markets.

The National Gardening Association, 180 Flynn Avenue, Burlington, VT 05401. National gardening advocacy group. Contact them to find out about gardening groups in your area. Publishes magazine and other literature.

Pesticide Action Network, 965 Mission Street, Room 514, San Francisco, CA 94103, (415) 541-9140. Publishes the quarterly *The Global Pesticide Campaigner.* Helps groups in the United States and abroad to implement sustainable agriculture.

Public Documents Distribution Center, Pueblo, CO 81009. Distributes government pamphlets, including several on food and related topics. Many free. Send for list.

Rodale Press, 33 E. Minor Street, Emmaus, PA 18049. Write for current publications list for books on gardening, self-help and nutrition. Includes classics such as *Encyclopedia of Organic Gardening.* Also sponsors Cornucopia Project, an education project to help agriculture toward self-sufficiency. Ads and notices in *Organic Gardening* magazine will lead you to other groups.

Society for Nutrition Education, 2001 Killebrew Drive, Suite 340, Minneapolis, MN 55425, (612) 854-0035. For professionals. Publishes journal.

3

Alcohol, Mood-Altering Drugs and Smoking

BY MARIAN SANDMAIER

1992 Update by Marian Sandmaier and Martha Wood.

As much as we would like it to be otherwise, all of us encounter stress in our daily lives. At one time or another, each of us struggles with work pressures, problems in our relationships, health concerns, loneliness, financial worries. Without thinking too much about it, many of us often respond to these pressures by pouring ourselves a drink, lighting a cigarette or taking a mood-altering pill; whether we're conscious of it or not, in each case we're using a drug to deal with what's bothering us.

Whether we use alcohol, pills or tobacco only occasionally or to the point where we feel dependent on them, we owe it to ourselves to find out more about the substances we're taking in.*

ALCOHOL

More of us are drinking than ever before, with two-thirds of adult women and about 80 percent of teenage girls now using alcohol regularly. Whereas society once frowned upon and even punished women for drinking, alcohol is now available to us—at times even pushed on us—in a

---

*Due to lack of space we will discuss only legal mood-altering drugs.

dizzying range of social and business situations. Now that more of us are working outside the home, we have both more opportunities to drink and more money of our own to spend on alcohol. The multibillion-dollar alcohol industry has been quick to take advantage of women's changing social and economic status with an aggressive advertising campaign geared to the "female market." In magazines as diverse as *Women's Day* and *Glamour*, we can scarcely turn a page without being offered a new kind of drink and with it the subtle promise of increased status, sophistication or sexiness. It is perhaps not surprising that in the United States alone, more than six million of us experience problems with alcohol use.

You just don't get many messages that say: hey, take this stuff seriously. You look at the beer commercials on TV or just your own social life where you get offered drinks coming and going, and you just see alcohol as another way to have a good time. No big deal. I think of all the times I got drunk at parties in college, and never once did it occur to me that I was overdosing on a drug. And now I come home from work every day and sit down with my two drinks before dinner, and if I was really honest with myself I would have to admit that in some small way I'm dependent on it.

We often forget that alcohol is a powerful, potentially addictive drug. Whenever we have wine with dinner, a vodka and tonic at a party or a couple of beers with the late movie, we are consuming a central nervous system depressant that slows down all our body's major functions. Alcohol diminishes motor coordination, judgment, emotional control and reasoning powers. Recent research indicates that women become intoxicated after drinking smaller amounts of alcohol than needed to produce intoxication in men. In having sex with a man, it is easier to forget protection and risk an unwanted pregnancy. In heavy-drinking situations we also may become more vulnerable to rape or other physical abuse. Sexist assumptions linking alcohol use to women's sexual availability remain in force: In one recent study, subjects rated drinking women as easier to seduce and more willing to engage in sex than nondrinking women.

Excessive drinking over a period of time not only leads to physical addiction but increases the risk of heart attack, stroke, brain damage, liver disease and several cancers. People who both smoke and drink are at particularly high risk for developing cancers of the upper respiratory and digestive tracts.[1] Chronic alcohol abuse appears to exact a particularly harsh physical toll on women. Women develop alcoholic liver disease after a comparatively shorter period of heavy drinking than men, and the death rate of female alcoholics is 50 to 100 percent higher than that of male alcoholics.

Women who drink very heavily during pregnancy—at least six drinks per day—may give birth to babies with *fetal alcohol syndrome*, a pattern of irreversible abnormalities that include mental retardation, prenatal and postnatal growth deficiencies and joint defects. As little as two drinks per day during pregnancy has been associated with lesser defects, notably lower birth weight in newborns. At present, no safe level of alcohol use during pregnancy has been established.[2]

In a society that judges women more harshly than men for dependence on alcohol, women tend to hide and deny their alcohol abuse rather than seek the help they need. Internalizing our culture's condemnation, alcoholic women suffer more guilt and anxiety than alcoholic men, have lower self-esteem and attempt suicide more often. Many women with drinking problems also become addicted to mood-altering pills prescribed by physicians who misdiagnose their alcoholism as "nerves" or depression (see p. 59 for getting help).

IF YOU DRINK

- It is a good idea to eat something before or while drinking. Sipping drinks, rather than gulping them, also slows down the rate at which the alcohol enters the bloodstream. A woman weighing between 100 and 140 pounds should allow about two hours for her body to metabolize or "burn up" each drink; a woman weighing between 140 and 180 should allow at least one hour between drinks. (A "drink" consists of three to five ounces of wine, twelve ounces of beer, or one ounce of hard liquor. Each contains the same amount of alcohol.)

- If you've been drinking, don't drive. Even small amounts of alcohol seriously interfere with judgment, coordination, vision and reaction time, all of which are crucial for safe driving.

- Avoid using alcohol within a few hours of using *any* other drug, including over-the-counter medications. When taken together, alcohol and many other drugs dangerously multiply each other's effects, with results ranging from headache, nausea and cramps to loss of consciousness and even death. It is particularly dangerous to mix alcohol with another central nervous system depressant, such as a barbiturate or tranquilizer.

- Sometimes the body is especially vulnerable to alcohol. When you're feeling sick or tired, for example, alcohol can affect your system more powerfully than usual. Women may be particularly vulnerable to alcohol's effects just prior to menstruation,[3] so it is a good idea to avoid using alcohol to relieve premenstrual discomfort. And during pregnancy, the safest course is not to drink at all.

- Avoid using alcohol as a problem solver. Many recovering alcoholic women report that they first began drinking heavily to cope with a specific crisis, such as a divorce or job loss, or to relieve chronic depression or anxiety. Such escape drinking keeps us from dealing with our underlying difficulties and tends to make us increasingly dependent upon alcohol—to the point where we can become addicted to it.

MOOD-ALTERING DRUGS

Unlike alcohol, mood-altering drugs, such as tranquilizers, antidepressants and sedatives, have long been marketed as *medicines*. They also have been primarily aimed at—and used by—women. In the nineteenth century, patent medicines containing dangerously large amounts of opiates were sold to women for relief of "female troubles." Today, physicians prescribe two-thirds of all legal psychoactive (mood-altering) drugs to women. Approximately 2 million women are estimated to have used these drugs daily for a year or more.

Prescription psychoactive drugs have justifiable and effective uses in certain short-term crisis situations, for truly disabling depression or anxiety and for some physical ailments. But too often, physicians prescribe these powerful, often addictive drugs to "treat" the ordinary stresses of daily life: boredom on the job, rambunctious children, loneliness, marital difficulties. With older women, the onset of menopause or a husband's death often becomes a reason to prescribe these drugs. More than one in four elderly women report taking these drugs, compared to one in six elderly men. Much of this "medicalization" of normal life problems is encouraged by the aggressive American drug industry[4] (see Chapter 25, "The Politics of Women and Medical Care"). Drug ads in medical and psychiatric journals often suggest that women are particularly unable to withstand the stresses of daily life without chemical relief.

I was in therapy when I got a new job in another state, and I talked with my psychiatrist about how nervous I was about the move and all the changes it would bring. She was very sympathetic about the problems involved in moving and adjusting to a new job. Then I watched as she took out her pad and wrote out prescriptions for a hundred Valium, a hundred Nembutal and a hundred Ritalin. "These might come in handy," she said as she handed me the three slips. At the time it never occurred to me not to get the prescriptions filled—that I might not need three hundred pills to survive the move.

Minor Tranquilizers

The minor tranquilizers (e.g., Valium, Librium, Serax, Equanil, Miltown) are designed to relieve anxiety and tension without significantly interfering with mental or physical functioning. Although their classification as "minor" distinguishes them from the "major" tranquilizers used primarily in the treatment of psychosis, there is nothing minor about the effects of these drugs or their abuse potential. Use of this term, encouraged by the drug industry, confuses both physicians and patients.

By far the most commonly prescribed of the minor tranquilizers are the benzodiazepines, which include Valium (diazepam) and Librium (chlordiazepoxide). Valium, an effective muscle relaxant as well as an antianxiety drug, is one of the most commonly prescribed drugs *of any type* in the United States, with women its primary users.

Although the benzodiazepines have long been considered one of the safest types of depressant drugs, negative effects reported for Valium and Librium include drowsiness, decreased muscular coordination, confusion, skin rashes, nausea, constipation, menstrual irregularities and changes in sexual drive. With Valium, paradoxical effects also have been reported, including insomnia, a reduction in REM (dream-producing) sleep, irritability, hostility and even rage. Still more alarming, Valium is the drug most frequently reported in connection with emergency-room visits caused by drug misuse or overdose.

In recent years, the addictive potential of the benzodiazepines has become increasingly apparent. The 1979 Senate hearings on problems associated with mood-altering drugs revealed that those who take the benzodiazepines regularly for more than four months are at the highest risk for addiction. In doses averaging only fourteen milligrams per day, withdrawal symptoms have been reported when benzodiazepines have been abruptly discontinued.[5]

New self-help approaches for gradually ending dependence on tranquilizers are being developed, with an emphasis on megavitamin therapy, nutrition, exercise and relaxation techniques. If you want to try this kind of program, be sure to get information about reliable methods[6] and the support of a knowledgeable person. Never try to kick a tranquilizer habit suddenly—or alone.

Barbiturates

Prescribed by physicians primarily to treat insomnia and anxiety, these depressant drugs include amobarbital (Amytal), butabarbital (Butisol), pentobarbital (Nembutal) and secobarbital (Seconal). Considered the most dangerous central nervous system depressants used in medicine today, barbiturates have a considerably higher potential for addiction and overdose than do the minor tranquilizers. They are also a major factor in many suicides, suicide attempts and accidental drug poisonings.

Although small doses of barbiturates will usually induce sleep, their effectiveness as sleeping pills lasts only about two weeks. At that point physical tolerance begins to develop, which means that it takes increasingly large doses to produce the same effects. Also, even with small doses, barbiturate-induced sleep often leads to grogginess, headache and a decrease in motor performance for several hours.

We cannot emphasize strongly enough the potential hazards of barbiturate use. Once you have developed a physical tolerance, the margin between a sleep-producing dose and a fatal dose is dangerously narrow. Barbiturates are also extremely hazardous in combination with alcohol: as little as two drinks taken with a moderate dose of barbiturates can cause an overdose. Finally, withdrawal from barbiturates must be undertaken gradually and under competent medical supervision, as abrupt discontinuation of these drugs can cause possibly fatal seizures.

Sedative-Hypnotics (Nonbarbiturate)

Among the most commonly prescribed of these sleep-inducing drugs are methaqualone (Quaalude), flurazepam (Dalmane), glutethimide (Doriden) and methyprylon (Noludar). Originally hailed as safer alternatives to the barbiturates, these drugs have been shown to pose many of the same risks of physical tolerance, addiction, dangerous withdrawal symptoms and overdose. Dalmane and Quaalude are among the most frequently named prescription mood-altering drugs in connection with drug-related emergency room visits. Both Quaalude and Doriden are stored in the body's fat tissue and are difficult to expel from the system, so that a person may apparently recover from the adverse effects of one of these drugs only to have the stored drug released into the system later, causing further complications.

Shirley Zeiberg

Common side effects of these drugs are headache, hangover and dizziness; less often reported effects include nausea, vomiting, blurred vision and paradoxical nervousness and excitement. All these drugs are extremely dangerous in combination with alcohol.

Antidepressants

The most widely prescribed of these drugs are the tricyclic antidepressants, including doxepin (Sinequan), imipramine (Tofranil), amitriptyline (Elavil), desipramine (Norpramine, Pertofran) and nortriptyline (Aventyl). Although they are considered effective for some types of depression, improvement is usually not apparent for several weeks. There is also evidence that antidepressants may not always be the crucial factor in relieving depression: In one study, 60 percent of patients improved after taking Tofranil, while 40 percent improved with a placebo, or sugar pill.[7]

Common side effects of tricyclic antidepressants are dry mouth, constipation, urinary retention, blurred vision, weight gain and drowsiness. When these drugs are stopped abruptly after prolonged use, nausea and headache may result.

Amphetamines

Amphetamines, or "pep pills," are highly addictive stimulant drugs usually prescribed for weight loss,* chronic fatigue and sleep disorders. Common brand names are Benzedrine and Dexedrine. These drugs have such a high potential for abuse and dependence that they are now accompanied by a written warning to physicians: "Should be prescribed or dispensed sparingly." They also have been shown to have so little value in long-term weight reduction that several states have banned their use for this purpose.

Low doses of amphetamines temporarily decrease appetite, relieve drowsiness and increase heart rate, blood pressure and breathing rate. Physical tolerance can develop within a few weeks of regular use, requiring increasingly large doses. With higher doses, some people report feelings of intense excitement and overconfidence; others become irritable and anxious. Common effects include sweating, insomnia, blurred vision, dizziness and diarrhea. Hazards of high doses also include risk of vascular damage or heart failure from a sudden increase in blood pressure, severe appetite loss and resulting malnutrition, and a general weakened condition that invites infection.

---

*In 1978 the Food and Drug Administration disapproved the use of amphetamines for weight loss, but many doctors still prescribe them.

SAFE USE OF DRUGS

- Before accepting a prescription for *any* drug, mood-altering or otherwise, ask your doctor: What is this drug for, and what are some nonchemical alternatives to it? Exactly how does this drug work on my body and mind? What are the risks, benefits and possible negative effects? Can I become addicted to this drug? How does it interact with other drugs, with certain foods and with alcohol? What are the specific risks of using this drug during pregnancy? How do I take the drug—when, how often, for how long, with food or not? How do I store the drug?

- If a prescribed drug comes with a patient information brochure, read it and follow instructions carefully. If there is no brochure, ask your doctor or pharmacist to show you the information on prescribing and adverse effects that the government requires drug companies to provide for each drug, or check the *Physician's Desk Reference* in your library. If any of this information is difficult to understand, ask to have it explained to you in layperson's terms. Be aware that brochures do not always list all side effects.

- Pay attention to your physical and emotional response to *any* drug you take. Even over-the-counter drugs can have unpre-

dictable and hazardous effects and should always be used with caution.

- Although it may seem like a helpful gesture, avoid sharing pills with family members or friends. A drug that is safe for one person may have unpredictable and harmful effects on someone else.

- Never take any mood-altering drug within a few hours of using alcohol or any other drug. A mixture of alcohol and tranquilizers, barbiturates or other sedative drugs can be an especially dangerous, even fatal, combination.

- Avoid taking mood-altering drugs during pregnancy. Minor tranquilizers, barbiturates and amphetamines have been associated with birth defects in newborns.

- When accepting a prescription for any mood-altering drug, make an appointment with your doctor for a reevaluation within one month. At that point, fully discuss with your physician the risks and benefits of the drug before accepting a refilled prescription or an increase in the dosage. Since extended use of many drugs can produce dependence and other harmful effects, it is important to explore nonchemical ways of coping with the stresses you are facing (see "Stress and Tension," p. 67).

Drugs and Alcohol: Getting Help

Our use of alcohol or mood-changing pills can become such a part of our daily lives that sometimes we don't notice when it has become a problem. Here are some questions you can ask yourself.

- Has someone close to you sometimes expressed concern about your drinking or drug use?
- When faced with a problem, do you often turn to alcohol or pills for relief?
- Are you sometimes unable to meet home or work responsibilities because of pills or alcohol?
- Has your drinking or pill use caused any problems in relationships with family, friends or co-workers?
- Do you often take a pill or have a drink to get going in the morning?
- Do you find you have to take increasing amounts of pills or alcohol to achieve the same effects?
- Have you had distressing physical or psychological reactions when you've tried to stop drinking or using drugs?

- Have you—or has anyone else—ever required medical attention as a result of your drinking or pill use?
- Have you often failed to keep the promises you have made to yourself or others about controlling or cutting out your drug use or drinking?
- Do you ever feel guilty about your drinking or pill use or try to conceal it from others?

If you have answered "yes" to any of the above questions, your drinking or pill use is probably interfering with your life in serious ways and you should seek help. You can overcome alcohol and other drug problems, and the sooner you get help, the easier it will be to free yourself from dependence on these substances.

I was positive I didn't have a drinking problem. After all, I only drank beer and wine, I never drank till after five o'clock, I still had my kids and I wasn't on skid row. But I needed alcohol to blot out something—some reality about myself and my life that I couldn't stand to feel. And I could say all I wanted about being "just a social drinker," but the truth of it was I couldn't stop on my own. I needed help.

Few people struggling with alcohol or drug problems can overcome them alone, without the support and help of others who have "been there." Probably the best-known self-help group for recovering alcoholics is Alcoholics Anonymous (AA), which holds group meetings in most communities across the country, including groups for women and for lesbians. Al-Anon and Alateen help the families and friends of problem drinkers. Women for Sobriety is a network of local support groups that focuses on the special issues and needs of women with drinking problems. Other newer self-help support groups for alcoholics include Rational Recovery and Secular Organizations for Sobriety, both of which focus on self-empowerment and personal responsibility as paths to sobriety. (See Resources for more information.)

In addition to these independent self-help groups, most local alcohol and drug treatment programs sponsor their own outpatient therapy and support groups. If you have a serious problem with alcohol or drugs, you may want to participate fully in one of these formal treatment programs, which provide medical care, individual and group therapy and a range of support services. It is important to emphasize that the aim of such treatment is not simply to "get you off drugs" but to help you better understand yourself and create a new life situation in which you won't *need* alcohol or pills to function. If there is a treatment program in your community designed specifically for women and staffed by women, you may find it particularly helpful. Other women may be more likely to understand your situation, your pressures and conflicts, and your practical as well as your physical and emotional needs. Child care also may be available at some programs.

To find an appropriate treatment program or support group, check your area council on alcoholism, your local women's center or community mental health center, the social services or health department of your city or county or the employee assistance program of your workplace, if there is one. (Check the yellow pages of your local phone book under "Alcoholism" or "Drug Abuse.")

After being that wiped out, I want it all. I'm fifty-one years old and I want everything that's due me as a person. I got off drugs to get a new life—and I'm going to have it.

SMOKING

By the time I was twenty years old I was up to two packs a day and a lot of the time I just felt rotten. I had a chronic cough and I would wake up in the middle of the night and cough and gag until sometimes I threw up. I felt my chest was so full of fluid I could almost scoop it out with a ladle. I always felt weak, like I had a cold I could never get rid of. What made me decide to quit was the thought that if I'm this bad off at twenty, what do I have to look forward to later?

More women smoke now than fifty years ago, for many of the same reasons that more of us are drinking. Although smoking has been slowly declining among adult women in recent years—about 27 percent of women currently smoke—those of us who do use cigarettes are more likely to be heavy smokers than in the past. Girls are beginning to smoke at younger ages than ever before, more than half before they are age thirteen. Among young people seventeen to nineteen, more girls than boys are now using cigarettes for the first time in history.[8]

For those of us who smoke, the news is not good. Women who smoke have more than a 5.5 times greater likelihood of developing lung cancer than nonsmoking women. Women's lung cancer incidence rates have increased 3 percent annually since the early 1980s. More women die of lung cancer than breast cancer in the United States, making lung cancer the leading cancer killer for women.

Compared to nonsmoking women, those who smoke cigarettes are more likely to suffer heart attacks, strokes and other serious cardiovascular disorders. Women who use oral contraceptives and also smoke are *ten times* as likely as female nonsmokers to suffer coronary heart disease. Cigarette smoking in women is also causally associated with cancers of the urinary tract, larynx, oral cavity, esophagus, kidney, pancreas and cervix. Women who smoke are also at greater risk for death from chronic obstructive lung disease and are more likely than nonsmokers to suffer from osteoporosis, chronic bronchitis, emphysema, chronic sinusitis, peptic and duodenal ulcer disease and severe hypertension. Smoking has also been linked with decreased fertility in women and with early menopause.

Passive smoking—that is, exposure to the cigarette smoke of others—is a serious health risk. Studies have shown that nonsmoking women exposed to their husbands' cigarette smoke were twice as likely to develop lung cancer as nonsmoking women with nonsmoking husbands. Other studies have shown that children of parents who smoke are at higher risk for respiratory ailments than children of nonsmoking parents and at increased risk for developing leukemia and lymphoma as adults.

Smoking and passive smoking during pregnancy poses serious risks for the unborn. Babies of women who smoked cigarettes during pregnancy are likely to be sicker and to weigh less at birth and appear never to catch up. Smoking during pregnancy also increases the risk of bleeding, premature rupture of membranes, miscarriage, premature delivery and neonatal death. Risk of sudden infant death syndrome (SIDS) may also be increased by smoking during pregnancy. Passive smoking may affect a child's intelligence, language and speech development, school performance and behavior.

I wish some of this information had been around when I was young. I started smoking back in the thirties when I was twelve years old, and I never knew there was anything wrong with it. They did tell us that smoking stunted your growth, but I was tall so I didn't care. I smoked all through my teens, twenties and thirties, and not a single person ever suggested that I stop.

Kicking the Habit

There is simply no "safe way" to smoke. Low-tar and -nicotine cigarettes do not lessen the risk of lung diseases, heart disease or fetal damage during pregnancy. The safest and healthiest course is simply to stop smoking. Difficult as quitting may be, more of us than ever are successfully freeing ourselves from addiction to tobacco. One out of every three women who has ever smoked has now kicked the habit, and since 1976 the percentage of woman who smoke has declined from 33 to 27 percent.

The results are worth it. Even if a woman is a heavy smoker, after quitting her risk of heart attack drops to near normal within two years. The risk of developing lung, kidney and laryngeal cancer drops gradually, nearly equaling that of nonsmokers after ten years. Although some of us fear that when we stop smoking we will gain unwanted weight, research shows that the average weight gain is only five pounds. Women who quit report that they have never felt better.

It's a great feeling to be able to do so many of the things that were just out of the question while I was smoking—running around the park, dancing for hours at a time, little things like enjoying the fragrance of my own clean hair. Just knowing that I'm healthier and my kids are probably healthier.

There's a great sense of accomplishment and power that comes from quitting—power to get ahold of your own life. But there's no way it's easy. I still identify with being a smoker. I still smoke in my dreams. If I thought I could go back to cigarettes and only smoke two or three a day, I'd do it in a minute. But I know I can't smoke that way. If I

smoked one, I'd smoke a pack, and I won't do that to myself anymore.

Studies indicate that the ability to quit smoking successfully depends largely on a strong commitment to stop, the belief that we *can* stop and support from others. There are a number of free or low-cost programs available to those of us who want to stop smoking, including those offered through local chapters of the American Cancer Society and the American Lung Association. Some of these programs offer special support groups for women. Other low-cost programs can be found through hospitals, health maintenance organizations, schools, businesses and community groups. Commercial smoking-cessation programs are also available, but they tend to be considerably more expensive.

We can participate in one of the formal programs offered in our community, or we can ask a friend or relative to stop smoking with us. And if we swear off cigarettes, then "slip" at some point along the way, we need to remember that nearly everyone does at one time or another. We need to try again—and again. It *is* hard to stop smoking. But it is also possible—and it is one of the biggest favors we will ever do for ourselves and our health.

NOTES

1. U.S. Department of Health and Human Services. *Fourth Special Report to the U.S. Congress on Alcohol and Health.* Washington, DC: U.S. Government Printing Office, 1981, pp. 47–59.

2. U.S. Department of Health and Human Services. "Surgeon General's Advisory on Alcohol and Pregnancy," *FDA Drug Bulletin*, Vol. 11, No. 2 (July 1981), pp. 9–10. Still holds true in 1992.

3. Ben M. Jones and Marilyn K. Jones. "Women and Alcohol: Intoxication, Metabolism and the Menstrual Cycle," M. Greenblatt and M.A. Schuckit, eds., *Alcohol Problems in Women and Children*, New York: Grune & Stratton, 1976, pp. 103–36.

4. Richard Hughes and Robert Brewin. *The Tranquilizing of America.* New York: Harcourt Brace Jovanovich, 1979, pp. 192–3.

5. Karl Rickels et al. "Long-term Therapeutic Use of Benzodiazepines. 1. Effects of Abrupt Discontinuation," *Journal of the American Medical Association*, Vol. 265, No. 15 (April 17, 1991), p. 1934.

6. See Bernard Green. *Goodbye, Blues: Breaking the Tranquilizer Habit the Natural Way.* New York: McGraw Hill, 1981.

7. Conan Kornetsky. "Drugs Used in the Treatment of Depression and Anxiety," in *Pharmacology: Drugs Affecting Behavior.* New York: John Wiley, 1976, p. 109.

8. U.S. Department of Health and Human Services. *The Health Consequences of Smoking for Women: A Report of the Surgeon General.* Washington, DC: U.S. Government Printing Office, 1980, p. 275.

RESOURCES

Alcohol and Drugs

Readings

Black, Claudia. *Children of Alcoholics: "It Will Never Happen to Me!"* New York: Ballantine Books, 1987.

Green, Bernard. *Goodbye Blues: Breaking the Tranquilizer Habit the Natural Way.* New York: McGraw-Hill, 1981. A step-by-step self-help program for gradually ending dependence on tranquilizers.

Jerome, Joan. *The Lost Years: Tranquillisers and After.* London: Virgin Publishing, 1991. An excellent self-help guide to avoiding, dealing with and recovering from tranquilizer addiction.

Kirkpatrick, Jean. *Goodbye Hangovers, Hello Life: Self-Help for Women.* New York: Ballantine Books, 1987.

McDaniel, Judith. *Metamorphosis: Reflections on Recovery.* Ithaca, NY: Firebrand Books, 1989.

Peele, Stanton, and Archie Brodsky. *The Truth About Addiction and Recovery.* New York: Simon & Schuster, 1991. A powerful, well-documented challenge to the notion of addiction as a disease and to the twelve-step ideology of recovery.

Roth, Paula, ed. *Alcohol and Drugs Are Women's Issues*, Vol. 1, *A Review of the Issues.* Metuchen, NJ: The Scarecrow Press Women's Action Alliance, 1991. A comprehensive review of the issues with a strong multicultural orientation.

——, ed. *Alcohol and Drugs Are Women's Issues*, Vol. 2, *The Model Program Guide.* Metuchen, NJ: The Scarecrow Press Women's Action Alliance, 1991. A step-by-step guide to replicating the model prevention and intervention program, developed by the Women's Action Alliance and tested at women's centers throughout the country.

Sandmaier, Marian. *The Invisible Alcoholics: Women and Alcohol Abuse*, 2nd ed. Blue Ridge Summit, PA: Tab Books, 1992. Explores why women drink, social attitudes, treatment needs and how and where to get help. Includes in-depth interviews with diverse women.

Wilsnack, Sharon, and Linda Beckman, eds. *Alcohol Problems in Women.* New York: The Guilford Press, 1984. Analysis of women's drinking patterns, consequences, treatment and prevention issues.

Audiovisual Materials

The Last to Know, a 45-minute 1984 film or videocassette. Available from New Day Films, 121 West 27th Street, Room 902, New York, NY 10001. A powerful feminist film on women's experience with alcohol and drug abuse.

Straight from the Heart: Stories of Mothers Recovering from Addiction, a 28-minute video. Six women of various ethnic and socioeconomic backgrounds support each other in a moving and powerful discussion about their addictions, ongoing recoveries, and how they got help. Available from Vida Health Communications, Inc., 6 Bigelow Street, Cambridge, MA 02139.

Organizations

Al-Anon Family Groups
P.O. Box 862
Midtown Station
New York, NY 10010
Sponsors self-help meetings for spouses and children of alcoholics. For information, literature and groups, contact your local Al-Anon office.

Alcoholics Anonymous
P.O. Box 459
Grand Central Station
New York, NY 10163
A worldwide self-help organization for recovering alcoholic women and men, with local chapters in most communities. Offers pamphlets for women, and for lesbians and gay men, and sponsors meetings for women and gays in some cities. To find meetings, contact AA headquarters or your local AA office (see phone directory).

National Association of Gay and Lesbian Alcoholism Professionals
204 W. 20th Street
New York, NY 10011
(212) 713-5074
A communication and support network. Publishes newsletter, bibliography and list of treatment resources for gay and lesbian alcoholics, and provides referrals to gay and lesbian groups of AA and Al-Anon.

National Black Alcoholism Council
1629 K St. NW
Washington, DC 20006
(202) 296-2696

National Clearinghouse for Alcohol and Drug Information
Box 2345
Rockville, MD 20852
A federal information service offering free publications on alcohol and drug abuse.

National Council on Alcoholism and Drug Dependence
12 West 21st Street, 8th Floor
New York, NY 10010
A national coordinating organization for local councils on alcoholism with publications on women and families. Local councils provide treatment referrals.

Rational Recovery
Box 800
Lotus, CA 95651
(916) 621-2667
Self-help groups nationwide that focus on self-empowerment through changing beliefs about self and drinking. An alternative to AA's spiritual emphasis.

Secular Organizations for Sobriety, National Clearinghouse
Box 5
Buffalo, NY 14215
(716) 834-2922
Self-help groups nationwide that emphasize personal responsibility and group support. No spiritual emphasis.

Wisconsin Clearinghouse on Alcohol and Other Drug Abuse
P.O. Box 1468
Madison, WI 53701
Offers low-cost, readable materials, including resources for lesbians and materials on fetal alcohol syndrome.

Women for Sobriety
P.O. Box 618
Quakertown, PA 18951
A national self-help organization for recovering alcoholic women. Write for referral to a local group.

Women's Alcohol and Drug Education Project
Women's Action Alliance, Inc.
370 Lexington Avenue, Suite 603
New York, NY 10017
(212) 532-8330
Offers a model prevention-intervention program on women's alcohol and drug problems for use in women's centers.

Smoking

Readings

American Cancer Society. "How Can We Reach You?" 1985. (Also available in Spanish.) Hazards and suggestions for breaking the habit. Available free from local units of the American Cancer Society.

Delaney, Sue. *Women Smokers Can Quit: A Different Approach.* 1989. Easy-to-follow book on cessation. Available from Women's Healthcare Press, 500 Davis Street, Suite 700, Evanston, IL 60201. $6.95.

Fielding, J. E., et al. "Smoking and Women: Tragedy of the Majority," *New England Journal of Medicine*, Vol. 317 (November 19, 1989), pp. 1343–5.

Janerich, Dwight T., Thompson W. Douglas, Luis R. Valela, et al. "Lung Cancer and Exposure to Tobacco Smoke in the Household," *New England Journal of Medicine*, Vol. 323, No. 10 (June 6, 1990), pp. 632–6.

March of Dimes. "Give Your Baby a Healthy Start: Stop Smoking." 1990. Health hazards of smoking to fetus and tips on stopping smoking. Free from local March of Dimes chapters.

Massachusetts Department of Public Health. *Women vs. Smoking: Our Health or Their Profits.* 1988. Conference proceedings. Available from Office for Nonsmoking, Massachusetts Department of Public Health, 150 Tremont Street, Boston, MA 02111. Free. Also available: "Parents' Smoking, Children's Health." 1989. (Available in Spanish.) Fact sheet on hazards of second-hand smoke. Also: "Women and Smoking." 1989. Pamphlet on special health risk for women who smoke.

Slattery, Martha L., Linda M. Robinson, Katharina L. Schuman, et al. "Cigarette Smoking and Exposure to Passive Smoke Are Risk Factors for Cervical Cancer," *Journal of the American Medical Association*, Vol. 261, No. 11 (March 17, 1989), pp. 1593–2598.

U.S. Department of Health and Human Services. *Clearing the Air: How to Quit Smoking.* Washington, DC: U.S. Government Printing Office, 1989. A readable guide with information on smoking-cessation programs. Available free from the Office of Cancer Communications, National Cancer Institute, Bethesda, MD 20892.

U.S. Department of Health and Human Services. *The Health Consequences of Smoking for Women: A Report of the Surgeon General.* Washington, DC: U.S. Government Printing Office, 1980.

U.S. Department of Health and Human Services. "The Health Consequences of Smoking: Nicotine Addiction." 1988. A report of the surgeon general. Available from: Office for Smoking and Health, Centers for Disease Control, 1600 Clifton Road, NE, Atlanta, GA 30333.

U.S. Department of Health and Human Services. "Smoking and Health: A National Status Report." 1990. A guide to national, state and local programs and projects. Available from Office for Smoking and Health, Centers for Disease Control, 1600 Clifton Road, NE, Atlanta, GA 30333.

U.S. Environmental Protection Agency. "Environmental Tobacco Smoke," Indoor Air Facts No. 5. Available from Public Information Center, U.S. Environmental Protection Agency, Mail Code PM-24B, 401 M Street SW, Washington, DC 20460. Free.

Audiovisual Materials

The Feminine Mistake, a 25-minute 1977 videocassette. A straightforward presentation of the dangers of cigarette smoking aimed primarily at young women. Includes an interview with a lung cancer victim. Available on loan from local units of the American Cancer Society and American Lung Association.

The Feminine Mistake: The Next Generation, a 30-minute 1989 videocassette. This film retains the most powerful images from the original version and brings the issue of women and smoking into the present. Available from Pyramid Film and Video, Box 1048, Santa Monica, CA 90406-1048.

First Time, Last Time, a 30-minute 1988 series of vignettes about women from teenage to middle age, discussing how they began smoking and their failures and successes at quitting. Available for free loan or purchase from your local chapter of the American Cancer Society.

The Lady Killers, a 40-minute British documentary featuring Bobbie Jacobson, author of two books on women and smoking. The video explores the reason why women smoke and barriers to quitting that are particular to women. Available from Communications Media, Yale Medical School, 333 Cedar Street, New Haven, CT 06510.

Organizations

Action on Smoking and Health
2013 H Street NW
Washington, DC 20006
A citizen's group working for legislation to reduce the health toll of smoking and protect nonsmokers' rights.

American Cancer Society
  3340 Peachtree Rd., NE
  Atlanta, GA 30026

American Heart Association
  7320 Greenville Avenue
  Dallas, TX 75231

American Lung Association
  1740 Broadway
  New York, NY 10019

The above three are national voluntary organizations that provide free or low-cost smoking-cessation programs and publish materials. Contact your local branch for information.

Americans for Nonsmokers' Rights
  2530 San Pable Avenue
  Berkeley, CA 94702

DOC: Doctors Ought to Care
  1423 Harper Street
  Augusta, GA 30912

4

Women in Motion

BY JANET JONES

With special thanks to Pat Lyga, Judith Stein and all the wonderful women who shared their experiences, feelings, thoughts, hard work and dreams and so made this chapter possible.

This chapter in previous editions was written by Janet Jones and Carol McEldowney.

1992 Update acknowledgment: Mary Lee Slettehaugh, Melpomene Institute.

A lot more of us women are out in the world moving around and *it feels good*. We are swimming, walking, dancing, jogging, power lifting, fencing and hiking. We play basketball, softball, soccer, rugby, badminton, racquetball, volleyball, lacrosse. We are bowling, skiing, gardening, canoeing, wrestling, skating, rock climbing. We play tennis, football, ice hockey, golf. We are boxing, surfing, scuba diving, motorcycle racing. We take archery, karate, yoga, judo, aikido, tai chi and gymnastics. We bike, sail, ride horses, race cars, take jazzercise and skydive. Times have changed!

North American women did not always exercise and do sports. The urban woman toiling long hours in factories, the pioneer woman, the slave woman, the poor white fieldworker—the lives of these women in the nineteenth century were so physically demanding that "exercise" as such was meaningless. For the middle-class woman, exercise was for the most part deemed "unladylike." She wore long, heavy dresses that allowed a minimum of movement and corsets that inhibited or impaired every organ in the torso, from lungs to uterus. Today only a few jobs are as physically demanding as those in the nineteenth century. Though many occupations are stressful and emotionally draining, almost none provides all the kinds of movement a healthy body, mind and spirit need.

Most women agree that over the past decade we have grown more active, both because of our increasing awareness of the health benefits of exercise and because the women's movement has brought a consciousness of our right to be vital, strong, confident people. All of us are not out there

Peter Southwick/Stock Boston

exercising all the time because there still are obstacles, both external and internal. But we are out there more often.

EXERCISE, SPORTS, PHYSICAL PLAY: WHAT THEY DO FOR US

Living is moving. Even when we lie still, all is in motion inside: the blood flows, the chest expands and contracts as we breathe, we digest food and eliminate wastes. The mind is full of thoughts, ideas, feelings, dreams. It is natural to want to move externally, too. We go to work, to the movies; we visit friends and shop. When we're forced to remain stationary, the urge to move increases. Hospital patients, confined to bed, look forward to the day they will be able to walk up and down the hall; prisoners locked in tiny, overcrowded cells demand the right to yard and exercise privileges; a paraplegic person whose specially equipped van is wrecked feels totally cut off from society. Women march in cities and towns every year to protest the violence against women that forces us indoors. Economically and psychologically, we need to be out in the world.

Exercise is good for every system in our bodies. Even women with chronic health problems like asthma or diabetes benefit from exercise.

The Cardiovascular System and Aerobic Exercise

When we move vigorously on a regular basis for twenty or more minutes at a time, the heart (a muscle) gets stronger and more efficient, pumping more blood with fewer strokes. Over time, this kind of *aerobic* exercise—that is, exercise that keeps us breathing hard while our blood is circulating rapidly—increases the actual number and size of blood vessels in our tissues and so increases their blood supply. When we exercise hard, blood circulates faster through these expanded vessels, bringing oxygen and nutrients to every part of us and taking wastes away more quickly. That's why we usually feel refreshed and invigorated afterwards.

The Respiratory System

Exercising makes us breathe more deeply and regularly as more air moves rhythmically in and out of the lungs. The lungs develop a larger capacity, opening the air sacs up to the top and way down to the bottom of each lung for better gas exchange. We end up taking in more oxygen, which is essential for each cell in the body. If we practice rhythmic patterns of inhaling deeply, holding our breath and exhaling all the air slowly, we strengthen the respiratory system while quieting the mind.

The Musculoskeletal System

Muscles increase in size when they are used on a regular basis. Strong back and abdominal muscles are better insurance than Blue Cross/Blue Shield against the lower back pain which plagues so many of us these days. The abdominals also help hold the stomach and intestines in place and are critical to good digestion and elimination. Solid leg muscles get us where we are going and help the heart: When they contract, they squeeze the veins and so push the blood toward the heart, usually against the pull of gravity. Well-developed biceps and triceps muscles in the arms allow us to carry more and to perform everyday tasks with less effort and more independence. For self-defense purposes, the more muscle power we have the better. When all our muscles are firm and flexible, they protect us in many ways from the stresses and strains of living.

When we exercise, our bones get stronger, too. As muscles contract they pull on the bones, which increases bone strength over time. Also the body lays down extra minerals in the bones along the lines of stress. So if you walk or run, for example, the long bones in your legs will be gradually reinforced to meet the added pressure from your feet hitting the ground over and over again (see also Exercise and Growing Older, p. 70).

The Reproductive System

Far from damaging our "internal organs," as women were taught until recently (it doesn't, for instance, hurt breasts or cause prolapsed uterus), exercise helps them. The more active we are the less premenstrual syndrome and menstruation interfere with our lives. Exercise eases cramps, so unless you have excessive bleeding, nausea or vomiting, you can go at it as hard as you want during this time of the month.* Exercise during and after pregnancy is highly recommended.

---

*Those of us who run over thirty miles a week, exercise or train heavily in other ways may find we menstruate less or not at all. Probably one or a combination of factors are responsible: intensity of effort, length of workout, fat loss, emotional stress, etc. If this is happening, try cutting back on your workouts to see if you will resume your cycles. Note that you can become pregnant during long periods of amenorrhea. See Melpomene Institute for Women's Health Research, *The Bodywise Woman: Reliable Information about Physical Activity and Health.* New York: Prentice Hall, 1990. See Chapter 12, "Anatomy and Physiology of Sexuality and Reproduction."

Stress and Tension

Living in a stressful society subjects us to incredible daily assaults. Oppressive working conditions, problems at home, transportation hassles and concern for our physical safety can cause frustration, anxiety, anger and fear. When our minds become tense, our bodies do too.

Backache in North America, for example, has reached epidemic proportions, largely because of so much tension and so little exercise.[1] Tense muscles in the neck can cause splitting headaches; in the leg, charley horses; in the gut, stomachaches. Overcontracted muscles restrict breathing, slow down or even cut off the blood supply in their vicinity by squeezing the vessels shut, and actually limit our strength and sap our energy.* So if you can answer your boss back, do it. If not, walk or run off the irritation and anger. Punch a pillow till you are exhausted. Boogie until three in the morning. Or let it go by relaxing every muscle in your body one after the other, listening to your breathing or imagining yourself in the most beautiful of all beautiful places.

I drink in the sky colors around me, concentrate only on breathing and the feel of my body moving, on the joy of being. The franticness of the day subsides.

While we work to change this oppressive society into a humane one we can all live in, soothing our nerves through physical or mental activity is an important and necessary release, and gives us more energy to work for the changes we need.

Many health practitioners suggest exercise as an actual treatment for depression. Some, looking into what joggers call "runner's high," are beginning to think that strenuous exercise increases levels of a natural narcotic-like painkiller in the blood.† This interest in endorphins may also lead to an explanation of why exercisers get restless and irritable when they are "grounded" due to illness or injury: they are actually suffering withdrawal symptoms! Altogether a very interesting area of investigation and ripe for new discoveries.

You may or may not be "flying" after a workout, but you will almost invariably feel better than you did before: calmer, less tired, most likely refreshed. Maybe it was the one good thing you did with and for yourself in a time of messy problems with no neat solutions. Maybe it was wonderful because you did it with friends or because your basketball team played its best game ever—win or lose. Maybe you took on a real adventure, and the risk was exhilarating—made you feel alive all over. Being physically active builds confidence, independence, greater peace *and* vitality of mind. You connect to your own body and at the same time sense yourself a part of a larger whole. You are one with the energy of the universe.

OVERCOMING OBSTACLES

This all-out pep talk sounds great, *but* there are real problems that keep us from becoming and staying physically active.

Economics

For every dollar men make, white women make about sixty-five cents, women of color and disabled women much, much less. Our paychecks go for food, shelter, clothing, transportation, medical care. Who can spend much on recreation? Many women cannot afford the money to join a club or a Y, or the time away from work. Accessibility, too, is a problem.

The facilities I use are pretty far from both my job and my home. It's too hard to get there every day in rush-hour traffic. Plus my best exercise time is other people's, too, so the place can be discouragingly overcrowded.

TV and automobile-induced passivity; hard, dirty streets; heavy traffic; pollution; lack of daylight hours before and after work and safety factors also take their toll.

The obstacles that confront us are all much more formidable for women of color. During hard times, those of us who have never had much in the way of public facilities will have even less. Carmen, a teenager, remarks

My mother walks for exercise. There has never been a dime available for her to go to an evening group of any kind.

I try to run around a lot and have fun in gym class because the way everything is getting cut, after-school sports may get dumped. The Y is down the street from my house, but there are too many gang fights so I never go there. Too bad, because I love games, love being a tomboy. It makes me feel I'm as good as anybody.

Last summer I spent hours on the bus every day going to a daycamp that turned out to be racist on top of being miles away. I've already started looking for a better one for next year, but, well, I'm not too hopeful. They keep closing things down.

---

*Unfortunately, these are only a few of the negative effects of stress on our bodies.
†See *The Bodywise Woman: Reliable Information About Physical Activity and Health.*

When we are face to face with survival, any kind of real health care for the body and soul—sufficient and nutritious food, regular exercise and good times—appears to be an extravagance. So the challenge is how we can all join together to fight not just the cutbacks but also the prevailing government attitude which says scraping by is enough. We need bread *and* roses.* Nothing less will do.

Family

If a mother wants to exercise, what happens to the kids? We may not have money for a sitter or have a husband, lover, friend or relative to leave them with while we go for a workout. Some places offer child care, but it is usually limited.

Getting Jody to her infant swim, then Michael to preschool gymnastics and later on Mary to her teen dance class takes all my spare time. When do I have time for me? During one of their sessions, if I'm lucky!

Old Myths and Prejudices

Even with a minimum of obstacles, many of us still don't exercise on a regular basis. This may be because of some old myths and prejudices that we need to throw out once and for all. We know well the long, cold stare and remarks like

- Big shoulder muscles are really ugly on a woman.
- Hey, fatty, you should get your exercise pushing away from the dinner table.
- You four girls are going to hog this court when we guys need a team practice? No way!
- Don't you know that sweating is unfeminine?
- You're fifty-one and you're taking up—*what?!*
- Keep on pitching like a man, sweetheart—we know you're a dyke!
- What are these crippled women doing here? If I looked like that I wouldn't be caught dead in a bathing suit.

We have internalized many of these negative attitudes about women and exercise.

For my brother, physical fitness is like breathing, but not for me.

Everyone and everything still come first—that old pattern of taking care of ourselves last if at all. Somehow we don't feel entitled to the time, still don't feel

*A slogan from a banner carried by young girls in a march during the great Lawrence, MA, textile mill strike of 1912. "Bread and Roses" was made into a poem by James Oppenheim and set to music by Caroline Kohlsatt.

WHAT WE CAN DO

We can exercise in the privacy and relative safety of our own homes—it's cheaper and we can do it at the most convenient times for us—alone or with family and friends. If your apartment is small, clear a space so your body doesn't feel hemmed in. Keep whatever equipment you like around for easy use. Hang a chin-up bar over the door opening and buy some dumbbells. Stretching, strengthening exercises, yoga, dance, karate techniques, jumping rope, running in place, stationary bicycling and rowing can all be done in your own living room or bedroom.*

Turn on the music. A steady upbeat makes you want to move; the slower rhythms are good for stretching, where the point is to hold to a count of ten to twenty (repeat at least once) with no bouncing. Stretch in quiet sometimes, though, so you can tune into your own rhythms, get a sense of what your body can and can't do. Visualizing how you want to feel and what you want your body to look like as you move on to more difficult feats is extremely helpful.

Women with older children can do physical things with their kids. Vanessa, a woman in a local black community, used to manage a dance school that her daughters started.

I got a lot of pleasure out of joining those classes. Later I took karate with my boys at the community school night program. Even with a tight schedule, my motto is: you make time for what is important to you.

*There is a lot of glamorous (and expensive) exercise equipment on the market that you don't need to buy in order to get fit. Start with what you can do with the basics and then invest later (if at all) when you know what you really want or need.

we're worth it. Moreover, my husband gives me very little support, and my girlfriend's husband actively discourages her.

An end to these old prejudices! We must start getting the exercise we want and need.

Carla jogs with her kids, especially on weekends, and this works well for them. If you jog with your children (from six years on), be sure it is *fun;* they will run *playfully* for long distances without tiring (miles and miles) and will prefer this to sprinting.

At my son's suggestion, I got a baseball mitt when he was eight, and we've played a lot of catch since then, in addition to the jogging.

Sonya missed her every-other-day run so much when her baby came she decided she couldn't wait six, seven, ten years.

After a few months, I put Charelle in a sturdy stroller and now I jog pushing her along. This way I can keep active and my daughter is getting a feel for movement right from the beginning!

Use bike paths in your area. If you live in the country, get together and make tracks for cross-country skiing, a network of paths to connect your houses.

Since many commercial clubs and health spas are unsatisfactory,* you may want to start an exercise group. For example, after working unhappily in a very competitive club in the city, two women in a suburb of Boston decided to go into business for themselves and set up a Creative Movement Center. They run a very personal set of classes for women with kids. Mothers bring their babies (four to fourteen months), toddlers (fifteen months to two-and-a-half years) and preschoolers and later

---

*Many commercial "figure salons" are making big bucks off women's interest in exercise and obsession with weight. They have little useful equipment and offer pitifully little variety in terms of classes. The ones with more equipment and variety are expensive. Almost all are depressingly diet oriented. The women who staff them are usually undertrained and grossly underpaid for the work they do. Too many of us are tricked into worrying about the number of inches we are told we should lose when we need to be much more concerned with getting strong and resilient and developing our powers of relaxation, endurance and coordination in ways that challenge us physically and mentally.

schoolers in for gym. During the baby class, the mothers exercise with their infants or help them exercise. This routine includes stretching and strengthening exercises, gentle bouncing on the trampoline, rolling the baby downhill on a foam mat, helping her/him hang on a bar or set of rings and other activities that develop self-awareness, balance and coordination. In midmorning, there is an aerobic dance class for the women, while two sitters watch their kids in the adjacent day-care room. The atmosphere is caring and noncompetitive. There is lots of movement and music, and every young participant is treated as a full individual. The equipment is simple: inexpensive foam mats, a wooden bar set between two posts, small and colorful hoops that the kids sit in or dance with.

We need more such groups around the country, perhaps run cooperatively to keep the fees low. With a little money, space and ingenuity women can make them happen. One single mother is planning to do just this for herself and her friends.

I feel so much better when I exercise, but it's tough being motivated alone. I'm sick and tired of funneling my hard-earned money into the local exercise spas when I can do it in my own living room on a thick rug with some weights, *a couple of exercise books or exercise records (even a video), music and common sense. We'll work out the child-care arrangements, taking turns or chipping in for a sitter.*

Think about raising money for the facilities, equipment and ongoing political work we need to do by organizing walk–run races, swimathons, exhibition games, a play day. What better way to create an upward spiral? The healthy energy we spend developing our bodies and spirits can help to fund the next cycle of growth for us all.

---

*Dumbbells, barbells, ankle weights. For dumbbells you can use sand-filled juice or coffee cans or jugs of water or make beanbags with pellets in them.

EXERCISE AND DISABILITY

Differently abled women are finding each other and the programs they need. One very fine adapted yoga program takes place once a week at an urban self-help center.* Linda spends her day in a wheelchair. Her leg muscles cannot hold her up, but her back muscles are okay. If she sits hour after hour with no chance to exercise, her back and abdom-

---

*People come to the class with a wide variety of disabilities, from multiple sclerosis to cerebral palsy, from angina to sickle cell anemia.

inal muscles will wither away, and she will become even more disabled. Because several of the women, like Linda, are in wheelchairs, they are encouraged to walk a number of steps with help and then spend time on mats breathing, stretching and doing visualization exercises. Loretta Levitz, the woman who developed and runs the program, explains:

I want people to stay as active as they can and then start reclaiming the parts of their bodies that the doctors usually consider lost. The group support is very important; so is healthy food.

Tosca, a woman with multiple sclerosis who has been a regular for a long time, explained that when she tries too hard and gets too frustrated, she blocks her own progress.

About a year ago, one of my legs started "tremoring," as it often does. In anger I hit it. Then my other leg began shaking, too, but I decided to pat that one instead. The leg getting the loving treatment stopped its movement almost immediately, while the "abused" leg kept right on shaking.
Relaxation and breathing have helped me expand my physical abilities, given me hope and renewed determination.

Swimming has always been a physical activity for those of us with differing abilities. Women of all ages come to an adapted swim class at one local YWCA with many differences, from blindness to cerebral palsy, and each goes at her own pace. The instructors help their students get over fear of the water and then proceed to teach swimming and water safety skills. It is liberating to be free of the "hardware"—canes, crutches, wheelchairs—and into a medium that buoys you up. The women tell each other about events of their week with great humor and caring.

Across town at another facility, the pool coordinator and special-needs coordinator have made people of all ages with special mental, emotional and physical needs a priority. Their sessions run for two-and-a-quarter hours twice a week with support group first, then stretch and swim time. All the pool activities there emphasize the *whole* person, not just swim lessons.

Jean, a mentally disabled woman, loves the pool now that she has overcome her fear.

Swimming is great. I like the way the water feels and the fun we have in it.

Unfortunately, the local medical establishment takes faint interest in programs like these, and seems to think that these people might as well accept their limitations and forget it. Society's attitudes and economic priorities cause problems: class cost, odd-hour scheduling, transportation hassles and limited wheelchair accessibility keep more people from coming.

EXERCISE AND FAT

Our access to movement is limited by the prejudice we encounter (see chapter 1, "Body Image"). The ridicule, hostility and fear that greet us every time we walk down the street keep a lot of us immobilized in our homes. Learning to move around in public despite the harassment we face, learning to relax and take up all the space our bodies occupy instead of always trying to look smaller—these are victories over the people who want us always to feel ashamed of our size.

Some Guidelines on Movement for Fat Women*

- Choose something that looks like fun. Don't worry about whether it's "good" for you or not, or if you do, think about improving your circulation and heart tone.
- Forget about losing weight or "firming flab."
- Find a place where you already see big women exercising, or do it at home.
- Go with a friend. Pick someone about your size or similarly new to the activity. Don't start out with a "jock."
- Give yourself leeway to be good or not so good at something.
- Get together with other fat women to find facilities. (Swimming is great, but locker rooms and bathing suits can be humiliating. A group of women in San Francisco rent a city pool a few hours a week for a fat women's swim, which makes all the difference.)
- Try walking, depending on your neighborhood; bowling, which requires no special clothes; social or ballroom dance classes, where you can have a friend as a partner.
- You have a right to remain physically inactive if you choose.

EXERCISE AND GROWING OLDER

Our need for exercise continues, even increases, as we grow older. Some say it is essential. As our bodies age, we can lose flexibility, muscle strength

---

*From Judith Stein, cofounder of Boston Area Fat Liberation. See also, Pat Lyons, *Great Shape: The First Fitness Guide for Large Women*, Palo Alto, CA: Bull Publishing Co., 1990.

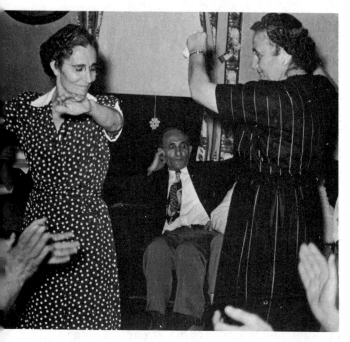

Varkey Sohigian

She runs about ten miles every day, walks a lot and dances, too. The people in her apartment building used to think she was crazy, but now they encourage her with, "Go, Ruthie!" She wishes they would get into it also, but so far very few have. She explains that women of her generation have many fears about their bodies, many don'ts and can'ts. Ruth guards her independence with a determined spirit, doing what feels right to *her*.

I need my sleep. I rest my arthritic leg when it bothers me, but I never miss that daily run.

Those of us in our sixties, seventies, eighties, nineties who are not out running ten miles do not need to let her example make us feel defensive but can let it inspire us to do something at home, at our social center or local Y. For instance, Miriam, living in a complex for the elderly in Pittsburgh, attends an exercise class in one of the lounges several times a week and goes walking regularly.

EXERCISE AND ILLNESS

After surgery or a long illness, we need exercise. Even in hospitals patients are encouraged to get out of bed as soon as possible. When we're ill, exercise gets the blood circulating, prevents painful bedsores and stimulates the respiratory system as well. If you are bedridden, it's important to get help with exercising the moveable parts of your body; even tensing and relaxing your muscles in a methodical way will help. Do some deep breathing at least once every hour.

Those of us who live in institutions would benefit from as much physical activity as possible, although we rarely get a fraction of what we need. Prisons, mental hospitals, nursing homes and similar institutions with their understaffing, heavy reliance on drugs and/or lockups remain inert if not crippling places. As Crystal tells it:

I've been in the nuthouse twice and jail once. If you let out how you feel in a physical way—and believe me, you need to—they just drug your ass, that's it. Or put you in max. I lost my body in there, and my mind.

OPTIONS

There are a lot of possibilities for fitness. Pick an activity that gives you pleasure, one you already enjoy or something new. Suit your exercise to your work. For stultifying jobs with a lot of sitting, pick an activity that excites you and gets your blood moving. If your work is physically exhausting, relax and stretch. Take breaks during the day (or

and aerobic power. Joints can become stiffer because the fluid in them can begin to dry up, joint space can narrow and bones weaken.* Muscles may sag more readily, and our minds, taking in all the ageist propaganda, may say, "Well, it's all downhill from here." We mustn't buy that line! Being active (perhaps with a longer warm-up period) will keep joints supple, although the first movements at the beginning of a workout may be more painful than in younger years. We can walk, swim, jog, lift weights, take up a new sport. Pay attention to your body; go slow but *don't* let your muscles and bones, heart and lungs deteriorate and your confidence with them. A friend, Woodie, took scuba diving recently to celebrate her fifty-fourth birthday:

Why wait? I said to myself. It's something I've always wanted to do.

Maybe we can't be as undaunted as Ruth Rothfarb, who at eighty ran her first marathon (Ottawa, 1981), but what a role model! At the end of the 26.2-mile course, her legs were tired, but

It was the greatest day of my life! I worked all my life in a store. I always liked the outdoors and enjoyed long walks, but there was never time for more. Eight or nine years ago I started jogging, and for the last five I have been competing.

---

*The gradual loss of calcium from the bones is called osteoporosis (see page 544).

night shift), too—stretch, walk around. A few wise employers provide company space and/or programs for employee fitness. Many more should be encouraged to do so—for everyone, not just VPs. Watch out for stereotypes: certain races, body types, "disabled" people can't do this or naturally excel at that. Never restrict your options based on other people's say-so. You can set modest health-oriented goals for each week, train seriously or go for a much more spontaneous kind of play—whatever keeps you moving. You may want to pick an aerobic activity first,* then add others according to your interests. Ask someone who has a lot of experience with the activity you choose, or read books to find out what it *is* and *isn't* doing for your body.† Just as walking, biking or running do little to develop our arms, torso and neck, so stretching and weightlifting need a supplementary aerobic exercise. Extra abdominal and back exercises are always in order. Some of us find it reasonably easy to be motivated alone. We turn inward more and prefer performing only for ourselves. Others of us need the push and encouragement of a group or TV show to get going and stay going. Some of us love team activities in which the social aspect—playing together—is very important. And new games are fun for everyone.‡

WALKING

Walking is excellent for all women who can use their legs. If you move along briskly, walking will do what running does: improve your circulatory and respiratory systems, increase muscle and bone strength, calm the nerves. It's great in sunshine, but a walk in the rain or snow can be equally terrific when you're dressed for it. Walk to work, or if that's too far, get off the bus two stops away. Go to the store on your feet, not on your behind; climb stairs instead of riding the elevator. Carrying a small pack on your back (three to five

pounds) adds a lot of benefit to brisk walking. Start slow, build up. After a while, you'll be going for an hour with no tiredness. Set a pace that feels good to you and develop an easy unbroken rhythm with the right stride for your leg length. Keep your feet pointing straight ahead and let your arms swing naturally at your sides (which means not carrying a pocketbook). Walking, like dancing and running, is primal movement. Women have been doing it for hundreds of thousands of years over fields and deserts, mountain slopes and city streets. It is free and requires no equipment (besides good shoes). Many of us who are older or fat have discovered that walking keeps the body active but does not stress it.

Unfortunately, physical safety is always a concern for women. Walk or run when and where there are a lot of people. If this isn't possible, go with a friend or a dog. When running or walking alone, assess your surroundings. Act confident. Keep an eye on any man who makes you feel uncomfortable—intuition is often right. Have a plan of action ready if a threatening situation develops. (See Martial Arts, page 74.)

JOGGING/RUNNING

Jogging and running do for you what walking does, but at a faster pace: your heart, lungs and all your systems get more of a workout. You can run purely for fun, for the good it does you physically, mentally and spiritually. Or you can get into a serious training program for competing in races or marathons.* Some people are bored by running; for others, it is a positive addiction. Mary, who is visually impaired, loves it. On weekends she runs with a friend:

---

*Contact your local chapter of The American Heart Association for pamphlets such a *Exercise and Your Heart.*

Forms of aerobic exercise include walking, jogging/running, swimming, biking, skipping rope, hiking, cross-country skiing, some forms of dance and group sports like basketball and soccer.
†Like *Sports for Life* by Robert Buxbaum and Lyle J. Micheli, Boston: Beacon Press, 1979. As far as we know, a whole popular book on activities and exercises for people with differing abilities has yet to be written, but Glorya Hale's *Source Book for the Disabled,* New York: Bantam Books (also Philadelphia: Saunders), 1979, does include a section on physical activity.
‡See *The New Games Book,* Andrew Fluegelman, ed., Garden City, NY: Dolphin, 1976, and *More New Games,* Dolphin, 1981. The new games books are full of new and old games that you can play "their" way or your own way with all ages, groups, and numbers of people—outdoors and in. The energy in the pictures and directions is infectious—it makes you long to head for a wide-open field and romp.

---

*Women's physiques are built so that we do very well at endurance sports like running. It's ironic that an official tried to literally run Kathy Switzer out of the Boston Marathon in 1967, and the Olympic Committee only recently gave women official permission to run in marathons. Our finishing times are improving with every race, and when it comes to the ultramarathons, we hang tough. A woman even finished at the head of the whole pack in one hundred-miler. See Ernst Van Aaken, *Van Aaken Method,* Mountain View, CA: World Publications, 1976, and Joan Ullyot, *Women's Running,* Mountain View, CA: World Publications, 1976.

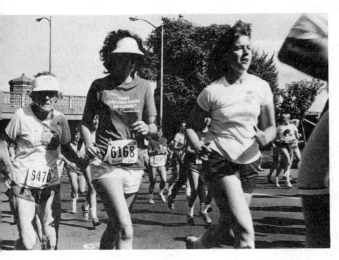

Sarah Putnam

We talk the miles away, getting caught up on each others' news over a five-mile course instead of a coffee cup.

Running does put pressure on the weight-bearing parts of the body: feet, ankles, knees, hips, spine. For this reason, well-fitted, well-padded running shoes (not sneakers) with good arch supports* are critical; the more protection between you and the ground, the better. Run on earth if it's even, tar-based pavement if necessary, concrete as little as possible. Keep your strides a comfortable length and low enough to the ground so you keep pounding to a minimum. Your feet should hit the ground heel first and roll forward to the toes. Develop a rhythm but don't let it limit you. Vary your pace and gait from time to time. Think light and lift your torso up off your pelvis and legs as you move along. Let your arms swing easily at your sides, shoulders relaxed, head steady but floating on the neck.

At least twenty minutes of jogging or running a few times a week, *plus* warm-ups, cool-downs and additional muscle-building exercises, will do it for fitness and keep injuries to a minimum for most people. Beyond this the risks are greater, as with any sport. Know what you are getting into. Look for good information on shoes, beginner's schedules, tips for running in different seasons, training for long-distance and injuries.

SWIMMING

Swimming—an especially good choice for larger women—is probably the most full-body and least physically stressful exercise going, once you know how to do it. Nonswimmers may have to overcome fear of the water, which is sometimes difficult, but the rewards are great. The water buoys you up, taking weight off aching backs, arthritic hips, bad knees, tired feet, weakened legs. You can do laps (twenty to thirty minutes several times a week) and get an excellent workout for a wide variety of muscles and your cardiovascular system even if you don't swim very fast. A lot of pools now offer aquatic exercises which put you through your paces whether you know how to swim or not.

If people are sensible and pools and beaches well guarded, swimming is a safe activity. While there are disadvantages to pool swimming—such as chlorine, membership or admission fees and crowds—most are well organized for lap swims at peak times and schedule swim classes to help you improve your skills.

As Lynn tells us:

Water is relaxing and calming for me, and some days very sensuous as well. The noise and distractions of the day just go as I tune into my own body and thoughts.

Water is really irresistible, maybe because our bodies are 70 percent water themselves and because we float in it for nine months before birth. Unless traumatized by some unhappy accident, children take to it fast. Mothers bring their infants as young as two to three weeks to the pool!* Play-

---

*Or even special arch supports (called *orthotics*) made from a mold of your own foot by a chiropractor, podiatrist or orthopedist.

*Claire Timmermans describes the whole process in *How to Teach Your Baby to Swim*, Briarcliff Manor, NY: Stein & Day, 1976.

Jowale Willa Jo Zollar of the dance troupe Urban Bush Women.   Cylla von Tiedemann

ing in the water is a joy, too—watch how long kids will keep busy, jumping in, sitting on the bottom, racing each other, playing catch, inventing new games all the time.

EASTERN DISCIPLINES

Eastern cultures have long understood that exercise involves body, mind and spirit, and that is why yoga, which means "union," is such an integrating experience. Everything you do as you practice yoga strengthens, stretches and relaxes your whole being. During half an hour to forty-five minutes of many poses you can stimulate all the major organs of the body. (For more, see Yoga, p. 92.)

Tai chi also originated in the East. It involves rhythmic body movements which put you in touch with your energy and the energy around you. You focus on balance and weight distribution. You are strong, not rigid; relaxed, not limp. You begin to heal yourself as you move. With calm and graceful motion you dance. It can also be a method of self-defense.

MARTIAL ARTS

Women continue to train in martial arts schools (run by women and men) at karate, aikido, judo, jujitsu. We develop self-defense skills, and with them confidence, a new physical presence and a mental awareness. We also enjoy the sports aspects. For instance, sparring in karate (controlled fighting with light or no body contact) is tremendously exciting, sometimes scary but often a tension releaser. Certain patterns and moves we learn in martial arts are very satisfying as art form, as fighting dance, as challenging sport, as meditation. Workouts often put a lot of stress on muscles, tendons, ligaments—especially in joint areas. Stretch properly beforehand. Don't get recklessly carried away in the thrill of learning how to strike or throw or in an effort to prove your seriousness to men in the class. Women's schools are or should be supportive of the slow and steady method for everyone—encouraging women with differing abilities to join and helping them to adapt standard techniques to what fits their situations best. These schools also need to help us deal with our feelings about all the violence around us and the political implications of what we are doing. Organizing a women's group inside a male school is useful for the same reasons—it may keep us going when we would otherwise drop out.

DANCE

Turn on the radio or put on your favorite record and move. Don't worry about the latest "steps," don't be shy, just get your body going. Dance for the sheer joy of it or dance off the effects of a long, frustrating day. Do it alone or with friends—at home or out on the town. Take a class in modern, jazz, African, belly, improvisational, ballet or aerobic dance. Or keep right on inventing what gives you pleasure. It's a great way to express emotion and moods physically without words. Stretch well before you start, know your limits and really get into it. Each time your body comes more alive, grows stronger, more coordinated and balanced. No matter what happens, no matter how depressing life becomes or how many hours we put in fighting against the injustices of the times, we must never forget to dance. We can dance (and sing) on the picket line, we can dance as we march and rally, we can dance as we celebrate our victories. Emma Goldman knew it when she proclaimed, "If I can't dance to it, it's not my revolution!"

BIKING, HIKING, SKIING, RACQUETBALL AND MORE

The beat goes on. Biking is terrific—you're outdoors with legs, hearts, lungs pumping hard and a helmet on! More and more people are riding to work. Hiking is excellent, too. In certain areas of the country we can enjoy it all year round while the rest of us switch in the winter to snowshoeing or cross-country skiing—equally great exercise. Racquetball has become a big favorite very fast; often, prime court time (i.e., before and after regular work hours) is at a premium. Gerry, though, signs up ahead of time for courts with reasonable fees, fitting it into her busy schedule.

I love the fast pace, the intensity of the game that wipes out all my problems for an hour—you don't have to excel at racquetball to have a lot of fun.

Tennis needs no introduction—it's a fast, total body sport, but your participation in it can suffer from cost and space factors, too. Badminton can be *much* more than a halfhearted backyard game. The equipment isn't expensive and you do not necessarily need a specially constructed area to play on. Jumping rope can be a super conditioner for lungs, heart, arms, legs.

WEIGHTS

No chapter on women's fitness these days would be complete without a word on pumping iron: weight-lifting, weight training, body building. A male preserve no longer, women are buying weights (barbell and weight set), an instruction book and are doing it at home. Others join a health club, a gym or a Y with a Universal or Nautilus (machines with weights on them). Some of us lift to be fit, feel strong, get to know our bodies, or for the sheer challenge of it; others to be more powerful (and protected from injury) at the sports we play or to be able to handle our jobs with less fatigue and more independence; a growing number to compete in body-building contests. If you start your program with a book, follow *all* the advice. Stretch before you begin heavy lifting and don't overdo it. Before you go the health club route, check out the program thoroughly, especially the instructors—they should be trained in anatomy and physiology as well as in how to use the equipment.

GROUP SPORTS

More and more of us are participating in group sports—practicing more often and developing our skills more seriously than ever before, whether in school or city (town) leagues. Basketball, volleyball and softball have always been and continue to be very popular; soccer, rugby and ice hockey are relatively new and growing. The challenge, excitement and great satisfaction come when you're out there on the court or field or ice as a part of a group with everyone playing hard and you make it all click. There is nothing like it. And who would miss the socializing afterward—the jokes, the stories about last year and plans for next season.

Make sure you find the right team for you. Some are very competitive—winning is all. Others are more fun-oriented; every woman gets to play in every game, people take turns playing different positions and help each other improve. You might want to check out the coach; she or he often sets the tone for the whole team. While stiff competition can be exhilarating and we are inspired by women who excel, it is more important for women of all races, ages, economic backgrounds and abilities to have a chance to enjoy a game than to produce a female sports elite. Big-money male athletics, with its superaggressive dog-eat-dog approach, reflects the values of our society at large. It need not be our model.

Some team sports give your body a well-rounded workout—some don't. Basketball, soccer, rugby and hockey are great for cardiovascular fitness and general body strength. They are strenuous, so you usually need to build up to them. Softball and volleyball are less rigorous. If you play a sport where you stand around waiting for the ball to come to you, some aerobic activity would be a good adjunct. Pregame warmup for all group sports is essential.

Getting good court or ice time is still hard; in most places the men's teams always get first choice. The same goes for softball—fields are hard to come by, especially in the city, so you usually have to be on a registered team in order to reserve a field for practice. Pickup games with a group of friends on Sunday morning are fast becoming impossible. Fees for joining a league are escalating at an alarming rate and in some communities you pay extra for lights and umpires.

SCHOOL SPORTS: THE POLITICS OF ACCESS

Title IX of the Educational Amendments Act, 1972, despite its imperfections and late-in-the-day appearance, has been an important piece of civil rights legislation for women in school and college sports. The law applies to all educational institutions that receive federal funds for anything. For athletics its goal is to "secure equal opportunities for men and women while allowing schools and colleges flexibility in determining how best to provide such an opportunity."[2] The result (of Title IX and other laws as well) has been that "hundreds of thousands of young women are competing in organized contests under the same circumstances that their fellow male students have [enjoyed] for many years"—with at least better uniforms, equipment, training, medical services, facilities, transportation, publicity, scholarships, awards, excitement and new respect for themselves, from other women and from the men.[3] There have been negative results, too: males taking over previously all-female teams; merging of programs so women who once ran their own, if meager, show find themselves administrative assistants to male athletic directors; men snatching up jobs coaching the new women's teams because the pay has suddenly become worth their while; and overcrowded facilities. Much controversy still exists over mixed teams—should highly skilled women play on "male" teams if they want to? Should all the guys who ask be allowed to join the girls' volleyball or field hockey teams?*

Certainly it is imperative that we know our legal rights in this area as in others. Sometimes all you have to do is get to know the male coaches and persuade them to share or remind a male administrator that he is violating the law to end an injustice. Other times filing a grievance with your regional office of the Office for Civil Rights of the Department of Education (DE), or going to court will be necessary. But we must never rely on government mechanisms to do things for us by themselves. The DE is woefully understaffed, and already Title IX, along with all civil rights legislation and the DE itself, is under serious attack in Washington. Budget cuts (national and local) are starting to take their toll at the elementary, secondary and college levels with the possibility that women's sports programs are going to be cut by the general abandonment of nonprofessional athletics before we ever get where we should have been in the first place. College sports will probably find a way to survive. But what will happen to the undefeated basketball team at an inner-city high school which proudly celebrated with the first female sports banquet in the city? How long will there be money for a coach, equipment, uniforms, transportation? How long can even one young

woman on the team dream of a college athletic scholarship, which was unheard of for any girl a mere ten years ago? If the high school forecast is for heavy clouds, it's downright gloomy for junior high and elementary. We need to support our local school system's sports program, perhaps organize a sports event to highlight the problem.

TAKING CARE OF OURSELVES

Just as you make space to move in, wear clothes that are loose or very flexible for full range of motion—sweatpants and jackets, loose shorts, T-shirts, jerseys or leotards, socks or bare feet.* For activities that make you sweat, cotton next to your skin is good because it's soft and absorbent, and it "transmits perspiration and heat away from your body."[4]

If you have or suspect any physical limitation, consider some kind of health checkup before beginning a rigorous exercise program.† Some physical problems—heart disease, high blood pressure—may not be symptomatic, and some types of exercise may aggravate them.

For every form of exercise, start slowly and build up, in general and during each session. Muscle growth comes from pushing each muscle involved slightly beyond what you forced it to the previous time. Stretching for flexibility is based on the same principle. Take care. When you're cold, stiff or out of shape you can tear a ligament or tendon (which can take a long time to heal) or permanently damage a muscle by driving it too violently or for too long. If you want to get into an activity that puts a lot of stress on joints, be sure that the surrounding muscles are strong (and coordinated) enough to support them; otherwise there will be trouble. Work up to exercising at least several times a week for at least twenty minutes. A once-in-a-while basketball-shooting spree or fling on the living room rug is of no benefit and could be dangerous. Make sure the equipment you use is in good shape.

Taper off any period of vigorous exercise slowly. Never flop down after an energetic run, for ex-

---

*Some states, like California, have further refined the rules with a state athletic code that regulates student teams, all-boys teams, all-girls teams and coed teams. See Bonnie Parkhouse and Jackie Lapin, *Women Who Win: Exercising Your Rights in Sports*, Englewood Cliffs, NJ: Prentice-Hall, 1980, pp. 49 ff. For more on this and Title IX in general, see *Out of the Bleachers*, Stephanie Twin, ed., New York, NY: Feminist Press, 1979.

---

*You don't need to be seduced by ads for expensive designer running outfits. Look for comfortable, well-tailored clothes designed for your sport. Plain old cotton sweats are often fine.
†When consulting with any medical or health professional (chiropractor, exercise physiologist, acupuncturist, physical therapist, trainer, phys. ed. teacher, doctor, fitness instructor, etc.), find out what their views on physical activity are and how much they know about it. A negative attitude may result in their being of little use or support to you. Try to do this when you call to make an appointment. Sports medicine is becoming more sophisticated at last (and more expensive), but get more than one opinion for anything serious. No matter whose advice you take, *always experiment carefully on your own—you know your body better than they ever will.*

Jean Raisler

drates. Don't worry about extra salt unless you eat no animal products of any kind, but be sure to get enough potassium and iron. Drink plenty of water, especially if you are sweating and/or the weather is hot or cold. Cut down on junk food, cigarettes, alcohol and drugs. For women who are using exercise to help lose weight, remember that aerobic activities are the ones that "burn up" the most calories.*

Get enough rest. You may need more when you start working your body harder. Or you may find exercising gives you more energy!

Expect some stiffness. If you're really pushing your muscles they're bound to hurt the following day(s). But don't pamper yourself and stop. The best remedy is moderate exercise: this will increase circulation which will help carry away the accumulated lactic acid causing the stiffness. Moist heat and massage applied to the sore muscle(s) are helpful as relaxants and they also increase blood flow, bringing fresh nutrients and speeding waste removal. As you keep exercising, your body will gradually become accustomed to working harder and the discomfort will disappear. Alternate hard and easy days.

INJURIES

Occasionally you will stretch the ligaments of a joint too far, maybe even tear them (a sprain) or pull a muscle or a tendon in much the same way (a strain). Unless the injury is severe, you can treat it yourself. As we get more in touch with our bodies we are often able to sense what we can heal by ourselves and what needs professional help. For a sprain, elevate and rest the injured part, applying cold immediately and for the next twenty-four to seventy-two hours. This minimizes pain and swelling. At the end of this period you can switch to moist heat. Begin gentle movement as soon as possible; when you are ready to start full-scale exercising again, bind it evenly (not too tight) for support and go easy. If in the meantime you are climbing the walls, be physical with the rest of your body; swimming might be a possibility, for example.

Back trauma is not nearly as easy to deal with. The advice of doctors is so contradictory (they continue to push complete inactivity, drugs and surgery) that women are forming groups to provide emotional support, to figure out where the problem lies, and to share information on how to get relief from pain and on the best ways to promote healing. Back care really means a commitment to

ample, without some transitional activity, such as walking. You need time for your heartbeat, breathing and temperature to adjust; you need to keep your blood flowing well in order to remove the wastes that have accumulated in the muscles during the run and bring them fresh supplies of oxygen and glucose. Sudden relaxation on rare occasion may make you dizzy.

Don't linger outside if you have been exercising in the cold—that will cause undue stiffness. Put something warm on. A hot bath or shower is ideal (after your circulation has returned to normal): It will relax your body, keep your blood flow up and wash away the sweat. A hot bath before exercising will increase flexibility. In hot weather, be reasonable. Acclimatize yourself and watch out for dehydration.

Don't eat heavily before or after exercising. The stomach and intestines require a large blood supply to digest food, and exercise diverts blood from the digestive tract to the muscles you're using. These organs' attempts to function actively with less blood than they need may cause pain. For most people exercise decreases appetite. Make sure when you do eat to include a variety of healthy foods (see Chapter 2, "Food") to meet the demands of greater physical activity. If you participate in endurance sports, eat more carbohy-

*See *Exercise and Your Heart* and other pamphlets available from your local chapter of the American Heart Association.

overall health through good posture, nutrition, relaxation and sensible but invigorating exercise.

Many headaches and nervous stomachs and much fatigue come from tension, boredom or depression. They can usually be driven off by some exhilarating activity, but any time you are "not yourself," take care. Lack of concentration for physical (a fever or overtiredness, for example) or psychological (anxiety over a personal problem, for example) reasons are injury-prone times.[5]

CONCLUSION

In the end we must deal with some depressing but upfront questions for the nineties. Will we lose the few decent facilities we've got? Will girls' school sports be budget-cut to death? Will women's competitive moneymaking sports continue to be almost all white? Will we let men convince us again that none of this matters because we've never had what it takes anyway? Will the national and state governments allow big business to pollute the air so badly that we won't be able to play and exercise outdoors? Will the ultimate chemical spill in the sky (or on the ground) end it all?

No! Working together we will hold the line and win back what we have lost. We will have a recreation center in every neighborhood where people of both sexes and all races will share the space equally. We will demand that our jobs be restructured in ways that are constructive for us physically and mentally. We will see to it that jogging is safe any time of the day or night. Our kids will grow up healthy with outstanding gym programs in decent public schools. Working together we will help to create a time when the spirit of the land is people before profit. But we must begin now to fight for it with the energy that comes from strong yet relaxed bodies and minds, with love and respect for each other and ourselves.

NOTES

1. See Hans Kraus. *Backache, Stress and Tension.* New York: Simon & Schuster, 1965; Pocket Books, 1969.

2. Bonnie Parkhouse and Jackie Lapin. *Women Who Win: Exercising Your Rights in Sports.* Englewood Cliffs, NJ: Prentice-Hall, 1980, p. 19.

3. Bonnie Parkhouse and Jackie Lapin. *Women Who Win,* p. 21.

4. Maggie Rollo Nussdorf and Stern B. Nussdorf. *Dress for Health: The New Clothes Consciousness.* Harrisburg, PA: Stackpole, 1980, pp. 62–3.

5. Thomas Fahey. *What to Do About Athletic Injuries.* New York: Butterick, 1974. Both this book and Hans Kraus's *Backache, Stress and Tension* are useful for the prevention and care of injuries.

RESOURCES

Books and Journals

Lyons, Pat. *Great Shape: The First Fitness Guide for Large Women.* Palo Alto, CA. Bull Publishing Co., 1990.

Melpomene Institute for Women's Health Research. *The Bodywise Woman: Reliable Information about Physical Activity and Health.* New York: Prentice-Hall, 1990.

The Melpomene Journal. Available from The Melpomene Institute (see below).

Nelson, Mariah Burton. *Are We Winning Yet? How Women are Changing Sports and Sports are Changing Women.* New York: Random House, 1991.

Reith, Kathryn. *Playing Fair: A Guide to Title IX in High School and College Sports for Athletes, Coaches, Parents and Friends.* New York: Women's Sports Foundation, 1992.

Women's Sports and Fitness (Journal), 1919 14th St., Suite 421, Boulder, CO 80302. (303) 440-5111.

Organizations

Melpomene Institute
1010 University Avenue
St. Paul, MN 55104
(612) 642-1951

Women's Sports Foundation
342 Madison Avenue, Suite 728
New York, NY 10173
(800) 227-3988.
A nonprofit, educational organization that promotes and enhances the sports experience for all girls and women. Send for their literature list. Also publishes *Headway: The Women's Sports Foundation Newsletter.*

5

Health and Healing: Holistic Practices and Systems

By Pamela Berger and
Nancy P. Hawley, with
Jane Pincus

With special thanks to Rose
Dobosz, Jon Kabat-Zinn, Pamela
Pacelli, Billie Pivnik and Susan
Reverby.

*1992 Update with help from Claire
Monod Cassidy, Savitri Clarke, Mary
Fillmore, Lori Ponge and Linnie
Smith.*

Many women today are excited by a compelling range of holistic healing methods that complement and challenge conventional biomedicine and broaden our options for health care. Some holistic approaches currently practiced, like massage, herbal medicine and visualization, are traditional female healing practices in use for centuries. Women have used them in their simplest forms, soothing and caring for members of their families and communities, applying herb poultices to wounds, assisting one another during labor and birth, attending to people through long illnesses and handing this knowledge down from mother to daughter.[1] In our society a cool washcloth for a headache, a massage for an aching back or a kiss to a child's bruised knee are simple examples of how we communicate positive healing energy; our confidence that we can "make it better" has a calming effect. The very fact that people think generously and kindly toward others is an important step in the healing process.

I think in terms of chicken soup and ice cubes. As a child I felt so reassured when my mother or grandmother cared for me. I felt so good lying in bed. The power of mother as healer, the oldest mode of care, can't be transformed into the setting of a doctor's office.

Other nonbiomedical healing methods, like acupuncture and yoga, originated in distant societies. Some of us are using these approaches alone, others in combination with biomedicine. They can help us stay healthy when we are well, cure some illnesses and enable us to live more

A late Medieval woodcut of an abbess as pharmacist.
(from *A History of Women in Medicine*, K.C. Hurd-Mead)

79

comfortably with disorders for which there are no known cures. The alternatives have often helped where the conventional methods of drugs and/or surgery could not.

We can learn to practice some holistic approaches ourselves with the help of books and knowledgeable friends. We can go further by apprenticing to teachers and practitioners and, in some cases, by taking coursework leading to diplomas and licensing. Or sometimes we find one or two methods helpful at certain times in our lives, use them, and go on without having or wanting to use them again.

MEDICINE

Grandma sleeps with
my sick
            grand-
pa so she
can get him
during the night
medicine
to stop
    the pain

        In
    the morning
        clumsily
        I
    wake
        them

Her eyes
look at me
from under-
                neath
his withered
arm

    The
    medicine
    is all
        in
    her long
    un-
        braided
                hair.

ALICE WALKER [1968]

UNDERLYING ASSUMPTIONS OF HOLISTIC HEALING APPROACHES

Holistic healing accepts the idea that the body, mind and spirit form an integrated whole and that the individual is deeply connected to her environment, her community and her world.

Holistic approaches to healing are based on certain underlying assumptions: first, that we are healthy when our body/mind/spirit exist in a dynamically balanced state of well-being. Though we are physically made up of cells, tissues, organs, and so on, no parts of us can be understood as isolated entities; all interconnected, they are harmoniously related.

Second, we have a great capacity for self-healing. Our cells are always engaged in the process of self-renewal, for our bodies continuously break down and build up structures, with tissues and organs replacing their cells in an ongoing process (with the exception of brain cells). We experience the physical body repairing itself in many ways, as, for instance, when scraped skin heals itself in a few days, or when the eye tears and washes away a foreign particle. In addition, we may consciously use the mind to focus healing energies on those aspects of our being that are hurt or feel unbalanced, or, we can use physical touch, as with massage, to help us relax, release tension and relieve pain. Part of our role in the healing process is to secure the information and support we need to enable us to return to a state of ease.

Third, in the broadest sense, our interactions with our family, community and world affect and shape our health. Positive, loving, supportive relationships with our family and friends help us keep healthy and give us opportunities to nurture and heal others and to receive love and nurturance, which strengthen us. Our health also depends on our larger social, economic, political and ecological environment, which affects us through the nutritional content of our foods, the potential dangers of the various products we buy and are exposed to, the energy sources we use, the air we breathe and particularly the financial and educational resources available to us. It is as crucial to try to achieve a balance between the individual and her surroundings as it is to balance body, mind and spirit.*[2]

Implicit in these premises is a particular way of defining healing and of thinking about how healing takes place. Though it is often important and sometimes necessary to seek help from health professionals, they are not responsible for healing us.

Healing comes from within. Every culture evolves a set of remedies that are given for dis-ease: some

---

*For example, Joanna Macy, a teacher, meditation instructor and organizer for social change, believes that deep despair about nuclear war keeps many of us from working effectively against it. She runs workshops in which people go through the process of acknowledging this despair with each other and feeling it as fully as possible. As a result, many become re-energized, reconnect with others and are moved to greater commitment and social action.

are thought to "cure," while others comfort, take away pain, overcome dysfunction or disability.... But no remedy, in and of itself, will restore good health.[3]

We, ourselves, play a significant role in making the treatment work through our willingness to be healed. While sound health practices can promote well-being and be a source of pleasure in their own right, they do not guarantee longevity or freedom from illness.

Though the words "heal" and "cure" are often used interchangeably, they are not synonymous. Sometimes no cures exist for particular diseases, yet people feel "healed," that is, able to reconcile themselves, accept and live with the effects of asthma, polio or even a terminal illness. Illness can provide opportunities for self-examination, growth and change, as seen in the experiences of the following two women:

I was in my forty-fourth year when I began experiencing what I called "fatigue." Weeks of "good nights' rest" did not change my stiffness and pain on arising. I had a three-year-old daughter, two teenage sons, a husband and a part-time job; I loved them all; I had no time to be sick or feel pain. When I found myself holding the wall as well as the banister to creep down the stairs one step at a time, I had to admit to myself that something was wrong. My wrists and fingers hurt; my elbows, knees and ankles; my back, legs and neck. An orthopedic surgeon told me that I had osteoarthritis.

Now I had to allow myself the luxury of time for exercise classes; a regime of exercise and aspirin soon made life more possible. I still only resentfully recognized that I probably would never be completely pain-free again.... Some days the distance from car to store or bed to bathroom seems the longest and most painful ten miles I could ever walk. Nevertheless, some days are better than others. I have learned to rest on the bad days and to insist on some daily rest even on the good days.

Most important, in seeking to understand why I denied the pain so adamantly when I first felt it, I entered therapy and learned how forcefully I had been denying emotional pain. My life is qualitatively different now—and better, even though lived with pain—as a result of my reevaluation of how I feel about myself, my goals, and my relations with others.

In the words of a woman who has since died of cancer:

A lot of people think dying suddenly in their sleep is a great blessing. I've realized that all I learn while dying is important; dying suddenly would be like reading a good book and leaving out a very important

part. I'm not for exaggerating: of course I do take pills to make myself more comfortable ... but I don't feel pain is wrong. I don't feel it's out of the flow. It's hard—like childbirth.

Many holistic methods present healing as taking place with the help of some form of *energy* that comes from a source within ourselves, from both within and without, or from a god or universal being.

As the acute stage of my asthma passes, I relax and further ease my breathing, reduce wheezing by feeling warmth and light flow through me, part of an energy I imagine to be universal energy of which we are all a part. As I am able to breathe fully again, I picture myself giving that energy back into the larger cosmos. In a concrete way this interchange enables me once again to be available to family, friends and co-workers.

I want to pray, but I don't believe in God. I'm going to pray "To whom it may concern"!

Both the setting and the practitioner influence the outcome of any specific therapy, whether biomedical or holistic. Trust, comfort, safety and good communication all play a role.

SOME PROBLEMS WITH HOLISTIC METHODS AND PRACTITIONERS

While the perspective common to many holistic modes of healing would seem to promise us a richer way of practicing health care than does the conventional biomedical system, holistic practices and practitioners have some of the same drawbacks.

Limited Availability

The majority of the approaches discussed as follows are available only to relatively few people. Most can be found only in large cities, and they are often expensive. In some rural areas, however, native healers continue to practice. Insurance companies and government aid, which provide low- and moderate-income people with access to the costly medical system, discriminate against many who choose nonmedical alternatives. Some alternative practices may have started out as informal, low-budget enterprises but often, in the process of making themselves "legitimate" and acceptable to insurance companies, they become more professional, hierarchical and expensive. Insurance companies also require licensing, which means that many compassionate, highly skilled but unlicensed practitioners are excluded from coverage. As a result, many holistic alternatives are available mainly to middle- and upper-middle-class people.

Risks of Professionalization

Just as with biomedicine, you can learn a lot from professionals who have information you may need to stay well. However, we live in a time of excessive dependence on experts, which means we often turn to professionals for things that they are not trained to do or that we could do better for ourselves. Some alternative practitioners, like conventional doctors, are setting themselves up as experts in such a way that they keep power for themselves, are unwilling to share their knowledge with you and try to get you to keep returning to them for additional services.

Lack of Social and Political Awareness

When holistic approaches identify the locus of healing only in the individual, as biomedical practice often does, they disregard political and social factors like poverty and racism as major sources of ill health. For instance, a practitioner might prescribe rest, exercise and change in diet, and not attend to the fact that the problem is caused by a dangerous on-the-job situation. All practitioners should be aware of the social causes of illness.

Blaming the Victim

Implicit in the practice of holistic healing is that you have a certain responsibility for keeping yourself healthy and for helping yourself get better. While trust in our capacity for self-healing is a welcome change from biomedicine's dependence upon outside intervention, some writers and practitioners of holistic health place *too much* emphasis on the individual's responsibility for her own sickness and health. They seem to imply that if you get sick or if you don't get well, it's your fault—your "wrong thinking," lack of will, personality defect (i.e., a "cancer personality") or insufficient faith in the practitioner. From several books on holistic health:

We should not fool ourselves into thinking that disease is caused by an enemy from without. We are responsible for our disease.[4]

The only tyrant you face is your own inertia and absence of will—your belief that you are too busy to take your own well-being into your own hands and that the pursuit of self-health through a wellness-promotive lifestyle is too hard, complicated or inconvenient.[5]

This kind of thinking disregards political and social factors that affect health. And sometimes, no matter how much we try to stay healthy, we become ill. It is both cruel and useless to blame ourselves or let others blame us for getting sick.[6]

Sexism

Holistic does not automatically mean nonsexist or feminist. Like biomedicine, many of these methods originated in male-dominated cultures. Although a large portion of holistic healers are women, it is wise to remember that both male and female practitioners may treat women disrespectfully, even harmfully.

Possible Ineffectiveness

Sometimes alternatives provide no more help than biomedicine. They can also be harmful and outright dangerous when practiced by "quacks." Just as the vast majority of biomedical therapies have not been evaluated for effectiveness and safety, so also few alternatives have been adequately tested in comparison with no treatment.

CHOOSING HOLISTIC METHODS AND PRACTITIONERS

Keeping both the advantages and limitations of holistic practices in mind, we can formulate guidelines for choosing and using practices and practitioners.

- Speak to other people who have been helped by a certain practice. Ask about the particular practitioner they used. Ask about negative as well as positive experiences with both method and practitioner.
- Seek out other women in your community who are also interested in getting information about how to approach and heal a certain illness. Form a research group. Get your local library to order books pertinent to your interests and to subscribe to women's health and holistic health publications. If there is a women's health center in your area, ask them for information.
- Call some of the national boards and information services listed at the end of this chapter. They may be able to tell you whether or not they think their approach is effective for your problem, and they may be able to recommend practitioners in your area.
- It may be important to you to know whether the method you want to use is based in any way on a sexist philosophy; whether it is organized hierarchically or dominated by white males with

patriarchal attitudes; whether it excludes or limits women or minority practitioners or clients; whether it is responsive to community needs (e.g., offering free classes, located near public transportation and in a building that is wheelchair accessible).

The best health care practitioners do not emphasize the conquest of disease, but see themselves as facilitating the healing process and helping you maintain your health. It is important to find someone with whom you feel comfortable, who works in partnership with you and whose ideas make sense to you. Ideally you should come away from every encounter feeling more confident in your ability to promote healing in yourself and supplied with the tools you need to make changes in your life.

- Good practitioners listen carefully and are interested in the ways you present your health concerns. Expect practitioners to be willing to try different approaches and teach you the skills you need to maintain or improve your health.
- Good practitioners must be well trained in their own healing methods. While a license or training certificate indicates a certain amount of knowledge and standardized training, no piece of paper ever guarantees a person's ability to heal. Apprenticeship is the usual mode of training in some systems.
- If your practitioner is in training, make sure that s/he receives supervision from someone more experienced.
- You may want to look for practitioners who have sliding fee scales or who are willing to barter services if you are unable to pay the full rate. A willingness to compromise on fees may indicate either a commitment to accessibility or inexperience, or both. Often practitioners are able to charge less when, as part of a group, they receive a salary (rather than a fee-for-service arrangement) and share expenses with others.
- Practitioners should be knowledgeable about other approaches to healing and willing to refer you to other practitioners if necessary. Beware of practitioners who think their treatment is the only good one.
- You may often want to combine the least invasive of biomedical diagnostic techniques with the best that a holistic method has to offer. It's important to look for practitioners who are open to any information you may bring from biomedicine, and who will evaluate it with you and with any consultants they might need.
- Beware of practitioners who offer miraculous cures. Even though you want definite answers, don't accept promises of magic any more than you would from biomedical practitioners. Occasionally immediate and dramatic results do occur, but many holistic methods require time and patience.
- Scrupulously avoid practitioners who directly or indirectly blame you for getting sick or not responding to treatment. They may be more concerned with their reputations than your well-being.
- Good practitioners should be especially sensitive to the larger social, political and economic issues that affect women's health.

We need to keep talking with one another, checking out, evaluating and reevaluating methods and practitioners. By doing so, we can make sure that they continue to be viable alternatives for us.

In the end, our own resources are the central issue.

I asked my friends for recommendations for a yoga teacher and several suggested one man. When I went to meet him, a voice inside me told me this man was not the teacher for me. I said to myself, "I really want to do yoga; this teacher has been highly recommended; perhaps it's because I don't get along well with men." But that voice kept saying, "I don't want to." I contemplated the matter by sitting down, closing my eyes and just being quiet. The thought kept rolling through my mind, getting stronger and more persistent: This is not the right teacher for me. *I dropped the idea of studying yoga with him.*

In general, be as informed and assertive as you can. Balance the isolation of the one-on-one therapeutic encounter by joining or forming self-help groups of women who share your health problem or who want to learn more about the method. Work for changes that would make holistic healing methods available to more people (e.g., suggesting that your practitioner adopt a sliding scale, pressing your insurance company to cover alternatives). There are many sincere, skillful, compassionate holistic practitioners and healers. We must look for them, ask them to share their skills with us, tell our friends about them and find ways of using them without becoming unnecessarily dependent upon them.

HOLISTIC APPROACHES

In this section we describe some holistic healing approaches and give information and guidelines so that you can look further on your own. Because so many alternatives exist, we sampled those most generally useful, most widely available and most familiar to us.

When you use a holistic approach for the first time you may have to change habits—the way you eat, the way you move, even the way you think about things. Learn as much as you can about the method you choose. Understanding the terms the practitioner uses—professional jargon, as in biomedicine, is often mystifying—can make you a more active participant in your care.

If you are used to going to biomedical doctors, it may feel strange to try something new. Family, friends and acquaintances can sometimes make it tougher by telling you that what you are doing is weird.

I tripped on the sidewalk and hurt myself so badly that I couldn't walk or work. I was taken to the hospital and had X-rays. The head orthopedist looked at the X-rays and told me that there was nothing wrong with my foot. But I still couldn't walk. At that point I decided to see a chiropractor. I didn't know anything about chiropractors except that they were an alternative to medical doctors. My sister was the only one I knew who had used a chiropractor.

When I went to the hospital to pick up my X-rays, I told them I was going to visit a certain chiropractor. "Don't go to him; he's a Communist," they said.

"I don't care what his political beliefs are if he can help me," I answered.

I made an appointment and after he adjusted my back and foot I could walk again in comfort.

Doing something new can feel strange.

I went for my first massage to someone recommended by a friend. Though apprehensive at first, I was quickly reassured by her strong, soothing hands.

Many women, not wanting to leave the biomedical-care system entirely but finding that it does not meet their needs for preventive "whole person" care, combine holistic approaches with conventional ones.

How do I integrate different health-care models in my life? I go to MDs mostly, but I understand their limits. I've done "talk" therapy and get (and give) massages. I take baths for aching muscles—water relaxes. Once in a while I experiment with herbs. I think about the food I eat, take some vitamins and have done some work with the Alexander Technique, which has helped chronic back and shoulder aches. I take my baby to doctors sooner than I take myself. Mainly I need sleep!

Here are some ways that people we know have combined methods.

- Chronic back pain: diagnostic X-rays, chiropractic adjustments, appropriate exercise and nutritional supplements, household help and childcare from friends and women's groups.

- For profuse and erratic bleeding around the time of menopause: acupuncture, vitamin A, figuring out when bleeding occurs (especially at times of stress), endometrial biopsy or dilation and curettage.
- Insomnia: diet changes, meditation, more exercise, psychotherapy, yoga, massage by friends, soporific herbal teas, warm milk at bedtime, occasional use of sleeping medications.
- Asthma: diet changes, massage, yoga, acupuncture treatments, psychotherapy, meditation, bronchial dilators, talking with family and friends.
- Cancer: diet changes, meditation and visualization, radiation therapy, chemotherapy, surgery, being able to talk about hopes, fears and worries with family and friends.
- Inoperable brain tumor: drugs, diet changes, yoga, meditation, psychotherapy, discussions with family and friends about feelings and treatment, radiation therapy.

Just as there is no one right way to keep healthy, there is no one right way of healing or acceptable path to follow. Bringing ourselves back into balance can mean something as simple as treating a cold by resting or as complex as totally altering our diet and other life habits to cope with severe chronic illness such as hypertension or arthritis. A method may work for one person or health problem but not for another. Sometimes it is possible to figure out which approach helps the most; at other times it is not so clear. We have to evaluate and make decisions about each situation as it arises; our own experience and intuition and the wisdom of trusted friends, family members, teachers and professionals will be our best guides.

Meditation

Meditation gives us the opportunity to be with ourselves. A simple definition of meditation is "the intentional paying of attention from moment to moment." In the words of a woman who has been meditating and teaching meditation for fifteen years:

Meditation in its essence is different from every other human activity, but its essence is contained in every activity. Meditating, each one of us touches base with our deepest concerns, with the truth of our aliveness. . . . You could say it is acknowledging the radiant core of our being . . . our godliness, our buddha nature, or whatever you like to call it—speaking out.

Meditating at its best doesn't remove us from living, numb us to stressful situations to stop us from acting effectively. It puts us in touch with the moment and helps us respond directly. If we have meditated recently we are more likely to be alert and resourceful when we are called upon to help someone.

People begin to meditate for different reasons—because it feels good in itself or because they want to feel calm, to diminish physical or mental stress or pain or to get through a spiritual crisis. You might approach meditation only for practical reasons—to relax or reduce stress—and then discover that something happens that makes you want to go deeper, to attain a different level of consciousness.

Although meditation practices have been directly or indirectly related to healing for millennia,[7] only in the last two decades have health practitioners in this country understood its potential and begun teaching people to use it for a variety of specific conditions. Meditation helps us slow down breathing and heart rate, reduce oxygen consumption, lessen muscular tension, change brain-wave patterns and respond calmly to stressful situations, thereby lowering the risk of having a heart atack or a stroke.[8] Meditation reduces stress.[9]

There are many ways to meditate. Though you can meditate while you stand, walk, dance or jog, many people sit or kneel in a quiet environment. Some meditate while carrying out daily activities such as washing the dishes.[10] Repeating a word or sound over and over again can calm your mind; concentrating on your breathing can help focus your attention. You can meditate at home indoors or outdoors, or in formal settings—churches, synagogues, zendos, ashrams and other places of worship. You can practice alone or with others in a common meeting place.[11]

You might feel best learning meditation practice by yourself, with guidance from a book or tape or you might want a religious or secular teacher to work more closely with you. However, if you expect to rely on a teacher to provide answers or a group to offer prescriptions for living, you're on the wrong track.

The role model of women was really questionable in the group I belonged to. The hierarchy was composed of men, and the leader set the standards for behavior. Women were expected to play traditional and outdated roles. I objected to the lack of morality and to people not taking responsibility for their actions. For instance, heavy drinking and sexual promiscuity were encouraged, while closeness with one other person was not. Yet the whole meditation practice of being with yourself was inspiring and wonderful.

The group provided a lot of security, especially during times of transition in my life. I felt less alone. But it was a bit of a cop-out because the group pre-sented a single view of the world, one that was unaccepting of other perspectives.

Since I left the group I have felt more balanced and better able to cope with making decisions in my life. While the group dynamics were distressing to me, the experience of meditation has helped me pull my life together.

When properly practiced, meditation can help us pull our lives together.

My early-morning meditation is part silence, part chanting. Sometimes I actively pray while I sit looking out the window at the rising sun. It's important for me to meditate every morning, if only for ten minutes to touch base with myself. I am continually surprised at how I get upset more easily on the days I don't meditate. Sometimes during the day when I'm silent or alone I find myself automatically feeling the tranquility I experience during meditation. This calmness helps me. Though usually my meditations are rather ordinary, on some days they are profound.

Visualization*

We all create images in our minds, sometimes consciously, sometimes without being aware of it. We picture how we would like a future event to turn out or how we want our relationships to change. Images fill our dreams; some of them last into the next day.

David and I made love last night beautifully, ecstatically, delicately. Then I dreamed about creating a strong, beautiful simple child? Jewel? I held it in my hand. And woke this morning perfectly content. So rare.

Positive images make us happy and carry us through difficult times.

Many women are finding that visualizing a certain symbol, scene or process has a positive healing effect on their bodies. Midwives have long used images and relaxation exercises to help women in labor relax, diminish fear or tension and open up. The earliest records of visualization techniques used in healing date back to Babylonia and Sumeria; other ancient peoples used these techniques as well. In our day, Canadian Eskimos, Navajo Indians and some Latin peoples (to mention only a few) use forms of healing based on visualization.[12] Placebos (substances with no known pharmacological action) can profoundly affect the course of a disease. People using a pla-

---

*Though visualization is now being used for everything from decreasing drug dependence to the improvement of athletic ability, we concentrate on visualization used in conjunction with meditation to help heal specific conditions.

cebo often get better just because they *believe in it*—the pills, charm, talisman or ritual. Perhaps one way placebos work is by helping the person visualize herself as healing; perhaps the placebo itself represents a visible symbol of healing.

Visualization works in a general way by helping people relax. We can also use visualization techniques to affect the involuntary systems of the body, increasing blood flow to one particular area or slowing down the heartbeat. We can also use visual images to help minimize or control pain.[13] In the words of a scientist who had several operations for cancer:

The two years since I've had the last operation have been the most productive of my life. I've had the opportunity to investigate healing in a way that I never did before. At first, when I felt the pain, I kept looking for an outside figure, a god figure to help me, to care for me, to make it better. Then I said to myself, "Who's the most caring, best mother you know?" And I said, "I am." So I pictured myself cuddling myself. When the pain came, I went to it as a mother would to a child. I said, "How can I help it? How can I go to it?" Now when it comes, I say, "Poor baby." I tried to treat myself in a loving way. The more loving I was to myself, the more healed I felt. Now the pain is mostly gone.

Visualization involves relaxing, feeling at one with the object, scene or process you imagine, letting it expand to fill your consciousness and become the only thing in your awareness. Hold your

mind upon it. Sometimes it helps to have someone guide you. Some people must practice this meditative visualization; it is a skill to be learned. Others do it more quickly.

An example of a healing visualization is as follows.

Relax and let your attention go to the particular body part causing discomfort or pain, or which does not function as it should. Focus your attention on this place and let yourself experience what it feels like right now. Don't feel pressured to achieve a specific goal. After a while, allow an image related to that area to come to your mind. It may be a detailed picture of what you think that part looks like, or it may be more abstract. Keep your mind focused until you are content with your image. Change it whenever you want. Now begin to visualize something happening within that part of your body to make it work better or start to heal. You might see energy, light or color flowing into it; imagine it becoming warm or cool. A powerful image could help you feel better right away.

Visualization has been formalized within biomedicine as *autogenic training.*[14] It is increasingly being used to modify bloodflow, slow the heartbeat and help us heal specific organs or conditions, such as ulcers, gastritis, gallbladder attacks, irritable colon, hemorrhoids, constipation, angina, headaches, asthma, diabetes, arthritis, low back pain, skin conditions and thyroid disease.[15] Cancer specialists use visualization in conjunction with drugs, surgery and radiation[16] to affect the cancer patients' attitudes toward living and dying, as well as to relieve the stress of the disease. Studies indicate that meditation and visualization techniques can help us strengthen the immune system and, therefore, the body's response to cancer and other disease.[17]

If visualization doesn't work, it may mean that you take in information in other ways than by using images—you might do it through your ears, so imagining sounds might be your way of "visualizing"; you might do it in terms of movement or spatial relations or touch. The possibilities are endless.

Biofeedback

Recently, lay people and practitioners have begun to use machines to help us monitor and influence our supposedly involuntary systems. Electronic devices connected to the body through wires and electrodes monitor certain physiological processes such as heart rate, muscle tension or brain waves, and convert them into signals that you observe on

One visual image: a strongly rooted tree.

Batik by Jane Pincus.

a screen or hear as a beep or sustained tone. (Smaller, simpler devices exist, which you can hold in your hand and use at home.) The sight or sound of the signal, indicating the rate of intensity of the process, encourages you to control it voluntarily. People use this technique to bring a variety of responses under control: heart rate, blood pressure, hand temperature, muscle tension, brain and sweat gland activity, genital responses, stomach motility, and so on.[18] It can help us deal with such diverse conditions as tension or migraine headaches, hypertension, insomnia, rapid heart rate, asthma and pain. For example, if you have Raynaud's syndrome (excessively cold hands caused by reduced blood flow) and go to a biofeedback session, the practitioner will explain how physiological conditions caused the symptoms, describe how to use the electronic thermometer and suggest general strategies you can use to regulate your internal activity and warm your hands. Early on s/he will adjust the machinery to register even small changes in the desired direction, indicating success. After you learn how to warm your hands with the machinery, you can practice without it at home. Training sessions take place from once a week to daily, and last from thirty to sixty minutes apiece for periods ranging from one week to three months or more. Insofar as you continue to practice the exercises, you continue to have increased control of the temperature of your hands.

Encouragement and good coaching are important. Be wary of anyone who sticks you in a room, hooks you up to a machine and then leaves you alone; if you have contracted for guided biofeedback therapy, see that you get it. Bring a friend along with you to observe the practitioner and the process. The experience may be useful to her or him as well as to you.

Though some people are put off by machines, biofeedback does convincingly indicate that we can indeed alter specific biological processes. Skilled biofeedback practitioners can teach people eventually to regulate their "involuntary" processes without the use of machines. They warn that overdependence on the machine can actually limit the application of your newly learned control. In other words, the machine simply teaches you a level of self-mastery you didn't have before.

Massage and Bodywork Techniques

Touching is one of the most natural ways we have to communicate and to comfort one another. Whether it's with a simple hug or a complete body rub, we can help one another feel better.

Foot rubs are my favorite kind of massage. They bring back childhood memories of my father rubbing

Christine Bondante

my feet; they feel so good to give and to get. My children often ask me to hold and rub their feet when I go into their rooms to say good night. Some of my friends and I exchange them as a way of being close and helping each other relax.

When done effectively, massage relaxes the body, releases muscle tension, improves joint flexibility, increases circulation and sensation and generally enhances our well-being. Massage and manipulative techniques involve prolonged and intense touching, pulling, pressing and rubbing. We can use many massage techniques on ourselves as well as on others.

Do not get a massage when you have phlebitis, skin disease, blood clots, redness, infections, or skin that has become thin due to burn or injury.

You don't need any special training to do general massage. Just get into a comfortable position and begin. Hold your friend's foot, head, hand, back, neck, shoulders. Ask her where she wants pressure, whether you are applying too much pressure or not enough. With your thumb or whole hand,* find and rub tender areas or sore spots. Alternate gentle stroking with deep kneading and use visualization, too, if you want to help the person relax even more. Avoid direct pressure on the spinal column; instead, press on either side. Breathe regularly and deeply while giving the massage.

---

*Massage is usually done with the hands, but sometimes feet are used, as in menstrual massage, illustrated in Chapter 12, "Anatomy and Physiology of Sexuality and Reproduction." Japanese massage is often done entirely or partly with the feet.

Michelle Fiorenza

cle tone in your body and how you communicate it to someone else, you have to be rooted in your own body and pay attention to what is happening to you all the time you are giving the massage. While I give everyone the same massage in the order of things I attend to, my touch feels different to different people. It was wonderful when a woman told me she not only knew where her body was during the massage, but was aware of mine as well.

One of my first experiences with emotional healing and massage happened in a small and simple apartment in Cambridge. I had gone to see the masseuse (who worked at her home) because my body was filled with tension and I wanted some relief. When I arrived, she suggested to me that I might be storing old emotional wounds in my body, as indicated by my posture. I asked her what she meant, a bit defensively. After all, I was doing yoga, walking and eating well. I just had a lot of tension, that's all.

She didn't give a mental explanation. Instead, she asked me to lie down, and she began to massage the vertebrae in my neck. Massage, hold steady, massage, hold steady. At first I felt only the degree of tension in my neck; gradually I experienced a lump forming in my throat, my chest heaving and a bunch of old sensations returning to mind. I began to cry, small jerky sobs at first, like the opening of a faucet that has been shut off for a long time. Then a burst of tears, and finally several minutes of sobbing.

I was both terrified and relieved—terrified to think that there was so much deep emotion behind a stiff neck and relieved to know that it could be unlocked and soothed. At that moment I made a decision to see what else I could learn from this mysterious body that walked around with me all day.

Many people who do massage see themselves as channeling energy through their bodies and hands to heal their family, friends and, if they are masseuses, their clients.

The massage methods most familiar to Westerners are Esalen and Swedish (generally wholebody, sometimes using deep pressure). Acupressure and shiatsu involve applying pressure to energy points along the same meridians (energy pathways) used for acupuncture treatments. Neuromuscular therapy works with muscle trigger points and the Bowen system with transverse muscle groups. Rolfing, Feldenkrais and the Alexander technique all emphasize realigning the body into a normal posture. Most practitioners combine techniques from several methods. Some masseuses incorporate the techniques of polarity therapy[19] or deep breathing and visualization.[20] Others use reflexology points and focus attention on feet[21] or hands. Still others include insights gained from bioenergetics or psychotherapy practices. A masseuse said:

The way you touch someone is more important than the actual system you use. Whether you see yourself as channeling energy or are concerned with the mus-

If at some point you decide you want a professional massage or want to take a course or apprentice yourself to someone, get names from friends, your local woman's center, health club, YWCA, or from a holistic health center if one exists in your area. Carefully select the person you go to for massages; recommendations from friends are often the best kind of referrals. Choose someone who uses techniques you like, and with whom you feel comfortable and can communicate well. Good two-way communication relaxes and energizes the masseuse as well. Note whether your therapist was trained at a nationally accredited school, whether s/he is certified and whether s/he is a member of the American Massage Therapy Association (Chicago) or the American Oriental Bodywork Therapy Association (New York).

You may not know what you want or what to expect the first time you make an appointment for a massage.

Some people come in with specific physical complaints or problems with body alignment; others just want a chance to stretch and relax, and others want to do emotional "work" along with the massage. Before we begin I work out an understanding with them about what they want.

Without any words, I begin to realize that my shoulders are getting a lesson in where they should be. The lesson feels very good, very soft and respectful of how they would be if I let go of the tension I begin to notice in them. But the massage is a lesson, not just a pat on the back. . . . The masseuse's hands are really asking my back questions and getting answers. The communication is clear and direct. As the hour comes to an end, I feel very good all over.[22]

Acupuncture

Acupuncture is the healing art central to the practice of traditional Chinese medicine. Developed and used over at least the last 2,000 years, acupuncture is now also accepted in some places in the West as a method for maintaining health and healing illness. In acupuncture the practitioner stimulates specific points on the body by inserting needles, applying heat (thermal therapy); pressing, massaging (acupressure) or by a combination of these.

Chinese medicine, intimately tied to the classical Chinese philosophy of Taoism, aims to maintain or restore balance in the body to ensure health. Central to the beliefs of Taoism is the notion that the body has the power to repair and regenerate itself or to restore its own equilibrium. Acupuncture is thought to stimulate or awaken these natural healing powers within the body.[23]

Acupuncturists often state their diagnoses and methods of treatment in terms of Yin and Yang. The terms Yin and Yang denote what the ancient Chinese saw as twin polarities that regulate humans and the universe. Though Taoism describes Yin as "negative" (e.g., earth, moon, coolness, moisture, quiescence, things female) and Yang as "positive" (e.g., heaven, sun, warmth, dryness, movement, things male), the terms are equivalent to modern physicists' calling protons "positive" and electrons "negative."[24] (A proton is not "better" than an electron. They are equally powerful forces.) Practitioners say that the Yin-Yang concept, though it is open to misunderstanding and misuse, does not imply bias against the female.

Unlike Western medical practitioners, the Chinese do not base traditional healing practices on the study of anatomy as we know it. Because Chinese people worshiped their ancestors, the dissection of a cadaver was not permissible. Instead of concentrating on the physiological or material structure of the body (muscles, nerves, bones,

Acupuncture Center of Washington

etc.), they focused on how we function—the dynamic aspects of the body, the "life force" that keeps the body alive and in healthful balance. They call this life force or vital energy *ch'i*. According to traditional Chinese medical theory *ch'i* circulates throughout the body along precise pathways or channels, the acupuncture meridians. The *ch'i*, which controls the blood, nerves and all organs, must flow freely along the meridians and be of a certain strength and quality if each organ is to function correctly. When the flow of *ch'i* is impaired, a person becomes susceptible to disease.

Trauma, improper nutrition, stress and many other factors can block or impair the flow of *ch'i*. In acupuncture, stimulating certain points along the meridians controls the flow of *ch'i* by attracting energy to a deficient area, dispersing an excess of energy or dissolving a blockage, thereby lessening pain or strengthening the body's ability to maintain health.

A traditional acupuncturist diagnoses the body's imbalance by a variety of techniques: questioning, observing, examining the tongue, listening (to breathing, voice, etc.), reading the pulses.* Often the practitioner takes a complete health history and looks for ways in which changes in diet, exercise, etc., could complement the acupuncture treatments. Many acupuncturists in the United States cooperate with biomedical physicians, and may ask you to get a diagnosis from one of them.

In my initial encounter with acupuncture, the acupuncturist was attentive and caring; even before I saw her, when I was just inquiring on the phone, she was taking notes. She sounded interested in my problem (heavy menstrual bleeding). She thought that she could help me heal it. I had a good impression of her as a person and a healer.

When I walked into the acupuncturist's office for the first time there was an herb burning that smelled like pot to me, and the first thing that went through my mind was, What am I doing here? These are really "New Age" healers; this is more than I bargained for. I started to feel very nervous. I asked her what the smell was, and she told me that it was an herb called moxa [common mugwort] which they use to heat the needles and which adds to the treatment's effectiveness. I was ready to try something new, but I was also mistrustful.

After I sat down, the acupuncturist asked me a series of questions having to do with digestion, elimination, menstruation, sleep patterns, level of energy, emotional state, pain, other illnesses, diet, lifestyle. This was a lengthy initial question period. Now each time I come she asks me how I've been feeling that week, if there is anything out of the ordinary. She takes my pulse and looks at my tongue, skin, eyes. After gathering all this information, she adjusts the treatment to meet the specific needs I have that week.

During treatments the acupuncturist stimulates the appropriate acupuncture points with sterilized hair-thin stainless steel needles. Needles vary in length from half an inch to several inches for use in different parts of the body. When the needle is inserted, you may feel a slight prick, tingling, numbness, pain or nothing at all.

Part of the initial high of starting acupuncture was that I had expected it to be very painful because my image of it was that they used these big long needles

and stuck them into people. When she actually did it, she used very small needles. The prick was quite mild and I got an almost euphoric feeling.

Acupuncture treatments have really minimized my problems with asthma. But I won't deny that the needles hurt as she was putting them in. Once in place, they didn't hurt anymore.

The needles are so small that they rarely cause bleeding. Anywhere from two to fifteen needles can be used. The hands, forearms, lower legs, feet, back, abdomen and ears are the most common places to insert needles. Often the acupuncturist inserts the needle far from the symptomatic area or what you would think of as the site of the disease, because the meridians s/he wishes to affect run the length of the body. S/he can direct the *ch'i* to bring back balance and harmony within the body from many places on the meridian. For acute ailments few treatments—sometimes just one—are needed. Chronic ailments usually require more treatments, but some people experience relief right away. Others initially feel worse and only begin to experience improvement after many sessions:

I am sixty years old and have severe arthritis, especially in my hands, feet and hips. I had been pushing this pain out of my mind while I was taking care of my husband. He was very sick and if he knew I was in pain he would have wanted to go to the hospital. After he died I was very depressed, and when I went for psychological counseling the counselor suggested that I try acupuncture for the arthritis. He researched it and got me in touch with the acupuncturist. The first few treatments were very painful. I even screamed out. We went through hell together. The acupuncturist told me that chronic pain like mine was deep-seated and harder to take care of. I had to go twice a week for a long time. It was expensive for me, and when after eight treatments I didn't feel any better, I didn't know what to do. Meanwhile, I had been put on a special arthritis diet by a nutritionist who worked with the acupuncturist. I decided I would go on with the acupuncture treatment, and when I got to sixteen treatments I started to feel a little better. By twenty weeks I had found the acupuncture really helped me. Now the treatments have tapered off, one every two or three months, when I start getting sore. So it was definitely worth continuing with them. You either sink or swim, and I didn't feel like sinking.

In the West, acupuncture has been effective in the treatment of menstrual disorders (amenorrhea, excessive bleeding, pain, premenstrual syndrome), fertility problems, gastrointestinal disorders, urinary and respiratory problems

---

*Reading the pulses is one of the primary diagnostic procedures. Acupuncturists use this method to diagnose the subtle fluctuations in the flow of energy along the meridian circuit. In Chinese medicine, the practitioner takes the pulses at three finger positions on each wrist and at two depths for each finger position. Each of these twelve positions corresponds to a functional organ system of the body. By palpating these pulses, the experienced practitioner can discover both the energy imbalances within the body at the time of diagnosis and some indication of past conditions as well as potential difficulties.

(asthma, allergies), hemorrhoids, constipation, insomnia and chronic fatigue. It is also effective in treating osteoarthritis localized in specific joints, muscle contraction and migraine headaches. Various neuralgias and pain related to nerve injury can also be helped. Some acupuncturists will treat patients suffering from anxiety or severe depression, usually when the person is under the care of a psychotherapist as well.

As helpful as acupuncture can be, when not practiced properly it can cause infection or nerve, vessel or organ damage. Make sure that the acupuncturist uses sterilized needles because a number of blood diseases can be transferred by skin puncture, including hepatitis and AIDS. Even though you may have a condition that acupuncture can successfully treat, you may not be able to find a formally trained and experienced acupuncturist. There is as yet no national board for licensing acupuncturists, but certain states do or will soon have a certification procedure. At present, you might try finding out about licensing procedures for acupuncturists in your state through your state board of registry in medicine. You may also check to see whether your practitioner was trained in Asia or in one of the more than twenty-five accredited training programs in the West.

Chiropractic: One Method of Body Alignment and Adjustment

While the extraordinary flexibility of our bodies allows us to move with ease, it also makes it possible for our bodies to become unbalanced. The connective tissues that enclose our muscles and bones and give our body shape can become distorted by the ways in which we habitually sleep, walk, or sit, as well as by accidents. We can get into the habit of pushing the head forward as we walk or tightening the knees when we stand. Emotional stress also creates physical tensions, which over time change the shape of our bodies. We accommodate to the distortions, but the longer we remain out of alignment, the more our movement becomes restricted. The resulting chronic muscle tension can affect us emotionally as well as physically; we sometimes lose our range of emotional responsiveness as we lose the flexibility of our physical movements.

Many methods can help us readjust and realign our bodies: chiropractic, Rolfing, the Alexander Technique and the Feldenkrais method are some of them. Space does not permit a discussion of all these methods; we have chosen chiropractic because it is the most widely available.

Chiropractors believe that the human body works at its fullest potential only when the nervous system functions smoothly. The spinal column (the bony vertebral column which covers and

protects our brain stem and spinal cord) is the "lifeline of the nervous system."[25] Chiropractors make adjustments (move the vertebrae) in the spine to restore proper nerve function and nerve flow from the brain to muscles and organs of the body, making normal motion possible again. Spinal misalignments result from a number of causes: trauma from car, bike, motorcycle or walking accidents; physical strain from overexertion or from sitting too long in one place; muscle tension from extreme mental stress; even poor diet or overuse of drugs.[26] When proper nerve function is restored to all areas of the body, the organs will function more completely, too. For instance, after adjustments have been made on the specific vertebrae associated with your adrenal glands, allergies connected to adrenal functioning may improve. Chiropractors can help with hands and feet. Many women visit chiropractors for preventive health care.

When I was pregnant, I visited my chiropractor once a month to be sure my back was aligned properly as my belly expanded and my weight shifted.

There are two distinct groups of practitioners within chiropractic. Believing that spinal misalignments cause diseases, the "straights" restrict their practice to spinal adjustments alone. The "mixers" have expanded their practice and offer other natural forms of treatment—suggestions about diet, exercise, meditation, visualization—in addition to spinal manipulation. The debate continues between these two groups. Some of these chiropractors use X-rays and some don't.

As with other alternative approaches to healing, women tell a range of stories about their experiences with chiropractors.

I went to see a chiropractor recommended by several friends. He helped me with a specific back injury from running, but after a while I didn't like his attitude. Even though I was no longer having back problems he suggested I keep coming more often than I wanted to. When I asked why, he said, "Well, there is always something to adjust."

"True," I said, "and I often feel better, but I can't afford the money."

So I looked and found another chiropractor who was willing to see me periodically for preventive care and in any crisis, too.

I've seen three different chiropractors over the last twelve years. I've enjoyed seeing each of them and have learned a lot about how to help myself heal. Each visit was not expensive, but you are expected to return regularly. All three chiropractors emphasized how important it is to prevent illness, and to be aware that sometimes slight illnesses, emotional upsets and even changes in seasons can throw your whole body off.

Yoga

I get up in the morning and do the exercise "Salute to the Sun" (actually a series of twelve postures). Whether I have a few minutes or a longer time to practice yoga, I benefit from the fullness of this exercise. I am cheered by the thought of saluting the sun. I am easily moved beyond the awkwardness of my body and the sleepy nature of my mind as I get into the movement of this exercise. After a while I am ready to welcome the day.

The aim of yoga is to renew the body, focus the mind and still the emotions. Yoga is a Sanskrit word that essentially means union. Underlying yoga practice is the belief that "the body and mind are part of the continuum of existence, the mind merely being more subtle than the body."[27]

The basic aspects of yoga practice include *asanas, pranayama* and *meditation.* All the exercises emphasize awareness—awareness of the moves and the breathing, of areas of flexibility and tightness, and of applying your mind to the task.

Asanas

Asanas are physical postures that help stretch and limber the body.

Before yoga my main experiences with exercise had been in gym class or in modern dancing. These exercises were a variety of stretches to strengthen or loosen a particular part of my body and were usually done in short repetitive motions. In contrast, when doing yoga postures I was asked to move slowly into

Jane Pincus

the posture, hold it still for some time, and then gradually release. This way of exercising has dramatic effects on my mind. I often begin in some turmoil, filled with the concerns of my day. As I focus my attention on my movements and my breathing, I experience my mind slowing down and relaxing. The practice gives me some distance from my problems. Doing the postures releases new energy, relaxes me and allows for another perspective to emerge.

Pranayama

Pranayama are breathing exercises that increase the flow of oxygen, thereby relaxing your whole being.

The first time I did yoga breathing exercises I was amazed at the capacity of my lungs. I watched my belly fill up, my chest expand, the air move into my shoulders. I realized I never had experienced a complete breath before—and I was in my thirties at the time!

Jana had us breathing deeply after the asanas. *"You are light," she'd say, drawing out the word "li-i-ght." "Take the light into your body, down your spine. . . . Be aware ("avare," in her Eastern European accent). We'd hold one nostril shut with one finger and breathe through the other, holding the breath, and then breathe out. It made me feel strong, calm and luminous.*

Meditation

Although the postures and breathing exercises are valuable in and of themselves, they also prepare you for meditation, or a practice of conscious relaxation that enables you to experience a coming together of the physical, mental and spiritual aspects of yoga. The breathing exercises and meditation are accessible to anyone, and no matter what your physical restrictions, you can do them.

Studies demonstrate the benefits of regular yoga practice. These include physiological changes such as reduced blood pressure, lowered pulse rates, diminished stress, increased joint movement and improved hormonal functioning.

We can learn yoga on our own by using books, records and tapes. However, there is no substitute for a good teacher who can give us individualized help with the various techniques. Yoga classes are taught in local YWCAs, adult education programs, college extension courses and dance centers. Whether you practice for fifteen minutes a day or for more extended times, it is important to practice regularly.

The problems with yoga are the problems of any healing method applied improperly. Don't push through the pain to complete the exercise no matter what. Be cautious and proceed at your own pace, trusting your limits. In all these practices, you must pay attention to the fine line between simply exerting yourself and pushing beyond your limits—and this is different for everyone. Beware of perfectionism and athleticism. Benefits come from your efforts rather than from reaching a specific goal.

Dance and Movement Therapy

Women have always danced for pleasure and relaxation. You find your own rhythm, experience control over your body and discover the freedom to move in new ways. Movement and dance also can be modes of healing, modes in which women today have a predominant influence. Dance and movement therapy are not recent innovations, though they have become more popular. Using movement rather than words, they treat a variety of physiological and psychological conditions, addressing a person's body, emotions, mental attitudes and relatedness to the world. The therapist, by observing you and moving rhythmically with you, is able to mirror not only your physical movements but also the *feelings* behind those movements. As you learn to identify certain details of your physical and emotional states while you move, you can learn to alter your movements so that you feel more comfortable with yourself and with the people around you.

I was incredibly timid and anxious, so shy that I had trouble making friends or having any social life at all. I went to a dance therapist who worked with me in her office, just moving, getting rhythms going. We began to breathe together, dance together, reach toward each other and move back. It was a way of communicating without needing to say anything. Once as we were moving I remembered my mother rocking me, and also the way I used to feel when she suddenly put me down to go take care of my brother. That memory released something in me and I started to cry. I never thought I could get such a feeling of release.

The therapist follows the person's lead rather than imposing a rigid set of strictures. S/he teaches exercises and techniques, but except for a few basics, the exercises suggested are natural outgrowths of the person's spontaneous discoveries about her body. Dance and movement therapists also use guided relaxation, role playing, breathing techniques and meditation as part of their treatment.[28] Dance and movement therapists in clinics and hospitals usually work as part of a team. Women often do movement therapy in groups to avoid the isolation characteristic of other modes and to be energized by the group as well as by the therapist. In the 1940s Marion Chace, a dancer,

Nona Charleston

was the first therapist to work within a hospital setting. She discovered that when traumatized soldiers could express their feelings through dance, they were able to leave the hospital more quickly. Chace set the path for other dance therapists to work with people who had a variety of severe psychiatric illnesses (e.g., children with autism, adults with schizophrenia) or who needed to counter the effects of powerful medications.[29]

Dance and movement therapists also work with people who feel overweight and/or have eating disorders. They support you in your efforts to make fundamental changes in the way you relate to food and your body. Their emphasis is on using dance and movement to let energy out rather than stuffing energy in. If you can learn enough about your body (e.g., sensations of hunger; differences between sensations of hunger and other feelings; ways of managing feelings other than eating, i.e., going for a walk, being with a friend, running), you can then learn to take better care of yourself without turning to diet programs that take a huge toll. (See Chapter 2, "Food," and Chapter 4, "Women in Motion.") In the words of a movement therapist:

As part of an exercise the group was physically lifting up a very large woman. This woman strongly believed that she always had to be supporting other people, but other people could not support her, especially because of her size. So the experience of being lifted up was a turning point for her. After this experience she could believe that she would be supported by people in other ways as well.

Energetic Healing

Though rigorous documentation does not exist, there are on record incidents of physical healing that cannot be explained in purely medical, physical or psychological terms.[30] Sometimes when a surprisingly rapid rate of healing or a total reversal of symptoms occurs, people attribute the healing to a nonphysical entity (spirit or deity), a group (prayer group, healing circle, church group), an individual (minister, shaman, psychic) or the person's attendance at a "miraculous" place (such as Lourdes). The techniques and rituals used in association with these incidents include meditation and prayer, touching with the intent to heal and visualization.

Insofar as the healer and the setting promote your belief in the efficacy of a ritual or activity, you may be able to make an extraordinary effort to heal yourself. As the healer communicates her/his concern through compassion, physical touch and a strong "healing" intention, you may be able to relax and let your body's healing energy take over. Like shamans in "primitive" societies and religious or faith healers in Western societies, modern psychic healers can mobilize the body's healing forces. Many healers emphasize the importance of "compassionate love" going from healer to person to be healed. They believe that the energy of compassionate healing love is greater than that of words. Religious healers speak of this "love" as the most potent factor in religious healing. Perhaps the emotional atmosphere these healers create, combined with physical touch and with people's faith in their own healing powers, makes possible any physical healing that takes place.

One noted psychic healer emphasizes that a healer should focus on the whole person, not just on the particular part to be healed. He warns people to be wary of healers who charge money and/or promise a cure, and he cautions against the sleight-of-hand tricks some "healers" use to reinforce their clients' belief in them. He also requires that all his clients be in consultation with a physician.

Therapeutic Touch, studied and taught by Dolores Krieger and Dora Kunz, is another technique for channeling energy through yourself to help the healing process in another person. The practitioner centers herself so that she feels peaceful and strong. She then moves her hands a few inches away and along the periphery of another person's body both to disperse blocked energy and to channel her healing energy into the other person's "field." According to Krieger and Kunz, the prac-

Ivory carving of Hygieia, ancient diety of health and healing.
Merseyside County Museums, Liverpool, England

titioner's hands, moving in this way, can bring about profound relaxation, relieve pain and facilitate healing. Therapeutic Touch has been effective in relieving stress-related conditions such as rashes, headaches, asthma, colitis, sleep disorders, high blood pressure, palpitations and angina.

From a woman who used Therapeutic Touch for the first time:

I have a long history of migraines. I went into the nurse's office as a migraine was just beginning. While I had heard about Therapeutic Touch, I had never tried it before. When the nurse offered me a choice of decongestants, pain relievers, Therapeutic Touch or some combination, I decided to try Therapeutic Touch. (After all, I knew what the drugs could and couldn't do for me.) After the session my head felt lighter and less congested.

From a nurse who began practicing Therapeutic Touch after twenty-five years of conventional medical nursing:

A woman had been to four or five doctors before she saw me. Her symptoms were back and leg pains with a lot of swelling on her ankles. She was told that she had no disc or circulatory problems, and was sent

94

home with a diuretic for the swelling. "Sometimes middle-aged women develop these problems," one doctor said.

I worked with this woman every three to four weeks for a year. With her energy back, she has returned to leading an active life with no physical restrictions. When she occasionally has pain, she returns for a single treatment.

Practitioners must develop sensitivity through repeated practice and must understand why they want to become healers. Healing is a power tool, and the healer must be sure s/he works in the best interests of the person being treated.

Check at alternative health centers and therapy organizations or through listings in alternative health journals to find both practitioners and classes. You can also learn and practice techniques in groups of women doing Therapeutic Touch. Once learned, it's a method we can easily use to help each other.

Homeopathy

Homeopathy is a system of medicine that uses remedies made from natural substances (animal, vegetable and mineral) and is based on "The Law of Similars", that is, "like cures like." Hindu sages in the tenth century B.C. had described the law, as had Hippocrates in 400 B.C.

Samual Hahnemann, a German physician, established the practice of homeopathy in the early 1800s. While translating medical texts he came upon a claim that cinchona bark (the source of quinine) cured intermittent fever because of its astringent and bitter qualities. Hahnemann did not find this plausible since he knew of other substances equally bitter that were not helpful in treating intermittent fever, so he decided to test the medicine on himself. He took the bark daily and soon developed the symptoms of intermittent fever, all of which disappeared when he stopped taking the drug. This was the first "proving," the testing of a medicine on a healthy person.

After experimenting on himself, Hahnemann enlisted the help of colleagues and friends to conduct "provings" of mercury, belladonna, arsenic, silver nitrate and other substances. From the findings he concluded that these drugs worked because of their ability to produce in healthy people the very symptoms of the disease state which they were used to cure. He further demonstrated that it was possible to cure without negative side effects by using a very small amount of the appropriate medicine. He felt that a person's inherent healing powers were so strong that only a small stimulus was needed to begin the healing process, to act as a catalyst to the body's own defenses. He

developed a special method of serial dilution (dilution of 1:10 to 1:100 repeatedly up to thousands of times). This, combined with succession (mechanical agitation), and the fact that with classical homeopathy only one medicine is given at a time differentiates homeopathy from herbal medicine.

I had been nursing my son, Michael, for a little over a year when I noticed soreness in my left breast while out doing errands with him. I didn't think much of it, but several hours later when we returned home, I began to have fever, chills and sweating, and my breast was throbbing with pain. It came on quickly and was so severe that I called a relative to come over and take care of Michael. When help arrived, I managed to drive the two miles to the office of my homeopath. Within minutes she had diagnosed the problem as mastitis and prescribed the homeopathic remedy "phytolacca" (poke root), which I took immediately. It was difficult to drive home. It seemed as if every inch of my body ached. Within an hour the pain began to subside. Relief swept over me— the remedy was working! By that evening I had only slight tenderness in my breast and was able to nurse my son without pain. I was happy to have gotten better so fast and to have avoided antibiotics.

Homeopathy is often effective in treating people with a wide variety of acute and chronic problems, including infectious disease, allergies, gynecological conditions, digestive problems, skin diseases, and even psychological and genetic disorders. According to a 1991 review of clinical research on homeopathy conducted by three Dutch epidemiologists, there have been 107 controlled clinical trials using homeopathic medicine, 81 of which showed the medicines were effective in treating common problems such as migraine headaches and dry cough. Fifteen of these trials demonstrating efficacy were considered well-designed studies with no obvious flaws.*

In a French study of women giving birth, those who took cauloplyllum during labor had a lower rate of dystocia ("difficult labor") than women given a placebo.† Another study demonstrated the effectiveness of oscillococcinum,‡ a homeopathic remedy now available in many health food stores and pharmacies, in the treatment of flu symptoms.

Since a burning sensation of the urethra was causing me considerable distress that day, Dr. Graham decided to concentrate on that. He handed me a packet of white granules to take right there in the

---

*British Medical Journal, February 9, 1991.
†Dorfman, P., et al. "Preparation for Childbirth by Homeopathy," Cahiers de Biotherapie, Vol. 94 (April, 1987), pp. 77–81.
‡From "Homeopathy," Cosmopolitan magazine, October 1974.

office (homeopathic medicines are often dispensed by the doctor, which means a big reduction in drug bills). Taken without water, the granules looked and tasted like sugar and melted on my tongue. Anyway, the burning sensation stopped—immediately. This seemed indeed like the miracle I'd come for.

During the years I have visited Dr. Graham we've grown to know and respect each other. He's . . . too concerned to ever dismiss any complaint of mine as "nerves." Physical examinations are infrequent: only once, when I had pleurisy, did he actually examine (and cure) me. Nor does he do extensive blood tests, electrocardiograms, biopsies or other laboratory work. "I may confirm a diagnosis that way," he explained, "but tests play no part in my primary diagnosis. That's always based on the patient's own description of symptoms."

In the United States, homeopathy is practiced by medical doctors, osteopathic physicians and other licensed health professionals, including nurses, physician's assistants, dentists, veterinarians, chiropractors, acupuncturists, naturopaths and psychologists. There is also a growing number of lay practitioners.

For chronic problems and/or serious health concerns you should consult a homeopathic practitioner rather than treat yourself with the homeopathic remedies. In some cases, remedies are easily inactivated or antidoted, so that it is important to get expert guidance on what special precautions you need to take. Once you become more knowledgeable about homeopathic remedies, first aid kits and books may also be useful in helping you to treat simple problems safely at home.

NOTES

1. Much of this healing work, however, was so taken for granted that little of it has been recorded in historical documents. See Muriel Joy Hughes, *Women Healers in Medieval Life and Literature*, New York: 1943, and Kate Campbell Hurd-Mead, *A History of Women in Medicine*, Haddam, CT: 1938.

2. Joanna Macy. "Despair Work," *Evolutionary Blues*, No. 1 (available from Evolutionary Blues, Box 4448, Arcata, CA 95521); also *Despair, Personal Power in the Nuclear Age*, Philadelphia: New Society Publishers, 1983.

3. Mary Howell. *Healing at Home*. Boston: Beacon Press, 1979, p. 87.

4. N. Muramato. *Healing Ourselves*. New York: Avon Books, 1973, p. 4.

5. D. Ardell. *High-Level Wellness: An Alternative to Doctors, Drugs and Disease*. Emmaus, PA: Rodale Press, 1977, p. 2.

6. See Louis Hay's *You Can Heal Your Life*, Santa Monica, CA: Hay House, 1984, and Bernie Siegal's *Love, Medicine and Miracles*, NY: Harper & Row, 1986, for examples of victim blaming.

7. Herbert Benson. *The Relaxation Response*. New York: William Morrow, 1975, pp. 75–98.

8. Herbert Benson. *The Relaxation Response*, pp. 70–1, Table 2.

9. A good resource on stress management and relaxation is *Charlesworth and Nathan's Stress Management*. New York: Ballantine Books, 1982, 1984.

10. Thich Nhat Hanh, *The Miracle of Mindfulness, a Manual on Meditation*. Boston: Beacon Press, 1976.

11. Helpful resources on meditation include *New Age Journal*, Diane Mariechild's *Motherwit* and Margo Adair's *Working Inside Out* (see Resources).

12. Robert T. Trotter, II, and Juan Antonio Chavira, *Curanderismo: Mexican American Folk Healing*. Athens, GA: University of Georgia Press, 1981.

13. Images stored in the cerebral cortex affect the autonomic nervous system, which controls sweating, blushing, blood vessel expansion and contraction and rate and force of heartbeat. The autonomic nervous system is also connected with the pituitary gland and adrenal cortex, which secrete hormones and steroids affecting thyroid and sex glands and metabolic processes.

14. W. Luthe. *Autogenic Therapy*. New York: Grune & Stratton, 1969, Vol. I, p. 1.

15. E. Peper and E.A. Williams, "Autogenic Therapy," in *Health for the Whole Person*, Boulder, CO: Westview Press, 1980, p. 134.

16. O. Carl Simonton, Stephanie Matthews-Simonton and James L. Creighton. *Getting Well Together*. New York: Bantam Books, 1978, pp. 183–5.

17. O. Carl Simonton, Stephanie Matthews-Simonton and James L. Creighton. *Getting Well Together*, pp. 127–48.

18. G.E. Schwartz. "Biofeedback and the Treatment of Disregulation Disorders," *Ways of Health*, New York: Harcourt Brace Jovanovich, Inc., 1979, pp. 362–68; and J. Kamiya and J.G. Kamiya, "Biofeedback," *Health for the Whole Person*, pp. 115–29.

19. Richard Gordon. *Your Healing Hands: The Polarity Experience*. Santa Cruz, CA: Unity Press, 1978.

20. Margaret Elke and Mel Risman. "Sensitive Massage," *The Holistic Health Handbook*, p. 175.

21. Lew Connor and Linda McKim. "Reflexology," *The Holistic Health Handbook*, p. 183.

22. Christina Robb. "A Sense of Touch," *The Globe Magazine*, November 15, 1981, p. 22.

23. Stephen Chang. "Acupuncture: A Contemporary Look at an Ancient System," *The Holistic Health Handbook*, p. 48.

24. Fritjof Capra. *The Turning Point*. New York: Simon & Schuster, 1982, pp. 79–80.

25. G.F. Rickeman, "Chiropractics," *The Holistic Health Handbook*, p. 173.

26. T.A. Vondarhaar. "Chiropractic in Theory and Practice," *The Holistic Health Handbook*, p. 173.

27. Judith Hanson Lasath. "Yoga: An Ancient Technique for Restoring Health," *The Holistic Health Handbook*, p. 36.

28. Billie Pivnik, "Dance Movement Therapy at New England Rehabilitation Hospital," *Spokes*, February 1977.

29. Another school of movement therapy is based on the work of Rudolf Laban (see *The Mastery of Movement*, Boston: Plays, Inc., 1971) and elaborated by Irmgard Bartenieff (see *Body Movement: Coping with the Envi-*

ronment, New York: Gordon and Breach, 1980). (Also see Fritjof Capra, *The Turning Point*, New York: Simon & Schuster, 1982, pp. 347–8.) Laban believed that we all express ourselves as we move, no matter what we are doing. Bartenieff, a physical therapist, applied many of Laban's ideas to people with physical problems. She works with people who have a variety of chronic illnesses (heart, brain and spinal cord diseases, multiple sclerosis, Parkinson's disease, etc.) and helps them with depression or simply teaches them to have fun.

Judith Kestenberg (*Children and Parents: Psychoanalytic Studies on Development*, New York: Langdon and Weed, 1983), a psychoanalyst, uses the Laban-Bartenieff system for analyzing movement in her studies of the movement patterns of people through life-cycle changes. Especially interested in facilitating healthy parent-child relationships, she and other dance therapists are now working with bonding between young children and their parents.

30. Here are a few examples: Stanley Krippner, "Psychic Healing," in *Health for the Whole Person*, p. 169, and other references to his work cited in Note 10; Dolores Krieger, *Therapeutic Touch: How to Use Your Hands to Help or Heal*, Englewood Cliffs, NJ: Prentice-Hall, 1979; Lawrence LeShan, *The Medium, the Mystic and the Physicist*, New York: Ballantine Books, 1982.

RESOURCES

Books and Articles

Adair, Margo. *Working Inside Out*. Berkeley, CA: Wingbow Press, 1984.

Bauer, Cathryn. *Acupressure for Women*. Freedom, CA: The Crossing Press, 1987.

Benson, Herbert, MD. *The Mind-Body Effect*. New York: Berkeley Publishing Corp., 1979.

———. *The Relaxation Response*. New York: William Morrow, 1975. A guide for reducing tension and stress for people with high blood pressure.

Berkeley Holistic Health Center. *The New Holistic Health Handbook: Living Well in a New Era*, Shepard Bliss, ed. Lexington MA: The Stephen Greene Press, 1985.

Bliss, Shephard, ed. *The New Holistic Health Handbook: Living Well in a New Age*. Lexington, MA: The Stephen Greene Press, 1985. Available from the Berkeley Holistic Health Center, 3099 Telegraph Avenue, Berkeley, CA 94705.

Borysenko, Joan. *Minding the Body, Mending the Mind*. Reading, MA: Addison-Wesley, 1987.

Capra, Fritjof. *The Turning Point: Science, Society and the Rising Culture*. New York: Simon & Schuster, 1982. This book shows how the revolution in modern physics foreshadows the new holistic approaches to health. It provides the philosophical underpinnings for the fundamental changes in our concept of healing.

Connelly, Dianne. *All Sickness is Home Sickness*. Columbia, MD: Centre for Traditional Acupuncture, 1987.

———. *Traditional Acupuncture, The Law of the Five Elements*. Columbia, MD: Centre for Traditional Acupuncture, 1979.

Cousins, Norman. *Anatomy of an Illness*. New York: W.W. Norton, 1979.

Crawford, Robert. "Healthism: The Medicalization of Everyday Life," *Journal of Health Services*, Vol. 10, No. 3 (1980), pp. 365–88.

Cunningham, D., and A. Ramer. *Spiritual Dimensions of Healing Addictions*. San Rafael, CA: Cassandra Press, 1988.

———. *Further Dimensions of Healing Addictions*. San Rafael, CA: Cassandra Press, 1988.

Davis, Martha, ed. *Research Approaches to Movement and Personality*. New York: Arno Press, 1972.

Donkin, Scott W. *Sitting on the Job*. Boston: Houghton Mifflin, 1986. Written by a chiropractor.

Downing, George. *The Massage Book*. New York: Random House, 1972.

Ehrenreich, Barbara, and Deidre English. *For Her Own Good*. New York: Doubleday, 1978.

———. *Witches, Midwives, and Nurses*. New York: The Feminist Press, 1973.

Feldenkrais, Moshe. *Awareness Through Movement*. New York: Harper and Row, 1972.

Fields, Rick, et al. *Chop Wood, Carry Water*. New York: St. Martin's Press, 1984.

Gawain, Shakti. *Creative Visualization*. New York: Bantam, 1979.

Gordon, Richard. *Your Healing Hands: The Polarity Experience*. Santa Cruz, CA: Unity Press, 1978.

Haas, Elson. *Staying Healthy with the Seasons*. Berkeley, CA: Celestial Arts, 1981.

Hoffman, David. *The Herbal Handbook: A User's Guide to Medical Herbalism*. Rochester, VT: The Healing Arts Press, 1987, 1988.

Howell, Mary. "Curing, Caring and Healing." Address to medical students at Duke University, Autumn 1980.

———. "A Paradigm of Healing." September 15, 1981. Available from the Boston Women's Health Book Collective.

Hughes, Muriel Joy. *Women Healers in Medieval Life and Literature*. New York: Kings Crown Press, 1943.

Hurd-Mead, Kate Campbell. *A History of Women in Medicine*. Connecticut: Haddam, 1938.

Hutchinson, Marcia. *Transforming Body Image*. Freedom, CA: Crossing Press, 1985. Visualizations for healing body image.

Hyatt, Richard. *Chinese Herbal Medicine*. New York: Schocken Books, 1978.

Iglehart, Hallie. *Woman Spirit*. New York: Harper & Row, 1983.

Jaffe, Dennis T. *Healing from Within*. New York: Alfred A. Knopf, Inc., 1980.

Juhan, Deane. *Job's Body*. Barrytown, New York: Station Hill Press, 1987. Resource on bodywork and massage with explanation of how and why they work.

Kaptchuk, Ted J. *The Web That Has No Weaver: Understanding Chinese Medicine*. New York: Langdon and Weed, 1983.

Kent, Anne Rush. *Bodywork for Women*. New York: Random House, 1973.

Krieger, Dolores. *The Therapeutic Touch: How to Use Your Hands to Help or to Heal*. Englewood Cliffs, NJ: Prentice-Hall, Inc., 1979.

———. *Living the Therapeutic Touch: Healing as a Lifestyle*. New York: Dodd, Mead, 1987.

LeShan, Lawrence. *The Medium, The Mystic and the Physicist: Toward a General Theory of the Paranormal*. New York: Ballantine Books, 1982.

———. *You Can Fight for Your Life: Emotional Factors in the Treatment of Cancer.* New York: M. Grans and Co., 1977.

Lock, Margaret, and Deborah Gordon, eds. *Biomedicine Examined.* Dordrecht, Holland: Kluwer Academic Publishers, 1988.

MacNutt, Father Francis. *Healing.* New York: Bantam Books, 1974.

Macy, Joanna. *Despair and Personal Power in the Nuclear Age.* Philadelphia: The New Society Publishers, 1983.

———. "Despair Work," *Evolutionary Blues*, No. 1. Available from Evolutionary Blues, Box 4448, Arcata, CA 95521.

Mariechild, Diane. *Motherwit, The Inner Dance and Crystal Visions.* Freedom, CA: Crossing Press, 1987.

Moskowitz, Richard. *Homeopathic Remedies for Pregnancy and Childbirth.* Berkeley, CA: North Atlantic Books, 1992.

Nissim, Rina. *Natural Healing in Gynecology: A Manual for Women*, New York: Pandora Press, 1986.

North, Marion. *Personality Assessment Through Movement.* London: MacDonald and Evans, 1972.

Panos, Maesimund B., and Jane Heimlich. *Homeopathic Medicine at Home.* New York: St. Martin's Press, 1980.

Parvati, Jeannine. *Hygieia: A Woman's Herbal.* Santa Rosa, CA: Freestone Publishing Collective, 1978.

Payer, Lynn. *Medicine and Culture.* New York: Penguin Books, 1988.

Pelletier, Kenneth R. *Mind as Healer, Mind as Slayer.* New York: Delta, 1977.

Pivnik, Billie. "Dance Movement Therapy at New England Rehabilitation Hospital," *Spokes* (February 1977).

Potts, Billie. *Witches Heal.* Hecuba's Daughters, P.O. Box 488, Bearsville, NY 12409, 1981. Herbal remedies.

Samuels, Mike, and Nancy Samuels. *Seeing with the Mind's Eye.* New York: Random House, 1975.

Schuster, Karolyn. "Dance Therapy: Moving with the Beat—Toward Health," *The Physician and Sports Medicine* (December 1978).

Seidman, Maruti. *A Guide to Polarity Therapy.* North Hollywood, CA: New Castle Books, 1986.

Simonton, O. Carl, Stephanie Matthews-Simonton and James L. Creighton. *Getting Well Again.* New York: Bantam Books, 1980. A self-help guide to dealing with the stress of cancer.

Sobel, Dava, and Arthur C. Klein. *Arthritis: What Works.* New York: St. Martin's Press, 1989.

Sobel, David S., ed. *Ways of Health: Holistic Approaches to Ancient and Contemporary Medicine.* New York: Harcourt Brace Jovanovich, 1979. Compilation of well-documented articles on health and healing.

Stein, Diane. *All Women Are Healers.* Freedom, CA: The Crossing Press, 1990.

Stein, Howard. *American Medicine as Culture.* Boulder, CO: Westview Press, 1990.

Stone, Randolph. *Health Building.* Sebastopol, CA: CRCS Publications, 1985. Polarity, therapy and diet.

Teish, Luisah. *Jambalaya.* New York: Harper & Row, 1985.

Tennov, Dorothy. *Psychotherapy: The Hazardous Cure.* New York: Abelard-Schuman, 1975.

Thrash, Agatha, and Calvin Thrash. *Home Remedies.* Available from Thrash Publications, Rt. 1, Box 273, Seale, AL 36875. Resource on use of herbs, clay, heat and cold.

Tierra, Michael. *The Way of Herbs: Simple Remedies for Health and Healing.* Santa Cruz, CA: Unity Press, 1980.

Trotter, Robert T., II, and Juan Antonio Chavira. *Curanderismo: Mexican American Folk Healing.* Athens, GA: The University of Georgia Press, 1981.

Ullman, Dana. *Discovering Homeopathy.* Berkeley: North Atlantic Books, 1991.

Ullman, Dana, and Stephen Cummings. *Everybody's Guide to Homeopathic Medicines.* LA and NY: Jeremy Tarcher/St. Martin's Press, 1991, revised edition.

Verbruege, Martha H. "The Social Meaning of Personal Health: The Ladies' Physiological Institution of Boston and Vicinity in the 1850s," in S. Reverby and D. Rosner, eds., *Health Care in America, Essays in Social History.* Philadelphia: Temple University Press, 1979.

Westcott, Patsy, and Leyardia Black. *Alternative Health Care for Women.* Rochester, VT: Thorsons Publishing, 1987.

Periodicals

East/West Journal
Box 1200
Brookline Village, MA 02147
(617) 232-1000

Holistic Health Review
Human Sciences Press
72 Fifth Avenue
New York, NY 10011

Medical Self-Care Magazine
349 Healdsburg Avenue
Healdsburg, CA 95448
(707) 431-1100

Prevention Magazine
33 East Minor Street
Emmaus, PA 18049
(215) 967-5171

Well-Being Magazine and Vegetarian Times
P.O. Box 570
Oak Park, IL 60303
(208) 848-8100

Yoga Journal
2054 University Avenue
Berkeley, CA 94704
(510) 841-9200

Associations and Organizations

American Association of Acupuncture and Oriental Medicine
50 Maple Place
Manhasset, NY 10030

American Dance Therapy Association
2000 Century Plaza, Suite 108
Columbia, MD 21044
(410) 997-4040

Berkeley Holistic Health Center
3099 Telegraph Avenue,
Berkeley, CA 94705

Boiron Borneman Homeopathic Pharmacy
1208 Amosland Road
Norwood, PA 19074
(800) BLU-TUBE
Offers homeopathic medicines, homeopathic medicine kits, books.

Homeopathic Educational Services
2124 Kittredge St.
Berkeley, CA 94704
(800) 359-9051
Offers books, study tapes, homeopathic software, homeopathic medicines and homeopathic medicine kits.

Kripalu Yoga Center
Box 793
Lenox, MA 01240

The National Center for Homeopathy
801 N. Fairfax St., Suite 306
Alexandria, VA 22314
(703) 548-7790
Provides information on homeopathy, including homeopathic study groups, books and a monthly newsletter.

The National College of Chiropractic
200 E. Roosevelt Road
Lombard, IL 60148-4583
(708) 629-2000

The National College of Naturopathic Medicine
11231 SE Market Street
Portland, OR 97216

6

Psychotherapy

By Nancy P. Hawley, with
Wendy Sanford

With special thanks to Judy
Norsigian and Norma Swenson.

*1992 Update acknowledgments: Jean
Baker Miller, Rachel Lanzerotti, Joan
Ditzion, Judith Herman, and
Catherine Riessman.*

When we feel depressed, anxious or hopeless or when we realize that certain problems keep repeating themselves in our lives, it can help immensely to talk about it with supportive friends and family. Sometimes, however, those closest to us are not able or willing to talk about what's wrong, offer too much advice, are too much a part of the problem or can't give us enough time and focused attention. We may then carefully choose a trained psychotherapist who will offer the objectivity, skill and attentiveness necessary to help us deal with emotions and complex problems.

In an ideal therapeutic situation you feel safe talking about the most intimate details of your life. As you and the therapist get to know each other, s/he listens carefully and helps you identify your problems and your strengths and develop the skills you need to uncover your feelings, experiment with solutions to problems, change your life or learn to live with the unalterable.

One evening, while I was nursing my one-month-old daughter, a friend criticized my character—at length. In fact, she tore me to pieces. That night I had a powerful dream: As I went up a steep hill all my possessions fell away from me. Once at the top, I slid back down, and at the bottom, in a gutter at a crossroads, lay a magazine. It was the story of my life, but it had just a short introduction; the rest of the pages were blank. As I stood there, everything I'd lost miraculously tumbled back down around my feet. I woke up. A few days later I decided to see a therapist, a psychiatrist who had counseled my brother. He seemed "safe," was like a wise turtle. And he already knew something about my family. Therapy turned out to be a revelation. Each session those first four months led to discovery. I sat and faced him; he asked me useful questions. I laid my life out. All those events I'd never thought much about before were brought together, were in fact connected, formed patterns, a whole. I was at the center, the one responsible. This was the beginning of my conscious wish to change myself and of my belief that I could.

Before consulting a therapist—or while you do—it makes sense to check for physical causes of confusion or depression, such as certain medications like birth control pills, certain combinations of medications (see, in particular, Chapter 23, "Women Growing Older") or exposure to toxic substances at work or in the home. Sometimes an improved diet, more exercise or simply more sleep can make a person feel better emotionally. Often a physician will refer a woman for psychiatric treatment when he or she cannot identify a physical cause or treatment for a problem, or because s/he learned in medical training that many of women's physical problems are "all in their heads." Sometimes therapy is just right; sometimes, despite what doctors or even family and friends tell us, it is not what we need.

Women must approach psychotherapy with caution.[1] Many mental-health professionals, especially male psychiatrists and psychologists, have distorted ideas about women based on their training, inadequate information about women's psychological development as it differs from men's[2] and the realities of most women's lives. Discussing sex bias in therapy, three women professionals wrote:

Clinical theories of personality specify women's innate nature as passive, dependent, masochistic, and childlike, and psychological treatment has often aimed at reducing her complaints about the quality of her life and promoting adjustment to the existing order.[3]

A well-known study revealed that psychologists see positive adult qualities and "healthy" male qualities as *the same*, while they portray the "healthy" woman in very different terms: for instance, as more submissive, suggestive, emotional and illogical.[4] The many therapists who hold such stereotypes are of little use to women and can do a lot of harm.

Rarely do mental-health professionals realize how women's disadvantaged status is directly damaging to our mental health. They are more likely to see women's emotional problems as internally caused (intra-psychic) than men's, and fail to perceive the external reality and stress of women's lives.* Consequently, they are more likely to prescribe psychoactive drugs to women than to men, and women are twice as likely as men to receive electroshock. Practices like these draw women into a web of inappropriate psychotherapy, drug dependence and reduced self-esteem.

The medical model dominates most psychotherapy today. Most therapists who are not physicians have physicians as their teachers, supervisors or superiors in institutional settings. In the medical model the client is the "patient," who by implication is sick; the therapist is the "doctor," who by implication will "cure" the patient. (A nonmedicalized alternative is to see the client as having the sources of healing, insight and wholeness within her, and the therapist as a facilitator of a process by which s/he uncovers these.) The doctor-patient relationship carries a power imbalance which can work against women in therapy, especially when the therapist is male and/or misuses this power.*

Tragically, in the extreme, this power imbalance can lead therapists to physically and psychologically abuse women. Some have colluded with family members to lock us away in mental institutions (where women are the majority of patients) when we refuse to comply with society's norms for us. Some have molested and raped us in the name of "therapy."† Most widely, they have used myths about woman's supposedly passive, masochistic nature to keep us "in our place." Their underlying motivation is often a fear that we will gain and use our full powers. While extremes such as these by no means represent the majority of women's experiences, they illustrate the potential for the misuse of power, which occurs with considerable frequency when women consult mental-health professionals. By far the greatest damage done to women is accomplished through the subtle ways in which women are encouraged to stay in positions of service to men rather than to realize our fullest potential.

There are approaches to therapy that avoid some of the possible abuses. In co-counseling (reevaluation counseling), people learn counseling techniques in a teacher-led group, then take turns "counseling" one another as equals, and for no money.

Co-counseling is based on the belief that human beings are born with a tremendous intellectual potential, natural zest and lovingness, but that these qualities have been blocked and obscured as a result of accumulated distressing experiences which begin early in life. The belief is that any person can recover from these hurtful experiences by the natural healing process of emotional discharge—through laughing, crying, trembling, raging, yawning, for example. Co-counselors' basic aim is to assist each other in recovering and in using this natural healing process.

Therapists with a *feminist* approach (whether they name it this or not, because it is the attitude,

---

*Consider, for example, this observation by an incest survivor: "Therapists buy into their client's denial of incest—if the client doesn't mention it—it never comes up because most therapists are just as afraid to get into it as their client. Either because it threatens them or they are just plain ignorant of the issue. They aren't aware of how certain behavior patterns, responses could indicate an incest experience, so they can't help her bring it to the surface."[5]

*It is difficult to bring complaints against a therapist or to sue for malpractice, because your protests themselves may be misinterpreted as signs of your "mental instability." Other forms of medical malpractice are usually quite visible; it's hard to *prove* you're mentally or emotionally damaged.
†Recently, women have been organizing to stop sexual abuse by therapists. See Boston Associates to Stop Therapy Abuse (BASTA) and Therapy Exploitation LinkLine (TELL) in Resources.

not the label, that's most important) seek to help us find and use our strengths. They are aware of the power imbalances in the therapy relationship and try to use respectfully the power they do have. They are likely to recognize social, political and economic influences upon our emotional well-being. The first to raise mental-health issues which traditional therapists have ignored—incest, rape, wife battering, child abuse, alcoholism*—they are also likely to be more understanding of women in their interpretations. (For a discussion of lesbians and therapy, see p. 190.) Fortunately, there are now more feminist therapists in urban areas.

By no means is every woman therapist a feminist, and a few male therapists have a feminist approach. Also, women can encounter many of the same problems with their therapist, whether feminist or not. To find a good therapist, talk with friends who have had positive therapy experiences, look in women's newspapers, call a local women's center or the local NOW (National Organization for Women) office.

In choosing a psychotherapist, check the guidelines listed on pp. 82–83 for choosing any practitioner. We suggest that you look for those therapists who are able to go beyond the limitations of conventional medical training or supervision or who do not come out of this tradition at all. It may take a while to find someone with whom you can work well. In the exploratory session, feel free to ask about the therapist's goals, training, fees and attitudes toward women. Shop around if you can. (Cost is a factor here. While therapists at clinics affiliated with prepaid health plans or at community health centers are more reasonably priced, your choice in terms of variety and sometimes quality is more often limited. The more nonconventional therapists may not be covered by insurance.†) It's worth taking the time to find someone whose training, style and personality are suited to what you need.

I've gone to a variety of therapists for shorter and longer periods of my adult life, by myself and with family members. The first time I went, I chose to see a woman, but men have helped me as well. The best of these therapists had these features in common:

They were gentle, friendly and respectful.

They listened well and understood what I was saying.

They accepted the way I presented issues and didn't alter them to fit some theory.

Their own life problems didn't usually get mixed up with mine; when that happened they were able to acknowledge the fact.

They helped me define my problems and see my way to making the changes I wanted to make.

They were open to my criticisms of them.

They cared that I succeeded without claiming responsibility for my success.

Working with the help of therapists who had these qualities, I felt stronger as a person after each session and clearer about my life.

APPENDIX

Different Kinds of Psychotherapists

The most important thing to keep in mind when selecting a therapist is that the particular title someone has earned is no guarantee of the kind of attitudes s/he holds. Each category contains people with a full spectrum of attitudes and beliefs about women. The specifics about different specialists are useful to know, but ultimately you must trust your perceptions and not under- or overestimate the title's meaning.

Counselors

Counseling programs exist in schools of education and psychology. Talented counselors can be extremely helpful. They are often more flexible and less dogmatic than therapists with extensive formal training, though there are also lots of problems they haven't been trained to tackle. They must be willing to refer you to someone else when necessary. Marriage and family counselors and pastoral counselors are particular kinds of counselors many women consult.

Clinical Psychologists

Clinical psychologists hold master's degrees or doctorates from graduate schools of psychology, education and social science. Although not medically trained, many of them follow the medical model for therapy. A lot of psychological testing is developed and administered by clinical psychologists; these tests set guidelines for "normal" behavior which other therapists often use to evaluate a person's mental health.

---

*Growing awareness of the effects of sexual abuse and of growing up in alcoholic and other dysfunctional families has resulted in many groups and services for sexual abuse survivors and adult children of alcoholics. Look for groups and therapists that listen carefully and do not blame a woman for behaving the way society teaches us to behave. (Some codependency groups and literature have this "blame the victim" approach.) See *Too Good For Her Own Good*, by Claudia Bepko and Joann Krestan, New York: HarperCollins, 1990, for more discussion.
†Furthermore, some women have hesitated to use the mental-health benefits included in their individual insurance policies, as employers have denied women (and men) jobs because they have psychiatric histories of depression and other mental health problems.

Social Workers

Social workers are trained in schools of social work to do either psychiatric, medical or community social work. (Some people with the title of social worker [e.g., in welfare offices and mental hospitals] do not actually have social work training.) Social workers practice in hospitals and schools or privately, doing casework, group work and community organization. Though they often have a medicalized orientation, they do tend to place emphasis on the entire family rather than just the individual. Unfortunately most social workers are overworked and underpaid; although they can be helpful, caring and insightful, they are often not taken seriously or given power within the medical hierarchy. In the last several years most states have licensed social workers to practice independently, which gives them more control over their work.

Psychiatrists

Psychiatrists have gone through medical school, are licensed physicians and can prescribe drugs. Their special training process prepares them to work with people who are severely disturbed and may require hospitalization. If you need medication or hospitalization, you will need at least to consult with a psychiatrist. However, for most problems which people bring to therapy, it is not accurate to assume that psychiatrists' training makes them better therapists. With rare exceptions, they bring a medical bias into therapy work and with it the reinforced sexism and authoritarianism which come with medical training.

Psychoanalysts

Psychoanalysts (almost all in the United States are psychiatrists first) receive training in a psychoanalytic institute for a specialized type of individual therapy work that involves many sessions per week and often many years of therapy. This work, which involves slowly taking your personality apart and building it back up again anew, is lengthy and expensive. Make sure that any psychoanalyst you see is fully credentialed and not just a bona fide member of the local psychoanalytic institute. Classical psychoanalytic theory has been the source of most of the distorted ideas about women that pervade all medical training. At the same time, there are some feminist analysts trying to change this.[6]

Special Approaches

Family therapists (who may have previous degrees as psychiatrists, psychologists, nurses, social workers or counselors) attend training programs at the growing number of family therapy institutes across the country. They work with different kinds of family groups, and assume that whatever problems arise result from interactions within the family rather than from the individual alone.

Finally, there are many *specific therapy training programs* that develop their own professional criteria—often in experimental therapies such as Transactional Analysis, Transpersonal Therapy, Gestalt, Psychodrama, Psychosynthesis, Neurolinguistic Programming (NLP), Ericksonian Therapy and the body-oriented therapies, such as Bioenergetics, Psychomotor or Primal Scream.

Some therapists, influenced by feminist and holistic perspectives, are doing exciting new work. Transpersonal therapists are working with meditation; psychotherapists are using biofeedback; psychoanalytically oriented psychiatrists are studying family therapy and finding it full of possibilities; family therapists are learning hypnosis and visualization. The communication between traditionally trained therapists and alternative therapists has increased greatly in the last fifteen years. We look forward to the continuation of this trend.

NOTES

1. See Dorothy Tennov, *Psychotherapy, the Hazardous Cure* (New York: Abelard-Schuman, 1975) for an insightful discussion of the effects of psychotherapy on women. See also Phyllis Chesler's *Women and Madness* (New York: Avon Books, 1972), and Jean Baker Miller's *Toward a New Psychology of Women*, rev. ed., (Boston: Beacon Press, 1986).

2. See *In A Different Voice: Psychological Theory and Women's Development* by Carol Gilligan, (Cambridge, MA: Harvard University Press, 1982).

3. Elaine Hilberman Carmen, Nancy Felipe Russo, and Jean Baker Miller. "Inequality and Women's Mental Health: An Overview," *American Journal of Psychiatry*, 138:10 (October 1981), p. 1324.

4. I. K. Broverman, D. M. Broverman, F. E. Clarkson, P. S. Rosenkrantz and S. R. Vogel. "Sex Role Stereotypes and Clinical Judgments of Mental Health," *Journal of Consulting and Clinical Psychology*, No. 34 (1970), pp. 1–7.

5. From an interview with lesbian incest survivors in *Off Our Backs: A Woman's News Journal* (October 1982), p. 17.

6. See Judith V. Jordan's *Women's Growth in Connection: Writings from the Stone House* (New York: Guilford, 1991); Joan Zilbach's "Female Adolescence: Toward a Separate Line of Development," in Max Sugar, ed., *Female Adolescent Sexuality* (New York: Brunner Mazel, 1992); and Joan Zilbach's "In the 'I': The Eye of the Beholder: Towards a Separate Line of Development in Women," Slavson Memorial Lecture, American Group Psychotherapy Association, February 6, 1987.

RESOURCES

Bass, Ellen, and Laura Davis. *The Courage to Heal: A Guide for Women Survivors of Child Sexual Abuse.* New York: Harper & Row, 1988.

Bepko, Claudia, ed. *Feminism and Addiction.* New York: Haworth Press, 1991.

Bepko, Claudia, and Joann Krestan. *Too Good for Her Own Good: Breaking Free From the Burden of Female Responsibility.* New York: HarperCollins, 1990.

Berry, Carmen. *When Helping You Is Hurting Me.* New York: HarperCollins, 1989.

Black, Claudia. *Double Duty.* New York: Ballantine Books, 1990.

———. *It Could Never Happen to Me.* Denver, CO: MAC Publications, 1981.

Boston Lesbian Psychologies Collective, eds. *Lesbian Psychologies.* Urbana: University of Illinois, 1987.

Braud, Marjorie, ed. *Women, Power, and Therapy.* New York: Harrington Press, 1988.

Breggin, Peter. *Toxic Psychiatry.* New York: St. Martin's Press, 1991.

Brody, Claire M., ed. *Women's Therapy Groups: Paradigms of Feminist Treatment.* New York: Springer Publishing Co., 1987.

Caplan, Paula L. *The Myth of Women's Masochism.* New York: Signet, 1987.

———. *Don't Blame Mother.* New York: Harper & Row, 1989.

Chamberlin, Judi. *On Our Own: Patient-Controlled Alternatives to the Mental Health System.* New York: McGraw-Hill, 1978.

Chesler, Phyllis. *Women and Madness.* New York: Avon Books, 1972.

Conrad, Peter, and Joseph W. Schneider. "The Medical Model of Madness: The Emergence of Medical Illness," *Deviance and Medicalization: From Badness to Sickness.* St. Louis, MO: C.V. Mosby, 1980.

Ernst, Sheila, and Lucy Goodison. *In Our Own Hands: A Book of Self-Help Therapy.* Los Angeles: J.P. Tarcher, 1981.

"Gays and Lesbians in Therapy," *Family Therapy Networker,* Vol. 15, No. 1 (January–February 1991).

Fine, Michelle, and Adrienne Asch, eds. *Women with Disabilities: Essays in Psychology, Culture and Politics.* Philadelphia: Temple University Press, 1988.

Gilligan, Carol. *In a Different Voice: Psychological Theory and Women's Development.* Cambridge, MA: Harvard University Press, 1982.

Goodrich, Thelma Jean, ed. *Women and Power: Perspectives for Family Therapy.* New York: W.W. Norton, 1991.

Goodrich, T. J., C. Rampage, B. Ellman, and K. Halstead. *Feminist Family Therapy.* New York: W.W. Norton, 1988.

Greenspan, Miriam. *A New Approach to Women and Therapy.* New York: McGraw-Hill, 1983.

Herman, Judith Lewis. *Father–Daughter Incest.* Cambridge, MA: Harvard University Press, 1981.

———. *Trauma and Recovery.* New York: HarperCollins, 1992.

Jack, Dana Crowley. *Silencing the Self: Women and Depression.* Cambridge, MA: Harvard University Press, 1991.

Johnson, Karen, and Tom Ferguson. *Trusting Ourselves: The Sourcebook on Psychology for Women.* New York: The Atlantic Monthly Press, 1990.

Jordan, Judith V., et al. *Women's Growth in Connection: Writings from the Stone House.* New York: Guilford, 1991.

Lerner, Harriet G., *The Dance of Anger,* New York: Harper and Row, 1985.

Leupnitz, Deborah Anna. *The Family Interpreted.* New York: Basic Books, 1988.

McGoldrick, Monica, Carol Anderson and Fromma Welsh, eds. *Women in Families.* New York: W.W. Norton, 1991.

Miller, Jean Baker. *Toward a New Psychology of Women,* rev. ed. Boston: Beacon Press, 1986.

Napier, Nancy J. *Recreating Your Self: Help for Adult Children of Dysfunctional Families.* New York: W.W. Norton, 1990.

Peele, Stanton, and Archie Brodsky. *The Truth About Addiction and Recovery.* New York: Simon & Schuster, 1991.

Sanford, Lynda T. *Strong at the Broken Places: Overcoming the Trauma of Childhood Abuse.* New York: Avon, 1992.

Tennov, Dorothy. *Psychotherapy, The Hazardous Cure.* New York: Abelard-Schuman, 1975.

Tesmer, Kathryn. *Breaking the Silence.* Santa Rosa, CA: ACAT Press, 1989.

Wegscheider-Cruse, Sharon. *Another Chance: Hope and Faith for the Alcoholic Family,* rev. ed. Palo Alto: Science and Behavior Books, 1989.

Zilbach, Joan J. "Female Adolescence: Towards a Separate Line of Development," in Max Sugar, ed., *Female Adolescent Sexuality.* New York: Brunner Mazel, 1992.

———. "In the 'I': The Eye of the Beholder: Towards a Separate Line of Development in Women." Slavson Memorial Lecture, American Group Psychotherapy Association, February 6, 1987. For copies: Joan J. Zilbach, 36 Amory Street, Brookline, MA 02146.

Organizations

BASTA: Boston Associates to Stop Therapy Abuse
528 Franklin Street
Cambridge, MA 02139
(617) 661-4667
Responds to the needs of those abused in sexual ways by psychotherapists and other human service/health care providers. Offers a variety of services (e.g., support groups, one-day workshops, advocacy and consultation) for female survivors, male survivors and secondary victims (friends and family of survivors). Provides training for professionals.

Therapy Exploitation Link Line (TELL)
(617) 964-TELL
Victim support group, self-help model, meets monthly. Free.

7

Environmental and Occupational Health

Environmental Health by
PATRICIA LOGAN
Occupational Health by
LETITIA DAVIS, MARIAN
MARBURY, LAURA PUNNETT,
MARGARET QUINN, CATHY
SCHWARTZ AND SUSAN
WOSKIE (all are members
of MassCOSH Women's
Committee)

With special thanks to Judy
Norsigian, the Shalan Foundation
and the thousands of women
around the country working in
community groups and fighting
toxics.

*1992 Update by Reggie Kenen and
Lin Nelson. Acknowledgments: Joan
Bertin, Katsi Cook, and Maureen
Paul.*

We live in a small town. One morning a neighbor came over and said, "Don't drink the water," just after my husband and I drank two cups of coffee made from tap water.

We had been drinking it for years, and we didn't know how long it had been contaminated. Then our neighbor said just how bad it was, how many milligrams of the chemicals were in it. No one knows where it came from or who caused it. I felt very angry. You pay your taxes—they get higher every year—and you've got people sitting down there in their offices letting things get that bad.

Everybody should have pure, clean water to drink. But what could I do about it? I don't know enough. And anyway, what about everything else? When you eat your chicken, how do you know if you get pure meat? Or what's in your vegetables? Or what's in your bottled *water?*

Where and how we live and work affects our health in some obvious and not so obvious ways all the time. Sixty to 90 percent of all human cancers and high percentages of other lung, heart, nerve and kidney disease as well as reproductive problems, birth defects and even behavioral disorders are now thought to be environmentally caused.[1] ("Environment" here includes our diet and living habits.) Environmental hazards have increased tremendously in the last forty years. To the accidents, stress and disease which people have always encountered, twentieth-century society has added toxic chemical and radioactive substances. Through their manufacture, processing, distribution, use and disposal, these substances create a severe and unreasonable risk of injury to our environment and to our health.

CHEMICALS

Between 50,000 and 75,000 chemical substances are in common commercial use in this country,

105

Lionel J-M Delevingne/Stock Boston

especially in farming, forestry and the chemical, drug and manufacturing industries. About a thousand new chemicals appear each year. The vast majority of these chemicals have not been tested for their potential ill effects, yet they are in our food, water, air, clothing, homes and workplaces. American industry generates 560 million tons of hazardous wastes each year—that is more than two tons for every U.S. citizen.[2]

Our sewers are loaded with acid and chemicals. You can see them cooking in there, coming right up in my cellar. I called the city officials and they said they have nothing to do with it anymore. It's up to the state. The state people came and took samples from the sewer. I have yet to hear the results. That was five months ago.

I have been going to the doctor for the past 30 years. I've got breathing problems, kidney and bladder trouble, my kid has a heart condition, my husband can't breathe. Every morning I get up I know I am going to get that "sweet air" from the sewer disposal, and then I say, what's going to be next?[3]

RADIATION

Available evidence suggests that low-level radiation from normally functioning nuclear power plants and weapons facilities and testing contaminates our environment and our bodies in slow

stages. Mining of uranium and disposing of the milling wastes (called tailings) and the spent fuel create even more hazards. Waste from a nuclear reactor or weapons plant remains radioactive for as long as 250 centuries.

Our immediate community has been threatened by the effluent from one of the largest uranium mines in this hemisphere. For many months this effluent contaminated our public water supply—our people drank, cooked with, and bathed in this water, which had radiation in excess of recommended exposures. It took litigation and thousands of dollars of taxpayers' money to remove this community from that contaminated water supply.

In 1978 I lost a very good friend and neighbor of twenty-five years to pancreatic cancer. I had maintained an almost bedside vigil for six months prior to her death. During her final weeks we spoke of the many people in our neighborhood who had succumbed to the ravages of cancer. We wondered if the number of deaths was unusually high, even though cancer is proclaimed the number two killer.

Only time will tell, I guess, and then the burden of proof will be on whom?

In the ultimate accident at a nuclear power plant, a meltdown, thousands would die immediately of lethal radiation exposure; tens of thousands would die within two or three weeks of acute radiation sickness; hundreds of thousands of cancers would occur five to thirty years afterwards. And of course, nuclear war itself is the ultimate environmental hazard. The United States alone has over 30,000 nuclear warheads and can kill every human being on earth twelve times over.

PERVASIVE RISKS, UNEQUAL BURDENS

Today environmental hazards are so widespread that none of us can totally avoid them. Even snow in Antarctica carries residues of polychlorinated biphenyls (PCBs), dichlorodiphenyltrichloroethane (DDT) and lead.*[4] Human breast milk contains high levels of some toxins and human sperm samples contain PCBs.

Although we encounter the most concentrated and dangerous hazards in the workplace, our general environment creates a toxic burden for everyone and an added burden for workers.

- Lead and gases from car exhaust; particles, ash and smoke from factories; emissions from chemical and nuclear plants; and drift from pesticide spraying contaminate our air.
- Pesticides applied to crops, herbicides sprayed on forests and industrial chemicals flushed from factories and leaking from dumps contaminate our water.
- Pesticides, fertilizers, preservatives and additives pollute our food. Lead can concentrate in food grown near roadways. Hormones and antibiotics added to cattle feed, pesticides sprayed on rangeland and low-level radiation accumulate in animal fats to be passed up the food chain to people who eat animal products.
- Typical household cleaners and appliances can produce toxic fumes and dusts. With the energy crisis, increased weatherproofing of homes traps and concentrates toxics like radioactive radon gas (from concrete foundations containing uranium tailings) and the fumes from formaldehyde (used in products like permanent-press fabrics, foam insulation, carpets, drapes and plywood). Even low levels of formaldehyde vapors, carbon monoxide and other air pollutants in the home may disrupt moods and impair mental abilities.

We are involuntarily exposed to some environmental health hazards no matter who or where we are. Toxics don't discriminate—they cross regional, sex, class and racial lines. In these cases economic power determines how much we can protect ourselves. Some people can afford to move away from a chemical dump or nuclear power plant; some can buy bottled water or food without additives or get better health care. Others at this point in our country's history cannot.

The burdens of the toxic economy are shouldered more by some than by others. The Commission for Racial Justice (United Church of Christ) conducted an extensive study that found three out of the five largest commercial hazardous waste landfills are located in mostly black or Hispanic communities; three out of five black and Hispanic Americans live in communities with uncontrolled toxic waste sites; about half of all Asians/Pacific Islanders and Native Americans live near uncontrolled waste sites.[5] The clear identification of this environmental racism and the limited response of the mainstream environmental movement to this reality have inspired new thinking and action on environmental justice.[6]

Nor are environmental health hazards simply an urban problem. Rural people face heavy exposure to pesticides and herbicides, especially since agribusiness has taken over food production. Native Americans live with persistent low-level radiation from the uranium mining that has taken over more and more of their land. Some companies have targeted their reservations for toxic-waste dump sites.[7]

In addition, pesticides, drugs and industrial chemicals and processes banned as too dangerous in the United States are exported for manufacture or use in developing countries where regulations are nonexistent or not enforced. This pattern of dumping hazardous products, waste and production activities is symbolized by the Union Carbide nightmare in Bhopal, India—the 1984 "holocaust unprecedented in the annals of man-made industrial disasters."[8] Seven years after the toxic gas leak from the Union Carbide pesticide factory in Bhopal, 400,000 victims continued to suffer from untreatable or fatal illnesses. A 1990 study showed that the death rate for these victims is twice that of those unexposed to the gas. Union Carbide, a large multinational, has paid a mere $470 million to date.*

As women, we have had little to say about what we need or want. We have been targeted by industry and advertising as the consumers, not the producers, of the new technology that creates environmental hazards. Yet women have been on the frontlines in the struggle to curb hazards.

Official government and business statements about environmental hazards are almost universally reassuring. "Don't worry, no long-term dan-

---

*PCBs, once widely used in adhesives, paints, lubricants, electric insulators and printing inks, can cause everything from skin discoloration to liver disorders to cancer; DDT causes cancer and endangers wildlife; lead damages the nervous system.

---

*For more information, contact the Bhopal Action Resource Center, Suite 9A, 777 United Nations Plaza, New York, NY 10017.

gers have been scientifically proved." They put profit and prestige before people's health. Today we face the tragic consequences of trusting the reassurances of earlier decades—about DDT, for instance, or atomic testing. We who are writing this chapter believe that we *must* be concerned about environmental hazards whether or not they are at present conclusively "proven" dangerous. We don't want ourselves, our loved ones or anyone anywhere in the world used as guinea pigs in long-term safety experiments. We know our bodies, our workplaces and our communities better than any scientist does.

THE HEALTH EFFECTS OF ENVIRONMENTAL HAZARDS

At Love Canal* they told us to go home and tend our gardens. But women are no longer at home tending their gardens because both have become unsafe.

There are many effects of Love Canal chemicals, like central nervous system disease, including nervous breakdowns, migraine headaches and epilepsy. We have not conducted a survey on cancer to see if the rate is abnormally high here, but we have found many women throughout the neighborhood with breast and uterine cancer. There are many cancers, and they are not just in middle-aged women. One twelve-year-old child had a hysterectomy. We have many people with urinary problems, brain damage, and the list goes on. We have to wonder what the future holds: Cancers and other diseases may not surface for years.

To understand environmental health, we must understand that *everything* is connected—our body systems and organs, our life habits, our work and our wider environment. Environmental hazards can attack a particular organ or body system, directly damaging it and/or leading to further complications. While scientists generally test substances in labs one at a time, in real life our bodies always deal with more than one hazard at once. The combined interaction of two or more hazards to produce an effect greater than that of either one

---

*From the 1920s to the 1950s, the Hooker Chemical Company buried metal drums filled with tons of chemical wastes in the excavations in the Love Canal neighborhood of Niagara Falls, New York. In 1953 they covered the dump and sold the land to the Board of Education, which built a school on the site. Over the years the drums rusted and chemicals seeped, mixed and were spread by flooding and underground streams. Toxics killed plants, grass and wildlife, sickened local residents and caused birth defects and spontaneous abortions. In August 1978, the government declared Love Canal a national emergency area.

ENVIRONMENTAL HEALTH TERMS

Carcinogen (car-*sin*-o-jen)
A substance or agent that causes cancer, a condition characterized by usually rapidly spreading abnormal cell growth.

Mutagen (*mew*-ta-jen)
A substance or agent that causes changes (mutations) in the genetic material of living cells. When a mutation occurs in the egg or sperm (germ cells), it can be passed on to future generations. Recent research suggests that because genetic material controls the growth of cells, mutagens may either immediately or after a latency period cause abnormal cell growth, which becomes cancer.

Teratogen (teh-*ra*-to-jen)
A substance or agent that can cross the placenta of a pregnant woman and can cause a spontaneous abortion or birth disabilities and developmental abnormalities in the fetus.

All carcinogens are mutagens. Most mutagens are carcinogens. Many mutagens are also teratogens.

---

alone is called *synergism*. The amount of exposure, route of exposure and the toxic substance(s) we are exposed to determine whether we will feel acute or chronic effects.

An *acute effect* is a severe immediate reaction, usually after a single, large exposure—like the nausea and dizziness of pesticide poisoning or the pulmonary edema (a blistering of the air sacs in the lungs) from the burns of toxic gases like ammonia or chlorine. A *chronic effect* is a recurrent or constant reaction usually after repeated smaller exposures. Chronic effects can take years—the *latency period*—to develop. For instance, exposure to asbestos causes lung disease

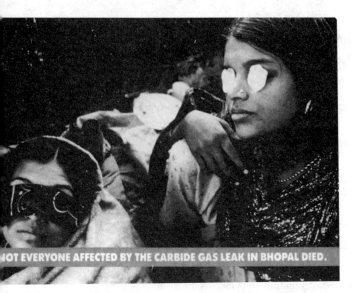

NOT EVERYONE AFFECTED BY THE CARBIDE GAS LEAK IN BHOPAL DIED.

Bhopal Group for Information and Action

years later, and most cancers and progressive liver diseases develop only after fifteen to forty years. Many scientists think we will see more and more problems as the toxics introduced after World War II "come of age."

We can absorb toxic substances in three ways: through the skin, through the digestive system (eating or drinking) or through the lungs. Often toxics cause damage on first contact—burns, rashes, stomach pain, for example. Once in the bloodstream, they can damage many internal organs and systems.

In general, toxics affect women and men in the same ways: Anyone can have an allergic reaction or liver damage, chronic headaches or respiratory problems, mental retardation or lung cancer. Environmental hazards put extra stress on our bodies and compound any other health problems that we might have.

Reproductive Health Hazards

A reproductive hazard is any agent that has harmful effects on the male or female reproductive system and/or the development of a fetus. These hazards can be chemicals (like pesticides), physical agents (like X-rays) or work practices (like heavy lifting).

Reproductive health hazards are probably the most controversial issues in environmental health. Because women bear children, reproductive hazards are too often considered "a woman's problem" involving pregnancy alone. This view ignores two important facts: that men are also affected by reproductive hazards, and that reproductive health means more than having healthy babies. All through life, men and women need

healthy sexual and reproductive systems. As it is, reproductive hazards are often used as excuses to penalize women workers and permit management to avoid cleaning up the workplace.

Infertility in either sex, a spontaneous abortion early in pregnancy or a baby with birth disabilities can all be early signs of a toxic environment. These can be important signals that something is wrong, since other signs like cancer can take a fifteen- to forty-year latency period to develop.

How Reproductive Hazards Affect Men

A recent government study found PCBs in every human sperm sample tested.[9] Environmental toxics can disrupt the production of male hormones in the testes, causing loss of sex drive and impotence. They can also cause problems with sperm production. A toxic agent can disturb sperm cells at any one of several stages of rapid growth, causing problems with fertility through a total lack of sperm, low sperm production or malformed sperm. Toxics may be causing an overall decline in sperm counts in American men.[10]

In addition, some reproductive hazards are mutagens. When a mutation occurs in sperm cells, men can pass damaged genes on to future generations, which can result in spontaneous abortions or disabilities in future children.

- Men exposed to lead have decreased fertility and malformed sperm.[11]
- Some believe that there have been higher rates of birth disabilities in the children of Vietnam veterans exposed to Agent Orange. This herbicide was contaminated with dioxin, considered a highly toxic man-made substance. Some studies dispute this claim.*[12]
- DBCP (dibromochloropropane), a pesticide, was found to cause dramatically decreased sperm counts in men who work with it or in its manufacture. The men in one California factory noticed that none of them had fathered children since they started working there, and demanded fertility tests. Many were found sterile.[13]

How Reproductive Hazards Affect Women

When toxic substances disrupt the reproductive hormones, they can cause menstrual disorders, sterility or loss of sexual drive.[14] Toxic substances may also directly damage the ovaries, eventually resulting in early menopause or ovarian disease. And, as with sperm cells, environmental mutagens can damage the genetic material in a wom-

*For a report of a major epidemiological study by Colin Norman, see "Vietnam's Herbicide Legacy," in *Science*, Vol. 219 (March 11, 1983), pp. 1196–97. The Centers for Disease Control in Atlanta offer a contradictory view based on a later analysis of the available data.

ENVIRONMENTAL HAZARDS AND OUR BODY SYSTEMS*

Body System/Function	Acute and Chronic Effects	Some Common Causes
Skin—Body's first line of protection from the environment; can be initiated directly; toxics can also penetrate skin to enter bloodstream	Redness, dryness, itching	Solvents, plastics, epoxies, metals
	Redness, burns, blisters	Ultraviolet and unfrared radiation, acids
	Severe acne (chloracne)	PCBs, dioxin
	Skin cancer	Mineral oils, ultraviolet radiation, X-rays, arsenic
Respiratory system (nose, throat, lungs)—Transfers oxygen to the blood; lungs, nose, throat can be burned or scarred directly; toxics can also be absorbed from lungs into bloodstream	Sneezing, coughing, sore throat, wheezing, congestion	Gases, ammonia, solvents, formaldehyde, cotton and mineral dusts, beryllium, metal oxide
	Burning, fluid build-up (pulmonary edema)	Ammonia, nitrogen oxides, sulfur dioxide, chlorine, kerosene
	Chronic lung disease (bronchitis, emphysema)	Asbestos dust, soft coal dust
	Lung cancer	Mineral oils, chromium, asbestos, cigarettes
Cardiovascular system (heart and blood vessels)—Pumps and carries blood throughout the body; damaged when deprived of oxygen	Irregular heartbeat	Carbon monoxide, barium, organophosphates, glues and solvents, heat and cold, carbon disulfide, cigarettes
	Arteriosclerosis	
	Coronary heart disease	
Gastrointestinal system (stomach, intestines)—Digests ingested toxics either breaking them down or passing them on to the bloodstream	Nausea, vomiting, diarrhea, constipation	Pesticides, chloroform, cyanide, fluonide, solvents, lead
Liver and kidneys—Toxics pass into the blood from the digestive system and are carried to the liver and kidneys, which work to break them down and pass them from the body; they can be inflamed, scarred or even poisoned in the process	Jaundice	Carbon tetrachloride, vinyl chloride
	Hepatitis (inflammation of liver)	Tetrachlorethane, chlorinated hydrocarbons, anesthesia
	Acute kidney disease	Lead, mercury, carbon monoxide, arsenic, high-voltage electricity
	Chronic kidney disease	Lead, carbon disulfide, alcohol
Central nervous system (brain, nerves)—Toxics can reduce oxygen to the brain and interfere with communication between nerves and other body systems, causing disorders	Behavioral disorders, confusion, lethargy, depression, anxiety, headache, irritability	Noise, metal poisoning (lead, mercury), stress, kepone, carbon disulfide, pesticides
	Learning disability or impairment, depression of central nervous system	Acetates, brominated/chlorinated chemicals
	Oxygen deprivation, brain damage	Asphyxiating gases, carbon monoxide
	Nerve function disorders	Organophosphate pesticides, mercury, lead, arsenic, manganese
Immune system—Minimum exposures to toxics can tax and suppress the body's ability to fight disease or poisons; some believe dysfunction of the immune system allows cancer to develop	Burning, nausea, headaches, psychosis, allergic reactions	Epoxy resins and plastics, hexachlorophene, nickel compounds, mercury compounds, formaldehyde
Circulatory system (blood)—Absorbs toxics from digestive system, lungs or skin and carries them to other organs	Anemia	Lead
	Leukemia	Benzene, ionizing radiation

ENVIRONMENTAL HAZARDS AND OUR BODY SYSTEMS*

Body System/Function	Acute and Chronic Effects	Some Common Causes
Reproductive system—Toxics can harm the reproductive organs themselves, cause direct damage to eggs, sperm or a developing fetus or cause mutations in eggs and sperm that can be passed on to later generations	Infertility or reduced fertility	Lead, carbon disulfide, ionizing radiation
	Decreased libido	Carbon disulfide, estrogens (in men)
	Menstrual changes	Carbon disulfide, estrogens, lead, PCBs
	Birth defects	Anesthetic gases, mercury, lead, DDT

*Compiled from *Work Is Dangerous to Your Health* by Jeanne Stellman and Susan Daum (New York: Vintage, 1973); and *We're Tired of Being Guinea Pigs* by Maxine Kenny, Juliet Merrifield et al. (New Market, TN: Highlander Research and Education Center, 1980).

an's eggs, with the same effects—spontaneous abortion or birth disabilities. Recent animal studies show ovary damage from polycyclic hydrocarbons (used in the petrochemical industry), alkylating agents (used in cancer treatment) and ionizing radiation. Exposure to lead, PCBs and vinyl chloride can cause menstrual changes.

The Developing Fetus and Young Children

The fertilized egg and the fetus can sometimes react to toxics that do not apparently harm an adult.

Some toxins affect the first three months of pregnancy, so early that the woman may not be aware she is pregnant. During the first two weeks, the fertilized egg is so sensitive that an environmental hazard powerful enough to damage it will also destroy it. From the fifteenth to the sixtieth day of a pregnancy, the cells of the fetus multiply and differentiate into specific organs and systems. A toxin can disrupt this process, and there is no second chance for the system to establish itself. If the effect is very strong, the pregnancy often ends in a spontaneous abortion (miscarriage). If the fetus survives, the child may have a low birth weight or physical, developmental or behavioral problems, some of which may not show up until years later.

The most common way that a fetus is exposed to toxics in the environment or workplace is through the mother's direct exposure. However, because semen is one place where toxics accumulate, having intercourse during pregnancy with a man who has had occupational exposure to toxics can cause birth disabilities.[15] (Pregnant couples might consider ways of making love other than intercourse; men exposed to environmental hazards may want to use condoms some or all of the time.)

The developing fetus and young children are particularly susceptible to certain environmental hazards because their cells are dividing and growing rapidly. Yet the government still sets standards for "safety" levels of toxics based on effects on adults.

Some toxics can concentrate in breast milk, posing poorly understood risks to newborns. The Environmental Protection Agency has reported that about 30 percent of U.S. women have PCB levels that exceed the FDA's "acceptable daily intake" levels for other foods. The World Health Organization, along with a growing number of researchers, has acknowledged that few women anywhere in the world are without some trace levels of industrial contaminants in their milk.[16] Still, because breastfeeding is so beneficial to babies, it is probably best to nurse—especially if a woman avoids exposure to high-risk foods, such as Great Lakes fish, and avoids quick weight loss (which mobilizes the body's fat stores, putting an infant at higher risk). Experts are struggling to develop a clearer advisory on this subject.[17]

Other Effects

Environmental mutagens also pose dangers for the entire human species. Damaged genetic material, whether it causes visible damage or not, contributes its permanent changes to the total human gene pool. A mutation rate increased by the effects of chemical and radioactive toxins could not only produce a general decline in human genetic health, it could threaten human existence.

TACKLING THE ENVIRONMENTAL HEALTH CRISIS

As women we are learning to be both more aware of environmentally caused problems and more confident about the power of such awareness. Often in the past we have just "accepted" a miscarriage or infertility or a chronically sick child. Now, instead of accepting, we're investigating. And when we do, we often find that the problems are environmentally connected. It's important not to just accept physicians' statements that "this is normal" or that we are "just being emotional." Environmental damage is often hard to prove. Persist. Don't just remain frustrated with the doctor. Find a new one. Find someone you can talk to about it.

And keep on learning to be more alert to things that can go wrong with your body because of environmental exposures. Don't discount your own knowledge of yourself, your own power.

We can begin to minimize the effects of some environmental hazards by avoiding voluntary exposures* and staying as healthy as we can. Yet the larger problems with environmental hazards can seem overwhelming and confusing. Taking action often seems too complicated—there is too much bureaucracy, too much chemistry and biology to learn and the polluters have too much power. "Surely someone is taking care of it all," we say. No one is. "It's all too impossible to deal with," we say. It's not.

Environmental health is basically a community issue, one we cannot fight alone. Luckily, we don't have to. Recent polls have shown that the vast majority of Americans are concerned increasingly about environmental conditions—from polluted water to toxic landfills—and they say they are willing to make sacrifices (e.g., pay higher taxes) to ensure a safer environment. The thousands of grassroots groups emerging across the country are evidence of this newfound determination. Because the manufacturers and agribusiness interests will not regulate themselves—and the Reagan and Bush administrations have done little to challenge business-as-usual pollution—we need a new era of environmental democracy with intense citizen involvement.

Strategies

Citizen action against environmental health hazards can take many routes. (See Resources for more information.) Experienced activists agree on some basic points:

1. The first step is education. What hazards are manufactured, used, stored or transported in your community and how do they harm people? Where do they come from? Become familiar with what's in use in your area and what the effects are. Pass on what you learn. Try working with existing community groups, bring in speakers, write letters to newspapers, show films, and set up information tables.

2. Keep a log of any changes in your health and

try to correlate them with what industries are doing in your area.

3. Talk to your neighbors. Work with other people. Many citizens' groups get going when people realize that they're not alone, that others are also being affected. Do a citizens' health survey.

4. Monitor your own "backyard." Watch for odd smells, bubbles or oozes in the air, land or water. Watch for sick and dying wildlife and pets. Watch for oil drums abandoned in fields or trucks dumping at night. Watch for "invisible" hazards, too: Radiation can't be seen, but the industries manufacturing it can be. Pay attention to reproductive patterns in your community. Government agencies may try to dismiss your results as nonscientific, but this information can be very helpful in showing patterns, establishing that there is a problem, keeping facts and history clear, activating citizens and helping health professionals know—later—what to focus their studies on.

5. When industry or government presents you or your group with information, statistics or data on a substance and its effects, always ask who paid for the study. The answer should help you to evaluate the data. Demand that information be presented in terms you can understand, not in the jargon of "experts."

6. Use the consumers' tool: the boycott. Find out where pollutants come from and what products they're used in and refuse to buy them. Women especially have enormous power as consumers.

The Citizens' Clearinghouse for Hazardous Waste (CCHW), the National Toxics Campaign (NTC), the Labor Institute and the COSH groups (see Resources) all help grassroots groups with legal options, conducting surveys, getting a company to accept a "neighbors' inspection" and using national data systems and community Right-to-Know provisions. Increasingly, coalitions of environmental, labor and other social justice groups are pushing beyond Right-to-Know (the basic right of access to certain information about on-site toxics) to Right-to-Act (the right to refuse work, change production activity or enforce an emergency shutdown).

Women's Activism

Women have always been active in exposing and working to eliminate environmental health hazards.

▪ Ellen Swallow, the first woman student admitted to MIT, created the interdisciplinary study of nutrition, air and water pollution, architecture, waste disposal and occupational health and safety. In 1892 she named this study "ecology."

---

*For example, avoid unnecessary X-rays, especially during pregnancy. Hair dyes have been shown to be mutagenic and carcinogenic. The coal-tar food dyes cause allergic reactions.

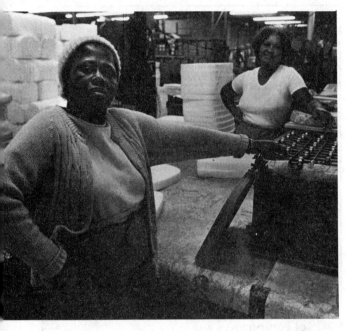

Earl Dotter

the water department. They proved the toxicity of the uranium as a heavy metal rather than as a radioactive element, forcing the local government to take action.

- On Earth Day 1980, the Chemical Control Company dump exploded in Elizabeth, New Jersey, forcing people from Elizabeth east to Staten Island to stay indoors while the chemicals burned. For years before this, residents had complained of respiratory and other health problems, suspecting the heavy concentrations of chemical manufacturers and the chemical dump as the cause. A citizens' group, led by Sister Jacinta Fernandes and other community women, had conducted health surveys, marched and held speakouts. Their pressure had forced cleanup of the worst chemicals from the dump *before* it exploded. Without their work, the fire would have been even more devastating.

As the women's health movement has shown, we must take charge of our bodies, our health, our environment and our lives.

Any average man or woman can do what we did. You can write press releases, push government, get things done. If you keep hammering the nail, eventually it's going to go in. I was "just a housewife." I'm proof that you don't need special talent or experience. I don't think people understand that. If I can get up and address five hundred people, believe me, anyone can. If something has to be done, there are ways to do it. You don't need a college education—just determination.

WORK CAN BE HAZARDOUS TO OUR HEALTH

The work we do affects our health not only while we are working but throughout the rest of the day, on weekends and vacations and even in the years after we have left the job. The consequences of hazardous working conditions are severe. More than 100,000 workers die each year from known job-related diseases, and more suffer from other diseases not yet recognized as resulting from exposures on the job. Over 16,000 American workers are killed every year in workplace accidents, and thousands more are disabled. We cannot take poor working conditions for granted as "just part of the job." We have to think about them—why they exist, what they might be doing to us and how they can be changed.

Workplace safety and health are usually associated with traditional "men's work," like mining, construction and heavy manufacturing. Women in the paid labor force have tended to be concentrated in "women's work," such as cleaning, nurs-

- Rachel Carson, in 1962, wrote *Silent Spring*, the book that exposed the widespread use and dangers of pesticides in our environment. Her work brought this problem to public attention, led to the ban on DDT in the United States and marked the beginning of the American environmental movement.
- Lois Gibbs organized the Love Canal Homeowners' Association and, with the women of Love Canal, forced the state of New York to recognize the problems. They signed petitions, did health surveys, embarrassed government and industry officials, picketed, blocked buses and testified in Washington. Because of their work, the government evacuated 1,000 families, purchased their homes and established a safety plan for the workers on site, a retroactive tax break and a health fund to cover future problems.
- Bonnie Hill and seven other women correlated their miscarriages with the spraying of 2,4,5-T, a herbicide, near their homes in rural Alsea, Oregon. Their protests to the EPA led to the emergency ban in 1979 on the chemical for most uses in the United States.
- Polly Heran, a member of the local water board of Rocky Flats, Colorado, discovered that the water supply had double the normal amount of uranium. The community is near a uranium mine and a nuclear weapons facility. Ms. Heran, along with a group of housewives, studied the issue. When they could not get the local authorities to act because there was no "conclusive" information on the radioactive effect of the uranium, they threatened to boycott and bankrupt

SOME COMMON WORKPLACE HAZARDS

Potential Safety Hazards	Potential Health Hazards
No machine guards	Dusts, mists, gases, vapors, smoke
Faulty switches, exposed wiring	Heat, cold, dampness
Dangerous floors, doors, exits, aisles, stairs	Radiation
Cranes, lifts, hoists	Noise, vibration
Poor lighting	Stress
Explosives	
No fire extinguishers	
No protective gear for emergencies	
Poor maintenance of equipment	
Lack of training in safe work practices and first aid	
Speedup	
No first aid equipment	

ing, teaching, garment making, clerical and "service" work. These jobs are not so safe either.

I had worked at the hospital for four years as a housekeeper when I got sick with hepatitis. I found out that a patient on my floor had hepatitis and nobody had bothered to tell me what precautions to take. I filed a claim for worker's compensation and the hospital fought my claim! I never thought that a thing like that could happen. I was working in a place that was supposed to care about people's health and they never told me anything about protecting my health.

The growing number of women in heavy industry and construction jobs generally face the same, often dangerous conditions that men face. But women often feel pressure to prove that they are "as good as" the men they work with, and when they speak up about health and safety they're seen as "too weak to take it." Yet the problems we are concerned about also affect men, and women's vocal presence in these traditionally male workplaces is bringing a change in the way people think about health and safety issues.

Women have special concerns because of our social and economic situations. Sexist job discrimination puts a large majority of women into low-paying and stressful occupations. Many women carry the double duty of paid work *and* responsibilities at home, which makes it more difficult to get involved in after-work meetings about working conditions. Women often have low seniority or jobs that place them in caretaking roles or require close working relationships with their bosses, making them hesitant to bring up complaints about hazards. In addition, only 16 percent of women workers belong to unions, which makes organizing more difficult.

Minority women are more often stuck with dead-end, "no transfer" jobs that expose them to more dangerous conditions for longer periods of time than their white counterparts. Poor, black, rural women are prime candidates for the high-risk poultry industry. In North Carolina, the 70,000 rural women in the poultry industry endure unsafe machinery, speed-up on the assembly lines, dull knives, slippery floors, and sexual harassment.[18]

Seventy percent of all migrant farmworkers are black and Latino. These workers face appalling working conditions, including exposure to pesticides that have well-documented harmful health effects.

Recognizing Hazards in the Workplace

Management is supposed to provide a safe workplace, but this task is frequently low on its priority list. Improving conditions often costs money, and in addition management may be afraid of giving up, or appearing to give up, control. Who controls the workplace is often an important, if unstated, issue in workplace health and safety struggles. If workers become knowledgeable about work processes and practices in order to make them safer, we are then more likely to question in general why and how things are done.

Recognition is the first step in eliminating hazards. You don't have to be an expert, but you do have to be persistent and thorough. A good way to begin is by talking with the people you work with. You and your co-workers are the best qualified to identify what the hazards and dangerous jobs are.

Some hazards are obvious. Just using your eyes, ears and nose will help you pick out safety hazards such as obvious dust or fumes and excessive noise. Recognizing hidden hazards is often more difficult. See if there is any pattern in who gets sick in your workplace. Talk to people or use a simple questionnaire to ask about mild symptoms, headaches, frequent illnesses, coughs, etc. These activities will not only help identify problems, they will also help to build awareness and interest among fellow workers about job conditions.

Learn about the chemicals and other substances you work with. A trade name such as Wite Out is not useful; you need to know the names of the actual chemicals in the product (in this case,

---

METHODS FOR CONTROLLING WORKPLACE HAZARDS

1. **Substitute.**
   Can a different substance or equipment (chemical or process) be used that will be safer?
   Clerical workers can use a water-based correction fluid to correct typing instead of a solvent-based fluid.

2. **Change the process.**
   Can the job be done in a completely different and safer way?
   Retail salesworkers are usually required to stand for most of the workday. This can lead to leg pain and varicose veins. If stools are provided and clerks encouraged to rotate sitting and standing, this stress will be reduced.

3. **Mechanize the process.**
   Is automating an operation the best answer to a dangerous job?
   Garment workers often have to lift large bundles of material and bins of finished products. If mechanical lifting devices are provided and used, the back and shoulder strain caused by manual lifting will be avoided.

4. **Isolate or enclose the process.**
   Can the hazardous job be removed to a different area or time where fewer people would be exposed? Can the worker be isolated from the operation or can the process be completely enclosed?
   Hospital workers are often exposed to irritating fumes when soldering parts. If ventilating hoods are installed, the fumes will be exhausted away from the breathing zone of the worker.

5. **Improve housekeeping.**
   In many operations strict housekeeping is essential to keep toxic materials from being reintroduced into the air or to prevent safety hazards.
   Textile workers can be exposed to cotton dust that causes brown lung disease. Strict housekeeping can keep dust levels down and keep obstacles out of the work areas and exits to prevent accidents.

6. **Improve maintenance.**
   Is equipment regularly serviced and repaired?
   Teachers and clerical workers often use photocopy machines. If poorly maintained these machines can give off irritating ozone gas.

7. **Provide personal protective equipment.**
   When other methods fail, or as a backup, can respirators, gloves, aprons or other protective clothing be used?
   Household workers often use toxic chemicals, such as drain cleaners, oven cleaners, pesticides and detergents, for example. Rubber gloves can protect the hands and arms from irritation and prevent the chemicals from being absorbed into the blood by the skin.

8. **Institute administrative controls.**
   When other methods don't work, can people be rotated through stressful or dangerous jobs to minimize their exposure?
   Clerical workers often work with VDTs (video display terminals). Considerable back, neck and eye strain can occur. With frequent rest breaks and job rotation, some stress can be relieved.

COMMON HAZARDS IN WOMEN'S OCCUPATIONS

Type of Work	Common Hazards	Health Effects
Household workers: over 859,000	Cleaning substances (drain and oven cleaners, bleach, aerosol sprays, waxes), pesticides	Irritation or burns of skin, eyes or lungs, allergies
	Lifting, falls, infections from children, electrical shock, noise	Muscle soreness, slipped disc, torn ligaments, bursitis
Clerical workers: over 14.7 million	Stress, video display terminals (VDTs)	Headache, heart disease, eyestrain, neck and back pain
	Poor air quality and ventilation, toxic substances from photocopy, duplicators, correction fluids	Nausea, colds, respiratory problems, eye, nose and throat irritation / Cardiovascular disease
	Noise	Anxiety, hearing damage
	Poor lighting and chair design	Varicose veins, neck and back pain, eyestrain
Hospital workers: 3.7 million	Infections	Infection from patients, utensils, specimens
	Lifting and falls	Back strain, slipped disc, torn ligaments
	Radiation	Tissue damage, genetic changes from X-rays and chemical hazards
	Chemical hazards (sterilizing gases, anesthetic gases, drugs)	Skin and respiratory irritation, liver, kidney, nervous system damage, cancer, reproductive problems
	Stress, electric shock	Headaches, heart disease, gastrointestinal problems
Retail salespersons: 4.1 million	Standing, lifting, stress	Leg pain, varicose veins, back and shoulder pain, headaches, irritability, high blood pressure
	Safety hazards (blocked aisles, exits; poorly designed equipment)	Accidents
	Poor ventilation	Colds, respiratory problems, eye, nose and throat irritation
	Infection	Communicable diseases
Artists: 115,000	Solvents	Dizziness, dermatitis, damage to liver, kidneys, nervous system
	Paints, solder	Damage to kidneys, liver, lungs, reproductive system, from heavy metals
	Clays, glazes, welding fumes, fumes from firing	Lung damage
	Poor equipment maintenance; poor ventilation	Accidents, fire
Health care lab workers: 240,000 Lab technicians and related support staff: 1,872,000	Handling biological specimens or animals	Infection
	Toxic chemicals, including carcinogens	Organ damage, changes in genetic material, reproductive problems, cancer
	Radiation in specimens, radioisotopes, machinery using radiation	Tissue changes or genetic changes, reproductive problems

COMMON HAZARDS IN WOMEN'S OCCUPATIONS

Type of Work	Common Hazards	Health Effects
Textile, apparel and furnishings machine operators (includes sewers and stitchers): 949,000	Chemicals (fabric treatment, dyes, cleaning solvents)	Skin and lung irritation, damage to liver, kidney and nervous system, dermatitis
		Asthma, respiratory disease
	Synthetic fiber and cotton dust	Hearing loss
	Noise	Wrist and hand inflammation
	Vibration	Heat stress, colds
	Heat, cold, poor ventiliation	Accidents, electric shock
	Unsafe equipment	Back and shoulder strain, varicose veins
	Lifting, standing, sitting	
	Stress	High blood pressure, headaches, anxiety
Electrical and electronic technicians: 47,600	Solvents	Dermatitis, dizziness, damage to nervous system and organs such as liver
	Acids	Skin burns and irritation
	Sitting and standing, fine work under microscope, repetitive work	Back and shoulder pain, varicose veins, headaches
	Stress	Heart disease, gastrointestinal problems
	Solder fumes, poor ventilation	Eye, nose and throat irritation, lung disease
Meat wrappers: number unknown	Lifting	Shoulder and back strain
	Standing	Low back pain, varicose veins
	Repetitive motion	Swelling and inflammation of the hands
	Plastic wrap fumes	Asthma, eye, nose and throat irritation, nausea, flulike symptoms
	Cold, cuts, slips, falls	Numbness, circulation problems
Hairdressers and beauticians: 672,000	Standing	Low back pain and varicose veins
	Chemicals (hair sprays and dyes, aerosol sprays, cosmetics and other preparations)	Lung disease, reproductive effects, cancer, allergies, skin irritation
Laundry and dry cleaners: 269,000	Laundry: soaps, bleaches, acids	Irritation or burns on hands, irritation of eyes, nose or throat
	Dry cleaning: solvents	Dermatitis, dizziness, damage to nervous system or liver
	Both: lifting	Back injuries, strains, hernias
	heat	Heart disease
	contamination	Exposure to whatever chemicals or biological materials are on clothes

trichlorethylene) because almost all information on chemicals is organized by the scientific chemical name. The federal Hazard Communication Standard provides workers with certain rights of access to information—that is, management is supposed to provide training, appropriate labeling, inventories of chemicals and material safety data sheets (MSDSs) for each substance of exposure. However, the reality is otherwise. Employees too often do not know or act on their rights. Employers often intimidate workers into not asking the right questions. Manufacturers often do not tell the whole story about the substances they distribute.

A few thoughts about what to do:

- Find out how the Hazard Communication Standard affects your workplace—there are exemptions.
- Use whatever legal rights you have to the fullest. Management may try strong-arm maneuvers and the manufacturer may cry "trade secret," but certain information is rightfully yours.
- You also have rights to any exposure data your employer might have collected; also, you and/or your union have rights of access to your company medical records. Using these and other sources—for example, a survey conducted by you and fellow workers—will strengthen your understanding of your working conditions.
- Check with the Association of Occupational/En-

vironmental Health Clinics to find knowledgeable medical resources in your region. (Few physicians are sufficiently trained about toxic exposures.)

Work and Stress

In the garment shop where I work, a lot of us who've been sewing there for a while have been having pains in our hands or our legs. The union is collecting information to see if some jobs are worse than others (like hemming or making linings). We're hoping that we can find out whether there are any changes that would help, like changing the height of the tables or the angle of the machines. Anything that would make the job more comfortable would help my general level of tension! Between the noise from the steam presses, working fast enough to make a good rate and bending over the machine all day without enough light, I'm lucky if I get out of there without my shoulders all bunched up and a splitting headache at the end of the day.

Management often tells us that stress is our fault, that we shouldn't bring our personal problems to work. But work conditions can *create* stress, which goes home with us and affects our personal lives, too.

Stress can result from physical factors, such as repetitive hand motions, poor seating conditions, excessive noise, heat or cold, eyestrain or general work overload. Other causes of stress range from relations with the boss and our co-workers, to sexual harassment, to worry about safety and health hazards. Many women have jobs with low pay and no chance of promotion or retraining because of sexual and racial discrimination in employment and limited educational opportunities. Women who have children or want to must worry about maternity leave, child care and loss of seniority.

Most women in jobs traditionally held by men have to deal with not being very welcome or ac-

Ellen Shub

cepted at the workplace, at least at the beginning. A black woman who works as a union carpenter's apprentice said:

It's difficult not to become paranoid that every insult or putdown comes from people's racist or sexist attitudes, even when you know that all apprentices get dumped on a lot.[19]

Stress can cause serious medical problems (see p. 116–17). We won't end stress on the job as long as job exploitation or racial oppression continue, but we can win some improvements, such as increasing the availability of information about the substances we work with, obtaining adequate staffing and securing a say in decisions that affect our work conditions.

One of the most stressful things about our job at the phone company was the "clacker" that would start going CLACK CLACK CLACK whenever all the incoming lines were busy. The idea was to make us work faster. But it would make my stomach tie into knots and my hands get sweaty whenever I heard that thing. So one day I got a big group of us to go in to the supervisor and say that we just couldn't work like that. There were so many of us that he had to give in.[20]

Though today many companies have "stress management" programs for employees, these programs define stress as an individual problem and allow the company to avoid changing the conditions that cause stress on the job.

"Protecting" Women Out of the Workplace

The distinction between protection and discrimination is often a fine one. For example, some states passed legislation after World War II limiting the number of pounds a woman could lift or the number of hours she could work on the job. While these laws were supposed to protect women from undue stress, the result was that women lost their jobs to returning servicemen.

Over the past decade many companies have instituted policies that prohibit women of childbearing potential from working in areas where they might be exposed to chemicals that would be harmful to fetuses. The reason given for these policies is the need to "protect the unborn child"; the result is that women have lost access to jobs that were only recently opened to them. It is no coincidence that such policies do not exist in companies or institutions that employ a largely female labor force, such as hospitals or the electronics industry. When studies found that anesthetic gases cause spontaneous abortions, hospitals didn't ban women workers from operating rooms.

Nicole Hollander

Instead they installed devices that eliminated the problem.

Exclusionary policies ignore the fact that women are not pregnant most of their lives and that many exposures that may be harmful to a fetus are also harmful to an adult. Barring women from jobs instead of cleaning up the workplace diverts energy and attention from the real issue: the need to protect all workers from reproductive and other health hazards. Women's presence on the job may in fact raise awareness about hazards.

On my job as a field service technician, three women have become pregnant during the last year and were immediately transferred to other jobs within the company for the duration of their pregnancies. Their doctors, three different doctors, recommended this precaution because of the strong cleaning solvents that we use. Their situation has drawn everyone's attention to the possible dangers that we face on our jobs. Both men and women have been discussing symptoms they believe to be job-related. This is the first time in the nine years that I have been here that the issue has become a major concern.

In 1991 a landmark Supreme Court case regarding working women's rights and workers' health was won by the United Auto Workers, supported by a coalition of labor, environmental and women's groups. The victory: The "fetal protection" policy (FPP) of Johnson Controls (a battery company) was found to be in violation of the Civil Rights Act of 1964. Most interpret this decision as a blow to FPPs and a new wedge for fuller protection for all workers—rather than removal of some workers. For details of this case and related issues, contact the ACLU/Women's Rights Project.

If you are pregnant, it becomes more urgent to remove yourself from possible hazards. One possibility is to request a transfer to a safe job with the same pay, benefits and seniority. If you have a union this should be written into your contract. You may need to leave the workplace if there are no jobs without hazardous exposures available.

Management will usually want you to leave without pay, but you may have certain rights to job transfer or paid leave under the pregnancy disability amendment to the federal Civil Rights Act. Under this law, women "disabled by pregnancy" must be treated the same as other temporarily disabled workers, like those who have had heart attacks or accidents. ("Disabled" is a legal term meaning that one is unable to work.) Some states also have pregnancy disability acts.

Male co-workers often think that reproductive hazards are just a woman's problem and must be educated to realize that this isn't true. Women are not expendable in the workplace, just as men are not expendable in the family. Job conditions should enable us to be both working people and parents. The United States is one of the few industrialized countries that fail to provide leave and monetary compensation for childbirth.

Legal Rights to a Safe Workplace

The major law dealing with workplace hazards is the federal Occupational Safety and Health Act, which requires employers to make their workplaces safe and free of health hazards "as far as possible." The law (first passed in 1970) established the Occupational Safety and Health Administration (OSHA), which sets standards for workplace conditions and inspects workplaces to see if the standards are being met. OSHA can impose fines on employers who violate standards and order them to clean up. Workers have a right to file complaints with OSHA calling for inspections and to ask NIOSH (see Resources) and state agencies to do health hazard evaluations.

Although the passage of the act was a victory for working people, OSHA alone unfortunately cannot solve all our problems. For example, few OSHA standards cover hazards found in jobs traditionally held by women, and OSHA has seldom inspected offices, hospitals or other predominantly female workplaces.

The Reagan and Bush administrations both have constricted OSHA, but there are still certain rights and provisions, such as the Hazard Communication Standard, you can make use of. Workers and organizations around the country have scored significant victories by making wise use of existing laws and by pushing for new protections.

Here are several laws you should know about:

- *State workers' compensation laws:* All states have workers' compensation laws which cover workers who are injured on the job or become ill as a result of work. These laws provide for the payment of medical expenses and part of lost wages.
- *State health and safety laws:* Some states have their own health and safety laws which are par-

Coal-mining workers. *Marat Moore*

ticularly relevant to state and local government workers who are *not* covered under OSHA.

- *State and local Right-to-Act laws and proposals:* Connecticut passed the first Right-to-Act law. Efforts to pass similar legislation in New Jersey, New York, and Michigan are underway.
- *Civil Rights Act:* Gives women "disabled" by pregnancy the same rights as other temporarily disabled workers, and possibly offers some protection against policies excluding women from jobs on the basis of "protecting their health."
- *National Labor Relations Act:* Provides some legal protection for concerted worker protests or job actions against unsafe working conditions. The act covers both unionized and nonunionized workers.

Women Taking Action

The Lowell mill girls struggled against hazardous conditions in the 1840s. In 1909, thousands of women in the garment industry in New York City went on strike to protest sweatshop working conditions and low wages. In 1943, 200 black women "sat down" at their machines in a tobacco plant in North Carolina in response to the death of a co-worker on the job, which the women saw

as being the result of years of exposure to excessive heat, dust and noise. In 1979, women led a strike to improve health and safety conditions and end sexual harassment at a poultry farm in Mississippi. With a long history behind us, we continue to take action.

The process of workers coming together over a particular health and safety problem often starts informally. A woman who worked as a word processor at a major Boston bank contacted 9 TO 5 (an affiliate of Working Women) with concerns about her equipment, specifically the noise from the printers. She and her six co-workers met and discussed the problem with 9 TO 5 and came up with some reasonable solutions. The women met with their supervisor and presented these solutions to him. At first he stalled, but they kept insisting, and eventually the company bought printer covers to reduce the noise. As one woman said, "While this may seem small, it is a big step for us. We've begun to talk together about our common concerns and now our supervisor is nervous that we may get together again on other issues."

I work as a printer, the only woman with six men. One of the men developed sore, red, cracked hands and arms. We all knew it was from the chemical he had to use on the job and that there was an inexpensive piece of equipment that could be used so that the work wouldn't have to be done by hand. But he was being "macho man" and didn't want to complain. I encouraged him to speak up because I knew that sometime someone else might have to do that job. I got a book about chemicals from a COSH group and brought it to work. We looked up the chemical he was using. We found it does cause dermatitis and serious liver damage if exposure is great enough. So he complained, but he didn't get anywhere. When he came back we were so mad we stopped working and gathered together reading the book again. The boss saw us and the next day told us he ordered the equipment we wanted. It was very exciting to do something together about a work problem for the first time.

Whenever possible it is most effective to form an ongoing workers' health and safety committee. Instead of just responding to emergencies, a committee can work preventively, uncovering potential problems before anyone gets hurt. A committee will have the task of approaching management, and there are lots of ways to get management's attention even when they don't want to listen.

I was working in a supermarket as a meat wrapper. You know, behind the windows at the meat counter. We take the cut-up meat and wrap it in plastic. The plastic comes off a big roll that we cut to size by pulling it against a hot wire. A bunch of us were having asthma attacks and getting acne real bad. The health and safety committee met and decided that it was from the fumes of the plastic when it melted. We talked to our supervisor and he basically said, "Don't worry, ladies, it's all in your head." So we got mad and decided to try a new approach. We planned it so on one busy Saturday we all came to work with respirators on. After about an hour behind the meat counter with the customers staring at us in shock, the manager decided we were serious and agreed to meet with us and discuss what could be done.

Committees can gather information, educate themselves and their co-workers, help set priorities and provide leadership and persistence to get things changed. Also, in groups we are less likely to be singled out as "troublemakers" and subjected to special harassment or even fired. A health and safety committee is most effective as part of a union. When you have a union, the company *has to*, by law, talk to the union—negotiate—about health and safety.

Our work has more impact on our physical and mental health than we often acknowledge. Getting involved in improving working conditions is one more way that we as women can take control of our lives.

One of the best periods of my life was when we were on strike. We were all like one big family. Once I took a stand on what I knew to be right, I never felt freer in my life.

NOTES

1. The Environmental Defense Fund and Robert H. Boyle. *Malignant Neglect.* New York: Vintage Books, 1980, p. 5. See also Erik P. Eckholm. *The Picture of Health: Environmental Sources of Disease.* New York: W.W. Norton and Co., Inc., 1977, p. 90.

2. G. Cohen and J. O'Connor. *Fighting Toxics: A Manual for Protecting Your Family, Community and Workplace.* Washington, DC: Island Press, 1990.

3. "Citizens Spoke Out on Chemical Control," *On CUE*, Vol. 4, No. 6 (July 1980), p. 1. (*On CUE* is the newsletter of the Coalition for a United Elizabeth, 135 Madison Avenue, Elizabeth, NJ 07201.)

4. Carol Sue Davidson. "Antarctic Lore," *The Cousteau Almanac: An Inventory of Life on Our Water Planet.* New York: Doubleday, 1981, p. 285. Tom Conry. "Chemical of the Month: Lead," *Exposure*, No. 13 (December 1981), p. 6.

5. Charles Lee. *Toxic Waste and Race in the US.* New York: Commission for Racial Justice, United Church of Christ, 1987.

6. *Race, Poverty and the Environment: A Newsletter for Social and Environmental Justice.* Vol. 1, No. 1, April 1990. San Francisco: Earth Island Institute.

7. *We Speak for Ourselves: Social Justice, Race and Environment.* Washington, DC: Panos Institute, 1990.

8. David Weir. *The Bhopal Syndrome.* San Francisco: Sierra Club Books, 1988.

9. Robert Richter. *A Plague on Our Children*, p. 39.

10. Jane E. Brody. "Sperm Found Especially Vulnerable to Environment," *The New York Times* (March 10, 1981). Michael Castleman. "Why Johnny Can't Have Kids," *Mother Jones* (April 1982), pp. 14–18.

11. Vilma Hunt. *Work and the Health of Women.* Boca Raton, FL: CRC Press, 1979, p. 155.

12. Constance Holden. "Agent Orange Furor Continues to Build," *Science*, Vol. 205 (August 24, 1979), pp. 770–2. See also Clifford Linedecker with Michael and Maureen Ryan, *Kerry: Agent Orange and the American Family.* New York: St. Martin's Press, 1982.

13. Daniel Ben-Horin. "The Sterility Scandal," *Mother Jones* (May 1979), p. 61.

14. See *Reproductive Health Hazards in the Workplace* (Office of Technology Assessment, U.S. Congress, 1985) for a helpful overview of reproductive effects.

15. Maureen Paul. "Reproductive Fitness and Risk," *Occupational Medicine: State of the Art Reviews*, Vol. 3, 1988, p. 323.

16. National Women's Health Network. *Turning Things Around: A Women's Occupational and Environmental Health Resource Guide.* Washington, DC, 1990.

17. Barbara Reale. "Breast Milk Contamination: An Issue for Nurses," *Health Watch* (newsletter of the Nurses Environmental Health Watch) (Summer 1986).

18. Press release from the Center for Economic Alternatives (1987), 207 W. Main Street, Ahoskie, NC 27910.

19. *Connections*, Network of Women in Trade and Technical Jobs, Boston, MA, February 1982.

20. "Women at Work—Their Dual Role." Women's Occupational Health Resource Center, Columbia University.

RESOURCES

Environmental Health

Readings

General

Berger, John. *Environmental Restoration: Science and Strategies for Restoring the Earth*. Washington, DC: Island Press, 1990. Examines need and capacity for restoration of environmentally degraded land and resources. Good case studies.

Cousteau, Jacques-Yves, and the staff of the Cousteau Society. *The Cousteau Almanac*. New York: Doubleday, 1981. Good political and economic background on local and global environmental pollution; many articles focus on specific incidents.

The Data Center (a nonprofit library and research center). *Toxic Nightmare—Environmental Perspectives*. Three volumes of selected magazine and newspaper articles crucial to environmental activists, researchers, journalists and other concerned citizens. Data Center, 464 19th Street, Oakland, CA 94612.

Diperna, Paula. *Cluster Mystery: Epidemic and the Children of Woburn, MA*. New York: C.V. Mosby, 1985. Connects personal drama with the politics of science as parents, citizens and scientists come to terms with a growing problem—environmentally induced childhood disease.

Elkington, John. *The Poisoned Womb: Human Reproduction in a Polluted World*. New York: Penguin Books, 1985. $5.95. Helpful overview of reproductive toxicology.

Epstein, Samuel S. *The Politics of Cancer*. San Francisco: Sierra Club Books, 1978 (paper). A comprehensive study of environmental carcinogens and how government has and has not regulated them.

Freudenberg, Nicholas. *Not in Our Backyards: Community Action for Health and the Environment*. New York: Monthly Press, 1984. Helpful case studies of community struggles, ideas for coalition building and resources for action.

Kane, D. N. *Environmental Hazards to Young Children*. Phoenix, AZ: Oryx Press, 1985.

Kazis, Richard, and R. Grossman. *Fear at Work: Job Blackmail, Labor and the Environment*. Philadelphia: New Society Publishers, 1991. Key analysis of how management creates labor vs. environment tension with threats of plant closure and job loss. Offers important analysis of how workers and environmentalists can work together for environmental safety and economic justice.

New Solutions: A Journal of Environmental and Occupational Health Policy. $40 subscription. New Solu-

tions, P.O. Box 2812, Denver, CO 80201 (303) 987-2229. A vital new publication that connects workplace and general environmental concerns and bridges the territories of citizen and scientist. Edited jointly by the Oil, Chemical and Atomic Workers and the Work Environment Program, University of Lowell, MA.

Norwood, Christopher. *At Highest Risk: Environmental Hazards to Young and Unborn Children*. New York: McGraw-Hill, 1980. A readable and inclusive overview on how environmental hazards are even more toxic to the developing fetus and to young children.

UNICEF. *Children and the Environment: State of the Environment 1990*. UNICEF and the United Nations Environmental Program, 3 United Nations Plaza, New York, NY 10017. Global view of environmental and workplace hazards to children; educational and organizational approaches to change.

Chemicals

Ashford, Nicholas, and Claudia Miller. *Chemical Exposures: Low Levels and High Stakes*. New York: Van Nostrand Reinhold, 1991. Key analysis of chemical sensitivity, diagnosis and treatment issues and recommendations for improved prevention and care.

Brown, Michael. *Laying Waste: The Poisoning of America by Toxic Chemicals*. New York: Pantheon Books, 1980 (paper).

California Department of Consumer Affairs. *Clean Your Room! A Compendium on Indoor Air Pollutants*. Sacramento, CA: Department of Consumer Affairs, 1982. $15.00. The most thorough, recent information. Write to DCA, P.O. Box 310, Sacramento, CA 95802.

Crook, Sherry. "How to Survive with or in Spite of Chemical Poisoning." By the founder of Injured Workers of New York and executive director of the National Coalition of Injured Workers. 1989. Send $5 to S. Crook, IWONY, 68 North Street, Camillus, NY 13031.

Davis, Earon, and Valerie Wilk. *Toxic Chemicals: The Interface Between Law and Science*. Washington, DC: Farmworkers' Justice Fund, 1982. (2001 S Street NW, Washington, DC 20009.)

Epstein, Samuel S., Lester O. Brown and Carl Pope. *Hazardous Waste in America*. San Francisco, CA: Sierra Club Books, 1982. A comprehensive book which surveys the sources and dangers of hazardous waste, including case studies, laws, a directory of 8,000 dumps, how to locate undisclosed dumps and solutions to the problem.

Freedberg, Louis. *America's Poisoned Playgrounds: Children and Toxic Chemicals*. Washington, DC: Youth News and the Conference on Alternative State and Local Policies, 1983.

Nader, Ralph, Ronald Brownstein and John Richards, eds. *Who's Poisoning America: Corporate Polluters and Their Victims in the Chemical Age*. New York: Charles Scribner's Sons, 1981.

Regenstein, Lewis. *America the Poisoned: How Deadly Chemicals Are Destroying Our Environment, Our Wildlife, and Ourselves—and How We Can Survive!* Washington, DC: Acropolis Books, 1982.

Weir, David. *The Bhopal Syndrome*. San Francisco: Sierra Club Books, 1987. $8.95. Important analysis of the world's worst industrial accident at the Union Carbide pesticide plant in Bhopal, India, 1984. Examines "mini-Bhopals," "slow-motion Bhopals" and the question, Where will it happen next?

Citizen Action

Cohen, Gary, and John O'Connor. *Fighting Toxics: A Manual for Protecting Your Family, Community and Workplace.* Washington, DC: Island Press, 1990. Must-have guidebook providing analysis and resources on organizing strategies, corporate campaigns, neighborhood inspections, media relations, environmental law and preventive tools. From the National Toxics Campaign.

Earthworks Group. *50 Simple Things You Can Do to Save the Earth.* Earthworks Press, 1989. Box 25, 1400 Shattuck Avenue, Berkeley, CA 94709. Also *Kids* version.

Erickson, Brad. *Call to Action: Handbook for Ecology, Peace and Justice.* San Francisco: Sierra Club Books, 1990. $14.95. Links environmental action and analysis to challenges in communications, education, militarism, economic and social justice.

Gibbs, Lois, with Murray Levine. *Love Canal: My Story.* Albany, NY: State University of New York, 1982. How "just a housewife" took on the local, state and federal government—and won. Great for inspiration and ideas.

Highlander Research and Education Center. *We're Tired of Being Guinea Pigs!* New Market, TN: Highlander Research and Education Center, 1980 (paper). Geared specifically to Appalachian areas, but adaptable to other locales.

Hynes, H. Patricia. *Earth Right: Every Citizen's Guide.* Rocklin, CA: Prima Publishing, 1990. By the founder of the Institute on Women and Technology, this book addresses "what you can do in your home, workplace and community to save our environment." Encompassing the big picture of ozone depletion and global warming, the book offers tactics and resources.

Race, Poverty and the Environment. A newsletter for social and environmental justice. $8/four issues from Earth Island Institute, 300 Broadway, Suite 28, San Francisco, CA 94133-3312. Key resource on environmental racism, examining racial/class patterns of exposure to toxics, lead, waste and inequitable government/industrial "solutions." Special issues on women.

We Speak for Ourselves: Social Justice, Race and Environment. The Panos Institute, 1990. $6.85 (includes handling) from the Panos Institute, 1717 Massachusetts Ave, NW, Suite 301, Washington, DC 20036, (202) 483-0044. Chronicles the connection between environmental degradation and oppression; profiles lessons and victories.

What Must We Do: A Grassroots Offensive Against Toxics in the 1990's. Special report of *The Workbook*, Vol. 14, No. 3 (July/Sept 1989). Southwest Research and Information Center, P.O. Box 4524, Albuquerque, NM 87106. Excellent assessment of what needs to be done.

Consumer Products

Dadd, Debra Lynn. *Nontoxic, Natural and Earthwise: How to Protect Yourself and Your Family from Harmful Products and Live in Harmony with the Earth.* Los Angeles: Jeremy Tarcher, 1990. Helps you protect yourself and the environment. Evaluates foods, cleaning products, cosmetics, appliances, office and art supplies, building materials, clothing. Includes do-it-yourself formulas and mail-order sources.

Guide to Hazardous Products Around the Home. Household Hazardous Waste Project, 1031 E. Battlefield, Suite 214, Springfield, MO 65807. (417) 889-5000. Layperson's manual of substances, health effects, precautions, substitutions.

Mason, Linda. *The Healthy Home: An Attic-to-Basement Guide to Toxin-Free Living.* Emmaus, PA: Rodale Press, 1989. Full of useful tips, especially on pest control.

Pim, Linda R. *The Invisible Additives: Environmental Contaminants in Our Food.* Toronto: Doubleday and Co., 1981.

Rousseau, David, W. Rea and Jean Enright. *Your Home, Your Health and Your Well-Being.* Berkeley: Ten Speed Press, 1991. Guide to designing or renovating houses and apartments to be free of outdoor and indoor pollution.

Steinman, David. *Diet for a Poisoned Planet: How to Choose Safe Foods for You and Your Family.* New York: Harmony Books, 1990.

Pesticides

Carson, Rachel. *Silent Spring.* Greenwich, CT: Fawcett Crest, 1962 (paper). The book that started it all by explaining the effects of DDT. Twenty-fifth anniversary edition.

Journal of Pesticide Reform. Northwest Coalition for Alternatives to Pesticides, P.O. Box 1393, Eugene, OR 97440. Also provides information packets, factsheets, and networking support.

NYCAP News (New York Coalition for Alternatives to Pesticides), 33 Central Avenue, Albany, NY 12210. (518) 426-8246. Excellent publication providing assessment of health effects, regulatory activity, citizen efforts, new resources, and networking information. Very informative on how to minimize pesticide use in schools and workplaces.

Thorpe, K. *Pesticides in the Schools.* Information package from National Coalition Against the Misuse of Pesticides, 701 E Street SE, Suite 200, Washington, DC 20003.

United Farm Workers. *Food and Justice.* A newsletter about the impacts of pesticides on farmworkers, communities, and consumers. UFW, Old Highway 58, La Paz, Keene, CA 93570.

Van Strum, Carol. *A Bitter Fog: Herbicides and Human Rights.* San Francisco: Sierra Club Books, May 1983. Tells the story of Van Strum's struggles as a mother-turned-activist to confront the agribusiness interests which want to tame forests while poisoning the people.

Weir, David, and Mark Schapiro. *Circle of Poison: Pesticides and People in a Hungry World.* San Francsico: Institute for Food and Development Policy, 1981 (paper).

Radiation

Bertell, Rosalie. *No Immediate Danger: Prognosis for a Radioactive Earth.* Summertown, TN: The Book Publishing Co., 1985. $11.95. A careful and clear analysis of the radiation/health connection, examining military and industrial policies and coverups. Explores the key role of women in challenging the nuclear powerfuls.

Brodeur, Paul. *Currents of Death*. New York: Simon & Schuster, 1989. Examines the science and politics of electromagnetic radiation.

Gofman, John W. *Radiation and Human Health*. New York: Pantheon Books, 1983. Exhaustive examination of the effects of radiation hazards. Club Books, 1981.

Nuclear Information and Resource Service, *Radiation Packet*. Washington, DC: NIRS, 1981. Explains what radiation is, where it comes from and health effects. Includes bibliography and resources.

Physicians for Social Responsibility, Inc. *Medical Hazards of Radiation Packet*. Watertown, MA: PSR, 1981 (paper). A collection of photocopied articles on radiation and health. (Write to PSR, 19 Garden St., Cambridge, MA 02138.)

Wasserman, Harvey, and Norman Solomon. *Killing Our Own: The Disasters of America's Experience with Atomic Radiation*. New York: Delacorte Press, 1982. Examines people's atomic exposure in and around the military, civilian power, uranium mining, X-rays. Provides "the basics of radiation and health."

Technical References

Bloom, Arthur. *Guidelines for Studies of Human Populations Exposed to Mutagenic and Reproductive Hazards*. White Plains, NY: March of Dimes Defect Foundation, 1981. Conference proceedings on how to investigate exposed populations. Case studies of children.

Blumenthal, Daniel. *Introduction to Environmental Health*. New York: Springer Publishing Co., 1985. Covers infectious agents, radiation, chemical exposures, air pollution; reviews legislation, hazardous waste management, regulatory activities.

Casarett, Louis J., and John Doull. *Toxicology: The Basic Science of Poisons*, 2nd ed. New York: Macmillan Publishing Co., 1980.

Gordis, L., ed. *Epidemiology and Health Risk Assessment*. New York: Oxford University Press, 1988.

Gosselin, R.E. *Clinical Toxicology of Commercial Products*, 5th ed. Baltimore: Williams & Wilkins, 1984.

Legator, Marvin, B. Harper and M. Scott. *The Health Detective's Handbook: A Guide to the Investigation of Environmental Health Hazards by Nonprofessionals*. Baltimore: The Johns Hopkins University Press, 1985. Provides assistance in developing community organization and investigation of environmental hazards. Guidance on survey design, data collection and analysis, evaluating evidence, legal tools and strategies for effective application of findings.

National Research Council. *Biologic Markers in Reproductive Toxicology*. Washington, DC: National Academy Press, 1989. Technical research review on reproductive function, pregnancy, fetal neurodevelopment.

Shepherd, Thomas H. *Catalog of Teratogenic Agents*, 3rd ed. Baltimore: Johns Hopkins University Press, 1980.

Sherman, J. *Chemical Exposure and Disease: Diagnostic and Investigative Techniques*. New York: Van Nostrand Reinhold, 1988.

Women and the Environment

Biehl, Janet. *Rethinking Ecofeminist Politics*. Boston: South End Press, 1991. $10.00. A feminist and ecological activist critically examines weaknesses she finds in much ecofeminist thinking.

Caldecott, Leonie, and Stephanie Leland. *Reclaim the Earth: Women Speak Out for Life on Earth*. London: Women's Press, 1983. Women from around the world link feminism and ecology.

Diamond, Irene, and Gloria Orenstein. *Reweaving the World: The Emergence of Ecofeminism*. San Francisco: Sierra Club Books, 1990. $14.95. Collection spanning different approaches to women and the environment, including analysis of reproductive technologies, women's health and movement strategies.

"Earthkeeping/Earthshaking: Feminism and Ecology." Heresies, No. 13 (1981). Heresies, P.O. Box 1306, Canal Street Station, New York, NY 10013. Classical collection of ecofeminist writings.

Hynes, Patricia, *The Recurring Silent Spring*. New York: Pergamon Press, 1989. Feminist analysis of Rachel Carson and women/environmental links, with focus on reproductive politics.

———. *Reconstructing Babylon: Women and Technology*. Bloomington, IN: Earthscan/Indiana University, 1990. Key analysis of women, technology and environment.

King, Ynestra. *What Is Ecofeminism?* New York: Ecofeminist Resources, 339 Lafayette Street, New York, NY 10012, 1990. Key document analyzing how the oppression of women, racism, economic exploitation and the ecological crisis interconnect.

———. *Ecofeminism and the Reenchantment of Nature*. Boston: Beacon Press, 1992. Explores the philosophical, historical and political foundations of women and environment connections. Examines current activism.

Merchant, Carolyn. *The Death of Nature: Women, Ecology, and the Scientific Revolution*. San Francisco: Harper & Row, 1980. An academic, historical account of the rise of science from a feminist perspective.

Nelson, Lin, Regina Kenen and Susan Klitzman. *Turning Things Around: A Woman's Occupational and Environmental Health Resource Guide*. Washington, DC: National Women's Health Network, 1990. $9.95. Analysis and guide to resources covers occupational hazards, reproductive health, multiple chemical sensitivity, hazards in the home and community/global strategies. Sections on health care, legal and governmental resources. Includes bibliography and organizations listed by state.

Ratcliff, Kathryn Strother, ed. *Healing Technology: Feminist Perspectives*. Ann Arbor, MI: University of Michigan Press, 1989. $14.95. Examination of reproductive technologies, health care, occupational/ environmental technologies and conditions. Offers feminist agenda for action in age of technology.

Shiva, Vandana. *Staying Alive: Women, Ecology and Development*. London: Zed Books, 1989. Path-breaking work on women, land, natural resources and development policy. Physicist, philosopher and feminist,

Shiva examines the women of the "Chipko movement" and challenges the oppressive forces of the United States' and other aid programs.

Women and Environments. WEED Foundation, 736 Bathurst Street, Toronto, Ontario, Canada M5S 2R4. Important quarterly publication exploring the many ramifications of built and natural environments on women. International focus.

Women's Resource Center. *Women and Technology: Deciding What's Appropriate.* Missoula, MT: WRC, 1979 (paper). Raises tough and important questions and talks about health technology and potentially hazardous technology. Write to Women's Resource Center, 315 S. 4th E., Missoula, MT 59801.

Zeff, Robbin, Marsha Love and Karen Stults, eds. *Empowering Ourselves: Women and Toxics Organizing.* Citizens' Clearinghouse for Hazardous Waste, P.O. Box 6806, Falls Church, VA 22040. From the work of activist women around the country, sections on health effects, stress, women in leadership, personal growth, building organizations.

Audiovisual Materials

For Export Only: Pesticides and Pills. Available from Richter Productions, 330 W. 42nd Street, New York, NY 10036.

In Our Own Backyards: Uranium Mining in the United States. Available from Bullfrog Films, Oley, PA 19547.

In Our Water. The story of well-water contamination in New Jersey. Available from New Day Films, 121 W. 27th Street, Suite 902, New York, NY 10001.

The Killing Ground. The story of improper chemical-waste dumping. Available from ABC Learning Resources, 1330 Avenue of the Americas, New York, NY 10019.

Our Hidden National Product. The siting of a hazardous waste facility. Available from Durrin Films, Inc., 1748 Kalorama Road NW, Washington, DC 20009.

A Plague on Our Children. Two-part film on 2,4,5-T, PCBs, DDT, and Love Canal. Available from Time/Life Multimedia, Time and Life Building, Room 32–48, New York, NY 10020.

For audiovisual lists on environmental issues, contact

The Video Project
5332 College Avenue
Suite 101
Oakland, CA 94618
(800) 4-PLANET

The Media Network
121 Fulton Street
5th Floor
New York, NY 10038
(212) 619-3455

Organizations

All of the following organizations provide information on issues involving environmental health. Many, as noted, provide newsletters.

Arkansas Reproductive Health Monitoring System
University of Arkansas
804 Wolfe Street
Little Rock, AR 72202-3591
(501) 375-3925

Association of Occupational and Environmental
Health Clinics
1030 15th Street NW, Suite 410
Washington, DC 20005

(202) 682-1807
Network of clinics, current medical information.

Center for Ecology and Social Justice
Institute for Policy Studies
1601 Connecticut Avenue NW
Washington, DC 20009

Center for Science in the Public Interest
1501 16th Street NW
Washington, DC 20036
(202) 332-9110
Special project: Americans for Safe Food.

Citizens' Clearinghouse for Hazardous Wastes, Inc.
P.O. Box 6806
Falls Church, VA 22040
(703) 237-2249
Founded by Lois Gibbs, this group provides technical and organizing assistance to citizens facing a hazardous waste problem. Newsletter: *Everyone's Backyard.*

Commission for Racial Justice
United Church of Christ
105 Madison Avenue
New York, NY 10016-7451
(212) 683-5656
Special project on people of color and the environment.

Environmental Action
1525 New Hampshire Avenue NW
Washington, DC 20036
Information packets, fact sheets, referrals for citizens' groups, particularly good for information on laws and regulations. Newsletter: *Exposure* (bimonthly).

Environmental Consortium for Minority Outreach
1001 Connecticut Avenue NW, Suite 827
Washington, DC 20036
(202) 331-8387
Works to reverse environmental racism and promote the rights of people of color within the environmental movement.

Environmental Defense Fund
444 Park Avenue South
New York, NY 10016
Litigation on environmental issues, including environmental health and consumer welfare. Bimonthly newsletter.

Environmental Health Network
P.O. Box 1628
Harvey, LA 70058
(504) 362-6574
Publishes *Profiles on Environmental Health.* Provides technical assistance to health providers and communities.

First Environment Project
Katsi Cook, Project Director
226 Blackman Hill Road
Berkshire, NY 13736
A project of the Akwesasne Mohawk Nation, a Native American community in the Northeast, which seeks to analyze and reduce the impact of toxics in the community. Publishes a newsletter.

Friends of the Earth
530 Seventh St. SE
Washington, DC 20003
National lobbying group on environmental issues.

Greenpeace
1436 U Street NW
Washington, DC 20009
(202) 462-1177
Information, advocacy, international network.

Hazard Evaluation System and Information
Service (HESIS)
State of California Department of Health Services
2151 Berkeley Way
Berkeley, CA 94704
Detailed information on toxics in laypeople's terms.

Health/Rights: Collaborative Project on Reproductive
Health Hazards
c/o American Civil Liberties Union
132 West 43rd Street
New York, NY 10036
(212) 944-9800
Joint effort of environmental, labor, women's, social justice and civil liberties organizations.

Mothers and Others for a Liveable Planet
Natural Resources Defense Council
420 W. 20th Street
New York, NY 10011
(212) 727-2700
Newsletter focusing on children and the environment.

National Center for Environmental Health Strategies
1100 Rural Avenue
Voorhees, NJ 08043
(609) 429-5358
Focused on multiple chemical sensitivies or ecological
illness.

National Center for Hazard Communication
University of Maryland/University College
University Boulevard at Adelphi Road
College Park, MD 20742-1663
(301) 985-7881
Publishes *Exposure* and other educational materials on
occupational and environmental hazards.

National Coalition Against the Misuse of Pesticides
701 E Street SE, Suite 200
Washington, DC 20003
Health, environmental, legal and community groups
lobbying and educating on pesticides. Newsletter.

National Toxics Campaign
37 Temple Place
Boston, MA 02111
(617) 482-1147
Key national organization, excellent how-to resources,
helping to build labor–environment coalition.

National Women's Health Network
Committee on Occupational and Environmental Health
1325 G Street NW
Washington, DC 20005
(202) 347-1140
Resource guide, information, referral and advocacy.

Nuclear Information and Resource Service
1346 Connecticut Avenue NW, Suite 405
Washington, DC 20036
Resource guides, fact sheets, referrals on radiation and
health. Newsletter: *Groundswell* (bimonthly).

Nurses Environmental Health Watch
33 Columbus Avenue
Somerville, MA 02143
(617) 666-4829
Provides information on occupational/environmental
hazards to health providers and concerned citizens;
special resources on hazards in health care settings.

Occupational and Environmental Reproductive Hazards Clinic and Education Center
University of Massachusetts Medical Center
55 Lake Avenue North
Worcester, MA 01655
(508) 856-2818
Key clinical/educational facility; mostly serves MA, but
clinic director Dr. Maureen Paul will provide information to others.

Organization for the Advancement of
Environmental Health
P.O. Box 3159
Ann Arbor, MI 48106-3159
(313) 662-5516
Publishes *Environmental Health News*. Special focus on
chemical sensitivity.

Pregnancy/Environmental Hotline
30 Warren Street
Brighton, MA 02135
(617) 787-4957

Reproductive Toxicology Center
2425 L Street NW
Washington, DC 20037
(202) 293-5137

Sierra Club
930 Polk Street
San Francisco, CA 94109
(415) 996-2211
One of the oldest environmental groups. Periodicals and
books.

Women's Community Cancer Project
c/o The Women's Center
46 Pleasant Street
Cambridge, MA 02139
Concerned about possible environmental causes of cancer; linked with national network of cancer activists
and environmental organizations.

Women's Foreign Policy Council
1133 Broadway, Suite 923
New York, NY 10010
(212) 691-7316
Advocacy of women's environmental action. Planner of
Women's Global Assembly on the Environment.

Working Group on Community Right-to-Know
U.S. Public Interest Research Group
215 Pennsylvania Avenue SE
Washington, DC 20003-1107
(202) 546-9707
Publishes *Working Notes on Community Right-to-Know*.

Urban Environment Conference
1314 14th Street NW
Washington, DC 20005
Focuses on urban environmental health, particularly among black and Latino people.

Worldwatch Institute
1776 Massachusetts Avenue NW
Washington, DC 20036
Papers on environmental health with a global perspective.

WorldWIDE—World Women in Environment
1331 H Street NW, Suite 903
Washington, DC 20005
(202) 347-1514
Global networking and advocacy organization for women working to restore the environment. Key planner for 1991 Global Assembly of Women and 1992 Environmental Meetings in Brazil. Publishes *WorldWIDE News* and *Directory of Women in Environment*.

Government Agencies Regulating Toxic Substances

Consumer Product Safety Commission
Washington, DC 20207
(800) 638-8326 (toll-free hotline for information on product safety)
(301) 492-6800 (hotline number for DC area)
Consumer goods, particularly household items.

Environmental Protection Agency
Public Information Center
401 M Street NW
Washington, DC 20460
(800) 555-1404
Chemical and nuclear hazards in the general environment.

Nuclear Regulatory Commission/Office of Public Affairs
Washington, DC 20553
(202) 492-7715
Regulating and licensing of nuclear facilities.

Occupational Safety and Health Administration
200 Constitution Avenue NW
Washington, DC 20210
(202) 523-9700
Chemical and nuclear hazards in the workplace.

Occupational Health

Readings

Bureau of National Affairs. *Pregnancy and Employment; The Complete Handbook on Discrimination, Maternity Leave, and Health and Safety.* BNA Special Report, 1987. $65. Bureau of National Affairs, 9535 Key West Avenue, Rockville, MD 20850. Check library, union, COSH group and others to see if they have this document on reproductive hazards, maternity leave, legal rights, corporate practices.
———. *Working Women's Health Concerns: A Gender at Risk?* 1989. BNA, 9535 Key West Avenue, Rockville, MD 20850.
Chavkin, Wendy, ed. *Double Exposure: Women's Health Hazards on the Job and at Home.* New York: Monthly Review Press, 1984. Excellent analysis of hazards faced (electronics, nursing, office, farmwork, housework, etc.) and strategies for change.
CLUW, Coalition of Labor Union Women, "Ban the Hazard, Not Women!" 15 Union Square, New York, NY 10003. (212) 242-0700. Helpful educational pamphlet on "fetal protection" controversy and union strategies for protecting reproductive health.
———. *Is Your Job Making You Sick? A CLUW Handbook on Workplace Hazards.* CLUW, 15 Union Square, New York, NY 10003. (212) 242-0700. Helpful resource on problems and solutions—model surveys, hazard checklists, sample letters.
Cullen, M. *Workers with Multiple Chemical Sensitivities.* Occupational Medicine State of the Art Reviews, P.O. Box 1377, Philadelphia, PA 19105-9990. (215) 546-7293.
DeMatteo, Bob. *Terminal Shock: The Health Hazards of Video Display Terminals.* Toronto: NC Press Ltd., 1985. Covers workstation design, stress, lighting, radiation, and so on.
Kenen, Regina. *Reproductive Hazards in the Workplace: Mending Jobs, Managing Pregnancies.* Binghamton, NY: Haworth Press, 1992. Examination of hazards in various worksites, assessing risks and making decisions, agendas for change and guides to legislation, agencies and resources.
Klitzman, Susan, Barbara Silverstein, Laura Punnett and Amy Mock. "A Women's Occupational Health Agenda for the 1990's." *New Solutions: A Journal of Environmental and Occupational Health Policy.* Vol. 1, No. 1 (Spring 1990). Review of work conditions, proposals for protecting women's health, job rights.
LaBotz, Dan. *A Troublemaker's Handbook: How to Fight Back Where You Work—and Win!.* Detroit: Labor Notes, 1991. $17 from Labor Notes, 7435 Michigan Avenue, Detroit, MI 48210.
Levy, B.S., and D. Wegman, eds. *Occupational Health: Recognizing and Preventing Work Related Diseases.* Boston: Little, Brown, 1988.
Lofgren, Don. *Dangerous Premises: An Insider's View of OSHA Enforcement.* Ithaca, NY: Cornell ILR Press, 1989. From an investigator's viewpoint, learn about solvents, asbestos and lead, among other hazards.
MassCOSH Women's Committee. *Confronting Reproductive Health Hazards on the Job: A Guide for Workers.* Massachusetts Coalition for Occupational Safety and Health, 555 Amory Street, Boston, MA 02130. (617) 524-6686. Based on years of shop-floor experience, this booklet presents helpful information on the hazards, worker rights and effective strategies.
NIOSH. *Occupational Diseases: A Guide to Their Recognition.* National Institute for Occupational Safety and Health Publication 77–181. $5.25. A very informative guide to work-related disease. Describes the wide range of occupational health hazards, their harmful effects and their legally permissible exposure limits. Superintendent of Documents, U.S. Government Printing Office, Washington, DC 20402. #017–033–00266–5.
Occupational Safety and Health Reporter. A publication of the Bureau of National Affairs, 9535 Key West Avenue, Rockville, MD 20850. This information-packed weekly may be available at local libraries, COSH groups (see Organizations section), unions, clinics or public health schools.

Office of Technology Assessment. *Reproductive Health Hazards in the Workplace.* 1985. OTA-BA-266. OTA, U.S. Congress, Washington, DC 20510. Detailed documentation of research on reproductive hazards and the role of regulation, workers' compensation and litigation. Revised and available from The Science Information Resource Center, E. Washington Square, Philadelphia, PA 19105.

Organizing for Health and Safety. Labor Research Review No. 16. Chicago: Midwest Center for Labor Research, Fall 1990. $8 from Midwest Center, 3411 W. Diversey Avenue, Suite 10, Chicago, IL 60647. Helpful and encouraging review of the frontlines in the struggle for workplace health; includes case studies, role of COSH groups, labor–feminist alliance, AIDS at work, and so on.

Paul, Maureen, ed. *Occupational and Environmental Reproductive Hazards: A Guide for Clinicians.* Baltimore: Williams & Wilkins, 1992.

Philadelphia Project on Occupational Safety and Health. *Getting Job Hazards Out of the Bedroom: The Handbook on Workplace Hazards to Reproduction.* 1988. PHILAPOSH, 511 N. Broad Street, Suite 900, Philadelphia, PA 19123. (215) 924-SAFE.

Proctor, Nick, et. al. *Chemical Hazards of the Workplace,* 2nd ed. Philadelphia: J.B. Lippincott, 1988. Widely used handbook covering 440 of the most common industrial chemicals.

SEIU Health and Safety Dept. *The AIDS Book: Information for Workers.* Service Employees International Union, 1313 L Street NW, Washington, DC 20005. One of the most widely used resources.

Stein, Z., and Maureen Hatch, eds. *Reproductive Health Problems in the Workplace.* Occupational Medicine State of the Art Reviews. Philadelphia: Hanley & Belfus, 1986. One of the key texts; directed to researchers, providers.

Stellman, Jeanne, and Mary Sue Henifin. *Office Work Can Be Dangerous to Your Health.* New York: Pantheon Books, 1983. Key book providing info on VDTs, office design, office machinery and so on.

Women's Health Unit. *Family, Work and Health.* November 1988. Massachusetts Department of Public Health, 150 Tremont Street, Boston, MA 02111 (617) 727-7222. Focus on reproductive hazards and family care issues; profiles of chemical and electronic industries.

———. *Women in the Workplace: Conference Proceedings,* Vol. 1, *Occupational Health Issues.* Massachusetts Department of Public Health, 150 Tremont Street, Boston, MA 02111. 1986. Addresses range of worksites, with special section on women of color.

Wykle, Lucinda, W. Morehouse and D. Dembo, *Worker Empowerment in a Changing Economy: Jobs, Military Production, and the Environment.* New York: Apex Press, 1991. Examines "job versus environment" dilemma and proposes "Superfund for Displaced Workers" as one way to protect workers in the toxics economy from corporate blackmail.

Audiovisual Materials

A Price for Every Progress: The Health Hazards of VDTs. Available from Labor Institute, 853 Broadway, Room 2014, New York, NY 10003. (212) 674-3322.

Breath Taken: The Landscape and Biography of Asbestos. Photo/essay exhibit and video. Available from the Center for Visual Arts in the Public Interest, 348 Congress Street, Boston, MA 02210.

Hazardous Inheritance. Health care professionals and workers on reproductive hazards. Available from Cambridge Documentary Films, Cambridge, MA.

It Didn't Have to Happen: Preventing Cumulative Trauma Disorders. Available from Labor Occupational Health Program, 2521 Channing Way, Berkeley, CA 94720.

It's Everybody's Business: Spill Drill. Interactive video program on workers' response to spill threatening plant neighbors. Available from International Chemical Workers Union, 1655 W. Market Street, Akron, OH 44313. (216) 867-2444.

More Than We Can Bear: Reproductive Hazards in the Workplace. Available from New Horizons Press, Publications Office, P.O. Box 337, Croton-on-Hudson, NY 10520. (914) 271-6500.

Not By Chance. On developing workplace health and safety committees. Available from AFL–CIO, 815 16th Street, Washington, DC 20006.

Trust in Training. On worker-directed health and safety training. Produced by the Oil, Chemical and Atomic Workers Union. Available from New Horizons Press, Publications Office, P.O. Box 337, Croton-on-Hudson, NY 10520. (914) 271-6500.

Organizations

AFL–CIO
815 16th Street NW
Washington, DC 20006
(202) 637-5000
Publications, technical assistance, advocacy and referral to appropriate projects and unions.

Center for Safety in the Arts
5 Beekman Place
New York, NY 10038
(212) 227-6220
Information, technical assistance, newsletter and training.

Coalition of Trade Union Women (CLUW)
15 Union Square
New York, NY 10003
(212) 242-0700
Education, advocacy and printed resources on women's occupational safety and health and workplace rights.

COSH groups: Coalitions or Councils or Committees on Occupational Safety and Health. COSH groups are made up of union locals, workers and prolabor health and safety professionals and lawyers. They can provide technical assistance, informational fact sheets and worker education. They have experience in working with unions and other worker groups setting up health and safety committees at the workplace. There are about thirty COSH groups around the country, and they will be very responsive to your request for information and other help. In addition, some COSH groups are in touch with similar groups in other countries. For information about COSH groups and publications, contact:

NYCOSH
275 7th Avenue, 18th Floor
New York, NY 10001
(212) 627-3900

Labor Occupational Health Program
Institute of Industrial Relations
University of California
Berkeley, CA 94720
(415) 642-5507
Publishes *LOHP Monitor*, good resource on VDTs, new technologies, AIDS, worker rights, literacy.

National Association of Working Women
614 Superior Avenue, NW
Cleveland, OH 44113
(216) 566-9308 or (800) 522-0925
Information and support on office hazards and solutions.

National Coalition of Injured Workers
12 Rejane Street
Coventry, RI 02816
(401) 828-6520
Vital network of injured worker groups (NY, MA, CA, LA, etc.) and related organizations concerned about occupational and environmental health. Key resource on workers' compensation.

National Tradewomen's Network
54 Mint Street, Suite 400
San Francisco, CA 94103
(415) 543-3077
Works on behalf of women in nontraditional blue-collar jobs such as construction and technical trades.

Office Technology Education Project
241 St. Botolph Street
Boston, MA 02115
(617) 526-8324
Publications, hotline, newsletter, advocacy.

White Lung Association
901 Broad Street
Newark, NJ 07012
Information, technical assistance on asbestos hazards and rights of asbestos victims.

Workables for Women
Oak Valley
Clinton, PA 15026-0214
(412) 899-3555
Supplier of personal protective equipment for women in the trades and nontraditional work.

Trade unions and local/regional labor councils: Check with local unions and councils for information on the key concerns, resources and activities in your area. Some local unions have health and safety projects/officers, and several of the national offices of unions have health and safety programs: for example, the Communication Workers of America (Washington, DC); Service Employees International Union (Washington, DC); Steelworkers (Pittsburgh); United Auto Workers (Detroit); Oil, Chemical and Atomic Workers Union (Denver).

Legal Resources and Agencies

Bargaining for Equality. A guide to legal and collective bargaining solutions for workplace problems that particularly affect women. Has a health and safety section. From The Women's Law Project, P.O. Box 6250, San Francisco, CA 94101.

Equal Employment Opportunity Commission (EEOC)
Enforces the federal Civil Rights Act, including the pregnancy disability amendment. For the office nearest you, look under "EEOC" in the federal-government listings of the phone book.

National Labor Relations Board (NLRB)
1717 Pennsylvania Avenue NW
Washington, DC 20570
Handles unfair-labor-practice charges of discipline or discharge of workers for engaging in activities around health and safety at work. For the office nearest you, look in the phone book under "Federal Agencies." If it's not there, contact NLRB for information. If you are not covered by the NLRB (if you are a public employee, for example) you will be covered by a state agency. Call your state department of labor to find out.

NIOSH (National Institute for Occupational Safety and Health)
4676 Columbia Parkway
Cincinnati, OH 45226
(800) 356-4674
NIOSH is the research partner of OSHA. It publishes criteria documents for many chemicals, and other useful documents. It may recommend standards to OSHA and conduct health hazard evaluations at workplaces.

OSHA (Occupational Safety and Health Administration)
U.S. Department of Labor
200 Constitution Avenue NW
Washington, DC 20210
(202) 523-9700
The federal agency responsible for setting workplace standards and enforcing them. The agency inspects workplaces, responds to worker complaints and has the power to fine companies that are in violation of the law and to require correction of the violation. Some states have state OSHAs that are administered by state government rather than federal government. Public workers are not covered by OSHA. Your state department of labor can tell you where the OSHA office closest to you is, and where to go for help if you are not covered by OSHA. You can get a free copy of the OSHA standards by requesting one.

Women's Bureau
U.S. Department of Labor
200 Constitution Avenue NW
Washington, DC 20210
Work and Family Clearinghouse (800) 827-5335
Information to employers, employees and unions on developing work and family programs (child care, elder care). Ask for *A Work and Family Resource Kit*. Single copies are free with self-addressed label to the Women's Bureau.

Workers' Compensation
Each state has an agency responsible for handling worker's compensation claims. Look in the state government section of the phone book under "Workers' Compensation" or "Industrial Accidents." If you don't find it there, try calling your state department of labor and asking for the name of the agency responsible.

Right-to-Know and Right-to-Act

To obtain a packet about federal, state, and local Right-to-Know and Right-to-Act legislation, contact AFL–CIO Health and Safety Department, 815 16th Street, Washington, DC 20006.

NLRB Decisions. Several NLRB decisions have come down enforcing unions' rights to health and safety information from the company and enforcing unions' rights to take experts into the plant to do inspections.

OSHA Rules on Access to Employee Exposure and Medical Records. Guarantees access of employees and unions to certain company records regarding exposure and medical records. For a free copy of this OSHA standard, call your local OSHA office or write for a copy (29CFR 1920.20) to OSHA Office of Information, 200 Constitution Avenue NW, Washington, DC 20210. (202) 523-8151.

8

Violence Against Women

By Dina Carbonell, Lois Glass, Suzanne Gosselin, Carol Mamber and Jill Stanzler (all members of Boston Area Rape Crisis Center, who wrote sections on rape, battering, incest and child abuse); Alice Friedman, Margaret Lazarus, Lynn Rubinett, Lena Sorensen, Denise Wells and Nancy Wilbur (all members of Alliance Against Sexual Coercion, who wrote the introduction, sexual harassment and activism box); Terrie Antico (self-defense); Wendy Sanford (prostitution).

With special thanks to Freada Klein, Boston Area Rape Crisis Center and Andrea Fischgrund.

This chapter is an expansion of previous chapters on rape, written by Gene Bishop, Roxanne Hynek and Judy Norsigian; and on self-defense, written by Janet Jones and Carol McEldowney.

1992 Update by Margaret Lazarus and Rachel Lanzerotti.

In this society violence against women occurs with shocking frequency.*

- FBI statistics indicate that every fifteen seconds a woman is beaten by her husband or boyfriend.
- Every six minutes, a woman is forcibly raped. One in three American women is sexually assaulted during her lifetime.
- One-fifth to one-half of American women were sexually abused as children, most of them by an older male relative.

- Nearly one-third of female homicide victims are killed by their husbands or boyfriends.
- A 1987 *Ms.* survey on date and acquaintance rape found that one in four women they surveyed were victims of rape or attempted rape, 84 percent of those raped knew their attacker, and 57 percent of the rapes happened on dates.

Every day we see real and imagined violence against women in the news, TV shows and movies, in advertising, in our homes and workplaces. It becomes a fact of life.

I have never been free of the fear of rape. From a very early age I, like most women, have thought of rape as part of my natural environment—something to be feared and prayed against like fire or lightning. I never asked why men raped; I simply thought it one of the many mysteries of human nature.[1]

---

*This chapter focuses on male violence toward women. While there are instances of female-to-male and female-to-female violence, they are relatively rare, and factual information is hard to obtain. In battering cases involving women assaulting men, the usual pattern is for a woman to act in self-defense or to strike out after having endured chronic abuse, often for years.

In the broadest sense, violence against women is any violation of a woman's personhood, mental or physical integrity or freedom of movement, and includes all the ways our society objectifies and oppresses women. Over the past decade, activists have made the definition more specific in order to facilitate organizing efforts around certain forms of violence. They have identified at least thirty specific forms of violence against women, ranging from sterilization abuse to prescription-drug abuse to pornography to violence against women in prisons, from self-hatred to economic and class oppression.*

Every form of violence threatens women with physical or psychological violation and limits our ability to make choices about our lives. Sexual violence is particularly insidious because sexual acts are ordinarily and rightly a source of pleasure and communication. It is often unclear whether a sexual violation was done out of sexual desire or violent intent or whether these motivations are even distinguishable, because violence itself has become eroticized in this culture.

Thirty years ago, most forms of violence against women were hidden under a cloak of silence or tacit acceptance. As more and more women talked with each other in the recent wave of the women's movement, it became apparent that violence against us occurs on a massive scale, that no woman is immune, and that family, friends and public institutions have been cruelly insensitive about it. Over the past fifteen years, women in communities throughout the country have mobilized to offer direct services to women who have encountered violence, to educate people about the range and nature of the violence and to develop strategies for resistance. This chapter reflects the important work of some of these women.

---

*We do not address the subject of pornography primarily because we disagree with one another and/or have not come to any clear positions yet on some crucial aspects of this issue. However, a few things all of us agree upon:

- We abhor all pornography that we find violent or degrading to women.
- We believe it important to protest the existence of this type of pornography, though we would not seek government censorship.
- We protest the fact that a huge pornography industry is making billions of dollars by objectifying, degrading and dehumanizing women, children and sometimes men. The work women are doing to expose this industry is central to our understanding of violence against women in cultures throughout the world.

We recognize that some of us will find offensive what others view as erotica and vice versa and that not all pornography represents "violence against women." But this need not keep us from speaking out against what we believe is degrading to women and, ultimately, everyone.

BLAMING THE VICTIM

Women who have been raped, battered, sexually harrassed or sexually assaulted in childhood report these emotions most frequently: guilt, fear, powerlessness, shame, betrayal, anger, denial. Guilt is often the first and deepest response. Anger often comes only later, which is not surprising because our socialization as women allows us so little sense of a right not to be violated.

We feel guilty about violence done to us because society tells us that we caused it or brought it on ourselves in some way—a clear case of "blaming the victim." Most of us heard from our parents, "Boys will be boys, so girls must take care," the message being that we can avoid unwanted male attention provided *we* are careful enough. If anything goes wrong, it's *our* fault. Blaming the victim releases the man who commits sexual violence from the responsibility for what *he* has done. By making us feel guilty, it discourages us from fighting back. *WOMEN ARE NOT GUILTY FOR VIOLENCE COMMITTED BY MEN ON OUR BODY, MIND AND SPIRIT. THIS VIOLENCE HAPPENS BECAUSE OF MEN'S GREATER POWER AND THEIR MISUSE OF THAT POWER.* As one battered woman wrote of her husband's violence, "I may be his excuse, but I have never been his reason."

MEN, WOMEN AND POWER: WHAT VIOLENCE AGAINST WOMEN REALLY DOES TO US

One man's violence against one woman may *seem* to result from his individual psychological problems, sexual frustration, unbearable life pressures or some innate urge toward aggression. Though each of these "reasons" has been used to explain and even justify male violence, they hide the truth. *Men use violence against women to exert and maintain their power and control over us.* When a battering husband uses beatings to confine his wife to the home and prevent her from seeing friends and family or pursuing outside work, he exerts dominance, hostility and control. When a boss sexually harasses his employee, he exerts his power to restrict her freedom to work and improve her position. When men rape women, they act out of a wish to punish or dominate, a desire that is often eroticized.

Whether or not an individual man who commits an act of violence views it as an expression of power is not the point. The fact that so many individual men feel entitled to express their frustration or anger by being violent to so many individual women illustrates the power men as a group hold over women as a group. In this distorted way even the most powerless men benefit from sexism.

Thousands of daily acts of violence throughout the country create a climate of fear and powerlessness that limits women's freedom of action and controls many of the movements of our lives.[2]

I learned not to walk on dark streets, not to talk to strangers or get into strange cars, to lock doors and to be modest.

I came to the vocational school instead of tne regular high school because I thought I'd like the electronics shop. But during orientation I met the two girls who are now in electronics and heard how they get teased and harassed. I'm taking cosmetology. It's all right, I guess.

The threat of male violence continues to keep us from stepping out from behind traditional roles and boundaries. It literally "keeps us in our place."

RACE, CLASS AND VIOLENCE AGAINST WOMEN

Public violence—rape and sexual harassment in particular—serves as a tool for keeping down or punishing women deprived of power by racism and other forms of discrimination. White men often use sexual violence as a means of asserting racial dominance over women of color. A married black woman who was fired for refusing to sleep with her supervisor said:

On many occasions Mr. —— said to me, "For a colored girl, you are intelligent." I told him that if he has to refer to a color or race concerning me, I considered myself "black." He replied, "I don't believe in black or all that stuff. To me you're colored, and that's it." One day he made a comment concerning my, as he called it, "voluptuous" shape. When I asked him politely to discontinue making such comments that include sexual overtures, he replied, "Why not? For a colored, you're very stacked, light-skinned and pretty."

It can be difficult for a woman of color to tell whether violence or harassment is prompted by her sex or race or both. In rape, the double jeopardy is even worse.

The man who raped me was white, and the cops here are all white. I didn't report it. I just told a few people I trusted. It helped, but I still feel scared, knowing he's out there and that nobody would do anything about it.

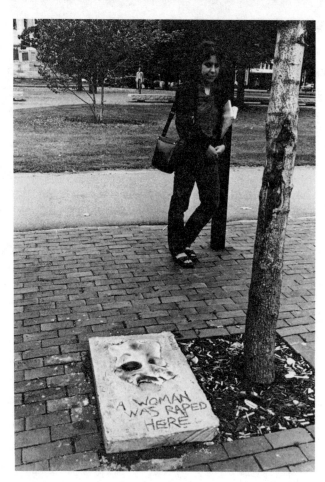

Ellen Shub

People in positions of power (usually white, affluent men) dismiss violence done to women of color as insignificant.[3] In addition, a woman of color in the United States faces a heightened vulnerability if she is not fluent in English or is not a citizen, because it is easier for men to take advantage of her and harder for her to get help.

Other forms of discrimination create other special vulnerabilities. People rarely take acts of violence as seriously if the woman is poor, old, a prostitute, a lesbian, a woman with physical or intellectual limitations or institutionalized. This is true for all women whose "male protectors" are nonexistent, invisible or socially less powerful than other men. Open lesbians have been raped by men or groups of men angry at their social independence. ("All she needs is a good fuck.") Older women have less freedom to fight sexual harassment at their jobs or to leave a battering husband, because age discrimination means they won't easily find other ways of supporting themselves. Older women and disabled women are frequently raped.

RESISTING VIOLENCE: PREVENTION VERSUS AWARENESS

Most safety advice offered to women is based on the "blame the victim" mentality: "Don't go out alone at night." ... "Don't wear sexy

133

clothes." ... "Don't be friendly to strangers." ... "Stay out of risky situations." As if what *we* do is decisive. The argument goes: Because it is women's behavior—our seductiveness or carelessness—that "invites" violence or allows it to happen, then it is up to us, by changing our behavior, to prevent it. Women sometimes tend to accept this view because it offers a false but desperately wanted sense of security. We think we can perhaps avoid violence by staying in or by being accommodating to an angry mate. We pay close attention to every detail about a woman who was raped and try not to be like her. Protective measures like self-defense may help individual women (see p. 144). However, what we do doesn't decrease the incidence of men's violent acts.

When we take steps to protect ourselves, we want it to be with full awareness that the true responsibility for preventing and eradicating violence belongs to men. *Men must stop committing violence against women, stop each other from doing it, stop condoning it in others and stop blaming women for it.* This is the most important and appropriate form of prevention.

THE LEGAL SYSTEM

As women have brought each form of violence against women to public attention, reform in laws and protocol has been one important goal. There have been a few gains: see pp. 145–46 for specific accomplishments in legal reform. It may now be

> Golda Meir said, when legislators in Israel proposed a curfew on women in an attempt to lower the incidence of rape: "But it is the *men* who are attacking women. If there is to be a curfew, let the *men* stay home."

slightly easier to report and prosecute rape, battering and cases of sexual assault against children; court and police personnel have been sensitized in some areas, and women and children are less often blamed; rape convictions have risen somewhat; emergency protection for battered women is more often available; some women who were sexually harassed have won back pay, damages and changed policies. Changing the laws has educated the public and made it possible for women to say, "I was violated and I want the assailant held accountable." Yet turning to the legal system is time-consuming, risky, expensive and traumatic, and it is available only *after* sexual violence has been committed. We have no idea whether or not better laws deter men from assaulting women. Furthermore, the legal system doesn't work the same for everyone. Women of color, poor women, divorced women and lesbians, for example, are believed and respected even less than white, financially stable, married, heterosexual women in court. White, married, middle-class (respectable) men are rarely prosecuted. Because of the limi-

SUMMARY OF MYTHS THAT SUPPORT VIOLENCE AGAINST WOMEN

| Type of Myth | How the myth gets applied to each specific form of violence | | | |
	Rape	Battering	Sexual harassment	Child sexual assault
Victim-blaming	Women invite by their dress or behavior; women lead men too far; women want it and/or enjoy being raped.	Women invite by their behavior; women pick violent partners; women stay so they must like it.	Women invite by their dress or behavior; women sleep their way to the top or for good grades.	Little girls are seductive; mothers set up incestuous relationships by their own failure as sexual partners.
Not a common problem or not a real issue	It's only done by perverts leaping from bushes.	Wives are violent, too.	It's just mutual attraction.	It isn't harmful to girls.
Male perpetrator isn't responsible for his actions	Rapists are psychopaths; rapists are provoked.	Batterers are alienated at work or unemployed or grew up in violent homes, or are alcoholic.	Most harassers don't intend harm; they're just complimenting women.	Male relatives had no choice because their sexual needs were unmet by their wives or they're psychopaths.
Racist assumptions	Black men rape white women; black women are looser about their sexuality; Hispanic women are hot lovers.	Black and Hispanic families condone violence.	Black women are looser; Hispanic women are hot lovers.	Black and Hispanic families condone sexual activity between adults and children.

Source: Copyright 1981, Freada Klein. Use with permission only.

tations of the legal system, every woman must make her own decision to report or prosecute her case.

RAPE

Rape is any kind of sexual activity committed against a woman's will. Whether the rapist uses force or threats of force is irrelevant. Men use different kinds of force against women, from pressuring us for a goodnight kiss, to withdrawal of econmic support from wives, to using weapons. Rape is always traumatic. When we are raped, survival is our primary instinct and we protect ourselves as best we can. Some women choose to fight back; others do not feel it is an option. If you were raped and are now reading this chapter, you did the "right" thing because you are alive.

Here are several facts which disprove common myths about rape. Rape is more likely to be committed by someone we know than by a stranger (acquaintance rape and marital rape). Two-thirds of reported rapes are planned and more than half occur indoors, usually in the woman's own home. Nine out of ten rapes occur between members of the same racial group. Most rapists lead everyday lives, go to school, work, have family and friends.

Emotional Reactions to Rape*

Rape hurts in every way. No two rapes are exactly alike, and no two women respond with exactly the same reactions in the same sequence. Differences in our culture, ages, personalities and the responses we get from others will influence how we respond.

Initial Responses

Immediate responses can range from numbness and disbelief, causing a woman to appear calm and rational, to extreme anxiety, fear and disorganization.

When he left, I fell into a deep sleep. As I was falling asleep, I told myself that when I got up in the morning I would have trouble remembering what happened to me.

I just sat on the floor and cried. When my husband came home, he asked me what was wrong. I was so upset I couldn't answer.

---

*Other forms of violence provoke many of the same emotions as rape does. We do not have room to discuss emotional reactions fully in each part of the chapter and hope that going into some detail here will be helpful to readers looking for support and understanding after being submitted to other kinds of violence as well.

I called up a friend and in a real calm voice asked her if she could come over. I was fine till she got here, and then I broke down and cried.

You deserve support for however you respond to rape. What is important is that you do what you feel you have to do and then, once you're ready, go to a hospital or doctor for care.

How people treat you when you seek medical care or report a rape makes a big difference in how you will feel. Medical providers and police are often insensitive and blaming.

I was telling the doctor about what had happened. He seemed kind and concerned, but after the exam was over, he asked what I was doing out so late at night by myself.

The officer I spoke to didn't seem to trust me because I was acting so "emotional," as he said. His rough questions felt almost like being raped again.

As a woman of color I was not able to allow myself to feel and express my reactions to the rape because I didn't feel safe from racist responses at the hospital, the police station, the counseling center.

Two major goals of feminists organizing around rape have been to get training programs into hospitals and police departments to teach personnel to respond more sensitively, and to make sure women going for care after a rape have the company of an advocate—a woman who is there specifically to give you support and get you fair treatment. If there are no such programs in your area (and even if there are), bring a friend with you if you possibly can. If anyone tries to make you feel guilty about the rape, s/he is buying into the myths that say that being raped is the woman's fault.

Second Phase

Once you are in a safe environment, you will often allow yourself to feel the full impact of what has just happened. You may be in physical pain from bruises, genital lesions, nausea or stomachaches. You are also likely to feel depressed, angry, afraid, humiliated and unable to sleep.

The responses we receive from loved ones can influence us during this time. Culture has a strong influence. If we are black we may not receive the respect we deserve, because black women are stereotypically seen as personifying sexual freedom and abandon. Cultures with strong religious prohibitions against non-marital sex may ostracize us. If we are Latina, we may find that our loved ones judge us as dishonored, because of a strong emphasis on virginity; we may therefore find it hard to speak about the rape. It's hard not to feel both worthless and at fault when those close to us tell us we are.

During this time, try to find friends, family or counselors who can support you as you discuss the feelings that you are experiencing.

Third Phase

In the third phase you may go through a period of "calm before the storm." It may last for weeks, months or years. You may feel as if the trauma has passed. Unfortunately, this is usually a temporary period of apparently calm readjustment. One woman stated, "I thought it was all over; then I saw a man who looked like the rapist. Again I have begun to think about it, but this time I was obsessed with it."

During this calm period, we forget. Then something happens—a joke about rape, a pregnancy test or a court appearance. Again we feel that we lack control over our lives, just as we felt when we were raped.

Fourth/Final Phase

Finally we may be able to discuss our deeper feelings with others. Many women who speak to someone during the initial crisis choose to discuss the rape again at this time. Many women join support groups to meet with other women who are also trying to understand this experience. To get rid of guilt feelings and regain a strong self-image, we must direct our anger outward at the rapist and at a society that not only allows rape to continue but also blames women for its occurrence. After a rape we may lose faith in our environment as a safe and predictable one, but we *can* regain a strong sense of ourselves in the world.

Medical Considerations

If you have been raped, the first thing you may want to do is take a shower or bath and try to forget what happened. Do whatever feels most comfortable, but consider two things. First, it is very important both physically and emotionally that you receive medical attention as soon as possible, even if you have no obvious injuries. Second, don't bathe or shower if you think you may later decide to prosecute, as you will wash away evidence that may be crucial to your case.

If possible, call a friend, relative or local rape crisis counselor who can give you comfort, support, and act as an advocate on your behalf in the hospital. If you feel reluctant to go because you may not be able to afford it, be aware that a hospital emergency room should not turn you away because you can't pay.

At the hospital, you have two basic concerns: medical care and the gathering of evidence for a possible prosecution (you can refuse to be exam-

ined for evidence if you are absolutely sure that you will not want to prosecute). Physical injuries to *any* part of the body can result from a rape; therefore, a thorough examination is necessary. That examination should include and/or result in:

1. *A pelvic exam.* (If you are raped vaginally; see p. 565 for a pelvic exam description. You will get a rectal exam if you were raped anally.) In collecting evidence, the doctor will look for the presence of semen. *(It is also possible to be raped vaginally with no semen or sperm present.)* S/he will also comb your pubic hair for the possible presence of the man's pubic hair, ask you to describe your physical and emotional condition and may take your clothing, so take an extra set with you.

All this medical evidence will be available to others, including the police, only with your written permission. You or the person with you at the hospital should check the record for accuracy and objectivity as soon as possible after the exam, while the doctor is still present.

2. *Examination and treatment of any external injuries.*

3. *Treatment for the prevention of sexually transmitted disease (STD).* The doctor will give you two shots of antibiotic in your buttocks. If you don't want this, be sure to say so. (Some women may not want to be given an antibiotic without an STD being diagnosed; however, it is used as a preventive measure.)

4. *Treatment for the prevention of pregnancy.* If you suspect that you will become pregnant as a result of the rape, the doctor or nurses may offer you DES (the "morning-after pill"). This drug has serious effects, so before deciding to take it, read about its dangers and ineffectiveness on p. 293–94. A pregnancy or STD resulting from rape cannot be detected until six weeks later.* Although you may feel physically recovered shortly after the rape, making a follow-up visit, which would include tests and treatment for STD and a pregnancy test if indicated, would assure you that you are taking care of yourself. If you find that you are pregnant and are considering abortion, see Chapter 17.

Legal Considerations

It is never easy to decide whether to prosecute a rapist. Of the 10 percent or less of rapes that are reported, fewer still are prosecuted. In some states you can report a rape anonymously or without prosecuting (for police records). Whether you report it or not, write down everything that you can remember, so that if you do report or prosecute later your statement will be accurate.

---

*Even though some pregnancy tests are accurate within seven days, some STDs are not detectable until six weeks later, so it is a good idea to return for a six-week checkup.

As you are deciding whether or not to prosecute, here are several things to keep in mind:

1. The police and the legal system very often make prosecuting a rapist a more difficult, painful experience for the woman than it should be. It will help tremendously to have a friend or rape crisis counselor with you throughout the process.

2. Chances of conviction are low: 20 to 40 percent in most states.

3. A trial can last from six months to two years, so you need to be prepared to continue thinking and talking about the rape for a long time, including giving an account of the event over and over while people judge whether you are telling the truth.

4. You will have to prove that you were sexually assaulted against your will and that the man used force or threatened force against you.

5. Rape is considered a crime against the state, so you will be a state's witness for the district attorney's office. You will not have a private lawyer unless you arrange for one to advise you and consult with the district attorney assigned to you. (For more on the legal process in your state, call a rape crisis center or the district attorney's office.)

WOMAN ABUSE

Woman abuse, often referred to as battering, is the most common and least reported crime in the United States.[4] Battering happens to women of every age, color, class and nationality. It is done by the men we married who beat us, by our sons and nephews who bully us and slap us around and by male relatives who verbally harass and degrade us. Twenty-five percent of American families have a history of woman abuse.[5]

PROTECTING OURSELVES AND EACH OTHER FROM RAPE

Authors' note: Listing these tips reminds us how angry we are that we have to protect ourselves from men's actions. Yet until men stop or are forced to stop raping women, we will need to take precautions. (The following are much more useful against a stranger than against an acquaintance or husband.)

When possible, *the most effective protection comes from being with other women.* Arrange to walk home together, set up a greenlight or safe house program in your neighborhood (see p. 145), get to know each other on a street or in an apartment building.

Where You Live
Keep lights in all the entrances; keep the windows locked and in place; have strong locks on every door; be aware of places where men might hide; don't put your full name on your mailbox; know which neighbors you can trust in an emergency; find out who is at your door before opening; say, "I'll get the door, Bill!" when going to the door.

On the Street
Be aware of what is going on around you. Walk with a steady pace; look as if you know where you are going; don't carry a lot of stuff; dress so you can move and run easily; walk in the middle of the street; don't walk through dark places or a group of men; if you fear danger, yell "Fire," not "Help" or "Rape"; carry a whistle around your wrist.

Transportation
Always check the backseat of your car before getting in; while driving, keep doors locked; don't stand near groups of men on public transportation; look aware and don't fall asleep; if you don't know where you are going, ask the driver and sit near the front.

"Legal Weapons" as Protection
A lighted cigarette, a plastic lemon or spray can filled with ammonia, a cheap heavy ring worn on the inside of your hand, a hatpin or an umbrella are all useful.

Body Basics
Use your elbows; if using fists, aim for his face; use your voice in his ear; use your teeth; if you kick, aim at his knees or genitals; pull his hair and clap your hands over his ears; keep your hands and arms close to you.

Hitchhiking
Don't hitchhike if you can possibly avoid it; it is just too dangerous. If you do, check the door handle, keep the window open and never ride with more than one man.

These tactics can help you but they are not foolproof. Practice tactics for the situations that make you feel most at risk and least powerful. Try to remain calm and to act as confident and strong as you can.

Adapted from *How to Start a Rape Crisis Center* (1972) by the Rape Crisis Center of Washington, D.C.

Examples

Battering takes many forms. The majority of women who are battered are abused repeatedly by the same person. As time passes, these beatings often increase in frequency and severity.

I have had glasses thrown at me. I have been kicked in the abdomen, kicked off the bed and hit while laying on the floor—while I was pregnant. I have been whipped, kicked and thrown, picked up and thrown down again. I have been punched and kicked in the head, chest, face and abdomen on numerous occasions.

I have been slapped for saying something about politics, having a different view about religion, for swearing, for crying, for wanting to have intercourse.

I have been threatened when I wouldn't do something I was told to do.

I have been threatened when he's had a bad day—when he's had a good day.[6]

Other women are abused less regularly, yet the abuse still affects our self-esteem and our children.

My very upper-middle-class, WASP father hit my mother drunkenly on an occasional Saturday night. Sunday morning she would explain away her bruises. I lived my whole childhood under this shadow—the possibility of violence, the sounds in the night and the toll it took on me that she put up with it.

Some of us have listened to verbal abuse for years and have begun to believe the degrading lies we hear.

Researchers have attempted to understand why violence within families is so prevalent. It is clear that men receive permission from law courts, police and other men to batter.

The fact that men all around the world, of every conceivable class, color, religion and ethnic group beat their wives shows that something more is sick than these individuals. Something has got to be wrong with the societies these men live in that they are allowed to beat women. . . . How can we explain former Prime Minister of Japan Sato having been given the Nobel Prize for Peace although his wife has publicly declared that he beat her?[7]

Many men learn violence at home; many men who batter saw their fathers abuse their mothers and many women who are abused have grown up in families where male power was never questioned and physical punishment "in the name of love" was accepted. When our families teach us to accept male power in all its forms, the message is difficult to defy.

What makes the problem so complex is that the men who do the battering are the people with whom we have been close or intimate, perhaps the fathers of our children. We may still be bound by love and loyalty. We remain at home not only because the men won't let us leave or make it as difficult as possible, but also because we hope that this episode will be the last one, that things will get better, that our men will change. We make excuses for their behavior.

Before I left I used to say, "Yeah, he punched and kicked me, but I'd said something to make him mad." Or "He only hits me when I argue." Now I see that everyone has a right to get angry—it's natural—but he had no right to express his anger so violently, to hurt me.

We don't leave home because, what will we do with the children? How will we live and support ourselves? Where will we go?

We rarely get adequate protection from clergy, courts or police, who often do not take us seriously.

I went early in our marriage to a clergyman, who after a few visits told me that my husband meant no real harm, he was just confused and felt insecure.

Things continued. I turned this time to a doctor. I was given little pills to relax me and told to take things easier. I was "just too nervous."

I turned to a friend, and when her husband found out, he accused me of either making things up or exaggerating the situation. She was told to stay away from me.[8]

Many battered women have had similar experiences of being challenged, patronized or told that our problems are insignificant. In the face of such inexcusable treatment we must remember that *no woman deserves to be verbally abused or beaten. Every woman deserves to have her story taken seriously.*

What to Do[9]

Try to stay calm during an attack; save your anger for a time when you are safe from physical attack. Remember, no matter what he says to you, that you are a valuable and worthwhile person.

- Defend and protect yourself, especially your head and stomach.
- Fight back only if you judge that it won't make him hurt you more.
- Call for help. Scream or, if you can get away, run to the nearest person or home, say you are being hurt and that you need help.
- Call the police, or have someone else do it; the police have a responsibility to protect you.

- Call your local crisis hotline to find out about a battered women's shelter in your area.
- Get away. If it is unsafe to stay at home, call a neighbor, friend or a cab. Find shelter and take your children with you, either then or, if it would be safer, the next day. Your personal safety and your children's welfare are primary; you can handle custody and property matters after you leave.

There *are* alternatives to staying in a battering situation. More and more women are leaving men who batter, and finding help in making a new life despite economic hardships. Over the last decade, women in every state have been organizing to help women leave abusive situations, to provide shelter and a more responsive legal system. Women have found the courage to tell their stories publicly. *We are not helpless, and we are not alone.*

SEXUAL HARASSMENT

Sexual harassment is any *unwanted* sexual attention a woman experiences. It includes leering, pinching, patting, repeated comments, subtle suggestions of a sexual nature and pressure for dates. It can also take the form of attempted or actual rape. Sexual harassment can occur in any situation where men have power over women—welfare workers with clients, doctors with patients, policemen with women drivers, teachers with students.* This section focuses on workplace harassment because it has been the most widely studied so far.

In the workplace, the harasser may be an employer, supervisor, co-worker, client or customer. Any unwanted sexual attention causes anxiety and embarrassment, but when it occurs at work, our jobs are threatened.

Recent surveys reveal that the majority of women will experience workplace sexual harassment at some point during their working lives. Eighty-eight percent of the 9,000 women answering *Redbook* magazine's questionnaire in 1976 had received unwanted sexual attention on the job. A 1991 survey of 4,450 women in the United States and Canada by *Ms.* found that 43 percent of the women experienced sexual harassment at work or in an academic environment. In addition, both studies confirm that no one is immune from sexual

---

*Sexual harassment in schools and universities has recently been defined as a form of sex discrimination under Title IX of the Education Amendments of 1972. Teachers or administrators barter for sexual favors with grades, scholarships and recommendations for college or graduate school. Students use sexual harassment to force women out of courses or majors like auto mechanics in high school and engineering in college.

Here are some things that battered women and their children need most frequently: emergency food, shelter, clothing; economic assistance and job training; advocacy with the legal, medical, police and welfare systems; school transportation, child care by caring adults; safety plans; a chance to think and get advice about separation, divorce, child support, child custody, housing, other relationships, choosing a lawyer; support of other women, often in a group run by a shelter, hotline or community center.

harassment—women of all ages and races and holding all types of jobs were affected.

Joan is a forty-three-year-old black woman who works as a waitress in a bar and restaurant. She likes her job because it's close to home and it gives her a steady income to support her children. She often feels isolated, though, as many of her co-workers are white and have racist attitudes.

A customer who comes in every day during the lunch rush begins to flirt with Joan, making suggestive comments about her clothing and physical appearance. Unnerved by his comments, she tries not to show it because she doesn't want to lose any tip money. Often he grabs at her and touches her when she walks by.

After several weeks of this treatment, Joan can't take it anymore. She feels so anxious at work that her stomach hurts, and she starts to call in sick more and more. She knows she needs to figure something out or she'll eventually lose her job. She's afraid if she complains she'll get blamed because she's friendly and attractive-looking.

Chris is a thirty-four-year-old Latina who works as a secretary in a large hospital. Chris has excellent organizational skills and is proud of her ability to take initiative and keep her office running smoothly.

Chris's boss depends on her a lot to take care of business and is appreciative of her work. He begins asking Chris out to lunch or for drinks after work as a way to thank her. Chris is uncomfortable with these invitations but doesn't feel able to say no. The other secretaries begin to wonder why Chris is spending her lunch hour with the boss and feel angry about it.

One evening as Chris is getting ready to leave, her boss comes in and asks her to have a drink with him. Chris finally tells him that it makes her uncomfortable to socialize with him outside the office, that it does not seem appropriate to her. He tells Chris that he thinks she is too impressed with herself and it is

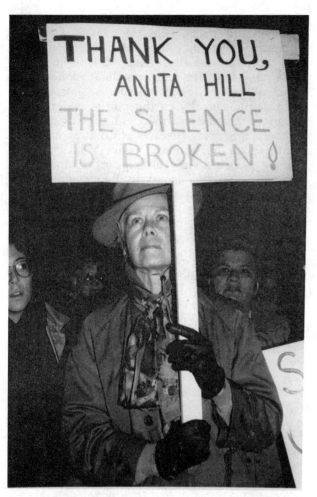

Demonstrator in support of Anita Hill, who challenged the nomination of Supreme Court Justice Clarence Thomas in 1991.   Ellen Shub

inappropriate for her to tell him what she will or won't do.

Theresa is an eighteen-year-old white woman who works as an assembler at a big electronics company in her town. It's her first full-time job after graduating from high school, and she's happy because the pay is pretty good since the company is unionized.

Soon after she begins work, one of the men who work near her starts to ask her a lot of questions about her personal life: what she does after work, if she has a boyfriend, where she lives, etc. Theresa doesn't want to talk to him about these things, but she wants to be friendly and sociable with people at work. Soon his questions become even more personal, and he starts to talk with her about his sexual relations with women. When Theresa tells him that she feels uneasy and asks him to stop, he laughs and says that if she can't handle a little friendly conversation, then she isn't ready for the working world.

Sexual harassment is another powerful way for men to undermine and control us. There is an implicit (and sometimes explicit) message that our refusal to comply with the harasser's demands will lead to work-related reprisals. These can include escalation of harassment; poor work assignments; sabotaging of projects; denial of raises, benefits or promotion; and sometimes the loss of the job with only a poor reference to show for it. Harassment can drive women out of a particular job or out of the workplace altogether.

Socializing at work often includes flirting or joking about sex. Although it may be a pleasant relief from routine or a way to communicate with someone we are "interested in," this banter can become insulting or demeaning. We have had little power to define this line for ourselves. It becomes sexual harassment when it creates a hostile, intimidating or pressured working environment.

There is such a taboo in many workplaces against identifying sexual harassment for what it is that many of us who experience it are at first aware only of feeling stressed. Headaches, anxieties, resistance to going to work in the morning—it often takes us a while to realize these symptoms may come from being sexually harassed. Sexual harassment can make us question our right to work, our competence, our appearance or attractiveness, our right to look and dress as we please or to go out with whomever we choose. We often respond by feeling isolated and powerless, afraid to say no or to speak out because we fear either that we somehow are responsible or that we won't receive help in facing possible retaliation. But when we take the risk and talk with other women, we often find that they are being harassed, too (or have been), and have had similar responses to ours.

INCEST AND SEXUAL ABUSE OF CHILDREN

Traditionally, incest has been defined as sexual contact that occurs between family members.* Most incest occurs between older male relatives and younger female children in families of every class and color. Because it happens within the family context, an incestuous relationship is one over which a child or young woman has no control. A trusted family member uses his power—as well as our love and dependence—to initiate sexual contact, and to insure that the relationship continues and remains secret.

My barter with my brother was that he could do sex on me to practice for his girlfriends. I consented not

---

*Each state defines incest differently. In this chapter, we will be discussing *social* attitudes and definitions regarding incest and sexual abuse of children, not legal ones.

WHAT YOU CAN DO IF YOU ARE SEXUALLY HARASSED

Authors' note: It's crucial to realize that every situation is different. What kind of strategy you choose will depend on many factors, including how much you can afford to risk losing your job and whether you feel you can get support from your coworkers. (Race and class differences sometimes isolate workers from each other, for instance.)

1. Remember that you are not to blame. Sexual harassment is *imposed* sexual attention. No matter how complicated the situation is, the harasser is responsible for the abuse.

2. Document what happens. Keep a diary; save any notes or pictures from the harasser—don't throw them away in anger. Write down specific dates, times, places, kinds of incidents, your responses, his answers, any witnesses.

3. *Generate support for yourself before you take action:* Break the silence, talk with others at your workplace or school and outside, ask for help in working out a response. They may feel more responsible then for backing you up if your response to the harasser fails.

4. Investigate your workplace's or school's policy and grievance procedure for sexual harassment cases. Know its overall records before you act. If possible, know the record of particular administrators, managers, union stewards or officials, personnel or equal-opportunity counselors or others you may need to involve to get your complaint heard.

5. You may discover others who have been harassed who can act with you. Collective action and joint complaints strengthen your position. Some who have not been harassed may join in collective action. Try to use organizations that already exist, such as your union or employee organization, a local rape crisis center or women's organization or an advocacy organization for your particular racial or ethnic group to help you strategize and carry out a collective response.

6. Let the harasser know as clearly, directly, explicitly as possible that you are not interested in his attentions. If you do this in writing, keep a copy of your letter.

7. Evaluate your options. What do you want from any action you take? What are your primary concerns and goals? What courses of action are available to you? What are the possible outcomes, including the risks of each course of action?

8. First consider taking actions *within* your workplace or school, strategizing with others to be as creative as possible; think about lawsuits only as a last resort.* But remember that sexual harassment is illegal because you may be able to use that fact to strengthen your position.

Source: Alliance Against Sexual Coercion (no longer in existence).

---

*The specific legal options for sexual harassment include filing charges of sex discrimination with your state's Human Rights Commission or the Federal Equal Employment Opportunity Commission. In addition, women have used unemployment compensation, civil or criminal assault, rape laws, union grievance procedures and workers' compensation. Students have used the federal law, Title IX of the Education Amendments of 1972. See pp. 136–37, Legal Considerations, for the problems and limits of legal strategies.

---

because I enjoyed it but because I was afraid to be alone when my parents went out. . . . I never even thought of talking about it. That just couldn't be done.

Sexual abuse of children is most often committed by family friends who have access to children within their family setting. Abuse is also perpetrated by people normally trusted by parents—doctors, dentists, teachers and baby-sitters. Despite popular myths, "stranger danger" poses much less threat to boys and girls. Yet parents teach us to expect danger from strangers, not from trusted authority figures, and the violation of this trust is often frightening and confusing.

Incest and sexual abuse of children take many forms and may include sexually suggestive language; prolonged kissing, looking and petting; vaginal and/or anal intercourse and oral sex. Because sexual contact is often achieved without force, you may not show signs of physical abuse. If you were very young when the abuse occurred, you may have scars from vaginal or anal lacerations. You may remember chronic sore throats and stomach pain if the abuse involved oral sex. Some of us became pregnant or contracted an STD.

It is difficult to talk about incest or sexual abuse of children. Some of us may never have told anyone, though the abuse may have continued for years. We never mentioned how we dreaded family gatherings, where a particular uncle or family friend would come after us. For some of us, exploring our bodies with an older brother turned into a sexual encounter, and we ended feeling oddly abused. Sometimes a father, uncle or teacher abused our sisters and we didn't find out for years, because our sisters were also afraid to tell. Every survivor has her own story. Many of us have kept our stories secret for years.

Feminist Insights

For many years "experts" wrote quantities of non-feminist material on incest and child abuse. They blamed mothers for abandoning their children to sexually deprived husbands and accused young girls of being seductive or of fantasizing about a sexual relationship with a male relative. Feminists have challenged these victim-blaming views: Incest and child abuse occur primarily because men have power and women and children do not. They are means by which fathers, uncles and significant family contacts bolster their low self-image by taking advantage of the powerlessness of children. Men can put these motives into action because family structures allow them to misuse their power.

Incest Survivors

Those of us who are incest survivors know that the effects of this abuse are lifelong. We often blame ourselves long after the abuse has ended—for not saying no, for not fighting back, for telling or not telling, for having been "seductive," for having trusted the abuser. Often there was no one to confirm that someone treated us cruelly and that this abuse was truly terrible.

For the next twenty years I will probably continue to walk around and ask other women, "What was your childhood like?" Hearing women say that no one touched them sexually at that young an age helps me realize that something in my childhood was really wrong.

Many of us have difficulty with sexually intimate relationships because of the memories they revive. Many of us desire sexual intimacy yet have difficulty trusting. Some incest survivors feel comfortable with sex yet know that something is vaguely wrong.

It's been really hard to figure out how this has affected me with men. I've had a hard time figuring out who is safe and who isn't. Now the only way I will sleep with someone is if I can have complete control. I need permission to feel uncomfortable with certain sexual acts.

Sometimes blaming ourselves takes other forms. Many teenagers with a history of incest "sleep around" to feel accepted, or run away. Many teenage and adult survivors feel depressed and don't know why and/or turn to drugs and alcohol to mask the pain. Some of us feel worthless.

I often feel hopeless and suicidal. My father treated me with such violence that this is the only way I know to treat myself. I'm learning better ways now, but it's difficult.
I have been a drug addict. I have been anorexic. I have been a compulsive eater. Food was the only thing I could control and trust when people in my life failed me.

Getting Help

To heal the emotional scars of incest or early sexual abuse, we need to tell our stories to people who understand deeply what we have experienced. Talking with others in counseling or support groups for women with a history of incest breaks the silence, helps us to gain perspective and know we are not alone, and eases the pain. Women who have taken advantage of these tools feel healthier and stronger.

I now have a lot of compassion for myself, because I know the implications of the abuse that occurred in my life. I owe myself all the understanding, patience and acceptance I can find—a ton of it.

Some women find that they need to confront the family member who abused them. This is a frightening task but may also be rewarding.

I feel empowered by letting him know I am aware that the incest occurred. I feel empowered by the fact that I didn't ask him if he remembered, I just told him. I knew he would deny it. I just wanted to say, "This happened." I did not expect results. Telling him was the total opposite of all that happened— what was invisible is now out in the open.

Those of us with a history of incest need to know that whatever we do or don't do, we have done okay because we have survived a childhood that wasn't like a childhood at all.*

SELF INJURY

Self injury, much more common among women than men, occurs when we consciously injure ourselves by cutting, hitting, burning, etc. Because of

*See especially Judith Herman's *Father-Daughter Incest* (Cambridge, MA/London: Harvard Univeristy Press, 1981).

the shame surrounding self injury, women often keep this problem secret and do not reach out for support from others. Self injury is not usually done with the intent of suicide.

Why do women self injure? According to one group of women who self injure:

There are many reasons why we self injure. No one reason seems to explain why. Some self injury acts as a way to block out emotional pain caused by childhood abuse or other trauma. Many of us say that the physical pain evoked by self injury somehow diminishes intense emotional pain. Some medical studies say that self injury releases endorphins in the brain which function like a pain decreasing narcotic. These endorphins may reduce the level of anxiety and provide relief from emotional pain.

Self injury can also be a way to express anger and other feelings that were forbidden to be expressed in any other way. Self injury can replay an abusive experience in order to regain control.

Many of us who self injure are also survivors of ritual or cult abuse. Those of us who were abused in this way are usually programmed by our abusers to hurt ourselves if we disclose any information about the abuse. Cults also program their victims to mark their bodies in a certain way so they can be identified should the person leave the cult.

Some of us use self injury as a way to draw attention to the pain of our abuse. Sometimes we view our physical scars as symbols of our hidden emotional pain.*

Many mental health professionals are uninformed about this problem, so women who self injure may find it helpful to contact a support group to find out what approaches other women have tried to stop injurious behavior. Support groups solely for self injury are rare, but groups for women who have been abused by others are more common and may provide useful suggestions. See Resources.

SELF-DEFENSE

As much as self-defense may help in certain situations, the most important step in ending violence against women is to stop men from doing the violence and allowing it to be done.

In recent years the experiences of women who have been practicing self-defense have changed our ideas about what self-defense is and how we

---

*From: "Women and Self Injury," available from the Independent Living Center of the North Shore.

can use its techniques. We have discovered that self-defense study actually includes any activity—assertiveness training, exercise, sports—that promotes self-confidence, self-knowledge or self-reliance. We have also discovered that skills we once associated almost exclusively with self-defense can benefit other areas of our lives. Self-defense classes teach us to shift our self-awareness so that we remember that we are the sources of our own energy and the initiators of our own actions. Instead of freezing in the face of assault, we learn to mobilize our thoughts, assess the situation, make a judgment about the level of danger, choose the response we wish to make and then make it. We can use this self-awareness in other common life situations when it may seem that someone else is in control: medical examinations, job interviews, confrontations with authority, communication with a difficult person. One woman states:

I have experienced such profound changes in my self-image and in the way that I see the world and relate to people that I really can't separate my study of self-defense from the rest of my life.

Inner and Outer Obstacles

Several myths can prevent us from defending ourselves effectively against a physical assault: that the assailant is invulnerable, that greater physical strength will decide who is to win in an assault situation, that we don't know how to defend ourselves. Yet women have defended themselves against attack in many instances. One woman frightened off three adolescent males who were following her along a city street by turning quickly and letting out a bloodcurdling yell. Another stopped a would-be assailant with a kick to the midsection. A young girl sitting on the train found a wayward hand on her knee. She took the man's wrist in her grasp, raised his hand high in the air and said loudly enough for the entire car to hear, "Who does this belong to?" He got off at the next stop. There are hundreds of such stories. We don't see them on TV, we don't read them in the newspapers, but stop in at any self-defense class run by and for women and you'll hear them. We often attribute such escapes to luck or good fortune, and we don't take credit for our own courage and resourcefulness. It is important to our self-confidence to reclaim those successes.

There are people around us, particularly the men in our lives, who may consciously or unconsciously seek to discourage us from learning self-defense. As we begin to learn physical techniques, we feel the stirrings of a fledgling self-confidence. We know how to break a hold, to avoid a grasp, to stay on our feet and keep our emotional and physical balance. Yet when we practice these techniques on men we know, we often fail, both because we have eliminated the element of surprise and because their resistance to our new skills undermines us. It is important to practice with people who support our efforts to become stronger.

We need to be on guard against the ideas that "a little knowledge is a dangerous thing" and that fighting back only makes matters worse. Although compliance is sometimes a prudent response to assault, it does not guarantee that a situation will not get worse. *In fact, studies have shown that women who use active resistance and who act quickly are more likely to avoid rape than those who use passive or no resistance.*

Up to this point we have had little experience in the uses of self-defense by battered women. Street techniques, which depend upon surprise and causing damage, don't work so well against repeated assault by men we live with. Yet other skills developed in the practice of self-defense may be useful, such as learning to overcome the inner obstacles that come up when we are faced with a violent situation. If we feel more self-confident, we may begin to think about resisting the battering situation in some way, about fighting back or leaving it.

We need to develop guidelines for adapting physical techniques for use by women with different physical capabilities: elder women, physically challenged women, injured women, women who are pregnant and others. Furthermore, we need to support the work of safehouse networks, temporary shelters, rape crisis centers and other organizations committed to our safety, because without them, self-defense is a piecemeal approach to women's security.

TODAY AND TOMORROW*

NO WOMAN IS SAFE
UNTIL ALL OF US ARE SAFE

Over the past twenty-three years, we have directed our collective anger into many kinds of action opposing violence against women.

- We organized consciousness-raising groups and discovered that our experiences of dominance by men were common and shared.
- We demanded that the public listen to us by demonstrating in large groups, holding public speakouts, creating films, radio and TV shows, street theater, dramatic productions, books, pamphlets, newspapers and articles.

- We set up educational programs for thousands of law enforcement and health professionals.
- In the spring of 1989, the Wisconsin Student Association, with urging from women's groups at

---

GUIDELINES FOR SELF-DEFENSE TRAINING

Finding a Self-Defense Class
Check YWCAs, community schools, adult education programs, women's publications, women's centers.

Choosing a Class
1. Observe a class.
2. After class, question the instructor about hypothetical defense situations, particularly those that you fear most.
3. Talk to the women students in the class, presenting the same hypothetical situations to them. Steps 2 and 3 will indicate whether or not the instructor teaches application of techniques to situations that women face.
4. When talking to the instructor and the students, try to determine how much awareness there is about issues of violence against women and about other safety resources in the area. Try to find a really complete approach to women's safety.

Training Without a Teacher
1. Read books on the subject; many written by women provide good guidelines for building self-confidence.
2. Strengthen your body with good nutrition and regular exercise, preferably with some combination of aerobics and weight training.
3. Working with friends to give feedback or in front of a mirror:

- Practice walking with strong, even strides, looking as if you know where you're going.
- Practice loud yelling, accompanied by ferocious facial expressions.
- Tell someone to take his hands off you, giving a coherent message through a combination of words, tone of voice and facial expression.
- Act out "what-if" situations, discuss various responses and drill the best ones.

---

*Throughout history women have protected themselves and each other from men's violence by fighting back, offering shelter, nursing and caring for each other. Unfortunately this chapter has no room for this proud history. Please refer to the Resources.

the University of Wisconsin, successfully pressured Miller to remove their sixteen-page pamphlet advertisement that appeared in the college paper, the *Daily Cardinal*. This pamphlet encouraged college men to "scam babes" and to drink Miller beer during spring break. The Wisconsin Student Association voted to encourage a boycott of Miller until the pamphlet was pulled; they achieved a great success against sexist advertising when Miller pulled the ad and sent out over one hundred apology notices to all colleges that received the pamphlet.

- Women defaced billboards advertising a moisturizer called Self-Defense because it made a mockery of work against violence through its slogan, "A pretty face isn't safe in the city." Ads were quickly withdrawn from the market.
- Women have supported each other through the process of taking offenders to court.
- Women organized in support of women of color assaulted by white men. Women held benefits for the legal defense of JoAnne Little, a black woman, and Inez Garcia, a Latina, who killed the men who raped them, and Yvonne Wanrow, a Native American who killed a known child-molester when he came after her and her children.
- Women of color formed organizations such as the Committee to End Sterilization Abuse and worked with white women, winning new regulations to attempt to control sterilization abuse.
- By 1979 as many as a thousand organizations were providing services around the country to assist women who had been raped. Some of these were autonomous rape crisis centers created and staffed by women.
- In 1974 a group of feminists doing legal-aid work in St. Paul, Minnesota, opened Women's House, the first U.S. refuge for battered women and their children. Current estimates suggest that there are more than 1,000 hotlines, shelters and programs for battered women. The National Coalition Against Domestic Violence, launched in 1977, now attracts over 600 service providers and activists to its conferences. Parallel coalitions of service groups exist in more than thirty-five states.
- Neighborhood groups have formed networks of refuges, called *safehouse* or *greenlight* programs because participating homes are identified by green lights, where women harassed or attacked in the streets can find safety.
- We have worked for legal reform on many fronts. Since 1974, forty-nine states have revised their rape laws in order to make it easier for women to report the crimes and obtain convictions. (Mississippi is the lone holdout.) By mid-1982, eleven states treated rape by a husband or co-habitor (marital rape) the same as rape by a

June Austin

stranger. Some thirty states permit marital rape charges under some circumstances—for instance, in some states the pair must be legally separated. Forty-nine states have now revised their statutes covering battering; thirty-six of these specifically include protective orders for victims. Legislation has been used creatively: Fourteen states impose taxes (usually on marriage licenses or divorce filings) whose revenues are earmarked to fund services for battered women. Unfortunately these may not hold up in federal court as constitutional.

- We learned from feminists in other countries. The 1976 Tribunal of Crimes Against Women, held in Brussels and attended by women from all over the world, expanded the definition of violence against women to include dowry murders* and genital mutilation. European feminists inspired both safehouses and "Take Back the Night" marches, which rally thousands of women yearly in cities across the United States to protest violence against women.
- Some men have participated in this movement. Men have formed a few groups in which men help batterers to deal with their violence (for example, Emerge, in Boston). Other men have worked for legislation, written articles or made films. Some men have begun to hold each other accountable, legally and socially, for their violence, recognizing that men who do not take action support the system that promotes violence against women. They talk about their socialization in relation to women, question the extent and consequences of male dominance, listen to and respect the women around them.

---

*Men marry women for their dowries and then kill them. This still happens in India.

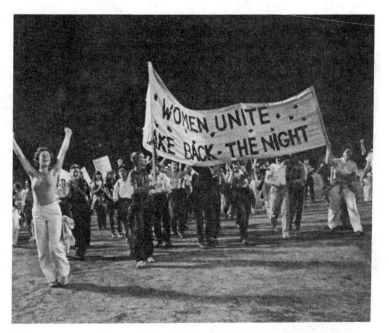

Bonnie Burt

Currently there is a backlash against the very actions which have helped and strengthened so many women. Conservative pressure groups claim that measures to protect women of all ages and to stop male violence undermine traditional family values. Funding is increasingly harder to get—especially since current budget priorities do not favor social services. Many shelters, rape crisis centers and other services are being forced to close for lack of funding.

We must continue to express our outrage loud and clear by keeping alive all the services to women, and by continuing to speak out. We will continue to teach our daughters to demand equality for themselves and others; we will teach our sons to question sexism and violence, to respect women as equals and fight all forms of dominance. We will continue to support one another in protecting ourselves with ingenuity, strength and pride. We applaud women who say no to male violence, who offer support to a friend, who protect each other, who fight back, who survive.

APPENDIX: PROSTITUTION

About 1.3 million women in this country earn all or part of their living as prostitutes. Contrary to the ugly stereotypes of prostitutes as fallen women, dope addicts or disease carriers,* prostitutes are women at work—supporting children as single parents, trying to save money to go to

*Only about 5 percent of STDs in the United States is spread by prostitutes.

school, surviving economically in a job market that underpays women at every economic level. Many are housewives or secretaries moonlighting as prostitutes to make ends meet.

Once politically voiceless and isolated from other women, over the past twenty years prostitutes have organized for support and political action.* As they speak out and write about their lives,† they expose the many forms of violence that prostitutes experience:

1. The poverty that forces women—especially poor women, women of color and runaway teenagers—into work as hookers (many women have no access to other jobs); the sexist job discrimination that means that even middle- and upper-class women can earn more in prostitution than in other jobs available to them; the fact that a great number of incest victims become prostitutes.

2. Police harassment.

3. Intimidation and beatings by pimps, to whom many prostitutes must give their earnings in return for protection. Many of them fear for their lives.

4. Lack of police protection against other crimes: streetwalkers especially, those women without jobs in safer massage parlors or houses, who are often raped, beaten and left unpaid.

5. The arrest and prosecution of prostitutes while clients (most of them are white, middle-aged, middle-class married men) go free.

6. The racism and class bias that lead to the arrest and imprisonment of far more prostitutes of color and poor women than white women, even though the invisible majority of hookers are white and middle class.

As a middle-class white woman, trained as a registered nurse, I could work in a private call business instead of hitting the streets. I was arrested but never did time in prison; the system isn't aimed at putting me in jail. Women of color have less easy access to places like upper-class hotels, where if you're black and alone you're automatically tagged as a hooker. So they're in the streets and in the bars, where they are more visible and more vulnerable to exploitation and arrest—and they're the ones who end up in jail.‡

*Examples of such groups are COYOTE (Call Off Your Old Tired Ethics) in San Francisco and PUMA (Prostitutes Union of Massachusetts). For more information, contact the National Task Force on Prostitution, P.O. Box 26354, San Francisco, CA 94126. Ask for their newsletter, *Coyote Howls.*
†See, for instance, *Sex Work*, edited by Frédérique Delacoste and Priscilla Alexander (Pittsburgh: Cleis Press, 1987).
‡Prison life in itself is brutal. This, combined with the lack of job opportunities once a woman gets out, makes prison hard to avoid again for many women. Seventy percent of women in prison today were first jailed for prostitution.

Some feminists have been critical of prostitutes for reinforcing sex-role stereotypes by allowing themselves to be sex objects. Prostitutes point out that they are no different from most women in having to sell their services to men. In the words of an ex-prostitute:

I've worked in straight jobs where I've felt more like I was prostituting my being than in prostitution. I had less control over my life, and the powerlessness wasn't even up front. People didn't see me as selling myself, but with the minimum wage so little and my boss so insulting, I felt like I was selling my soul.

In a world where women have so little power, nearly all women depend in some way on men's money, protection, favor. Many who are not hookers, for example, feel they must have sex when their man wants to because he provides financial or emotional security. From feminist Karen Lindsey:

The question of whether or not to sell ourselves to men is a false one: the real question is how *to sell ourselves in the way that is least destructive to ourselves and our sisters. That is not a decision any one of us can make for any of the others. . . . Prostitutes don't need our condescension. What they need is our alliance. And we need theirs.*[10]

Prostitutes have organized in this country and Europe (including the famous French Prostitutes Strike in 1975) to demand *decriminalization*, the abolition of all laws against prostitution. (Legalizing prostitution isn't enough. In West Germany, where women work in government-run houses, prostitutes feel they have traded illegal pimps for a legal one: They have little control over their working conditions and still turn over a big part of their income in fees.) With decriminalization, prostitutes would have more control over their work and the money they earn. Most of all, they would no longer go to jail for providing a service that society itself puts in such high demand and for choosing the highest-paying work available to them. A longer-range goal is, in the words of a PUMA member, that "no woman should have to be a prostitute because she has no alternatives." From a British prostitute: "The end of women's poverty is the end of prostitution."

NOTES

1. Susan Griffin. *Rape—The Power of Consciousness.* San Francisco: Harper & Row, 1979, p. 3.
2. A study reported in 1981 revealed that women far more than men report that fear curtails their daily activities. The most fearful women are the elderly, the poor and members of racial/ethnic minorities. Stephanie Riger and Margaret Gordon. "The Fear of Rape: A Study in Social Control," *Journal of Social Issues*, Vol. 37 (1981), pp. 71–92. See also: Brenda Seery and Michelle Clossick. "Violence Survey What You Told Us," *Ms.* magazine, Vol. 1, No. 5 (1991), pp. 35–43.
3. A study in 1980 found that black women were less likely to have their rape cases come to trial and to result in conviction than white women. G.D. LaFree. "Variables Affecting Guilty Pleas and Convictions in Rape Cases—Toward a Social Theory of Rape Processing," *Social Forces*, Vol. 58 (1980), pp. 833–50.
4. "Breaking the Cycle," *Newsletter of the Vermont Governor's Commission on the Status of Women*, September–October 1980.
5. Mildred Daley Pagelow, "Factors Affecting Women's Decisions to Leave Violent Relationships," *Journal of Family Issues*, Vol. 2, No. 4 (December 1981).
6. "Letter from a Battered Woman," in *For Shelter and Beyond*. Boston, MA: Massachusetts Coalition of Battered Women Service Groups, 1981, p. 6.
7. Lisa Leghorn. "Social Responses to Battered Women." Paper presented at the Wisconsin Conference on Battered Women, October 2, 1976.
8. "Letter from a Battered Woman."
9. Several of the "during an attack" suggestions have been adapted from Milwaukee Task Force on Battered Women, *Battered Women: A Handbook for Survival*, rev. ed., 1978; and from Jennifer Baker Fleming, *Stopping Wife Abuse* (Garden City, NY: Anchor Press/Doubleday, 1979), pp. 32–33.
10. Karen Lindsey. "Beginning to Demystify the Oldest Profession," *The Second Wave*, Summer 1976.

RESOURCES

Books

Armstrong, Louise. *The Home Front: Notes from the Family War Zone.* New York: McGraw-Hill, 1983.
———. *Kiss Daddy Goodnight: Ten Years Later.* New York: Simon & Schuster, 1987.
Backhouse, Constance, and Leah Cohen. *Sexual Harassment on the Job.* Englewood Cliffs, NJ: Prentice-Hall, 1981. Case studies, history, analysis of the problem and action plans for management and unions are covered.
Barry, Kathleen. *Female Sexual Slavery.* Englewood Cliffs, NJ: Prentice-Hall, 1979. Cross-cultural evidence documents the international slave trade connected to prostitution, genital mutilation, rape, battering, incest and pornography.
Bart, Pauline, and Patricia O'Brien. *Stopping Rape: Successful Survival Strategies.* Elmsford, NY: Pergamon Press, 1985.
Bart, Pauline, et al., eds. "Violence Against Women," special issue of *Gender and Society*, Vol. 3, No. 4 (December 1989). Available from Sage Publications, 2455 Teller Rd., Newbury Park, CA 91320.
Bass, Ellen, and Laura Davis. *The Courage to Heal: A Guide for Women Survivors of Sexual Abuse.* New York: Harper & Row, 1988.
Blume, E. Sue. *Secret Survivors: Uncovering Incest and*

Its Aftereffects in Women. New York: Ballantine Books, 1991.

Bowker, L., and L. Maurer. "The Medical Treatment of Battered Wives," *Women and Health,* Vol. 12, No. 1 (1987), pp. 25–45.

Brady, Maureen. *Daybreak: Meditations for Women Survivors of Sexual Abuse.* New York: HarperCollins/Hazelden, 1991.

Brendtro, M., and L. Bowker. "Battered Women: How Can Nurses Help?" *Issues in Mental Health Nursing,* Vol. 10, No. 2 (1989); pp. 169–80.

Butler, Sandra. *Conspiracy of Silence: The Trauma of Incest.* Volcano, CA: Volcano Press, 1985.

Candib, Lucy M. "Violence Against Women: No More Excuses," *Family Medicine,* Vol. 21, No. 5 (September/October 1989), pp. 341–42.

———. "Violence as a Gender Issue," in M. K. Hendricks-Matthews, ed., *The Society of Teachers of Family Medicine Violence Education Monograph.* Kansas City, MO: STFM Publications, 1992.

Cantrell, Leslie. *Into the Light: A Guide for Battered Women.* Edmonds, WA: The Charles Franklin Press, 1986.

Courtois, Christine A. *Healing the Incest Wound: Adult Survivors in Therapy.* New York: W.W. Norton, 1988.

Davis, Angela. "The Dialectics of Rape," *Ms.* (June 1975), 74ff. The author relates the case of JoAnne Little to the history of rape and racism in the United States.

———. *Violence Against Women and the Ongoing Challenge to Racism.* New York: Women of Color Press, 1988.

Davis, Laura. *Allies in Healing: When the Person You Love Was Sexually Abused as a Child.* New York: HarperCollins, 1991.

———. *The Courage to Heal Workbook for Women and Men Survivors of Child Sexual Abuse.* New York: Harper & Row, 1990.

DeSalvo, Louise. *Virginia Woolf: The Impact of Childhood Sexual Abuse on Her Life and Work.* New York: Ballantine Books, 1989.

Estrich, Susan. *Real Rape.* Cambridge, MA: Harvard University Press, 1987.

Farley, Lin. *Sexual Shakedown: The Sexual Harassment of Women on the Job.* New York: McGraw-Hill, 1978. An analysis of the origins of sexual harassment in the economic system and in women's subordinate status within society.

Gil, Eliana. *Treatment of Adult Survivors of Childhood Abuse.* Walnut Creek, CA: Launch Press, 1990.

Herman, Judith L. *Father-Daughter Incest.* Cambridge, MA/London: Harvard University Press, 1981.

Jones, Ann. *Women Who Kill.* New York: Fawcett Crest, 1988.

Lederer, Laura, ed. *Take Back the Night: Women on Pornography.* New York: William Morrow, 1980.

Levy, Barrie. *Dating Violence: Young Women in Danger.* Seattle, WA: Seal Press, 1991.

Lobel, Kerry, ed. *Naming the Violence: Speaking Out About Lesbian Battering.* Seattle, WA: Seal Press, 1986.

Mackinnon, Catherine A. *Sexual Harassment of Working Women: A Case of Sexual Discrimination.* New Haven, CT: Yale University Press, 1979.

Martin, Del. *Battered Wives.* New York: Simon & Schuster/Pocket Books, 1983.

Massachusetts Coalition of Battered Women's Service Groups. *For Shelter and Beyond: An Educational Manual for Working with Women Who Are Battered.* Provides practical information on counseling and advocacy, and covers a range of issues that confront service providers in shelters. Available from MCBWSG, 107 South Street, Suite 504, Boston, MA 02111.

Mattz, Wendy, and Beverly Holman. *Incest and Sexuality: A Guide to Understanding and Healing.* Lexington, MA: D.C. Heath/Lexington Books, 1987.

Miller, Alice. *Banished Knowledge: Facing Childhood Injuries.* New York: Doubleday, 1990.

———. *Thou Shalt Not Be Aware: Society's Betrayal of the Child.* New York: Penguin/Meridian, 1990.

NiCarthy, Ginny. *Getting Free: A Handbook for Women in Abusive Relationships.* Seattle, WA: Seal Press, 1986.

———. *The Ones Who Got Away: Women Who Left Abusive Partners.* Seattle, WA: Seal Press, 1987.

Randall, Margaret. *This Is About Incest.* Ithaca, NY: Firebrand Books, 1987.

Lerner, Gerda. "The Rape of Black Women as a Weapon of Terror," in Gerda Lerner, ed., *Black Women in White America: A Documentary History.* New York: Vintage Books (1972), pp. 172–93.

Rush, Florence. *The Best Kept Secret: Sexual Abuse of Children.* Englewood Cliffs, NJ: Prentice-Hall, 1980. Rush documents the history of sexual abuse of children by reviewing the Bible, myths, fairy tales and popular literature.

Russell, Diana E.H. *The Politics of Rape: The Victim's Perspective.* New York: Stein and Day, 1984.

———. *Rape in Marriage. Expanded and Revised.* Bloomington: Indiana University Press, 1990.

———. *The Secret Trauma: Incest in the Lives of Girls and Women.* New York: HarperCollins, 1986.

Sanford, Linda Tschirhart. *Silent Children—A Book for Parents About the Prevention of Sexual Abuse.* Garden City, NY: Anchor Press/Doubleday, 1980.

———. *Strong at the Broken Places: Overcoming the Trauma of Childhood Abuse.* New York: Random House, 1990.

Schechter, Susan. *Women and Male Violence: The Struggles of the Battered Women's Movement.* Boston: South End Press, 1982. A description of the origins and evolution of the contemporary battered-women's movement and a critical analysis of major developments.

Seery, Brenda, and Michelle Clossick. "Violence Survey: What You Told Us," *Ms.,* Vol. 1, No. 5 (March/April 1991), p. 35.

Survivor Newsletter Collective. *For Crying Out Loud: A Newsletter for Women Survivors of Child Sexual Abuse.* Survivor Newsletter Collective, 46 Pleasant Street, Cambridge, MA 02139.

Warrior, Betsy. *Working on Wife Abuse.* 46 Pleasant Street, Cambridge, MA 02139. Continually updated since the mid-1970s, this directory is an extensive resource list of organizations and individuals working against battering. Other practical materials, such as sample forms and policies of shelters, are also included. (Available by writing to the Women's Center at the Pleasant Street address.)

Warshaw, Robin. *I Never Called It Rape: The Ms. Report on Recognizing, Fighting and Surviving Date and Acquaintance Rape*. New York: Harper & Row, 1988.

White, Evelyn. *Chain Chain Change: Black Women Dealing with Physical and Emotional Abuse*. Seattle, WA: Seal Press, 1985.

Wise, Sue, and Liz Stanley. *Georgie Porgie: Sexual Harassment in Everyday Life*. New York: Pandora, 1987.

Wisechild, Louise M., ed. *She Who Was Lost Is Remembered: Healing from Incest Through Creativity*. Seattle, WA: Seal Press, 1991.

Articles

Bowker, L., and L. Maurer. "The Medical Treatment of Battered Wives," *Women and Health*, Vol. 12, No. 1 (1987), pp. 25–45.

Brendtro, M., and L. Bowker. "Battered Women: How Can Nurses Help?" *Issues in Mental Health Nursing*, Vol. 10, No. 2 (1989), pp. 169–80.

Candib, Lucy M. "Violence Against Women: No More Excuses," *Family Medicine*, Vol. 21, No. 5 (September/October 1989), pp. 341–42.

Seery, Brenda, and Michelle Clossick. "Violence Survey: What You Told Us," *Ms.*, Vol. 1, No. 5 (March/April 1991), p. 35.

Magazines and Newsletters

The Cutting Edge
P.O. Box 20819
Cleveland, OH 44120
A newsletter by and for women who self injure.

Spare Rib
Spare Rib Ltd.
27 Clerkenwell Close
London, England EC1ROAT
A British feminist magazine, which is a good source of articles describing protests over violence against women in the media.

Survivorship
318 Mission No. 19
San Francisco, CA 94110
A newsletter for survirors of ritual abuse.

Audiovisual Materials

After the Montreal Massacre, a 27-minute 1990 film. A documentary about the 1989 shootings at the University of Montreal, situating the massacre in the context of violence against women and a backlash against feminism. Interviews survivors and other students. Available from Women Make Movies, 225 Lafayette Street, Room 212, New York, NY 10012, (212) 925-0606.

Breaking Silence, A Film on Incest and the Sexual Abuse of Children, a 58-minute 1985 16-mm film/video. Available from New Day Films, 121 West 27th Street, Suite 902, New York, NY 10001, (212) 645-8210.

The Confrontation: Latinas Fight Back Against Rape, a 37-minute 1983 black-and-white 16-mm film/video. Available from Women Make Movies, 225 Lafayette Street, Room 212, New York, NY 10012, (212) 925-0606.

Dating Rights: Gang Rape on Campus. Available from Filmakers Library, 124 East 40th Street, New York, NY 10016.

Delores, a 50-minute 1988 film. Addresses the problem of domestic violence in Latino communities through a dramatization of relationships in a Hispanic family. Available from the Cinema Guild, 1697 Broadway, Suite 802, New York, NY 10019. (212) 246-5522.

In Need of Special Attention, a 17-minute film, with training manual, designed to assist emergency room staff in establishing protocol for battered women. Available from ODN Productions, 74 Varick Street, Room 304, New York, NY 10013; and 1454 Sixth Street, Berkeley, CA 94710. Other films also available.

Not A Love Story, a 69-minute 1981 film about the content of pornography and its relationship to physical acts of violence. Not as open to sexuality, particularly lesbian and gay sexuality, as other films, but still a good discussion starter. Rated X. Available from the National Film Board of Canada, 1251 Avenue of the Americas, New York, NY 10010.

Rape/Crisis, an 87-minute film/video. An award-winning docudrama on the roots of sexual violence in our culture. Available from the Cinema Guild, 1697 Broadway, Suite 802, New York, NY 10019. (212) 246-5522.

Rape Culture, a 33-minute 1975 film. Uses excerpts from Hollywood movies and interviews with feminists and convicted rapists to illustrate the role of societal forces in promoting rape. Widely used. Available from Cambridge Documentary Films, P.O. Box 385, Cambridge, MA 02139. (617) 352-3677.

Rape: The Boundaries of Fear. Available from Barr Films, P.O. Box 7878, Irwindale, CA 91706.

Rape: Face to Face, a 55-minute video. Made by men. Available from Filmmakers Library, 124 East 40th Street, New York, NY 10016.

Rethinking Rape, a 26-minute 1986 film/video on acquaintance rape and its causes. Available from Film Distribution Center, TLPO Box 8293, Kirkland, WA 98034.

Still Killing Us Softly, a 30-minute 1987 film. About images of women in advertising. Explores violence and stereotyping. Available from Cambridge Documentary Films.

To Have and To Hold, a 20-minute film. Features interviews with men who have been Emerge's counselors and clients. Produced and distributed by Emerge, 18 Hurley Street, Cambridge, MA 02141.

Waking Up to Rape, a 35-minute 1985 16-mm film/video. Available from Women Make Movies, 225 Lafayette Street, Room 212, New York, NY 10012, (212) 925-0606.

We Will Not Be Beaten, a film or video. Features interviews with staff and residents of a shelter. It is a powerful analysis of the dynamics of battering, institutional response and the role of shelters. Available from Transition House Films, 120 Boylston Street, Boston, MA 02116.

Why Am I Hiding? Available from Rape Victim Advocates, 222 South Morgan Street, Chicago, IL 60607.

Organizations

Association of American Colleges, Project on the Status and Education of Women
1818 R Street NW
Washington, DC 20009

Coalition Against Trafficking in Women
Calder Square
P.O. Box 10077
State College, PA 16805-0077

Education Wife Assault
427 Bloor Street West
Toronto, Ontario, Canada
M5S 1X7
(416) 968-3422

Emerge
18 Hurley Street
Cambridge, MA 02141
(617) 547-9870
First men's group working with batterers, produced many useful materials, including a monograph, "Working with Men Who Batter."

Independent Living Center of the North Shore
583 Chestnut Street
Lynn, MA 01904
(617) 593-7500 Voice/TTY
Publishes the pamphlet "Women and Self Injury" and offers support groups.

Model Mugging
801 Lighthouse Avenue
Monterey, CA 93940
(408) 659-2041
An innovative course that teaches women to defend themselves in simulated rape situations against an instructor dressed as a mugger (with protective clothing and equipment). Contact Model Mugging for a program near you.

National Clearinghouse on Battered Women's Self-Defense
524 McKnight Street
Reading, PA 19601
(215) 373-5697

National Clearinghouse on Marital and Date Rape (NCOMDR)
Women's History Research, Inc.
2325 Oak Street
Berkeley, CA 94708
(415) 524-1582
Offers phone consultation, document search, date rape packet, state law chart, speakers and internships.

National Coalition Against Domestic Violence
(202) 293-8860

National Coalition Against Sexual Assault (NCASA)
P.O. Box 21378
Washington, D.C. 20009
(202) 483-7165
A national membership organization, NCASA sponsors annual conferences and publishes a newsletter. Regional representatives facilitate the exchange of information and resources.

National Domestic Violence Hotline
1 (800) 333-SAFE

Violence Against Women Act Task Force
NOW Legal Defense and Education Fund
99 Hudson Street
New York, NY 10013
(212) 925-6635

Washington, D.C. Rape Crisis Center
P.O. Box 21005
Washington, DC 20009
As one of the first rape crisis centers in the United States, this center played an important role in fostering communications between projects. Publishes *How to Start a Rape Crisis Center*, an excellent resource for new programs. $5.00.

Relationships and Sexuality

Introduction

BY WENDY SANFORD, WITH
PAULA BROWN DORESS

NEW FACE

I have learned not to worry about love;
but to honor its coming
with all my heart.
To examine the dark mysteries
of the blood
with headless heed and
swirl,
to know the rush of feelings
swift and flowing
as water.
The source appears to be
some inexhaustible
spring
within our twin and triple
selves;
the new face I turn up
to you
no one else on earth
has ever
seen.

ALICE WALKER

Loving is essential to our lives. Most of the people we love we are not sexually involved with; some we are. Sexual relationships are intense, puzzling, frustrating, energizing, potentially oppressive and potentially freeing. They enable us to learn about ourselves and our lovers and to get close in ways we never expected. They raise issues of power and vulnerability, commitment and risk. Sexual relationships can be painful; a long-time union breaks up, a love affair promises much and then fizzles, a lover dies, a marriage turns abusive. Yet most of us want and need intimacy, so that we usually recover from the hurt and try again.

This unit looks closely at our sexual relationships. What do they give us? How can we make them more what we want? What is unique to sexual relationships with men? With women? How can we understand our sexuality better and enjoy it more? How can we change the social structures and attitudes about age, disability, sex roles, sexual orientation, which keep us from freely loving others and ourselves?

PROLOGUE: SEXUAL ORIENTATION

Over the past three decades more and more women have spoken openly about their choice, as lesbians, of women lovers and partners. Encouraged by the women's movement to be more open about sexuality, many women who are mainly involved with men have also begun to speak of their sexual feelings or fantasies about women. That every woman is innately heterosexual is a myth.

More than thirty years ago, research by Kinsey showed that most people have both heterosexual and homosexual feelings. A woman might have played around sexually with girls and boys in her childhood or fallen in love with her best girlfriend in high school, then married a man. Another who had been involved with men for thirty years may find herself choosing women at fifty. Some women are sexually and emotionally intimate with both women and men through their lives.

As we come to understand that most people have some same-sex feelings, we begin to accept a lot of things we were taught to fear. In our families and schools people either didn't mention lesbians or gay men at all or joked cruelly about them; they made us feel hesitant about some of our closest female friendships.

When I was seven or eight, I had this best friend, Susan. We loved each other and walked around with our arms around each other. Her older sister told us not to do that anymore because we looked like lesies. So we held hands instead.

We became aware that society penalizes lesbians through job discrimination and violence. In these and other ways, our culture teaches us an irrational fear and hatred of homosexuality in ourselves and others (*homophobia*). Homophobia insults those of us who are lesbian and bisexual and makes our lives unnecessarily difficult. It also hurts those of us who are heterosexual. Fear and prejudice turn us against lesbian friends and family members, depriving us of important relationships. Homophobia makes us fear and dislike aspects of our own personality and looks that are not "feminine" enough (assertiveness, muscular build, body hair, deep voice). It causes us to deny attractions that are natural to us and may prevent us from choosing the sexual partners who are right for us. And it divides us from each other as women.*

With time, familiarity and friendship we can unlearn homophobia.

The main thing that finally helped me start letting go of my homophobia was getting to know a few lesbian women. As we became friends, the myths I'd heard about lesbians—that they are mannish, oversexed, undersexed or out to seduce straight women—fell away. They were just like everyone else.

Once I admitted to myself that I do have sexual feelings for women, I didn't feel so alarmed by lesbians anymore. It was as if they had represented something in myself I was scared of.

Even after I became a lesbian at thirty-five, I found that I had big doses of homophobia inside me. Sometimes I'd wake up after having sex with a woman I loved and have an attack of thinking that the wonderful thing we'd done was "queer." Or I'd get upset when other dykes seemed "too obvious" in public. Slowly I've become prouder and more deeply affirming of lesbians and lesbianism—that is, of myself.

Many heterosexual women believe they know no lesbians personally. However, chances are we all know a number of lesbians who simply don't feel safe being open about it.

OPENING UP HETEROSEXUALITY TO CHOICE

Some lesbians today are asking their heterosexual sisters to reconsider the naturalness of heterosexual preference. Can heterosexuality be a free choice when we are taught such a deep fear of loving women? Can we comfortably assume that women are naturally drawn to men when we consider the many cruelties that drive us to seek protection from men and punish us for being alone: rape and sexual harassment, consistently lower pay for women workers, the lack of economic protection for widows, the derision of "old maids," the fact that prostitution is often the only available work that pays enough to support a family? If it is unsafe anywhere to be a woman without a man, then heterosexuality is not so much natural as *compulsory.**

Compulsory heterosexuality may make us feel desperate when we're not with a man, and cause us to jump into the arms of men who are available but not good for us. It means we never have a chance to make a real choice, to ask ourselves whether we would be happier with a man, a woman or alone. Free to ask these questions, we might well end up choosing to be with men, but we would be responding to what we genuinely want and not to what society tells us we ought to want.†

---

*Homophobia is politically useful for those who want to preserve the traditional forms of family life and to suppress any alternatives.

---

*See Adrienne Rich's important and challenging article, "Compulsory Heterosexuality and Lesbian Existence," in her *Blood, Bread, and Poetry*, New York: W.W. Norton, 1986.
†Chapter 11, "Sexuality," seeks to break down false separations by including experiences with both men and women. We wrote two separate chapters on relationships because it first seemed to us that lesbians and heterosexual women encounter different pressures and possibilities. But we learned from each other that we face many similar issues, whether our partners are women or men.

FEAR OF LESBIANS AND OUR UNITY AS WOMEN

Some women hesitate to join feminist projects because friends and family assume that being a feminist means one is a lesbian. Ultraconservative political and religious groups play on these fears by portraying all feminists as overbearing man haters and actual or would-be lesbians. Using homophobia as a tool to divide us and turn us against each other, they rob us of our energy and unity as a movement of women trying to build a more just society for everyone. On the other hand, some lesbians struggling for legitimacy and acceptance suggest that "straight" women are less feminist than lesbians or that "true" feminists wouldn't ally themselves with men in any way. As a collective of women with varied sexual choices, we hope all women will feel safe enough in this society to become less condemning of each other's choices. We urge more heterosexual women who share feminist goals and visions to identify themselves openly as feminists. The women's movement will become a stronger force for social change when women of all sexual orientations can find friendship, growth and power within it.

9

Working Toward Mutuality: Our Relationships with Men

By Paula Brown Doress
and Peggy Nelson
Wegman

With special thanks to Catherine
Cobb Morocco, Sandy Rosenthal
and Elizabeth Matz.

*This chapter in previous editions was
called "Living with Ourselves and
Others—Our Sexual Relationships,"
by Paula Brown Doress and Nancy P.
Hawley.*

What do we value about our relationships? Some women's voices:*

The best thing is that we have a long, intimate history together and still feel connected to and admiring and turned on to each other. I consider it a minor miracle as I look around me. I have learned that my husband has many of the same weak feelings—fragile feelings—that I used to think were female—just as he has learned that I have certain kinds of strengths that he doesn't have. The crucial thing is to take time to build up confidence and trust and comfort and kindness. [forty, married twenty years]

Even with all my wonderful friends and my job, which I love, and my dancing and my cat and everything else, life used to be very lonely. Simple little details could suddenly seem so hard . . . like finding someone to go to the laundromat with. Now that I love Mark I really don't live much differently than I did before, but life feels quite different. We are committed to each other in a way that transcends the

little daily ups and downs. Having him there, even with all the fights and issues we have yet to resolve, is like a big, soft cushion between me and the roughness of life. [single, mid-twenties]

The hard thing about widowhood is that I have lost the person I held hands with in life. I was extremely important to my husband. . . . When I was unhappy I could always go to him and talk to him, and when I was happy he had a smile from ear to ear. He gave me unlimited support throughout my whole married life. I don't have that anymore. That's a very, very important loss. I've made up for it by relying more on other close people in my life. I have a close friend that I can call at the drop of a hat and say, "Something is bothering me and I have to talk to you about it," and I'm extremely close with my children. I need about a dozen close people to fill in for the loss of that one special relationship. [sixty-eight, widowed three years]

He has a deep, keen interest in what I do, in my work and my interests, that no other man I've been involved with has ever had. It's absolutely essential that the man I love be tuned in to feminism and able to live that out in a day-to-day way. The mutuality, the give and take and the constant questioning of gender stereotype is critical. And it's not just on an intellectual plane, either; it's also about the mun-

---

*This chapter is one of the chapters most based on our experiences as white middle-class women. We hope you will find it useful and provocative as you think about your relationships with men, but we don't pretend to speak to or for women with very different kinds of experiences.

dane stuff like taking care of the house and doing the dishes, not just who does things but who thinks about what has to be done. [thirties, married one year]

The best thing about my marriage is that I have a real friend. When you've done a lot of things together you have a commonality of ethics, a way of looking at the world that is terribly important, so I trust my husband a lot. [sixties, married thirty-nine years]

THE PERSONAL IS POLITICAL

We want to be close to other people—to matter to them, to know that they will be there when we need them, to feel safe, loving and loved—this closeness is essential to our well-being. Most women seek to fulfill much of this need for closeness through intimate sexual relationships with men. As we grew up, many of us learned one pattern or model for these relationships: Our families and communities expected us to marry and have children; men would earn the most money, have the most important jobs and be more logical, while we would cook and "keep house" and be more aware of feelings and relationships. This was the way things had to be, and when our lives fit this pattern we would automatically be happy.

But during the past twenty-five years, with the recent wave of the feminist movement, we began to question these assumptions and affirm one of the basic principles of the feminist movement— that our lives, work, ideas, perceptions and wishes are important, as important as those of men, and that society should be reorganized to reflect and support this belief. We saw that most heterosexual relationships in this culture reflect those old assumptions about women and men. In talking with each other, at first tentatively, about our lives, our dissatisfactions, frustrations and sometimes anger began to crystalize and became newly articulated feelings that affected each of our lives differently: Some of us worked with our husbands or lovers at changing what went on between us; longstanding relationships that just couldn't change in response to our new visions broke up. Some of us lived with each other in communal living situations, decided not to marry or chose to live only with women. Although our examination of male–female relationships led to a variety of "solutions," some women came to equate feminism with hating men and rejecting marriage and family, and many of these women became reluctant to identify with the women's movement.

However, many of us were committed to finding ways to live out our feminist beliefs without having to give up intimate relationships with men. Frustration and anger don't mean that we want

to end these relationships; instead, they make us determined to change them.

When I work on women's issues, I have an appropriate outlet for my angry feelings, and I direct my anger at the source of what oppresses women and not only at individual men in my life. Often I am less angry toward men than a lot of women who shy away from being associated with feminism.

We are not proposing any fixed model of "The Ideal Couple Relationship." How we talk together, how we play and fight and work and make love grow not from any external prescription but from who we are. We do propose that the price of the intimacy we build together should not be our own richness as individuals, that we see each other not simply as two halves of a whole, each with our own immutable territory, but as two separate, whole people who have chosen to touch closely, to build something together, to intertwine—enriching one another, rather than detracting from the potential ways that each may grow. Working toward an egalitarian relationship is not a matter of creating a one-time grand design that will guide us for years to come, but a slow and continuing process of negotiation, compromise and renegotiation.

Changes will occur, for the most part, slowly and in very small steps. In an efficiency-minded, goal-oriented culture heavily influenced by technology, these small, slow processes of fixing and adjusting are neither taught nor valued. We live in a disposable age: When it breaks, throw it out and get a new one. When *we* speak of commitment, we don't mean the traditional pressure to be "committed" to a relationship at all costs, which has often meant letting go of our needs or putting up with an empty or abusive relationship. We have in mind a true commitment to a process of working on the relationship, which may make things harder for a time as we attempt to make them better. It involves risk taking, constant questioning and not always waiting for the right moment to bring up a problem. It also means being willing to change as we are asking our men to change. We cannot always be sure how things will evolve; despite our most valiant efforts the relationship may end, and sometimes that may be for the best. Although there may be many other sources of tension between a woman and a man—personality differences, family history, ethnic and class differences, illness, economic hardship—this chapter focuses on the tension that comes from living in a culture based on inequality and limiting role definitions between the sexes. When we work toward an equal relationship we are, in effect, swimming against the tide.

Our culture stresses the importance of the individual rather than of the group and teaches us to believe that our personal circumstances and problems arise from qualities within us, from our own individual histories, our personalities and our conscious choices. As a result, most of us tend not to see the ways in which gender, race and class affect personal choices. The feminist insight that "the personal is political" expresses our belief— that what seem like personal problems are often symptoms of larger social problems.

This chapter is about our vision and about how our culture's values, expectations and structures affect our intimate relationships with men. In earlier editions of *Our Bodies, Ourselves* we focused on alternatives to couple relationships. In this edition we look at what goes on *within* heterosexual couple relationships because that is still the way so many women live.

BEING SINGLE

Some women prefer being single, either fitting lovers into our lives without living with them and settling down together or living with no romantic attachments at all. For those of us who want to make a major commitment to work, who have finished grieving the end of a relationship or who have already raised families, being single can be positive, creative and peaceful.

I simply don't plan my life around a man even when I am in love. There are so many other things that I want to do, too. I've had two husbands. I also have three grown kids. Naturally I still think about them, but not like when they were little. I can really focus on what I want to do now.

Now *ALONE* Is a Bed Partner

Now Alone *is a bed partner, is a
precious gem,
is a bandit she wants, is a woman with
silver hair,
is better than a man.*

*Alone was a gift she didn't recognize
when it first
arrived. She locked it in the bedroom
and stayed
downstairs. She wouldn't let it come
to meals.*

*She knew the sweet faces of her friends,
she didn't
trust* Alone *who slept in her mirror, in
her voice,
in the hollow where her hands covered
her eyes.*

*Alone was patient and when she took its
hand, it gave her
songs and poems, drawings and slow
breath, a peace
larger than sunset. Everyone felt it.
The children*

*drew around her as if she were the
hearth.*
*Alone moved in as no one else could,
unpossessive,
leaving space for women and men to
interact with her. Now*

*Alone is there in the morning and
welcomes her home
and wants nothing from her and gives all
of itself
to her and never turns her away.*

JUDITH W. STEINBERGH

However, being single can be hard because in our society, couples are the norm.

A single woman . . . is not buttressed by a family and the responsibilities of a family. . . . She has made a choice that cuts her off from a lot of things most people consider life, for the sake of something else, something both chancy and intangible. No wonder anxiety is the constant attendant of such a one![1]

A survey of single women and men in thirty-six states found that the best aspect of being single was freedom and the worst, loneliness. Men and women who wrote comments for the survey agreed that being single is more difficult for a woman than a man because

- Women have less sexual and social freedom.
- Divorced women more often have responsibility for children.
- Women are more vulnerable to physical abuse.
- Women earn less money and have less social mobility.
- Women have been socialized to feel stigmatized by not being attached to a man.

Only one-third of single men and one-fifth of single women in the study liked or desired the single life. The rest regarded it as a waiting period, a special, limited time to do things they'd never done or a time to look for a new partner.[2]

There are powerful social pressures to be in a couple, especially one kind of couple—married, heterosexual, racially alike. The pressure starts early. Storybooks and movies of our girlhoods ended with romantic marriage and perpetual bliss. Relatives asked us at age three or four who our boyfriends were and at twenty when we were going to marry and have children. Recently it has

from "Sylvia" by Nicole Hollander

become more socially acceptable not to marry and not to have children, but the pressure to be part of a couple persists. Indeed, the idea of the "relationship" has taken on some of the mystique formerly reserved for marriage and the nuclear family. Even after divorce or the death of a partner, friends assume we are seeking another relationship. Lesbians and heterosexual women alike often believe that we have to be in a couple to be fulfilled.

When I think of the hours I've spent in bars and at parties trying to meet someone, I am bitter about such wasted energy. I could have started my own business or earned a degree in that time.

Our communities are organized on the premise that the family will meet nearly all our needs for intimacy and continuity. Close friends may organize their social life only around couples.

When I got divorced, I kept all my women friends, but I noticed they would only invite me to lunch. At dinner when their husbands were home they had couples over. It was as if at night I became another species altogether.

There are economic pressures to be in a couple. Women experience severe wage and salary discrimination and are often financially insecure and overworked.

I am part of a circle of friends who have been single for most of the past ten years. We moved fairly easily in and out of relationships or were involved in several at a time. Now all of a sudden everyone is coupling off. You know, I think it's the economy and the state of the world. Many of my friends are teachers and social-service workers who are being laid off and losing their pensions and health insurance, too. When people are scared they want to be with someone else.

It can be hard to imagine being older and single.

I love my life the way it is now—the freedom to be with different partners or not with any, living by my own rhythms, feeling strong and happy with myself. But sometimes when I wake up in the middle of the night I see myself old and alone, and it is terribly scary and empty.

Ageism makes us fear growing older, because we assume that old people don't have friends or community, that someone who's not with a partner will be totally alone. For many of us it is literally dangerous to be alone because of violence and sexual harassment.

Afraid to be alone, we often jump into relationships only to discover that we have chosen too quickly: Our partners aren't good for us; we have given up too much of what we really wanted and our very neediness lessens our relative power within the relationship.

Community is especially important to us as single women. We can develop strong, intimate friendships which stay with us throughout life and make being alone and growing old much less frightening.

I hope I'll be growing old together with Dan, but since he is considerably older [eighteen years] than me it is possible that he will die before me. Then I imagine growing old with Margie, who has been my best friend for the past fifteen years. I like thinking of us as old women together.

We live in a time when it is acceptable for women to work and live in more varied ways than ever before. It is important to acknowledge that many women feel lonely, and for us to give one another support both for our lives as single women and for our efforts to find a partner. Although we don't want to be pressured to find someone and get married, neither do we want friends to assume that we love being single. It is up to us to let people know if we *are* interested in meeting someone. Loving ourselves more when our community values us, we are more likely, when and if we go out looking for a partner, to find a person who will be right for us. Surrounded by the affection and caring of friends and family, we become less vulnerable to exploitative relationships, more able to resist the emphasis on being or becoming part of a couple.

When I broke up with my lover I luckily had a circle of warm affectionate friends who would give me a hug or a pat on the back. Yet I felt the lack of that very intimate whole-body contact. I didn't want to rush precipitously into a new relationship just because I felt so hungry to be touched. One answer was to get a massage every other week for several months.

When my younger sister got engaged, my parents bought each of us a beautiful set of cookware. They said they loved us both and wanted to support the life choices that each of us was making by getting us each something for our homes. I felt so affirmed because I understood they were saying, "This is your life, and we value you and your choices."

Here is what she loves deeply
*   her work she drives into with the sun*
*   polishing wet roads to chrome,*
*   her son who waits, feigning sleep*
*   in his crib until he can caress her face,*
*   her golden-haired, blue-eyed, hell-bent,*
*   anti-authoritarian daughter who says*
*   shit at the right time,*
*   her husband who has left her*

here is what she loves, but once removed
*   her men with tongues, who put their mouths on*
*   hers,*
*   who make her laugh deeply into the night, who*
*   take her*
*   to bed during sesame street, who take her*
*   children*
*   to school, or haven't met her children, or never*
*   met a child at all, her men who juggle, who*
*   paint*
*   day after day landscapes that have never left the*
*   mind,*
*   who walk her on winter beaches, and fly her*
*   into*
*   the chambers of coral reefs.*

here is what she likes with an embarrassing relish
*   the luminescent stars and comets she's stuck on*
*   her*

ceiling, the thought of toads in her husband's
*   lover's*
bed, her bell bird clanging a pottery sea bell
*   sound,*
her shells, colored powders, beach stones, sheep
*   bones,*
ropes of feathers, long Indian skirts, filmy violet
*   scarves,*
snow over the lakes to ski on, her children's bare
*   bodies,*
summer with a wind in the moors, the stitching
*   of night*
with the loon's pointed sound

here is what she needs and keeps her
a net of women so strong that when she falls
from the tightrope she walks day after day
sometimes with easy precision, sometimes
with wire cutting her feet into bands,
sometimes with a fatigue so great
her dreams have to hold her, that when she falls,
her women friends tighten their almost
invisible web, and she bounces and breathes,
bounces and weaves every fiber of their strength
into her own body, bounces and is free in a way
that will let her bounce against them again,
she bounces and soars, a dark bird
against the stadium lights, swoops to the crowd
and is off, a speck in the cranberry dawn.

JUDITH W. STEINBERGH

EXPLORING MAJOR AREAS OF TENSION IN HETEROSEXUAL RELATIONSHIPS

Toward Shared Power in Relationships

All kinds of power come into play in our relationships—personal, physical, spiritual, social, economic and political.* However, women and men belong to groups that have different degrees of power. The resulting imbalance inevitably influences the way we think, act and relate to each other. How people perceive and treat us outside our relationships inevitably affects how we feel within them. Until recently the "ideal" heterosexual relationship has been a marriage in which a man supports a woman economically and shares his status with her. In return she is responsible for the personal and household services that enable him to perform his role in society without such "menial" distractions. In contrast we envision a relationship in which each partner would support the other, so both play a role in the world outside the home as well as in the home, and one partner does not gain power at the expense of the other.

---

*A crucial part of our personal/political power is having control over our bodies and our lives through reproductive and sexual choice (see p. 714).

Social and Economic Power

We think of politics as having to do with power relationships among large-scale groups and nations, but there is a politics of intimate relationships as well. However strong our commitments to each other and to treating one another as equals may be, it is naive to think that widely held social attitudes and pervasive institutional practices will not affect what goes on between us. For example, a conflict within a heterosexual relationship is not simply a conflict between two persons who are everywhere regarded as social equals, but between two people who have different standing before the law (especially if married) and different rights and privileges.* Most societal institutions are thoroughly permeated with the assumption that the rights of men should take precedence over the rights of women. Because money is the most common source of power in this society and frequently symbolizes social power, it is not surprising that the person who brings economic resources into a family or a relationship has increased power.†

This society values and rewards men's work a great deal more than women's work. Most women cannot bring in an equal amount of money, for we earn on the average only 71 percent of what men earn.[4]

Men automatically hold the power in a relationship because they usually earn more money. If a man abuses this power imbalance, he may show it during the early stages of a relationship by making a woman feel indebtedness to him and implying that she should "repay" him with sexual favors. If he does this, watch out. In the words of a forty-year-old divorced woman:

A man took me out, and on the second or third date he wanted to sleep with me. So I told him I didn't want to be that intimate on so short an acquaintance. And he grumbled and said, "I just want to know if there's a pot of gold at the end of the rainbow."

Some men imply that paying for dates is burdensome, but may be reluctant to give up the control that goes with paying when offered a chance to share expenses. Others may be more flexible. A single woman in her twenties told us:

I believe in paying my share when I go out with a man. The man I'm involved with now earns a lot more money than I do, and he enjoys spending it on things that are fun. We often end up arguing about what kinds of things both of us can afford, which he feels limits us to what I can afford. Sometimes we compromise and he treats so we can do something special.

It is important to most people to be economically independent. As women we are socialized to see paid work as secondary to our job as wives and mothers, and believe that work and parenting are mutually exclusive choices. Or else we find work that we can balance with child care, usually low-paid "women's" occupations, for example, elementary-school teaching, secretarial work or waitressing, which pay far less than "men's" jobs.* When a woman cannot earn as much as a man, she (and he) are more likely to see her work as less important, more dispensable when children come, less important when a move is contemplated, less worth disrupting the family routine for. Even in couples that start out with egalitarian ideals and plans, the woman usually adapts more and more to the man. Because of this economic imbalance, a man may simply assume that it is his right to take charge. If a woman wants to make changes, she has to change his ideas as well as this conventional pattern. From a woman in her thirties:

When I buy something, even if it's for the house, I'm often afraid to tell Ron. He gets upset and says, "We can't afford it." But what he really means is that I shouldn't have bought it without consulting him. I get afraid to tell him because I think that since he earned the money, it's not really mine, even though he couldn't be out earning it if I weren't here running the house and taking care of the kids.

Sometimes I think getting a job and earning some money myself is the only thing that will resolve the conflict. But I get a strong message from Ron that he doesn't want me to work even though we could use the extra income. He's afraid that then he would have to deal with me differently.

This is not a simple disagreement about how to spend money, but raises the issue of decision-making power within the family.

When we were first married, I earned much less than Zach but enough to support myself. But from the time when our first child was born seven years ago, I have worked only part-time and my salary is very low. We could not find part-time work for both of us that paid well enough to support us. Neither of us

---

*We still need the Equal Rights Amendment to be equal before the law.

†In studies of married couples, wives who worked in paid employment were found to have greater power in family decision making than nonearning wives.[3]

*Because of a combination of sex discrimination and sex-role socialization, 40 percent of all women in the workforce are segregated into ten "women's occupations". These are so poorly paid—even teaching—that a woman supporting even one child and herself on the *average* salary of these occupations would be living below the poverty level.

wanted to have the children in full-time day care when they were young. Now that the children are both in school, I want to earn a living again. All along, Zach has regarded my work as equally important to his own but, in truth, I have more often left work to stay home with a sick child than he has, and while his identity comes largely from work, mine comes primarily from being a mother. I want to change this now and get on an equal footing.

It's going to be a long time before women get equal pay *or* equal work. Meanwhile we must insist in our relationships that the contribution of both people be equally valued.

Developing Our Personal Power

By "personal power" we mean self-reliance, assertiveness, the ability to earn a living, independence, self-confidence; many of us were taught to find a man with these qualities and literally attach ourselves to him ("If you can't be one, marry one"). In this way, we would become complete. Creating an intimate relationship with a man was not to be simply a way to enrich our lives but the foundation of our identities as whole adult people. Whom we are close to became confused with who we are. And so we faced a paradox: To feel stronger, many of us followed the best-traveled route and found a man, yet we were stepping into a role which only served to undermine our inner strength.

And what of physical strength? Many women have been taught that to be physically strong is unfeminine, and a man's greater physical strength can pose an unspoken threat of intimidation that causes all sorts of problems, from feeling overpowered in a sexual encounter to being intimidated in an argument. Because we live in a society where violence or the threat of violence is ever present, it is not surprising that we have such feelings. When we refuse to accept the cultural image of women as lacking in physical strength and competence, learn new skills and become physically stronger, our self-esteem grows.

One of the things I plunged myself into at age fifty-four was to take Tae Kwon Do (a Korean martial art). I had always been fascinated by martial arts but never had enough nerve to try it. I was stirring up long years of status quo; one more unorthodoxy didn't matter, I reasoned. All through our marriage I was never able to stand up to my husband, and I felt taking a martial art might perhaps help me to become more assertive. My husband was totally put off by my taking up such a "masculine" activity. But I have persisted.

Women are often tentative, prefacing statements with a little laugh and apologies about how

Greg Wenzel

little we know about the subject under discussion, whereas men learn to present their strongest points and to remain silent about their reservations.

One of the hardest things for me to do is hold my own at points when we really disagree about something. I might start out knowing just what I think but then, the more I listen to William argue his point (he is always so sure of himself), the less sure I feel of mine and the more confused I get about what is true. Sometimes I wind up crying when what I really want to do is fight for myself. Then, later on, I feel angry; a sort of smoldering resentment sets in, and I don't even want to sleep with William at those times. It's because I still feel angry about not being able to hold my own in the fight and I know I can hurt him by withholding sex.

Although physicians and mental-health professionals in conventional sex and marriage books often "scold" women for withholding sex when we are angry about something else, they fail to recognize that it is often the best indirect way of exercising power when more direct ways are blocked.

Women are taught to be uncomfortable with the idea of having power. (It is as unladylike as being physically strong!) Often when we do what is expected of us, we abdicate our power almost entirely.

I always arranged my life around Larry. When we were first together I was beginning a career in teaching. But soon he got a job offer in another city, and so we moved there. Then he wanted to have children, which I didn't really care about. But he wanted them badly, so it seemed all right to me. Then we moved again, this time to a fancy house in a fancy suburb, but I had no car—he took it—and I was quite lonely. The children became the center of my life, and I loved them and my husband deeply. Several times I thought of returning to school part-time to get my certificate. But Larry was not willing for me to do that; he did not want the responsibilities for the house and the children to fall on his shoulders. And he said he was glad to support us, which I think he really was. Then, one day when the children were still quite young (our son was not even a year old), I learned something that terrified me ... that for more than a year Larry had been having affairs with other women. They were all women whom he met in his job as a supervisor, professional women, very bright and competent and unattached and ten years younger than I was.

When I confronted him, he said that he found me dull, always talking about the house and the children—of course, since that was my world!—and that these other women were far more interesting, as they had professional lives and were more worldly and more knowledgeable than I was about things that interested him in his work. He did not say, but I think it is true, that he also hated my asking him to be more involved with the children and the house. He ran to these women whenever I criticized him, looking for the things in them that he discouraged me from developing in myself. When I was younger, I did not see any problem with my shaping my life around Larry. Now I know I have paid a very high price.

When I started working on my graduate degree I was ambitious to become really well known in my field and fantasized being an adviser to members of Congress or even the President. Then I got involved with Dave and began to spend more and more time with him. He wanted total support for his work and since we were in the same field I could help him a lot and be learning at the same time. But I definitely put my own ambitions on the back burner for about two years. I began to be more attached to the idea of staying in the city when I finished school so I

wouldn't have to leave Dave, and I even began to fantasize about a less demanding job, maybe even just three days a week.

When we broke up all my options opened up again and I could reconsider my early ambitions. It was scary to consider the possibility of being as successful as my fantasies.

Traditional Roles and Getting Beyond Them

Roles are like parts in a play. We learn how to be a sexual partner, a wife or a mother by following scripts that we learned as children. The scripts save us the trouble of creating our lives from scratch each and every day, but they may also lead us to drift into rigid roles without questioning them.

Certain qualities are usually reinforced as being appropriate to women or to men. When our behavior varies from the stereotype we may be punished: Whereas a male's assertive behavior is called "leadership," in a female it is called "aggressiveness." Nurturing may be labled "warmth" in a woman and "weakness" in a man.*

Each partner begins a relationship with a set of experiences and beliefs that shape her/his notions about masculine and feminine roles. Many of us grew up in families that followed conven-

---

*One study of mental-health professionals' attitudes found that when they were asked to list the traits of a healthy adult, a healthy man and a healthy woman, they equated traits listed for males with those for healthy adults; but the traits for a "healthy" woman differed from and often contradicted those for a healthy adult.[5] No wonder that women experience so much role conflict and difficulty reconciling contradictory expectations. (Thanks in great part to the women's movement, these attitudes and limitations are changing, but slowly.)

George Malave/Stock Boston

SOME CONSEQUENCES OF ACCEPTING THESE ROLES

The conventional role structure, in which the woman functions as a support system for the man, while receiving no support to earn a living and/or to develop herself, leaves us too vulnerable emotionally and economically. Thousands of displaced homemakers,[6] after nurturing others most of their lives, are then left without resources or marketable skills. (Most do have skills, unrecognized because of a combination of age and sex discrimination and because household skills are devalued when in fact they are similar to professional and management skills.) In today's world, where the divorce rate is one in two and where alimony has virtually disappeared (although the income gap remains), where women outlive their male partners, often by a decade or two (80 percent of surviving spouses are women) and where the inflation rate makes the old pattern of one salary supporting two adults and children an alternative available only to a small elite (only 7 percent of families conform to the old norm of husband as sole breadwinner), the traditional role of woman as support system to the man exists only at great risk to women.

From a very first meeting with a man, we may play roles. If we want to pursue the relationship, continue to see one another and spend time together, live together or get married and have children together, each step toward permanence, commitment and formalization of the relationship increases the pressures to assume conventional roles. Structures and arrangements that may have worked well for years can be challenged or shattered by having children.

If we leave our paid work, we lose not only our independent income but our status as a paid worker and our community of work friends. We lose our source of outside validation; we may feel less competent and respected, and become almost completely dependent on our partner and our child(ren). Even when we want to share work and child care equally, the shortage of good child-care services, the lack of well-paid part-time work and the severe sex discrimination limiting our earning powers as women all contribute to a gradual drift back toward conventional arrangements during the early parenting years.

We believe that as long as women do most of the child care, this will have a fundamental impact on our lives and opportunities and thus influence subsequent generations and *their* choices.

---

tional patterns. Others of us may have grown up in situations where death, divorce, emigration of one parent, war or a period of unemployment occurred and roles had to be shared or varied in nonconventional ways.

When I was growing up my father was away fighting in the war, and so my mother and I moved in with my grandmother and aunts. I grew up seeing women managing by themselves without men for years at a time.

Some parents mistakenly believed they were teaching us that we could do everything boys could do, but they really gave us a mixed message.

I grew up in a household where we believed there were no distinctions between boys and girls. We were always told that girls were equal and the five of us had exciting, far-reaching discussions and no-holds-barred, stimulating, intellectual arguments over dinner. But later I realized that while my father held court with us, my mother was clearing the table. At some point he would call for his coffee to be brought to him. This affected my marriage. I feel intellectually equal or superior to Steven, but it's hard for me to feel okay about doing anything for my own work and that demands or requires any adaptation by my family.

We are not taught gender roles simply out of sentiment and tradition, but because they fit us into existing social forms. As we struggle to change our relationships we must at the same time work to end sex discrimination at our workplaces, establish child care in our communities and end the legal inequities women still face. In this transitional time we have the task of fitting the kinds of relationships we want into a society that may not only fail to support our vision but often actively oppose it.

Making Changes

We can begin to take small steps to change fixed roles. We can devise an affirmative action plan, taking time for ourselves to build up our work skills, to work on something that interests us and brings in some income. We don't have to say no automatically to opportunities that require travel. We can leave an unsatisfactory relationship or work hard toward changing our partner's attitudes and the structure of the relationship.

The change began for me as I prepared for a full-time job when all the kids were finally old enough to take some responsibility. I knew then I had to have Matthew as an active partner, though he preferred being passive and having everything done for him. My therapist told me to make a list of all the jobs that a family required in order to run. It was pages long: it just grew and grew. When I got it all written out after several weeks, it was clear that I did about 95 percent of it. And then I got very angry that I was the one who kept everything working around here. I basically decided I was going to go on strike. We began slowly and painfully to work out a more equitable system in the distribution of housework and cooking and parenting. Matt . . . felt that he "couldn't" do things that he didn't want to do, so it was painful. But I told myself it was worth it because it was the beginning. I was getting ready to start business school.

In the six months before I started school, I determined that I would teach the kids how to run the washer and dryer, to cook simple meals, to scrub the kitchen floor, to clean a bathroom. We set up job lists and everybody had to do one thing a week: They would cook, and I would just be here if they needed help. And then I started business school full-time, and I was immediately overwhelmed. I was struggling. It was far more competitive than I had thought it was going to be. . . . I wasn't home after school, I had study groups late at night and on Saturday and Sunday. Things started to fall apart. Nobody liked it. The kids would grumble because other mothers didn't make their children do so much. We all need order in our lives, and it was chaotic for a while. By the time the first year had gone by, our job system was pretty well in place. This is really my break away from the house. I am no longer going to be here the way I have always been.

To create mutually supportive relationships rather than one in which one partner functions only as the support system for the other, we must realize that there is a difference between sharing *tasks* (taking turns calling for babysitters or paying the bills) and sharing *planning* (the overview—being *aware* of when sitters are needed, when a child needs to go to the doctor and what the long-term financial plans are).

Even when a woman and man both work, they fall into the pattern of the man doing long-term planning, because women until recently have not been in the habit of doing so and believe that men are better at it. Women develop skill at saving small amounts of money by couponing, saving pennies day by day but often not dealing with the larger question of their future economic security. Middle-class women are brought up with the assumption that there will always be someone there to take care of us, whereas women from working-class backgrounds often learn to be more self-sufficient, providing for themselves. But most women's incomes are so marginal that we can't put any money aside for the future. Middle-class women often find it hard to assume responsibility for planning because they can't envision a time when the coffers may be empty, and it is tempting to let someone else worry, just as our parents once did. When we try to take more responsibility, some in-laws, parents—perhaps even therapists—may accuse us of being emasculating. But many of us have found that when we take more responsibility for money matters, not only do our partners appreciate it but we have more control over our lives.

Understanding Some of the Barriers to Intimacy Between Women and Men

Intimacy is having someone in my life who I can get to know really deeply over time, who can get to know me and who I can be the best and worst of myself with.

There are many different facets to knowing each other well and communicating on a deep level, letting our vulnerabilities show and our secrets be known, trusting enough to depend on someone and to allow them to depend on us.

The quality of our intimacy is exquisite. It's like a river that runs between us, and we can tap into it whenever we want. To me it's a rich and wonderful thing that someone can be intimate with you in so many ways . . . as a lover, as a friend.

Commitment means working on the relationship even when the early passion and urgency have evolved into a deeper if less dramatic kind of loving, and sticking through the hard, awful, painful, lousy and deadening times (which can be dramatic in its own way!).

I'm still drawn to that rush of passion that I get early in a relationship, but now I'm old enough and I've been through enough with men to know that the rush doesn't last. We can rekindle it; there are times when I feel that passion with Don that always exists at the beginning, but I sure don't feel it twenty-four hours a day every day. It takes a lot of work and creativity to keep things sparking in a relationship. Sometimes I'm attracted to other men, but I think this has mostly to do with my fears about intimacy

Owen Franken/Stock Boston

and with wanting the rush . . . and trying to disperse some of the intensity of being with one person. As I get older, I'm more interested in whether this person is going to be with me. If the passion isn't there every night, it's okay.

Fearing Intimacy

We are all too often expected to merge our identities with our men's, taking *their* names, moving to where *their* jobs are and so on. We may fear too much closeness if in previous relationships we merged our own wishes, aspirations and identities with those of our partners to such an extent that we lost sight of what we wanted for ourselves.

I wanted to be a satellite to him, revolving around him in his world . . . to let his life, his work, his friends, his energy pull me along. I was so relieved not to have to work anymore to build my own identity. This is what ultimately suffocated him and me and the marriage.

Often we experience conflicts between dependency and self-sufficiency, between the security of being in a good relationship and our need to remain separate.

One thing that's clear about my second marriage is that, because I'm older and because of who Rob is, I am much closer to him than I was to my first husband. I am able to care for him much more deeply. And there are moments when he's away even overnight that are very painful to me. It's not "Oh, my God, I couldn't take care of myself," because I have and I can—but it's deeply, passionately missing somebody. And it's ironic because I had so strongly identified with the women's movement's "superwoman agenda" of being self-sufficient. Yet it's come home to me just how painful it would be

if something were to happen to Rob, how empty life would be. Not because my life isn't full in addition to him, but because I risked having a certain depth of commitment and feeling.

This society, which assigns active and dominant roles to men and passive or subordinate roles to women, exaggerates these conflicts. When we become conscious of men's greater power and prestige, we may fear the vulnerability that naturally comes with intimacy.

My work is lecturing and writing about pornography, child sexual abuse in battering situations and other areas of female sexual slavery. I live two truths all the time: I live in a male-supremist culture, yet I have a relationship with a man who is not a sexist. I used to feel that to be a totally strong woman and a feminist I should be alone, and I would feel guilty for having this real partner who loves me and helps me, whom I love and trust and depend on. But now I think, Why not just enjoy the special life I have and not worry about how I "should" be?

The stronger and more confident I feel about myself, the more able I am to be close to someone without fearing I'll lose myself.

We Learn Different Styles of Intimacy

Frequently women value talking as a way of being close, whereas many men express intimacy mainly through physical activity or sexual closeness.

My idea about being intimate, more than making love, is having long, deep conversations. My fantasies of love affairs are about conversations like that. You just keep on talking and every once in a while something important or interesting will get said. John's idea is that you don't talk until you have something to say. I want to talk about everything from every possible angle. He considers that gossipy, repetitious and intrusive. He's not secretive, but he wants to work things out for himself. His idea of intimacy is doing something together, like camping or canoeing. I sometimes think that John does not really know the part of me that I cherish most, and vice versa.

Society holds up "the strong, silent type" as a masculine ideal. Many men find self-disclosure very threatening;[7] showing one's softer side is not considered masculine. Although over the past several years some men have been trying to be more emotionally open, the male world continues to expect them to be goal oriented and to keep feelings concealed, and does not reward openness. Because our sexist culture does not value a personal, "fem-

Cary Wolinsky/Stock Boston

inine" style of relating to others, most men are not motivated to learn it.

A man I almost married said to me, "I'll bring home the money and you can do the rest," by which he meant all the child care, the housework, the endless small tasks and, most importantly, I came to understand, all the emotional work.

This arrangement has cost men dearly: Many otherwise "successful" men are emotionally impoverished. It costs the women as well, who turn to these men for intimacy and find them seriously lacking. Very often women are responsible for the emotional climate in which a couple exists and also, since many men have no or few intimate friends except for the women they are involved with, we end up having to give them a huge amount of emotional support. Again, a woman winds up doing "invisible" work. Her energy is sometimes so taken up with maintaining a relationship that she is diverted from her own personal achievement and development.

Most men have not yet caught up with women in terms of personal growth, knowing how to work on a relationship or knowing how to be a good friend. Some men have begun to meet together in groups to talk about these issues, to develop the skills necessary for intimate personal relationships and to learn how to pay more attention to their relationships with children, wives or lovers and friends, even though nothing in our society encourages them to do so.

When it works, intimacy makes us feel so good

that it enriches other parts of our lives and contributes to our energy and creativity.

MAKING IT WORK

In any long-term relationship with a man, problems and painful issues come up regardless of how "right" we are for each other, of how hard we have worked to build the relationship and even of how stable and solid we feel together. It can be frightening to look squarely at what is difficult and hurtful, for we want to believe that we chose a good partner, that we have made wise decisions; to become aware of aspects we were afraid to face, to admit deep conflicts may mean that we have made a major error. Sometimes, as we begin to get angry, we become afraid that if we do not immediately squelch this anger, it will rage out of control and lead us inevitably to the end of the relationship.

Yet avoiding confrontation is more likely to result in stagnation and resentment than in keeping the peace or making things better. *Conflict can be part of a creative process of working things out.* As a start we can identify the social aspects of our conflicts and avoid the common pitfall of blaming one another or blaming ourselves for everything that goes wrong.

Constantly Questioning Our Assumptions

We need to make a conscious and continuing effort to articulate what we really want in our intimate relationships with men, or the conventions of society will inevitably take over. One way to begin changing our relationships is to reconsider the kind of men we (think we) are looking for and our patterns of relating to men when we first meet

Owen Franken/Stock Boston

them. Making changes at the beginning of a relationship may help us to shift the balance that gets set up in our future relationships.

I thought I was marrying this very exciting man, and I didn't see that his dynamism was an expression of the control he needed to have. I just saw the excitement, the energy. I didn't realize that it would make me feel smaller in the process. I learned that it's not just how "wonderful" the other person is, but how they make you feel. Now I pay a lot of attention to how I feel with someone at the beginning of a relationship. If I feel distinctly less wonderful in a man's presence, I don't care how sparkling or brilliant he is—I'm not interested.

My wish in my yearbook was to marry a Marlboro man. I grew up in a family of Marlboro men. But I figured out eventually that I didn't want that anymore. Max is very intense and verbal. He is about my height and weight. From the back we even look alike. He's very emotionally accessible—and vulnerable. We have a great deal of fun together. And it's very easy to talk to him. But sometimes I look at him and think, You're so much a friend and a peer . . . I wonder if you are strong enough for me to lean on.

Many of us want our partners to be friends and peers. The men's liberation movement has been an important ally in building this consciousness among men.

Only in the feminist men's movement did I finally find men with a commitment to grapple with sex roles, and it has made an immeasurable difference. Yes, in the past I did find other men willing to change to make our relationship work, but only after arguing and buttressing the points over and over from ground zero. After a while you just want to be with someone who truly has the same values you do and not have to fight that war at home.

As a relationship develops, we must continue to be aware of our assumptions. The danger in taking small things for granted is that they are often attached to larger issues. A seemingly small gesture, like choosing a last name when we decide to get married, can serve as a statement right from the start that we want to have a different kind of connection to a husband than that implied when a woman automatically takes his last name as her own.

I had been married once before, had changed my name and then changed it back, and I knew I didn't want to go through that again. I gave up an important part of myself, which didn't feel like a comfortable way to begin a relationship of equals. When

Sam and I decided to get married, we wanted a new beginning. We thought about somehow combining our last names, but we couldn't come up with one that we liked. The decision to choose an entirely new name has had a lot of meaning for both of us. The name itself is rich in meaning for me. . . . It is from the language that our grandparents spoke, and it means "rebirth" or "renewal." . . . The process of choosing it was very moving. I didn't stop using my original name. I still use it as a middle name, and I like it to be very visible. People often ask about our name, and when I tell them how and why we did it, it's like offering them a new option, a new way to deal with old assumptions. This name is a gift.

But many of our relationships began on a very different footing. We didn't question them until years after patterns were set. We may be scared to change or to have our partners change. If we were raised to believe that men should be strong and silent, we may feel uneasy when our partners express vulnerability, even though we have been asking them to talk about their feelings. We may want them to share caretaking chores but fear that they will encroach on our role, neglecting their paid work or being "unmasculine."

After fifteen years of being a full-time homemaker, I decided to go to school. My husband and I divided up all the jobs and responsibilities so I could finish school and work at a fairly demanding job full-time. Everything was working out fine, I thought, until one day Jim made some passing remark about one of our daughters and some problem she was having with her boyfriend. I was shocked to realize that something was going on I knew nothing about. I was no longer the "nerve center" of the family. That was a loss, because for many years knowing all those details had been my source of power within the family. Yet on balance the change has been good for all of us. Being the nerve center was holding me back from developing other parts of myself, and as I moved out into the world, Jim grew a great deal closer to the kids.

And we renegotiate these arrangements as time goes on.

We have been married forty-one years, but because of the women's movement, there have been some recent changes in our relationship. My husband is a great theoretician. He may have read a hell of a lot more about the women's movement than I have, but to get him to cook dinner is a struggle!
By now we have struggled through the business about making dinner five or six times—different times at which decisions were made and they're acted on for a time, then something happens like he

Cheryl Boudreaux

goes away for three weeks, and when he comes back he's tired and he doesn't take the thing up again. So we have to negotiate the whole thing over again. At one point he said, "You know, the truth is I'm just lazy. It's just so much more comfortable not to have to do it." He can recognize that, but it doesn't prevent it from happening again. But the thing that makes it work is that he's open to being challenged about it. And from what I've heard and read about it, an awful lot of men are not.

Paying Attention to Each Other

So many things vie for our attention: work, friends, children, our various activities and chores. A new love eclipses almost everything else, but before too long the balance changes and it gets squeezed in between the children's needs, the laundry, the car's transmission and evening meetings.

An intimate relationship, while often background and sustenance to the rest of our lives, must at times have our full attention.

Several evenings a week since we married eleven years ago, we sit in the living room, each of us in our own favorite chair, and we have a glass of wine after the kids are in bed. And we talk ... about the day, about ridiculous details of what happened at work, about some problem we've been having or whatever. Sometimes it's hard to take the time ... the dishes need washing or there is a good show on TV or I just don't feel like it. But this, more than any other single thing, has kept us from getting too far apart without touching base.

We have long dry spells between us.... Sometimes I look at him, especially when he's upset about something and very silent and withdrawn, and it feels like I forget what I was ever drawn to in this

man. And then we take a morning off from work or we stay up until two A.M. trying to work out some big crisis, and then we might end up making passionate love, and then I remember, Oh! So this is what I love about you! But it's not the lovemaking so much as really talking about something other than whether today is garbage collection day or which check I forgot to enter in the checkbook. It's seeing "into his soul," into the person I am so close to.

Although raising children can bring us closer, often their presence distracts us or just cuts into the time we have alone together.

One of the hardest things for us since having kids is just getting enough time alone together. When I can't get a sitter, Bob feels neglected, and I'm sure I've failed, even though I know there's no reason why it should just be up to me to arrange our time alone. When we do have a sitter, the kids complain. Both of us come from working-class families where the kids were always included in everything, so it's easy for us to feel guilty when we do something by ourselves.

What we do when we want to be alone together is get in the car. We go for long drives without the radio on, and we talk. That's a way that we can relax, something we enjoyed doing even when we were eighteen years old. But we have to work at it. The kids take up an enormous amount of time and energy that we used to have just for ourselves. Both of us realize that now that I have a career, too, it would be easy for us to drift into our careers as the kids leave home and to have nothing left between the two of us. It's a danger that we have to pay attention to. In thinking about our future years together, we have considered buying a shack or a beachhouse, something that we could afford, and we would go there on weekends and work on it together. It's relaxing, it's being outdoors and it's doing something we enjoy doing together. And we know from past experience that this is how we can stay close.

Some couples have an annual celebration to affirm their commitment, to review their contract and renew their vows.

There is no one "right" way to nurture a relationship; each of us must find what works best for us.

Enjoying Separateness

When partners in a couple go on separate vacations or see separate friends, other people often take it as a sign that something is wrong. Sometimes one member of a couple may be threatened when a partner's life excludes him/her in some way.

Vaughn Sills

I have been seeing a man for almost a year now. I like him a great deal, but he is unable to understand my way of life. He is retired and enjoys just sitting with his feet up for the first time in his life. But I have a new volunteer job, and so I have a number of activities that to me are really stimulating. And these very things, which I've always wanted to do, make it seem to him like I can't stay home and am always running around.

I remember years ago wanting so badly to go to a party we were invited to. But Carl really couldn't stand those people; he refused to go. What I really wanted was to go alone, and I would have had a grand old time, but in those days if you did such a thing people would surely have gossiped that you were on the brink of divorce! Several years ago our

college-age daughter said to me, "Well, why don't you just tell them next time that Daddy really doesn't enjoy parties very much, but that you'd love to come!" I have done this several times now; recently I even went out to dinner alone with a couple I particularly like. It's so much better than missing the parties and resenting Carl or dragging him along and having him sulk and then having to leave earlier than I want to. I resent it far less now when he watches sports on TV, which I dislike. I think that I wasted many years not doing what I enjoyed because sometimes it was different from what we enjoyed.

Martin and I have been together for thirteen years. By together I don't mean married; it has always seemed sort of ridiculous to me to have the state involved in what is really a personal contract. And beyond that, I think that when you get married you begin to make a lot of assumptions and you don't even realize you're doing it. I use my relationship with Martin as a solid base to move out from. . . . I have a very active life independent of him . . . work and political meetings and seeing my friends. He and they are equally important to me—neither alone would be as good.

While some women think that avoiding legal marriage is a safeguard against falling into conventional roles, most want the commitment that marriage symbolizes.

Sometimes when we are involved with a man, we fail to develop certain of our abilities. We may be lulled into thinking that there will always be a man to take care of us. We avoid learning skills like money management, home repairs, strenuous physical tasks.* As a result we may think of ourselves as weaker or less competent than we really are.

I know that I've gotten through the worst times as a single parent, and I've survived and flourished. Being alone and having to learn certain skills, like putting up a Christmas tree alone when your husband used to do it, wasn't something that gave me so much pleasure, but the fact that I did it was another small incident that showed I could manage, and there's a certain satisfaction in just being able to manage your life. Being able to manage your house and raise kids and work outside the house— it's a sense of accomplishment. Learning new skills,

---

*Many men in turn look to women for the kinds of caretaking they may associate with mothering, like the provision of balanced meals, day-to-day household management and the maintenance of general emotional well-being. The difficulty men have in coping without a woman to take care of them in these ways is suggested by their much higher and earlier remarriage rate after divorce or widowhood and also by their higher mortality and morbidity rates after these same life crises.

171

Some co-authors, family and friends at the 20th-anniversary celebration of the publication of Our Bodies, Ourselves.

Ellen Shub

like putting up storm windows, taking the car to the mechanic and negotiating with him, managing your finances, deciding where you're going to have a vacation and with whom—it's all just learning to rely on your own strengths.

Keeping some distinct turf for ourselves, whether it's separate checkbooks or separate vacations, separate friends or not rushing into living together, does not have to threaten our relationship. In fact, it can be renewing to us and contribute to the vitality and growth of what goes on between us.

One of the reasons we have lasted together is that we have always lived in places where each of us could really build a whole life for ourselves—in terms of friends, work, interests—and not have to depend on each other for more than the other could give.

Having Other Friendships

Sometimes couples tend to close in on themselves. We may come to attach less importance to other friendships and let them drop. Yet it is unrealistic to expect that one person can meet all our needs. Other friendships are crucial to our emotional well-being, our happiness, our growth.

Having deep friendships with other people creates a garden in which all of our potential can grow and flourish. We get a broader idea about who we are or can be and call upon different strengths. We are richer, more complex. What we learn through our intense friendships with others—about how to be close, how we seem to other people, how to fight constructively, what we enjoy—we can then weave back into our lives with our partners. Sometimes we have deep friendships with men, but more often with women. By expanding our intimate circles we relieve some of the pressure on our main relationships, and when times are hard other people can then give us support, nurturance and understanding. We don't have to depend only on our partners.

It's so much easier for me living communally because there are other people one can turn to and I'm not Ed's only source of support. When you live alone with someone, you tend to get locked into roles, to divide the work in half and each take part, and there's far less fluidity than you have in a group. And also, when I've lived in a group there's always been an observer to say, "Hey, I see this going on," which helps us to stop the argument we're in and to look at it.

Sometimes Robert falls completely apart. He drags around the house in his bathrobe, doesn't shave, feels sick and talks endlessly about it and generally comes unglued. This almost invariably happens when I am under the most pressure at work or when the kids are in shreds and demanding extra attention. I get so enraged at Rob for getting weak just when I need him that I yell and scream and berate him

172

. . . just what he doesn't need—to be kicked when he's down. What I generally do is call up a friend I really love and trust. She has known me for six years and knows how to help me talk about things so that I get a better perspective on them. Having her to lean on when I feel overwhelmed or down also helps me to be less angry at Rob for falling apart at those times. I can go back to him able to say what I want to say much more clearly, having talked about it with Marie.

Many women have developed strong friendships with other women in the support and consciousness-raising groups that have proliferated over the past twenty years. Women have always gotten together to talk with each other about the details of their personal lives. Though both women and men have considered these gatherings to be idle and unimportant, trivial "chatting," what we are really talking about is the fabric of our lives. By spending time with other women, we see the potential power of articulating and clarifying what is going on in our lives. We learn that many of the issues we struggle with in loving and living with men are not unique to us.

The six of us have been meeting every week, or sometimes every other week, for almost five years. Many times I've gone to a meeting with one perspective and come out with another . . . we talk about work and children, lovers and husbands, friendships, our parents and anything else that is important to us. My husband said once that he thought he owed the fact that our marriage was still in existence to my group. In fact, he's right, even though this goes directly against the stereotype some people have that the main activity of women's groups is to go around busting up marriages. Our group helped me work for what I really wanted. I had spent years treading on eggshells. He felt very insecure professionally and really couldn't get his act together at work. I was doing better, and at one point, when I had the chance to get a major promotion that would have made my salary much higher than his, he threatened to leave the relationship if I took it. I was frightened. I wanted to preserve the marriage rather than get ahead professionally. The women in my group knew that my career was important to me, and that I was very, very good at it. They helped me to look hard at whether those were terms I could ultimately feel good about . . . that I should always walk a step behind him. They also thought that he was bluffing . . . that he was scared that if I really began to feel how competent I was and how valued by other people, that I would leave him. I did take the promotion, and it didn't destroy our marriage. I am stronger now and stand up for what is good for me, and I say to him, "This does not mean that I don't love you, but I won't buy into your fear."

Support groups are helpful at all ages. Sheila is sixty years old and has been married for thirty-seven years.

I've been a member of a women's group for seven years now, and I think we came together out of a feeling that here we were, middle-aged. We didn't really fit into the women's movement totally. And yet there were things we wanted to talk about, and that was the only place they were getting talked about. We could recognize many of the things these women were talking about. And we looked at our lives and how not having a women's movement when we were younger had made an impact on our lives.

Some men, seeing the value of these groups, have set up their own. Other support groups include both men and women, such as single-parent; postdivorce and widow/widower groups, and groups that deal with a particular problem, such as alcoholism or drug abuse.

Getting Help

When problems are very resistant to change and talking to each other and to friends gets us nowhere, when we feel that we've gone around and around on the same issues with no improvement and are completely overwhelmed, then we may believe that our problems are much worse than they ever were. But often it is simply that we get to a point where we are no longer willing or able to put up with a situation which has been going on for a long time. Profound changes can grow from these most desperate moments.

A few months ago things got to the point where, even though I loved Richard a lot, I just couldn't go on with this marriage the way it was set up. Richard refused to go to a therapist with me. In desperation I talked to two friends, each of whom has known us a real long time. And those conversations led to a mind-blowing realization that everything we did in our marriage had been set in the first six months of our relationship. I knew that I couldn't go on that way, so I told Richard how I felt. We stayed up all night talking and crying, then we slept and in the morning we cried again. He said he didn't want to lose everything he had ever loved and that he would try to change, and I said I would try but I couldn't promise and we would see. Right now things are much better between us and we are really trying to make it work.

But sometimes we get stuck in patterns which make it difficult for the two of us alone to make changes, or sometimes we just don't know how. Talking with friends may not always help enough. At this point, we may turn to therapy for help in understanding our own feelings and changing our behavior.

Therapy has helped me to focus on things I do over and over with men that result in my not getting what I need. For example, when I started therapy, I didn't realize how hard it was for me to ask for certain things. I didn't feel strong enough or confident enough to fight for myself. I found it hard to feel close, and I didn't understand how learning to get what I wanted would make me feel closer. It was a circle. . . . Now that I feel confident enough and aware enough of this pattern, it has changed.

We can use therapy to help improve communication about painful issues.

He didn't feel totally comfortable with my handicap, and he would say so, and that made me terribly angry. I couldn't look at my anger at all, which made him very upset, and then he would clam up. I needed a place to feel safe to deal with all this. So we decided to go into couples' therapy. It helped for me to be able to relax and to hear what he was saying to me. He would say to me, "I love you, but I don't like how that part of your body looks." And a lot of it was really my feeling, that I didn't like how it looked either.

But therapy for women can be a double-edged sword. Most often the woman initiates the move to see a therapist, whereas the man may resist or refuse to go. But if we accept the cultural conditioning which teaches us that our job is to maintain emotional relationships, to take care of and give to other people, to be sensitive and work out problems, then turning to a therapist implies that we have "failed" at our role. Tragically, traditional therapy has often reinforced this perception (see Chapter 6, "Psychotherapy"). It is important to find a therapist whose definitions of health and normalcy are based on a worldview that sees women as having a full range of options, not on the premise that women's only or main role is to "service" men and take care of children.

After the first few months of couples' therapy, the therapist said to Matt, "So, you think the problem is that Anna is crazy just because she wants to go back to school, and if she would get 'better,' things would be okay again? Well, let me show you how you fit into Anna's problem." Then we began to look into Matt's part of it, how he wouldn't help take care of our four kids, how he needed to change for us to be able to work things out. For me that was enormously freeing. For the first time I saw that I wasn't the "crazy" one. And I began to feel that I could stay in my marriage and still grow and change in the ways I wanted to.

Not all relationships survive these profound changes. When a breakup seems likely, we have to ask ourselves which is more acceptable to us: the cost of leaving things as they are or the risk that, in trying to improve the relationship, we may lose it.

Knowing When to Leave

Many of us struggle along for years in relationships that are not rewarding or affirming, wanting to make them better but not succeeding, and not yet convinced that we would be better off if we left. We may come again and again to the brink of leaving and then back off. This is not because things are not quite "bad enough"; even women whose men are violent toward them or are alcoholics or drug abusers or have incapacitating emotional problems often find themselves staying or struggling with whether or not to leave or how to leave. (See Chapter 8, "Violence Against Women," for a fuller discussion of domestic abuse.) What holds us back? We may, even with all the problems, still love our partner and be reluctant to lose him; we may feel loyal to him and perhaps not want to hurt him. Perhaps we think that breaking our commitment is a great personal failure, that we will be harshly judged by friends and family. We may try to stay together "for the good of the children" or may dread the prospect of being alone. And there is often the very real fear that we will not be able to support ourselves, and perhaps our children, financially. Yet many women do ultimately decide that they want to end their relationships.

At first Phil seemed to revel in my accomplishments, my growing self-confidence. But I also grew more able to challenge him where he didn't want to be challenged. I have wanted more from him: more involvement with the children, more sharing of paid jobs and housework. I want him to value my strength as I have come to value myself more. His response has been to have a string of affairs, all with women who are much younger than I am and, as you might guess, totally undemanding, unthreatening, willing to accept him precisely as he is.

My relationship with Greg ended when I said that it was no longer working for us and that nothing we were doing was making it any better. He was not a person with whom I could fully engage. We never really learned to fight well together . . . not just having arguments but learning to compromise well. I felt turned off sexually, attracted to others, and the pleasure of being with him was gone. I would come home and not want to tell him what was exciting that day . . . I preferred to tell other people who seemed more "simpatico." What was hardest about the divorce was that the family part of our relationship was good. . . . It was painful to let go of the father of my kids. It was scary to give my own needs so much weight.

The man I was living with began to undercut everything I did—to devalue my work, to be jealous of my friends and my small successes. When I got bogged down in a project, rather than encouraging me he would point out how the project was probably ill-conceived and not of much use anyway. The longer things went on, the more of my good creative energy went into trying to make the relationship work, and the less energy I had for my work and the rest of my life.

When I was first thinking about getting out of my marriage, I would think, Well, I get a lot of satisfaction out of being a parent and I'm very close to my kids. I get a lot of satisfaction from my friendships and I have a really good work situation. My relationship isn't so good, but maybe you just can't have everything. My husband had some serious problems, so I felt I couldn't blame him or just leave him. I never stopped to consider what it was doing to me to be spending years of my life with someone who was giving me so little. After a while I built up so much resentment that I just wasn't able to treat him in a loving way. And I began to be afraid that I would lose my capacity to love someone. I knew that I had a potential for loving that wasn't getting expressed. Yet it was a leap to assume that getting out of our marriage meant that I would have a good relationship again.

If you wind up just accommodating your partner to prevent fights rather than having some hope that it's worth sitting down and trying to work things out; if your relationship is based on evasiveness, deception and withholding; if it is characterized by stagnation and a lack of room for change and growth or if it just doesn't seem that your life is better in the relationship than it would be out of it, then it is time to consider ending it. You don't need to do this in isolation. There are good books on the subject (see Resources). Turning to friends, particularly ones who are willing to talk openly about their divorces or hard times with their partners, can be an excellent source of support and insight. Individual or group therapy can help, as can support groups. Much as we know it is important to work very hard to build a relationship, it is also important to leave before we are damaged by it.

Though it may seem to be contradictory to advocate paying attention to our relationships and at the same time trying to be a separate person and seek other friendships, these multiple aspects of our lives can and do enrich rather than detract

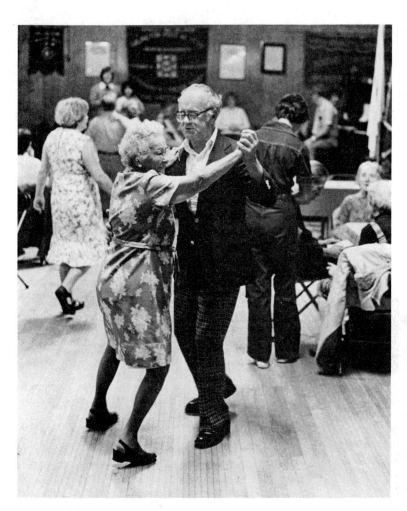

Patricia Hollander Gross/Stock Boston

from one another. They also provide a balance that stimulates our growth and promotes our joy and well-being—our capacity for independence along with our capacity for intimacy.

We have been married for thirteen years. . . . Daniel is not my best friend. We are quite different in many ways, have different friends, interests and so on. There are ways in which I'm not even as intimate with him as I am with some of my women friends. But ever since I met him, I have not felt the excruciating loneliness that was the core of my life for twenty-six years. Being with him, knowing that we are partners in life, has permitted me to grow from an extremely unhappy, lonely person with little self-esteem and a lot of self-hatred into a happy, fulfilled and self-loving woman. My identity is not derived from him, but being with him has enabled me to create a major transformation in myself.

NOTES

1. May Sarton. *Plant Dreaming Deep*. New York: W.W. Norton, 1983, p. 91.

2. Jacqueline Simenauer and David Carroll. *Singles: The New Americans*. New York: New American Library, 1982.

3. R.O. Blood and D.M. Wolfe. *Husbands and Wives: The Dynamics of Married Living*. New York: Free Press, 1960. See also Philip Blumstein and Pepper Schwartz, *American Couples: Money, Work and Sex*. New York: William Morrow, 1983.

4. U. S. Department of Labor, 1988.

5. I.K. Broverman, et al. "Sex-Role Stereotypes and Clinical Judgments of Mental Health," *Journal of Consulting and Clinical Psychology*, Vol. 34 (1970), pp. 1–7.

6. Laurie Shields. *Displaced Homemakers*. New York: McGraw-Hill, 1981. Available from Older Women's League, Washington, DC.

7. Sidney Jourard. *The Transparent Self: Self-Disclosure and Well-Being*, 2nd ed. New York, Van Nostrand, 1971.

RESOURCES

Arendell, Terry. *Mothers and Divorce: Legal, Economic and Social Dilemmas*. Berkeley: University of California Press, 1986.

Bernard, Jessie. *The Future of Marriage*. New York: Bantam Books, 1972.

Crawford, Linda, and Lee Lanning. *Loving: Women Talk About Their Love Relationships*. Minneapolis: Midwest Health Center for Women, 1981.

Edwards, Harriet. *How Could You?: Mothers Without Custody of Their Children*. Freedom, CA: The Crossing Press, 1989.

Ehrenreich, Barbara. *Hearts of Men: American Dreams and the Flight from Commitment*. Garden City, NY: Anchor Press/Doubleday, 1983.

Fleming, Jennifer Baker, and Carolyn Kott Washburne. *For Better, For Worse: A Feminist Handbook on Marriage and Other Options*. New York: Charles Scribner's Sons, 1977.

Gettleman, Susan, and Janet Markowitz. *The Courage to Divorce*. New York: Simon & Schuster, 1974.

Gilligan, Carol. *In a Different Voice*. Cambridge, MA: Harvard University Press, 1982.

Hailey, Elizabeth Forsythe. *A Woman of Independent Means*. New York: Avon Books, 1979. Fictionalized account of a strong woman told through her letters.

Hertz, Rosanna. *More Equal Than Others: Women and Men in Dual-Career Marriages*. Berkeley: University of California Press, 1986.

Lear, Martha Weinman. *Heartsounds*. New York: Pocket Books, 1980. Autobiographical account of a woman's relationship with a husband who is suffering from a serious and eventually fatal heart condition.

Lindsey, Karen. *Friends as Family*. Boston: Beacon Press, 1981.

Malos, Ellen, ed. *The Politics of Housework*. New York: Schocken Books, 1980. Anthology includes the ground-breaking article of that same title by Pat Mainardi.

Miller, Jean Baker. *Toward a New Psychology of Women*. Rev. Ed. Boston: Beacon Press, 1986.

Miller, Stuart. *Men and Friendship*. Boston: Houghton Mifflin, 1983.

Mininni, Darlene, MPH. *Sex Talk: The College Student's Guide to Sex in the '90s*. New York: Good Friend Press, 1991.

Peterson, Nancy L. *Our Lives for Ourselves: Women Who Have Never Married*. New York: G.P. Putnam's Sons, 1981.

Rich, Adrienne. *On Lies, Secrets and Silence*. New York: W.W. Norton, 1979.

Robertson, Christina. *A Woman's Guide to Divorce and Decision Making*. New York: Fireside, 1988.

Rubin, Lillian B. *Just Friends: The Role of Friendship in Our Lives*. New York: Harper & Row, 1985.

———. *Intimate Strangers*. New York: Harper & Row, 1983.

Scarf, Maggie. *Intimate Partners: Patterns in Love and Marriage*. New York: Ballantine Books, 1987.

Segal, Lynne. *Slow Motion: Changing Masculinity, Changing Men*. New Brunswick, NJ: Rutgers University Press, 1990.

Simenauer, Jacqueline, and David Carroll. *Singles: The New Americans*. New York: New American Library, 1982.

Stack, Carol B. *All Our Kin: Strategies for Survival in a Black Community*. New York: Harper & Row, 1974.

Steinbergh, Judith W. *Lillian Bloom: A Separation*. 1980. Available from Hot Mama Poetry Collective/Wampeter Press, Box 512, Green Harbor, MA 02041. These fine poems chronicle a woman's separation from her husband, her pain and anger and her growing sense of competence and joy as a woman and a mother.

Tannen, Deborah. *You Just Don't Understand: Women and Men in Conversation*. New York: Ballantine Books, 1990.

Triere, Lynette, with Richard Peacock. *Learning to Leave: A Woman's Guide*. New York: Warner Books, 1982.

Vaughan, Diane. *Uncoupling: Turning Points in Intimate Relationships*. New York: Vintage Books, 1987.

Women in Transition, Inc. *Women in Transition: A Feminist Handbook on Separation and Divorce*. New York: Charles Scribner's Sons, 1975.

10

Loving Women: Lesbian Life and Relationships*

By the Lesbians Revisions Group, including BARBARA A. BURG, LOLY CARRILLO, SASHA CURRAN, J. W. DUNCAN, BUFFY DUNKER, DEANNA FORIST, D. HAMER, B. J. LOUISON, JUDY NORRIS, GWENDOLYN PARKER, MARIANA ROMO-CARMONA, LYNN SCOTT, ANN SHEPARDSON and several women who must, with sadness and anger, remain anonymous to protect our jobs, family relations, living situations or parenthood.

With special thanks to the Cambridge Women's Center for use of their archives, Jill Wolhandler, the Lesbian Mothers Group (at the Cambridge Women's Center) and to the hundreds of lesbian women who wrote letters in response to the previous lesbian chapter.

This chapter in previous editions was called "In Amerika They Call Us Dykes" and was written by a Boston Gay Collective.

1992 Update by Amy Alpern, with help from Mary Bowe, Holly Ellison, Brenda Reeb and Wendy Sanford.

Being a lesbian for me is about the joy and wonder of loving women. It means being woman-identified, making women my priority. It is a way of life, so much more than a matter of who I want to sleep with.

In many communities, a lot of the activist work that is being done to free all women from oppression is being done by lesbians. Not having this big emotional or economic dependence on men makes us able to do that. If you're not trying to get so much from men, you can often be more objective, assertive

and powerful. That's the freedom we have to shape the world.

Sometimes when I talk positively about being a lesbian, heterosexual friends say they hear me criticizing their choice to be with men. That's not true. For me, part of what's essential in being a lesbian is caring for other women, and this includes women who have made choices other than mine.

The chapter on lesbians in the original *Our Bodies, Ourselves* drew letters from women all over the country telling about their experiences and asking for advice, news, contacts, support. So much has happened for lesbians since that original chapter appeared that several lesbians decided to work together in bringing the chapter up-to-date.

---

*Although this edition of *Our Bodies, Ourselves* includes lesbian voices throughout, the Collective decided also to have a separate chapter for a more careful focus on issues and information that specifically affect lesbians.

Ranging in age from twenty-four to seventy-six, we come from diverse backgrounds and experiences.

In revising the chapter we want especially to reach out with information and support to women who are newly exploring their lesbian identity and to lesbians who find themselves isolated from other lesbians, geographically or otherwise. We also want to give heterosexual women a clearer picture of our lives.*

In the past fifteen years the U.S. lesbian community has grown and flourished. Lesbians are numerous in every ethnic group, economic class and political persuasion. We are factory workers, teachers, translators, doctors, high school and college students, clergy, shopkeepers, flight attendants, politicians, labor leaders, athletes. Some of us have physical disabilities, some have or plan to have children, some are sure we don't want children and find this a freeing choice, some have relationships that last a lifetime, some are celibate. Some of us are married to men and cannot easily leave our marriages, yet we identify ourselves as lesbian and even make primary commitments to women.

Although most historical records leave lesbians invisible, research is uncovering a lesbian culture dating back to ancient times. We have been present, out and struggling for centuries. Despite periods of intense persecution, we have continued to choose and to love one another, and to challenge patriarchy by the very fact of our emotional independence from men.

We who are writing this chapter are excited by this heritage. Although we are grateful to live in a time and place where lesbians can love and live somewhat openly, prejudice and oppression are still a daily fact of our lives. We hope the chapter will help other lesbians—our sisters—grow in understanding, pride and power.

COMING OUT

Coming out is the process of coming to accept and affirm our lesbian identity and choosing how open we want to be about it. It can involve many stages—admitting to ourselves that we are les-

Shay Ogelsby

bian, getting to know other lesbians, telling friends and family, marching in a gay-rights demonstration, being open at school or work. Many of us will never be free to do all these. We spend a lot of energy deciding whether, when, how and to whom we want to come out. When/if our society one day freely accepts lesbians, we will be able to use that energy in many other ways.

Coming Out to Ourselves

Each of us has her own story of growing lesbian awareness. Because we grow up in a culture that assumes everyone to be heterosexual, becoming aware of our identity and accepting it is often a gradual process. Coming out to ourselves can happen at any age or stage in life.

At fourteen I already knew I was different. All my girlfriends talked about was boys, and I wasn't interested. I dated a few guys but mostly I skipped the social events. I picked out any strong women I could find and hung around with my coaches a lot. I was in trouble all the time—fighting with my parents, dealing drugs, drinking. I see now it was because I realized I was different and didn't know what to do about it. [For more on lesbian teens, see Lesbian Youth in Resources.]

I didn't think about becoming a lesbian until at twenty-five I just fell in love with a woman and had to deal with it. As long as I was with her it was pretty simple, but when we broke up three years later, I finally had to ask myself, "Am I really a lesbian?"

I think I was always gay, but it took me seventy years to realize it.

---

*None of the present writers worked on the 1973 chapter, "In Amerika They Call Us Dykes." In fact, it provided crucial support and inspiration for several of us when we first came out as lesbians. We have written a chapter quite different in focus and tone from the original one, using briefer stories so as to make room for more topics. See Resources for many books in which lesbians talk personally at great length, or write to Lesbian Liberation, The Women's Center, 46 Pleasant St., Cambridge, MA 02139.

After my divorce I dated men and even slept with a few, but something was missing. I was celibate on and off for five years, mostly glad of the clear space and solitude, but at times in despair that I'd never let anyone really close. I felt a strong political and personal commitment to women and a fascination for lesbians, but it scared me to think that maybe I wanted to love a woman—my parents would explode, my ex-husband would try to get custody of our kids, my friends might think I was out to seduce them. I was also afraid it would be a choice against men instead of for women. Finally one day I said to myself, "For now, I am a lesbian," and some important piece of my identity clicked into place. I'm glad I chose to be a lesbian before I had a woman lover.

When I went to college there were only two other black students on the entire campus, and they came from comfortable middle-class families. I felt as out of place with them as I did with the middle-class white students. It was about this time that I began to become aware of an attraction to women, which I kept trying to suppress.

Since I was out of my element socially, I always came on as tough and aggressive to cover up, and people started accusing me of being a dyke. I was terrified that my fantasies were showing in some way, and I began dating to cover up, to show that I wasn't "like that." Now I realize that the accusations were intended to bring me into line and make me behave "like a lady," and it worked. I knew that being a black woman gave everyone the right to walk on me (or try to, anyway), and I thought that being a black lesbian was some sort of capital crime. It was this more than anything else that made me steer clear of women who showed an interest in me.

The women's movement came along about the time I finished college. The movement gave me support because I could see other women having the courage to change their lives. Their example gave me the courage to see that I was cheating myself by pretending to be straight. I finally did come out sexually with a black woman I met at work. I reasoned that if a racist society wanted my head, they'd get it because I was black, and being gay wasn't going to make all that much difference. My life has been much fuller since then and a lot happier.

At first many of us try to deny our lesbianism. It contradicts all the expectations our families and society have for us—and, often, the expectations we have had for ourselves. All we've ever heard about lesbians is negative. We may not even know any open lesbians.

In my little town in upstate New York I didn't know there were other dykes around at all. When I fell in love with a woman and became lovers with her at sixteen, she was the only person I knew who was gay. It was hard to say to myself, "I am a lesbian," when I didn't know any.

Stereotypes of lesbians may scare us away.

I was fascinated by the idea of loving a woman, but totally turned off by what I thought lesbians were supposed to be like. I didn't want to be a man or look like one.

We may want to reject our lesbianism because our sexist upbringing has taught us that women are inferior or because we know life will be hard or complicated for us as lesbians in certain ways, though satisfying in others.

Many of us have painful memories of trying to deny our feelings for women—dating men, getting married, consulting psychiatrists who tried to "cure" us, becoming dependent on alcohol or other drugs.

I was afraid that if I touched other girls I would like it and keep on touching them. So I became repulsed at the idea. I'm angry that I held the feelings down for so long that now I have a hard time just relaxing and touching someone I love.

Coming out to ourselves means primarily letting go of the guilt, self-hatred and fear learned from living in a homophobic society. (Homophobia is the irrational fear and hatred of homosexuality in ourselves and others.) Coming out means loving ourselves as women and as lesbians.

When you first come out, it's like you're telling yourself something you don't want to believe. "You kissed that girl, didn't you? It felt good, didn't it? So what's wrong with it?" You finally begin to be honest with yourself. After that the rest of your life opens up.

A month after I said to myself, "Okay, I'm a lesbian," and had my first female lover, I suddenly started to go dancing a whole lot, to take bubble baths, swim nude at night, wear soft, slinky shirts.

When I came out, I didn't know any Asian lesbians in my city. It was like juggling three worlds. I was raised in a very traditional Chinese family. I didn't know I was an American citizen until all of a sudden at eighteen I realized I was here to stay and had to deal with this country as reality. A few years later I realized my sexual preference was for women, despite all the traditional Chinese expectations and the extreme homophobia of Chinese culture, along with all the other social expectations out there in American society.

I gradually began to integrate all the three together: I tried to maintain my Chinese identity and to integrate that with feeling strong as a woman,

179

tracing it basically through feelings of closeness with my grandmother, who was the matriarch of the family. I tried to pick out strong women in my personal past and to combine the traditions there that could help me to be strong as a woman and help me be able to feel strong about being a lesbian. So although I am not out to my family, I don't feel like I'm going to be put out on the mountain to die.

Coming Out to Friends and Family

Letting other people know we are lesbians is usually more problematic. If we decide to be openly lesbian we become visible targets for physical and psychological harassment. We may be labeled sick, kept away from children, fired from our jobs. Yet if we keep our lesbianism hidden we face insults and embarrassment when people assume we are heterosexual: Gynecologists want us to use birth control, friends want to fix us up with men, men make passes at us. We live with the fear that others will find out. We feel cut off from many of the people we love.

I want my family and friends to know I'm a lesbian because I want to be honest with them. I don't want to be hiding something from them, especially something so central to my life, something I'm glad about and proud of.

Many of us come out to friends first, choosing the ones who seem likely to be the most accepting.

One friend I came out to said, "I'm happy that you're in love. But I also feel that it's wrong, that you should have those feelings for a man." Once she said the negative part she seemed to let it go. From then on I asked my friends for their negative as well as positive responses, so they wouldn't try to be good "liberal" friends and hide the homophobic feelings that most everyone has somewhere.

My best friend for thirteen years broke off our friendship several months after I told her, and I haven't heard from her in ten years. No matter how well you know someone, you can never know exactly what to expect from them when you come out.

Not being out to family is often particularly painful.

It's hard at family events when everyone is very heterosexual and brings their families and I'm not able to bring my lover. My aunts all ask when I'm going to marry.

Most parents have a hard time with the news.

I look at my parents as being totally isolated. Who can they talk to about their daughter being lesbian? In this society people make very harsh judgments about gay people, and a judgment about a kid is taken as a judgment about the parents. My parents feel that they are responsible for the person I am, and they can get into guilt trips about what they "did wrong."

Thinking lesbianism is something wrong and that it has a cause, parents may blame themselves.* Many react at least at first with anger, guilt, shame, hurt, fear. Some react with violence: They send lesbian daughters into therapy for a "cure," put them into mental institutions, kidnap and send them for deprogramming, disown them. Others don't take their daughter's choice seriously, and keep hoping she'll meet a nice man and *really* fall in love. Some are more accepting.

My mother's reaction was exceptional. She said, "I don't understand it at all, but I'm glad you're happy."

Coming out to family is usually a process that takes several years. Some parents do come to an understanding, even if they refuse any contact at first; some do not. Coming out makes family relationships more honest and sometimes more close than they would be if we kept living a lie. We may even be pleasantly surprised, as a lesbian grandmother reported: "One of my nineteen grandchildren said, 'I love telling my friends about my gay granny.'"

Beyond Friends and Family

Coming out publicly—to our employers, doctors, therapists, supervisors, teachers or clergy—is risky. These people have the power to make our lives extremely difficult. Job discrimination, a problem for all women, hits lesbians hard. If we are openly lesbian, we are likely to be the last hired and the first fired. And if we hide our lesbianism in order to find a job, we fear being found out. Many lesbians keep totally "closeted" in the public eye, living a scrupulously careful double life.

Yet an increasing number of lesbians today are more open at work about their lesbianism. In certain parts of the country lesbians and gay men

---

*A Kinsey study concluded that there is *no* cause for homosexuality, neither heredity nor environment (including parents' actions). Looking for a cause usually implies the homophobic assumption that there is something wrong with being lesbian or gay. Who looks for causes of heterosexual orientation?

Ellen Shub

have fought against job discrimination and won. Employers in all fields need to learn that we'll work better at our jobs when we can be honest about who we are.

The more that lesbians are able to be visible, the more of a chance people have to see us realistically, to notice our support of each other and to feel our strength. Our increasing visibility in numbers enables us to work more effectively against job discrimination and other kinds of oppression that have made many lesbians keep hidden.

I want us all to announce, "We're Lesbians!" all at the same time. People would be shocked to discover they know lots of lesbians, that they like us, respect us. If people were really aware of how many of us there are, they'd have a much harder time seeing us as abnormal.

I don't think I'm an alarmist when I say that I find it is more often not safe to be obviously out. In my experience homophobia is as intense and pervasive as racial and sexual prejudice, plus it is still legally *and socially reinforced. I don't think the answer is to act closeted. I think it is to be aware of the risks, evaluate them, prepare for them and then take them.*

FINDING OUR COMMUNITY

Contact with other lesbians is crucial but often difficult to achieve.

My friend and I have been together for five years. We have not "come out" as gay. We have always felt that all we need is each other, but now we are beginning to feel very alone and isolated. When you constantly live a secret, you begin to feel as if you are not real. We need contact with other gays so we can say to someone, "Look! We love each other and we do exist!"

I didn't think there were any older lesbians in the whole city. Then two friends of mine gave a party and invited all the lesbians they knew over forty years old. It made me feel entirely different to look around

181

that room and see how many we were. Now we meet every month.

As late as the 1950s most lesbians were extremely isolated from each other.

Unless you knew someone who knew someone else, the only place to meet lesbians was in the bars, and maybe you didn't like the bar scene. There were few books except lurid novels where lesbians were miserable and usually died unhappily, no newspapers that I knew of, no groups to go to. I was hungry for contact.

Thanks to the many lesbians and gay men who have struggled for our right to live and love openly and with pride, we now have many networks and organizing tools for reaching out to one another. Although the bars offer a place for some lesbians to meet openly and relax together, it has been important to create gathering places that are not built around alcohol and night life, and reflect all the different interests lesbians have. Daughters of Bilitis (DOB), founded in the 1950s, was the first to provide a place for lesbian women to get together for sociability and discussion. Later, organizations such as Lesbian Liberation and Radicalesbians focused on the politics of lesbianism and feminism. Some cities now have groups for young lesbians and gays, for lesbians of color, for older lesbians, for lesbians with disabilities and for lesbian mothers. The National Gay Task Force and the Lesbian Legal Defense Fund focus on the struggle to challenge the courts and change the laws and social mores that oppress us. The Gay and Lesbian Alliance Against Defamation monitors video and print media and the presentation or absence of lesbian and gay images and issues. We have newspapers, independent publishing houses, record companies, bookstores, restaurants, and professional, religious and cultural organizations and centers (see Resources). We have festivals and dances. Every summer in cities throughout the country lesbian and gay-pride marches commemorate the anniversary of the Stonewall Riots of 1969.* The 1987 lesbian and gay march on Washington drew some 200,000 to 600,000 people. Today militant activist groups like Queer Nation use humorous and/or confrontational tactics to promote lesbian and gay visibility. (As we did with *dyke* in the early 1970s, reclaiming *queer* gives positive and proud connotations to a word once used as an insult.)

Groups and events offer chances to take that

---

*After gay men fought back during a 1969 police invasion of the Stonewall Inn bar in New York's Greenwich Village, gay activists started the lesbian- and gay-liberation movement.

RURAL LESBIANS

Meeting other lesbians in a small town or rural area can be very hard.

This is one section of the country where nothing different is accepted. It is a backwoods area. There aren't a lot of gay women here. If there are more, they are well hidden from the rest of us.

Some suggestions:
1. Read books and/or listen to records by and about lesbians. (See Resources for mail-order women's bookstores.) They can make you feel good about being a lesbian.
2. Contact the nearest lesbian or gay organization (no matter how far away!). Check guides such as *Gaia's Guide* or *Places of Interest to Women*, or contact national lesbian and gay groups (see Resources). Organizations not near you may be able to tell you about nearby groups or give you the name of a woman who could put you in touch with other lesbians in your area.
3. Become involved in women's political activities. Is there a women's center near you, maybe in a university? Any feminist groups? Many lesbians are politically active and most women's groups have lesbian members.
4. Go to women's events such as concerts, conferences and festivals. Many women's music festivals are held in the summertime in rural areas. Listings of upcoming festivals appear in women's and gay newspapers. Even if these events are not close to you, you might meet other lesbians from your area there, or someone who knows someone.

Remember, you are not alone.

---

first step in getting to know other lesbians, though we may feel shy.

The first time I headed for the lesbian support group at the Women's Center I walked around the block four times and went home. I was scared to come out to a whole new group of people. The next month my need for friendship and support won out over my fears, and I went in.

Despite and perhaps even because of our increased visibility, attacks upon us and efforts to silence us continue. Across the country, documented antilesbian and antigay hate crimes have increased. As of 1991, only three states had passed lesbian and gay civil rights bills; the majority of state legislatures continue to deny us the same protection under the law that other citizens receive. For eight years Karen Thompson fought in the courts until she finally won the right to visit and participate in the care of her lover, Sharon Kowalski, who was brain injured in a 1983 auto accident.[1]

RELATIONSHIPS

Knowing that we love women and acting on that is usually an exhilarating experience. Being outside the dominant culture can give lesbians a certain freedom in shaping the kinds of relationships we want. Some of the choices, dilemmas and possibilities that come up parallel those of our heterosexual sisters; some do not.

Pressure to Be in a Couple

This society expects women above all else to find, fall in love with and have a relationship with a man. Lesbians look instead for a woman lover, often maintaining a tremendous emphasis on being part of a couple.

We're so conditioned to think we're only half a person without somebody else.

The only thing that we have in our heads is: you meet a woman, you feel for her, you enter into a relationship, you relate only to her. It's been the downfall of many intimacies.

Often we have to struggle to feel okay if we're not in a couple.

When I'm around lesbian couples for any length of time I feel this sense of creeping desperation, like something's wrong with me because I'm not in a relationship. The pressure makes you latch on to anybody instead of thinking the thing through.

Choosing Not to Be in One Major Relationship

Some lesbians choose to be single—to have many lovers or none, but not one primary lover.

Being on my own lets me find out what my needs are, and find out who I am and just get a better sense of myself.

I like not being answerable to anybody. One reason to be single or celibate is to have clarity about what

Ellen Shub

you want in your life. You make emotional and physical space. What you want is not dependent on what somebody else wants.

When I was in a couple we had to spend so much time hassling out all the little details of everything. Everything had to be a compromise—everything, from the most minute detail to the biggest thing—and it seemed like such a waste of energy most of the time.

When I'm on my own, my security comes from myself and the connections I have with different people. In a relationship, my security depends so much on that relationship and on that one other woman.

It's amazing how much energy it frees up for me. I feel great; I feel a real surge of power!

Not being in a relationship has given me time to reconnect with my friends in a really intimate way.

There are so many more women in my life now, so much room for so many more women.

I found I can get a good deal more work done and am more creative.

I like the feeling of trying to create something new.

In choosing not to be in a couple, we do not distance ourselves from others. We still want, and have, intimate friendships. Some are sexually intimate with friends.

It's very hard for me to draw the line between friends and lovers, so I sleep with some of my very close friends. I find that really satisfying. A lot of the time I sleep with very close friends without having sex, which I find equally satisfying.

We may choose intimacy without sex because we like our friendships as they are.

The lesbian community has completely copied the heterosexual community in thinking that relationships, to be really intimate, to be really close and to supply the affection that's needed in a person's life, have to be sexual. I don't think that's true. I think you can have really good relationships, intimate and the most binding, without sex. Bringing sex into a relationship does not necessarily improve it.

How well being single works for us depends at least partly on our ability to avoid slipping into feeling dependent on particular people for our feeling of well-being. We often look for the happiness of somebody else liking us, valuing us, and we would do well to find that satisfaction in liking ourselves.

Having One Primary Lover

Many of us choose to be in an intimate sexual relationship with one other woman, whether or not we live together and even if we sleep with other women from time to time. We build a relationship—planning our work and play so we can count on spending time together, helping each other through personal changes and difficulties, working through conflicts. We might stay together as lovers for a few months, a few years or a lifetime.

I like being with someone who follows all the threads of my life, even the most mundane.

When I hear another lesbian talking about being involved as lovers and friends with lots of women, it excites me. I know that by choosing to be with one woman I am missing out on a certain kind of emotional adventure. But for my lover and me there is a kind of adventure I prefer at this point. Finally, after a few years, we are able to say to each other, "I need you," and know what that means. It doesn't mean, "I'm hopeless on my own—I can't let you go," but does mean risking a certain kind of interdependence that I haven't known before.

Keeping a long-term primary relationship alive and well takes work, and straight society doesn't do anything to make it easier. Fortunately, lesbians in long-term couples have begun writing

about it. See the Resources for books and other resources on both the emotional and legal issues.

Intimacy

Models

Whatever kinds of relationships we are in, our families and the media offer us mostly heterosexual models for intimacy, and limited ones at that. Although it is freeing to be without models and sexist role stereotypes, there can also be a lot of uncertainty about how to proceed.

When I was married at nineteen, I knew exactly what I was supposed to do forever. I didn't have to think about it. When I entered into my first lesbian relationship I didn't have any idea. It's scary. I don't know where I'm going half the time; there's no one to turn to and ask, "Is this right?" because nobody knows—there isn't any "right." Without role models, how we live has to come from our gut, and mostly I like it that way.

Being lesbian gives me a chance to do things differently from heterosexual couples I've seen. I'd like to be less possessive than they often are. But when it comes to my lover being sexually involved with another woman (or a man), it hurts. I've decided that I've got to be up front about my very human need for sexual dependability.

I am always surprised how many of my lesbian friends have ex-lovers as best friends. I wonder if it is because the community is so small, if women have a harder time letting go or if women simply are able to maintain better relationships with each other. It is not the same for my straight friends.

Family Patterns

Many of the issues in lesbian friendships and sexual relationships have more to do with the ups and downs of intimacy than with the fact that we are lesbians.

In my family no one ever got outwardly angry. There were no fights, only "discussions." So when a lover or close friend blows up at me my first reaction is panic. I know I want to fight more openly and not get so quiet with my anger, but it's hard.

My parents lived and worked together twenty-four hours a day until they died. My lover Lou's family was more traditional; her father was away all day working or being with his male friends and his wife spent a lot of time with her sisters. Lou saw her parents enjoying separate time, and she needed that.

Tia Cross

I had trouble accepting that she wanted to be without me sometimes. We struggled over these differences until we could help each other feel safe doing things differently from how our families did.

I went from a mother who spoiled me to a classic butch role where I had no responsibility for any housework. About ten years into living with my lover Roz I realized I had a lot of growing up to do. I saw I was no different from any male if Roz was the one who did all the work around the house.

Separateness

Every one of us who loves another woman has grown up in a sexist society that devalues women and fails to give us a strong sense of identity. Women's "role" in relationships has traditionally been to give in, give over, bend, care for our loved ones. Although there are endless differences between any two women, there is a certain closeness that comes from being the same sex—similar body, similar socialization. We can slip into being so close that there isn't enough breathing room. We may have to work to find a healthy balance between closeness and distance, to define ourselves assertively and to encourage each other to grow as individuals.

It's critical that my lover and I really understand our boundaries, where we want to say no and where we want to say yes. If I don't build my own privacy right away into a relationship, then the next thing I know I'm either spacing out or leaving.

If you get involved with a woman who lives far away or has to move for a job, you can't either of you assume the other is going to give up her home, friends or job so you can be together. You both know how important all these are. My lover right now lives in another state. I hate the separation but I value her independence as I value my own.

Lesbian Battering

Despite the appealing image of love between women as somehow free of the painful misuse of power that plagues so many heterosexual couples, it has become clear over the past few years that lesbian relationships can be marked by physical, verbal or emotional abuse. Abuse can take many forms. Even if your lover does not actually physically harm you, you may be experiencing abuse in a relationship if you feel frequently insulted and demeaned by your lover, or frightened by her physically or emotionally, if she uses intimidation of any kind to control what you do or how much time you spend with your family or friends, if she rages at you and blames you for problems in her life that you have nothing to do with. Even if you love each other, this kind of treatment is abusive, and you may want to seek help in getting free of the relationship.*

The battered women's shelter movement has struggled with the long-hidden problem of lesbian battering. Initially, many lesbians who fled abusive relationships with women lovers found their problems misunderstood or overlooked by shelter workers. In an effort to improve this situation, some shelter staff and boards around the country have had trainings to counter their homophobia and heterosexism, in order to help the shelters better serve lesbian women.

Butch–Femme

Many lesbians out and active during the 1950s and before followed a strict dress and behavior code, especially in social situations; they chose either a butch role (masculine, aggressive) or a femme role (feminine, receptive). Butches were supposed to initiate sexual relationships, and femmes were supposed to continue their passivity even in bed, allowing butches to make love to them but not reciprocating. Feminist lesbians sometimes criticize butch–femme lesbians for imitating heterosexual models and perpetuating sexism. Others have responded:

I was a femme, a woman who loved and wanted to nurture the butch strength in other women. Although I have been a lesbian for over twenty years and embrace feminism as a world view, I can spot a butch fifty feet away and still feel the thrill of her power.

---

*One place to start might be the Lesbian Caucus of the Massachusetts Coalition of Battered Women's Service Groups, 107 South Street, 5th Floor, Boston, MA 02111, at (617) 426-8492; or HAWC (Help for Abused Women and their Children) of Salem, MA, (508) 744-6841 (hotline) or (508) 744-8552 (office). For an important discussion of lesbian battering, see *Naming the Violence: Speaking Out Against Lesbian Battering* by Kerry Lobel, ed., and National Coalition Against Domestic Violence Lesbian Taskforce, Seattle, WA: Seal Press, 1986.

Contrary to belief, this power is not bought at the expense of the femme's identity. Butch–femme relationships, as I experienced them, were complex erotic statements, not phony heterosexual replicas. They were filled with a deeply lesbian language of stance, dress, gesture, loving, courage and autonomy. . . . Butch–femme was an erotic partnership, serving both as a conspicuous flag of rebellion and as an intimate exploration of women's sexuality.[2]

Some women say that butch–femme is a thing of the past, but many lesbians have spoken up recently to say this isn't true. Although the codes are less strict nowadays, in one way or another many lesbians continue to explore the butch–femme evocation of assertiveness and receptivity, its celebration of "difference in women's textures"[3] and its particular forms of courageous eroticism.

Oppression and Support

Heterosexuals can hold hands in public, go anywhere together, be welcomed as a couple by their families and at religious services, celebrate their relationships openly, make decisions for each other in times of sickness and provide for each other's material well-being in case of death. Lesbians can take none of these commonplace things for granted.

In the faculty room where I work, I hear the other teachers talking about their relationships . . . nothing real heavy, but they do give each other a lot of support. Since being out to them would mean losing my job, I can't let off steam all day; if Ann's sick and I'm worried about her I can't get any comfort at work. If we have a big decision to make, I can't ask for help in sorting it out. All this makes our lesbian friends terribly important, especially the ones who talk with us about our relationship.

Throughout all eras lesbians have supported each other's relationships despite oppression. Today in simple daily ways we can ask our friends how their relationships are going, give each other a chance to talk about fights, commitment, jealousy, work, housework and all the other things people need to talk about. And many of us are creating our own rituals, where friends and family (sometimes blood relatives, sometimes alternative families) come together to celebrate important events: to affirm our identities as women and lesbians, to honor commitments between women.*

We could also gather around each other on other occasions: to mark our children's comings and goings or the endings as well as beginnings of relationships.

Loving each other—as friends, lovers and family—is a source of power, joy, struggle and growth. We look forward to loving more openly, more bravely, more outrageously and more deeply, in as many ways as we can create.

SEXUALITY*

Part of loving women is feeling sexually attracted to women. What we do with this attraction is as varied as we are. Through sex we may express love, friendship, lust, nurturance, need, a sense of adventure, delight in our own bodies. We may kiss and hug a lot, caress our lover's body for hours or have a "quickie." We may play with her nipples or clitoris, explore her vagina with our fingers or our tongues, touch our own bodies, too. We may have orgasms, not have orgasms, use erotic pictures, share fantasies, play sex games, laugh while making love, sleep together without genital sex. There is no one way to be sexual as a lesbian, and no "right" way.

Books and movies always show men and women being sexual together, with certain roles that everyone expects. For lesbians, even what "having sex" means isn't so clearly defined. For me and my lovers it's always been teaching each other, learning together, making it up as we go along. That's how I like it. I feel like anything is possible.

Sex with my male lovers was always okay. But with Paula I'm amazed at the intensity. I want to touch and be touched, make love all the time, be rough, be gentle, penetrate her, feel her moving on me. I think I'm finally feeling the fullness and depth of my sexuality. I had always suspected there must be more to it, but hadn't figured out how to find it.

In finding out what turns my lover on, exploring her body, tasting her, learning her odors and textures, I am growing to love myself more, too.

There are also problems, of course, one of which is the myth that lesbian sex is problem free. We can run into trouble by expecting sex with women to be "blissful, intuitive, spontaneous and never dull."[4]

Making love with a woman for the first time

---

*Lesbians are also pushing religious groups to celebrate lesbian relationships and life events. Others are creating their own rituals. See *Ceremonies of the Heart* by Becky Butler, ed., Seattle, WA: Seal Press, 1990.

*To enjoy sex with another woman without risking human immunodeficiency virus (HIV) transmission (the cause of AIDS) see Safer Sex in Chapter 15, "AIDS, HIV Infection and Women." For specifics about women's sexual response, see Chapter 11, "Sexuality."

Joy Schneider Kendra

usually involves a lot more than what happens sexually. We may feel suddenly freed as sexual beings. We may feel exhilarated and joyful and terrified out of our skins. It can take months and even years to learn about our shifting patterns in sex, what we like and what our particular stumbling blocks are.

Making love with a woman, we have at least a basic idea of what would feel good to her. However, we may wrongly expect that because she has a body like ours, we should know what pleases her.

The more women I sleep with, the more I realize you can't assume what you like is what she likes. There are tremendous differences. All kinds of stuff needs to be talked about and often isn't.

I have a real hard time getting started in sex, but once I'm started I have an easy time coming. My lover loves to get started but has a hard time coming and gets real frustrated. We have trouble talking about it.

We had a wildly passionate sex life for a year and a half. When we moved in together, sexuality suddenly became an issue. It turned out our patterns were very different. My lover needs to talk, to feel intimate in conversation, to relax completely before she can feel sexual. I need to touch and to make a physical connection first before I feel relaxed enough to talk intimately. I'd reach out for her as we went into the bedroom and she'd freeze. We battled it out for months, both feeling terrible, before we figured out what was going on.

In this age of AIDS and other sexually transmitted diseases (STDs), negotiating with our women lovers about safer sex—*before having sex*—is absolutely necessary. It is a dangerous myth that lesbians are not at risk of passing STDs or HIV infection to each other. We *are* at risk. Never having had to negotiate about birth control with a woman partner, we may feel awkward bringing up safer sex, but it's crucial.

I couldn't believe it when she told me that none of her other lovers had ever asked if she had been exposed to any diseases before they slept together.

See Chapter 14 and Safer Sex, p. 338, for more information.

Because women are so deeply socialized not to be sexually assertive or to seek pleasure openly, it can be a revelation to learn with a lesbian lover how to talk freely about what you both want in sex.

When I make love with a woman, the challenge is to be honest more often; to say what I am really feeling; to explore when I'm not feeling present instead of pretending that I am; if I am spacing out, to ask what's the fear.

"We can come to lesbian sex with . . . a legacy of heterosexual role models harmful to women. Whether we have been heterosexual or not, those ideas creep in anyway."[5] We may bring the following to lovemaking:

- The belief that we don't like sex much and are perhaps undersexed or "frigid."
- The feeling that sex is okay but not very profound.
- The assumption that we owe it to our lovers to have sex when they want to.
- Distrust of our sexual responses—the conviction that we can't orgasm in sex with a partner.
- Little experience in being assertive or taking the lead in sex.
- Shyness about touching ourselves in sex because we think (or we think our partner thinks) she should do it all.
- A focus on performance in lovemaking, including orgasm as a goal every time.
- Emotional scars from having had our bodies used or abused sexually.

Some of us may suspect our own impulses and preferences when they seem to follow a male model. We may feel uncomfortable with lust, for instance, or with acting aggressively, having fantasies of dominance or using erotic materials. Yet these may be aspects of sexuality which we would enjoy. A dildo, for instance, is not necessarily a "penis substitute"; it gives us pleasure if we enjoy being penetrated in sex. As lesbians we have a chance to move away from male-defined sexuality and to reclaim all the dimensions of sexuality that deepen our intimacy, pleasure and love.

Some lesbians practice sadomasochism (S/M), that is, eroticizing the consensual exchange of power with the goal of safe, sane, consensual sex.*

Finding time and energy for sex, if we want it, isn't always easy.

I was with a group of five lesbian couples last summer, all close friends. Ten women, and we all wish we made love more frequently than we do. Does it have to do with having kids (some of us are mothers), or that the excitement has gone from the relationship, or are we taking in negative stuff from what society thinks of lesbians?

It's all there: How are you feeling about your work? About the people you work with? Or about the fact that the house hasn't been vacuumed in two weeks, and the car needs something done to it? Gosh, it really would be nice to have a little time for sex now and then.

We need to feel free to be sexual, whatever form that takes for us. We are learning as women to balance what we give to others by taking time for ourselves: Maybe we also have to affirm the need for taking time for sexual pleasure.

People say lesbians don't have much sex. Well, I know a whole lot of lesbians who have a whole lot of sex, and good sex, at that!

If you or you and your lover(s) have problems with sex, you may want to join a lesbian discussion group or seek counseling. (See the appendix in Chapter 11, "Sexuality.") Most important, we can probably help each other as friends more than we do now, by bringing sexual problems and issues into our conversations. "How's your sex life?" may be a timely, kind and enormously helpful question to ask.

LEGAL ISSUES

As lesbians, we struggle—along with other minority groups—for the legal rights and protections we deserve. This dilemma is compounded for poor lesbians, lesbians of color, lesbians in prisons. Most legislators, judges and lawyers in the American judicial system are white heterosexual men who exercise this society's bias against lesbians and other peoples different from themselves.

In the last thirty years, we have won some changes. A few states, like Massachusetts and Wisconsin, have passed lesbian and gay civil rights laws. Some cities have passed domestic partnership laws, which offer legal rights to registered partners (same or opposite sex). Lesbians have won a small but growing number of child custody and job discrimination cases. Some lesbian and gay couples are suing for the right to marry. Co-adoption by same-sex couples has happened in California, and cases are pending elsewhere. Some judges and lawyers are becoming less biased—a few are even open lesbians. Our increased visibility and openness help to bring these changes.

Lesbians face many legal issues beyond those that are addressed in this chapter, such as protection of the rights of lesbians in prison, legal defense after police raids of bars and public gathering places, protection from housing discrimination, recourse for lesbians committed to mental institutions by homophobic relatives. (See Resources for groups and books that may be helpful.)

Relationship Rights and Contracts

Because relationship laws are oriented toward marriage, lesbian lovers are in a legal vacuum in defining our rights and responsibilities to each other.* Lesbians today are exploring various ways of establishing and protecting our relationships.

If you are in or entering into a relationship that you think will last for some time, you and your lover can protect yourselves by working out a formal written agreement or contract about expenses, purchases, work and so on.

Where property is involved (unlike matters involving children), courts may well consider a notarized contract binding. However, court proceedings are painful and costly, and the outcome in lesbian and gay cases is not predictable. If you wish to separate and cannot solve property disputes, consider couples therapy or mediation

*For both sides of the debate about S/M in the lesbian community, see *The Lesbian S/M Safety Manual* by Pat Califa, ed., Boston, MA: Lace Publications, 1988, and *Against Sado-Masochism: A Radical Feminist Analysis* by Robin Linden, Darlene Pagano, Diane Russell, and Susan Star, eds., East Palo Alto, CA: Frog in the Well, 1982.

*Whether or not "marriage" is what we would want, there are some important legal and financial benefits not available to us because we can't legally marry: We can't get health insurance coverage on each other's policies, for instance, or provide for each other in sickness or death through Social Security or death and disability benefits. Domestic partnership laws can change some of this. A useful resource is *A Legal Guide for Lesbian and Gay Couples* by Curry F. Hayden and Denis Clifford, Berkeley, CA: Nolo Press, 1991.

first, as they often help you to continue to treat each other more decently.

Many of us who are lesbian lawyers encourage women to agree in their contract to community arbitration, thus avoiding the sexist, homophobic legal system.

Medical Rights

In time of sickness or death, the law will automatically entrust your nearest blood relative with decisions and leave your lover powerless to choose a course of treatment or a burial site or dispose of your property. Your family may listen to your lover, but they are not obligated to do so. You and your lover can try to guarantee each other control in medical situations by giving each other power of attorney, by writing a health care proxy where possible, by setting up a guardianship to take effect in case of incapacity and/or by writing each other into your wills (see Legal Issues in Resources).

Parenthood

Court proceedings are both more necessary and far less predictable in situations involving children, be they children from a heterosexual marriage that has ended, or adopted or born to us as single mothers or as lesbian partners. The court can step in at any time to do whatever it thinks is in the best interest of a minor child, even despite previous court orders or written agreements.

Custody

Some lesbians have fought successfully for custody of their children in the past few years, often with the legal and emotional backing of other lesbians. In many states now, homosexuality alone is not supposed to be used to determine one's fitness as a parent. But winning custody as a known lesbian is still difficult or impossible in many communities. (See the box Seeking Custody for some guidelines.)

Sharing Parenthood with a Lover

It is a good idea for two lovers who have or adopt a child (or if one lover "adopts" her partner's child) to write up a contract stating each partner's responsibilities and intentions, particularly with regard to custody and visitation rights after separation or the biological mother's death. Put provisions in each of your wills for your lover to be the child's guardian. The courts do not have to honor your contract or will, but such documents will nevertheless demonstrate a social–psychological basis for your partnership and establish your clear intent to parent together.

SEEKING CUSTODY

Even if you think you may want your children to live with their father, it is often wise to establish custody at first so that you can retain control over that choice. If you do not want to live with your children but would like the option of spending time with them periodically, be sure the divorce/custody agreement includes specified visitation rights. If visits are left up to the children's choice, their father may pressure them into staying away from you.

It is invaluable to have a sympathetic lawyer, even if you don't expect that your sexual orientation will be an issue in the divorce and custody negotiations. Try if at all possible to find a lawyer who accepts lesbianism, has experience in custody cases (preferably with lesbian mothers) and is known and respected by the local court. Such an ideal person is often not available but worth looking hard for. Lesbians with limited financial resources and/or who live in nonurban areas may get some advice and assistance from the Lesbian Mothers' National Defense Fund or another lesbian organization (see Resources).

Prepare for a custody case with extreme care. You must demonstrate to the court as conclusively as possible that you are a competent, caring and dependable mother. A social worker may assess your mothering and present evidence at the hearing. You must seem reasonable, friendly and cooperative to the social worker no matter what you are feeling. Keep records of events that will document your concern for your children: medical and dental care, school conferences and reports, clothing and food expenditures. Record your interactions. Gather as much support from friends around you as you can during this stressful time, but if you have a lover, much as you want to, it is best not to move in together now. You may think of taking your children to another state, but this could be dangerous: The Uniform Child Custody Act makes it difficult to escape court involvement, and an attempt to take them away will reflect unfavorably on your case. Finally, expert witnesses like child psychologists are expensive but may be essential in case the opposition brings in its own "experts."

Alternative Insemination

Many lesbians are turning to artificial insemination as a form of conception that doesn't require having sex with a man. Chapter 18, "New Reproductive Technologies," mentions the legal considerations that may arise, and describes insemination techniques.

Far more health-care providers are now willing to inseminate lesbians and single women. If you find one who is willing to do so, s/he may contact the Sperm Bank of California to obtain semen. See Resources for this and other lesbian friendly insemination programs in the United States.

MEDICAL CARE*

Perhaps the most serious health issue for lesbians is that too often we don't feel comfortable or safe seeking care when we need it (until an emergency arises) because of the ignorance, antiwoman and antilesbian attitudes we encounter in most of the medical system. As a result of the women's and gay rights movements, a few more enlightened and unprejudiced providers are available—usually nurses, occasionally physicians, most often in urban areas where large lesbian communities exist and especially in women-controlled health centers. But most of us depend on providers who know little about our special issues, such as our risk of AIDS, or which STDs we are most likely to catch.

I went to the clinic hemorrhaging badly. The doctor, who knew I was a lesbian and not trying to get pregnant, insisted I was having a miscarriage.

A growing number of health care providers are lesbian or sensitive to lesbians' health care needs, but there are also insensitive practitioners who can put us into uncomfortable situations. If we don't come out to them, they may try to persuade us to use birth control, or question us about intercourse. Yet if we tell them we are lesbian, we may get lectures, snide remarks and voyeuristic questions. ("What do lesbians do in bed anyway?") Our lesbianism may become the focus of the visit, and our medical problems may never be seriously addressed. We also risk having our lesbianism documented in our medical records, which are supposed to be confidential but are not always kept that way.

I would not come out in a medical situation unless there were compelling reasons to do so, because in the "patient" role I have so little power and am especially vulnerable to harassment. So I practice in advance how to maintain my privacy and still get the care I need—ways of refusing to answer offensive or unnecessary inquiries, and of asking direct, specific questions about what I need to know. For instance, if a practitioner says, "No sex for a month," I can ask whether I should avoid sexual arousal itself or just vaginal penetration. The book Lesbian Health Matters! [see Resources] has helped me invaluably in dealing with medical visits.*

You may find a lesbian-sensitive provider by asking lesbian friends or using a lesbian/gay health service, a feminist women's health center, a regional lesbian/gay service guide, community center or hotline.

Alcoholism

Because oppression creates extra stress in our lives, and because often bars are the only public places where we can get together openly with other lesbians, a lot of lesbians drink. Drinking becomes a problem for anyone who can't control when and/or how much she drinks. If this seems true for you or a friend, please consult Chapter 3, "Alcohol, Mood-Altering Drugs and Smoking." A growing number of alcoholic support and recovery programs are willing to deal openly with lesbians, and the more progressive ones respect lovers as family members. Many chapters of Alcoholics Anonymous and Alanon have lesbian meetings. Within the lesbian community we can all become more conscious about alcoholism. We can create drug-free spaces and serve inexpensive nonalcoholic drinks at the bars to support recovering women and others who have problems with drinking.

Mental Health

Almost everyone runs into times of emotional confusion, and a lesbian in this society faces extra emotional stress. We may get help by turning to friends who listen well; by being in a women's or lesbian support group; by asking an objective third person to mediate between us and a lover, co-worker or housemate; by trying to take better care of ourselves physically. When these sources of help aren't enough, we may choose to work for a time with a trained psychotherapist.

Good therapy can be a tremendous help. Finding good therapy, however, is not always an easy job for any woman. Historically, psychiatry has been sexist, antihomosexual and male-dominated. Its goal for women has been that we adapt ourselves to our role in society. In 1973, the American Psychiatric Association removed homosexuality

---

*Particular health and medical problems as they affect lesbians appear throughout the book.

from its list of illnesses to be "cured," but many conservative therapists still consider it abnormal. Be wary of a therapist who sees your sexual preference as the source of your problems and therefore fails to take your real problems seriously.

Fortunately today there are more openly lesbian therapists (mostly in urban areas so far) and more heterosexual therapists who are feminist and/or see lesbianism as a valid way of life. To find someone, check with friends, a women's center, the YWCA or in women's journals and newspapers. Sometimes it's important to see a lesbian, who will be more likely to understand your experiences from the "inside." A lesbian therapist said, however,

I don't care who my therapist sleeps with as long as she or he doesn't think sleeping with women is sick. Just because a therapist is a woman or even a lesbian doesn't mean she'd be the best one for you to work with.

In your first interview, don't hesitate to ask about the therapist's views, training and beliefs. You can ask yourself: Do I feel comfortable talking to this person? Does s/he listen to me? Is the therapist willing to recognize the importance of political and social factors, like sexism and homophobia? Does s/he have a merely tolerant attitude toward lesbians or is s/he genuinely positive and affirming?* It's worth putting energy into finding someone you can work well with. If as the therapy progresses it feels oppressive in any way, bring this up with the therapist, and if you can't work it out together, leave.

Sometimes frightened or angry parents pressure or force a young lesbian into therapy—or, worse, into a mental institution—in hopes of changing her sexual orientation. A young rural lesbian said, "My parents stopped giving me money for school when I came out to them. They said, 'We'll pay for a psychiatrist but nothing else.'" Obviously therapy in such a situation is a mockery and a punishment.

WE ARE EVERYWHERE

Lesbians *are* everywhere. In every possible ethnic group, occupation and geographical location, we are beginning to identify ourselves more openly and to discover our common issues. To conclude this chapter, lesbians in four different kinds of

*See Chapter 6, "Psychotherapy," for general guidelines in choosing a therapist. See also *The Lavender Couch: A Consumer's Guide to Psychotherapy for Lesbians and Gay Men*, by Marny Hall, Boston: Alyson Publications, 1985.

groups have spoken of their special experiences and concerns.

Older Lesbians

A forty-five-year-old woman in her first lesbian relationship said:

I have a whole different feeling about aging since I met Ruth. Partly it's loving her and feeling so loved and so fully known for the first time. Also, as she and other lesbians teach me about being strong, being your own person, I feel more optimistic about growing older.

A lesbian in her seventies said:

Many women have a false security. A woman will say, "I'll always have my husband to take care of me." No, she won't. There's no security for any animal, any organism in the natural world. But lesbians are accustomed to the reality of life. That keeps them flexible and more prepared for the later years. It's partly the rigidity that people nurture within themselves that makes their old age hard for them. Most lesbians don't have the luxury of being rigid.

When asked about the disadvantages of being lesbian and old, this woman said, "You've asked the wrong person. For me there are no negative aspects to it at all."

Like most older women, lesbians resent the various stereotypes about aging. We object to the patronizing way the young often assume that we are weak and helpless. We also object to being seen as wise, serene, above the passions of youth. People generally don't want to think of older women as sexual beings; an old lesbian, with the sexual connotations of the word, is considered even more unacceptable. We are still quite human, emotionally alive and sexually active and proud of that.

Any older woman can find herself isolated and unable to find satisfying, sustaining work. This is even more true for older lesbians, because homophobia operates in addition to ageism and sexism. Therefore, it's necessary for us to find and develop a family—if not our own, a family of friends, homosexual and heterosexual, old and young, with whom we can share, care, love and encourage. This is especially important for older lesbians who are single, have lost a lover or live in remote areas where it's hard to find support.

For some single older lesbians who feel that there isn't much time left, a scary question is "Can

*Poverty, ageism and racism are probably the most significant factors in making old age hard for many women. (See Chapter 23, "Women Growing Older.")

I ever find a lover?" It takes courage and initiative.* If a lover is considerably younger, age difference can be an issue. Some women feel that wide age differences are inappropriate ("I should act my age" or "I won't be able to keep up with her"); others feel that age doesn't matter.

Alice and I grew up in different worlds—she in the fifties and I in the twenties. So much has changed, especially for women. What she wants for her life is not what I ever wanted or expected for mine. As long as both of us notice, respect and understand these differences, we do well together. In a way, the age span is good—it makes us see that we can't be everything for each other, that we need friends our own age.

Older lesbian couples need to be prepared for some special situations. See Legal Issues (p. 188) for strategies to make sure that close relationships are honored in times of sickness or death. We must face the inevitability of death, and talk together about dying, loneliness and pain. See Chapter 23, "Women Growing Older," for more on this and on taking control of our death.

An older lesbian who is out, strong, independent and unafraid can find support from younger women who may welcome such a role model. But we also need support for our fears, dependencies and weaknesses.

It's good to mix older and younger lesbians. When younger people get together more often with older lesbians and see that they're not doddering and so on, they'll be aware that there's not that much difference, and perhaps it will make it easier for them as they grow older.

Lesbians of Color—Our Rich Variety

The fabric of our lives as lesbians of color is as dense as a tapestry, woven of the hundred shades and hues of our variety. It is difficult to tease out a thread and let it stand for the whole. For some of us, the brilliance of our color is the tapestry's dominant theme.

I was with two friends of mine one morning—one is Dominican and the other is from the Philippines. We were all in the bathroom getting ready for work and we each touched the others' hair. One thick, one

---

*An unusual resource for finding a lesbian friend is The Wishing Well, Box 1328, Novato, CA 94948. This is a quarterly publication with self-descriptions (by code number) of lesbian women wishing to meet others, as well as letters, ads, resources, etc.

Ellen Shub

wavy, one kinky. I kept smiling during the day when I thought about it.

Sometimes I get almost a physical charge from being black. I hear a beautiful black woman singing, and I feel like jumping up and down for joy. I think, How powerful, that's me.

The Women of Our Tradition

Our eyes are often drawn to the images of the renegade women we have known, women who haven't fit our culture's ideal for women—an aunt, a cousin, an old friend of the family. Often, despite their differences, these women were (and are) not cast out of their community; as part of an oppressed culture in the United States, our friends and families may rely on each other too much not to encourage and accept anyone—regardless of gender—who is spirited. Some of us, however, draw more pain than strength from these outsiders in our culture, some of whom must have been lesbian. Although they might have lived with a sister or a friend, their lives were still seen in terms of their role within the family. Mother, father or brother had a considerable say over what they did. The silence that veiled whatever intimate relationships they enjoyed obscures our heritage as lesbians of color.

Our Particular Oppression

Homophobia, woman hating and distortion of our self-image as women are woven into our lives and cultures. The stark fact of our oppression as lesbians and as women may not differ from what our white sisters experience. But the expression, the contradictions, the meanings and contexts may all be vastly different, both from our white sisters and among ourselves.

Coming to womanhood as a Third World woman, regardless of your sexual preference, you have to deal with certain stereotypical images of Third World women that are prevalent in this society. If you're a lesbian, it's even more difficult to struggle against these images. For a black woman, the images of the strong black woman who can carry everybody on her back or the earthy, sexy vamp are hard to fight against. Those images are unreal, confining and racist, to say the least. Many people expect you to fit into some preconceived idea they have about what a black woman is supposed to be. They deny whole sides of you as a woman.

I remember the sting of words like maricón *[fag]* and tortillera *[lesbian]. I began to realize these words had something to do with me. But they didn't speak for me, for my feelings as a human being. The Catholic Church had placed me in all-girl schools all my life and taught me to love others. Now it was wrong. This was a time of incredible contradictions.*

Coming out to my family meant I risked losing not only them as loved ones but a whole safety net, a barrier between me and a hostile world. It made it more frightening, but the need I had for my family made the desire to be honest more pressing as well.

Creating Ourselves

As lesbians of color, we are women moving between two or more cultures or value systems, none of which fully sees or accepts us. As African-American, Latin, Asian or American Indian women, we each carry within us the traditional expectation of womanhood in our culture. At the same time, we live within the greater Anglo-American society, which through its schools, mass

Long-time lesbian-feminist activists Audre Lorde, Barbara Smith and Beverly Smith.   Tia Cross

media and political and economic systems teaches us another brand of ideal womanhood. Both images are predominantly heterosexual. We must face this denial of our love for women in a society where the color of our skin and the language of our people as well as our identity as women who love other women are all strikes against us, tools used to separate us from one another.

Our struggle to survive and grow as lesbians of color becomes the difficult task of always balancing all the elements of who we are and who we choose to become. We can explore our past and our diverse cultures and draw from each those qualities and traditions that will most enrich and strengthen our lives.

As women, and especially as Latina women, we have been programmed to be caretakers. Especially as lesbians, because we have never married, we often have to take care of everybody else, everybody else's family, everyone's needs. I'm taking care of myself now, too. I am affirming my life.

Our Experience in a White Community of Women

As lesbians we are drawn to the growing lesbian community and culture of women in this country—to bars, concerts, support and political groups. Many white sisters reading this can share the feeling of excitement we've had entering these places, where it's safe to be open in our love and care for other women. Yet there is a painful contradiction. It is in these, the places where we expect to feel most accepted and supported, that we often meet with barriers of misunderstanding and ignorance from white sisters unfamiliar with our lives and needs as women of color. Much of the structure of the women's community excludes us and makes us invisible. The language and approach are largely those of a white culture, not our own.

I was doing some volunteer legal work for a women's music-archives group. Almost all the music in the collection was by white women. I'd name women of color whose music I loved, and they kept saying their collection was "feminist." I said I questioned how they defined "feminist," since in reality it kept translating to "white."

Some people in the women's community give me a hard time about my nails—the length and color. My feelings about color and adornment are wholly different from theirs.

At a drumming concert a lot of the women began beating time (not even on the beat, mind you) on their knees. I know they wouldn't presume to sing along unless asked to with, say, Holly Near. It's a subtle thing but spoke clearly to me about a lack of respect for a culture.

Many of us feel that as soon as we stop talking with white women about our experiences as women of color or about racism, that part of us ceases to be in their eyes. It can be lonely, disheartening and infuriating. A sharing of the load is welcome.

A white friend of mine broke into a conversation I was having with two other women about racism among lesbians. She defended what I was saying. When we talked later, I said what an easing it was not to have to struggle alone. A patch on her face that turns red when she's excited blazed bright. "You shouldn't have to fight. We should do it. We should do it!" Tears came to my eyes with the relief I felt.

We need to talk, to be unafraid to confront each other about our misperceptions and our fears. The conversation must be not only between us and our white sisters but among ourselves as well. As members of oppressed groups, we have been divided by suspicion and ignorance about other peoples of color and even about our own. Sometimes when we look at another woman of color we see reflected in her the oppression of our culture, our language, our ways, and we experience a fear of looking at ourselves.

Whenever I saw other Asian women on the street or at a gathering, we wouldn't look at each other directly and would actually be embarrassed, as though we weren't supposed to be there. It showed me how effective racism is in destroying bonds between people.

Those of us who are or have been involved in interracial relationships and friendships are sometimes torn by the pressure to separate, by the fears that have always divided our peoples. When we talk openly with other women who are different from us, we see the common patterns of gender, class and racial oppression and can begin to find our unity.

We are reclaiming our right to join as women and lesbians of color, celebrating our heritage and our rich tradition. At the same time, we recognize the importance of a common struggle waged by all women, particularly lesbians. We must remember that our common roots span continents, races and languages. Our conversation has just begun.

Lesbians with Physical Disabilities

Disabled lesbians are a large and growing group that the lesbian community acknowledges but doesn't yet fully embrace. We are all colors and races, all cultures, shapes, sizes and ages. Some of our disabilities are hidden, some are very visible. Some of us are born differently abled; some of us acquire a disability suddenly and unexpectedly, or over time.

For a long time we have been isolated from each other in our dual identity as lesbians and disabled women.

From my perceptions and from other disabled dykes I've talked to, there are lots of reasons differently abled dykes hesitate to come out as lesbians. Being someone who is physically different in appearance leaves me already open to ridicule and stares. Lesbians are attacked all the time for being different. Why choose to get hurt twice if you can avoid it? Also, people think disabled women are sexless. If I came out at work I don't know if they'd be upset or just laugh. They'd say, "How can you be a lesbian if you have no sex?"

Today more and more of us are coming out, and our networking is working. At the Michigan Women's Music Festival in the late 1970s, some of us exchanged names and started a mailing list. The Disabled Lesbian Alliance helps us keep in touch. There is also the National Rainbow Alliance of the Deaf, for lesbians and gay men, which has chapters all over the United States.

Loving women is sometimes part of coming to accept ourselves as women, which can be hard to do if we don't fit the description of what a woman is "supposed" to look like.

I was disabled by an accident before I became a lesbian. As a woman in a wheelchair I felt something less than a person. But my nurse, who is a lesbian, told me I could have a strong self-image. She said that we are taught to hate ourselves because we are women and that we can love ourselves instead. I started spending time with lesbians. The closer I came to lesbianism the more I began to like myself.

Lesbians are often more accepting of us and our bodies than men are. But even lesbians often hold us at a distance.

Some women are uncomfortable just being around a disabled woman; others are comfortable with being a friend but can't consider a sexual relationship. I feel like my sexuality is taboo.

Sexually we are often stereotyped as sexless or overly needy.

When I tell people Janet is my lover they look at her like they're thinking, Poor thing! or She must be a nurse! or Maybe she's a pervert who gets off on sex with a disabled woman. They can't imagine that she loves me and the disability is only one thing about me.

Although it is common for those of us who spend time in institutions or hospitals or with daily attendants to have sexual relationships with our primary caretakers, it isn't necessarily a "nursing" relationship. Our lovers take care of us no more than we take care of them. We may have to make special arrangements for sex or give our lover certain information about our sexuality, but every sexual relationship in the world is shaped by both individuals' wants, needs and capabilities.

I felt weird because I had to explain what my sexual needs were to anyone I wanted to sleep with until I realized that everyone has to explain what their needs are in order to get them met. I don't have sensation in my pubic area, but since there is no set standard to what lesbian lovemaking is, it leaves a whole world of sexuality and sensuality open to explore.

Once we have accepted our dual identity, we would like to be able to live it more easily. But many people we meet have a hard time with it.

People on the street will deal with my disability sometimes, but no matter how butch I am or what buttons I have on, they won't deal with me as a lesbian.

In health care, heterosexual physicians will look at our disability but are rarely sensitive about lesbianism and thus do not see us as whole people. Feminist or lesbian health care services will welcome us as lesbians, but the facilities are usually inaccessible. We wind up most of the time being seen as either lesbian or disabled but not both.

The lesbian community is committed at a certain level to including all kinds of women. Lesbians usually look for wheelchair-accessible spaces in which to hold concerts and community events and offer signing there for the deaf and hearing-impaired. Yet this risks being tokenism if a tremendous amount more is not done.

There's been both sensitivity and a lack thereof in this community. We can confront other lesbians about things that wouldn't even come up in the heterosexual world—like not just getting wheelchair access to concerts but being able to sit with our friends. Yet where were other lesbians when we picketed inaccessible movie houses? Our power and strength are used for lesbian issues at lesbian rallies, but few women rally for us.

It is time for the lesbian community to hear our voices. Don't segregate us from our other sisters. We all need each other.

Lesbian Mothers

When the rest of the world pretends we don't exist or tells us we can't exist, we as lesbian mothers need to say to each other, "Yes, come on and join us!"

Many of us were mothers before we knew we were lesbians. Some of us have become mothers since. Either way, being a mother is full of wonder and work. Although being a *lesbian* mother adds some unique satisfactions and special difficulties, the main issues we live with as our children grow are shared by most mothers in our society.

Our situations as lesbian mothers are varied. Some of us live with our children; some do not. Some of us are out to our children; others are not. Our support systems vary: Many of us are single parents; some are coparents; we receive very different amounts of support from friends, the child's father and/or blood relatives. Some of us live in neighborhoods where we can be relatively open about being lesbians, and others among us have to keep our lesbianism hidden from adult and child neighbors alike.

The heterosexual world of parent–teacher conferences, visits to pediatricians and birthday parties rarely recognizes that we are both lesbians and mothers. Even within the lesbian community we often feel like an invisible minority. While our need to come out of isolation and make ourselves known has sometimes brought us loss and pain, it has also created experiences of joy and understanding in support groups and in many friendships.

Today more and more lesbians are choosing to have or adopt children, either as single women or in couples. For books about this choice and about lesbian parenting, see Resources.

Susan Butler

195

Coming Out

Should I tell my kids I'm a lesbian? When? When I have a lover? If she moves in? It is such a big part of my life that it feels crazy to hide it from them.

Being out or closeted with our children is a personal choice that ends up being based on the reality of each lesbian mother's life. All of us must weigh our concern for protecting our children from a society that validates only heterosexual nuclear families against our need to be honest and open.

Being out to our children may bring problems. Children may feel they have to hide our lesbianism and resent it.

If they [other kids] knew about my mom I'm afraid they wouldn't like me. Sometimes I feel like I'm in the closet, too, and I'm not even gay.

Our sons may feel that our choice of women implies a rejection of them. A seventeen-year-old remembers:

My mother told me she was gay when I was twelve. It made me feel very different from everyone else. I thought that if you were a lesbian, then you didn't want boys around. My mother said that wasn't true, but about six months later I went to live with my father. Now that I'm older, I view it differently and I've also proved to myself that it didn't matter as much as I thought. I'm moving back home now.

For many of us, the rewards of coming out to our children outweigh the problems.

A lot of women in my lesbian mothers group have said that their kids were relieved to finally have it [our lesbianism] said instead of thinking it anyway and wondering why it couldn't be said.

I have been out to my daughter as long as I have been out to myself. I heard her at four telling a communal sister that girls could fall in love with girls and it was okay for boys to fall in love with boys. Where is the revolution? Sometimes it's right in our own backyards.

I think for those of us who are out to our kids, there are great results. Because we make ourselves open to our kids in this one area we are open to them in a lot of ways. We dare to be different, and sometimes it hurts to be different. That we share that with them creates a very special relationship. It also helps them understand prejudice. They begin to see that a kid who calls another kid some name about their religion or race is probably being as bigoted and narrow-minded as someone who calls their mother a dyke.

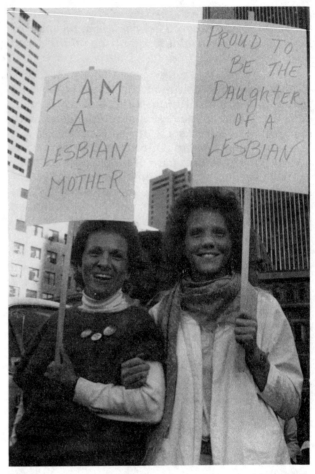

Ellen Shub

They can make connections that many people are never able to make.

For all of us who are considering coming out to our children, finding support during this time can help us move toward a healthy, strong identity as a lesbian and a mother. Some of us think it is good for our kids to have a lesbian mother because they see the options; they do not grow up believing the world to be heterosexual; and they have, right in the family, someone who is willing to be different. The better we feel about ourselves and our choices, the more we have to share with our kids and each other.

Custody

Some of us have not been able to choose whether or not we will live with our children.

Having come out as a lesbian has been real difficult for me because my child was taken away by his father. I was granted visitation rights and because I didn't know to make it specific, I've gone for six months without seeing him. It takes that long sometimes for legal proceedings to work themselves out.

196

It's amazing how the men—the fathers—get such special treatment. I mean, a battering husband is not treated the way a lesbian mother is. At the same time, though, it was being a lesbian and stepping out as a strong woman that made me able to withstand what followed.

Some of us live with the constant fear of losing our kids, and we shape our lives—coming out, jobs, lovers and living arrangements—with this in mind. Our basic right to raise our children may be challenged in the courts at any time by the father, the grandparents, relatives, neighbors or social service agencies.

However, during the past few years an increasing number of lesbians have been winning their custody battles in court. Some of us are now able to live with our children freely. Sometimes a father will win custody but sooner or later send the children back because he doesn't want the work of raising them. In addition, children who voluntarily leave may return home when they are older and clearer in identity.

It is important to recognize that *not* living with our children may be what we need or want, though in this society it can be hard to admit. Some lesbians have left their children with their fathers, which is a courageous choice since so many people believe mothers should keep their kids. We need to be free to make the arrangements that are the most sensible and loving all the way around.

Sometimes I feel real guilty, like a lousy mother. You know: I should be able to handle it all. I should be able to raise two kids and not be overwhelmed all the time by being a mother. On the other side of that is that I feel real good that I could be clear about the decision that my younger son would live with his father. It has worked out for all of us.

Resisting Guilt

All mothers are made to feel guilty about not being "good enough," and we may feel extra guilty if we think that our lesbianism makes our children's lives harder. If we are divorcing, our children express the anger and feelings of dislocation that nearly all children experience after their parents separate. We have to remember that they would be sad and angry at this time even if we weren't lesbians. All children, especially as teenagers, will have problems, because that is the nature of growing up. It is difficult to let go of the guilt because society's disapproving view of lesbians supports and reinforces it. It helps to look at our heterosexual friends: Their children have nightmares, stay home sick from school, keep their rooms a mess, fight with their friends, get depressed, get furious at their parents, think they

have the worst luck a kid has ever had—just like our kids do.

Support

So much of what we need as lesbian mothers, whether we stay with our kids or not, is the same as if we weren't lesbians.

I'm a single mother, and that's the most important factor in what makes it hard for me to be doing all that I'm trying to do.

My lover and I both work full-time. One of our daughters is in day care and the other's in kindergarten. It's a scramble. Some days, family life feels like an endless negotiation about who's going to be where, when.

For all of us, help from friends is one thing that makes it easier to get through a day. Women who share a living space or live near each other can take some responsibility for each other's kids.

In my communal lesbian house, the other women were comothers to my daughter. Everyone did one night of child care a week. Everyone also took on part of the child's rent so I didn't have to pay double.

In other cases, women have built stable, regular relationships with our kids and cared for them on a regular basis, such as one afternoon a week or one weekend a month. In this way we have a break we can count on, a chance to relax a little, pull ourselves together, go out with our friends or just be alone. Still another kind of support comes when groups or gatherings of women make plans for child care so mothers aren't the only ones with responsibility for arrangements. For us, the importance of adequate child care and reasonable locations and hours at lesbian events cannot be overestimated.

Some of us have also been part of ongoing groups where we tell about our feelings and experiences as mothers. It has helped to know that other lesbian mothers live with problems similar to ours, to realize the problems aren't our fault, to strategize new approaches and share the daily surprises and delights we get from our kids. Here are a few things that the mothers in one group had to say about it.

What I've always wanted for my children is a wider network of caring adults, and we're making one in this group. It's not enough just to come in and talk about being lesbian mothers; we include our kids, having parties for us all, going to the beach together. . . . The kids must at some point look around the room and say to themselves, "All these kids have lesbian mothers," and feel less isolated. . . . It is wonderful finding out how many lesbian mothers there are. I used to think there must be two or three in the whole city.... The group is a place where neither we nor our kids have to hide any part of our lives.

NOTES

1. Karen Thompson and Julie Andrzejewski. *Why Can't Sharon Kowalski Come Home?* San Francisco: Spinsters/Aunt Lute, 1988.
2. Joan Nestle. "Butch-Fem Relationships: Sexual Courage in the 1950s," *Heresies*, Sex Issue, Vol. 3, No. 4, Issue 12 (May 1981), p. 21.
3. Joan Nestle. "Butch-Fem Relationships: Sexual Courage in the 1950s," p. 22.
4. Tacie Dejanikis, in *Off Our Backs*, November 1980, p. 25.
5. Tacie Dejanikis, in *Off Our Backs*, p. 25.

RESOURCES

Readings

Special thanks to the women at New Words Bookstore, Cambridge, MA, for their help with the 1992 update.

General

Allen, Paula Gunn. "Beloved Women: Lesbians in American Indian Cultures," *Conditions: Sixteen (1991)*, pp. 84–106.

Anzaldúa, Gloria, ed. *Making Face, Making Soul/Haciendo Caras: Creative and Critical Perspectives by Women of Color*. San Francisco: Aunt Lute Foundation, 1990.

Baetz, Ruth. *Lesbian Crossroads: Personal Stories of Lesbian Struggles and Triumphs*. Tallahassee, FL: Naiad Press, 1988.

Balka, Christie, and Andy Rose, eds. *Twice Blessed: On Being Lesbian, Gay, and Jewish*. Boston: Beacon Press, 1989.

Bechdel, Alison. *New, Improved! Dykes to Watch Out For*. Ithaca, NY: Firebrand Books, 1990.

Beck, Evelyn Torton, ed. *Nice Jewish Girls: A Lesbian Anthology*. Boston: Beacon Press, 1989.

Berzon, Betty. *Positively Gay: New Approaches to Gay Life.*, rev. ed. Studio City, CA: Media Mix, 1984. Deals with coming out, relationships, lesbian mothers, older lesbians, parents of lesbians and more.

Blumenfeld, Warren J., and Diane Raymond. *Looking at Gay and Lesbian Life*. Boston: Beacon Press, 1988.

Cruikshank, Margaret, ed. *The Lesbian Path: Women Loving Women*, rev. ed. San Francisco, CA: Grey Fox, 1985.

Geok-lim, Shirley, Mayumi Tsutakawa and Margarita Donnelly, eds. *The Forbidden Stitch: An Asian American Women's Anthology*. Corvallis, OR: Calyx Books, 1989. A collection of writings by Asian-American women, some of whom are lesbians.

Grahn, Judy. *Another Mother Tongue: Gay Words, Gay Worlds*. Boston: Beacon Press, 1984.

Hutchins, Loraine, and Lani Kaahumanu, eds. *Bi Any Other Name: Bisexual People Speak Out*. Boston: Alyson Publications, 1991.

Lorde, Audre. *Sister Outsider*. Freedom, CA: Crossing Press, 1984.

Love, Barbara, and Sidney Abbot. *Sappho Was a Right On Woman: A Liberated View of Lesbianism*. New York: Stein and Day, 1972. A classic. One of the first positive books.

Martin, Del, and Phyllis Lyon. *Lesbian/Woman*. Volcano, CA: Volcano Press, 1991. This 1972 classic affirmation of lesbian lives by the founders of Daughters of Bilitis (DOB) has been updated for its twentieth anniversary.

Moraga, Cherrie, and Gloria Anzaldúa, eds. *This Bridge Called My Back: Writings by Radical Women of Color*. Latham, NY: Kitchen Table Press, 1984. An excellent anthology of essays, poetry and conversations by Asian, African-American, Latin and American Indian women, many of whom are lesbians.

Penelope, Julia, and Sarah Valentine, eds. *Finding the Lesbians: Personal Accounts from Around the World*. Freedom, CA: Crossing Press, 1990.

Penelope, Julia, Sarah Valentine, and Susan J. Wolfe, eds. *The Original Coming Out Stories*, expanded edition. Freedom, CA: Crossing Press, 1989.

Pharr, Suzanne. *Homophobia: A Weapon of Sexism*. Little Rock, AR: Chardon Press, 1988.

Pratt, Minnie Bruce. *Rebellion: Essays 1980–1991*. Ithaca, NY: Firebrand Books, 1991. Important essays.

Ramos, Juanita. *Compañeras: Latina Lesbians (An Anthology)*. New York: Latina Lesbian History Project, 1987. Short stories, essays, poems, oral histories and art by U.S. and Latin-American lesbians.

Rich, Adrienne. *Compulsory Heterosexuality and Lesbian Existence*. Denver: Antelope Publications, 1982. A now classic and often-cited pamphlet.

Silvera, Makeda, ed. *Piece of My Heart: A Lesbian of Colour Anthology*. Toronto, Ontario: Sister Vision (Black Women and Women of Color Press), 1991.

Lesbian History

Cruikshank, Margaret, ed. *Lesbian Studies: Present and Future*. New York: Feminist Press, 1982. A wonderful collection of articles about lesbians in academia, and aspects of research about our lives.

Duberman, Martin, Martha Vicinus and George Chauncey, Jr., eds. *Hidden from History: Reclaiming the Gay and Lesbian Past*. New York: Penguin/Meridian, 1990.

Faderman, Lillian. *Odd Girls and Twilight Lovers: A History of Lesbian Life in Twentieth-Century America*. New York: Columbia University Press, 1991.

Humphrey, Mary Ann. *My Country, My Right to Serve: Experiences of Gay Men and Women in the Military, World War II to the Present*. New York: HarperCollins, 1990.

Nestle, Joan. *A Restricted Country*. Ithaca, NY: Firebrand Books, 1987. Outstanding mix of historical, personal and erotic essays.

Weiss, A., and G. Schuller. *Before Stonewall: The Making of a Gay and Lesbian Community*. Tallahassee, FL: Naiad Press, 1988.

Older Lesbians

Adelman, Marcy, ed. *Long Time Passing: Lives of Older Lesbians*. Boston: Alyson Publications, 1986.

Copper, Baba. *Over the Hill: Reflections on Ageism Be-*

tween Women. Freedom, CA: Crossing Press, 1988.

MacDonald, Barbara, and Cynthia Rich, eds. Look Me in the Eye: Old Women, Aging and Ageism. San Francisco: Spinsters/Aunt Lute, 1983.

Rich, Cynthia. Desert Years: Undreaming the American Dream. San Francisco: Spinsters/Aunt Lute, 1989.

Sang, Barbara, Joyce Warshow and Adrienne Smith, eds. Lesbians at Midlife: The Creative Transition. San Francisco: Spinsters, 1991.

Lesbian Youth

American Friends Service Committee. Bridges of Respect: Creating Support for Lesbian and Gay Youth. Philadelphia: AFSC, 1989.

Brett, Catherine. S.P. Likes A.D. Toronto, Ontario: Women's Press, 1989. A novel.

Garden, Nancy. Annie on My Mind. New York: Farrar, Straus & Giroux, 1982. A novel.

———. Lark in the Morning. New York: Farrar, Straus & Giroux, 1991. A novel.

Heron, Ann. One Teenager in Ten. Boston: Alyson Publications, 1983.

Scoppettone, Sandra. Trying Hard to Hear You. Boston: Alyson Publications, 1991. A novel.

Wernette, Tim. "Exploring Sex with Someone of Your Own Sex," Ruth Bell, Changing Bodies, Changing Lives: A Book for Teens on Sex and Relationships. New York: Random House, 1987 Rev. Ed. Includes the voices of many lesbian and gay youths.

Young, Gay and Proud! U.S. edition prepared by Sasha Alyson. Boston, MA: Alyson Publications, 1980. A supportive guide covering many concerns of lesbian and gay youths, including special health concerns.

Health-Related Material

Boston Lesbian Psychologies Collective. Lesbian Psychologies: Explorations and Challenges. Urbana: University of Illinois Press, 1987.

Bradford, J., and C. Ryan, National Lesbian Health Care Survey. Washington, DC: National Gay and Lesbian Health Foundation, 1987.

Hall, Marny. The Lavender Couch: A Consumer's Guide to Psychotherapy for Lesbians and Gay Men. Boston: Alyson Publications, 1985.

O'Donnell, Mary, et al. Lesbian Health Matters!: A Resource Book About Lesbian Health. Santa Cruz, CA: Santa Cruz Women's Health Collective, 1979. $6.00. Available from Santa Cruz Women's Health Center, 250 Locust Street, Santa Cruz, CA 95060. An indispensable handbook on problems of the current health care system, gynecological exams, alternative fertilization, menopause, alcoholism and feminist therapy.

Shernoff, M., and W. Scott. The Sourcebook on Lesbian/Gay Health Care. Washington, DC: National Gay and Lesbian Health Foundation, 1988.

Relationships

Becker, Carol S. Unbroken Ties: Lesbian Ex-Lovers. Boston: Alyson Publications, 1988.

Berzon, Betty. Permanent Partnerships: Building Gay and Lesbian Relationships That Last. New York: E. P. Dutton, 1988.

Butler, Becky, ed. Ceremonies of the Heart. Seattle, WA: Seal Press, 1990. Describes commitment ceremonies of several lesbian couples.

Johnson, Susan. Staying Power: Long-term Lesbian Couples. Tallahassee, FL: Naiad Press, 1990.

Sexuality

Bad Attitude. Named Bad Attitude because "that's what women who take their sexuality into their own hands are told they have." Includes lesbian erotic fiction, poetry, reviews and photographs. S/M focus. Bimonthly.

Bright, Susie. Susie Sexpert's Lesbian Sex World. San Francisco: Cleis Press, 1990.

Califa, Pat, ed. The Lesbian S/M Safety Manual. Boston Lace Publications, 1988. This guide to S/M safer sex includes a national list of lesbian S/M support groups.

———. Macho Sluts. Boston, MA: Alyson Publications, 1988. S/M erotic fiction.

Corinne, Tee, ed. Intricate Passions: A Collection of Erotic Short Fiction. Austin, TX: Banned Books/Edward-William Publishing Company, 1989.

Linden, Robin, Darlene Pagano, Diana Russell and Susan Star, eds. Against Sado-Masochism: A Radical Feminist Analysis. East Palo Alto, CA: Frog in the Well, 1982.

Loulan, JoAnn. The Lesbian Erotic Dance: Butch, Femme, Androgyny and Other Rhythms. San Francisco: Spinsters, 1990.

———. Lesbian Passion: Loving Ourselves and Each Other. San Francisco: Spinsters/Aunt Lute, 1987.

———. Lesbian Sex. San Francisco: Spinsters/Aunt Lute, 1985.

On Our Backs: Entertainment for the Adventurous Lesbian. Features erotic photos and fiction, often controversial; this publication thrives on the taboo. S/M focus. Bimonthly.

Sexuality and Sexual Abuse

See Chapter 8, "Violence Against Women," for more resources.

Bass, Ellen, and Laura Davis. The Courage to Heal: A Guide for Women Survivors of Child Sexual Abuse. New York: Harper & Row, 1988.

Kelly, Liz. Surviving Sexual Violence. Minneapolis: University of Minnesota Press, 1988.

Maltz, Wendy, and Beverly Holman. Incest and Sexuality: A Guide to Understanding and Healing. Lexington, MA: Lexington Books, 1987.

Legal Issues

Boggan, E. Carrington, et al. The Rights of Gay People. New York: American Civil Liberties Union, 1983. Available from ACLU, 132 West 43rd Street, New York, NY 10036.

Curry, F. Hayden, and Denis Clifford. A Legal Guide for Lesbian and Gay Couples. Berkeley, CA: Nolo Press, 1991.

National Attorney's Directory for Lesbian and Gay Rights. $15.00. Available from Gay and Lesbian Advocates and Defenders (GLAD), P.O. Box 218, Boston, MA 02112. (617) 426-1350. GLAD will also do attorney referrals over the phone.

Partners: Newsletter for Gay and Lesbian Couples. Available from P.O. Box 9685, Seattle, WA 98109. (206) 784-1519. Has national and international legal information on adoption, child-custody cases, personal stories, relationship issues. Keeps you updated on legal information.

Thompson, Karen, and Julie Andrzejewski. *Why Can't Sharon Kowalski Come Home?* San Francisco: Spinsters/Aunt Lute, 1988.

Lesbian Mothers

Hanscombe, Gillian E., and Jackie Forster. *Rocking the Cradle: Lesbian Mothers—A Challenge in Family Living.* Boston: Alyson Publications, 1982.

Lorde, Audre. "Man Child: A Black Lesbian Feminist's Response," in *Sister, Outsider.* Freedom, CA: Crossing Press, 1984. A sensitive article about raising a son within the lesbian community.

Pies, Cheri. *Considering Parenthood.* San Francisco: Spinster, 1988.

Pollack, Sandra, and Jeanne Vaughn, eds. *Politics of the Heart: A Lesbian Parenting Anthology.* Ithaca, NY: Firebrand Books, 1987.

Rafkin, Louise. *Different Mothers: Sons and Daughters of Lesbians Talk About Their Lives.* San Francisco: Cleis Press, 1990.

For Family and Friends

Elwin, Rosamund, and Michele Panese. *Asha's Mums.* Toronto, Ontario: Women's Press, 1990. For children.

Fairchild, Betty, and Nancy Howard. *Now That You Know: What Every Parent Should Know About Homosexuality.* New York: Harvest, 1981.

Federation of Parents and Friends of Lesbians and Gays, P.O. Box 27605, Washington, DC 20038. (208) 638-4200. Write for their booklet: *About Our Children* or other publications.

Griffin, Carolyn Welch, Marion J. Wirth and Arthur G. Wirth. *Beyond Acceptance: Parents of Lesbians and Gays Talk About Their Experiences.* New York: St. Martin's Press, 1986.

Newman, Leslea. *Gloria Goes to Gay Pride.* Boston: Alyson Publications, 1991. For children.

———. *Heather Has Two Mommies.* Boston: Alyson Publications, 1989. For children.

Rafkin, Louise, ed. *Different Daughters: A Book by Mothers of Lesbians.* San Francisco: Cleis Press, 1987.

Valentine, Johnny. *The Duke Who Outlawed Jellybeans and Other Stories.* Boston: Alyson Publications, 1991. For children, with lesbian and gay characters.

Lesbians and Battering

The Lesbian Caucus of the Massachusetts Coalition of Battered Women Service Groups. *Voices of Battered Lesbians.* New Words. Audiocassette. $5.95. Available from author, 107 South Street, 5th Floor, Boston, MA 02111. (617) 426-8492.

Lobel, Kerry, ed., and National Coalition Against Domestic Violence Lesbian Taskforce. *Naming the Violence: Speaking Out About Lesbian Battering.* Seattle, WA: Seal Press, 1986.

Fiction

Write to publishers, presses and bookstores for current book lists. Our list is only a taste of what is available.

Alther, Lisa. *Other Women.* New York: Signet, 1985.

Arnold, June. *Sister Gin.* New York: The Feminist Press, 1989.

Brown, Rita Mae. *Rubyfruit Jungle.* New York: Bantam, 1977.

Davis, Jill, ed. *Lesbian Plays.* London: Methuen, 1987.

Forrest, Katherine V. *Murder at the Nightwood Bar.* A Kate Delafield mystery. Tallahassee, FL: Naiad Press, 1991.

Gearhart, Sally Miller. *The Wanderground: Stories of the Hill Women.* Boston: Alyson Publications, 1980.

Gomez, Jewelle. *The Gilda Stories.* Ithaca, NY: Firebrand Books, 1991.

Lorde, Audre. *Zami: Another Spelling of My Name.* Freedom, CA: Crossing Press, 1982.

Miller, Isabel. *Patience and Sarah.* New York: Ballantine, 1990.

Nestle, Joan, and Naomi Holoch, eds. *Women on Women: An Anthology of American Lesbian Short Fiction.* New York: Penguin Books 1990.

Rule, Jane. *Desert of the Heart.* Tallahassee, FL: Naiad Press, 1990.

———. *Memory Board.* Tallahassee, FL: Naiad Press, 1989.

Sarton, May. *Mrs. Stevens Hears the Mermaids Singing.* New York: W. W. Norton, 1975.

Schulman, Sarah. *People in Touble.* New York: Penguin Books, 1991.

Wilson, Barbara. *Gaudi Afternoon.* A Cassandra Reilley mystery. Seattle, WA: Seal Press, 1990.

Also look for reissues of the 1950s novels by Ann Bannon and Paula Christian. Other writers to look for: Dorothy Allison, Jane Chambers, Jan Clausen, Sarah Dreher, Camarin Grae, Andrea Freud Lowenstein, Judith McDaniel, Valerie Miner, Leslea Newman and Monique Wittig.

Poetry

Because there are so many fine poets currently in print, we will list only names: Paula Gunn Allen, Gloria Anzaldúa, Robin Becker, Becky Birtha, Olga Broumas, Stephanie Byrd, Chrystos, Cheryl Clarke, Jan Clausen, Michelle Cliff, Sandra Maria Esteves, Elsa Gidlow, Judy Grahn, Joy Harjo, June Jordan, Willyce Kim, Irena Klepfisz, Joan Larkin, Audre Lorde, Cherrie Moraga, Barbara Noda, Pat Parker, Adrienne Rich, Kate Rushin, Chocolate Waters and Fran Winant.

Periodicals

This is a representative sample. Periodicals listed for "feminists" or "women" regularly feature lesbian-related articles.

Bridges
P.O. Box 18437
Seattle, WA 98118
A journal for Jewish feminists and our friends.

Common Lives/Lesbian Lives
P.O. Box 1553
Iowa City, IA 52244

Conditions
P.O. Box 56
Van Brunt Station
Brooklyn, NY 11215
A magazine of writing by women, with an emphasis on writing by lesbians.

Dykes, Disability, & Stuff
P.O. Box 6194
Boston, MA 02114

Gay Community News (GCN)
62 Berkeley Street
Boston, MA 02116
(617) 426-4469
The weekly for lesbians and gay men.

Hot Wire. The Journal for Women's Music and Culture
5210 Wayne
Chicago, IL 60640

Lesbian Connection
c/o Helen Diner Memorial Women's Center/Ambitious Amazons
P.O. Box 811
East Lansing, MI 48823
Free to lesbians.

Lesbian Contradiction. A Journal of Irreverent Feminism
584 Castro Street, Suite 263
San Francisco, CA 94114

Lesbian Ethics
LE Publications
P.O. Box 4723
Albuquerque, NM 87196

Ms.
P.O. Box 57132
Boulder, CO 80322
The "new" *Ms.* without ads.

Off Our Backs: A Woman's News Journal
2423 18th Street NW, 2nd Floor
Washington, DC 20009

Out/Look: National Lesbian and Gay Quarterly
2940 16th Street, Suite 319
San Francisco, CA 94103

Sinister Wisdom
P.O. Box 3252
Berkeley, CA 94703
A journal for the lesbian in the arts and politics.

Sojourner: The Women's Forum
42 Seaverns Avenue
Jamaica Plain, MA 02130
(617) 524-0415

Trivia, a Journal of Ideas
P.O. Box 606
North Amherst, MA 01059

Visibilities: The Lesbian Magazine
P.O. Box 1258
Peter Stuyvesant Station
New York, NY 10009

Presses and Publishers

Alyson Publications
Department B-19
40 Plympton Street
Boston, MA 02118

Aunt Lute Foundation/Spinsters Book Company
P.O. Box 41687
223 Mississippi Street
San Francisco, CA 94141

Cleis Press
P.O. Box 8933
Pittsburgh, PA 15221
or P.O. Box 14684
San Francisco, CA 94114

The Crossing Press
P.O. Box 1048
Freedom, CA 95019

Firebrand Books
141 The Commons
Ithaca, NY 14850

Kitchen Table: Women of Color Press
P.O. Box 908
Latham, NY 12110

Naiad Press
P.O. Box 10543
Tallahassee, FL 32302

New Victoria Publishers
P.O. Box 27
Norwich, VT 05055

Sister Vision: Black and Third World Women of Colour Press
P.O. Box 217
Station E
Toronto, Ontario, Canada M6H 4E2

Womyn's Braille Press
P.O. Box 8475
Minneapolis, MN 55408

Bookstores

Write for current book lists. These businesses will do mail order.

Judith's Room
681 Washington Street
New York, NY 10014
(212) 727-7330

New Words
186 Hampshire Street
Cambridge, MA 02139
(617) 876-5310

Old Wives Tales
1009 Valencia Street
San Francisco, CA 94110
(415) 821-4675

Archives/Special Collections/Information Clearinghouses

This list is a sampling, as more regional archives are being established.

Lesbian Herstory Archives (LHA)
P.O. Box 1258
New York, NY 10016.
This is an extensive collection of material about lesbian lives. Write for information about the archives and subscribe to the newsletter, which is an invaluable source of information about their holdings.

West Coast Lesbian Collections
P.O. Box 23753
Oakland, CA 94623
The West Coast counterpart to the LHA.

Women's Collection—Special Collections Department
Northwestern University Library
Evanston, IL 60208-2300
Extensive holdings of lesbian periodicals, posters and records.

Guides to Meeting Places/Business/Resorts

Gaia's Guide International, 16th ed.
Sandy Horne, ed.
New Montgomery Street
San Francisco, CA 94105

Gayellow Pages
Frances Green, ed.
Renaissance House
P.O. Box 292
Village Station
New York, NY 10014
National edition and five regional editions.

Places of Interest to Women: The Women's Guide: USA & Canada
Ferrari Publications
P.O. Box 16054
Phoenix, AZ 85001

Van Gelder, Lindsy, and Pamela Robin Brandt. *Are You Two . . . Together?: A Gay and Lesbian Travel Guide to Europe.* New York: Random House, 1991.

Audiovisual Materials

In the Best Interests of the Children, a 16-mm film. A sensitively presented film about eight lesbian mothers and their children. Available from Iris Films, P.O. Box 5353, Berkeley, CA.
Pink Triangles, excellent film about lesbian and gay oppression; good consciousness raiser for schools and community groups. Available from Cambridge Documentary Films, P.O. Box 385, Cambridge, MA 02139.
Straight Talk About Lesbians, a slide/tape presentation produced by Liz Diamond. Available from Women's Educational Media, 36 Colwell Avenue, Brighton, MA 02135.
Woman-Loving Women, a slide/tape presentation produced by Patricia A. Gozemba and Marilyn Humphries. Available from Lavender Horizons, P.O. Box 806, Marblehead, MA 01945.

Organizations

Alcoholics Anonymous (Gay AA groups)
P.O. Box 459

Grand Central Station
New York, NY 10007
Write for a referral to a local group to General Services.

Boston Alliance of Gay and Lesbian Youth (BAGLY)
P.O. Box 814
Boston, MA 02103
(800) 42BAGLY
Support group for gay and lesbian youth

Custody Action for Lesbian Mothers
P.O. Box 281
Narbeth, PA 19072

Disabled Womyn's Educational Project
P.O. Box 6194
Boston, MA 02114

Lambda Legal Defense and Education Fund (LLDEF)
666 Broadway
New York, NY 10012
(212) 995-8585

Lesbian Mothers' National Defense Fund
P.O. Box 21567
Seattle, WA 98112

National Association for Gay and Lesbian Alcoholism Professionals
204 West 20th Street
New York, NY 10011
(212) 713-5074
A communication and support network. Publishes newsletter, bibliography and list of treatment resources for gay and lesbian alcoholics, and provides referrals to lesbian and gay AA and AL-Anon groups.

National Center for Lesbian Rights
1663 Mission Street
San Francisco, CA 94103
(415) 621-0674
A nonprofit, public interest law firm dedicated to preserving and increasing the legal rights of lesbians and gay men. Write for a list of books on topics.

National Domestic Violence Hotline
(800) 333-7233.
This organization makes referrals to lesbian or lesbian-friendly support and shelter services.

National Gay and Lesbian Task Force (NGLTF)
1734 14th Street NW
Washington, DC 20009
(202) 332-6483
Write for referrals and publication lists.

SAGE (Senior Action in a Gay Environment)
208 West 13th Street
New York, NY 10011
(212) 741-2247

Alternative Insemination

Chicago Women's Health Center
3435 North Sheffield
Chicago, IL 60657
(312) 935-6126
This home- or office-based insemination program serves mostly lesbian women, but is also open to single het-

erosexual women. Facilitated support groups are available monthly.

Feminist Women's Health Center
580 14th Street NW
Atlanta, GA 30318
(404) 874-7551

Due to the legal restrictions (home insemination is illegal in Georgia), this program provides only office-based alternative insemination. The program is open to lesbians and single heterosexual women.

The Fenway Community Health Center
7 Haviland Street
Boston, MA 02115
(617) 267-0900

An insemination program where lesbians and single women can access frozen and tested donor sperm and are instructed on how to inseminate at home. Support groups are available for women considering insemination, as well as for women currently inseminating.

Routh Street Women's Clinic
4228 North Central Expressway, Suite 201
Dallas, TX 75206
(214) 748-0498
(800) 880-0498

Home or office insemination for women without a male partner or with an infertile male partner.

The Sperm Bank of California
3007 Telegraph Avenue, Suite 2
Oakland, CA 94609
(415) 444-2014

This nonprofit organization features donor screening, semen testing and home or office insemination programs. The program is accessible to all women and men regardless of marital status, sexual preference, race, income and geographical or national residence.

11

Sexuality

By Wendy Sanford, with
Nancy P. Hawley and
Elizabeth McGee

With special thanks to Paula Brown
Doress, Jane Pincus, Janice Irvine,
Bonnie Engelhardt, Shere Hite and
the women of Boston Self-Help,
including Frances Deloatch, Mary
Fitzgerald, Jean Gillespie, Oce,
Rosemarie Ouilette, Marsha Saxton,
Janna Zwerner and Joan Lastovica.

*This chapter in previous editions was
written by Jenny Mansbridge, Ginger
Goldman, Nancy London, Nancy
Hawley, Elizabeth McGee and Wendy
Sanford.*

*1992 Update by Amy Alpern, with
help from Diana Chace, Brenda Reeb,
Wendy Sanford and Marsha Saxton.*

Our powers to express ourselves sexually last a lifetime—from birth to death. Whether or not we are in a sexual relationship with another person, we can explore our fantasies, feel good in our bodies, appreciate sensual pleasures, learn what turns us on, give ourselves sexual pleasure through masturbation. Taught to be embarrassed or ashamed of our sexual feelings, we have spent a lot of energy denying them or feeling guilty. We are learning to experience our sexuality without judging it and to accept it as part of ourselves.

We are all sexual—young, old, married, single, with or without physical disability, sexually active or not, heterosexual or lesbian. As we change, our sexuality changes. Learning about sex is a life-long process.

When we have relationships with other people, sexuality is pleasure we want to give and get, communication that is fun and playful, serious and passionate. It can be a tender reaching out or an intense and compelling force that takes us over. It can get us into situations that delight us and ones we wish we could get out of. Sex can open us to new levels of loving and knowing with someone we love and trust. It can be a source of vital energy. Misused, it can hurt us tremendously.

At times, sexual awareness and desires are quiet and other parts of our lives take center stage. Then, after a month or a year or ten years, the sexual tide may come flowing in.

Although the majority of women currently explore sexuality in relationships with men, many (at least 10 percent) do so with women. Our aim here is to affirm and support *all* women's choices of whom to love, and to invite you to understand and enjoy your own sexuality more fully.

The 1992 update of this chapter includes some small changes in the text and significant changes in the Resources. Please consult Chapter 15, "AIDS, HIV Infection and Women," for important information on ways to enjoy sex with a partner without risking transmission of the deadly human immunodeficiency virus (HIV).

SOCIAL INFLUENCES

Society shapes and limits our experiences of sexuality. We learn, for instance, that if our looks don't conform to the ideal—if we are fat, old or disabled—then we have no right to be sexual. If we are women of color, stereotypes often picture us as being more sexually available and active than we are or want to be.

The 1960s sexual revolution has had mixed results. Although it did encourage people to be less restricted about sex, it has also made many women feel we *ought* to be available to men at all times. And the double standard still prevails. Women are not really free, sexually or otherwise, as long as we remain socially and economically unequal to men. (A dramatic example of this is the way men continue to use sexual violence as a weapon against women.)

Finally, nowhere in the world have women had full access to services crucial to our enjoyment of sex—sex education, protection from unwanted pregnancy and sexually transmitted disease, abortion when we need it. Current efforts by conservative political groups threaten to limit our access even further, in an attempt to squeeze *all* our sexuality back into the confines of marriage and motherhood.

Breaking the Silence

When the women's movement surfaced again in the late 1960s, women began speaking in small groups about sexual experiences and feelings. Talking more openly about sex with our friends or in small groups is not always easy at first, and shyness comes and goes, but we have much to learn from each other. Such discussions can be funny, painful and healing. We can affirm each other's feelings, help each other challenge society's distortions of our sexuality, encourage each other in our sexual adventures and learn together to be more assertive about our own sexual needs and desires.

Over the past twenty years, we have begun to redefine women's sexuality according to our own experiences and not what male "experts" have imagined. Wanting to do more than merely react to sexist patterns that we don't like, we ask: What do *we* want? What images, fantasies, practices unlock the powerful erotic forces within us? We are delving deeply into our own sexual imaginations and our satisfying sexual experiences with men and/or women for a fuller vision of what sex can be. We are working for a society free of male/female inequalities, sexual violence, homophobia and media misuse of sex, so that our sexuality can be a source of refreshment, play, passion, connection and energy.

Ann Popkin

GROWING UP

I watch my daughter. From morning to night her body is her home. She lives in it and with it. When she runs around the kitchen she uses all of herself. Every muscle in her body moves when she laughs, when she cries. When she rubs her vulva, there is no awkwardness, no feeling that what she is doing is wrong. She feels pleasure and expresses it without hesitation. She knows when she wants to be touched and when she wants to be left alone. It's so hard to get back that sense of body as home.

Childhood experiences and memories shape our sexuality. It is most helpful, but rare, for our families to talk comfortably about sex. From the embarrassment, what *isn't* said, the "don'ts" that come as our fingers start to explore vulva, vagina and clitoris, we may learn to think of sex as forbidden, dirty and shameful.*

When we become teenagers our developing bodies are usually a mystery to us.[†] We discover that what the media, and most people, consider beautiful falls into a narrow range. We lose respect for our uniqueness, our own smells and shapes. We judge ourselves in relation to others. We come to feel isolated. ("Could anyone else be as ugly, dull, miserable as I?") An ad for sanitary napkins reinforces our aloneness and shame: "When you have your period, you should be the only one who knows."

---

*Sexual abuse, which one in three females experience by the age of eighteen, can seriously affect our sexuality. See Resources and Chapter 8, "Violence Against Women."
†See *Changing Bodies, Changing Lives: A Book for Teens on Sex and Relationships* by Ruth Bell, et al., New York: Random House, 1987, for lots more on teenagers' experiences.

It takes time—sometimes years and years—and positive experiences to get rid of these shameful, negative feelings. Many of us with young children want to help them grow up feeling good about their bodies and their sexuality, though sometimes it is hard to move beyond our own upbringing.

The other day I was taking a bath with my almost-three-year-old daughter. I was lying down and she was sitting between my legs, which were spread apart. She said, "Mommy, you don't have a penis." I said, "That's right, men have penises and women have clitorises." All calm and fine—then, "Mommy, where is your clitoris?" Okay, now what was I going to do? I took a deep breath (for courage or something), tried not to blush, spread my vulva apart and showed her my clitoris. It didn't feel so bad. "Do you want to see yours?" I asked. "Yes." That was quite a trick to get her to look over her fat stomach and see hers, especially when she started laughing as I first put my finger and then hers on her clitoris.

Thanks in part to the women's movement, many of us with grown children and grandchildren talk with them more freely about sex now than we once would have. "Growing up" sexually never ends.

FANTASIES

Sometimes when I'm making love with myself or someone else, I think about the ocean roar and feel the waves swirling about me. Perhaps this means that I'd rather be floating in the sea than be in my bed. But it's also a way of heightening the experience for me. The fantasy makes me feel loose, easy, fluid. It makes me more relaxed. I usually have the fantasy just before orgasm, and it helps me let go.

Today as I stretched out before my run, I closed my eyes and imagined my lover's naked body floating a few inches above me. I could feel her breasts on my face and in my mouth, our bodies reaching out, drawing close and then wrapped together. The images and feelings sailed me through an hour of strong running.

A fantasy before I made love to a plumber I know: I was entertaining myself one night by imagining I was dancing with a stillson wrench (the most enormous wrench I ever saw, very businesslike!), and it turned into the plumber. He said, "Well, men are still good for something!" We were fixing the pipe while we were dancing, and the scene changed. We were swimming in a sea of rubber doughnuts (the connector between the tank and the bottom parts of the toilet), and the doughnuts got stuck over our arms

and legs. The scene changed again, to the beach, where we fell asleep.

I used to have a fantasy that I was a gym teacher and I had a classful of girls standing in front of me, nude. I went up and down the rows feeling all their breasts and getting a lot of pleasure out of it. When I first had this fantasy at thirteen I was ashamed. I thought something was wrong with me. Now I can enjoy it, because I feel it's okay to enjoy other women's bodies.

I had the fantasy of making love with two men at once. I pictured myself sandwiched between them. I acted on this one, with an old friend and a casual friend who both liked the idea. It was fun.

Nearly everyone has fantasies, in the form of fleeting images or detailed stories. They express depths within us to learn about and explore. In fantasy we can be whatever we imagine. Yet it can be difficult to accept sexual fantasies.

I was scared they would take me by surprise, tell me things about myself that I didn't know, especially bad things.

I imagined I was sitting in a room. The walls were all white. There was nothing in it, and I was naked. There was a large window at one end, and anyone who wanted to could look in and see me. There was no place to hide. There was something arousing about being so exposed. I masturbated while having this fantasy, and afterward I felt very sad. I thought I must be so sick, so distorted inside, if this image of myself could give me such intense sexual pleasure.

We have been brought up to think that sex should be "one way." We often decide we are bad or sick for imagining something different, or feel disloyal when we fantasize about someone other than the man or woman we are with. Yet our fantasies treat us to *all kinds* of erotic experiences. It takes a while to learn that this is okay, and that we can enjoy these stories and images without having to act on them.

What about rape fantasies? Some people say that if we fantasize about having sex forced on us, that means we want to be raped. This is untrue: Totally unlike actual rape, fantasizing about rape is voluntary and does not bring us physical pain or violation. For those of us who grew up learning that "good girls" don't want sex, a fantasy of being forced to have sex frees us of responsibility and can be highly erotic. It can allow us the feeling of being desired uncontrollably.

In one of my juiciest fantasies a woman and a man tie me up and make love to me and to each other.

206

There is something extremely erotic in imagining being that powerless. In real life my lover and I do at times feel totally vulnerable to what the other does or wants. This fantasy lets me play around with the power dynamics that are sometimes so intense between us.

We may distrust fantasies that seem to play into male pornographic images of women as submissive or masochistic, and imagine that in a less sexist future fantasies of dominance would come to us less often. Yet this is difficult to predict. For now it seems important to accept that all kinds of fantasies may be erotic for us and free up our vital sexual energies.*

SEX WITH OURSELVES: MASTURBATION

Masturbation is a special way of enjoying ourselves.

As infants, touching and playing with our bod-

---

*If you repeatedly have fantasies that disturb or scare you, they may be a sign that you need help. Talk about them with a friend whom you trust to be wise and empathetic or a trained counselor or therapist.

ies, sometimes our genitals, felt good. Then many of us learned from our parents, and later from our schools and churches, that we were not to touch ourselves sexually. Some of us heeded their messages and some did not. But by the time we were teenagers most of us thought masturbation was bad, whether we did it or not. We felt guilty if we did masturbate, or we "forgot" it or never discovered masturbation at all.

I never even knew about masturbation. When I was twenty-one, a man-friend touched me "down there," bringing me to orgasm (I didn't know that word either). Then I had a brilliant thought—if he could do it to me, I could do it to me, too. So I did, though it was a long time before I could feel a lot of pleasure and orgasm.

Masturbation allows us the time and space to explore and experiment with our own bodies. We can learn what fantasies turn us on, the kinds of touch that arouse and please us, what tempo and where. We can learn our own patterns of sexual response without having to think about a partner's needs and opinions. Then, if and when we choose, we can tell our partners what we've learned or show them by guiding their hands to

Ann Popkin

the places we want touched. As women who have for so long been taught to "wait for a man to turn us on," knowing how to give ourselves sexual pleasure brings us freedom.

I used to think masturbating was okay only if I didn't have a lover and only for a quick release. Now I see it's part of my relationship with myself, giving myself pleasure. My rhythms change. Sometimes I masturbate more when I have a lover. Sometimes I'll go for weeks without doing it.

For me at seventy-three, masturbation is better than a sexual relationship, as most of the time I'm more interested in nonsexual pursuits. Sustaining a relationship with all the time and thought involved would be a nuisance.

We can enter a sexual relationship knowing more about what we want. We aren't totally dependent on our partners to satisfy us, which can be a freedom for them, too. After menopause, masturbating also helps us avoid the drying up of vaginal tissues that can come with age.

Not everyone enjoys masturbating.

I have tried masturbating because I learned about it, not out of natural desire. Sometimes it seems like a chore. I feel like I should take the time to explore my body but I quit after a few minutes because, quite frankly, I'm bored. It just doesn't seem to have the effect another person would.

If masturbating doesn't bring you pleasure, trust your own preferences and don't do it.

Learning to Masturbate*

If you have never masturbated and want to, we invite you to try. You may feel awkward, self-conscious, even a bit scared at first. You may have to contend with voices within you that repeat, "Nice girls don't . . ." or "A happily married woman wouldn't want to. . . ." You may fear losing control of yourself or you may feel shy or guilty about giving yourself sexual pleasure. Many of us have these feelings, but they change in time.

Some suggestions: Find a quiet time when you can be by yourself without interruption. Make yourself as comfortable as possible: You are expecting a lover, and that lover is you! Take a relaxing bath or shower. Rub your body all over with cream, lotion, oil or anything else that feels good. Slowly explore the shape of your body with your eyes and hands. Touch yourself in different ways. Put on music you like, keep the lights soft, light a candle if you want. Think about the people or situations you find sexually arousing. Let your mind flow freely into fantasy. Let your body relax.*

Women have many ways of masturbating. We can moisten our fingers (with either saliva or fluid from the vagina) and rub them around and over the clitoris. We can gently rub or pull the clitoris itself; we can rub the hood or a larger area around the clitoris. We can use one finger or several. We can rub up and down and around and around, and try different kinds of pressure and timing. Some of us masturbate by crossing our legs and exerting steady and rhythmic pressure on the whole genital area. We may insert something into the vagina—a finger, peeled cucumber, dildo. We may rub our breasts or other parts of our bodies. Some of us have learned to develop muscular tension throughout our bodies.

At sixteen I gave up masturbation for Lent. Since I defined masturbation only as touching my genitals in a sexual way, in those six weeks I learned that I could have wonderful orgasms through a mixture of fantasy and quietly tensing up and relaxing the muscles around my vagina and vulva.

Still other ways of masturbating include using a pillow instead of your hands, a stream of water, an electric vibrator.†

I can direct our shower nozzle so the water hits my clitoris in a steady stream. I have a real relationship with that shower! I wouldn't give it up for anything! It's nice when I get up for work and don't have time for sex with my lover but do have a little time for the shower. Those few minutes are real important for me.

As you get sexually aroused, your vagina will become moist. Experiment with what you can do to feel even more. Open your mouth, breathe faster, make noise if you want or move your pelvis rhythmically to your breathing and voice.

As you are getting more aroused you may feel

*See *The Hite Report* by Shere Hite, New York: Dell, 1987, for many examples of how women masturbate. See also *For Yourself: The Fulfillment of Female Sexuality* by L. G. Barbach, New York: Doubleday/Anchor Books, 1981; and *Sex for One: The Joy of Selfloving* by Betty Dodson, New York: Crown Books, 1987.

*Such a relaxed and special atmosphere isn't always possible—or necessary! Desire can overtake us at the most unexpected moments. We can find ourselves sexually aroused and masturbate while cooking a meal, traveling on a bus, working at a desk, riding a horse or bicycle, climbing a tree.
†Vibrators are sold at many drug and department stores, often as body or neck massagers. For mail-order catalogs, see Eve's Garden International, Ltd., or Good Vibrations Catalog in Resources.

your muscles tighten. Your pelvic area will feel warm and full.

For me the most pleasurable part is just before orgasm. I feel I am no longer consciously controlling my body. I know there is no way I will not reach orgasm now. I stop trying. I like to savor this rare moment of true letting go!

It's this letting go of control that enables us to have orgasms. If you do not reach orgasm when you first try masturbating, don't worry. Simply enjoy the sensations you have. Try again some other time.

Masturbating opens me to what is happening in my body and makes me feel good about myself. I like following the impulse of the moment. Sometimes I have many orgasms, sometimes I don't have any. The greatest source of pleasure is to be able to do whatever feels good to me at that particular time. I rarely have such complete freedom in other aspects of my life.

PHYSICAL ASPECTS OF OUR SEXUALITY

Sounds, sights, smells and touch can arouse our sexual feeling, as do fantasies, a baby sucking at the breast, the smell of a familiar body, a sexy picture, a dream, touching our own bodies, a lover's breathing in our ear, brushing against someone or hearing the person we love say, "I love you."

When I'm feeling turned on, either alone or with someone I'm attracted to, my heart beats faster, my face gets red, my eyes are bright. My whole vulva feels wet and full. My breasts hum. When I'm standing up I feel a rush of weakness in my thighs. When I'm lying down I may feel like doing a big stretch, arching my back, feeling the sensations go out to my fingers and toes.

No matter what arouses our sexual feelings or how we express them, if we continue to receive sexual stimulation our bodies go through a series of physical changes, sometimes called *sexual response*. Although these changes may feel different each time, they follow certain basic patterns that are helpful to know about.*

Early on in sexual excitement, veins in the pel-

vis, vulva and clitoris begin to dilate (open) and fill with blood, gradually making the whole area feel full. (This is called *vasocongestion*.) In the vagina this swelling creates a "sweating" reaction, producing the fluid that makes the vaginal lips get wet—often an early sign that we are sexually excited. At the same time, sexual tension rises throughout the body as muscles begin to tense up or contract (*myotonia*). We may breathe more quickly, nipples may become erect and hard, the whole body feels alive to touch.

Orgasm

Enough stimulation of or around the clitoris and (for some women) pressure on the cervix or other sensitive areas cause pelvic fullness and body tension to build up to a peak. Orgasm is the point at which all the tension is suddenly released in a series of involuntary and pleasurable muscular contractions that expel blood from the pelvic tissues. We may feel contractions in the vagina, uterus and rectum. Some women describe orgasms without contractions.

Orgasm can be mild like a hiccup, a sneeze, a ripple or a peaceful sigh; it can be a sensuous experience, as the body glows with warmth; it can be intense or ecstatic, as we lose awareness of ourselves for a time.

Orgasm may feel different with a finger, penis, dildo or vibrator in your vagina and different when you masturbate from when you make love with another person. It may feel totally different at different times even with the same person.

Often we become aroused at times when we can't get additional stimulation and reach orgasm. Although sexual tension subsides eventually without orgasm, it takes longer. When we get sufficiently aroused and don't have an orgasm, our genitals and/or uterus may ache for a while.

Quite a number of women have never had an orgasm. With all the publicity about orgasms in the past years, many of us who don't orgasm believe we're missing something pleasurable. We can try to reach orgasm by masturbating, reading books about it,* asking a partner to help, joining what is sometimes called a preorgasmic women's group.† A fifty-three-year-old woman wrote to our Collective that after reading an earlier edition of this book she had masturbated and reached orgasm for the first time in her life. Yet it's important that orgasm doesn't become one more performance pressure.

---

*The following description comes primarily from the groundbreaking laboratory research of William Masters and Virginia Johnson in the 1960s, with a number of modifications in response to more recent findings and especially to women's criticisms and additions to the Masters and Johnson model. For more details, see Sexual Arousal and Orgasm in the appendix to this chapter, p. 228.

---

*See Dodson, Barbach and Hite books in Resources.
†Sexual, physical or emotional abuse (past or present) may impair a woman's ability to have orgasms. Also, not being able to reach orgasm with a partner may be a clue that the relationship itself has problems and needs to change in some way.

When I try too hard to have an orgasm it usually doesn't work and I end up frustrated and bored. For me it's best if I relax and let it happen if it's going to.

Some women can reach orgasm twice or more in quick succession (which men cannot do). Knowing that multiple orgasms are possible has made some of us feel we ought to have them, that we are sexually inadequate if we don't. Men may expect it, too; one woman wrote that a man she knew was considering a divorce because the woman he was married to didn't have multiple orgasms. Yet one orgasm can be plenty and sometimes sex without orgasm is pleasurable. Seek whatever feels best to *you*.

The Role of the Clitoris

It may be arousing to stroke any part of our bodies, exciting to have our thighs caressed or our necks nibbled or our breasts sucked. However, the clitoris—the organ that is the most sensitive to stimulation—has a central role in elevating feelings of sexual tension.

Until the mid-1960s, most women didn't know how crucial the clitoris was. Even if we knew it for ourselves, nobody talked about it. Medical texts and marriage manuals (written by men) followed Freud's famous pronouncement that the "mature" woman has orgasms only when her vagina, not her clitoris, is stimulated. This theory made the penis very important to a woman's sexual satisfaction (what brought a *man* sexual release supposedly satisfied women, too). Following Freud, psychoanalytic theories belittled women's enjoyment of masturbation as "immature" and labeled lesbian sex as a pale imitation of the "real thing." In the 1960s, sex researchers found that for women *all* orgasms depend at least in part on clitoral stimulation, although some women respond to internal pressure as well.

Learning about the clitoris increased sexual enjoyment for countless women and freed many of us from years of thinking we were "frigid." Our ability to give ourselves orgasms and to show our lovers how to please us has been one of the cornerstones of a new self-respect and autonomy and has therefore been politically as well as personally important for women.

The clitoris is sometimes called the *joy button*, which implies that it is one small spot. In fact, the clitoris has several parts to it. The glans (or tip, the part you can see) attaches to the shaft, which runs along internally from the glans toward the vaginal opening. The clitoris connects to a branching interior system of erectile tissue that runs through your genital area. (Erectile tissue responds to sexual arousal by filling with blood, becoming erect and hard. A penis also contains

erectile tissue.) During sexual excitement, the clitoris swells and changes position. (See Chapter 12, "Anatomy and Physiology of Sexuality and Reproduction," for a fuller description of the clitoris.)

You or your lover can stimulate your clitoris in many different ways—by rubbing, sucking, body pressure, using a vibrator. Any rubbing or pressure in the pubic hair–covered mons area or the lips (even on the lower abdomen and inner thighs) can move the clitoris and may also press it up against the pubic bone. Although some women touch the glans to become aroused, it is often so sensitive that direct touching hurts, even with lubrication. Also, focusing directly on the clitoris for a long time may cause the pleasurable sensations to disappear. As women grow older, the hood of skin covering the clitoris may pull back permanently, so that if you are past menopause you may need lots of extra lubrication in order to tolerate having your clitoris rubbed.

Vagina-to-penis intercourse gives only indirect clitoral stimulation. As the penis moves in and out of the vagina it moves the inner lips, which are connected to the clitoral hood, and therefore may move the hood back and forth over the glans. When the inner lips become swollen and firm they can act as an extension of the vagina, hugging the penis as it moves back and forth and further increasing clitoral friction.* To reach orgasm during vagina-to-penis intercourse, many of us need *direct* and sometimes prolonged clitoral stimulation both before and during intercourse.

Many women making love to other women focus less exclusively on vaginal penetration and give more (and longer) stimulation to the clitoris. Many women who make love with men in their sixties and older (when erections happen less frequently) find that sexual pleasure increases, partly because penetration by the penis is no longer the focus of lovemaking. As more women begin to explore lovemaking beyond vagina-to-penis intercourse, it's likely that more of us will orgasm more often with our partners.

The Role of the Vagina, Uterus and Cervix

Women have the potential to respond to sexual arousal throughout the entire pelvic region. When we are aroused, the erectile tissue around the outer third of the vagina becomes full, and nerves in that area become more sensitive to stimulation and pressure. When the muscles around this part of the vagina (pubococcygeus muscles) are strong

---

*Some feminists criticize this Masters and Johnson theory as an attempt to justify penis-in-vagina intercourse as the norm for lovemaking. See, for example, *The Hite Report*, by Shere Hite, p. 247.

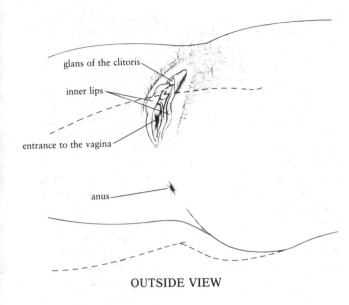

glans of the clitoris

inner lips

entrance to the vagina

anus

OUTSIDE VIEW

MAJOR AREAS OF CHANGE DURING SEXUAL AROUSAL AND ORGASM.
(The dotted lines indicate most of the changes that take place. See the illustration below.)

- *The blood vessels through the whole pelvic area swell, causing engorgement and creating a feeling of fullness and sexual sensitivity. (The blood vessels in this drawing actually represent only a fraction of what's there.)*
- *The clitoris (glans, shaft and crura) swells and becomes erect.*
- *The inner lips swell and change shape.*
- *The urethral sponge and the bulbs of the vestibule enlarge.*
- *The vagina balloons upward.*
- *The uterus shifts position.*

Please see the diagrams in Chapter 12 for other views.

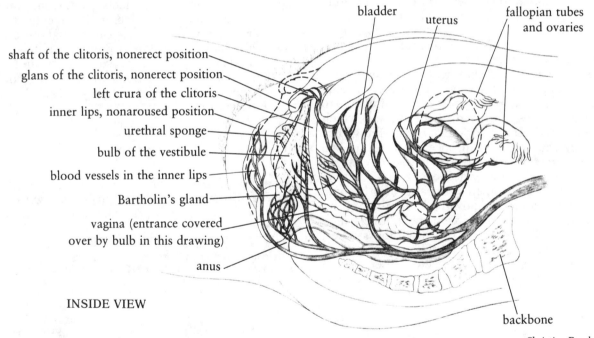

bladder

uterus

fallopian tubes and ovaries

shaft of the clitoris, nonerect position

glans of the clitoris, nonerect position

left crura of the clitoris

inner lips, nonaroused position

urethral sponge

bulb of the vestibule

blood vessels in the inner lips

Bartholin's gland

vagina (entrance covered over by bulb in this drawing)

anus

INSIDE VIEW

backbone

Christine Bondante

and well exercised, many women find they orgasm more easily (see Kegel exercises, p. 406). Childbearing increases the venous system in the pelvis, often making arousal quicker and stronger.

Two researchers have recently identified what they call the *Grafenberg spot* (G-spot), a sensitive area just behind the front wall of the vagina between the back of the pubic bone and the cervix. They say that when this spot is stimulated during sex through vaginal penetration of some kind, some women orgasm with a gush of fluid from the urethra, which is not urine. This is at present a controversial theory among sex researchers. It's a relief for those women who feel a urethral gushing of liquid during orgasm to find an explanation for this apparent ejaculation, and for some others to find what may be another source of pleasure. However, if a G-spot orgasm becomes an ideal for women to live up to or is used to reinstate so-called vaginal orgasms as superior, it will become a new source of pressure, making us feel inadequate or unaccepting of our own sexual experiences.

Further up in the vagina, the cervix and uterus are crucial to orgasm for a number of women. Although the inner two-thirds of the vagina and the cervix itself have little sensitivity, a penis, finger or dildo pressing repeatedly on the cervix "jostles" the uterus and indeed the whole lining of the abdominal cavity (peritoneum). This can create a different kind of feeling internally before and during orgasm. If you have had a hysterectomy, you may have to learn to focus on different kinds of sexual stimulation and feelings, because the cervix and uterus are no longer there.[1]

Who Defines Orgasm? The Politics of the Great Orgasm Debate

Although Masters and Johnson asserted that all orgasms are physiologically the same (clitorally induced, with contractions occurring primarily in the outer third of the vagina), women today are speaking up about orgasms that don't fit the Masters and Johnson model. For example, one such orgasm is brought on by penetration of the vagina and feels "deep," or "uterine." The buildup sometimes involves a prolonged involuntary holding in of the breath, which is released explosively at orgasm. No contractions seem to be involved.

It's not surprising that women experience a range of orgasms. But a new debate is stirring among sexologists, researchers and feminists as to how many types of orgasm there are and which kind is better or stronger or more satisfying. The danger is that people will once again set up one kind of orgasm as the norm, just as the vaginal orgasm was for so many decades.

The debate on women's sexuality has become increasingly professionalized: A number of researchers, many of them women, have claimed this as their field of expertise, wielding studies, scientific language and statistics to make their points. We are wary of these new "experts." Are they trying to tame our sexuality by making it respectable? To make themselves a professional reputation? Might male or male-oriented researchers, threatened by women's new sexual autonomy and assertiveness, have a bias toward reasserting women's dependence on men for sexual satisfaction? In modern society professionals have enormous power to shape our understanding of ourselves. Much so-called scientific debate ends up defining women for society's purposes rather than enabling us to arrive at our own chosen development. Women doing sex research must constantly ask what people are going to do with the results and whether their efforts may be used against women in a society where women do not have adequate social or political power.

It is crucial that women have accurate information about our sexuality, and some form of research is necessary. We believe that the information we need comes most usefully and powerfully from women talking about our experiences in settings of our own making.

There is no one "right" pattern of sexual response. What works, what feels good, what makes us feel more alive in ourselves and connected with our partners is what counts.* Our sexual patterns, too, will change at different points in our life. If the "models" proposed by sexologists and researchers (*or* feminists) don't fit our experiences of orgasm, then we must trust ourselves and learn more from each other.

VIRGINITY

A virgin is someone who hasn't had sexual intercourse. Although men are virgins in this sense before they have had sex, the main pressure to *be a*

---

*Many women with spinal cord injuries have no feeling in the pelvic area, yet they report experiencing orgasm and its sensations elsewhere in their bodies. Clearly we all have lots more to learn about sexual responses.

Shirley Zeiberg

virgin is on women. Today we experience conflicting pressures about virginity.

My mother told me it's a gift I can give only once, so I'd better hold on to it.

The day I left the Church was the day I had an argument in the confessional with the priest about whether having intercourse with my fiancé was a sin. I maintained it wasn't; he said I would never be a faithful wife if I had intercourse before marriage. He refused me absolution and I never went back.

I've done everything else I can do—even oral sex, which personally seems to me as close as you can get to someone. But I feel like I'll be "dirty" if I lose my virginity. Why does that one act make such a difference?

Among my girlfriends during senior year of high school, I was the only virgin. This caused me embarrassment and teasing from my friends. I was branded as a nice girl, chicken, weird, etc., even though I did all the same things they did except have sex.

The idea of virginity is an old one. People in early Greece and Rome used it to refer to a woman (or a goddess) who was autonomous, on her own, not "owned" by any man. Later it came to mean only sexual virginity and, ironically, to reflect the prevailing view of women as man's property. Remaining a virgin until she married guaranteed that a woman would uphold the family honor by passing from father to husband like unspoiled goods. Because there was no dependable birth control, it guaranteed also that babies would be born only to married couples.

Many parents today are less concerned about preserving their daughters' actual virginity than about how soon or with whom they have intercourse. Some parents respect and encourage a daughter's decisions about sex. But in many other families, the message is still "Stay a virgin!"* We may "do everything but" have intercourse and feel confused—though technically virgin, we may have become as emotionally and physically involved as we would have with intercourse. If we start having intercourse, we may feel troubled, guilty or ashamed about having "lost" our virginity. This may keep us from enjoying sex then or later, from asking for what we want or from feeling free to say no later on if we want to. It may keep

us from finding out about birth control and using it.

Meanwhile, schoolmates and the media may pressure us to be sexually available, a pressure as strong these days as the more traditional pressure to remain a virgin.

We must be free to have sex *or not*, as we think best. Having sex usually brings many changes in the relationship and in our life. Because it is often a big decision, it makes sense to think about it, talk it over with friends and the person we're involved with, choose a method of birth control if necessary. We may well want to say no to someone who is pushing us to have sex when we don't want to.*

It might be helpful to think of *virginity* differently. Instead of virginity being something we "lose" or have to "save" for someone, it could mean our physical, spiritual and emotional wholeness, our self-respect and bodily integrity, our freedom to make a choice. When we make choices about sex out of this feeling of self-respect and virginity, we will more likely put ourselves into situations we can be glad about. We are virgins with each new lover, sometimes even with the same lover, and in each new phase of our lives.

A NEW UNDERSTANDING OF CELIBACY

Traditionally, *celibacy* meant choosing not to marry. Today many people use it to mean not having sex for a certain period of time.† It can mean no sex with someone else or no masturbation as well. Sometimes we choose celibacy in response to our culture's overemphasis on sex, as a break from feeling we must relate to others sexually all the time: "I was tired of having to say yes or no."

Or it's a personal adventure.

I'm exploring myself as a sexual person but in a different way. My sensitivity to my body is heightened. I am more aware of what arouses my sensual interests. I am free to be myself. I have more energy for work and friends. My spirituality feels more intense and clear.

As part of a religious commitment (for nuns, priests and others), celibacy offers a freedom to use one's energy for other people, not so much because lovemaking drains energy but because sexual relationships necessitate commitments,

---

*This is especially true for young Latina women. In Puerto Rico, for instance, many families have a physician verify a daughter's virginity before she entertains proposals for marriage.

*For more on virginity and first intercourse, see *Changing Bodies, Changing Lives* by Ruth Bell, et al.
†See *The New Celibacy* by Melanie Brown, New York: McGraw-Hill, 1989, for a fuller discussion of this expanded view of celibacy.

time and attention. Yet religious celibacy has often been misunderstood or ridiculed. A nun wrote to the Collective as follows:

For many religious women sex means so much that we use it as a gift of our life in the service of all people. Not to engage in an active sex life or to marry is for the purpose of being free to be of service. It is painful and depressing when others speak of this gift as though to have made this decision is necessarily to have a warped personality.

When we choose celibacy, we can experiment with any form that offers what we want.

I spend part of each day in yoga and meditation. Sometimes I go for days without thinking about my sexual identity at all. I masturbate only when inspired, which is seldom these days. Yet in meditation last week I found myself having an orgasm. It was ecstasy!

In couple relationships, we may choose celibacy when we want some distance or solitude or when we just don't want to have sex for a while. This can be awkward and requires careful communication if a partner isn't feeling the same way.

I say to my woman lover, "I don't feel like making love this month, and I may not next month." Now, who does that? Is it okay? Am I allowed? The last thing we were ever taught was that it was okay to try what we want.

Some couples choose celibacy together, which allows both people to explore other dimensions of loving. It can help us get out of old sexual patterns, expand our sensual/sexual focus beyond genital sex if we want to and make us feel more self-sufficient and independent, which can strengthen the relationship.

Sometimes we are faced with celibacy when we *don't* choose it—after a breakup or divorce or when a partner or lover dies. Sometimes being a parent to a new baby enforces a time of virtual celibacy. Painful if we don't want it, celibacy sometimes surprises us with its own satisfactions.

BISEXUALITY

Today many women are entering or at least thinking about sexual, intimate relationships with both men and women.

I ask myself: Is it possible to be bisexual, or is it some kind of New-Age fantasy that I can have a man lover and a woman lover?

I've been in lesbian relationships for ages. Then suddenly last year I fell in love with a man. A total surprise!

When I first started getting involved with women as well as men, I wanted to be more intimate with them as an extension of being friends.

Sometimes thinking of ourselves as bisexual is a safe stopping place in a transition from one identity to another.

For years I said to myself and my friends, "I think maybe I'm bisexual," meaning, "I'm probably a lesbian but I'm scared to death to admit it."

Yet for many of us bisexuality is not transitional at all.

I've tried to define myself using labels of lesbian, straight, bisexual, and I didn't feel that any of them were mine. I think of it in terms of people I could love, not sexes I could love.

Being lovers with people of both sexes opens our eyes to social and political realities that may be new to us. If we were sexually intimate only with men before, a relationship with a woman may introduce us to the world of lesbian experience, with its particular satisfactions and oppressions. We soon find that we have to be more careful in public than we ever dreamed of being; we may become aware of homophobia for the first time. Our friendships may take on new dimensions.

Sleeping with a woman for the first time allowed me to feel much more with my close women friends. Many times I'll have sexual feelings and not say anything, but they make me feel closer and more caring. I'll hug and kiss a friend and she'll have no idea what's going on inside me—the feeling of arousal is wonderful—like an opening, a blossoming.

If we have been exclusively lesbian, being lovers with a man puts us temporarily into the dominant heterosexual culture: We have the privilege of "fitting in," of being able to show our love freely in public. There also may be more struggles with sex-role stereotypes than we are used to and, before menopause, the unfamiliar need for birth control.

Invisibility is a problem. Few people know we exist, because we don't "fit" into either the heterosexual or the lesbian world. When we are open, both worlds judge us.

I'm cautious about talking about it, fear being judged, being told, "Your sexuality is wrong!"

Heterosexual friends may be shocked and

scared when we have a woman lover (see Coming Out, p. 178). Lesbian friends may be mistrusting, too, afraid that we may in the future slip back into the safer heterosexual role and hurt lesbians who have fallen in love with us. If we as lesbians become lovers with men as well, other lesbians often see us as disloyal. ("My lesbian friends have an incredible scorn for bisexuals.")

When I'm having troubles with a man and tell a lesbian friend, she usually gets a look in her eye that means, "What did you expect, being with a man?"

All these judgments isolate us. And we may feel pressure to choose: "I've had people press me to say I'm 'more' one than the other." As more women feel comfortable and safe in being open about bisexuality, we will create more of a community for ourselves, and we will further challenge both heterosexual and lesbian assumptions about who and how women can love.

SEX IN A RELATIONSHIP

Currents of sexual attraction and passion crisscross our lives and pull us into new relationships, deepen the ones we're in, teach us about ourselves. We may act on them with a look, smile, touch, kiss, or we may not want to. When we make love with someone familiar or new, woman or man, we are often at our most open, most vulnerable and also our most powerful. Sex can be dramatic, dull, comforting, scary, friendly, funny, passionate, frustrating, satisfying.

Sex doesn't take place in a vacuum. We take struggles about other things—power, money, mutuality, competition—into bed with us.

Sex in relationships can vary in meaning and intensity.

Sometimes I make love to get care and cuddling. Sometimes I am so absorbed in the sensations of touch and taste and smell and sight and sound that I feel I've returned to that childhood time when feeling good was all that mattered. Sometimes we tumble and tease. Sometimes sex is spiritual—High Mass could not be more sacred. Sometimes I make love to get away from the tightness and seriousness in myself. Sometimes I want to come and feel the ripples of orgasm through my body. Sometimes tears mix with juices mix with sweat, and I am one with another. Sometimes through sex I unite with the stream of love that flows among us. Sex can be most anything and everything for me. How good that feels!

I enjoy sex with Mike more than I have with anyone. When we get aroused, we make the most beautiful

Owen Franken/Stock Boston

music together! Still, sex often feels difficult for me. When I feel good about myself and close to him, when the pressures of our children and my work and friends are not demanding a lot of my energy, our sex is very fluid and strong. When I feel angry, sad, depressed or very childlike and needy, or any combination, or busy with other people in my life, I have a hard time being sexually open with Mike. We've talked about this, and he experiences a lot of the same ups and downs and distractions as I do.

Deborah's and my lovemaking has been strong, deep and varied since the first night we slept together. I've felt so sure of my sexuality with her, and increasingly trusting of the rhythms of our desire. Yet last year when I went to live with her in her city away from my friends, work, women's group, my own turf, I suddenly became frighteningly dependent on whether she wanted to make love with me or not. When she did, it was wonderful because I was in touch with such deep places of need and sexual vulnerability in myself that our lovemaking was profoundly moving. But when she didn't—when she wanted to go to sleep or get up and do some work or go for a run or make some calls—I felt awful. I'd lie there feeling that I wanted sex "too much," afraid to tell her, angry, hurt, worried that she'd feel guilty. I finally dared to say something to her, only because our trust was deep enough for me to risk it. I cried as though a dam had broken. I began to see that when I'm away from my own world, the power in our relationship gets out of balance. Feeling out of touch with my own sources of strength and identity, I needed her to want me, as though her desire for me would actually make me exist. Sex and orgasm weren't the issue; identity was. We pulled out of this difficult time with a new respect for the power dynamics in our sexual loving.

COMMUNICATING ABOUT SEX

Sexual Language

The true language of sex is primarily nonverbal. Our words and images are poor expressions of the deep feelings within and between us.

Few words in the English language feel appropriate for sex because they convey attitudes and values very unlike how we actually feel. Clinical, "proper" terms—vagina, penis and intercourse—seem cold, distant, tight; slang terms—cunt, cock, fuck, ass—seem degrading or coarse; euphemisms like "making love" are vague. We use different words with lovers, children, friends and doctors. Though sex is a natural way of expressing ourselves, we have no natural way of talking about it. Many of us are trying to put together a sexual language with which we are comfortable.

How to Say What We Really Want

There are certain issues we all face in a sexual situation, whether it's with a date, longtime lover or spouse: How do I feel at the moment? Do I want to be sexually close with this person now? In what ways? What if I don't know—can I say I'm confused? Then can I communicate clearly what I want, what I don't want? Do I feel comfortable saying it in words or letting him/her know some other way? What are the unspoken rules? Is there enough trust and caring between us for this person to listen to my feelings and respect them if I feel differently from him/her?

Often the question is whether or not to make love. When we want to ask someone to make love with us, we may have to overcome certain inhibitions, for we have been brought up to think that men, not women, should initiate sex. We have to get used to the possibility of being turned down. When we *don't* want to make love, we often face (in men primarily) the assumption that "women don't really mean it when they say no." Or someone interprets our not wanting sex as a sign of rejection or frigidity. The more complex truth lies somewhere between the extremes of "good girls don't initiate sex" and "liberated women always want it": Often we do, often we don't. Sometimes we love being coaxed into it, sometimes we hate feeling pressured. All we can do is try to be as fully aware as possible of our feelings at the moment, to be honest with ourselves about them and to practice saying them, with clarity and no apologies, to the men or women we are with.

Communication about our sexual needs is a continuous process. A woman who had found the courage to talk with her lover about their sexual relationship said in angry frustration, "I told him

what I like once, so why doesn't he know now? Did he forget? Doesn't he care?"

Even in the most loving relationships, asking for what we want is hard.

- We are afraid that being honest about what we want will threaten the other.
- Our partner seems defensive and might interpret our suggestion as a criticism or a demand.
- We are embarrassed by the words themselves.
- We feel sex is supposed to come naturally and having to talk about it must mean there's a problem.
- We have been making love with the same person for years (sometimes several decades) and it feels risky to bring up new insights.
- We and our partner aren't communicating well in other areas of our relationship.
- Even with a willing partner, we may as women feel a deep inhibition about asserting our sexuality openly and proudly, which is what we'd be doing if we proclaimed our erotic needs and wishes.
- We don't know what we want at a particular time, or we need to react to something our partner does. The barriers can be inside us, not just between us and our partners.

How do we work on better communication in sex? Making love is one of the special times when we have more than words to use to reach each other. Taking a partner's hand and putting it in a new place, making the sounds that let him/her know we are feeling good, speeding up or slowing down our hip movements, a firm hand on the shoulder meaning "let's go slow"—there are many ways of communcating if we will use them.

I've liked just saying, "Watch," and showing.

We were both really excited. My lover began rubbing my clitoris hard and it hurt. It took me a second to figure out what to do. I was afraid that if I said something about it, I would spoil the excitement for both of us. Then I realized I could just take my lover's hand and very gently move it up a little higher to my pubic hair.

We can practice saying what feels good while exchanging massages, for example, when the atmosphere is less intense. But communicating about sex doesn't happen overnight, and it doesn't always work no matter how hard we might try.

EXPLORING LOVEMAKING

We have many ways of getting and giving pleasure—touching, caressing, looking, teasing, kissing, massaging, licking, sucking, penetrating.

Joy Schneider Kendra

My lover and I can spend hours—when we're on vacation or the kids are away on a weekend morning—looking at each other, stroking and cuddling each other, pulling and pushing and feeling our bodies stretch together. If we go past a certain point, we'll both know we want to "make love," but actually we have been making love the whole time.

What we do in sex is a matter of personal preference and ingenuity, whom we are with, how much love and understanding we feel, how comfortable we both are with our bodies, how each of us feels that day. At its best, lovemaking takes its shape as we and our partners move together by mutual (often unspoken) agreement. Sexual equality is as important in bed as it is everywhere else.

Some sexual activities are riskier than others. See Chapter 15, "AIDS, HIV Infection and Women," for more on safer sex.

Touching and Sensuality

Massages, back rubs, foot rubs, head rubs—these are wonderful anytime. As part of lovemaking, they can make sex slower and more sensual.

Sometimes it's a thrill to make love fast, whenever and wherever the desire hits. Other times I like to take time to emphasize every little sensual detail. We'll eat something delicious together (not too much or I'll get full and sleepy). We'll put on music, light a candle, take turns rubbing each other with oil or lotion, roll around a lot, caress each other every-

where, let our excitement build up slowly, let orgasm happen if it does. It's like a long sexual dance.

Eric likes me to rub his feet and suck his toes. I think that gives him as much pleasure or more than anything else we do in sex.

Tender touching can be a way of making love.

We always sleep right up next to each other naked. There's always a lot of touching and feeling, so even though we don't have intercourse that often, I consider us having sex all the time.

When a couple has problems in sex, it may turn out that they have been focusing entirely on each other's genitals, and not taking time or learning how to touch and stroke each other lovingly all over. Many men are more focused on genitals than women are and need to learn the pleasures of touching.

One lover told me with great puzzlement at first that I made love slower than any woman he knew, and he didn't just mean it took me a long time to come. Later he got used to my "style" and said he liked it.

Oral Sex

We can suck or lick our partner's genitals, which when done to a woman is called *cunnilingus* (slang: going down, eating, eating out) and when done to man is called *fellatio* (slang: going down, blow job). Sometimes oral sex is more intimate than any other kind of lovemaking. For some of us, it brings orgasm more surely than other ways of making love.

We're really into oral sex and he's always ready and willing. He'll say, "Do you want to have an orgasm?" And he'll go down on me. It's terrific.

To enjoy oral sex it helps to like our partner's genitals and feel good about our own. Yet we are often ashamed of our "private parts."

For ages I thought my lover was doing me a favor when he did oral sex on me. I couldn't imagine that I tasted good. Finally he convinced me that he loves doing it. Also, I tasted my juices and they're not bad!

At first I was repulsed by the idea of going down on a woman. I thought we smelled bad, that vaginas were nasty. It was a little pungent and intimidating in the beginning (though less so than a penis had been!). I soon learned to lose myself in the wonderful textures, tastes and formations of a woman's genitals. I realized that lesbian sex is about loving myself, overcoming my hatred of my own body.

217

One of the pluses of oral sex with men is that we won't get pregnant. But with men or women, the risk of getting HIV/AIDS or another sexually transmitted disease still exists. And, like everything in sex, it's good only if we want to be doing it.

Often a guy I'm dating will say, "If you won't have intercourse, just give me a blow job." But if I didn't want him in my vagina, I probably don't want him in my mouth. Oral sex can feel like rape to me if I'm not in the mood to be doing it.

My husband likes me to do oral sex on him. Sometimes it's incredibly erotic for me to have his penis moving in my mouth. Since I don't enjoy swallowing his semen, I usually spit it out or let it flow out on the sheets, and that's fine. Sometimes, however, blowing him makes me gag—I don't want his penis filling up my mouth at all. Then we do something else. Or we get in a position where I have more control, like being on top of him with the base of his penis in my hand.

What feels good in oral sex differs from time to time.

I like tongue, lips, moisture, not too much sucking and pulling, and time for exploring—my lover's got to be willing to stay with it for a while.

It can be done rather crummily! I hate it when I feel like he's eating me up with his teeth or when the pressure's too hard and it hurts or when he moves around from place to place and doesn't keep the stimulation steady.

For me there's no right or wrong place, just the places I want concentrated on on a particular day. I'm getting better at telling my lover where it feels best.

Anal Stimulation

The anus can be stimulated with fingers, tongue, penis or any slender object. For many of us, it is a highly sexually sensitive area.

I like having something small in my anus during lovemaking—no pressure or movement, just there.

Having the area around my anus licked during oral sex is a real turn-on. And anal intercourse when I'm in the mood is incredibly sexy. I love the sensations deep inside me and the thrill of doing something so unusual.

The anus is not as elastic as the vagina, so be gentle. If you have anal intercourse (penis in

anus), go slowly, wait until you're relaxed and use a lubricant—saliva, secretions from the vagina or penis or a water-soluble jelly such as K-Y Jelly. Unfortunately, anal bacteria can cause serious vaginal infections and cystitis, so if you want your partner's finger(s) or penis in your vagina after being in your anus, be sure they have been washed well first, and have a male lover use a condom. Also be careful using your tongue (sometimes called *rimming*), as you may get a stomach infection or a sexually transmitted disease.

Anal sex is a very risky activity for HIV/AIDS transmission. The delicate tissue in the rectum is prone to small tears that make an entryway for the AIDS virus. Latex barriers (condom, gloves) *must* be used. See Chapter 15, "AIDS, HIV Infection and Women."

Anal intercourse isn't for everyone.

My husband wants to have anal sex a lot because he likes the tight fit and the exoticness of it. Once it happaned and I almost didn't know it was happening. There was lubrication and everything was right and it felt fine. At other times I've really not wanted it and a few times it's been almost painful and I've stopped it. I wish I liked it better because I'd love to give him that pleasure, but I have to be honest—I just don't enjoy it.

In our one great try at anal intercourse I ended up jumping three feet in the air and squealing like a stuck pig. This so terrified him that he completely lost his erection, and we laughed and laughed. I don't think it ever really got in or anything—somehow we hadn't quite worked out the logistics of it.

Masturbating in Lovemaking

When my fiancé asked if he could help me masturbate I thought it was kinky at first. Then I showed him how I do it and he showed me how he does. We watch each other to see what feels good. He has trouble sometimes having orgasms inside me, and I know it's a relief to him that he can openly bring himself to orgasm after intercourse.

My lover rubbed her breasts and clitoris while I made love to her yesterday. After I got over feeling a little inadequate (I should be able to do it all!), I found it was like having another pair of hands to make love to her with. It was a turn-on to both of us.

When one person in a relationship wants sex or orgasm more than the other, masturbation is a possibility. Here are some different views.

It's typical for my husband to want to make love at night, but I'm too tired. Then by morning I'm very horny and he wants to get up. I always tease him in the morning, ask whether he jerked off or not. Sometimes he did. Sometimes I'll be going off to sleep and feel the bed shaking.

I guess I'm old-fashioned enough to say that no husband of mine is going to have to masturbate because I wouldn't satisfy him.

Masturbation is such a private thing, and I want to keep it for when I'm alone with myself. Also, doing it with someone else would be the ultimate in showing that I'm a sexual person, and maybe I'm shy about that.

It's a relief to me to know that either of us can give ourselves an orgasm if that's what we want. It helps make coming less the center of sex for us, and frees both of us from feeling we have to "do it right" or the other person will be frustrated.

Intercourse

When you make love with a man, you will probably want to have intercourse—to feel his penis in your vagina. Think of intercourse as reciprocal—you open up to enclose him warmly, you surround him powerfully and he penetrates you. It can be infinitely slow and gentle, hard and thrusting, or both—at its best, an exceptional part of lovemaking.

Your bodies and minds, your most private parts, have tremendous contact, and you connect intimately, profoundly.

I can so clearly remember moving in and around him and him in me, till it seemed in the whole world there was only us dancing together as we moved together, as we loved together, as we came together. Sometimes at these times I laugh or cry and they are the same strong emotions coming from a deep protected part of me that is freer now for loving him.

When I was trying to get pregnant, I found intercourse especially exciting because of the possibility that this *might be the time his sperm met my egg. It was as if my vagina was beckoning his penis to come in for an intimate hug. I felt expansive and open in my whole body.*

For intercourse to give you pleasure you must feel aroused, sexually excited, your vagina wet and open. Often it takes women longer—sometimes much longer—than men to become aroused. If you are sexually inexperienced or angry with your partner or have a partner who practices only the "in and out" of intercourse and not the lovemaking that surrounds it, then penetration (especially when your vagina is dry) can be boring, unpleas-

Suzanne Arms

ant, even painful. Do whatever gives *you* the most pleasure. Sometimes you will feel open and ready for intercourse immediately; more often you will want your partner first to touch, rub, kiss or lick your vulva and clitoris, using his hands, mouth or penis.

Certain positions will feel more exciting to you than others (and may differ each time you make love). The "man on top" is not a "naturally" better position at all. You can sit or lie upon him or lie side by side. Sit up with your legs over his and his penis in you; or he can enter you from behind and reach around to caress your clitoris. If you want deep penetration and pressure on your cervix, choose positions that make these more possible. We are all different shapes and need to find positions that suit us.

Intercourse is about pleasure and connection for *both* of you and not necessarily orgasm. Many women don't orgasm during intercourse. Sometimes trying to have an orgasm makes you self-conscious and tightens you up. On the other hand:

Sometimes it's exciting to strive for orgasms—if I don't strive I won't get them, and they feel so good!

If you are not ready for orgasm and the man is highly aroused when you begin intercourse, he might reach orgasm too soon for you if he moves back and forth inside you and you move your pelvis against his quickly. Both of you can slow your movements until you become more excited yourself. Experiment with holding your bodies still for a time when he enters you, then begin to move together slowly. Moving slowly can help men learn to delay ejaculation, which can make intercourse more pleasurable for both of you.

Pressure of the penis on the cervix can be the

key to orgasm for some women, as are clitoral and vulval stimulation.

I love rubbing his penis against my clitoris and vulva. It gives both of us great pleasure and always brings me to the verge of orgasm.

It is best if you can communicate with words or movements what feels best to you. Yet sometimes talking about it is neither easy nor possible.

He would come almost instantly when we began to make love after marvelous kissing. A little while later we'd make love again, when I'd be more aroused— aching for him, in fact. I never knew how to alter this pattern, never dared talk about it and later on found out that he had resented "having" to make love twice.

Over time you and your partner can learn your mutual rhythms of desire and arousal and explore what gives each of you the most pleasure.

After Lovemaking

The hour or so after active lovemaking can be a special time.

After sex we talk tenderly, laugh deeply, whisper, cry, sleep like babies in each other's arms. Some of the most important conversations in our relationship have come in those satisfied and intimate moments.

Some Possible Variations

- Changing roles. The one who usually initiates sex can be more receptive, the quieter one more vigorous or noisy. It can take a while to get comfortable with these changes.

I have real difficulty taking the initiative in sex, even though I know my husband would like it. Growing up I was taught that sexually aggressive women are less civilized, and I can't seem to shake my inhibition. Also, what if I initiate and he says no? What a risk; yet he takes it all the time.

- Making love in different places or positions. (Many of us find, however, that toward the end of lovemaking one or two positions are best for orgasm.)
- Enjoying sexual fantasies while making love.

We've just started to talk about the fantasies we have during sex. At first it felt somehow "disloyal" that we needed fantasies when the other person was such a good lover. Now we figure, the more pleasure the better.

- Using sexually explicit materials such as books, magazines or photographs, welcoming the images or words that arouse us and free up our sexual energy.

There are times when Gwen and I want a little extra turn-on. Maybe we're tired, or preoccupied with work or kids, yet we'd also like to make love. Our own fantasies are usually plenty juicy enough, but when they're not, we'll read something sexy together and have a great time.

Unfortunately, most of the erotic material that's available today is based on men's fantasies, not ours. Most of it is pornography, which depicts women's bodies as depersonalized objects and instruments of men's sexual pleasure. The exotic positions usually shown do little for a woman's clitoral stimulation. All this can aggravate the differences between what women and men want in sex.

My husband has read porn magazines since he was fourteen. He gets lots of ideas from them and keeps wanting to try things in sex that don't arouse me and I don't like much. We are both pretty disappointed in our sex life at this point.

It can be important to distinguish between *erotica*, sexually explicit material showing sex that doesn't degrade anyone, and *pornography*, the materials that show someone (usually a woman) being forced or degraded. Women need to create more erotica of our own!*

- Playing games in sex. We can playact situations and fantasies that excite us, like being kids about to be caught or making love in a public place. We can dress up. We can be our child selves as well as our adult selves, our lusty, vigorous as well as our needy selves.

Sometimes when I'm feeling good I'll create a strip scene for my husband—and for me, since our mirror is strategically placed—and we both get very excited. Now he does it, too, standing in front of the bed, moving his body rhythmically, slowly taking off and throwing down his clothes. I love it. His strength and vulnerability come through at the same time.

In sadomasochistic (S/M) sex play the playacting is based on fantasy situations of dominance and submission. Partners act out roles like teacher–student, police–citizen, monarch–subject. One will enforce her/his will on the other,

---

*The Dodson and Friday books (see Resources) are erotic for many. For lesbian erotica, see the Resources in Chapter 10.

Peter Simon

often experimenting with activities involving physical pain, until the other gives the signal to stop. S/M is highly controversial among feminists and has caused debate and even division among lesbians. Women who support S/M point out that between partners who both *fully* want to be doing it, S/M play can increase sexual pleasure and open up hidden issues of power, which are present in most human intimacy. Others argue that dominance and pain infliction have no part in "healthy" sexuality. A major concern is that the many *real* inequalities in our society create a risk that S/M won't be just play, and that one partner will actually *be* dominant, while the other feels forced to acquiesce. S/M can camouflage truly oppressive behavior.

I was a battered wife. My husband, a professional with a good job, said he was into bondage. I bought into it at first. Toward the end he said that he could relate to me sexually only if he tied me up. At the end he was threatening to kill me. For him, bondage had to do with low self-esteem and wasn't a healthy expression of sexuality.

It's important to say *no* to anything you don't want to do. If you are confused or upset by pressure from a sex partner, discuss the situation with a friend who can help you decide how to respond.

A LIFETIME OF SEX

Over our lifetime we can have many changing feelings about our sexuality—how we want to explore it, with whom and so on. Here is what several women have to say about changes in their sexual lives.

Just in the last two years—after fourteen years of marriage—we've been able to talk to each other about sex. We experience a deep kind of uncrazy passion. When you are in love it's crazy passion—you want to swallow each other up and be swallowed. This, in contrast, is a relaxed openness. Anything goes, no hurry, free of guilt. We are more sexually connected than we've ever been in our lives and able just to be with each other.

I have trouble talking about sex right now because there isn't much. I feel closeness and deep connection with my mate, and still I'm disturbed. We used to always count on being able to make love, no matter what else was wrong. And that just isn't true anymore. I feel uneasy.

After twenty years of being married I find myself thinking a lot about a sexual relationship with a woman.

My divorce (at forty-five) has me feeling like a teenager all over again. I go on dates; get crushes; wonder whether to sleep with someone for the first time; wait passionately for the phone to ring, hoping it's my current lover.

I want companionship from time to time. Yet I don't want an intense, continuous relationship. That means I have sporadic and spontaneous encounters with men (some sexual, some not)—momentary intimacies. This is a new experience for me, and the newness of it sometimes makes me feel shaky.

Having a baby to take care of makes us both too tired to have sex much. Yet nursing my daughter, touching her soft skin, feeling her sleeping body on mine—these are very sensual for me.

We've been married thirty-two years. I have no doubt that we'll be together until one of us dies. Yet for the past ten years our libidos have been much lower than they used to be. It's possibly the effect of medications we are taking, my husband for a heart condition and I for high blood pressure. The ten years before that were my peak sexual years, and I don't think you suddenly go from a peak to a low. I don't mean we don't have sex; it just comes in spurts.

I've gotten so angry at him in fights we've had—little fights, big ones—that I could easier kill him than sleep with him. At first these feelings scared me. Now I know they pass and change and I feel loving again.

When Cindy and I moved in together I went through a period of having no erotic energy whatsoever. I panicked and thought I'd never feel that passion for her again. Surprise! It came back.

Louis Alexander

We're forty-eight and fifty, and we're both very private people, but ours is such a success story that somebody ought to hear about it.

I was a virgin when I married and, as such, had quite an undefined sexuality. It quickly became apparent that, while I enjoyed making love, I liked it a great deal less than my husband did. In fact, if he had his way, I am sure he would like to make love at least once a day, now as well as then.

We immediately exploded the myth of the vaginal orgasm and learned to use manual stimulation of the clitoris, which increased my pleasure. But I was terribly afraid of making my own wishes about frequency known; above all I was afraid that, like so many other men, he would "need" to have his sexual life supplemented by extramarital sex. I never called it "rape" when he wore down my resistance over and over again or misused his superior physical strength. I now know that I did sometimes look upon it as rape.

But it doesn't happen anymore. When I was forty, for many reasons not related to marriage and sex (and maybe a few that were), I went into a depression. Sexual activity virtually ceased for us. And when I began to come out of the depression about a year later, I continued to call the shots; that is, we made love when I wanted it, and only when I wanted it. My husband had been tender and forbearing all during the worst times, and he continued to be so.

The result is that he waits to make love until I'm ready, and our sex life has never been so good. I think even he has become willing to accept the trade-off: less frequency, more intensity. We try more daring things. But the most interesting development is that I have begun to ask to make love more often. It may have something to do with age—I understand that we women just continue to get better and better—but I think it has more to do with the fact that I was given—no, took—more space for myself. Now I make my wishes known, he respects them and I

We have been married for fifteen years. For several years we were passionate lovers. There was a lot of romance in our lives. Now there is less romance and very deep love and friendship. Sex is no longer the most important thing in our lives. We have sex less frequently and yet our lovemaking feels good in different ways than in those early years. We feel very warm, intimate and deeply trusting of each other.

Sally and I have been together seventeen years. Originally we had a sexual relationship. Then we broke up for five years and when we got back together it never became sexual again. I'm really glad because I can't conceive of a happier relationship. We cuddle and kiss; we hold hands on the bus; we are affectionate all the time. But we don't have sex, and I don't miss it.

After my marriage ended I got involved with a man I felt good about and I knew felt good about me. It wasn't until then that I discovered not only was I orgasmic, I was wild, abandoned, spontaneous, crazy, witty, funny, wonderful!

Jerry Berndt/Stock Boston

no longer fear losing him to a more highly sexual woman. Because I'm great in bed, and so is he.

We look forward to a lifetime of ups and downs and growth and change in how we live our sexuality. We will be fascinated to see how our daughters revise this chapter!

SEX AND PHYSICAL DISABILITIES*

Some of the women speaking about sexuality throughout this chapter have a physical disability, either invisible, like epilepsy, or evident, like cerebral palsy, spina bifida or paraplegia. Those of us with physical disabilities are feeling increasingly open and proud about being sexual people.†

Whether we get a physical disability during our life or grow up with it from birth, we too often find other people assuming that we are not sexual at all.

I never get comments from guys. To them I'm an asexual object. It's a side of me that men don't see.

When I went out with my first ever, very good-looking boyfriend, school friends were openly amazed that I had been able to capture such a creature. I was not seen to be a woman, so I did not really see myself as a woman.

Those of us with physical disabilities discover early and more painfully something that all women face: that our identity as women and as sexual beings is measured according to our looks and our desirability to men.‡

One day the gas man came to read the meter. As he was leaving the flat he asked if I was married. I told him I was, and then a funny look came into his eyes and he asked if I had sex. I was shocked. Then I was angry and said the first thing that came into my head. "Yes, do you?" He looked embarrassed and hurried away.

---

*See also the table on Sex and Physical Disabilities at the end of this chapter, pp. 231–33.
†Please see Chapter 1, "Body Image," for our reasons for speaking as "we" even though no one in the Collective has a physical disability and for more on popular stereotypes of women with physical disabilities. Our special thanks to the women of Boston Self-Help for their contributions to this section on sexuality and physical disabilities.
‡It is ironic that with most physical disabilities we are considered asexual, yet if we have a condition that makes us appear unintelligent—mental retardation, emotional or speech disability—we are often thought of as *overly* sexual. For instance, one argument against sex education for mentally retarded or deaf people has been that others didn't want to encourage their "natural promiscuity." This reveals an odd warp in our society's assumptions about sexuality.

Growing up with certain physical disabilities keeps us from getting in touch with many of the dimensions of our sexuality.

Friends have said to me that getting their period for the first time was an important moment in their growing sense of themselves as womanly and sexual. Because my disability required my mother to catheterize me several times a day, she was the one who discovered my period. I understand now why it was so important to me a few years later to learn to change the pads myself.

I spent several months in a body cast when I was eleven and twelve years old, just when my breasts were developing. They kept having to alter the cast around my chest to make room. When my father finally came to take me home from the hospital, he brought a little sunsuit I'd worn months before. There was no way I could get my breasts in there! It was a riot. The nurses helped me fix up a hospital johnny to go under the sunsuit. That was my introduction to puberty!

Yet we may develop some dimensions of our sensuality more than others do.

A nice thing about my disability as a child was that my parents and others held me a lot, touched me all the time when they were helping me dress, kept me on their laps. Touching is still a very sensual thing for me.

Certain disabilities such as multiple sclerosis and some spinal cord injuries can be so painful that there are times when we may want sex but can't stand to be touched. For the many times when the medical world can't ease the pain, some of us are turning to nonmedical alternatives like visualization, biofeedback or acupuncture (see Chapter 5, "Health and Healing: Alternatives to Medical Care").

Reclaiming our bodies for our own experiences of sexuality takes time and patience.

In my lesbian illness-support group we have to push past our own censored voices to discover what to do when the vulnerability of the body to pain and to medical manipulation numbs it to the touch of a lover.

I persist in feeling that my body is ugly when I'm naked. Yet my husband clearly loves making love with me. I asked him one day if I made love with a limp. "Yes," he said, "you make love with a rhythm like your walking rhythm. It's nice."

My lover, who is a paraplegic, has been subjected to enormous amounts of insensitive medical attention

223

all her life. Health-care professionals have handled her body again and again without allowing her control over the process. So obviously it is difficult for her to let go of control of her own body and to entrust a lover with this control. I need to honor her experience, to know that it is not my fault or my inadequacy as a lover—or hers—that is the reason for sexuality being an issue in our relationship. We have discovered that honest and loving communication, with no blame or criticism, leads us to finding several ways to experience sexual pleasure with each other.

With all the obstacles, many of us choose to be sexually active.

My ex-husband and I had four children and spent twelve years raising them. The sexual side of marriage was the most satisfying part of the relationship for me and, I think, for my husband, too. If we could have spent our lives in bed I think the marriage would have been a great success!

I prefer to relate sexually to women because they are far less judgmental of my "odd" body and are really far more into sensual expression than men.

I finally lost my virginity at twenty-eight, just before going to college. Even so, it took the guy in question six months of sensitive and gentle persuasion, and then the occasion was for me a joyful and enjoyable one, coupled with a sense of relief.

The logistics of lovemaking are often a challenge, especially with a severe disability. But the "problems" are often distorted or exaggerated because of the discriminative attitudes and factors we have to face, from others' fears or unrealistic expectations to physical spaces that are poorly designed for our needs. The cultural pressure for sex to be spontaneous is hurtful to those of us who need some accommodation to our disability.

There is that first moment when the mechanics of your bladder management are revealed. This is the major test. How will he react to a mature woman who wears plastic knickers and pads and requires help when going to the bathroom? Reflection on this count is painful and inhibiting. Time is an important factor, because a considerable amount of physical preparation is required for intercourse. Unexpected disturbances or visitors are impossible to cope with, as I am unable to get up quickly, dress and wash. Even when sexually aroused the spontaneity can soon disappear when your partner has to help empty your bladder and carefully clean and position you. . . . My sexual fantasies relate to spontaneous sexual behavior—sex in an elevator, in any room of the house and in numerous positions—on the floor, up against the wall, and so on.[2]

Tee Corinne

Some advanced sexual planning and open discussion may be necessary, and we need to use our imaginations and be open to whatever makes us feel good. This can be a model for all lovers whether or not they are disabled.

Whether one or both partners are disabled, often we depend on a personal care attendant (PCA) to help us prepare for sex. Having a PCA who affirms our sexuality and wants to help us is *crucial*. Then our lover has a choice about how much of the preparation to be involved in, and we can feel more independent in the sexual relationship.

Existing literature and counseling on sexuality and disability is often unsatisfactory for women.* Its terminology, for instance, can undermine our sexuality. If we experience sexual response and orgasm despite a lack of sensation in our pelvic region, for instance, we are said in medical liter-

---

*Most current literature and counseling about sex and physical disability focuses on men, penis-in-vagina intercourse and male concerns about performance and potency. Most books assume that sexual readjustment is easier for a woman, and stress how to be attractive to men rather than how to get sexual satisfaction. They deal almost exclusively with spinal cord injuries, and give little helpful information for women with other disabilities. Those of us who are blind or deaf find even less information. See Resources for a few suggestions.

ature to have *phantom orgasms,* as though they're not quite real. The emphasis on "achievement" of orgasm and on "performance" and "sexual adequacy" makes us more conscious of what we may not have rather than delighted by what we experience. The literature also focuses on sexual techniques and positions, when sexuality for *all* human beings involves above all affection, touching, communication, caring, sensuality and love.

We don't do much "hard-core sex," but find our greatest fulfillment in slow, deep touching and holding. We can't seem to get enough cuddling.

I have no sensation below my waist now, but for some reason my neck, ears and armpits are much more sensitive than they used to be, and stimulation there is really quite exciting to me.

I really like going down on my partner because I can totally control what's going on and I experience so much sensation in my mouth, whereas I can't control my vagina or feel anything there.

I have erratic, vague sensation in my vagina and clitoris. When I have an orgasm, I feel most of the pleasure in my knees—it's a nerve transfer thing, I guess. I'm probably the only woman in the world whose knees come. . . .

THE POLITICS OF SEX

It can be difficult, even painful, to be sexual in a sexist, violent society. We have blamed ourselves and been blamed if sex didn't go well. We have accepted cruel labels such as "frigid," "cold," "dysfunctional," "cockteaser" or "insatiable." Yet when we talk with other women, we learn that many others have had the same problems we suffer over in the privacy of our bedrooms.*

Sexism and Power

Men as a group have more power in our society than women do. Even if you feel equal to your husband, male lover, friends, colleagues or co-workers, our culture values men more. This supposed superiority (even though your sex partner may not *feel* superior at all) gets played out in sex in the following ways.

- You should make love when he wants to, whether you're in the mood or not.

---

*Most of the following factors affect heterosexual couples mainly but are often in lesbian relationships in some form. See Chapter 10, "Loving Women," for more on lesbians and sex.

- You should take care of birth control because condoms interfere with his pleasure.
- You should make yourself attractive to him when he gets home from work (this despite the fact that you have been working, too, inside or outside the home or both).
- You should make sure the kids don't interrupt while you are making love.
- You should have orgasms to show him what a good lover he is.
- If you don't have intercourse, you should at least relieve him of his sexual tensions by oral sex or masturbating him. (It's no more painful for a man to go without orgasm than for a woman.)

I always used to see myself as there for a man's pleasure. I would do anything to please him. Just recently, at twenty-three, I've realized that I have needs in sex and started to say something about it.

It's hard to say no to having sex with a guy when he's taken me out to dinner several times and given me so much.

I have a physical disability that makes me slow to feel sexual sensations in my genitals. With my husband I am finally going slow enough to get past my terror that I won't feel anything. But for five years I faked orgasms so men would think they were great lovers. I am angry now that I subjected myself to that kind of sexual pretense.

There are so many times I say yes when I don't really want to, just to avoid a long discussion about why not.

When I finally learned to have orgasms and wanted to make love more, my husband seemed to have less of a desire for sex. He wasn't used to my being so turned on and assertive. I think he missed the power he used to have in determining how our lovemaking would go.

Underlying all my sexual relationships with men was the assumption that my body somehow belonged to him, not me. I thought I owed my partner my sexuality and should muster it up for him when he wanted or needed it. It was not even as crude and simple as giving over my body to be fucked. I had somehow to give him my ardor as well, let him turn me on. In fairness to the men who were my lovers, I want to say that these were not superdemanding or overly macho men. Whether or not they thought I owed them my sexuality was irrelevant, because the assumption that I did was deep in the culture and deep in my own sense of myself. Only as I finally begin to feel my authentic and sexual passion as a lesbian take root and grow within me do I begin to understand the sexual need my partners used to bring to our lovemaking. I see it now less as a demand and more as a mix of excitement and desire and a powerful connecting instinct. I believe it is sexual politics, not male personality, which makes an erect penis seem to be a demand rather than a human expression of yearning and vulnerability.

We will have more satisfying sex and begin to know our full sexual potential only when we are in relationships (and eventually in a society) where sexual, racial and class prejudice and dominance are absent.

Sex-Role Stereotypes

Men are "supposed" to know more about sex, to initiate it, to have a stronger sex drive. Women are "supposed" to be passive recipients or willing students. Supposedly *they* want sex and *we* want love. Such rigid classifying of people by gender is false, silly and damaging.

Many men, for instance, seem to want sex more often than women do, and there is a myth that men have a stronger sex drive. Yet perhaps what's at issue is not male sex drive at all, but the fact that men are raised with few ways of expressing their emotions. Sex (i.e., intercourse and/or orgasm) is one of the few permissible ways for a man to be close to someone, the only acceptable place for men's tender, loving feelings. It may be this limitation, rather than an innate, irrepressible sex drive that prompts men to initiate sex so often and leads to the false notion that women are less sexual than men. The stereotype must also arise from a deep cultural fear of women's sexual passion and power.

Conventional Definitions of Lovemaking

Most people define sex mainly in terms of intercourse, a form of lovemaking that is often well suited to men's orgasm and pleasure but is not necessarily well suited to ours.

I have orgasms easily during intercourse. Sometimes I love his thrusting deep inside me. Sometimes I don't want the penetration, I want something else. But he feels if we haven't had intercourse, we haven't actually made love.

I feel shy to ask for more foreplay when I know what he's really waiting for is the fucking.

In high school we had long making-out periods and I had orgasms all the time. When we "graduated" to intercourse I stopped having them so easily because we stopped doing all the other things.

Standard (male) definitions call all the touching, licking, sucking and caressing that turns us on *foreplay* to the big act—*intercourse*. Most texts even call us *dysfunctional* or *frigid* if we don't reach orgasm *during* intercourse. This is not a female definition of female sexuality.

In one survey, 70 percent of women did not orgasm during intercourse, although most did during other kinds of sex play or masturbation.* Many of us have learned ways of increasing our satisfaction in intercourse. But the more basic answer seems to be to change our definitions of lovemaking.

Around the time when I learned I could have orgasms through oral sex but not intercourse, I was angry because so much emphasis had been placed on how to achieve them in intercourse. Why did I consume so much energy worrying about that when it seemed like you could just have a different concept of what sex is?

It took making love with women for me to see that all the other things—oral sex, having my breasts sucked, rolling around or just lying still and feeling the sensations, touching my lover and turning her on—all these are lovemaking for me. Now when I make love with men I do it more like making love with a woman—slower, more sensually and tenderly, sometimes without penetration at all.

Getting rid of the notion of foreplay and calling it *all* lovemaking may be difficult for some men to get used to. But it may be a relief to the many men who worry about keeping an erection long enough to satisfy a woman during intercourse.

Emphasis on Performance and Goals

Sex books focus on techniques and say little about feelings. We worry about being sexy enough, about "doing it" well enough to please our partners. Orgasms, too, can become a goal: Some partners work at it for hours, wanting to please us or to show they are good lovers.

Because my previous relationships with men involved orgasm-centered sex (his orgasm, that is), I have brought to my first woman lover lots of expectations about coming. If one of us doesn't come, I feel we haven't made love "well." I think I miss a lot of pleasure that way.

Perhaps it takes someone my age, sixty, who has lived through other times, to point out that this society's

---

*See *The Hite Report* by Shere Hite.

glorification of sexual orgasm borders on the excessive. It's almost enough to make a person flaunt her chastity!

The first few years we had a great sex life. We were very attracted to each other and I loved sex with Ralph. I didn't have orgasms and I didn't even know what an orgasm was. Then I learned about orgasms, partly by reading some of the new books and articles and partly by having one while masturbating. It felt so good that I wanted to have it with Ralph. The next two years were awful in bed. We had this goal—my orgasm—and it was like we'd look at our watches and say, "One, two, three, go," and work at it until we succeeded. Now, finally, we're back on an even keel. Usually I come, sometimes I don't. I let Ralph know which way I'm feeling. We can forget that goal and just do what feels good. But I wish I'd known everything I know now back when our feelings were so intense.

We may judge ourselves by new norms.

I feel vaguely guilty if sex isn't great all the time, as though if I'm a real woman I should have an incredible orgasm every time, instead of accepting that sometimes there will be little ones and sometimes big ones.

With sex coming at us from every direction in the media, we may worry whether we are doing it enough. If we're single, we "should" be finding more sex partners. If in a relationship, we "should" be making love a certain number of times per week.

Many couples these days report the "problem" of lack of interest in sex. This may reflect problems in the relationship or in ways of lovemaking. But what experts are calling insufficient interest in sex may actually be our own desires measured against today's escalated sexual standards. It may even be a reaction against the general hype about sex in the media, or simple skin hunger—the need to be touched by another human being without sex.

Objectification of Our Bodies in the Media

We bring negative feelings about our bodies into sex in a particular way. The media's "ideal" woman often robs us of sexual confidence.

For years I wouldn't make love in a position that exposed my backside to scrutiny, for I had been told it was "too jiggly." Needless to say, this prevented me from being sexually assertive and creative and limited my responses.

We have a good sex life with lots of variety, fantasies, games. The fact that my disability prevents me from bending my leg limits us in some positions, but we just try different ones. Yet I don't have orgasms with my husband, only in masturbation. I am still struggling with my body. When I am unclothed I still feel like parts of me are really ugly. I think that when I can finish mourning, cry out my anguish over the disability, then sex will get better for me.

If we like the way we look and feel good about our bodies, we feel better about making love.

One of the difficult things about being large is that more often than not other people are the problem, not me. Many times I have felt that people I know wonder at my friendship with my lover. They wonder how a thin person can make love to a large one. The idea, I suppose, is that large women aren't attractive. Nonsense, of course. I enjoy my body immensely when I make love, either to myself or my boyfriend. I never think about my largeness. I simply am it and positively luxuriate in it. I love my body when I make love. It is beautiful to me and to my boyfriend. For six years we have both exulted in good lovemaking.

Violence Against Women

It is a cruel fact of our lives that many men abuse women, often using sex as a weapon. Rape, an early experience of incest, sexual harassment by a boss or co-worker or teacher, battering in the home by the man we share a bed with: Any of these can devastate what sex could be for us. If we don't experience violence directly, the possibility leers at us from pornography, news stories, movies, crude jokes, and so on.

Sometimes when I hear about a rape that's happened, I can't make love with my husband, even though I love him and usually enjoy sex. I know he is a gentle person, but for a moment I don't see him, I see all the men who use their penises as weapons to dominate and hurt women.

Making love with Rachel I am sometimes swept over by a feeling of fierce protectiveness. Her body is so precious to me. I want women and nonviolent men to become stronger and stronger and to change the things in our world which make sexual violence possible.

We must work for a more equal, less violent society in which sex is used not for somebody else's profit or as an instrument of dominance, but in service of love—love of ourselves, love and friendship for others.

All of us as women face the troubling paradox of seeking to open ourselves to the deep vulnerabilities of sexual loving in a society in which we are often not safe.

APPENDIX

Sexual-Health Care

Sexual health is a physical and emotional state of well-being that allows us to enjoy and act on our sexual feelings. We all need to follow certain procedures of routine care to stay sexually healthy.

- *A gynecological exam.* (See p. 564.)
- *Care of infections.* (See p. 596 and pp. 606–10.) If you get an infection of the vagina or urinary tract, you need to do something about it immediately.
- *Douching.* Unless you are instructed by a doctor for a particular reason, you never need to douche (wash out the vagina). The vagina has a natural cleansing process. Frequent douching and the use of vaginal deodorants can change the acidic and alkaline balance in the vagina and lead to infections. Scents used in vaginal deodorants can also cause allergic reactions.
- *Genital cleansing.* Rather than douche or use vaginal deodorants, you simply can wash your genital area daily with warm water. Separate the outer lips and pull back the hood of the clitoris to clean away the secretions that collect around the glans. Our body secretions and smells are a natural part of us, and if you are in good health and wash regularly, you smell and taste good. However, some of us like to wash our genitals before lovemaking. Do what makes you comfortable.
- *Birth control.* (See Chapter 13.) If you do not want to be pregnant and you are having intercourse, you'll need to discuss with the man involved the use of birth control and who will use the selected method. If you cannot discuss it with him or he won't discuss it with you, perhaps the relationship is not ready for sex. Even if you are not having intercourse, if sperm is deposited anywhere near the vagina (even in the mons area), the sperm can swim into the vagina on vaginal secretions and up through the cervix to the uterus and fallopian tubes and join with an egg.
- *Prevention against STDs and HIV/AIDS.* (See Chapter 14 and Chapter 15, "AIDS, HIV Infection and Women.".)
- *Menstruation.* It's fine to have sex during your menstrual periods if it feels comfortable to you. Some of us have found that orgasm relieves menstrual cramps.
- *Pregnancy.* (See Chapter 19.)

Sexual Arousal and Orgasm

Here are some details left out of the text.

Excitement

The vagina becomes moist (lubricated) (see p. 230). It begins to expand and balloon and eventually the inner two-thirds double in diameter.

The inner lips swell and deepen in color.

The clitoris swells, becomes erect and is highly sensitive to touch.

The breasts enlarge and become more sensitive. The nipples become erect.

The uterus enlarges and elevates within the pelvic cavity.

The heart rate increases; breathing becomes heavier and faster.

A flush or rash may appear on the skin.

The muscles begin to tighten, especially in the genital area.

If stimulation continues, the inner two-thirds of the vagina continue to balloon. The outer third narrows by one-third to one-half of its diameter and is quite sensitive to pressure.

The entire genital area continues to swell, as do the breasts. (You may become increasingly aware of these areas of your body.)

The uterus elevates fully.

We breathe very rapidly; we may pant.

The muscles continue to contract.

With full arousal the clitoris retracts under its hood. Stimulation of the inner lips from manipulation or intercourse moves the hood of the clitoris back and forth over the glans.

Orgasm: The Release of Sexual Tension

For women, if sexual stimulation is interrupted, excitement may decline. This is especially true just before and during orgasm, when we need continuous stimulation. Direct or indirect stimulation of the clitoris (and/or, for some women, pressure on the uterus) leads to orgasm.

During orgasm, muscles around the vagina, uterus and rectum contract (the contractions cause the release of the blood trapped in the pelvic veins). For one-half hour or more after orgasm, if lovemaking doesn't continue, swelling decreases, the muscles relax and the clitoris, vagina and uterus return to their usual positions.

The Role of Testosterone in Sexuality*

Certain hormones play a role in sexual feelings, sexual activity and intensity of orgasm. The most influential is *testosterone*, sometimes called the *libido hormone* and also, erroneously, the *male hormone*. Testosterone, like estrogen, is present in

---

*Prepared by Edith Bjornson Sunley.

both men and women, though the proportions differ between the sexes. In women it is produced through the operation of both the *adrenals* (two small glands near the kidneys) and the *ovaries*, with the ovary probably the more important source.[3]

The role of testosterone in sexuality is illustrated in several ways. (1) When one adrenal is removed, women report a dramatic decrease in sexual interest, sensation and frequency of orgasm. (2) When ovaries are removed, many women report a similar loss.[4] Testosterone levels are lower in women after menopause or after ovary removal (oophorectomy) than in healthy young women with ovaries in place, showing that less testosterone is produced as ovarian function slows or stops. (3) A recent study of sexually active women showed a significant correlation between blood testosterone levels and sexual responsiveness and satisfaction.[5] Knowing the importance of testosterone, ovaries and adrenals can alert us to protecting our sexuality from unnecessary removal of the ovaries or adrenals.

Problems with Sex

At one time or another all of us have problems with sex. Read about the causes and treatment for the problem you are having, particularly if it is a severe one (see Resources).

Sexual problems in a relationship are relationship problems. Some common causes are: sexual ignorance, poor communication patterns, male and female role expectations, a lack of trust or commitment or unresolved conflicts. An abusive partner may use sex as a weapon to hurt or dominate you; in that case, the *abuse* is the problem.

How we think and feel about ourselves and sex powerfully affects how our bodies respond. Guilt, shyness, fear, conflict and ignorance, all can block or inhibit sexual responsiveness. If any of the following is a problem, we owe it to ourselves to explore further. We need not be in total agony or the worst on the block before we look for help. Sexual problems are common.

Problems with Orgasm*

Many of us experience difficulties reaching orgasm, either by ourselves or with a lover. Shame about exploring and touching ourselves keeps us from learning to bring ourselves to orgasm through masturbation. A variety of problems keeps us from having orgasms with another. Here are some of the reasons why:

- We don't notice or else we misunderstand what's

---
*See especially *For Yourself: The Fulfillment of Female Sexuality* by L. Barbach, New York: Doubleday/Anchor Books, 1981.

happening in our bodies as we get aroused. We're too busy thinking about abstractions—how to do it right, why it doesn't go well for us, what our lover thinks of us, whether our lover is impatient, whether our lover can last—when we might better be concentrating on sensations, not thoughts.

- We feel ourselves becoming aroused, but we are afraid we won't have an orgasm, and we don't want to get into the hassle of trying, so we just repress sexual response.
- We are afraid of asking too much and seeming too demanding.
- We are afraid that if our lover concentrates on our pleasure we will feel such pressure to come that we won't be able to—and then we don't.
- We are trying to have a simultaneous orgasm, which seldom occurs for most of us. It can be just as pleasurable if we come separately.
- We are in deep conflict about, or angry at, the person we are sleeping with. Unconsciously we withhold orgasm as a way of withholding ourselves.
- We feel guilty about having sex and so cannot let ourselves really enjoy it.
- We rush into sex—swept off our feet just like in the movies and swept under the rug when it comes to climaxes.

Lack of Interest in Sex: Sexual Aversion

For a few of us the conflicts about ourselves and sex are so deep we never have any interest in sex. We may even feel an extreme, unpleasant sensitivity to touch or may feel so ticklish that we can't relax. Our bodies are reacting this way for a reason and protecting us from sexual experiences we can't handle at this point. This may well be a time to look for professional help.

Painful Lovemaking

You may experience discomfort, even pain, with lovemaking for the following physical rather than emotional reasons.

Local Infection

Some vaginal infections—like monilia (yeast) or trichomoniasis—can be present in a nonacute, visually unnoticeable form. The friction of a penis or finger moving on your vulva or in your vagina might cause the infection to flare up, making you sting and itch (see p. 607). A herpes sore on your external genitals can make friction painful (see pp. 317–18).

Local Irritation

The vagina might be irritated by a birth control foam, cream or jelly you are using. If so, try a different brand. Some of us react to the rubber in a condom or diaphragm. Vaginal deodorant sprays and scented tampons can irritate the vagina or vulva.

Insufficient Lubrication

The wall of the vagina responds to sexy feelings by "sweating," giving off a liquid that wets the vagina and the entrance to it, which makes penetration easier. Sometimes there isn't enough of this liquid. Some reasons: You may be trying to let the penis in (or the man might be putting/forcing it in) too soon, before there has been enough stimulation to excite you and set the sweating action going; you may be nervous or tense about making love (e.g., it's the first time, or you're worried about getting pregnant); if you are using a rubber (condom) you may need to add lubrication. Be sure to give the vagina time to get wet. If you still feel dry you can use saliva, lubricating jelly (e.g., K-Y) or a birth control foam, cream or jelly. (Never use Vaseline or other oil-based lubricant with a condom or diaphragm. It will deteriorate the rubber.) Hormone deficiency can also cause dryness. After childbirth (particularly if you are nursing your baby or if your stitches hurt) and after menopause are two times when a lack of estrogen can affect the vaginal walls in such a way that less liquid is produced. Try the lubricants suggested above.

Tightness in the Vaginal Entrance

The first few times you have intercourse, an unstretched hymen (if you have one) can cause pain. And whenever you are tense and preoccupied the vaginal entrance is not likely to loosen up enough, and getting the penis in might hurt. Even if you feel relaxed and sexy, timing is important. If you try to get the penis in before you are fully aroused, you might still be too tight, though you are wet enough. So don't rush, and don't let yourself be rushed.

Pain Deep in the Pelvis

Sometimes the thrust of a finger or penis hurts way inside. This pain can be caused by tears in the ligaments that support the uterus (caused by obstetrical mismanagement during childbirth, a botched-up abortion, gang rape); infections of the cervix, uterus and tubes (such as pelvic inflammatory disease—the end result of untreated sexually transmitted disease in many women); endometriosis; cysts or tumors on the ovaries. All these may be treatable.

Clitoral Pain

The clitoris is exquisitely sensitive, and for many of us direct touching or rubbing of the clitoris (especially the glans, or tip) is painful (many men don't know this until we tell them). Also, genital secretions can collect under the hood, so when washing pull back the hood of the clitoris and clean it gently.

Painful Penetration: Vaginismus

If you have vaginismus, you experience a strong, involuntary tightening of your vaginal muscles, a spasm of the outer third of your vagina, which makes entrance by finger, tampon, speculum or penis acutely painful.

Vaginismus can be your body's defense against a sexual situation you can't handle or don't want to be in. It can also be the result of bad experiences, such as rape.*

Vaginismus can be treated successfully by a variety of methods, including sex therapy, psychotherapy and hypnotherapy. For aid in choosing an effective and trustworthy practitioner, see the following section, Helping Ourselves, or Chapter 6, "Psychotherapy."

Whatever the cause, if lovemaking is at all painful, don't put up with the pain! Find out what is causing it and do something about it. Until the problem is solved, figure out other ways to make love. The power that each of us has and the power that we have together to make our lives more satisfying is enormous.

Helping Ourselves

If you are feeling pain in your pelvic, genital or vaginal area, get a good gynecological exam to find out if there is a physical cause. Remember, however, that most doctors have not been trained to discuss sexual problems. Enlist the help of friends or a local women's group to find a sympathetic and competent nurse-midwife or physician.

Despite our knowledge about sex, despite the support of friends and partners, sometimes we cannot work through our difficulties. If you need someone to talk with, call your local women's health center, free clinic or the American Association of Sex Educators, Counselors and Therapists (AASECT) for the name of a recommended counselor or therapist in your area. Because there are men and women without adequate training who call themselves sex therapists, we believe that contacting AASECT is better than consulting your yellow pages or, often, your health practitioner.

When there are sexual problems in a couple relationship, it is often the woman who seeks help first. This may be because culturally it is easier

(text continued on p. 233)

---

*If you think you are suffering from vaginismus, read about it in *When a Woman's Body Says No to Sex: Understanding and Overcoming Vaginismus* by Linda Valins, New York: Viking Penguin, 1992; and in *The New Sex Therapy* by Helen S. Kaplan, New York: Brunner-Mazel, 1974.

SEX AND PHYSICAL DISABILITIES

Chronic Disease or Disability	Effects on Our Sexuality	Helpful Hints and Special Implications
Cerebral palsy (CP)	Muscle spasticity, rigidity, and/or weakness may make certain sex acts and self-pleasuring difficult to impossible for us. Contractures of our knees and hips may cause us pain under the pressure of a partner, and spasms may increase with arousal. Our genital sensations remain intact but some of us experience a lack of lubrication. Menstruation, fertility and pregnancy are not affected. During delivery, those of us with severe CP might need a cesarean section.*†	Nongenital lovemaking, different positions and propping our legs up on pillows may help ease spasms. We can use a vibrator to make love alone or with another person if our arms and hands are involved. A water-soluble lubricant can often help if our vagina lacks lubrication. Inserting spermicidal foam or a diaphragm may be complicated by spasms or poor hand control. Because of an increased risk of clotting, the birth control pill is not advisable for those of us taking seizure medication (anticonvulsants) or if our mobility is greatly restricted by severe CP.§
Cerebral vascular accident (CVA) (stroke)	We may have difficulties in sexual positioning and sensitivity because of impaired motor strength, coordination or paralysis. How much this affects our sexual functions will depend upon the severity of our CVA. Our sex drive may decrease, more commonly when our CVA occurs in the dominant side of the brain (for right-handers usually the left hemisphere with right-side paralysis). Menstruation and fertility are not affected, but there may be complications with pregnancy and delivery.*	If spasms or paralysis persist, we can use other lovemaking positions that do not require strenuous activity. Most persons who were sexually active before CVA remain active; thus one cannot generalize about sex drive and functioning. An understanding friend or partner will often be the best help during the long recovery process. The birth control pill is never good to use, especially if our CVA resulted from diabetes or circulatory disorders.‡§‖
Diabetes	Most of the medical literature is about male sexual functioning and the few reports show conflicting results. About a third of diabetic women in one study reported that their orgasms gradually got to be rarer and less intense. One possible explanation was that the threshold for orgasm increased because of damage to the nerve fibers in the pelvic region. A lack of vaginal lubrication and recurrent infections may make some lovemaking unpleasant.*	Some women say that using a vibrator allows them to reach orgasm because the stimulation is more intense. Poorly controlled diabetes may stop menstruation and cause fertility problems. Depending upon how stable our blood glucose levels are, pregnancy may be complicated and should be closely monitored. Birth control pills often aggravate other symptoms of our diabetes and should not be used because of possible cerebrovascular and cardiovascular complications.‡§‖
Renal failure	In chronic renal insufficiency, menstruation may stop or become extremely irregular. Many women become infertile and rarely carry pregnancies to term. We may have difficulties in becoming sexually excited and as in diabetes, our orgasms may become rarer and less intense. Sometimes we have a decrease in vaginal lubrication and breast tissue mass.*	Maintenance hemodialysis often brings on excessive and sometimes painful menstruation but may improve our sex drive, though not necessarily sexual functioning. Kidney transplants usually improve both our sex drive and sex function, and fertility improves dramatically. If our vagina is too dry, a water-soluble lubricant can help. Many of the drugs used to lower hypertension are likely to dampen our sex drive. The birth control pill is usually not advised.‡
Rheumatoid arthritis (RA)	Swollen, painful joints, muscular atrophy and joint contractures may make it difficult for us to masturbate or make love in some positions. Pain, fatigue and medications may decrease our sex drive, but genital sensations remain intact. Menstruation, fertility and pregnancy are not affected, but birthing may be complicated if our hips and spine are involved. However, symptoms may improve during pregnancy due to changes in our immune system. (For footnotes, see p. 233.)	To avoid pain and pressure on affected joints, we can be creative in sexual positioning. If our symptoms respond to heat, we can plan sex after a compress or a hot bath with our partner. Choose the best time, when you have the least pain and stiffness, for lovemaking. Try sex instead of corticosteroids—it is said to stimulate the adrenal glands and so increases output of natural cortisone, which alleviates painful symptoms. The birth control pill may not be good for us if we have circulatory problems or greatly restricted mobility.‡§

SEX AND PHYSICAL DISABILITIES

Chronic Disease or Disability	Effects on Our Sexuality	Helpful Hints and Special Implications
Systemic lupus erythematosus	Many difficulties are the same as in RA (above). However, because different people have quite different symptoms, often connected to other disorders, one cannot generalize. Research on the female sexual effects of lupus is scarce, despite the fact that nine out of ten people with lupus are women. Sometimes we also have sores in and around the mouth and vagina and a decrease in vaginal lubrication, so we may have pain during vaginal penetration.*	For helpful hints, see RA above. Also, we can use a water-soluble lubricant if our vagina is too dry. Choose birth control methods with extreme caution, especially if symptoms or complications other than RA exist. Birth control pills may not be advisable if we have circulatory or kidney problems or if our mobility is greatly restricted.‡§
Myocardial infarction (MI)	For those of us with very serious conditions, chest pain, palpitations and shortness of breath may limit our sexual activities. However, many of us can resume regular lovemaking once we can climb two flights of stairs at a brisk pace without causing symptoms. (The cardiac responses during step climbing and lovemaking are similar, the average being 125 beats per minute.)†	We should consult our physician to see when and if we can safely begin an exercise regime. We can use lovemaking positions that require little or no exertion, especially with our arms (for example, on our side or back). Go slow in the beginning to minimize stress and fear of stress, because the majority of sexual problems arise from anxiety and misinformation about this ailment. Birth control pills should not be used.‡
Multiple sclerosis (MS)	Depending upon the stage and severity of MS, our symptoms will vary and may come and go. Some of us experience difficulty in having an orgasm, decreased genital sensitivity, dryness of the vagina, muscle weakness, pain and bladder and bowel incontinence. There is no change in our menstrual and fertility patterns. Pregnancy and postpregnancy stress may increase MS symptoms, but the reports about this are conflicting.*†	Because sexual difficulties may come and go with other MS symptoms, it helps to be creative. Medication for spasms and topical anesthetics for pain may be helpful. If our balance is not good and we tire easily, we can use lovemaking positions that require little exertion. A water-soluble lubricant can help with a dry vagina. Some women say that intercourse is painful but having their clitoris stimulated feels good. The birth control pill is not good to use if you have paralysis or restricted mobility, but a recent study showed that it may help symptoms in early stages of MS.*‡§‖
Ostomy	Although much more is known about sexual functioning of men with ostomies, it appears that women are better off. Surgery should not impair our genital functioning or fertility and often makes it safe to become pregnant, because a disease process, such as cancer or ulcerative colitis, has been wiped out. However, a few women report pain during intercourse or a lack of vaginal sensations after ileostomy and colostomy surgery.	An ostomy is a hidden disability until our clothes are off; therefore, it may help to find a comfortable way to tell potential partners before sexual relations begin. The opening or appliance may be covered or secured before lovemaking, both for aesthetic reasons and for support so it does not get in the way. We can use lovemaking positions where we feel most secure that the bag will not get pulled out. If odors are a problem, we can bathe and empty the bag before making love. Consider alternatives and consult a physician if taking the birth control pill because sometimes it is not absorbed properly.‡
Spinal cord injury (SCI)	Our sexual functioning will depend on the location and severity of the injury, and there is great variation even for women with injuries at the same spinal level. Basically, if our injury is above the sacral area, there will be reflex sexual responses, and at or below this level (conus medullaris), our reflex responses will be disrupted. SCI may result in paralysis, spasticity, loss of sensation, incontinence, skin ulcers, pain and a dry vagina, sometimes complicating making love with yourself or another. We may con-	It can help to make love in ways other than vaginal penetration, which may be painful due to increased bladder infections, spasms, vaginal irritation and tearing and autonomic dysreflexia. Routine bowel and bladder programs can decrease the risk of "accidents" during sex, and a towel will help if there is any leakage. We can also tape our catheter down or move it out of the way so it does not get pulled out. Spasm medications and a water-soluble vaginal lubricant may be of some assistance. Pregnancy in- (continued)

SEX AND PHYSICAL DISABILITIES

Chronic Disease or Disability	Effects on Our Sexuality	Helpful Hints and Special Implications
	tinue to have orgasmic sensations or they may be diffused, either in general or to specific body parts, such as our breasts or lips. Our neck, ears and the area above the injury may become more sexually exciting. Arousal, self-pleasuring and lovemaking may increase spasms and the risk of incontinence. Although we may stop menstruating for several months after the injury, fertility is not permanently disrupted.†	creases the risk of thrombophlebitis and bladder infections, but many women have relatively healthy and painless births. Be on guard for signs of autonomic dysreflexia during labor and delivery, and of uterine prolapse afterward. Take birth control pills only with extreme caution, if at all, and never if taking antihypertensive medication or if you have circulatory problems.‡§‖

*The research literature is severely limited. Information presented here is only meant to be a guide because it is based on only one or two studies or clinical observations.
†Most of the literature concerning sexuality and this disability is male oriented, and many studies generalize their findings from men's to women's sexuality. Adequate research on sexual functioning (as opposed to reproductive functioning) has yet to be carried out with women.
‡Many medications are directly responsible for the negative effects on sexual functioning—often much more so than the disability itself! Examples of such drugs are antihypertensives, phenothiazines and so forth. Consult your physician/pharmacologist for alternative medications if you think you may have this problem. Be sure to inform your sexual-health-care provider about the medications and dosage you are taking when seeking contraceptive services.
§The diaphragm may not be a good method of birth control if you have poor hand control, recurrent bladder or vaginal infections or very weak pelvic muscles. If the use of your hands is limited, ask your partner or attendant to help insert the diaphragm. There are also devices available that can make it easier to insert the coil-spring diaphragm, but some hand control is required.
‖The IUD is not good to use for women with a loss of sensation in the pelvic area because of the risk that puncture or pelvic inflammatory disease may go unnoticed. Also, good hand coordination is needed to check the strings every month to make sure the IUD is still in place.
Note: Table prepared by Janna Zwerner.

for us to admit to our sexual concerns. It may also be because we too often assume that if sex is a problem, it's we who are in need of help. Sexual problems usually reflect or express relationship problems.

You may have a difficult time finding a good doctor or therapist. Those of us who are single or in lesbian relationships have even fewer resources than heterosexual couples. You may need to concentrate on working with friends or your partner or both, after reading the available books.

A Word About Men

Male Sexual Response

Sexual arousal in men, as in women, leads to vasocongestion (blood-engorged veins) and myotonia (muscle contraction). A woman's first reaction to arousal is vaginal lubrication, and a man's is penile erection. For both sexes the peak of sexual excitement is orgasm, which for a man includes ejaculation (when a fluid called *semen*, which includes sperm, spurts out of the penis). After orgasm a man has a period of a few minutes or even hours (longer as he gets older) when he cannot have another erection.

Male Sexual Problems

If we are having sex with a man who is having sexual difficulties, it is hard to have the kind of pleasure both partners would like. Further, his difficulties may complicate our own problems—even create some for us.

Men can suffer problems similar to ours and for many of the same reasons. The common male sexual problems are *premature ejaculation*, the inability to control the ejaculatory reflex; *impotence*, the inability to maintain, or even be aroused to, an erection; *dispareunia*, pain with intercourse; and *sexual aversion*, lack of interest in sex altogether.

Some sexual problems can be worked through with the help of good books and a caring partner, whereas others might call for professional help.

Sex Discussion Group for Women: Learning Together About Sex

In a women's sex discussion group, we can discuss factual information; explore our feelings; talk out problems; practice communicating (verbally and nonverbally); get help deciding how, when and with whom to share sexual feelings and learn alternative ways to get what we want sexually.

Here are some suggestions for organizing such a group: Meet together and explore what you want to discuss with each other. Draw up a list of topics and a flexible plan for discussions. Select some members of the group to find out more about local resources you might want to use—films you could see or persons who might want to meet with you and offer their specialized knowledge. Choose other members to consider what materials besides this chapter you might like to read together.

Topics you may want to discuss include childhood and adolescent memories of sexuality, your feelings about your body, differences in female and male socialization, masturbation, fantasies, the nature of female sexual response, virginity, homosexuality, lovemaking, intercourse, orgasm, feelings about touching and looking at your genitals, sexual-health care, birth control, abortion, sexual problems, relationship with yourself, relationships with other women, relationships with men, the sexuality of your children.

The following "journey" through one's own sexuality is a stimulating way to begin your discussion. Before your second or third meeting, two of you get together and draw up a list of questions beginning with first memories of sensual pleasure and affection (e.g., "What kind of touching did you get as a child from your parents?" "How did you feel?"). You will want to include questions about sexual language, your parents' relationship to each other and to you, sex play with siblings and friends (e.g., playing doctor), your first menstrual period, dating, petting, intercourse, orgasm, crushes on girlfriends, marriage, sexuality as an adult and so forth. When you all meet together again, the two of you take the rest of the group on the journey. Ask each woman to find a comfortable spot and close her eyes. The two of you alternate reading your questions very slowly, giving women time to remember. Leave a minute or two between questions. When the questions are finished, leave some more space before joining together to discuss your memories and reactions to them.

Early memories can be painful and upsetting for women who have experienced sexual abuse; be sure to talk about this in the group beforehand, and adjust your plan accordingly.

Consider activities you think would enrich your talking together. You might keep personal journals throughout the weeks you meet and share from them at a final meeting, make a collage of sex cartoons at the beginning of one week's meeting, see a porno flick or visit a bookstore that sells pornography, make a group list of all the street and slang terms you know for sex and include your lovers for a meeting or two.

NOTES

1. L. Zussman, S. Zussman, R. Sunley and E. Bjornson. "Sexual Response After Hysterectomy–Oophorectomy: Recent Studies and Reconsideration of Psychogenesis," *American Journal of Obstetrics and Gynecology*, Vol. 140, No. 7 (Aug. 1, 1981), pp. 725–31.

2. Jo Campling, ed. "Julie," in *Images of Ourselves: Women with Disabilities Talking*. London: Routledge and Kegan Paul, 1981, p. 17.

3. Christopher Longcope, "Steroid Production in Pre- and Postmenopausal Women," Chapter 2 in R. B. Greenblatt, V. Mahesh and R. McDonough, eds. *The Menopausal Syndrome*. New York: Medcom Press, 1974.

4. L. Zussman, S. Zussman, R. Sunley and E. Bjornson. "Sexual Response After Hysterectomy–Oophorectomy."

5. Harold Persky, et al. "The Relation of Plasma Androgen Levels to Sexual Behaviors and Attitudes of Women," *Journal of Psychosomatic Medicine* (1983). Reported at March 25, 1982, meeting of the American Psychosomatic Society.

RESOURCES*

Readings

To add to this brief list, you can get extensive bibliographies on all aspects of sexuality from SIECUS, the Multi-Media Resource Center and the Kinsey Institute for Sex Research (addresses in Organizations, below). Good sources of feminist books on women's sexuality are Down There Press (P.O. Box 2036, Burlingame, CA 94011), Naiad Press (P.O. Box 10543, Tallahassee, FL 32302), and for Spanish and English publications, Volcano Press (330 Ellis Street, Department BL, San Francisco, CA, 94102). The Sexuality Library at the Good Vibrations mail-order store carries the titles listed below (see Mail Order for address).

For information on HIV, AIDS and safer sex, see Chapter 15.

For books specifically on lesbian sexuality, see Resources following Chapter 10, "Loving Women: Lesbian Life and Relationships."

Barbach, L. G. *For Each Other: Sharing Sexual Intimacy*. New York: Doubleday/Anchor Books, 1983. Useful information for women who want to improve sexual intimacy with their partners. Includes practical information on sustaining sexual desire, communicating about sex and changing sexual patterns.

———. *For Yourself: The Fulfillment of Female Sexuality*. New York: Doubleday/Anchor Books, 1981. Written for the preorgasmic woman, a fine guide to female sexuality.

———, ed. *Pleasures: Women Write Erotica*. New York: Harper & Row, 1985.

Barbach, L. G., and Linda Levine. *Shared Intimacies: Women's Sexual Experiences*. New York: Bantam, 1981. This fine book includes lengthy, informative and explicit quotes from women in many kinds of sexual relationships.

Bell, Ruth, et al. *Changing Bodies, Changing Lives: A Book for Teens on Sex and Relationships*. New York: Random House, 1987. Filled with quotes from teenagers and young adults.

*Prepared by Amy Alpern with help from Diana Chace and Brenda Reeb. Thanks to Good Vibrations for the use of their book descriptions and to the staff at New Words Bookstore, 186 Hampshire Street, Cambridge, MA 02139.

Blank, Joani. *Good Vibrations: The Complete Guide to Vibrators*. Burlingame, CA: Down There Press, 1989. Discusses types of vibrators and ways to enhance pleasure, as well as various vibrator anecdotes. Written by the proprietor of San Francisco's vibrator store for women.

———. *The Playbook for Women About Sex*. Burlingame, CA: Down There Press, 1982. A sexual self-awareness workbook for every woman.

Bright, Susie. *Herotica: A Collection of Women's Erotic Fiction*. Burlingame, CA: Down There Press, 1988.

Brown, Melanie. *The New Celibacy*. New York: McGraw-Hill, 1989.

Calderone, Mary S., and Eric W. Johnson. *The Family Book About Sexuality*. New York: HarperCollins, 1990. Liberal in approach, it does neglect certain political issues about sex and is tolerant rather than affirming of homosexuality.

Chester, Laura. *Deep Down: The New Sensual Writing by Women*. Boston: Faber and Faber, 1989.

Corinne, Tee. *The Cunt Coloring Book*. San Francisco: Last Gasp, 1989. Forty-two different drawings of women's genitals are depicted in this unorthodox coloring book.

Dodson, Betty. *Sex for One: The Joy of Selfloving*. New York: Crown Books, 1987. An inspirational book from the "mother of masturbation." Dodson describes her Bodysex workshops, discusses masturbation for women and men and guides the reader through specific techniques designed to enhance the experience of self-love.

Friday, Nancy. *Forbidden Flowers*. New York: Pocket Books, 1975.

———. *My Secret Garden: Women's Sexual Fantasies*. New York: Pocket Books, 1987.

———. *Women on Top: Women's Sexual Fantasies of Power, Self-Exploration and Insatiable Lust*. New York: Simon & Schuster, 1991. Full of women's sexual fantasies, these three books are a kind of natural erotica for some.

Heiman, Julia, and Joseph LoPiccolo. *Becoming Orgasmic*. New York: Simon & Schuster, 1986. A personal growth program designed to put the reader in touch with her capacity for arousal and sexual pleasure. Includes good general information on female sexuality, communicating with partners and how to overcome anxieties about sex.

Heresies: A Feminist Publication on Art and Politics, Sex Issue, Vol. 3, No. 4, Issue 12. Provocative articles, poems, artwork on the theme that in women's sexuality, variety is the spice of life. Thoughtful treatment of lust, casual sex, celibacy, prostitution, sadomasochism and butch–femme. A classic from the pre-HIV awareness era. Available from *Heresies*, P.O. Box 1306, Canal Street Station, New York, NY 10013.

Hite, Shere. *The Hite Report*. New York: Dell, 1987. More than 3,000 women are surveyed about what they really do in sex.

———. *The Hite Report on Male Sexuality*. New York: Ballantine, 1987.

Irvine, Janice. *Disorders of Desire: Sex and Gender in Modern American Sexology*. Philadelphia: Temple University Press, 1990. Excellent analysis.

Kasl, Charlotte Davis. *Women, Sex and Addiction*. New York: Harper & Row, 1990.

Kirkpatrick, Martha, ed. *Women's Sexual Experience: Explorations of the Dark Continent*. New York: Plenum, 1982. Essays by diverse writers on women's sexual responses, teen mothers, American Indian women, African-American women, ageism in sexual counseling, woman abuse, incest and more.

Kitzinger, Sheila. *Woman's Experience of Sex*. New York: Penguin Books, 1985.

Ladas, Alice Kahn, Beverly Whipple and John D. Perry. *The G Spot and Other Recent Discoveries About Human Sexuality*. New York: Dell, 1983. This popular but controversial book met criticism in much of the scientific community for proclaiming a theory based on skimpy data. Many feminists criticize its authors' reinstatement of the old dichotomy between clitoral and vaginal orgasm. Other readers are more positive about the inquiry into women's varied experience of orgasms.

Mininni, Darlene. *Sex Talk: The College Student's Guide to Sex in the 90s*. Good Friend Press, 217 E. 82nd Street, Box 22, New York, NY 10028, 1991.

Nelson, James B. *Embodiment: An Approach to Sexuality and Christian Theology*. Minneapolis, MN: Augsburg, 1978. Nelson's feminist perspective on sex and sexual relationships makes this an unusual and helpful book for women who are thinking about sexuality and religion.

Off Our Backs, 1724 20th Street NW, Washington, DC 20009. A monthly women's news journal. Often runs excellent articles on sexuality.

Pond, Lily, ed. *Yellow Silk: Journal of Erotic Arts*. Verygraphics, P.O. Box 6374, Albany, CA 94706. Erotic poems, stories, essays, graphics, for women and men. The motto: "All persuasions; no brutality."

Sevely, Josephine L. *Eve's Secrets: A New Theory of Female Sexuality*. New York: Random House, 1987. The author challenges many assumptions about the female sexual response, demonstrates an unsuspected symmetry between women's and men's sexual organs, introduces a new theory of orgasm and provides a controversial discussion of female ejaculation. Available from Exodus Trust, 1523 Franklin Street, San Francisco, CA 94109.

Snitow, Ann, Christine Stansell and Sharon Thompson, eds. *Powers of Desire: The Politics of Sexuality*. New York: Monthly Review Press, 1983.

Stimpson, Catharine, and Ethel Person, eds. *Women, Sex and Sexuality*. Chicago: University of Chicago Press, 1980. Important essays from a feminist/academic perspective.

Valins, Linda. *When a Woman's Body Says No to Sex: Understanding and Overcoming Vaginismus*. New York: Viking Penguin, 1992.

Vitale, Sylvia Witts. "An Herstorical Look at Some Aspects of Black Sexuality," *Heresies: A Feminist Publication on Art and Politics*, Sex Issue, Vol. 3, No. 4, Issue 12, 1980. Available from *Heresies*, P.O. Box 1306, Canal Street Station, New York, NY 10013.

Walker, Alice. *The Color Purple*. New York: Harcourt Brace Jovanovich, 1982. A powerful novel that touches on many aspects of black women's sexuality.

Sexuality and Sexual Abuse

Please see the Resources in Chapter 8, "Violence Against Women," for a more extensive listing of books on sexual abuse. Below are listed a few books that address healing from the impact of sexual abuse on our sexuality.

Bass, Ellen, and Laura Davis. *The Courage to Heal: A Guide for Women Survivors of Sexual Abuse.* New York: Harper & Row, 1988.

Davis, Laura. *Allies in Healing: When the Person You Love Was Sexually Abused as a Child.* New York: HarperCollins, 1991.

———. *The Courage to Heal Workbook: For Women and Men Survivors of Child Sexual Abuse.* New York: Harper & Row, 1990.

Maltz, Wendy, and Beverly Holman. *Incest and Sexuality: A Guide to Understanding and Healing.* Lexington, MA: D. C. Heath, 1987.

Sex Research

Masters, William H., and Virginia E. Johnson. *Human Sexual Inadequacy.* New York: Bantam, 1981. Major research on the nature and treatment of sexual problems. The major drawback is the medicalized and performance-oriented approach to sex and sexual problems.

———. *Human Sexual Response.* New York: Bantam, 1981. Masters and Johnson's revolutionary research helped lead the way to more helpful understandings of women's orgasms, particularly the central role of the clitoris.

Sherfey, Mary Jane. *The Nature and Evolution of Female Sexuality.* New York: Vintage Books, 1972. This history-making study highlights the role of the clitoris in orgasm and the potential intensity of women's sexual drives and satisfactions. A feminist classic, sadly it is no longer in print.

Sex Therapy

Kaplan, Helen S. *The Illustrated Manual of Sex Therapy,* 2nd ed. New York: Brunner-Mazel, 1987.

———. *The New Sex Therapy.* New York: Brunner-Mazel (Quadrangle/New York Times Book Co.), 1974. Male and female sexual dysfunctions and their treatment, primarily according to the Masters and Johnson technique. Pictures are particularly fine.

Textbooks

Katchadourian, Heront, and Donald Lunde. *Fundamentals of Human Sexuality.* New York: Holt Rinehart & Winston, 1989. Fine general textbook on human sexuality as a biological, behavioral and cultural phenomenon.

McCary, James L., and Stephen P. McCary. *McCary's Human Sexuality,* 4th ed. Belmont, CA: Wadsworth Publishing Co., 1984. Highly readable general discussion of human sexuality.

Sex and Physical Disability

Bregman, Sue. *Sexuality and the S.C.I. Woman,* 1975. Available from the Sister Keanny Institute, 800 East 28th Street, Minneapolis, MN 55407, (612) 863-4205.

Duffy, Yvonne, . . . *All Things Are Possible,* 1981. A. J. Garvin and Associates, P.O. Box 7525, Ann Arbor, MI 48187. More than seventy-five differently abled women speak candidly about their lives. Chapters about parental attitudes, masturbation, relationships, sexual intercourse, lesbianism, birth control, childbirth and childrearing contain explicit descriptions and concrete suggestions for overcoming difficulties.

Organizations

American Association of Sex Educators, Counselors, and Therapists (AASECT)
435 North Michigan Avenue, Suite 1717
Chicago, IL 60611
(312) 644-0828
Can help you find resources for sex therapy in your area.

Information Service of the Kinsey Institute for Research in Sex, Gender, and Reproduction
313 Morrison Hall
Indiana University
Bloomington, IN 47405
Send for their list of bibliographies on many aspects of sexuality.

Multi-Focus, Inc.
1525 Franklin Street
San Francisco, CA 94109
(415) 673-5100
Distributes films, videos and slides on all aspects of sexuality. Send for free catalog.

SIECUS
130 West 42nd Street, Suite 2500
New York, NY 10036
(212) 819-9770
(617) 742-2100
SIECUS publishes a bimonthly journal, annotated bibliographies, brochures and other informational publications related to sexuality research, education and legislation. Full list and order form are available upon request.

Mail Order

Eve's Garden International, Ltd.
119 West 57th Street
New York, NY 10019
(800) 848-3837

Good Vibrations
1210 Valencia Street
San Francisco, CA 94110
(415) 550-7399
Vibrators and sex toys are available from both these stores. A wide range of book titles including many of those listed here are also available—from erotic titles to practical sexual advice that won't insult your intelligence.

PART III

Controlling Our Fertility

Introduction

BASED ON THE WORK OF
JOAN DITZION AND
JANET GOLDEN

Controlling our fertility is central to controlling our lives. The chapters in this unit present tools for understanding our fertility and making choices about whether and when to have children. We realize more every day that safe, affordable birth control and abortion, though absolutely crucial, are only part of our full reproductive freedom. All women must be free not only to prevent or end unwanted pregnancy, but also to have children when and how we choose. This means, for example, that no woman should be forced into abortion or sterilization because she can't afford to raise a child (as many poor women and women of color are today). It means that no woman should become infertile due to dangerous birth control methods or misdiagnosed or untreated sexually transmitted disease.*

The following "Principles of Unity" from the former Reproductive Rights National Network (R2N2) express the many facets of complete reproductive freedom:

We believe that as women we have a right to control our own bodies and that we must organize to secure that right in the face of attacks by church, state and the organized right wing. Therefore,

1. We support the right and access of all women, regardless of age or income, to abortion. We oppose the Hyde Amendment and any other attempt to cut off or restrict Medicaid funds for abortion, any legislation requiring parental or spousal notification, slanted "informed consent" ordinances and all other forms of restricting access to abortion.

2. We oppose all forms of sterilization abuse, including lack of informed consent, abuse of disabled persons, abuse in prisons and mental hospitals, industrial abuse and abuse resulting from the denial of abortion rights and the lack of safe, accessible forms of birth control. We support the HEW (now DHHS) regulations on sterilization abuse.

3. We stand for reproductive freedom, including not only abortion rights and freedom from sterilization abuse but also good, safe birth control, sex education in the schools, the right to conduct one's sex life as one chooses and an end to nuclear, chemical and occupational hazards to our reproductive systems.

4. We support each person's right to determine his/her own personal and sexual relationships regardless of the sex of the people involved. We oppose the breaking up of families by the state in order to punish a parent for his/her sexual or po-

---

*See also *Ourselves and Our Children* by the Boston Women's Health Book Collective, New York: Random House, 1978.

litical beliefs. We support the struggle for legislation guaranteeing civil rights to homosexuals.

5. Reproductive freedom depends on economics: equal wages for women, sufficient to support a family alone; a decent public health system; adequate welfare benefits; good housing; quality child care, and a public school system that meets children's needs.

6. We see our struggle for reproductive freedom as a worldwide one. We do not believe that overpopulation is a primary source of the world's problems. We oppose the racist population control policies of the U.S. government and agencies aimed at Third World peoples that limit their populations through forced sterilization and the distribution of dangerous drugs.

7. We are an activist network seeking to organize and educate women and men in health-care facilities, workplaces, unions, schools and communities in support of these principles.

8. We will work in a variety of ways with other groups to achieve these ends locally, nationally and internationally.

RIGHT TO LIFE

A woman is not a pear tree
thrusting her fruit in mindless fecundity
into the world. Even pear trees bear
heavily in one year and rest and grow the next.
An orchard gone wild drops few warm rotting
fruit in the grass but the trees stretch
high and wiry gifting the birds forty
feet up among inch long thorns
broken atavistically from the smooth wood.
A woman is not a basket you place
your buns in to keep them warm. Not a brood
hen you can slip duck eggs under.
Not the purse holding the coins of your
descendants till you spend them in wars.
Not a bank where your genes gather interest
and interesting mutations in the tainted
rain, any more than you are.

You plant corn and you harvest
it to eat or sell. You put the lamb
in the pasture to fatten and haul it in
to butcher for chops. You slice
the mountain in two for a road and gouge
the high plains for coal and the waters
run muddy for miles and years.

Fish die but you do not call them yours
unless you wished to eat them.

Now you legislate mineral rights in a woman.
You lay claim to her pastures for grazing,
fields for growing babies like iceberg
lettuce. You value children so dearly
that none ever go hungry, none weep
with no one to tend them when mothers
work, none lack fresh fruit,
none chew lead or cough to death and your
orphanages are empty. Every noon the best
restaurants serve poor children steaks.

At this moment at nine o'clock a partera
is performing a table top abortion on an
unwed mother in Texas who can't get Medicaid
any longer. In five days she will die
of tetanus and her little daughter will cry
and be taken away. Next door a husband
and wife are sticking pins in the son
they did not want. They will explain
for hours how wicked he is,
how he wants discipline.

We are all born of woman, in the rose
of the womb we suckled our mother's blood
and every baby born has a right to love
like a seedling to sun. Every baby born
unloved, unwanted, is a bill that will come
due in twenty years with interest, an anger
that must find a target, a pain that will
beget pain. A decade downstream a child
screams, a woman falls, a synagogue is torched,
a firing squad is summoned, a button
is pushed and the world burns.

I will choose what enters me, what becomes
flesh of my flesh. Without choice, no politics,
no ethics lives. I am not your cornfield,
not your uranium mine, not your calf
for fattening, not your cow for milking.
You may not use me as your factory.
Priests and legislators do not hold
shares in my womb or my mind.
This is my body. If I give it to you
I want it back. My life
is a non-negotiable demand.*

---

*Copyright Marge Piercy, The Moon Is Always Female, New York: Alfred A. Knopf, 1980.

12

Anatomy and Physiology of Sexuality and Reproduction*

BY ESTHER ROME

With special thanks to Nancy Reame.

This chapter in previous editions was written by Abby Schwarz, Esther Rome, Nancy Hawley, Barbara Perkins and Toni Randall.

1992 Update by Esther Rome, with help from Leah Diskin and Nancy Reame.

FINDING OUT ABOUT OURSELVES

In talking with other women about our bodies and learning the biological facts, we arrive at a new respect for the beings we are. We equip ourselves with information of use to us in our daily lives and become active participants in our own health and medical care.

It's important to become as familiar with the appearance of our sexual organs as we are with other parts of our bodies. We have found that with just a mirror we can see how we look on the outside. The women's self-help movement encourages us to look inside at our vaginal walls and cervix (lower part of the uterus). To examine ourselves, we use a mirror, flashlight and a clean plastic speculum, an instrument that we insert into the vagina and gently open up. We can do self-exams alone or with others, once or often. With practice we can see how the cervix and vaginal walls change with the menstrual cycle, with pregnancy or with meno-pause, and learn to recognize various vaginal infections.*

It has taken a while for some of us to get over our inhibitions about seeing or touching our genitals.

When someone first said to me two years ago, "You can feel the end of your own cervix with your finger," I was interested but flustered. I had hardly ever put my finger in my vagina at all and felt squeamish about touching myself there, in that place "reserved" for lovers and doctors. It took me two months to get up my nerve to try it, and then one afternoon, pretty nervously, I squatted down in the bathroom and put my finger in deep, back into my vagina. There it was, feeling slippery and rounded, with an indentation at the center through which, I realized, my menstrual flow came. It was both very exciting and beautifully ordinary at the same time. Last week I bought a plastic speculum so I could look at my cervix. Will it take as long this time?

---

*Anatomy is the physical shape and placement of our organs; physiology is how our organs work.

*This chapter touches on topics discussed throughout the book but not repeated in detail here. Please check the index if you wish to find out more about any of these subjects.

DESCRIPTION OF SEXUAL AND REPRODUCTIVE ORGANS: ANATOMY (STRUCTURE) AND PHYSIOLOGY (FUNCTION)

Pelvic Organs

The following description will be much clearer if you look at yourself with a mirror while you read the text and look at the diagrams. It is written as if you were squatting and looking into a hand mirror. If you are uncomfortable in that position, sit as far forward on the edge of a chair as you comfortably can. Make sure you have plenty of light and enough time and privacy to feel relaxed. You may want to see more with a speculum.

First, you will see your *vulva,* or outer genitals. This includes all the sexual and reproductive organs you can see in your crotch. Too often we confuse the vagina, only one part, with the whole area. The most obvious feature on an adult woman is the *pubic hair,* the first wisps of which are one of the early signs of puberty. After menopause, the hair thins out. It grows from the soft fatty tissue called the *mons* (also *mons veneris,* mountain of Venus, or *mons pubis*).* The mons area lies over the *pubic symphysis.* This is the joint of the pubic bones, which are part of the *pelvic bones,* or hip girdle. You cannot feel the actual joint, though you can feel the bones under the soft outer skin.

As you spread your legs apart, you can see in the mirror that the hair continues between your legs and probably on around your *anus.* The anus is the opening of the rectum, or large intestine, to the outside. You can feel that the hair-covered area between your legs is also fatty, like the mons. This fatty area forms flaps, called the *outer lips (labia majora),* which are more or less pronounced for different women. For some, the skin of the outer lips is darker. The outer lips surround some soft flaps of skin that are hairless. These are the *inner lips (labia minora).* They are sensitive to touch. With sexual stimulation they swell and turn darker if the skin is light colored. The area between the inner lips and the anus is the *perineum.*

---

*The formal medical term is included in parentheses if it is different from the English term. We are not including slang terms in the text. They often represent a male view of a woman's body and have been used to put women down. We can make up new words of our own, find old words with a gentler sound, like *yoni,* or use the common words, like *pussy* or *cunt,* in a more positive and loving way.

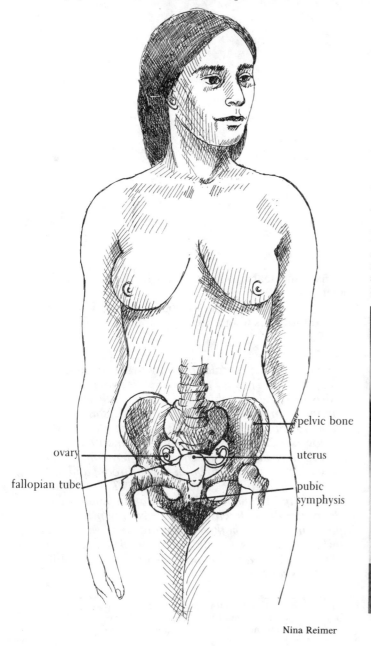

ovary
fallopian tube
pelvic bone
uterus
pubic symphysis

Nina Reimer

Ann Popkin

242

As you gently spread the inner lips apart, you can see that they protect a delicate area between them. This is the *vestibule*. Look more closely at it. Starting from the front, right below the mons area you will see the inner lips joining to form a soft fold of skin, or *hood*, over and connecting to the *glans*, or tip of the *clitoris* (*klit-or-iss*).* Gently pull the hood up to see the glans. This is the most sensitive spot in the entire genital area. It is made up of erectile tissue that swells during sexual arousal. Let the hood slide back over the glans. Extending from the hood up to the pubic symphysis, you can now feel a hardish, rubbery, movable cord right under the skin. It is sometimes sexually arousing if touched. This is the *shaft* of the clitoris. It is connected to the bone by a *suspensory ligament*. You cannot feel this ligament or the next few organs described, but they are all important in sexual arousal and orgasm. At this point where you no longer feel the shaft of the clitoris it divides into two parts, spreading out wishbone fashion but at a much wider angle, to form the *crura* (singular: *crus*), the two anchoring wingtips of erectile tissue that attach to the pelvic bones. The crura of the clitoris are about three inches long. Starting from where the shaft and crura meet, and continuing down along the sides of the vestibule, are two bundles of erectile tissue called the *bulbs of the vestibule*. These, along with

the whole clitoris and an extensive system of connecting veins and muscles throughout the pelvis, become firm and filled with blood (pelvic congestion) during sexual arousal. Some pelvic congestion, giving a feeling of fullness or heaviness in the pelvic region, can occur during the menstrual cycle right before your period comes. Both the crura of the clitoris and the bulbs of the vestibule are wrapped in muscle tissue. This muscle helps to create tension and fullness during arousal and contracts during orgasm, playing an important role in the involuntary spasms felt at that time. The whole clitoris and vestibular bulbs are the only organs in the body solely for sexual sensation and arousal.

Vestibular or Bartholin's glands are two small rounded bodies on either side of the vaginal opening and to the rear of the vestibular bulbs. They sometimes get infected and swell. You can feel them then. Once these glands were thought to provide vaginal lubrication for intercourse, though it is now known that they produce only a few drops of fluid.

Let's return to what you can see with the mirror. Keeping the inner lips spread and pulling the hood back again, you will notice that the inner lips attach to the underside of the clitoris. Right below this attachment you will see a small dot or slit. This is the *urinary opening*, the outer opening of the *urethra*, a short (about an inch and a half), thin tube leading to your *bladder*. Below that is a larger opening, the *vaginal opening* (*introitus*). Because the urinary opening is so close to the vaginal opening, it can become irritated from prolonged or vigorous sexual activity and may lead to some

---

*The glans of the clitoris is commonly referred to as "the clitoris." We will follow that convention, but please remember that the clitoris referred to here as "the whole clitoris" is really a much more extensive organ, consisting of the glans, shaft and crura, all described in the text.

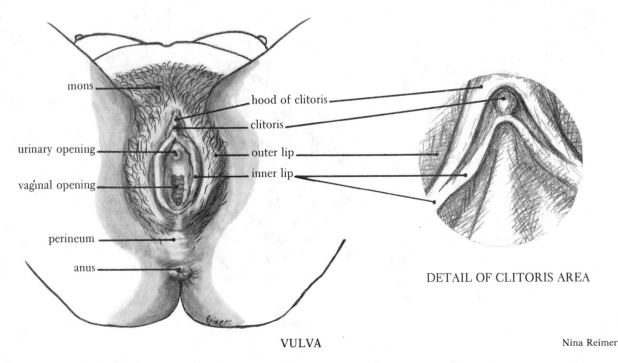

mons

hood of clitoris

clitoris

urinary opening

outer lip

inner lip

vaginal opening

perineum

anus

VULVA

DETAIL OF CLITORIS AREA

Nina Reimer

discomfort while urinating. Around the vaginal opening you may be able to see the *hymen*. When you were born, it was a thin membrane surrounding the vaginal opening, partially blocking it but almost never covering the opening completely. Hymens come in widely varying sizes and shapes. For most women the hymen stretches easily. Even after being stretched, little folds of hymen tissue remain.

SOME HYMEN VARIATIONS   Nina Reimer

Now insert a finger or two into your *vagina*. Notice how the vaginal walls, which were touching each other, now spread around your fingers and hug them. Feel the soft folds of skin. These folds allow the vagina to mold itself around what might be inside it: fingers, a tampon, a penis or a baby. Notice that your finger slides around inside the vagina as you move it. The walls of the vagina may be almost dry to very wet. Dryer times usually occur before puberty, often during lactation and after menopause, as well as during that part of the cycle right after the flow. Wetter times are around ovulation, during pregnancy and when sexually aroused. These continuous secretions provide lubrication, help keep the vagina clean and maintain the acidity of the vagina to prevent infections. Push gently all around against the walls of the vagina and notice where you feel particularly sensitive. For some women it is only the outer third; in others it is most or all of the vagina. Now put your finger halfway in and try to grip your finger with your vagina. It might help if you imagine you are stopping the flow of urine. You are contracting the *pelvic floor muscles*. These muscles hold the pelvic organs in place and provide support for your other organs all the way up to your diaphragm, which is stretched across the bottom of your rib cage. If these muscles are weak, you may have trouble having an orgasm, controlling your urine flow (urinary incontinence) or have prolapse of your pelvic organs. See p. 406 for ways to strengthen these muscles.

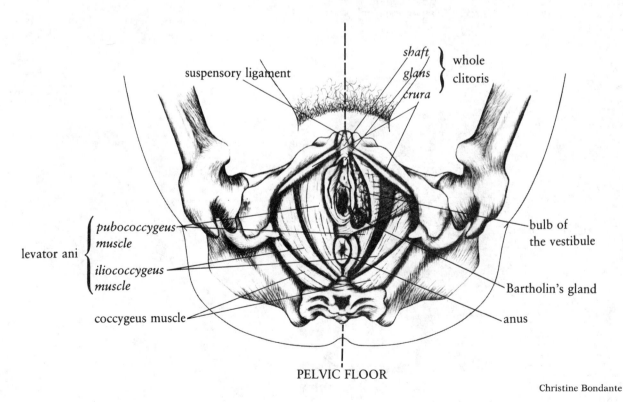

PELVIC FLOOR

Christine Bondante

There is only a thin wall of skin separating the vagina from the rectum, so you may be able to feel a bump on one side of your vagina if you have some stool in the rectum, a small hemorrhoid or perhaps a prolapsed organ pushing on your vagina.

Now slide your middle finger as far back into your vagina as you can. Notice that your finger goes in toward the small of your back at an angle, not straight up the middle of your body. If you were standing instead of squatting, your vagina would be at about a forty-five-degree angle to the floor. With your finger you may be able to just feel the end of your vagina. This part of the vagina is called the *fornix.* (If you are having trouble reaching it, bring your knees and chest closer together so your finger can slide in farther. However, some women still may not be able to do this.) A little before the end of the vagina you can feel your *cervix.* The cervix feels like a nose with a small dimple in its center. (If you've had a baby, the cervix may feel more like a chin.) The cervix is the base of the *uterus,* or womb. It is sensitive to pressure but has no nerve endings on its surface. The uterus changes position, color and shape during the menstrual cycle and during sexual excitement as well as during puberty and menopause, so the place where you feel the cervix one day may be slightly different from where you feel it the next. Some days you can barely reach it. The dimple you felt is the *os,* or opening into the uterus. The entrance into the uterus through the cervix is very

small, about the diameter of a very thin straw, and closed with mucus, which controls the entry of sperm. No tampon, finger or penis can go up through it, although it is capable of expanding enormously for a baby during labor and delivery. Most of us can see our cervixes easily during self-examination and can watch for changes if we examine ourselves fairly regularly.*

You probably will not be able to feel the rest of the organs except during orgasm. The nonpregnant uterus is about the size of a fist. Its thick walls have some of the most powerful muscles in the body. It is located behind the bladder, which is beneath the abdominal wall, and the rectum, which is near the backbone. The walls of the uterus touch each other unless pushed apart by a growing fetus or an abnormal growth. The top of the uterus is called the *fundus.*

Extending outward and back from the sides of the upper end of the uterus are the two *fallopian tubes* (or *oviducts;* literally, "egg tubes"). They are approximately four inches long and look like ram's horns facing backward. Inside are microscopic hairs (*cilia*) that propel the egg toward the uterus and the sperm toward the egg. The connecting opening from the inside of the uterus to the fallopian tube is as small as a fine needle. The

---

*See Suzanne Gage's photos of cervical changes during the cycle in *A New View of a Woman's Body,* by the Federation of Feminist Women's Health Centers, New York: Simon & Schuster, 1981.

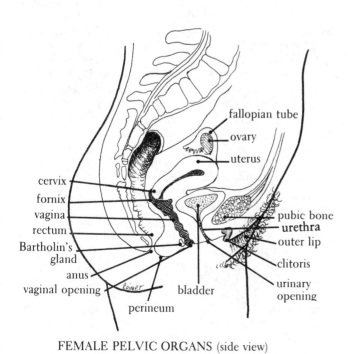

FEMALE PELVIC ORGANS (side view)

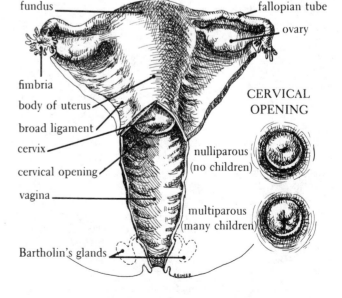

FEMALE PELVIC ORGANS

Nina Reimer

other end of the tube is fringed (fimbriated) and funnel shaped. The wide end of the funnel wraps partway around the *ovary* but does not actually attach to it. It is held in place by connecting tissues.

The ovaries are organs about the size and shape of unshelled almonds, located on either side and somewhat below the uterus. They are about four or five inches below your waist. They are held in place by connective tissue and are protected by a surrounding mass of fat. They have a twofold function: to produce germ cells (eggs) and to produce female sex hormones (estrogen, progesterone and many other hormones, only some of whose functions we understand). The small gap between the ovary and the end of the corresponding tube allows the egg to float freely after it is released from the ovary. The fingerlike ends (*fimbria*) of the fallopian tube sweep across the surface of the ovary and set up currents that wave the egg into the tube. In rare cases when the egg is not "caught" by the tube, it can be fertilized outside the tube, resulting in an abdominal pregnancy.

Parallels in Female and Male Pelvic Organs

All female and male organs, including sexual and reproductive organs, are similar in origin, homologous (developed from the same embryonic tissue) and analogous (similar in function). Female and male fetuses appear identical during the first six weeks in the uterus. The following are examples of corresponding organs:

Female	Male
Outer lips	Scrotum
Inner lips	Bottom side of penis
Glans of clitoris	Glans of penis
Shaft of clitoris	Corpus cavernosum
Ovaries	Testes
Bulb of vestibule	Bulb of penis and corpus spongiosum
Bartholin's glands	Cowper's glands (bulbourethral glands)

Breasts

When we look at our breasts in the mirror we will most likely notice that they are not the same size and shape.* Often the right one is smaller than the left. If we observe our breast shape over time we will also notice that they usually become droopier over the ___ as our skin becomes less elastic. This hap___s e___ fa___ter menopause. For some of ___ th___re are p___no___d changes during the mens___ual cycle, with the most fulln___s right

---

* For stories of how women feel about their breasts and many pictures of breasts, see *Breasts: Women Speak About Their Breasts and Their Lives* by Daphne Ayalah and Isaac Weinstock, New York: Summit Books, 1979.

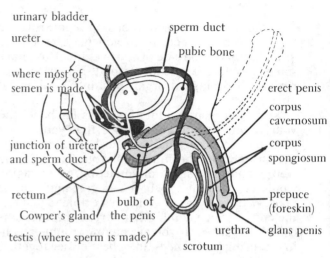

MALE PELVIC ORGANS (side view)
Nina Reimer

before our periods. Also, during pregnancy and nursing our breasts can enlarge considerably. Examining our breasts regularly can help us learn our usual patterns as well as detect anything out of the ordinary.

In the middle of the breast we notice a circle of darker skin. The color can be light pink to almost black. During pregnancy it may become larger and, in light-skinned women, darker. Sometimes the changes are permanent. This darker skin is made up of the *areola* and *nipple*. The areola may have small bumps on it. These are *sebaceous* or *oil glands*, which secrete lubricant that protects the nipple during nursing. Hairs often grow around our areolas and may increase over time or with the use of the birth control pill. Our nipples may stick out, lie flat or be inverted (go inward). Each may be different and all are normal. The nerves come into the nipple near the bottom of the areola. The only muscles in our breasts are directly under the nipple and areola. In response to cold or touch or sexual arousal, the areola may pucker and the nipples become more erect.

The inside of the breast consists of *fat, connective tissue* and a *milk-producing (mammary) gland*. The gland is made up of *milk-producing areas* and *ducts*, which during lactation carry the milk from these areas to the nipple. During the reproductive years, even when we are not nursing, these glands periodically produce small amounts of fluid that flow from the nipples.

With the great increase of sex hormones during adolescence, the glandular tissue in the breasts starts to develop and increase in size to about the amount of a spoonful. All women have approximately the same amount of glandular tissue at the same points in their reproductive life cycles. Most of the breast consists of fat over and between sections of the gland and connective tissue. The

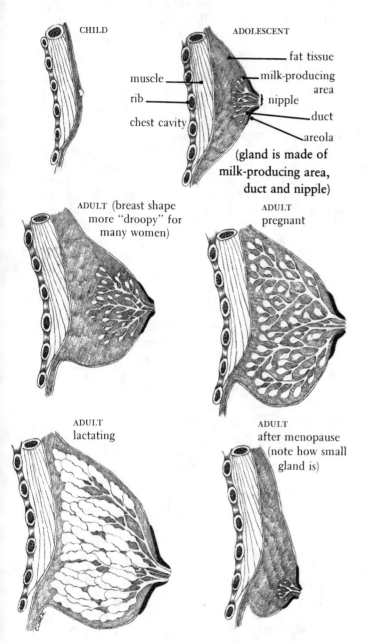

CHILD

ADOLESCENT

fat tissue

muscle

milk-producing area

rib

nipple

chest cavity

duct

areola

(gland is made of milk-producing area, duct and nipple)

ADULT (breast shape more "droopy" for many women)

ADULT pregnant

ADULT lactating

ADULT after menopause (note how small gland is)

Breast changes over a lifetime.　　　　Peggy Clark

amount of fat collected in the breasts is partly determined by heredity. This fat makes breast size vary and explains why breast size is not related to the sexual responsiveness of the breast area or to the amount of milk produced after giving birth. Because sex hormone levels change during the menstrual cycle, when starting and stopping birth control pills, during pregnancy, during lactation and after menopause, there can be variations in a particular woman's breast size and shape.

STAGES IN THE REPRODUCTIVE CYCLE

In childhood our bodies are immature. During puberty we make the transition from childhood to maturity. In women, puberty is characterized by decreased bone growth and by growth of breasts and pubic and armpit (axillary) hair. Ovulation and menstruation (menarche) start near the end of puberty, generally when we are about twelve and a half, though any time from nine to eighteen years is normal. To menstruate, a girl probably needs her body fat to be about one quarter of her total weight. This happens at just over one hundred pounds. In order to sustain menstrual cycles, a woman must maintain a slightly higher weight than when she first menstruated. Others theorize that her pelvis must reach a certain size. Menstruation and ovulation continue until the average age of forty-eight or forty-nine, with a range of between forty and fifty-five as normal. When they stop, menopause has occurred. The transition between the reproductive and postreproductive stages, called *menopause* or the climacteric, often takes place over as many as fifteen years.

This entire reproductive cycle is regulated by hormones, chemical messengers and initiators in the body. The levels of sex hormones are low during childhood, increase tremendously during the reproductive years and then become somewhat lower and in a different balance after menopause. The signs and symptoms of the transitional periods are thought to be caused by the changing levels of hormones.

During the reproductive years there are monthly fluctuations of hormones that determine the timing of ovulation and menstruation. This cycle, the menstrual cycle, regulates our fertility, allowing for the possibility of pregnancy a few days every month.

THE OVARIAN CYCLE: OVULATION

Both ovaries at birth contain about 1,000,000 follicles, which are balls of cells with an immature egg in the center. About 300 to 500 of the 400,000 present at menarche will develop into mature eggs.

Each month during our reproductive years, several (ten to twenty) follicles begin maturing under the influence of hormones (see Appendix). Usually only one develops fully and is able to be fertilized. Our bodies reabsorb the others before complete development. One of the cell layers in the follicle secretes estrogen. The follicle, with the maturing egg inside, moves toward the surface of the ovary. During ovulation the follicle and the ovarian surface opens over the egg, allowing it to float out. Around ovulation some women feel a twinge or cramp in the lower abdomen or back, sometimes with vaginal discharge, perhaps bloody. The symptoms can be severe enough to be confused with appendicitis or ectopic pregnancy. This is *Mittelschmerz* ("middle pain"). A few women have headaches, gastric pains or sluggishness. Other women feel better around ovulation. Cervical mucus changes at this time, too.

Just before ovulation the same cell layer in the follicle starts secreting progesterone as well as estrogen. After ovulation the follicle is now called a *corpus luteum* ("yellow body," referring to the yellow fat in it). If the cycle is interrupted by pregnancy, the hormones produced by the corpus luteum help to maintain the pregnancy. If no pregnancy occurs, the follicle is reabsorbed. After sev-

eral months only a whitish scar remains near the surface of the ovary. It is then called the *corpus albicans* ("white body") and eventually disappears entirely.

After ovulation the released egg is swept into the funnel-shaped end of one of the fallopian tubes (oviducts) and begins its several-day journey to the uterus, moved along by wavelike (peristaltic) contractions of the tube. Fertilization, the union of an egg from a woman and sperm from a man, takes place in the outer third of the fallopian tube (nearest the ovaries). This is also called conception and usually occurs within one day of ovulation. There is a growing number of women in whom the fertilized egg implants itself in the fallopian tube while en route to the uterus because the tube

The endometrium at four stages of menstrual cycle: the end of menstruation, ovulation, about five days after ovulation and menstruation.

Nina Reimer

248

has been scarred or unusually twisted by infection resulting from an IUD, endometriosis or pelvic inflammatory disease, although these are not the only causes of a tubal pregnancy. The midpoint of the tube is the most likely site, probably because the egg stops briefly there on its way. Tubal pregnancy requires surgery before the tube ruptures but may not require tube removal.

If the egg is not fertilized, it disintegrates or flows out with the vaginal secretions, usually before menstruation. You won't notice it.

THE UTERINE CYCLE

Cervical Changes

The kind of mucus produced by your cervix changes through the cycle in response to hormones. Although there are general patterns, you can follow your own cycle to find out what yours is by feeling the entrance to the vagina with your finger, looking at the secretions, being aware of sensations of vaginal wetness or dryness and recording these characteristics every day for several cycles. You may also wish to taste your secretions. They can be sour, salty or sweet, changing during the cycle in a pattern typical for you. If you looked at it under a microscope, the mucus would usually look like a maze of tangled fibers. It is extremely difficult for sperm and many other organisms to get through it. At ovulation, under the influence of estrogen, it changes to form longer strands, more or less aligned, which can guide the sperm into the uterus. The mucus is a kind of gatekeeper for the uterus. At this time it is profuse enough to coat the vagina and protect the sperm from the acid secretions produced there. After ovulation, as estrogen drops and progesterone rises with the approach of menstruation, your vagina gradually becomes drier. Menopausal women may find that following the changes in their cervical mucus is a simple way of monitoring their estrogen levels.

If you look at your cervix with a speculum, you may or may not be able to see the mucus change. You will probably notice that around ovulation the cervix is pulled up high into the vagina. It may also enlarge and soften and the os may open a little.

Endometrial Changes and Menstruation

Estrogen, made by the maturing follicle, causes the uterine lining (*endometrium*) to grow, thicken, form glands and increase the uterine blood supply (proliferative phase). This part of the cycle can vary greatly in length. Progesterone, made by the ruptured follicle after the egg is released, causes the glands in the endometrium to begin secreting embryo-nourishing substances (secretory phase). A fertilized egg can implant only in a secretory lining, not in a proliferative one. It takes the fertilized egg approximately five to six days to reach the uterus.

If conception has not occurred, the remaining follicle, or corpus luteum, will produce estrogen and progesterone for about twelve days, with the amount lessening in the last few days. As the estrogen and progesterone levels drop, the tiny arteries and veins in the uterus close off. The lining is no longer nourished and is shed. This is menstruation, the menstrual period or flow. During menstruation, most of the lining is shed; the bottom third remains to form a new lining. Then a new follicle starts growing and secreting estrogen, a new uterine lining grows and the cycle begins again.*

Any cycle that is more or less regular is normal. The length of the cycle usually ranges from twenty to thirty-six days, the average being twenty-eight days. (Menstruation is from the Latin *mensis*, for "month.") Some women have alternating long and short cycles. There are spontaneous small changes, and there can be major ones when a woman is under a great deal of stress. As you get older or if you have a baby, you may notice marked changes. An average period lasts two to eight days, with four to six days being the average. The flow stops and starts, though this may not always be evident. A usual discharge for a menstrual period is about four to six tablespoons, or two to three ounces.

The Menstrual Fluid

The menstrual fluid contains cervical mucus, vaginal secretions, mucus and cells and endometrial particles as well as blood (sometimes clotted), but this mixed content is not obvious since the blood stains everything red or brown. This regular loss of blood, even though small, can cause anemia. The fluid usually does not smell until it makes contact with the bacteria in the air and starts to decompose. Toward the end of the flow, some of the discharge may have an unpleasant odor.

Women in different cultures have handled their menstrual flow in many ways. Sometimes they don't use anything. Since earliest times, women have made tampons and pads from available materials, often washing and reusing special cloths or rags. Today, some women make them from gauze or cotton balls. Most women use commer-

---

*It is possible to menstruate without ovulating (anovulatory period) even after cycles have been established. In young women, anovulatory cycles average once a year, increasing to eight to ten a year as menopause approaches.

cial sanitary napkins and tampons. Directions come with the products. (Toxic shock syndrome, TSS, has been linked to the use of tampons and rarely to sponges and diaphragms.) Do not use tampons between your periods or ones that are more absorbent than you need during your period. Check the absorbency rating on the tampon boxes to help you select the lowest absorbency you need. A tampon is too absorbent if it is hard to pull out or shreds when you remove it or if your vagina becomes dry. Tampons can cause sores you probably are not able to notice on the vaginal walls when used under those circumstances. Some women experience vaginal irritation, itching, soreness, unusual odor or bleeding while using tampons. If you do, stop using them, use a lower absorbency or change brands to see if that helps. There is no premarket safety testing of tampons. Most research is done by the manufacturers who keep it secret. Although the law requires the U.S. Food and Drug Administration (FDA) to set uniform standards for the safety and performance of medium-risk medical devices including tampons, the agency has no plans to do so.*

Some women have rediscovered natural sponges (not cellulose), which are reusable and economical. Because the FDA does not approve sponges for this use, it will not allow them to be labeled as such.† A sponge is soft and comfortable and when damp takes the shape of your vagina, eliminating the dryness and irritation so common with commercial tampons. Unfortunately, because sponges grow in the oceans where so many pollutants are dumped, we don't know what the sponge has been exposed to, how much pollutant it has absorbed or whether residual pollutants may cause us problems. Almost no testing has been done.‡

Dampen the sponge before insertion. When you think the sponge is full, pull it out with your finger. Wash it well in cool water. Before reinserting, squeeze it to remove excess water. Some women tie a string onto the sponge, but as with tampons, the string may act as a wick for bacteria from outside the vagina. To make things simpler in public restrooms, carry an extra sponge in a plastic bag. If the sponge develops an odor, rinse it in a mild solution of vinegar and water. The sponge

In 1988, the Women's Environmental Network in London, England, launched a successful campaign to stop the processing of some paper products with chlorine. They targeted tampons, sanitary napkins and disposable diapers. Chlorine bleaches products whiter than do other bleaches. Thus manufacturers prefer it, thinking that the whiteness conveys an appearance of cleanliness even though the product functions no differently. But during the bleaching process the chlorine combines with other organic compounds to create about a thousand chlorinated organic compounds, one of which is the highly carcinogenic dioxin. While the paper products retain trace amounts of the dioxin, most of it is discharged with the waste water. When the paper products are disposed of in a landfill or an incinerator, the trace amounts are not destroyed and can become concentrated or dispersed. Once loose in the environment, the chlorinated organics travel to all continents.

In North America, the Women and Environments Education and Development Foundation (WEED) has started a campaign similar to the one in England. You can find out current details, including where to buy non–chlorine bleached products, from the foundation at 736 Bathurst Street, Toronto, Ontario M5S 2R4; (416) 516-2600; fax: (416) 531-6214.

does not have to be made sterile. (Tampons and napkins are not sterile.) However, if you have an infection, do not reuse your sponge. Discard the sponge when it begins to fall apart.

Other women are using a rubber menstrual cap, The Keeper, similar in appearance to a cervical cap, but worn near the vaginal opening in the same place as a tampon.* Some women use a diaphragm or cervical cap. All of these hold more than a sponge or tampon. You will learn from experience when yours is full. Then remove, wash and reinsert. A method developed and used by women in advanced self-help groups is menstrual extraction (see p. 358).†

Those of us who have limited sensation in the lower part of our bodies or are confined to wheel-

---

*Report any tampon-related problems you have to the U.S. FDA (see p. 676).
†Although the U.S. FDA was acting according to its rules and regulations, it concentrated on menstrual sponge distributors, all very small businesses, because of the political pressure on it to take some kind of action while the issue of TSS was prominent in the media.
‡Different researchers, using only a few sponge samples each, have gotten contradictory results. Try to get Caribbean or Florida sponges, since these grow in *generally* less polluted waters than Mediterranean sponges.

---

*For more information on The Keeper menstrual cap, write to The Keeper, Box 20023, Cincinnati, OH 45220.
†See *A New View of a Woman's Body* by the Federation of Feminist Women's Health Centers.

Sanitary product companies are always introducing "new, improved" products. Avoid *deodorized* or *scented* tampons, napkins and feminine deodorant sprays. Many women have allergic reactions to the chemicals in them. If any of them cause problems, stop using them immediately.

chairs often find all of these methods either irritating or difficult to use. There is no satisfactory solution to this yet.

Attitudes About Menstruation

Cultural, religious and personal attitudes about menstruation are a part of our menstrual experience and often reflect negative attitudes toward women. Consider for a moment the ways you have been influenced by attitudes and customs about menstruation. How did you first hear about it? How else have you found out about it: family, friends, advertising, lovers, books, films, teachers, nurses, doctors, taboos, slang, names, jokes? What particular experiences stand out in your mind? How did they make you feel? Are your current experiences different? How is menstruation a part of your life now?

Certain cultures have isolated women entirely or put them only in the company of other women, during their periods, because people thought menstrual blood was unclean and gave menstruating women supernatural powers, sometimes good but more often destructive. Women themselves may have started these practices to give themselves a

LEARNING MORE ABOUT YOUR CYCLE

A good way to start learning more about your own cycle and what is usual and normal for you is to keep a simple chart. Note the start of your flow on a calendar. Add whatever else you are interested in or make a separate chart or journal. Some things you might consider looking at more carefully are color, texture, taste, clots, cervical changes, breast changes, fluctuations in your general physical, emotional or sexual state. You may find no pattern where you thought there was one, or you may find that some changes occur at particular times in your cycle.

time for meditation or to give older women a chance to pass on special women's secrets to younger ones.

Our taboos include refraining from exercise, showers and sexual intercourse or hiding the fact of menstruation entirely. Notice the wording in ads for menstrual products to see how this is reinforced in our country.

In the belief that the whole menstrual cycle makes women unstable or less capable, some people deny jobs to women and treat us as inferior. Both women and men experience mood swings, but for women the changes are seen as a sign of inherent instability. This negative attitude leads us to deny admitting the changes for fear of being discounted. The idea that women lose a lot of time from work is largely unsupported. One study of nurses shows that they lost very little time because of menstrual problems.[1] Most women do not have any measurable difference in their thinking capacity throughout their cycles[2] or in their ability to perform tasks.[3] We still work where we are "needed"—at home, in factories, in offices—with no concessions in schedules or routines to take account of individual differences in our cycles. Men, however, who are much more prone to seriously incapacitating and unpredictable diseases, such as heart problems, continue in highly responsible positions (the presidency of the country, for example).

Feelings About Menstruation

Many of us were scared or even embarrassed when we first started to menstruate. We grew up with little or no knowledge about where the blood and tissue were coming from and why it came and why it sometimes hurt. Some of us thought we were dying when we first saw our menstrual blood. Some of us were desperately afraid that a teacher or boy would notice when we had our period. On the other hand, some of us felt inadequate if we didn't menstruate.

I used to worry about having my period. It seemed that all my friends had gotten it already or were just having it. I felt left out. I began to think of it as a symbol: When I got my period, I would become a woman.

Beginning and ending menstruation will always be different for each person—welcome to some, not to others. We do know that as we feel better about our bodies and learn more about ourselves, our experiences of our cycles can change. During times when we feel especially good about ourselves, we may experience our periods as self-affirming, creative and pleasurable. Or we may have contradictory feelings at the same time.

I really love getting my period. It's like the changing seasons. I feel a bond with other women. I feel fertile and womanly and empowered because of my potential to make a life. I even like the little aches I get because it's a reminder of having my period.

Some of us will pay less attention to menstruation and others will explore it further through art, songs, writings and new rituals. We want to be sure to tell both our daughters and sons about the many changes of the life cycle so that they can be comfortable and open about them in a way that we were not.

Menstrual Problems

Menstruation is a normal, healthy occurrence for many years of a woman's life. Yet many women, in very different cultures, experience menstrual problems that range from mild discomfort to acute pain. For those of us who have these problems either occasionally or regularly, it is important to recognize that they exist and to deal with them—arranging schedules so we can get more rest if we need it at that time, planning critical meetings for a time when we are not premenstrual, and so on.

Menstrual problems may well not be inevitable. We simply do not know enough about the interactions of our physical and emotional health and of our external environment (physical and social) and our internal environment (including cyclically changing body chemicals and heredity) to know why some have problems and others don't. We also don't know enough to understand why certain remedies work for some and not for others.

Standard medical views have not been helpful for women. How doctors categorize a woman's health problem often determines what medical treatment she receives and whether the doctor treats her respectfully. In the past, doctors have attributed cramps and other problems to a variety of physical and psychological causes. Medical remedies sometimes still include general painkillers (when other medication works better), hormones (sometimes in the form of birth control pills), tranquilizers, a "pat on the head," a hysterectomy or a recommendation to see a psychiatrist. Many doctors claim that a woman's cycle is complicated and mysterious and do not respect our self-knowledge. Researchers are finally working to understand some of the reasons for menstrual problems, but there is still much more to learn.

Premenstrual Syndrome (PMS)

Premenstrual syndrome (PMS) is the development of a wide range of symptoms for several days before and sometimes during the first day of most

or all of your periods. The symptoms then generally go away until at least ovulation. Researchers have not all agreed on a definition of PMS. Some researchers include only symptoms that completely disappear postmenstrually, whereas others include a severe premenstrual intensification of symptoms that exist all month.

All efforts to find a biological basis for PMS so far have failed. Nor have any of the medical treatments, such as progesterone, high-dose vitamins or minerals, oil of evening primrose or antidepressants, worked better than a placebo in well-controlled trials. Hormone suppressants have not had careful clinical trials. Many of these drugs are expensive and have serious side effects when taken in large doses over long periods of time. Self-help remedies can work. Some women find that making changes in their diets or increasing exercise makes a significant difference.* The placebo response rate is so high for PMS that uncontrolled trials make all remedies seem effective.

The number and severity of the symptoms alone do not distinguish those who report having PMS from those who don't report it. A recent investigation into the psychological characteristics of women with PMS, however, shows some interesting distinctions between the two groups. The women with PMS had lower self-esteem, were more likely to blame themselves for negative events, felt guiltier over being angry, avoided stressful events, were more likely to wish problems would go away rather than attempt to solve them, kept their feelings to themselves and felt more stress. This sounds pretty close to the prescription for being a good female. So the issue appears more to be not whether some women have different kinds of cyclical changes, but how our upbringing structures our response to the changes. This hypothesis fits nicely with reports of women who say they feel more energetic and creative premenstrually. One of the researchers concludes that by helping a woman increase her self-esteem, to learn more flexible and direct problem solving and to feel more comfortable with her anger, she may experience her premenstrual symptoms very differently. Thus the cure for PMS may lie in resocialization, not medicine.

Depression

Those of us who get depressed premenstrually find, when we think about it, that we are concerned with problems that have usually been there all the time. We just can't ignore them as well

*For more specifics on self-help remedies see *Self-Help for Premenstrual Syndrome* by Michelle Harrison, New York: Random House, 1985 and *Premenstrual Syndrome Self-Help Book: A Woman's Guide to Feeling Good All Month* by Susan Lark, Berkeley, CA: Celestial Arts Publishing, 1989.

during our premenstrual period. It is important to remember the problems that bother you, even if it means writing them down, so that when you are feeling better you don't forget to try to work toward solving them.

A week before my period comes I go through a few days of feeling more helpless, stuck or down about things in my life that have been there all along. Sometimes I appreciate being more in touch with the underside of my feelings. Other times it really gets to me. The voices inside my head which are overly critical of what I do get much more insistent when I'm premenstrual. Recently I've identified them more quickly. I'll start to get down on myself for not being a good enough mother, friend, worker, daughter and so forth, and I'll say, "Those are your critical voices—go easy on yourself!" It helps.

You might plan to get support for yourself for the times when you feel worst. Ask close friends to drop by, involve the rest of the family more in running the household or get a baby-sitter for the kids. You might start a self-help group by advertising in the paper. If fatigue is a problem, try to schedule time for extra sleeping or for energizing exercise.

Dysmenorrhea

You can do something about dysmenorrhea, the sometimes incapacitating cramping during your period. A particular constellation of symptoms, including cramping and often nausea and diarrhea, may be caused by an excess of a certain type of prostaglandin found in the uterus and perhaps "leaking" into the intestines. (Prostaglandins are substances found throughout the body, one of which causes contractions of the uterine and intestinal muscles.) With too much prostaglandin, the usually painless rhythmic contractions of the uterus during menstruation become longer and tighter at the tightening phase, keeping oxygen from the muscles. It is this lack of oxygen that we perceive as pain. But we don't know why some women have more prostaglandin in their uterus than others. Because the uterus is a muscle, relaxation exercises help, as does massage and sometimes biofeedback techniques. Anticipation often worsens the pain by making us tense up. Antiprostaglandins, a class of drugs developed for arthritis, constitute a medical solution that helps some women. In severe cases, you must take the drug before cramping begins; still, it may only lessen the pain. Some women find some of these drugs easier to tolerate than others. The most frequent complaint is upset stomach, which is often avoided by taking the drug with milk or other food. A few women have found that one drug ceases to be effective and that they must try an-

other.[4] Antiprostaglandins also reduce the amount of flow and shorten the period. We don't yet know how safe these drugs are for long-term, intermittent use, although they seem *relatively* safe so far.*

Endometriosis and pelvic inflammatory disease also cause menstrual problems, especially cramping. Today, as doctors are beginning to find some physical basis for menstrual distresses, they are prescribing drugs that treat the particular problems. We must understand that the doctors, diagnosing on the basis of symptoms, are *only treating symptoms* and do not know the underlying causes. Although various drugs, especially antiprostaglandins, show great promise, we are cautious because we don't want their use to turn out to be another DES or thalidomide story. We don't yet know the risks of taking these drugs over a lifetime. It is best to start with the least invasive treatments, often home remedies. Acupuncture has also helped women with all types of menstrual problems.

Home Remedies for All Menstrual Problems

Women have been sharing menstrual remedies for centuries. Some of us have gained new respect for our own knowledge after trying traditional remedies and exploring new ones. Listed here are only those most frequently reported to work. Try one or more of the following suggestions, and because *each woman is unique and has different reactions, pay attention to how the remedy you choose affects you.*

Food

Make sure the food you eat is varied, sufficient and balanced. You can be malnourished and not be underweight. Pay attention to the positive and negative effects of what you eat. Many women find it helps to eat *more* whole grains and whole flours, beans, vegetables, fruits and brewer's yeast and *less* or *no* salt, sugar, alcohol and caffeine (in coffee, tea, chocolate and soft drinks). Some of us avoid salt, white flour and caffeine for at least the week before our periods and find that it helps (see Chapter 2, "Food"). Also, you may need to eat small, frequent meals or snacks rather than two or three bigger meals.

Sleep

Get the right amount for *you.* Your rhythms may change during your cycle. Allow time for extra sleep if you need it.

---

*These include ibuprofen (Motrin), mefenamic acid (Ponstel), naproxen (Naprosyn), indomethacin (Indocin). Drug companies are continuing to develop new antiprostaglandins. Naprosyn has been linked to pituitary tumors and swollen lymph nodes. (M. Dowie et al. "The Illusion of Safety," Part I, *Mother Jones*, Vol. 7, No. 5 [June 1982], pp. 42–43.)

Exercise

See Chapter 4, "Women in Motion." Some yoga exercises, especially the cobra position, are particularly helpful. Experiment with different positions to find out what helps you, even if it only works temporarily.

Home Remedies for Specific Menstrual Problems

Cramps and Backache

Herb teas* can help. Raspberry leaf tea is one most consistently recommended. Brew one tablespoon for each cup. Some women take calcium and magnesium supplements in a two-to-one ratio for several days before the flow or all through the cycle. Start with 250 milligrams of calcium and half that of magnesium. (Take the tablets separately. Dolomite, calcium containing magnesium, may be contaminated with lead or arsenic. Taking these supplements for a long time in large doses may cause problems.) Heat on your stomach or lower back may help. Orgasm, with or without a partner, may work, but some research suggests an increased risk of endometriosis. Some women use nonprescription drugs such as aspirin, acetaminophen (e.g., Tylenol), ibuprofen or alcohol. Marijuana can be effective but may cause other menstrual problems. We encourage moderation in the use of all these drugs. All kinds of massage may work. See Menstrual Massage for Two People on p. 255 and look for others specifically for menstrual problems in yoga, Shiatsu, acupressure and polarity therapy books.

Depression, Tension, Moodiness, Bloated Feeling

Many women find vitamin B_6 or pyridoxine a great help. Start with twenty-five to fifty milligrams a day and try up to 100 milligrams a day. Discontinue if you get tingling or other signs of temporary nerve damage. See p. 38 for food sources of B_6. Use with a general B-complex for better absorption. Try to decrease sodium by eating less salt and increase potassium (see Chapter 2, "Food"). Some women use diuretics (plain water, water-reducing teas, foods—consult a book on using herbs—or drugs). Use them with caution; most diuretics except water deplete the body of potassium.

Tiredness or Paleness

Check your iron level for anemia.

Heavy Periods and/or Irregular Bleeding

Try eating foods or take supplements with vitamin C *and* bioflavinoids (also called vitamin P). Most foods with vitamin C also contain bioflavinoids. If this problem starts after stopping the Pill,* try vitamin A. Be cautious when taking more than 10,000 IU of vitamin A a day. If you start to feel nausea, skin irritation, itching, or other changes, discontinue using it; excessive vitamin A is toxic.

Amenorrhea

Another menstrual problem is amenorrhea (absence of menstrual periods). Primary amenorrhea is the condition of never having had a period by the latest age by which menstruation usually starts (eighteen); secondary amenorrhea is the cessation of menstruation after at least one period. Some causes are pregnancy, menopause, breastfeeding, too little body fat, dieting, starvation, heavy athletic training especially during early adolescence, previous use of birth control pills, use of some drugs, a congenital defect of the genital tract, hormone imbalance, cysts or tumors, disease, chromosomal abnormalities, stress or emotional factors. Because it is a frequent symptom of infertility,† medical textbooks and practitioners pay considerably more attention to amenorrhea than to PMS or painful periods, although these are far more common. Doctors once again focus more on a less common but more dramatic problem and pay little attention to the kinds of emotional adjustments we may go through and the kinds of support we need.

As a home remedy to bring on your period or for unusually light periods, you might want to try pennyroyal leaf tea (don't use the oil; it can be toxic). Brew one teapoon per cup. Also, weight loss of 10 to 15 percent below a healthy minimum can stop your periods; a return to *your* minimum weight will correct this. If you've taken the birth control pill, try supplements of B_6, folic acid and vitamin E and decrease the amount of protein you eat. Severe anemia can stop menstruation temporarily. For menopausal symptoms, see Chapter 23, "Women Growing Older."

---

*See also Chapter 13, "Birth Control." Irregular bleeding may come after sterilization and heavy bleeding with IUD use. Psychotropic drugs, either prescribed, such as Valium and Librium, or "street" drugs, can cause menstrual irregularities. Amphetamines and probably over-the-counter diet aids can increase menstrual flow and cramping.

†For a good description of medical treatments, see *Womancare* by Linda Madaras and Jane Patterson, New York: Avon Books, 1984.

---

*See *Hygieia: A Woman's Herbal* by Jeannine Parvati, Monroe, VT: Freestone Publishing, 1979, for more on herbs.

MENSTRUAL MASSAGE FOR TWO PEOPLE

For better balance put both hands on hips or one on a chair

Keep weight on outer leg

inner leg

Rock forward and back

Toes in the air

Direction of push →

Top ridge of pelvis

Esther Rome

Woman with Cramps

A. Lie flat on your stomach, with or without clothes. Place a blanket or pad under you for extra comfort.
B. Have your arms straight out or slightly bent at the elbows. Point your toes inward if possible.
C. Tell the other person what feels good and what doesn't. It should feel good.

Person Giving the Massage

A. Basic movement:
  1. Remove your shoes (or kneel and use the heel of your hand).
  2. Check to see if the woman is comfortable. You might gently shake her feet or legs to help her relax and to establish physical contact.
  3. Stand, placing your outer leg next to the head and *above* the shoulder of the woman on the floor.
  4. Put the *heel* of your inner foot against the edge of the top ridge of her pelvis, on the same side where you are standing (see diagram).

  5. "Hook" your heel as much under the bone as you can. If you are not sure where the pelvic ridge is, feel for it first with your fingers. It may be higher up on her back than you think.
  6. Keep both of your legs slightly bent.
  7. Gently push away from you, toward her feet, at regular intervals of once or twice a second.
    (a) When doing this, rock with your whole body by bending *only* at the *knee* and *ankle* of the leg you are standing on.
    (b) Move forward and back. Avoid a circular motion.
    (c) When you are pushing firmly enough the whole body of the woman getting the massage will rock, too.
    (d) Try not to push toward the floor with your inner foot. Keep your toes pointing upward to prevent this.
    (e) Keep your heel in contact with her pelvic bone so the woman getting the massage won't feel bruised.
  8. Increase the frequency and length of the push as long as the woman with the cramps says it is comfortable. You will probably need to work more vigorously than you first imagined.

B. When you feel comfortable with the basic movement:
  1. Move your heel from side to side to different spots along the ridge of her pelvis on the side you are standing next to. Avoid her spine.
  2. Stand on your other leg and repeat A and B-1.
  3. Change sides as often as you want. Continue with the massage until the woman's cramps diminish or go away.

APPENDIX: HORMONES OF THE MENSTRUAL CYCLE SIMPLIFIED

During the reproductive part of a woman's life, baseline levels of all the sex hormones are being continuously produced. In addition to those levels, there are fluctuations that establish the menstrual cycle. The main organs involved in the cycle are the *hypothalamus* (a part of the brain) and the *pituitary* and the *ovaries* (both glands). The hypothalamus signals the pituitary, which then signals the ovaries, which in turn signal the hypothalamus. The signaling is done by hormones secreted by the different organs and carried from one part of the body to another through the blood.

The hypothalamus is sensitive to the fluctuating levels of hormones produced by the ovaries. When the level of estrogens, primarily estradiol-beta-17,

255

drop to low levels, the hypothalamus increases gonadotropin-releasing hormone (GnRH). This stimulates the pituitary to increase follicle-stimulating hormone (FSH). This triggers the growth of ten to twenty of the ovarian follicles. Only one of these will mature fully; the others will start to reabsorb sometime before ovulation. The ones that reabsorb are called *atretic*.

As the follicles grow they secrete estrogens in increasing amounts. The estrogens affect the lining of the uterus, signaling it to grow, or proliferate (proliferatory phase). When the egg approaches maturity inside the follicle that will develop fully, the follicle secretes a burst of progesterone in addition to the estrogens. The estrogens probably trigger the hypothalamus to increase GnRH. This releasing factor signals the pituitary to secrete large amounts of both FSH and luteinizing hormone (LH). The FSH–LH peak

probably signals the follicle to release the egg (ovulation). Under the influence of LH, the follicle changes its function. Now called a *corpus luteum*, the follicle secretes decreasing amounts of estrogens and increasing amounts of progesterone. The progesterone influences the estrogen-primed uterine lining to secrete fluids nourishing to the egg if it is fertilized (secretory or luteal phase). Immediately after the peak that triggers ovulation, FSH returns to a baseline level. LH declines as the progesterone increases. If the egg is fertilized, the corpus luteum continues to secrete estrogens and progesterone to maintain the pregnancy. However, the corpus luteum is stimulated to do this by human chorionic gonadotropin (HCG), a hormone that is secreted by the developing placenta. HCG is almost chemically identical to LH, so it's not surprising it has the same function.

If the egg is not fertilized, the corpus luteum becomes a corpus albicans. In this process it produces lower levels of hormones, paving the way for the release of the uterine lining. At this point menstruation begins. When the level of estrogen reaches a low enough point, the hypothalamus release GnRH and the cycle starts again.

NOTES

1. Jean Garling and Susan Jo Roberts. "An Investigation of Cyclic Distress Among Staff Nurses," in Alice Dan et al., eds., *The Menstrual Cycle*, Vol. 1, New York: Springer Publishing Co., 1980, pp. 305–11.
2. Sharon Golub. "Premenstrual Changes in Mood, Personality and Cognitive Function," in *The Menstrual Cycle*, Vol. 1, pp. 237–46.
3. Effie A. Graham. "Cognition as Related to Menstrual Cycle Phase and Estrogen Level," in *The Menstrual Cycle*, Vol. 1, pp. 190–208.
4. Personal conversation with Penny Budoff, MD, based on her clinical experience.

RESOURCES

Readings

Abraham, Guy E. "Premenstrual Blues." Available from Optimax, P.O. Box 7000-280, Rolling Hills Estates, CA 90274. This 20-page 1982 booklet is a dietary and vitamin-supplement approach to PMS.

Armstrong, Liz, and Adrienne Scott. *Whitewash.* Toronto: HarperCollins, 1992. About the hazards of disposable sanitary products and diapers.

Ayalah, Daphna, and Isaac Weinstock. *Breasts: Women Speak About Their Breasts and Their Lives.* New York: Summit Books, 1979. Photos of breasts and women's feelings about their own.

Bell, Ruth, et al. *Changing Bodies, Changing Lives: A Book for Teens on Sex and Relationships.* New York: Random House, 1987. Excellent.

The menstrual cycle: the relationship between follicle development, hormone cycles, and endometrial (uterine lining) buildup and disintegration. The cervical mucus gets progressively wetter from the menstrual phase to ovulation, then becomes drier during the secretory phase.

Peggy Clark

Blume, Judy. *Are You There, God? It's Me, Margaret*. New York: Dell, 1970. A wonderful adolescent novel with a positive attitude about menstruation.

Buckley, Thomas, and Alma Gottlieb, eds. *Blood Magic: The Anthropology of Menstruation*. Berkeley: University of California Press, 1988. Includes study of women in Borneo who use nothing to absorb blood during menstruation.

Budoff, Penny. *No More Menstrual Cramps and Other Good News*. New York: G. P. Putnam's Sons, 1980. A medical approach to cramps and several other gynecological problems.

Costello, Alison, Bernadette Vallely and Josa Young. *The Sanitary Protection Scandal*. London: Women's Environmental Network, 1989. Available from The Network at 287 City Road, London EC1V 1LA, England. Environmental and health hazards of production, use and disposal of women's sanitary products and disposable diapers.

Dalton, Katharina. *Once a Month*. Pomona, CA: Hunter House, 1979. About PMS and progesterone treatment. Although PMS clinics have recommended this book, Dalton has a dreadful attitude toward women and no interest in changing women's roles.

Dan, Alice, et al. *The Menstrual Cycle*, Vol. 1, *A Synthesis of Interdisciplinary Research*. New York: Springer Publishing Co., 1980. Good research papers covering a variety of topics.

Dan, Alice J., and Linda L. Lewis, eds. *Menstrual Health in Women's Lives*. Urbana/Chicago: University of Illinois Press, 1992.

Delany, Janice, Mary Jane Lupton and Emily Toth. *The Curse: A Cultural History of Menstruation*. Urbana/Chicago: University of Illinois Press, 1988. A wide-ranging exploration of attitudes.

Federation of Feminist Women's Health Centers. *A New View of a Woman's Body*. New York: Simon & Schuster, 1981. Excellent drawings and photos. Text sometimes confusing.

Friedman, Nancy. *Everything You Must Know About Tampons*. New York: Berkley Publishing Corp., 1981. Just what it says.

Frisch, Rose. "Nutrition, Fatness and Fertility: The Effect of Food Intake on Reproductive Ability," in W. Henry Mosley, ed., *Nutrition and Human Reproduction*. New York: Plenum, 1978. A good introduction to Frisch's work. She continues to do research and publish on the trigger mechanisms for menstruation.

Gardner-Loulan, J., B. Lopez and M. Quackenbush. *Period*. Volcano, CA: Volcano Press, 1991. A good book for girls. Shows all kinds of body types.

Golub, Sharon, ed. "Lifting the Curse of Menstruation: A Feminist Appraisal of the Influence of Menstruation on Women's Lives," *Women and Health* (special issue), Vol. 8, Nos. 2 and 3 (Summer/Fall 1983).

———. *Periods: From Menarche to Menopause*. Newbury Park, CA: Sage, 1992. Comprehensive summary of research.

Harrison, Michelle. *Self-Help for Premenstrual Syndrome*. New York: Random House, 1985.

Hubbard, Ruth, et al., eds. *Women Look at Biology Looking at Women: A Collection of Feminist Critiques*. Cambridge, MA: Schenkman, 1979. Selections on menstruation and menopause.

Kolkmeyer, A. V. *The Clear Red Stone: A Myth and the Meaning of Menstruation*. Santa Fe, NM: Insight Press, 1982. For girls who have not yet menstruated or have just started.

Komnenich, Pauline, et al., eds. *The Menstrual Cycle: Volume 2: Research and Implication for Women's Health*. New York: Springer Publishing Co., 1980. Another good group of research papers.

Lander, Louise. *Images of Bleeding*. New York: Orlando Press, 1988.

Lark, Susan. *Premenstrual Syndrome Self-Help Book: A Woman's Guide to Feeling Good All Month*. Berkeley, CA: Celestial Arts, 1989.

Laws, Sophie. *Issues of Blood: The Politics of Menstruation*. New York: Macmillan, 1990.

Laws, Sophie, Valerie Hey and Andrea Eagan. *Seeing Red: The Politics of Pre-Menstrual Tension*. Wolfboro, NH: Longwood Publishing Group, 1985. Excellent political analysis of PMS.

Madaras, Lynda, and Jane Patterson. *Womancare: A Gynecological Guide to Your Body*. New York: Avon Books, 1984. What a readable popular version of a gynecological text would be.

Martin, Emily. *The Woman in the Body*. Boston: Beacon Press, 1987. Excellent. How we conceptualize our body processes based on our social organization.

Paige, Karen. "Women Learn to Sing the Menstrual Blues," *Psychology Today*, Vol. 7, No. 4 (September 1973), pp. 41–46. Investigates cultural context for menstrual problems.

Parlee, Mary Brown. "The Premenstrual Syndrome," *Psychological Bulletin*, Vol. 83, No. 6 (1973), pp. 454–65. One of the earliest and best critiques of Dalton's work. Classic

Parvati, Jeannine. *Hygieia: A Woman's Herbal*. Monroe, VT: Freestone Publishing, 1979. The only herbal specifically for women.

Peterson, Lorna. *PMS: The Premenstrual Syndrome*. Phoenix, AZ: Oryx Press, 1985. Annotated bibliography.

Rome, Esther R. *Premenstrual Syndrome (PMS) Examined Through a Feminist Lens*. 1983. For a copy send a self-addressed, business-size envelope with two stamps to BWHBC, P.O. Box 192, W. Somerville, MA 02144.

Rome, Esther R., and Jill Wolhandler. "Can Tampon Safety Be Regulated?" in Alice J. Dan and Linda L. Lewis, eds., *Menstrual Health in Women's Lives*, Urbana/Chicago: University of Illinois Press, 1992, pp. 261–73.

Rome, E. R., J. Wolhandler, J. Dieckmann and R. P. Kahn. "Tampons: Are They Safe?" Boston: Boston Women's Health Book Collective, 1990. Brochure. For a copy, send a stamped, self-addressed business-sized envelope plus 50¢ to BWHBC, P.O. Box 192, W. Somerville, MA 02144. Also available in Spanish: "Tapones Vaginales."

Shuttle, Penelope, and Peter Redgrove. *The Wise Wound: Eve's Curse and Everywoman*. New York: Richard Marek Publishers, 1978. Grove-Weidenfeld, 1988. A psychoanalytic but provocative approach to menstruation and menstrual problems.

Sloane, Ethel. *Biology of Women*. Albany, NY: Delmar, 1985. One of the few (only?) anatomy and physiology texts with a feminist perspective.

Snowdon, Robert, and Barbara Christian. *Patterns and Perceptions of Menstruation*. New York: St. Martin's Press, 1983. Comparison of menstruation in different cultures.

Taylor, Dena. *Red Flower: Rethinking Menstruation*. Freedom, CA: Crossing Press, 1988.

Taylor, Diana, and Nancy Woods, eds. *Menstruation, Health, and Illness*. New York: Hemisphere Publishing Co., 1991.

See Resources in Chapter 11, "Sexuality," for other readings.

See Resources in Chapter 23, "Women Growing Older," for other resources on menopause.

Audiovisual Materials

Culpepper, Emily. *Period Piece*, a 10-minute 16-mm color film. About attitudes, experiences and images of menstruation. Available from E. E. Culpepper, Director of Women's Studies, University of Redlands, Redlands, CA 92373. (714) 622-7624.

Feferman, Linda. *Linda's Film—Menstruation*, a 1974 18-minute color film. A lively film for teens and pre-teens. Available from Phoenix Films, 470 Park Avenue South, New York, NY 10016.

Mills, Sylvia V. *Is It PMS or Are You Really a Wreck?* and *Getting PMS Out of Your Relationships*, a set of two 1991 audio tapes on coping with PMS. Emphasizes ways to take care of yourself. Introduction mediocre but most is empowering. Available from S. V. Mills, World Trade Center, Suite 275H, San Francisco, CA 94111.

13

Birth Control

BY SUSAN BELL

With special thanks to Judy
Norsigian, Pamela Morgan, Ruth
Bell and Susan Reverby.

*This chapter in previous editions was
written by Abby Schwarz, Nancy
Hawley, Pamela Berger, Wendy
Sanford, Barbara Perkins and Ruth
Bell.*

*1992 Update by Susan Bell, with
Suzannah Cooper-Doyle, Judy
Norsigian and Felicia Stewart.
Special thanks to Jennifer S.
Edwards, Philip Hart, Rachel
Lanzerotti, Ken Legins, Alice
Steinhardt and James Trussell.*

Birth control is fundamental to our effort to understand our bodies, control our health care and have autonomy in our lives. In the United States, women raised the issue of birth control in the early twentieth century primarily as an effort to increase our reproductive freedom through greater access to contraceptives. Today we have numerous contraceptive methods, yet many of us are dissatisfied with the choices facing us, and we still get pregnant when we don't plan to. Worrying about pregnancy can prevent us from enjoying sexual intercourse with fertile men. We may dream of a contraceptive that is perfectly safe, 100 percent effective, easy to use, instantly reversible and free. Yet controlling birth involves more than having the "right" methods and techniques. Even with them, our decision to use birth control involves our feelings about ourselves, our sexuality and our relationships. Real reproductive freedom depends on having the personal, social and political power to choose freely whether or not to have children (see introduction to Part III, Controlling Our Fertility, p. 239).

Since the 1950s, the population control estab-lishment* has dominated the development and distribution of contraceptives. These organizations typically have been more interested in limiting the size of certain groups (especially poor and minority populations) than in helping individual women control their fertility. Joining the population control establishment's efforts are a scientific community whose research may not be reflective of women's needs, a medical profession that may view us as ignorant and incapable of taking an active role in controlling our fertility and the pharmaceutical industry seeking profits from new and improved products. Together, these groups control much of our reproductive health. A noted figure in population research writes, "Basically, current research goals in contraception are often set to meet corporate goals and the perceived needs of society rather than the expressed needs

---

*The population control establishment includes the U.S. government, through the Agency for International Development, for example; and private groups, such as the International Planned Parenthood Federation and the Association for Voluntary Sterilization. See Chapter 27, "Developing an International Awareness," for further discussion.

of individuals."[1] This perspective has resulted in racist practices, such as forced sterilization and the toleration (even espousal) of contraceptive methods with substantial risks: "The dangers of overpopulation are so great that we may have to use certain techniques of contraception that may entail considerable risk to the individual woman."[2] To protect women everywhere, we need to recognize this kind of mentality and protest against it.

SOME OBSTACLES TO BIRTH CONTROL OR USING IT WELL

Birth Control and Sex Information

Deeply felt antisex attitudes and shame about sex prevent many of us from seeking information. On a wider scale, these same attitudes serve to keep sex information from being distributed freely in schools and community organizations. Laws, medical practices and public school policies prevent us from getting the information and services we need, especially when we are young. Many recent studies have exploded the myth that giving teenagers birth control information makes them promiscuous.

In the 1960s and 1970s some legislatures and school boards reversed restrictive laws, and parents, teachers and community people started a few good sex education programs in several U.S. school systems. More recently, groups such as the Moral Majority, supported by the policies of conservative federal and state governments, have sought to reinstate the old restrictive laws or pass new ones and to stop existing sex education programs.

Birth Control—Who Protects Our Interests?

We would like to think that because a method is available through a doctor's office, a medical clinic or a drugstore, its safety and efficacy have been proven. The Food and Drug Administration (FDA) regulates the methods of contraception, deciding which ones are still experimental and which are legal to prescribe and sell, so we assume that they have been carefully tested before we use them.

All birth control methods must be tested first on animals and then on women before the FDA approves them for marketing. Often, drug companies test new methods on women in Third World countries or poor women and women of color in this country (see section on Depo-Provera, p. 292). When the effectiveness and safety of the method satisfy federal requirements, the FDA approves it for general distribution and marketing. However, the recent history of women's contra-

ceptives has shown that the long-term complications and negative effects are rarely thoroughly understood when methods are approved. FDA requirements take up to ten years of work before a drug is marketed, but it takes twenty years or more for some complications to become apparent. As a result, all women using the Pill or the intrauterine device (IUD), for instance, become subjects in prolonged experiments.

When we make careful choices about birth control and seek trustworthy advice, we find conflicting information and false reassurances. Much available evidence has been researched and published by the drug companies themselves and is biased accordingly. Advice from physicians is problematic, because many physicians depend on drug company literature and sales personnel for information. Even when physicians are aware of the complications and risks associated with a particular method, some of them hesitate to tell us about them because, as one Boston gynecologist explained in testimony before Congress, ". . . well, if you tell them they might get headaches, they will get headaches."[3] This paternalistic and condescending attitude keeps us from receiving the information we need to make a responsible choice about which birth control method best suits us. Furthermore, physicians often recommend their own favorite method, which may not be the best one for us. And it is alarming that many physicians' recommendations depend on the methods they have available at the time of our visit. Thus, many of us find ourselves with inadequate or downright dangerous methods, and some of us, unwilling to go through the hassle, end up using nothing at all.

Men and Birth Control

Most women and men in this society assume that the responsibility for birth control should fall on women. One reason for this is that women have more at stake in preventing pregnancy than men do, for we bear the children and, in this culture, are primarily responsible for raising them.

Placing *total* responsibility for birth control on women is unfair. It usually means that we must make arrangements to see a practitioner for an exam and a prescription, go to the drugstore, usually pay for supplies and make sure they don't run out. With the Pill or IUD, we feel the effects and, more seriously, take whatever risks are involved. If we don't have some kind of birth control and a man presses us to have intercourse, we must say no. If we become pregnant, it means that it's *our* fault. Total responsibility often creates anger and resentment that can't help but get in the way of our sexual feelings.

Many of us do not talk much about birth control

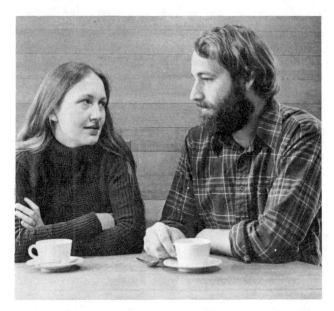

Page Bond

with our partners. Yet a man can share the responsibility of birth control in several ways. When no good method is available at the moment, a supportive partner will join us in exploring ways of lovemaking without intercourse.* He can use condoms and not just when we remind him to, help pay the doctor and drugstore bills, share in putting in the diaphragm or inserting the foam, check to see if supplies are running low. He can, if it is a long-term relationship where no children or no more are wanted, have a vasectomy. A man who truly shares responsibility for preventing pregnancy may gain our respect. We feel better about our relationship and use birth control better, as well.

Women and Birth Control

The increased availability and effectiveness of birth control methods can encourage friends, husbands, lovers to pressure us to have intercourse whenever they want. We need to be assertive about *our* desires: Being protected does not always mean we want intercourse. Many of us have found that we ourselves resist using birth control. What may appear to be personal reasons are actually due to social and political factors as well, such as poor sex education, a double standard of sex, inequalities between women and men. For instance:

- We are embarrassed by, ashamed of or confused about our own sexuality.

---

*There are many ways to have sex with a man, but this chapter is about how to prevent pregnancy when sex includes vagina-to-penis contact and intercourse.

- We cannot admit we might have or are having intercourse, because we feel (or someone told us) it is wrong.
- We are unrealistically romantic about sex: Sex has to be passionate and spontaneous, and birth control seems too premeditated, too clinical and often too messy.
- We hesitate to "inconvenience" our partner. This fear of displeasing him is a measure of the inequality in our relationship.
- We feel, "It can't happen to me. I won't get pregnant."
- We hesitate to find a practitioner and face the hurried, impersonal care or, if we are young or unmarried, the moralizing and disapproval that we feel likely to receive. We are afraid the practitioner will tell our parents.
- We don't recognize our deep dissatisfaction with the method we are using and begin to use it haphazardly.
- We feel tempted to become pregnant just to prove to ourselves that we are fertile or to try to improve a shaky relationship, or we want a baby so that we will have someone to care for.

WHAT CAN WE DO?

We can learn for ourselves and teach one another about the available methods. By speaking openly and by carefully comparing experiences and

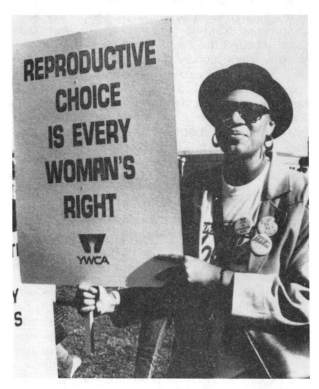

Ellen Shub

knowledge, we can guide each other to workable methods and good practitioners. We can recognize when a practitioner is not thorough enough in examinations or explanations and encourage each other to ask for the attention we need. By talking together we can also get a better handle on our more subtle resistances to using birth control. We can begin the long but worthwhile process of talking with our male partners about birth control, encouraging them to share the responsibility with us. We can join together to insist that legislatures, courts, high schools, churches, parents, doctors, research projects, clinics and drug companies change their practices and attitudes so that we can enjoy our sexuality without becoming pregnant. We can create self-help clinics and other alternative-health-care institutions where our needs for information, discussion and personal support in the difficult choice of birth control will be better met. We can use the good clinics that do exist. We can push for decent housing, jobs and child care so that we can choose birth control freely instead of being forced to use it by our circumstances. Whatever we choose to do, we can act together.

HOW PREGNANCY HAPPENS*

Pregnancy depends on a healthy egg, healthy sperm and favorable cervical mucus. Fertile (favorable) mucus begins in response to rising levels of estrogen in the first part of the menstrual cycle.

During sexual intercourse, sperm are ejaculated through the man's penis into the woman's vagina. If not blocked and in the presence of certain cervical mucus conditions, some of the sperm move, guided by the mucus, through the cervical opening (os), through the woman's uterus and into the fallopian tubes. If the sperm encounter an egg in the outer third of the fallopian tube, one may join with the egg. The process of an egg and a sperm uniting is called *conception* or *fertilization*. The fertilized egg takes several days to travel down the fallopian tube to the uterus, where after one-and-a-half to two days it implants in the uterine lining and develops over the course of the next nine months.

It is also possible for sperm to be deposited in or near the lips around the vagina during sex play. If fertile mucus is present, sperm can move into the vagina and follow the same route to join with the egg. (This is even possible if the woman has an intact hymen or has never had intercourse!)

The egg leaves the ovary *(ovulation) approximately two weeks before the beginning of the next menstrual period.** It can be fertilized for only about twelve to twenty-four hours. A woman can become pregnant from intercourse up to five days before ovulation if fertile mucus is present. Although unusual, *conception can happen after a woman has intercourse during her period* if the mucus begins during her menstrual flow, especially if she has an occasional short cycle.

The Sperm

Sperm are made in the man's testicles ("balls"). Sexual stimulation makes blood flow into erectile tissue inside the penis, causing the penis to become stiff, hard and erect. The drops of liquid (semen) that come from the penis soon after erection occurs contain many sperm. If stimulation is continued, the man usually has an orgasm. As orgasm begins, sperm travel up the sperm ducts, over the bladder and through the prostate gland into the urethra and then are propelled out of the urethra by rhythmic contractions, which are very pleasurable to a man. This is called *ejaculation*.

About 300 million to 500 million sperm come out in one ejaculation. This large number is needed to ensure conception; even under favorable conditions only about 200 sperm actually reach the egg.

Sperm move quickly and, depending on the cervical mucus, may reach an egg in as little as thirty minutes. Sperm cannot survive unaided in the acid environment of the vagina. Without cervical mucus to nourish and protect them, sperm die in one-half to four hours. As soon as cervical mucus appears (during or after menstruation), sperm can survive in a woman's body for three to five days.

For birth control to work, the process of conception must be stopped at some point along the way (see illustration).

CHOOSING A BIRTH CONTROL METHOD

Because there is no one perfect method, our choice of contraceptive will be something of a compromise. Safety and effectiveness are probably the most important factors. Convenience is also important to some. Most of us are healthy and fertile when we begin using birth control, and we want to stay that way. We need a method that is most likely to protect us from pregnancy, will not make us sick or infertile and, ideally, will protect us from sexually transmitted diseases (STDs) which

---

*See Chapter 12, "Anatomy and Physiology of Sexuality and Reproduction," for more details.

---

*A common misunderstanding is that the egg leaves the ovary at midcycle, halfway between menstrual periods. This is only true when the cycle is twenty-eight days long (something that cannot be known for certain until that particular cycle is over and menstruation begins).

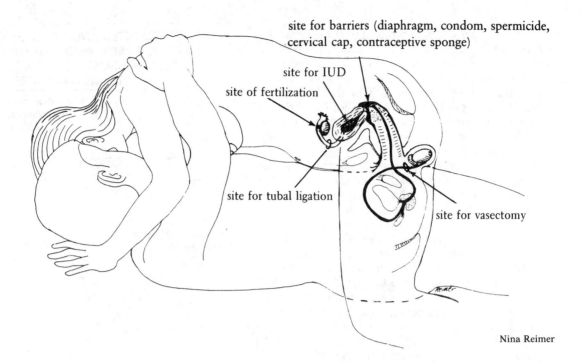

site for barriers (diaphragm, condom, spermicide, cervical cap, contraceptive sponge)

site for IUD

site of fertilization

site for tubal ligation

site for vasectomy

Nina Reimer

include human immunodeficiency virus (HIV) infection and AIDS.

The table at left on p. 264 compares the risk of death associated with different birth control methods, pregnancy and abortion. Be aware that this table does not take into account other factors such as social class, race and pregnancy history. Birth control methods differ in how much protection they give against STDs (e.g., gonorrhea, herpes, chlamydia and HIV) and pelvic inflammatory disease (PID). In general, barrier methods, especially condoms, provide good protection against most reproductive tract infections. *Note that inconsistent or incorrect use reduces the protection given by barrier methods.* The Pill provides some protection against PID; it increases the risk of chlamydia. Its effect on STDs remains unsettled. The IUD offers no protection against STDs and increases the chance of developing PID, especially in the first month after it is inserted.[4] (See Chapters 14 and 24 for more information on STDs and PID.)

When looking at *effectiveness* statistics in books and magazines, keep in mind that there is a difference between the *lowest expected failure rate,* which is based on consistent and correct use of the method, and the higher *typical failure rate,* based on records of actual use of the method over time. Typical user failure rates include accidents such as forgetting a pill, failing to put on the condom early enough and removing the diaphragm within six hours after intercourse; they also reflect factors such as frequency of intercourse and age of the woman. The typical failure rate will give

you a more realistic idea of how effective the method is and will invite you to consider the crucial question of how effectively *you and your partner* will use it. Recently, researchers have carefully reviewed studies of birth control effectiveness and, as a result of their reviews, they have revised their estimates of both lowest expected and typical rates of failure.[5] (See table at right on p. 264.)

The table on p. 264 gives both typical and lowest expected rates. A 5 percent pregnancy rate, or failure rate, means that studies in the past have shown that five women out of every hundred using that particular method have become pregnant the *first year* of using it. By contrast, heterosexually active women using no method at all have an 85 percent pregnancy rate. Note that this table does not differentiate among groups of women on the basis of age, social class and race. However, there *are* differences among these groups. Older women, for example, are more likely than younger women to use spermicides correctly and consistently and

If you think your method of birth control is making you sick, go to a clinic or health practitioner. If the clinic/practitioner doesn't give you an adequate answer, get a second opinion. Stop using that method, and be sure to use another one to avoid pregnancy.

less likely than younger women to conceive if they do not use a method of birth control. Thus, the typical failure rate of spermicides is lower for older women than for younger women and lower than the percentage reported in the table. Also, *after* the first year the failure rates for each method are likely to be lower, since women who conceive in the first year are no longer included in the statistical calculations.

The Collective favors certain methods of contraception over others and has chosen to place them first. Most of us who use or have used birth control chose a diaphragm, cervical cap or foam and condom, because they effectively prevent pregnancy, are safe and offer some protection against STDs and PID. The *safest* way to control our fertility is to use barrier methods of contraception with abortion as a backup in case of failure. If abortion is an unacceptable option for moral or religious reasons, then the overall safety of these methods, which are, in actual practice, less effective than the Pill and IUD, is reduced by whatever risks pregnancy and childbirth might bring. Obviously, health problems associated with pregnancy and childbirth vary greatly among women and depend upon overall health status, access to appropriate care before and after birth and social factors such as income and education. Beyond safety, we believe far greater use of barrier

RISK OF DEATH ASSOCIATED WITH BIRTH CONTROL METHODS, PREGNANCY AND ABORTION

	Chance of Death in a Year
Birth control pills (nonsmoker)	1 in 63,000
Birth control pills (smoker) (See Chapter 3 for other dangers of smoking.)	1 in 16,000
IUDs	1 in 100,000
Barrier methods	none
Natural methods	none
Sterilization:	
Laparoscopic tubal ligation	1 in 67,000
Hysterectomy	1 in 1,600
Vasectomy	1 in 300,000
Pregnancy:	
Terminating pregnancy:	
Illegal abortion	1 in 3,000
Legal abortion:	
Before 9 weeks	1 in 500,000
Between 9 and 12 weeks	1 in 67,000
Between 13 and 16 weeks	1 in 23,000
After 16 weeks	1 in 8,700
Continuing pregnancy	1 in 14,300

Source: This table was adapted from R. Hatcher et al. *Contraceptive Technology*, 1990–1992, 15th rev. ed. New York: Irvington, 1990.

LOWEST EXPECTED AND TYPICAL FAILURE RATES DURING THE FIRST YEAR OF USE OF STERILIZATION AND REVERSIBLE BIRTH CONTROL METHODS IN THE UNITED STATES

Method	Percent of women experiencing an accidental pregnancy in the first year of use	
	Lowest expected* (1)	Typical† (2)
Chance‡	85	85
Spermicides§	3	21
Periodic abstinence		20
Calendar	9	
Ovulation method	3	
Symptothermal‖	2	
Postovulation	1	
Withdrawal	4	18
Cap**	6	18
Sponge		
Parous women	9	28
Nulliparous women	6	18
Diaphragm**	6	18
Condom††	2	12
IUD		3
Progestasert	2.0	
Copper T 380A	0.8	
Pill		3
Combined	0.1	
Progestogen only	0.5	
Injectable progestogen		
DMPA (Depo-Provera)	0.3	0.3
NET	0.4	0.4
Implants		
Norplant‡‡		
(6 capsules)	0.2	0.2
Norplant-2		
(2 rods)	0.03	0.03
Female sterilization	0.2	0.4
Male sterilization	0.1	0.15

Source: This table is reprinted and adapted with the permission of The Population Council from James Trussell et al.,"Contraceptive Failure in the United States: An Update," *Studies in Family Planning*, Vol. 21, No. 1 (January/February 1990), p. 52.
*Among couples who initiate use of a method (not necessarily for the first time) and who use it *perfectly* (both consistently and correctly), this is the percentage expected to experience an accidental pregnancy during the first year if they do not stop use for any other reason.
†Among *typical* couples who initiate use of a method (not necessarily for the first time), the percentage who experience an accidental pregnancy during the first year if they do not stop use for any other reason.
‡The lowest expected and typical percents are based on data from populations where contraception is not practiced and from women who cease practicing contraception in order to become pregnant. These represent the percent who would conceive among women now relying on reversible methods of contraception if they stop using contraception altogether.
§Foams and vaginal suppositories.
‖Cervical mucus (ovulation) method supplemented by calendar in the preovulatory and basal body temperature in the postovulatory phases.
**With spermicidal cream or jelly

(Notes to table continued on p. 265)

methods should be encouraged because they offer protection against STDs and HIV. We must seek to change the attitudes and prejudices that have kept us from using these methods in the past. Even when women choose the Pill, IUD or long-acting hormonal methods, such as Norplant, barrier methods are important "companions" that help prevent STDs.

As you read, you will, of course, form your own opinions and make your choices. If you stop using one method, and you don't want to get pregnant, use another method.

THE DIAPHRAGM AND SPERMICIDAL CREAM OR JELLY

Before the diaphragm was invented in the nineteenth century, women had to depend on men (using condoms and withdrawal) to prevent pregnancy, and on crude abortion and infanticide for backup. The diaphragm was a major breakthrough, giving women responsibility over birth control and freeing us from unwanted pregnancies. It was popular until the 1960s—at one time, a third of all U.S. couples practicing birth control used it. By 1971, however, Planned Parenthood reported that only 4 percent of its clients were choosing diaphragms. What had happened?

In the late 1950s and 1960s, the drug industry, the medical profession, private foundations and the U.S. government began to pour money into researching, developing and distributing the Pill and the IUD, virtually excluding any research on the diaphragm and other barrier methods. Usually, these interests were more concerned with developing new technologies and/or making profits than with the health and well-being of women. Many of us believed the drug industry's and physicians' proclamations about Pill and IUD safety and hoped that the Pill and IUD would allow us more sexual spontaneity and protection against pregnancy than diaphragms.

Recently, many women have begun using the diaphragm again. Our more positive feelings about our sexuality and our increasing ability to communicate openly with the men we sleep with allow us to use the diaphragm more easily. Also, we have learned that diaphragms, correctly fitted and worn, prevent pregnancy, protect us against STDs and are safer than the Pill or IUD.

Yet there are still obstacles to diaphragm use. Only a practitioner can legally prescribe it. Some

Diaphragm, cap and sponge.   Phyllis Ewen

practitioners, especially physicians, do not include time for fittings in their schedules and often charge high fees for their services. A practitioner's attitudes about sexuality *can* affect her/his attitudes about certain methods of birth control and affect ours in turn. Many practitioners don't trust our ability to use a barrier method well; they frequently assume that IUDs or pills are better and that we wouldn't want to "mess" with the diaphragm. Research on barrier methods has increased in the past few years but continues to be inadequate: From 1980 to 1983 an average of $62 million was spent worldwide each year on contraceptive research. Of this amount, $2.9 million was spent on barrier method research.[6]

Description

A diaphragm, *which must always be used with spermicidal cream or jelly,* is made of soft rubber in the shape of a shallow cup (see illustration). It has a flexible metal spring rim (arcing, coiled or flat). When properly fitted and inserted, it fits snugly over your cervix, sitting in place behind the pubic bone and reaching back behind your cervix. It comes in a variety of sizes measured in millimeters, ranging from 50 to 105 millimeters, or two to four inches, depending on the size of your upper vagina.

How It Works

When the diaphragm is in place, holding spermidical jelly or cream up to your cervix, the sperm cannot go into your cervical canal. Sperm may move around the rim of the diaphragm and be killed by the cream or jelly. Some women also smear jelly on the outside of the diaphragm to help kill sperm remaining in the vagina. Always use a diaphragm with cream or jelly: *They* are the important contraceptives; the diaphragm exists only to hold them in the proper place.

††Without spermicides.
‡‡This figure differs from that in earlier versions of this table, because it includes women who were probably pregnant when they started Norplant. If these women were excluded, the failure rate would be 0.04.

Effectiveness

The diaphragm can have a failure rate as low as 6 percent if fit properly, its use carefully taught and used correctly and consistently. Most likely, the 6 percent failure rate exists because the diaphragm moves around a bit with frequent insertion of the penis, positions in which the woman is on top and expansion of the upper vagina during intercourse. The typical failure rate is higher, about 18 percent, which reflects not only imperfect use but also factors such as age and frequency of intercourse.

You can combine the use of the diaphragm with fertility observation (see p. 276). You can achieve almost 100 percent effectiveness with the diaphragm if your partner also uses a condom on your fertile days.

Reversibility

The diaphragm doesn't affect your fertility at all. Simply don't use it if you want to become pregnant.

Safety and Possible Problems

The diaphragm is almost completely safe. It cannot slide up inside us and disappear (as some of us may fear) because the vagina stops about an inch beyond the cervix. A particular cream or jelly may irritate your vagina or your partner's penis. Try a different brand if this happens. The diaphragm itself might push forward and cause cramps in your uterus, bladder or urethra. For some women, this can lead to urethritis or recurrent cystitis. The diaphragm could also push backward on your rectum, which can be uncomfortable, too. If this happens to you, it may mean that the diaphragm is the wrong size. Try out different types of diaphragms as well to see if one is less uncomfortable than another. Some women get recurrent yeast infections when using the diaphragm, which you can avoid by making sure that you wash and dry your diaphragm thoroughly between uses. (For possible negative effects of creams and jellies, see p. 274.)

Who Shouldn't Use the Diaphragm

If you have a severely displaced uterus (severe prolapse, for instance), you cannot use a diaphragm. If you have a protrusion of the bladder through the vaginal wall (cystocele) or other openings in the vagina (fistulas), you cannot use this method. If you have curvature of the spine (scoliosis) or an incompletely formed spinal cord (spina bifida), you may not be able to use the diaphragm. Women with chronic urinary tract infections or a history of toxic shock syndrome probably should not use the diaphragm.

If you don't feel comfortable touching your genitals and do not think you can get used to it, you would most likely have trouble using a diaphragm effectively. You may feel very squeamish and embarrassed the first time you put your finger into your vagina, but as you get used to it and realize that your body is yours to touch, you should get over any uneasiness about inserting the diaphragm. Starting or joining a self-help group may help you to discuss negative feelings about touching yourself.

How to Get the Diaphragm

The size of diaphragm you should use depends on the size and contour of your vagina and the muscle strength of the surrounding vaginal walls. In this country it is usually a doctor, nurse-practitioner or other women's health-care provider who measures (or fits) you for a diaphragm. If your uterus is tipped forward or backward slightly, the person fitting the diaphragm can choose one of the three kinds of metal spring rim (arcing, coiled or flat) to fit your particular anatomy. If one kind doesn't fit, try another kind.

Very important: When you have been measured and fitted, practice putting the diaphragm in and taking it out before you leave the practitioner's office, so s/he can tell you if you are doing it right. (Or go home, practice and come back in a few days with the diaphragm in place.) Reach in and see what it feels like when it is in correctly and get help immediately if you have problems, so that when you actually use it you won't be experimenting. Many practitioners neglect this important step.

The practitioner will have the diaphragm available right there or will give you a prescription for the proper size.

How to Use the Diaphragm

Somebody once said that if someone handed you a toothbrush with no instructions and you had never seen one before, you might not use it very well for a while. Like any tool, the diaphragm is simple to use once you've practiced with it. Putting it in and taking it out might feel awkward at first, but it will become easier and quicker every time. You must put the diaphragm in *within six hours** before intercourse or vagina-to-penis contact, because the creams and jellies may start to

---

*See Robert Hatcher et al. *Contraceptive Technology,* 1990–1992, 15th rev. ed., New York: Irvington, 1990, p. 218; see also Barbara Seaman and Gideon Seaman, *Women and the Crisis in Sex Hormones,* New York: Bantam Books, 1978.

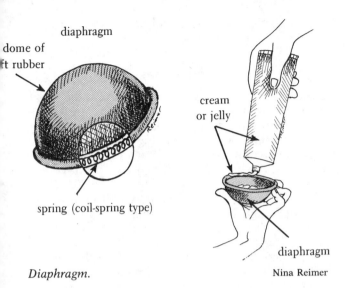

Diaphragm.

Nina Reimer

lose their spermicidal potency in the body after that time. The most conservative estimates say to put it in as close to intercourse as possible, but if you tend to get carried away with sexual intensity, it's probably best to insert the diaphragm in advance.

Preparation and Insertion

Put one teaspoonful to one tablespoonful of cream or jelly (three-quarters of an inch from the tube) into the shallow cup (see illustration above). Spread the cream around. (Some books say to put the cream on the rim also; others say that cream on the rim makes the diaphragm slip. An effective compromise might be to put cream around the inside of the rim and not on top of the rim.) Then squeeze the cup together by pressing the rim firmly between your thumb and third finger. If you have trouble, you can buy a plastic inserter (good only with a flat-spring diaphragm). You can squat, sit on the toilet bowl, stand with one foot raised or lie down with your legs bent. With your free hand, spread apart the lips of your vagina and

push the diaphragm up to the upper third of your vagina with the cream or jelly facing up. If you have not used tampons or reached into your vagina before, remember that it angles toward your back (see illustration below). Now push the lower rim with your finger until you feel the diaphragm lock into place. You should then reach in to make sure you can feel the outline of your cervix through the soft rubber cup. (For more protection, some women insert a little extra cream or jelly with an applicator when the diaphragm is in place, but this is *not* necessary.) When it's in right and fits properly, you should not be able to feel the diaphragm at all. Your partner probably won't either, although some men notice that the tip of their penis is touching soft rubber instead of cervical and vaginal tissue. (This is not painful.) *Never use petroleum jelly (like Vaseline) with a diaphragm, as it destroys the rubber.*

Leave the diaphragm in for at least six hours after intercourse, because it takes the spermicide that long to kill all the sperm. You can leave it in up to twenty-four hours, but not longer. Douching is unnecessary, but if you want to douche, you must wait six hours.

Subsequent Intercourse

If you have intercourse again, you *must* add more cream or jelly with an applicator. Put it into your vagina, leaving the diaphragm in place.

Removal

Remove the diaphragm by choosing a comfortable position, perhaps the same way you chose to insert it. If you have trouble reaching the diaphragm, try another position or bear down as if you were going to have a bowel movement. Slide a finger into your vagina and hook it under the lower rim of the diaphragm, either between the diaphragm and your vaginal wall or over the rubber dome. Pull the diaphragm forward and down. If you have long nails, take care not to rip the diaphragm.

Insertion of diaphragm.

Checking of diaphragm.

Nina Reimer

Care

Wash the diaphragm with mild soap and warm water, rinse and dry carefully, dust it with cornstarch if you wish (but never talcum powder) and put it into a container (away from light). Don't boil it. *Check it for holes* every so often by holding it up to the light or filling it with water and looking for leaks, especially around the rim. If you poke the dome with your finger, it will be easier to detect possible cracks along the rim.

Life of Product

Get your diaphragm size rechecked every year or two. You may need a new size if you gain or lose a lot of weight or have vaginal surgery and after pregnancy, abortion or miscarriage. The diaphragm will last at least a couple of years with proper care.

Cost

A diaphragm costs about twenty dollars.* The medical examination for the diaphragm can cost from fifty to a hundred dollars depending on whether you go to a clinic or a private physician and on how extensive the examination is.

Spermicidal jellies and creams vary in price from about nine dollars, depending on the size of the tube. A 3.8-ounce tube contains approximately twelve applications.

Advantages

It is a good method if you have intercourse with a partner who is cooperative and helpful about using it and/or if you have intercourse relatively infrequently, because it only has to be used around the time of lovemaking.

It is very effective if used well and every time. There are almost no side effects or dangers.

The diaphragm is helpful if you want to have intercourse during your period and don't want a heavy menstrual flow to interfere.

Using a diaphragm can be a good kind of body education. If you are unfamiliar with what your vagina feels like, using a diaphragm will teach you. In the long run, the more familiar you are with your body, the more you will enjoy sex.

Repeated studies indicate that the diaphragm with cream or jelly reduces your chances of getting gonorrhea or trichomoniasis infections in the vaginal canal. It increases your protection against

*In some federally funded clinics, diaphragm kits (including diaphragm and jelly) can be had for twelve dollars or even less.

PID and cervical dysplasia and may help clear up adenosis.

Disadvantages

If either you or your partner wants sex to be uninterrupted and absolutely spontaneous, putting in the diaphragm can be a hassle if you don't put it in long before you start having sex.

You must remember to use it every time, be sure not to run out of cream or jelly and have it with you when you need it.

The discharge of cream or jelly can be a nuisance, although it does not stain. Try different brands and, if necessary, use a pad or a tissue for leaking after intercourse.

Some people who enjoy oral sex find the taste of the jellies and creams unpleasant. One way around this is to wash carefully after putting in the diaphragm. Another is to put the diaphragm in after oral sex play and before intercourse. This is a definite interruption, however, and that increases the possibility that you won't put it in at all. Some women find they have more yeast and urinary tract infections while using a diaphragm.

Responsibility

After you are fitted, you and your partner can share the responsibility of insertion, although a lot of women do the whole thing themselves.

THE FEMALE CONDOM OR VAGINAL POUCH

Description

In late 1992 the FDA is expected to approve the first condom for women—the Reality or Femidom Vaginal Pouch (see illustration)—as an over-the-counter, nonprescription birth control device. The vaginal pouch consists of a soft, loose-fitting polyurethane sheath, which is closed at one end (this part covers the opening of the cervix). One flexible polyurethane ring is located at either end of the pouch, one at the closed end and one at the open end at the external edge of the sheath (this remains just outside the vagina after insertion). The ring inside (at the closed end) is used to insert the condom and also serves as an internal anchor. The ring outside the vagina covers the labia and keeps the pouch in place during intercourse. When in place, the vaginal pouch lines the vaginal wall, creating a covered passageway for the penis. Like the male condom, this is intended for one-time use. The pouch comes prelubricated and does not require precise placement over the cervix. (If not available in your area yet, contact Wisconsin,

Pharmacal Company, 919 North Michigan Avenue, Suite 2208, Chicago, IL 60611.)

Effectiveness

The Reality Vaginal Pouch is about as effective as the cervical cap and diaphragm in preventing pregnancy. It offers more protection against STDs and HIV infection than the cap or diaphragm.

Reversibility

Perfectly reversible. To get pregnant, just don't use it.

How to Use the Vaginal Pouch

Squeeze the inner ring and insert the pouch into your vagina just past the pubic bone, so that the inner ring covers your cervix. Check with your finger to make sure that the sheath is not twisted, so that it will be easy for the penis to enter into the vagina.

Advantages

The Reality Vaginal Pouch helps women to protect themselves against both pregnancy and STDs. In an era during which HIV infection among women is on the rise, this protection—although not 100 percent effective—is especially valuable. It will be particularly useful for women whose partners are unwilling to use condoms. Because the pouch can

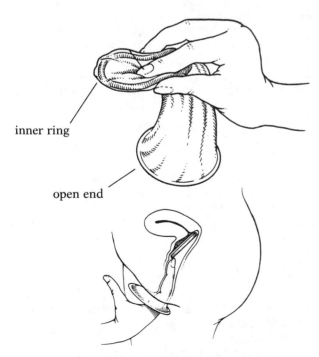

inner ring

open end

INSERTION OF REALITY VAGINAL POUCH.

be inserted long before intercourse, it does not break the flow of lovemaking in the way that the male condom can. In addition, for men who *are* willing to use a male condom but find it difficult to keep an erection while putting on a condom, the vaginal pouch helps to avoid what can be an awkward moment during lovemaking that includes intercourse. Also, an erection is not necessary for removal of the vaginal pouch.

The polyurethane lining in the vaginal pouch is stronger than the latex membrane used in male condoms. It is soft and thin and more resistant to oils. Lastly, as an over-the-counter product, the vaginal pouch does not require a visit to a clinic or practitioner's office.

Disadvantages

Some women may find the vaginal pouch a little cumbersome. Sometimes the outside ring is too noticeable. As with other female barrier methods, it does require that we are comfortable touching our genital area, although a little practice is usually all we need to overcome any awkward feelings.

THE MALE CONDOM (RUBBER, PROPHYLACTIC OR SAFE)

Description

Egyptian men wore condoms in 1350 B.C. as decorative covers for their penises. The condom was popularized for protection against conception and STDs (see Chapter 14) in the eighteenth century. It is a sheath, usually made of thin, strong latex rubber, designed to fit over an erect penis to keep semen from getting into the woman's vagina. A condom usually comes rolled up and unrolls to about seven and a half inches; the open end has a one-and-three-eighths-inch-diameter rubber ring around it to help keep it on the penis, and the closed end is either plain or tipped with a little nipple that catches the semen and helps to keep the condom from bursting. "Skin" condoms (made of lamb membrane) are more expensive but much thinner and offer less protection against STDs. Lubricated rubber condoms minimize the risk of tearing but tend to slip off the penis more easily and have to be used extra carefully. Condoms that are preshaped or contoured may increase sensitivity for some men; they may also be less likely to slip. Some condoms contain a spermicide, which kills most sperm on contact, offers more protection against STDs and is probably more effective than condoms without spermicide.

The condom is the only temporary means of birth control a man can use. Because it can be purchased over the counter or found on a drugstore shelf, or even purchased by mail, men don't need to visit a medical facility to obtain a prescription. Furthermore, women can also easily buy and carry condoms. It should not be surprising, therefore, to find that the condom is the most frequently used barrier method in the United States.

Once even more widely used, the condom, like all other methods, fell into disfavor when the Pill and IUD appeared. Men could share in the spontaneity and relative sexual freedom brought about by the Pill and IUD without having to experience their negative effects. Today, the condom is viewed much more favorably because people have learned more about heterosexual transmission of AIDS.[7] Current research on a new plastic condom as well as other improvements are likely to increase condom usage even further.

Effectiveness

A good-quality condom has a failure rate of about 2 percent when used as directed, but typically its failure rate is about 12 percent. We suggest combining condoms with a spermicidal foam, cream or jelly for close to 100 percent protection. Used with an IUD or diaphragm, condoms provide extra protection at ovulation.

Reversibility

Perfectly reversible. To get pregnant, just don't use condoms.

How to Use the Condom

The man or woman unrolls the condom onto the erect penis before *any* vagina-to-penis contact or intercourse—*not* just before ejaculation, because long before ejaculation the male may discharge a few drops with enough sperm to cause pregnancy.

Cautions

Leave space at the end of the plain-ended condom for the semen: One-half-inch of air-free space between the end of the penis and the condom will keep the ejaculate, which comes out fast, from bursting the condom. Catching air in the end may also cause bursting.

If you do not use a lubricated condom, use a lubricant to prevent tearing—spermicidal foam, cream or jelly or K-Y Jelly, but *never* Vaseline (petroleum jelly), which can corrode the rubber. Saliva is always available but may increase your chances of developing a monilia (yeast) infection. Apply the lubricant after the condom is on the penis.

One of you must hold the rim when you move away from him or he withdraws his no-longer-

Condoms.   Elizabeth Cole

erect penis after ejaculation; otherwise the condom might slip off and sperm could get into the vagina.

In case of accident, insert cream or jelly or foam into your vagina as quickly as possible. Do not douche.

Responsibility

The man uses the condom. It is much more enjoyable to use it if both partners join in putting it on. For a couple who have intercourse more than a few times, condoms are a good way for the man to share in birth control. In a shorter-term relationship, when you may not know whether you'll be having intercourse or not, condoms can be very convenient. But don't expect the man to have a condom in his pocket—you may be disappointed. If you don't know him well enough to be sure he'll have a condom, it makes sense for you to have some with you. But it is hard for many of us to pull out a rubber and suggest that the man use it.

Advantages

It is fairly cheap, readily available and easy to use.

It is a method of birth control that gives good protection against some STDs, including HIV infection, when used in *every instance* of vagina-to-penis contact. It also prevents partners from reinfecting each other with an STD, such as trichomoniasis, during the treatment period.

If the man tends to ejaculate too quickly, a condom may decrease the stimulation of his penis enough to help him delay ejaculation and prolong intercourse.

A condom catches the semen, so if the woman wants to go somewhere right after intercourse, she won't feel drippy.

You don't need a doctor's prescription to buy a condom.

Disadvantages

You have to use the condom right at the time of intercourse, which ruins the spontaneity of sex for some couples unless the woman puts it on the man and makes it a part of sex play.

It may lessen the man's sensation, as his penis doesn't touch the vaginal walls directly. Many men resist using condoms for this reason, forgetting the effects that women's birth control methods can have on a woman's enjoyment of sex. Some men say they do not feel such a great reduction in sensation.

The condom eliminates one source of lubrication for intercourse (the drops of fluid that come out when the man gets an erection), and the resultant friction can irritate a woman, especially during the entrance of the penis into her vagina. If this happens, use a lubricant or a lubricated condom, preferably lubricated with a spermicide.

How to Get Condoms

You can find condoms in drugstores, at family planning agencies or in vending machines. Many men say they were embarrassed the first time they bought condoms, particularly if the druggist asked, "What size?" and the man didn't know s/he was referring to the size of the package. Condoms are made in a standard size, they come in packages of three or twelve, and they cost about two to three and a half dollars for a package of three and six to eight dollars for a package of twelve, depending upon the brand. Some high-quality condoms are Ramses Rubber Prophylactics, Ramses X-tra, Trojans Rubber Prophylactics, Trojan-Enz Rubber Prophylactics. Some condoms are colored, but both men and women have reported that the dyes stain and cause burning and irritation. Some manufacturers are making ribbed or studded condoms, which they claim make intercourse more enjoyable for women, though some of us who have experienced them could not feel any difference.

Life of Product

Condoms have a shelf life of five years if kept away from heat. Because heat causes them to deteriorate, do not store them for very long in a wallet or pocket. If you carry them around, use the kind sealed in foil.

THE CONTRACEPTIVE SPONGE

Investigation to develop a contraceptive sponge began a few years ago, prompted by a number of factors: women moving away from using the Pill and IUD, a growing recognition by the medical establishment that women are seeking alternatives, a slight rise in publicly and privately funded research for improving barrier methods and producing new ones. In 1983, the FDA approved the sponge for general over-the-counter marketing.

Description

The disposable sponge is made of polyurethane, an artificial substance. It comes in one size, two and a quarter inches in diameter and three-quarters of an inch thick, with an indentation (dimple) in the center and a loop of tape attached (see photograph on p. 265).

How It Works

The sponge covers the opening of the cervix (os), where it collects sperm. It is held in place by the walls of a woman's vagina and the "dimple" covering the cervix. It also contains a spermicide (nonoxynol-9), which it releases slowly to kill sperm.

How to Use the Sponge

Wet the sponge with water and compress it. Then insert it into your vagina by hand or with an applicator. Once the sponge is inside your vagina, it expands in the space around the cervix, blocking the opening (os). It does not require an exact fit as the diaphragm and cervical cap do. You should *not* use the contraceptive sponge during menstruation. To reduce the risk of toxic shock syndrome during your period, use another method of birth control.

Once the sponge is in place, you can have intercourse as often as you like, without having to add any more spermicide. After intercourse, you *must* leave it in place for at least six hours; you *can* leave it in your vagina for up to twenty-four hours (one day). Take it out by pulling on the tape that is attached to it and throw it away.

Effectiveness

For women who have not given birth, the sponge is about as effective as the diaphragm: Its lowest expected failure rate is 6 percent and its typical failure rate is 18 percent. Its failure rate is much higher for women who have previously given birth.

Reversibility

There is no indication that the sponge will interfere with a woman's fertility when it is not being used. If you want to become pregnant, just stop using the sponge.

Safety

No long-term studies have been conducted on the safety of the material used in the contraceptive sponge. It is unclear whether the high concentration of nonoxynol-9, which is considerably more than that used with other barrier methods, poses any increased risks. Also unknown is the effect of polyurethane. The possible association between the sponge and toxic shock syndrome has not been adequately tested yet. About 2 percent of women using the sponge have reported allergic reactions. Some sponges have shredded while they are in place.

Advantages

The contraceptive sponge has most of the advantages of the diaphragm: safety and effectiveness, easy reversibility, encouragement for learning about your body, possible prevention of sexually transmitted diseases.

It remains effective for up to twenty-four hours, allowing vagina-to-penis contact and sexual intercourse to be spontaneous.

It comes in one size, so it doesn't need to be fitted.

You can buy it over the counter.

It doesn't leak, so it's less messy than most other barriers, and doesn't interfere with oral sex.

Disadvantages

Some women notice an unpleasant odor after intercourse.

About 2 to 3 percent of women in clinical trials report expelling the sponge, usually during a bowel movement.

Some women have difficulty removing the sponge or find that it tears or shreds.

Some women, such as those with a prolapsed uterus, cannot wear it.

Some women have more yeast infections while using the sponge.

THE CERVICAL CAP

The cervical cap was approved for marketing in the United States in 1988. It is a thimble-shaped rubber cap that fits snugly over the cervix. Like the diaphragm, it blocks sperm from entering the cervical opening. Usually, a small amount of spermicide is used on the inside of the cap to kill any sperm that might break through the suction seal. Used in some European countries, the cap was also used during the early twentieth century in the United States.* With the rise in use of the Pill and IUD, the cervical cap, like the diaphragm, declined in popularity. By the mid-1960s, U.S. companies had completely stopped producing it for contraceptive purposes.

The National Women's Health Network, feminist health groups and a small number of physicians and nurses spent nearly a decade campaigning for the cap and shepherding it through the long process of review by the FDA. In addition, much of the research on the cap has been conducted at feminist health centers across the United States. The availability of the cervical cap today represents a victory for women's health activists.

Description

The only cervical cap approved for use in the United States is the Prentif cavity rim, made of flexible rubber. It looks somewhat like a thimble with a rim and fits over the cervix the same way a thimble fits over your finger. It is about one and a half inches long and covers almost the entire cervix (see photograph, p. 265). Because cervices are different sizes, this rubber cap comes in four different sizes, from twenty-two millimeters to thirty-one millimeters in diameter (less than one inch to about one and a quarter inches). Other kinds of caps not approved by the FDA are the vault (or Dumas) cap and the Vimule cap. (The information below is about the Prentif cervical cap only.)

How It Works

Like other barrier methods, the cervical cap keeps sperm out of the uterus. The cap is designed to create an almost airtight seal around the cervical opening. Suction, or surface tension, hugs it close to the cervix, and sperm can't move past the edge of the cap the way they can with the diaphragm. The spermicide both inactivates sperm and strengthens the suction seal between the cap and the cervix.

Effectiveness

Research on the Prentif cap shows it is about as effective as a diaphragm. Its lowest expected failure rate is 6 percent; its typical failure rate is 18 percent. A certain percentage of failures may be due to the cap being dislodged during intercourse by the penis thrusting against the cervix.

---

*The idea of the cervical cap is thousands of years old. In ancient Sumatra, women molded opium into cuplike devices to cover their cervices. See Barbara Seaman and Gideon Seaman, *Women and the Crisis in Sex Hormones*, p. 190.

How to Get the Cap

You can get a list of practitioners and clinics that fit cervical caps from the Concord Feminist Health Center, 38 South Main Street, Concord, NH 03301, (603) 225-2739, or from Cervical Cap Ltd., 430 Monterey Avenue, Suite 1B, Los Gatos, CA 95030, (408) 395-2100.

The cervical cap must be fitted to your cervix by a trained practitioner. When it fits properly, a cap should completely cover your cervix and grip on to it firmly. Whenever you are fitted for a cap, be sure that the practitioner gives you time to try inserting and removing it. A cervical cap is somewhat more difficult to use than a diaphragm, since you have to be able to reach your cervix with your fingers to put the cap into place. With practice it becomes easy for most women.

How to Use the Cap

Most health workers advise using a small amount of spermicidal jelly or cream inside the cap. The cap should be filled about one-third full. If you use too much, it may break the suction. The spermicide should be spread around the inside of the cap but not on the rim. You may insert the cap up to forty hours before intercourse or vagina-to-penis contact. For backup, some women insert cream or jelly into their vagina if they have intercourse after the cap has been in place for a few hours, but some practitioners feel this may interfere with the cap's suction.

You *must* keep the cap in place for at least six to eight hours after intercourse. Douching is unnecessary, but in any case, never douche while the cap is in place, since this could dilute the spermicidal jelly or cream.

Practitioners debate how often to remove the cap. Although some believe the cap can be worn continuously for seventy-two hours (three days) or longer, the FDA regulations state that it should not be left in place for longer than forty-eight hours (two days) partly because of the lack of good data on failure rates with longer use and concern about toxic shock syndrome. Some women remove the cap once a day or every other day to allow cervical secretions to flow freely. This may help prevent infections and toxic shock syndrome.* During your period, remove the cap often or don't use it at all, in order to reduce the risk of toxic shock syndrome and because the menstrual flow may break the suction seal.

Some women help prevent odors by soaking the cap for twenty minutes in one cup of water mixed with one tablespoon of cider vinegar or lemon juice. After soaking, rinse and dry the cap before using.

For a month or two after you start using the cap, and whenever you have intercourse with a new partner, check it right before and after intercourse, and use extra spermicide in your vagina or have your partner use a condom for extra protection. Especially if the cap doesn't fit exactly right, and depending on the angle of penetration and your particular anatomy, the cap can become dislodged when a man's penis thrusts against your cervix. You may have to see if a different-size cap fits better or switch to a diaphragm.

Who Shouldn't Use the Cervical Cap

Many women, even those who can't wear the diaphragm, can use the cervical cap, but the existing sizes may not fit all women. If you have a cervical erosion or laceration, you shouldn't use the cap, because it doesn't allow the free flow of cervical secretions, which may be a cause of irritation. If you have a history of toxic shock syndrome, you should not use the cap.

If your cervix is very long or of an irregular shape, you may not be able to use the cap. Also, it is possible for a woman's vagina to be so long that she can't reach deep enough inside to place or remove the cap easily. Some women have found that a diaphragm inserter/remover (similar to a giant plastic crotchet hook) can help with removal. Ask your practitioner to write a prescription for an inserter/remover if you need one and the local pharmacy will not sell it over the counter.

Other reasons for not using the cervical cap are the same as those for not using the diaphragm (see p. 266).

Advantages

When used properly, the cap is very effective and you can insert it long before intercourse, which means it need not interfere with lovemaking.

The cap itself is relatively inexpensive, costing about $30, and the fee for the initial fitting can be $70 to $130. Because it requires so little spermicide, it's less messy than the diaphragm, and one tube will go a long way.

It provides some protection against gonorrhea and chlamydia.

Because of its size, the cap may be more comfortable than the diaphragm. It is a good choice for women who experience repeated urinary tract infections when they use a diaphragm if this problem is caused by pressure from the diaphragm rim. Cap users, however, also may have problems with urinary tract infections because of altered bacterial growth in the vagina.

---

*Some researchers have found high concentrations of *Staphylococcus aureus*, the bacteria involved in toxic shock syndrome, in women who have left the cap in for three days or more.

Like the diaphragm, the cap helps us get to know our bodies better.

Disadvantages

The cap is still not available everywhere, so depending on where you live, it may be difficult to obtain.

The cap comes in only four sizes, so it does not fit all women.

The cap may cause an unpleasant odor if you don't remove it fairly often.

Some women dislike the idea of trapping cervical secretions for as long as the cap is worn, because this may lead to infections.

Occasionally a partner feels discomfort if his penis hits the rim of the cap during intercourse.

You have to keep checking the cap carefully after intercourse to feel whether it has become dislodged. If the seal is broken, the cap's effectiveness is reduced.

Some women have trouble inserting and removing the cap.

(See the section below on possible negative effects of creams and jellies.)

JELLIES AND CREAMS

Spermicidal cream or jelly is really designed for use with a diaphragm or cervical cap (and can be used for extra protection with a condom). The lowest expected failure rate for spermicides used alone (jellies, creams, foams and vaginal suppositories) is 3 percent. However, recent studies, on which this estimate is based, are mostly about suppositories and foam. The failure rate of jellies and creams is probably higher than 3 percent. Some researchers believe that even the recent spermicide studies are of poor quality, and that the failure rate for all spermicides is higher than 3 percent. Using spermicides with condoms is wise.

Cream or jelly comes in a tube with a plastic applicator. Jellies are clear, creams are white. They are available without prescription at all drugstores. (See How to Get Foam, p. 276, for purchase hints.)

Deposited just outside the entrance to your cervix at the top of your vagina, cream or jelly keeps sperm from entering the cervix and kills them as well.

How to Use Jellies and Creams

For use with a diaphragm or cap, see the earlier sections. For use with a condom: As short a time as possible (under fifteen minutes) *before* vagina-to-penis contact or intercourse, you or your partner should fill the applicator, insert it into your

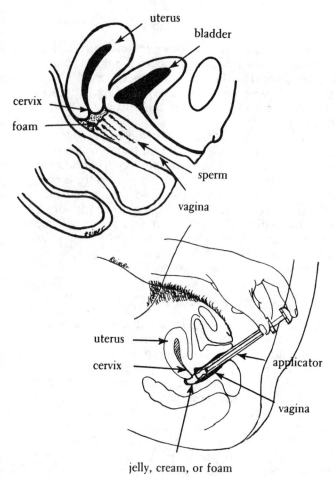

jelly, cream, or foam

How to insert sperm-killing foam, cream or jelly.

Nina Reimer

vagina and push the plunger. Use an additional full plunger for each additional act of intercourse. Leave the jelly or cream in for six to eight hours. If you want to douche, you must wait.

Possible Negative Effects

In 1981 a *much criticized* study linked spermicide use with birth defects.[8] Since then, better studies have found no such link.[9] Some brands sold in the United States at one time contained mercury. As a result of Japanese studies showing that mercury could cause kidney damage, it was removed. It is still found in some jellies and creams sold outside the United States.

Advantages

Like condoms, you can get cream or jelly on short notice. They increase your protection against gonorrhea and chlamydia.

Disadvantages

There can be problems of leakage, allergy or reaction to the smell or taste. Jelly may be less irritating but tends to be more gooey than cream.

FOAM–AEROSOL VAGINAL SPERMICIDE

Description

Foam is a white aerated cream that has the consistency of shaving cream and contains an effective sperm-killing chemical. It comes in a can with a plunger-type plastic applicator.

How It Works

Deposited just outside the entrance to your cervix at the top of your vagina, foam keeps the sperm from entering the cervix and kills them as well.

Effectiveness

Foam used alone consistently and correctly has an expected failure rate of 3 percent, but the failure rate among typical users is 21 percent. Researchers do not yet understand why foams and suppositories used alone appear to be more effective than barrier methods used with a cream or jelly. Some think that foams and suppositories work differently from creams and jellies that are used with a barrier. They may coat the vaginal walls and cervix better than the creams and jelly that are used with a diaphragm and cap.

We strongly recommend using foam in combination with a condom. When used together, their effectiveness approaches 100 percent. Foam is also very effective when used as a supplement during the first months of Pill use or as an extra precaution with an IUD.

Problems with effectiveness arise from using too little foam, not realizing that the container is almost empty, failing to shake the container enough, not inserting the foam correctly, or inserting it after vagina-to-penis contact has begun.

How to Use Foam

Insert no longer than thirty minutes before vagina-to-penis contact. If the foam is in a can, *shake the can very well*, about twenty times. The more bubbles the foam has, the better it blocks sperm. Also, the spermicide tends to settle in the bottom of the container, so it must be mixed. Put the applicator on top. When the applicator is tilted (Delfen) or pushed down (Emko and Koromex), the pressure triggers the release valve and the foam is forced into the applicator, pushing the plunger up. Some brands of foam come in preloaded applicators.

Lie down, use your free hand to spread the lips of your vagina, insert the applicator about three to four inches and push the plunger. Then remove the applicator *without pulling on the plunger*, or you may suck some of the foam back into the applicator. Insert one full applicator of Emko, Emko Pre-fil, or Because, or two applicatorsful of Delfen or Koromex. If you have never used tampons, you may want to practice inserting the applicator. You'll find that your vagina angles up toward your back, not straight up in your body. Your aim is to deposit the foam at the entrance of your cervix.

Wash the applicator with mild soap and warm but not boiling water before putting it away. You don't have to wash it immediately.

Cautions

Put in more foam every time you have intercourse or vagina-to-penis contact, no matter how recent the last time was. Leave the foam in for six to eight hours. If you want to douche, you must wait. If the foam is dripping and bothers you, use a mini-pad or tissue in your underpants.

Keep an extra can on hand. Some brands indicate when they're running out; others just come out of the can more slowly.

Use foam with a condom for maximum effectiveness of both.

Negative Effects

Foam (especially the suppositories) irritates some vaginas and some penises, leading to pain, itching or the sensation of heat.

Responsibility

Basically the responsibility is the woman's, but either you or the man can put it in.

Advantages

When used with a condom, it is a highly effective means of birth control.

It is quick, taking about thirty seconds to use.

It is less drippy than cream or jelly.

It helps to prevent gonorrhea and chlamydia.

Disadvantages

Alone, it is quite ineffective.

Using it can be a (brief) interruption if you do not treat it as part of sex play.

Many people think it tastes terrible; it must usually be inserted after oral sex play.

Some brands use aerosol cans, which environmentalists are against.

How to Get Foam

You can buy it in a drugstore without a prescription.

Although you don't have to see a health practitioner to get foam, have a checkup if you think you've been exposed to an STD.

Try different brands. If one causes irritation, another may be satisfactory.

Other Foaming Spermicides

There are two other types of foaming spermicides: suppositories and contraceptive film. Spermicidal suppositories (Encare Oval, Intercept, Koromex Inserts, Prevent, Semicid) and vaginal contraceptive film (VCF) can be used alone but *we strongly recommend that you use them only in combination with a condom.* To use a suppository, unwrap one and insert it into your vagina ten to thirty minutes before vagina-to-penis contact. To use VCF, make sure your hands are dry, place one paper-thin sheet on your finger and insert the film on or near your cervix fifteen minutes before vagina-to-penis contact. The spermicidal suppository or VCF will remain effective for no more than an hour. With repeated intercourse, you need to insert another suppository or VCF; you must leave it in your vagina for at least six hours after intercourse. Suppositories and VCF are considered to be as effective as spermicides with most of the same advantages and disadvantages of foam.

FERTILITY OBSERVATION (NATURAL BIRTH CONTROL)

We can learn to observe and understand our bodies' hormonal changes that are linked to fertility by observing three simple body signs: cervical mucus, basal body temperature and cephalad shift (cervix changes). In this way, we can accurately decide whether we are fertile (able to conceive) or infertile on a day-to-day basis. It takes only a few minutes each day to make and record our observations.

Most of us have heard of the rhythm method, notorious for its high failure rate. It tries to predict a woman's cycle based on information from past cycles. However, because no one has absolutely regular cycles all the time, it *fails* frequently. Bad experiences with rhythm have led many women to discount so-called natural methods of birth control; yet natural methods that work *have* been developed, and their scientific basis is well documented. *They should not be confused with the rhythm method.*

Using fertility awareness we learn that we are fertile only during part of our menstrual cycle and that we can recognize this time. Fertility observation has far-reaching implications: We can use it to learn basic body information even if we aren't interested in birth control, and to prevent or achieve pregnancy or to predict menstruation. Lesbians can also use it to achieve pregnancy using self-help methods (see Chapter 18, "New Reproductive Technologies").

The Three Fertility Signs

1. *Cervical fluid (mucus).* This is a daily method of identifying fertile and infertile times by simple observation, as the cycle unfolds. Cervical fluid tells when fertility begins and ends with each cycle, times of highest fertility and when ovulation is approaching. Fertility begins when cervical fluid appears and lasts through the evening of the fourth day past the cervical fluid peak (the last day of fertile cervical fluid). Ovulation occurs anywhere from two days before to two days after the mucus peak.

Cervical fluid identifies fertile and infertile days throughout the entire cycle, regardless of whether or not cycles are regular. It reflects the levels of estrogen and progesterone in the body.

2. *Basal body temperature (BBT).* BBT identifies infertile times after ovulation and confirms pregnancy. Temperatures are lower before ovulation and higher afterward. A sustained rise (up to three days) of at least four-tenths of a degree Fahrenheit confirms that ovulation has occurred. If BBTs remain elevated for more than seventeen days (if fever is not present), pregnancy is confirmed.

BBT confirms ovulation after it occurs and identifies postovulatory infertile days. It does not identify when fertility begins or which preovulatory days are safe for vagina-to-penis contact or intercourse.

3. *Cephalad shift (cervix changes).* The cephalad shift represents a change in the position and feel of the cervix. When fertile, the cervix becomes softer and higher, and the os (opening) widens. When cervical fluid changes from wet to dry, the cervix becomes firm, lower and less open.

Cervix changes alone do not tell when fertility begins and ends or safe or unsafe days for vagina-to-penis contact and intercourse. However, they offer a valuable way to confirm the accuracy of cervical fluid and BBT observations.

The three fertility signs are simple to observe and record, requiring no more than a few minutes each day.

Avoiding Pregnancy Through Fertility Observation

When preventing pregnancy, two uses of fertility awareness knowledge are available:

1. *Natural family planning (NFP).* This involves postponing all vagina-to-penis contact when fertile (about one-third of the cycle). Intimacy can be expressed in ways that prevent sperm (including that in early pre-ejaculatory fluid) from coming in contact with fertile cervical fluid on the labia or at the cervix.

NFP is acceptable to those who do not wish to use artificial means of contraception for religious, medical or philosophical reasons. NFP is most often taught by instructors and organizations affiliated with the Catholic Church.

2. *Fertility awareness method (FAM).* FAM offers the choice of postponing vagina-to-penis contact or using barrier methods when fertile. This non-religious approach enables contraceptive users to know when a barrier method failure is more likely to result in pregnancy so that contraceptives can be used even more carefully during these times. Women can also reduce barrier use with FAM knowledge because they can identify the two-thirds of the cycle that is naturally infertile. Although jelly or foam in the vagina can mask indications of fertility, some women report no problems in combining a barrier method with fertility observation, especially if using a condom.

*It is crucial for women to learn fertility observation methods directly from other women and to chart their observations daily.** It is *not* advisable to learn a method just by reading a book. Although a number of books in the Resources can be very helpful and are recommended, books (including this one) cannot give you the personal feedback, support and experience sharing you need. Check your local women's health center or write to the following nonreligious fertility awareness groups for more information: Ovulation Method Teachers Association (OMTA), P.O. Box 101780, Anchorage, AK 99510-1780; Fertility Awareness Network (FAN), P.O. Box 1190, New York, NY 10009. Both are feminist, prochoice groups that offer all fertility awareness options. For a free list of all fertility awareness books and groups (including which signs they teach, their philosophy and options for preventing pregnancy), send a stamped, self-addressed envelope to Fertility Awareness Services (FAS), P.O. Box 986, Corvallis, OR 97339 (FAS specializes in compiling all available fertility awareness information). If you are willing or want to hear Catholic morality mixed in with the information, most Catholic hospitals or churches can help you find a teacher.

Here are some issues to consider in choosing a group:*

1. Is the teacher a woman with experience herself? A male–female couple? A medical person? A nun or priest?

2. Does the format include participatory classes or groups and more than one meeting?

3. Is there an option to learn in an all-woman group? If all classes are open to men, is the orientation toward monogamous heterosexual couples? What efforts are made to ensure support for other sexual life-styles?

4. Can you get help from the teacher in the months or years after the training process is over?

5. Where does the registration fee go? (Are you unwittingly supporting a cause you would find offensive?)

6. What is the sponsoring organization's or teacher's position on birth control and abortion? Will they refer you to a facility that provides a full range of birth control options and/or abortion services? If you do not get straightforward answers to questions 5 and 6, be suspicious. If you hear the term *prolife* used, remember that this indicates an antiabortion philosophy.

THE OVULATION METHOD (AWARENESS OF MUCUS)

Thirty years ago, an Australian couple, Evelyn and John Billings, sought a method of child spacing that would be effective in preventing pregnancy and also acceptable to the Catholic Church—one that would reinforce the Catholic philosophy about sexuality, marriage and women. They developed the ovulation method, a way of interpreting the vaginal sensations of wetness or dryness and the consistency of the mucus discharge so as to determine whether you are fertile or infertile.

You may already be aware that you normally have a vaginal discharge that varies throughout your menstrual cycle. You may notice nothing for several days and then suddenly experience a discharge—a bubbling sensation, a stickiness or a feeling of your vaginal lips being wet. This is caused by mucus, made in the cells of the cervical canal in response to your hormonal changes. Here is a brief outline of the relationship of mucus to fertility (see the chart on p. 256).

1. *Menstruation.* A cycle begins on the first day of your period. Because menstrual discharge may mask mucus discharge, the menstrual period is

---

*Depending on which method you use, write down the day of your cycle; whether you feel wet or dry; describe the color and consistency of any external mucus, your temperature and changes in your cervix.

*Adapted from S. Bell et al., "Reclaiming Reproductive Control: A Feminist Approach to Fertility Consciousness," *Science for the People,* Vol. 12, No. 1 (1980), pp. 6–9, 30–35.

not necessarily safe for unprotected intercourse or vagina-to-penis contact.

2. *Dry days after menses (if any).* Most women have several days of dryness (no mucus) after menses. You may have no sensation of discharge, no mucus present at the vaginal opening, no noticeable discharge on your underwear, and your labia feel dry. Alternate evenings of these preovulatory (before ovulation) dry days are safe for intercourse or vagina-to-penis contact. This allows a day after intercourse to ensure that seminal fluid is not masking the beginning of fertile mucus. This has been found to be the most effective way to use these days for intercourse.

Note: You will almost always find something resembling mucus if you look *inside* your vagina. The mucus that promotes sperm survival is fluid enough to flow to the *outside* and should be checked outside only.

3. *Mucus days.* Fertility begins as soon as mucus appears. This usually occurs after having several dry days, although mucus can also begin during your period. Your fertile time begins when you feel a sensation of discharge from the vagina, see it on your underwear or wipe it off with toilet paper or your fingers. The mucus usually starts off with a day or two of sticky mucus, which becomes increasingly creamy, wet, slippery and sometimes like egg white. It also becomes more fluid and thinner as ovulation approaches. Some women can take a sample and stretch it between two fingers. *As soon as* mucus appears, it nourishes and protects sperm until ovulation. Therefore, to prevent pregnancy, postpone intercourse or use barriers from the time mucus appears to the evening of the fourth day after it changes to dryness or an infertile type of mucus.

The last day of mucus with any fertile characteristics is called the *mucus peak day.* Ovulation occurs anywhere from two days before to two days after peak day. You are fertile from the time the mucus appears until the evening of the fourth day after peak. The number of fertile days varies from cycle to cycle, although they usually last six to twelve days (about one-third of the cycle).

4. *Postpeak (luteal) phase.* After the peak day, your mucus will undergo a distinct change: You may become dry again or develop a thicker (sticky, tacky or gummy) discharge. In either case, a change is evident. These dry or sticky days signal the beginning of the luteal phase, the ten to sixteen days of dryness before your next period arrives. From the fourth day past the peak day until your period begins, you cannot conceive.

These descriptions cover the general pattern most women have. Although every woman is unique and may differ slightly from the classic mucus pattern description, every woman can easily learn to recognize her own pattern.

If you have a vaginal infection, you may not be able to tell the difference between cervical mucus and the discharge from your infection or with any medication you are using to treat it. During this time, you should rely on other methods of contraception. If you do not check your mucus on a given day or if you do not know what type it is, you should consider yourself possibly fertile.

THE SYMPTOTHERMAL METHOD

The symptothermal method (STM) employs the use of BBT and cervical mucus observation. Some consider it to also include rhythm method use. However, because mucus gives more accurate information about preovulatory infertile and fertile times, rhythm is no longer used by most fertility awareness groups.

If using the STM, fertility begins and ends according to the mucus (see previous section). With BBT, temperatures are low before ovulation and higher afterward. By taking your temperature on a basal body thermometer (which measures in tenths of a degree) each morning at the same time and recording it on a chart, you will see that your temperature rises slightly following ovulation and stays high until menstruation begins. (It falls as your period starts and stays low until the next ovulation.) Your fertile time ends *either* on the fourth day after the mucus peak *or* on the evening of the third day in a row of elevated temperatures, whichever is later. (Elevated temperature means four-tenths of a degree Fahrenheit above the highest of at least six preovulation readings after the first four days of menstruation.)

Effectiveness

Some health professionals rate all natural methods of birth control as poor. In most cases, they have confused the word *natural* with the word *rhythm*. Recent studies (based on women avoiding all vagina-to-penis contact on fertile days) indicate that the ovulation method and STM can be extremely effective when taught carefully, understood thoroughly and used correctly. When used consistently and correctly, the ovulation method's failure rate is 3 percent and the STM's failure rate is 2 percent during their first year of use. When the ovulation method is not used consistently and correctly, that is, when women and their partners have intercourse or vagina-to-penis contact during the fertile time or when there is misunderstanding of the rules or disagreement between partners about how to use the method, it has a higher failure rate. Failure is also more likely during periods of stress. A recent reinterpretation of the World Health Organization clinical trial determined that the failure rate during typical use of the ovulation method is 20.4 percent.

You can use fertility observation to *increase* the effectiveness of the IUD and barrier methods by avoiding any vagina-to-penis contact on fertile days.

Reversibility

Excellent reversibility. Just have intercourse on fertile days.

Responsibility

Basically the responsibility is the woman's. It requires cooperation from the man.

Advantages

It has no negative effects.

Many of us enjoy being more aware of our body's cycles and have found this knowledge useful in making many other health care decisions.

It can lead, during fertile days, to exploration of other ways to give and receive pleasure, such as mutual masturbation and oral sex. (Be sure to avoid *all* vagina-to-penis contact.)

The cooperation necessary for this method can bring understanding and closeness between partners.

Disadvantages

The major disadvantage is the risk of pregnancy if you are not committed to using it correctly.

It does not protect you against STDs, including HIV infection.

Pill packets.   Elizabeth Cole

It takes at least two to three cycles to learn and use confidently.

It may be impractical if you are not in a committed, cooperative relationship with your sex partner.

If you choose not to use a barrier method and instead abstain from intercourse and vagina-to-penis contact when you are fertile, it can be sexually frustrating unless you enjoy other forms of sex.

Mechanization of Fertility Observation

Numerous machines and devices are being developed to measure hormonal changes and to pinpoint fertility. They are based on the same principles as the ovulation method and the STM, but they're more expensive without necessarily being more accurate.

ABSTINENCE

There is nothing wrong with abstinence. In fact, sometimes it is just what we want. Abstinence means making love without having intercourse. It is the most effective form of birth control, has been used for centuries and is still very common. It has no physical side effects as long as prolonged sexual arousal is followed by orgasm to relieve pelvic congestion. Take care not to have any vagina-to-penis contact, as sperm can move inside your vagina and eventually reach the ovum.

BIRTH CONTROL PILLS

The FDA approved the Pill for marketing in 1960 without adequate testing or study. A synthetic pill almost 100 percent effective in preventing pregnancy when taken daily, it created tremendous excitement among the medical, scientific, pharmaceutical and population-control communities. Although medical literature confirmed dangers of the original Pill as early as 1962, very few professionals cautioned against using it too widely or too quickly; to do so meant fighting against the prevailing ideology, which supported rapid development and distribution of new drugs generally, and risking the charge of holding back progress. To women, it seemed like a wonderful alternative to the methods then available.

The Pill became a gigantic experiment: Within two years about 1.2 million American women used it, and by 1973 the number rose to an estimated 10 million.

Many women first heard about the dangers of the high-dose estrogen pill, when they read Barbara Seaman's book, *The Doctor's Case Against the Pill*, published in 1969 and again, updated, in

→ sim.
to copper
of para-
+ (Cindy
Perkins)

1979 (New York: Dell). Many elected to stop taking the Pill or to find another alternative. Efforts by women and consumer activists in the late 1960s, along with well-publicized congressional hearings, led to modifications of the Pill as well as special patient package inserts; since 1978 the FDA has required physicians and pharmacists to hand out comprehensive information sheets on its possible negative effects and complications.

Because many of the most serious negative effects are associated with high dosages of estrogen, drug companies reduced the estrogen content of the Pill and also began to develop progestin-only pills. The National Women's Health Network cautions that although pills with lower dosages of estrogen do seem to be *safer* than the pills produced in the 1960s, there are no data to support the claim that pills in current use have all the *positive effects* and none of the negative effects of higher-dose pills. Fortunately, current research will be answering some important questions about the Pill's long-term effects.

How They Work

To understand how birth control pills work, you need to know how menstruation works. Chapter 12, "Anatomy and Physiology of Sexuality and Reproduction," and its appendix describe what hormones are and how the female hormones, estrogen and progesterone, guide a woman's menstrual cycle.

The way the most widely used pills (combination pills) work to prevent pregnancy is outlined in the chart on p. 281, which puts an average menstrual cycle and the Pill cycle side by side. It shows how the Pill interrupts your menstrual cycle by introducing synthetic versions of the female hormones.

Combination birth control pills prevent pregnancy primarily by inhibiting the development of the egg in the ovary. During your period, the low estrogen level normally indirectly triggers your pituitary gland to send out follicle-stimulating hormone (FSH), a hormone that starts an egg developing to maturity in one of your ovaries. The Pill gives you just enough synthetic estrogen to raise your estrogen level high enough to keep FSH from being released. So during a month on the Pill, your ovaries remain relatively inactive and there is no egg to join with sperm. This is the same principle by which a woman's body checks ovulation when she is pregnant: The corpus luteum and placenta put estrogen into her blood, thereby inhibiting FSH. So in a way, using much lower levels of hormones, the Pill simulates pregnancy, and some of the Pill's negative effects are like those of early pregnancy. If ovulation occurs, it is because your body needed a higher dose of estrogen

than your Pill gave you to inhibit FSH or because you have missed one or more pills.

Synthetic progesterone, called *progestin*, is used differently in different varieties of the Pill. Progestin provides important contraceptive effects including increased thickness of cervical mucus, incapacitation of sperm, slowed movement of the egg and incomplete development of the uterine lining. The progestin-only pills are not quite as effective as combination pills in preventing pregnancy.

The *biphasic combination pill* (Ortho-Novum 10/11) has a constant low dose of estrogen (thirty-five micrograms); it provides less progestin during the first ten days of the cycle (half a milligram) and more in the next ten days (one milligram).

In the *triphasic combination pill*, the amount of progesterone (Ortho-Novum 7-7-7, Tri-Norynl) or both estrogen and progesterone (Triphasil) varies during each third of the menstrual cycle. It has a lower dose of estrogen than other combination pills and a lower dose of progesterone than the progestin-only pills. In all triphasic pills the progesterone slowly increases throughout the cycle. In Triphasil, estrogen also increases at midcycle.

Combination Pills

Effectiveness

The combination pills have a very low expected pregnancy rate of 0.1 percent, but in typical use, they show a failure rate of 3 percent. Pregnancy is more likely if you forget to take your pill for one or more days, if you don't use a backup method of birth control for your first packet of pills, or while taking antibiotics or anticonvulsants when experiencing vomiting or diarrhea and occasionally when you change from one brand of pill to another. (Under these conditions, use a backup method of birth control for the rest of your cycle to prevent pregnancy.)

Reversibility

If you want to become pregnant, stop taking pills at the end of a packet. Most women soon become fertile again. It may be several months before your ovaries are functioning regularly, and your first non-Pill periods may be a week or two late or missed completely. If your periods were irregular before taking the Pill, especially if you are a teenager, you may have irregular periods for up to one year or longer when you stop. It is a good idea to use another method of birth control for six to twelve months after you go off the Pill to allow your body to return to normal before you try to get pregnant.

Most women do have successful pregnancies after they go off the Pill. However, on average it

WOMAN'S MENSTRUAL CYCLE AND THE WAY THE COMBINATION BIRTH CONTROL PILL AFFECTS THAT CYCLE TO PREVENT PREGNANCY

Normal Menstrual Cycle*	Menstrual Cycle with the Pill
Day 1. Menstrual period begins.	*Day 1.* Menstrual period begins.
Day 5. An egg in a follicle (pocket, sac) in one of your ovaries has begun to ripen to maturity. The egg starts developing in response to a hormonal message (FSH) from your pituitary gland, which in turn has been triggered indirectly by the low level of *estrogen* (an ovarian hormone) at the time of your period.	*Day 5.* Take your first pill. In the pill, you take two synthetic hormones every day: *estrogen* and *progestin* (synthetic progesterone). *Estrogen:* The pill contains more estrogen than there usually is in your body on day 5—enough to stop the usual message from your pituitary gland (FSH) for an egg to develop. By taking this amount of estrogen every day for twenty-one days, you prevent an egg from developing at all that month. Therefore there is no egg to join with the sperm.
Days 5 to 14. The follicle in which the egg is developing makes first a little, then more and more estrogen. **1.** *Estrogen* stimulates the lining of your uterus to get thicker and the cells of your cervix to produce mucus that is receptive to sperm. **2.** As estrogen increases, it slows down and then cuts off FSH.	*Progestin:* A little *progestin* every day provides three vital backup effects: **1.** It keeps the plug of mucus in your cervix thick and dry, so sperm have a hard time getting through. **2.** It keeps the lining of your uterus from developing properly so that if an egg does ripen (if estrogen level of pill is too low for you or if you forget a pill) and sperm do join with the egg, the fertilized egg will not be able to implant.
Day 14. Ovulation: Estrogen peak and a spurt of progesterone occurring during days 12 to 13 indirectly trigger ovulation. Ripe egg is released from ovary, starts four-day trip down fallopian tube to uterus. Conception with sperm from the man must occur in first twenty-four hours.	**3.** It inhibits activation of enzymes that permit sperm to unite with the egg.
Approximately days 14 to 26. The ruptured follicle, now called *corpus luteum* ("yellow body"), makes two hormones for about twelve days: *Estrogen* continues. *Progesterone* increases and peaks about day 22: **1.** It makes your cervical mucus (plug of mucus in cervix) thick and dry, a barrier to sperm. **2.** It stimulates the glands in lining of your uterus to secrete a sugary substance and further thickens the lining.	*Days 6 to 25.* Continue taking one pill a day.
Approximately days 26 to 27 to 28. If pregnancy is prevented successfully, *corpus luteum*'s manufacture of *estrogen* and *progesterone* slows down to a very low level. This drop creates an "appropriate environment for reducing the excess layers of" the tissue lining your uterus.‡	*Day 26.* Take your last pill.† *Days 27 to 28.* The sudden drop in *estrogen* and *progestin* creates an "appropriate environment for reducing the excess layers of" the tissue lining your uterus.‡
Approximately day 29 to day 1. Menstrual period begins. Low level of *estrogen* (see days 26 to 28) will begin indirectly to stimulate pituitary's egg-development hormone (FSH) to start a new cycle.	*Day 29 to Day 1.* Menstrual period begins. Your period is lighter than normal, because of effect 2 of progestin in the pill.

*This is a simplified version of the menstrual cycle. See the appendix to Chapter 12 for a more thorough description.
†With the 28-day combination pill, you take pills without hormones in them from day 27 to day 5.
‡Emily Martin, *The Woman in the Body.* Boston: Beacon Press, 1987. p. 52.

takes two or three months longer for them to conceive than women who have not taken the Pill; roughly one-quarter of the women who stop taking the Pill require at least one year to conceive. If you have not conceived within one year of trying after going off the Pill, you might want to seek medical assistance (see Chapter 22).

Safety

Many of us are uneasy about taking a medication that affects almost every organ in our bodies each day for months and years, because its effects have not been conclusively tested. Yet some of us choose to take whatever risks are involved because we want a highly effective method and absolutely don't want to become pregnant.

A great deal of information exists on both the benefits and adverse effects of the Pill, as the following pages demonstrate. In most cases of Pill-related injury or death, women had not been examined carefully enough by the doctor who prescribed the Pill for them, had taken the higher-dose Pill, had not had checkups while taking the Pill or had not been told that they had some particular risks. Some women ignored pains that were, in fact, warning signals and sought help too late.

How Long to Take the Pill

If you are not now experiencing problems, you may want to enjoy the freedom of the Pill indefinitely. Yet if you take the Pill for many years at a time, you are in a sense part of a huge experiment on the long-term effects of daily hormone ingestion in healthy women. Researchers disagree on how long a woman should stay on the Pill. Also, taking periodic breaks from the Pill does *not* appear to improve your future ability to have a baby. Once you pass forty, you are at higher risk of Pill-related death if you have an additional risk factor (see Who Should Absolutely Not Use the Pill). Some researchers believe that complications and problems increase the longer you take the Pill.

Going Off the Pill

It is a sad fact that many women get pregnant in the first few months after going off the Pill because they feel awkward using another method of birth control, especially one of the safer barrier methods. We need discussion, information and support in making the switch to another method. It helps to have a partner or partners who understand and appreciate our desire to change to a safer form of contraception.

Warning Signals

Any problem lasting more than two or three cycles should be reported to a physician or medical facility. The following are symptoms of serious problems: severe pain or swelling in the legs (thigh or calf), bad headache, dizziness, weakness, numbness, blurred vision (or loss of sight), speech problems, chest pain or shortness of breath, abdominal pain. *Report these immediately*, for they are signs of heart attack, stroke or liver tumors and mean you should stop taking the Pill. (*Note on leg pain:* Some leg cramps may be caused by fluid retention induced by the estrogen in the Pill. Don't confuse this with severe leg pain, but also don't hesitate to call a medical practitioner if your leg cramps become painful.)

Who Should Absolutely Not Use the Pill

The Pill is dangerous for certain women. The FDA requires drug companies to publish a list of contraindications and conditions that prohibit the use of the Pill and include the list with your package of pills. Do not use the Pill if you have

- *Any disease or condition associated with excess blood clotting.* Bad varicose veins, thrombophlebitis (clots in veins, frequently in the leg), pulmonary embolism (blood clot that has traveled to the lung, usually from the leg), stroke, heart disease or defect, coronary artery disease.
- *Hepatitis or other liver diseases.* As it is the liver that metabolizes sex steroids (progesterone and estrogen), no one with liver disease should take the Pill until the disease is cleared up. Use a good alternative method of contraception because pregnancy can be a great strain on the liver. A woman who has had jaundice during pregnancy should not use the Pill.
- *Liver tumors; undiagnosed abnormal genital bleeding; cancer of the breast or of the reproductive organs; pregnancy; previous cholestasis during pregnancy.*

Who Is Strongly Advised Not to Use the Pill

Women with the following conditions are strongly advised not to use the Pill.

- *Severe headaches.*
- *Hypertension.* A woman with high blood pressure (hypertension) or mild varicose veins must take the Pill with caution.
- *Congenital hyperbilirubinemia (Gilbert's disease).*
- *Mononucleosis in the acute phase.*
- *Elective major surgery planned in the next four weeks.*
- *Major surgery requiring immobilization.*
- *Long leg casts or major injury to the lower leg.*
- *Impaired liver function at the present time.*
- *Women over forty with a second risk factor, such as diabetes or high blood pressure.* They run a statistically higher risk of thromboembolism and other complications when taking the Pill. Because such risks also increase during pregnancy, women over forty should consider a barrier method or sterilization—tubal ligation for you or vasectomy for your partner.
- *Smokers.* Smokers, especially women who smoke fifteen or more cigarettes a day and are over thirty-five years old, run a statistically higher risk of stroke and heart attack on the Pill (see table, p. 264).

Who Should Probably Not Use the Pill

Women with the following situations or conditions should probably not use the Pill or only with regular consultation with their practitioners.

- *Diabetes, prediabetes or a strong family history of diabetes.* Sugar metabolism is extensively altered in women on the Pill. The progestin tends to bind the body's insulin and keep it out of circulation, which increases a diabetic woman's insulin requirement. If you have diabetes or if close relatives are diabetic, practitioners recommend that you take a low-dose Pill with norethindrone-type progestin and have regular blood tests. Many doctors do advise diabetic women to take the Pill because pregnancy is especially hazardous to them.

- *Gallbladder disease.*
- *Sickle cell anemia or trait.* Black women planning to go on the Pill should have a sickle cell test. If it is positive, you should discuss the hazards of going on the Pill, which include an increased risk of intravascular blood clotting.
- *Lactation.* The Pill may dry up the mother's supply of milk, especially if administered soon after she gives birth. Even if it does not dry it up, the Pill decreases the amounts of protein, fat and calcium in the milk. Some estrogen will also come through in the milk. At present this is a controversial subject, because no one knows the long-term effects of this substance on children.
- *Pregnancy ended within the past ten to fourteen days.**
- *Weight gain of ten pounds or more while taking the Pill.**
- *Cardiac or renal disease or a history of these diseases.**
- *Conditions likely to make a woman unreliable at following Pill instructions.* Major psychiatric problems, alcoholism and mental retardation.
- *Family history of hyperlipidemia.*
- *Family history of the death of a parent or sibling (especially a mother or sister) due to heart attack before age fifty.*

It may not be wise for women with the following conditions to take the Pill: depression,* chloasma, or hair loss related to pregnancy or a history of such;* asthma;* epilepsy;* uterine fibromyomata;* acne; varicose veins; history of hepatitis (except for hepatitis A and mononucleosis) but normal liver function tests for at least one year; a woman who is a DES daughter.

Complications and Negative Effects

The Pill enters our bloodstream, travels through the body and affects many tissues and organs, just as natural estrogens and progesterone do. However, the hormones in the Pill are synthetic and have exaggerated effects on some women.

Although there is an FDA-required package insert, health workers and doctors must clearly explain the risks we take in choosing the Pill. Unfortunately, they don't always know themselves. Also, they sometimes believe that effects are psychosomatic and that telling us what might happen will influence our perceptions. This attitude is insulting and dangerous. Find out what the risks are before you get a prescription for the Pill.

---

*Starred conditions are contraindications to combination pills and may not be contraindications to progestin-only pills or may be less of a contraindication to progestin-only pills.

Many of us experience none or only a few effects from using the Pill. Some women have pregnancy-like symptoms during the first three months, but after that they don't notice anything. Also, many women choose to put up with mild effects in exchange for the Pill's convenience and effectiveness. If you want to use it, try it for a few months to see how your body responds.

The Pill and Cardiovascular Disease—Heart Attack and Stroke

Cardiovascular disease (heart attacks, strokes, pulmonary embolisms, other clotting disorders) is responsible for most Pill-related deaths. (This may be related to higher triglyceride [blood fat] and cholesterol levels in Pill users.)[10] The risk of death from these diseases is higher among Pill users than among women who have never used it; the difference is more pronounced for women taking higher-dose pills, women over the age of thirty-five and women who smoke. (In other words, the risk of circulatory disease is low for nonsmokers who are healthy and younger than thirty-five if they take low-dose pills.) Recent studies show that the risk of cardiovascular disease is not related to the length of time that you use the Pill and disappears when you stop taking it.[11] See list at left for warning signals.

The Pill and High Blood Pressure

Less than 5 percent of women on the Pill will develop hypertension (abnormally high blood pressure) and will be at greater risk for heart attack and stroke. The incidence of high blood pressure is higher for older women and increases the longer women take the Pill. Women who develop hypertension should stop taking the Pill; within a few weeks of stopping, blood pressure usually returns to normal. Women with a family history of hypertension or who already have high blood pressure are strongly advised by practitioners to choose some other form of birth control.

The Pill and Cancer

The relationship between Pill use and cervical cancer is not entirely clear. A number of studies, however, suggest that there may be some connection between the Pill and certain forms of cervical cancer. Because of this, practitioners strongly recommend that women taking the Pill have a Pap smear every year.[12]

There may be a relationship between skin cancer and the Pill, although researchers disagree and are currently studying this.[13]

Researchers disagree about the relationship between the Pill and breast cancer. Most studies show that women who take the Pill are not more likely to develop breast cancer than women who do not. Three recent studies indicated that there may be an increased risk of breast cancer after long-term use of the Pill. However, well-respected studies do not support these findings. Important questions remain about the effects of using the low-dose pill, especially its use before a woman's first full-term pregnancy, for more than four to eight years, before the age of twenty-five, or by women who have fibrocystic breasts.[14]

The sequential pill (which has been removed from the market) has been linked to cancer of the uterus. Several recent studies show that the high-dosage pill *protects* women from endometrial and ovarian cancer and that this protection lasts for at least fifteen years after they stop taking it. However, there are as yet no data showing that the low-dose pill offers the same protection.[15]

The Pill and Your Present or Future Children

Sex malformation or cardiac defects *do not* appear to be more common among babies of mothers who were taking the Pill while pregnant or who became pregnant within three months of stopping the Pill. They *do* appear to be more common among babies of mothers who smoke and were taking the Pill while pregnant. (They are also more common among those whose mothers took DES to prevent miscarriages. See Chapter 24.)

Don't use the Pill while breastfeeding (see p. 480).

Children who find pills and eat them may become nauseated. We do not know what harm this may cause. You should go to or call a medical facility if your child swallows more than a few pills.

Other Effects

Headaches
Around 5 percent of women on the Pill develop severe, recurrent or persistent headaches or more severe migraines.

Migraines are throbbing headaches that result from a problem in the circulation of blood to the brain. Migraines are painful. Further, *migraines can be a warning signal for impending stroke* and should cause a woman to switch to a lower-dose estrogen pill or to stop taking pills altogether.

Diabetes
In some women, the Pill, like pregnancy, can affect glucose tolerance (see also Who Should Probably Not Use the Pill, p. 282).

Depression
Possibly one in four women are more irritable, anxious or depressed on the Pill. These symptoms often continue instead of improving with succeeding cycles. Switching to a lower-dose pill may help. Vitamin B$_6$ supplementation can also help

(see p. 286). If you have serious depression, stop taking the Pill.

Change in Intensity of Sexual Desire and Response
Many women feel and act sexier as soon as their fear of pregnancy is removed. But some women on progestin-dominant, low-dosage estrogen pills don't feel like making love, orgasm less easily and complain about dry vaginas and less sensation in the vulva.

Nausea
This is a common early negative effect of the Pill. The estrogen in the Pill may irritate your stomach lining or make you feel sick to your stomach, just like a pregnant woman whose body is getting used to the high levels of estrogen that the placenta puts into her blood. Nausea usually goes away after three months; antacid tablets or taking the Pill with dinner usually gives relief and so does switching to a pill with twenty micrograms of estrogen (e.g., LoEstrin).

Vaginitis and Vaginal Discharge
Vaginitis is a vaginal inflammation that may be caused by infection with a fungus, trichomoniasis, bacteria or a virus. The Pill changes the normal vaginal environment. Its effect on vaginitis is unclear. It makes women more susceptible to chlamydia. Pills with high doses of estrogen make the vagina more susceptible to the yeast monilia (*Candida albicans*); lower-dose pills seem to have little or no effect. Vaginitis is treatable, but if it persists you may have to go off the Pill. Increased vaginal discharge is fairly common, can be due to estrogen and does not necessarily indicate infection—though if it is bothering you, you should have it checked.

Urinary Tract Infection
Some reports indicate that women on the Pill tend to have more infections of the bladder and urethra, the tube that leads urine out of your body.[16] More recent studies do not support this finding.

Changes in Menstrual Flow
Your periods will be lighter with most pills (estrogenic pills cause more normal flow). Occasionally your flow will be very slight or you will miss a period. If this happens and you have missed any pills or were late starting your pill pack, have a pregnancy test. Missing a period when you haven't missed a pill does not necessarily mean you are pregnant; sometimes it is due to taking pills for a long time or taking progestin-only pills. If you miss two periods in a row, consult a practitioner and have a pregnancy test.

Breakthrough Bleeding

This is vaginal bleeding or staining between periods. If there isn't enough estrogen or progestin in the pills you are taking to support the lining of your uterus at a given point in your cycle, a little of the lining will slough off. (This may also occur if you miss a pill.) With combination pills, it usually happens in your first or second pill cycle and often clears up after that, as your uterus gets used to the new levels of hormones. If breakthrough bleeding doesn't stop after a few months, see a practitioner to find out whether you need to try a different brand or whether you may have another problem. With progestin-only pills, this is very common. Breakthrough bleeding does not mean that the Pill isn't working as a contraceptive.

Breast Changes

Increased breast tenderness or fullness may occur, but it usually lasts for only the first three cycles. Switching to a pill with only twenty micrograms of estrogen can offer relief.

Skin Problems

The Pill may be associated with eczema, urticaria (hives or rashes) and, more rarely, chloasma, changes in skin pigmentation, sometimes described as "giant freckles" or pregnancy mask.

The progestin-dominant pill can cause or increase skin oiliness in some women. An estrogenic pill can decrease acne.

Gum Inflammation

The Pill, like pregnancy, can cause gum inflammation. Women on the Pill should brush their teeth extra carefully, use dental floss regularly and see a dentist every six months to a year.

Liver and Gallbladder Disease

The Pill is associated with an increased incidence of gallbladder disease and of liver tumors (both benign and malignant). Jaundice may be an early symptom of liver complications, so at the first sign of jaundice you should stop taking the Pill. Benign liver tumors are rare, but they can increase rapidly in size and may rupture spontaneously.

Epilepsy and Asthma

The Pill can aggravate existing epilepsy and asthma. Low-estrogen pills should be used, and the woman should stay under close medical supervision.

Virus Infections

A slightly higher incidence of bronchitis and viral illnesses among Pill users suggests that the Pill may affect your body's immunity.

Cervical Dysplasia

This problem, growth of abnormal cells on the cervix, is more common in women using oral contraceptives than in women not using the Pill.

Other Problems

The Pill also has been linked to pleurisy; suppression of bone growth in young women; arthritic symptoms (swelling of joints); visual disturbances, including discomfort or corneal damage among contact lens wearers; ulcers in the mouth; bruising; antagonism with Rifampin, a drug for tuberculosis, so that neither works as it should; lupus erythematosus, a disease of unknown origin that may be caused by an allergic reaction; abdominal cramping during the first three months; changes in thyroid function; photodermatitis (sunlight sensitivity with hypopigmentation); one form of hair loss, called alopecia; excessive hair growth (hirsutism); benign growths consisting of muscular tissue; autophonia, an ear or nasal disorder that causes increased resonance of your voice, breath sounds and so on; cervical ectropion, making a woman more vulnerable to chlamydia (most studies have found an increased risk of cervical infections with chlamydia among Pill users). There is no conclusive proof that the Pill causes these effects; nevertheless, if you should encounter one of these problems, consider that it might be connected with taking the Pill.

Beneficial Effects

Besides greater freedom from pregnancy, the Pill has a number of beneficial effects. Women taking it have shorter menstrual periods with less bleeding and cramping. Premenstrual tension tends to decrease. Iron deficiency anemia is less likely, probably because of decreased menstrual flow. Benign breast growths are less frequent. The Pill also protects against PID and probably protects against ovarian and endometrial cancer and functional ovarian cysts.

Nutrition and the Pill

The Pill alters the nutritional requirements of women who take it, which may contribute to some of the complications and negative effects. Pill use has been linked to increased requirements for vitamins C, B_2 (riboflavin), B_{12} and especially B_6 (pyridoxine) and folic acid (folate or folacin). Women who face the greatest nutritional risks are teenagers, poor women, women recovering from a recent illness or surgery or who have just given birth and women who have taken the Pill for two years or more who take brands with moderate to high estrogen levels. Because metabolic changes occur within the first few months after beginning the Pill, it is a good idea to have a physical exam and blood tests after you have used the Pill for six months and suspect you have any particular deficiencies.

Studies show that women on the Pill may have impaired glucose tolerance tests. This means that their carbohydrate metabolism is adversely affected, resulting in weight gain and/or elevated glucose and insulin levels (ranging from mild to diabetic). These alterations are most often seen when women take combination pills, especially those containing seventy-five micrograms or more of estrogen. Trying a low-dosage pill and eating wholesome foods may help to decrease glucose and insulin levels.[17]

While on the Pill, try to maintain a healthy nutritional balance:

1. Eat wholesome foods—especially those containing complex carbohydrates.
2. Reduce sugar intake.
3. Take vitamins, especially B-complex (but less than twenty-five to fifty milligrams of B_6 per day), C supplements and folic acid.

Doing the same thing for a few months after you stop taking the Pill is also a good idea, especially if you plan to become pregnant. A higher than average number of women who conceived within four months after discontinuing the Pill developed folic acid and B_6 deficiencies during pregnancy.

Water Metabolism and Weight Gain

The Pill alters water metabolism. Estrogen can cause weight gain due to increased breast, hip or thigh tissue, usually after several months on the Pill. Both the estrogen and progestin in pills can cause fluid retention, a temporary and usually cyclic effect that usually begins in the first month as a result of increased sodium. You may experience swollen ankles, breast tenderness, discomfort with contact lenses or a weight gain of up to five pounds. Changing to a pill with lower amounts of progestin or estrogen or reducing your salt intake moderately are ways of controlling water retention. (Diuretics are risky, so discontinue Pill use if the above methods do not work.)

Progestin-dominant pills (Ortho-Novum, Norlestrin, Ovral) can cause appetite increase and permanent weight gain because of the buildup of protein in muscular tissue. If you want to gain weight, this is helpful. Pill-related depression may also lead to increased appetite and weight gain.

How to Get Pills

As we have seen, certain physical conditions make taking birth control pills very dangerous, so *it is in your vital interest to have a careful exam before taking pills.* Don't borrow them from a friend. Be sure a health practitioner gives you an internal pelvic exam, breast exam, eye exam, Pap smear and blood pressure, blood and urine tests. The interview should include questions about you and your family's medical history of breast cancer, blood clots, diabetes, migraines and so on. If you were born between 1945 and 1970, find out if your mother took DES while she was pregnant. If so, you should have a colposcopy test because you might have adenosis, a condition that the Pill can aggravate (see the section on DES in Chapter 24). *Too many people prescribe and use birth control pills hurriedly; make sure you are carefully checked for each one of the contraindications.* When you are on the Pill, you should have an exam once a year.

How to Use Pills

Monophasic combination pills come in packets of twenty-one or twenty-eight pills. With the former, you take one pill a day for twenty-one days and then stop for seven days, during which time you will menstruate. With twenty-eight-day pills, which give you twenty-one hormone pills followed by seven different-colored placebos (without drugs), you take one pill a day with no pause between packets. You will have your period during the time that you are taking the seven different-colored pills. The twenty-eight-day pill is good if you feel you would have trouble remembering the on-and-off schedule of the twenty-one-day pill. There is no medical difference between them.

Most pill regimens start the first pill on the fifth day after your period starts, counting the day you start your period as day 1. (Some pills start on the first Sunday after your period comes or on the first day your period begins.) Take one pill at approximately the same time each day. If you feel nausea, take the pill with a meal or after a snack at bedtime. Here is an almost foolproof schedule: Take a pill at bedtime, check the packet each morning to make sure you've taken a pill the night before and carry a spare packet of pills with you in case you get caught away from home or lose pills. *Read the directions carefully.*

If You Forget a Pill

Take the forgotten pill as soon as you remember it, and take the next pill at its appointed time, even if this means taking two pills in one day. If you forget two pills, take two pills as soon as you remember, then take two pills the next day to catch up and use an additional method of contraception (foam, condoms) for the rest of that cycle. You may have some spotting. If you forget three pills or more, withdrawal bleeding will probably begin, so act as though you are at the end of a cycle. Don't make up the missed pills; stop taking your pills and start using a second method of birth control immediately. Start a new package of pills the Sunday after you realized you missed three or more pills, even if you are bleeding. Use an extra method of birth control from the day you realize you forgot the pills through two weeks of the next cycle.

If you miss a pill or two and skip a period, start using another method of birth control and get a pregnancy test. If you've been taking your pills correctly and you skip a period, it is unlikely that you are pregnant, but you may need a different brand of pill.

Protection

Your first packet of pills may not protect you completely, as an egg may have started to develop before you take the first pill. To be safe, use another method of birth control for the first two weeks. After this, you will be protected against pregnancy all month long, even during the days between packets. If you are taking antibiotics for an acute infection, or if you get sick and have vomiting or diarrhea, you should use another method of birth control for the rest of the cycle to be safe.

Responsibility

Birth control pills are primarily the woman's responsibility. You see the doctor, get examined, remember to take the pill, feel the effects and run the risks.

Advantages

You have almost complete protection against unwanted pregnancy.

Regularity of menstrual cycles—a period every twenty-eight days.

About 50 percent reduction in risk of PID.

Lighter flow during periods. This effect pleases most women, bothers some.

Relief of premenstrual tension.

Fewer menstrual cramps or none at all.

An estrogenic pill will clear up acne for some women.

You may enjoy sex more because the fear of pregnancy is gone.

Taking the Pill has no immediate physical relationship to lovemaking, which is especially relaxing if you are just starting to have intercourse and have a lot to learn about your body and a man's. Later on, when you are more comfortable with sex and more able to communicate openly with your partner(s), the interruptions involved in using a diaphragm or foam and condoms may not seem so prohibitive.

Disadvantages

Most of the disadvantages have been described under the section on effects. The only one to add is that you do have to remember to take a pill every day. Some women are forgetful or live lives that are too chaotic for them to remember to do so. Younger women who live at home and feel a need to hide their pills from their parents sometimes leave them behind or are unable to take them on time.

Differences Among the Several Brands of Pills

How do you and your medical practitioner determine which pill you should take? Be aware that different pills have different kinds, strengths and quantities of synthetic estrogen and progesterone in them. Pills with less than fifty micrograms of estrogen are associated with a significantly lower incidence of serious negative effects and are as effective as the higher-dose pills. Use of high-dose pills is much less common and the FDA recommends that companies stop marketing them. In 1987, only 3 percent of all prescriptions for the Pill were written for brands with more than fifty micrograms of estrogen. Practitioners have been prescribing pills with lower and lower doses of estrogen. Today, they typically begin by prescribing pills with thirty-five micrograms of estrogen. In addition, with more information about negative effects caused by progestin, practitioners often begin by prescribing pills with one microgram or less of progestin.

Monophasic combination pills containing thirty-five micrograms or less of estrogen are Loestrin 1.5/30, Loestrin 1/20, Lo/Ovral, Brevicon, Modicon, Ovcon-35, Norinyl 1 + 35, Ortho-Novum 1/35, Demulen 35 and Nordette. The lowest-dose pills are Loestrin 1/20, Brevicon, Modicon and Ovcon-35. Pills with less than thirty micrograms of estrogen (Loestrin 1/20) produce more spotting between periods. Biphasic or triphasic combination pills with thirty-five micrograms of estrogen are Ortho-Novum 10/11, Ortho-Novum 7/7/7, Tri-Norinyl, Tri-Levlen and Triphasil.

The effects of a particular pill are related to the amount and potency of the progestin relative to the estrogen in that pill. The low-dose pills producing the most androgenic (male) effects—for example, hairiness, acne and permanent weight gain—contain norgestrel (Nordette, Lo/Ovral). Low-dose pills producing the least androgenic effects contain norethindrone (Ovcon-35, Modicon, Brevicon).

It is not always possible to predict the estrogen or progestin potency by the dose, because the synthetic compounds vary in potency and effect. Also, each woman's body has its own normal estrogen and progesterone levels. You and your medical practitioner may want to experiment with different brands to minimize undesirable effects.

Progestin-Only Pills

Progestin-only pills are sometimes called *minipills*, but this term will not be used here in order to avoid confusion with the low-dose estrogen combination pill and with a pill that was taken off the market several years ago. Less than 8 percent of all women taking birth control pills take progestin-only pills.

Description

These pills contain small doses of the same progestins available in combination pills. Micronor and Nor-Q-D each provide 0.35 milligram of norethindrone, and Ovrette provides 0.075 milligram of norgestrel. They contain no estrogen. You take one a day continuously, starting on day 1 of your period, at the same time each day (particularly important), without stopping during your period, which may come irregularly.

Progesterone changes cervical mucus so that it blocks sperm, inhibits the egg's travel through the tubes, partially inhibits the sperm's ability to join with the egg and partially inhibits implantation. You may feel safer taking them knowing they have no estrogen and a very small dose of progestin and that they may have about the same rate of effectiveness as an IUD. On the other hand, the irregular cycles may get you down, or you may not wish to be one of the testers of a very new pill.

Effectiveness

The lowest expected pregnancy rate is 1 to 1.25 percent, higher than the combination pill. The typical failure rate is 3.0 percent. The pregnancy rate may be lower for women who switch from the combination pill to the progestin-only pill than it is for women have never taken the combination pill. Pregnancy rates are highest in the first six months, so using an additional method of contraception during this period is reasonable.

Contraindications

Women who absolutely should not take combination pills (see p. 282) should absolutely not take progestin-only pills. Women with the following conditions are strongly advised not to take progestin-only pills: acute mononucleosis, history of functional ovarian cysts or ectopic pregnancy, inability to take pills consistently and correctly, unexplained abnormal bleeding in the past three months, severe headaches, hypertension, elective major surgery or surgery requiring immobilization in the next four weeks, long-leg cast or major injury to lower leg.

Possible Effects

The progestin-only pills were developed in part to avoid estrogen-associated complications. Some women who had estrogen-related problems while taking combination pills are now using progestin-only pills. However, some of the negative effects seen with the combination pill also occur but are less common with the progestin-only pill: head-aches, change in weight, cervical erosion and change in cervical secretion, jaundice, allergic skin rash, chloasma, depression, gastrointestinal disturbances and breast changes. There may also be an increased risk of ectopic pregnancy. A common complaint is that menstrual bleeding is very irregular in amount and duration of flow and length of cycle.

RESEARCH AND DEVELOPMENT OF SYNTHETIC HORMONES

Most money for contraceptive research goes into projects to develop variations on the Pill that introduce synthetic hormones into a woman's body. We should view all of them *extremely cautiously* and judge them in light of lessons that we've learned from the Pill. Most likely, once the FDA approves a new product for marketing, it will be advertised widely as both safe and effective. But because all of these products are new, their long-term effects are *unknown*. Some products being developed are a once-a-month pill, progestin-coated vaginal rings and cervical devices.

Research is also being conducted on ways to synthesize a brain hormone, luteinizing hormone-releasing hormone (LHRH), to inhibit ovulation. LHRH acts directly on the pituitary gland to suppress fertility. Like other new hormone products, its long-term and short-term risks are unknown.

NORPLANT

Description

Norplant is a long-lasting contraceptive implant that is inserted in the fleshy part of a woman's upper arm, just under the skin, by a qualified, specially trained practitioner. It consists of six match-size flexible Silastic rubber capsules, each containing the synthetic progestin levonorgestrel, which is present in some birth control pills. This hormone is released slowly through the walls of the capsules until the capsules are removed. The capsules can be felt and sometimes can be noticed as ridges or bumps. Norplant is designed to last for up to five years.

How Norplant Works

No one completely understands how Norplant prevents pregnancy, although it is probably through a combination of inhibition of ovulation (so eggs are not released by the ovaries) and thickening of the cervical mucus (which impedes sperm activity). Other mechanisms may add to these contraceptive effects.

A set of six Norplant capsules.   The Population Council

Norplant begins working within twenty-four hours of insertion and provides highly effective protection from pregnancy for up to five years. After that, effectiveness is significantly reduced, and there is an increased risk of ectopic pregnancy, so that the capsules must be removed after five years. A new set can be implanted or another birth control method chosen if a woman still wants to avoid pregnancy.

Effectiveness

Norplant is extremely effective. The pregnancy rate is 0.2 percent in the first year of use, 0.5 percent for the second year, 1.2 percent for the third year and 1.6 percent for the fourth year. The overall pregnancy rate for five years of continuous use is 3.9 percent.

Women who weigh over 154 pounds have an increased risk of pregnancy beginning in the third year of use. This group of women can expect a 5.1 percent pregnancy rate after three years of use in comparison to a 1.2 percent pregnancy rate for all women.

Reduced Norplant effectiveness has been reported for women taking phenytoin (Dilantin) or carbamazepine, which are antiseizure drugs. If you take any prescription drugs, ask your practitioner if there is new information about the possibility of drug interactions.

Reversibility

Norplant can be removed at any time (although cost factors and the availability of a trained prac-

titioner may determine how freely a woman can make this choice). The pregnancy rates for women who have Norplant removed (and do not use any other method of contraception) are comparable to the pregnancy rates of women using no contraception. For Norplant, about 40 percent of women become pregnant in three months, and about 77 percent within one year.

Safety and Possible Problems

As of late 1991 more than 55,000 women in fifty countries had used Norplant in various studies, some lasting more than five years. (Outside of clinical trials about a million women have used this method.) Although accumulated data are still insufficient to detect rare or long-term adverse effects, there is no evidence of cardiovascular, respiratory or central nervous system problems in the short term. Also, the hormone found in Norplant has been used in combined oral contraceptives for over twenty years.

Because the long-term safety of Norplant has not been established, the National Women's Health Network opposed Norplant's approval by the FDA in 1990. At the same time, the reality remains that long-term safety of a hormonal method such as this one cannot be measured except through careful postmarketing studies. Furthermore, controlled clinical trials do not tell us about problems that might occur under ordinary, less rigorous circumstances.

Postmarketing surveillance of Norplant use is essential to learn more about possible long-term problems. Wyeth-Ayerst, the U.S. distributor, is required by law to report any unusual events associated with Norplant use to the FDA. In addition, since 1988 the World Health Organization (Geneva, Switzerland), the Population Council (New York City) and Family Health International (North Carolina) have been monitoring Norplant use in the first internationally coordinated surveillance of a contraceptive in developing countries. Their study involves sites in Bangladesh, Chile, China, Colombia, Egypt, Indonesia, Sri Lanka and Thailand.

In general, progestin-based birth control methods are not the first choice for breastfeeding women compared to nonhormonal methods. However, some nursing mothers do use Norplant, *but not earlier than six weeks after childbirth.* So far, studies have shown no major effects on the growth or health of infants whose mothers used Norplant beginning six weeks *after* childbirth. (In contrast, estrogen-based contraceptives should *never* be used by nursing mothers.)

Studies show no increased risk of birth defects in the infants of women who have used birth control pills prior to becoming pregnant, and there is no evidence suggesting that this risk is any different with Norplant use. There has been only one known instance of a birth defect, when a boy in one study was born with ambiguous genitalia. Although this condition was most likely *not* caused by Norplant, women who become pregnant while using Norplant should have their implants removed if they want to continue the pregnancy. A woman who becomes pregnant and chooses to have an abortion should discuss the question of Norplant removal with her practitioner.

Although Norplant does affect thyroid and adrenal functioning, lipid and lipoprotein metabolism and blood sugar level, so do oral contraceptives (the Pill), which sometimes produce greater changes. The long-term cardiovascular effects of Norplant are unknown. Because most birth control pills contain four to five times the level of progestin than is present in Norplant, it is assumed that progestin-related problems would be fewer with Norplant, which presents the lowest possible exposure to a hormone of any hormonal-based method.

Who Shouldn't Use Norplant

Women should not use Norplant if they have or have had blood-clotting problems, heart disease or stroke, acute liver disease (or liver tumors) or breast cancer (confirmed or suspected). In addition, women who suspect they may be pregnant, who are breastfeeding infants younger than six weeks or who have undiagnosed abnormal vaginal bleeding should not use Norplant. Because it is not known whether progestin-only contraceptives, such as Norplant, increase the risk of serious cardiovascular problems for cigarette smokers, it is advisable for women smokers to avoid Norplant or to quit smoking before using Norplant.

Conditions That May Make Norplant a Riskier Choice

Women should check in regularly with their health-care provider if they choose to use Norplant and have any of the following conditions: diabetes; high levels of cholesterol or triglycerides; high blood pressure; migraines or other headaches; epilepsy; abnormal mammogram; fibrocystic breasts; breast nodules; mental depression; gallbladder, heart or kidney disease.

How to Get Norplant

Many doctors, nurse-practitioners and family-planning clinics now offer or will offer Norplant. Make sure you get Norplant from someone who has had special training in how to insert the capsules, because improper insertion can make removal quite difficult. Ask your provider if s/he has attended a training course for insertion and removal of the implants or for referral to someone who has. Get as much information as possible *beforehand* and make sure that removal will be available on demand and for a fee you can afford.

Norplant should be inserted within seven days after a woman's period begins (to ensure she is not pregnant) and under sterile conditions (to avoid the possibility of infection). A local anesthetic is injected into the arm and may cause some initial pain. After a small incision is made, the six small capsules are placed one at a time, through this incision, just under the skin and in a fan shape. The procedure, done in a clinic or office, should take no longer than ten to fifteen minutes but may take more time in rare cases when there are problems. The incision is covered with a protective bandage that can be removed after a few days. Discoloration, bruising and swelling may occur in the area of the capsules for several days.

When in place Norplant should *not* cause pain or discomfort for more than a day or two. If there is pain, see your Norplant provider to make sure an infection is not present.

Cost

In late 1991, Wyeth-Ayerst, the U.S. distributor of Norplant, charged all purchasers (clinics, hospitals and practitioners) the same fee for one Norplant set (plus a few other items packaged along with the capsules): $350. Despite many pleas to adopt a public sector price for family-planning clinics that serve low-income women, Wyeth-Ayerst has refused to do so as of late 1991. (The company did agree, however, to set up a special fund to reimburse doctors and clinics for Norplant given to low-income women. How much this will help remains to be seen.) By October 1991, forty-eight states and the District of Columbia were providing Medicaid coverage for the implants and practitioner fees, as were over 400 insurance plans and 35 of the largest health maintenance organizations in the country.

In contrast, the U.S. Agency for International Development was able to purchase Norplant for use in so-called developing countries for only $23 per set from Leiras Pharmaceuticals. This Finland-based company, which manufactures Norplant, was able to obtain the marketing rights for Norplant outside the United States in part because of their agreement with the Population Council, the developers of Norplant, to offer a public sector price.

Norplant's actual cost to women can be higher,

because hospital pharmacies may mark up the price $50 to $75 more. In addition, there is the cost of insertion, with some doctors charging as much as $150 to $200. Removal will cost an additional $70 to $150. In 1991, the median physician fee for implants plus insertion was about $528.

If used for five years, Norplant will cost $500 to $700, while five years of birth control pills will cost $1000 to $1200. However, if used for only one year, Norplant is two to three times more expensive than birth control pills would be. It also involves a large one-time up-front expense, whereas the purchase of pills is spread out over a long period. (Please note that women who want birth control for only one year probably should not use Norplant, but there are times when a woman unexpectedly will discontinue the method.)

An additional cost for women who experience unpredictable bleeding with Norplant (see below) is the expense of panty liners or sanitary pads.

Removal

Norplant capsules should be removed at the end of five years, although they can be removed earlier at your request. Make sure your provider is trained in performing removals; if not, ask to be referred to a trained provider. By the end of 1992, there should be trained practitioners in most parts of the United States.

Removal is more difficult than insertion. Although removal can be a simple process taking no more than fifteen to twenty minutes, complications do occur in rare cases. In some studies, one or more of the capsules could not be removed with the first attempt and required a return visit. The Population Council reported that such problematic removals occurred in 7 percent of the cases in controlled clinical trials (many of which took place outside the United States). The rate of problem removals in the United States will depend upon the quality of services women can obtain.

Key to successful removal is proper insertion. When the capsules become embedded in deeper tissue, they are harder to remove. Some women develop more scar tissue around the capsules than other women.

After removal, a woman should keep the insertion site clean, dry and bandaged for at least several days to avoid the possibility of infection.

Care

No special care is necessary for Norplant, although a woman should not wet, bump or strain the insertion site for a few days after the procedure.

Complications and Negative Effects

- *Irregular bleeding.* The most common problem associated with Norplant is erratic, unpredictable bleeding. In the first year of use about 75 percent of Norplant users report some irregularity in menstruation, from amenorrhea (no bleeding) to excessive bleeding (but rarely enough blood loss to produce anemia). Bleeding irregularities usually decrease during the first year of use. For many women, their periods return on a regular basis. If regular periods do return and then a woman misses a period, she should get a pregnancy test.

  Irregular bleeding is the most common reason given for discontinuing Norplant use. This sometimes requires frequent use of menstrual pads. You should consider the importance of this likely inconvenience in making a decision about trying Norplant. Some clinics recommend that a woman try a month or two of the progestin-only pill (see Progestin-Only Pills, p. 287) before using Norplant. If irregular bleeding should occur and be too disruptive, then Norplant might be a poor choice for her.

- *Headaches, acne, weight changes and breast tenderness.* All of these are common effects of Norplant (and any other hormone-containing method of birth control). Weight gain is far more common than weight loss. Depression, nervousness, hairiness and nausea are also associated with Norplant use. Although usually not severe, sometimes these problems are disruptive enough to make a woman seek Norplant removal.

- *Functional ovarian cysts.* Norplant use increases the risk of functional ovarian cysts, which are usually symptom-free but may cause lower abdominal pain. These cysts usually go away spontaneously but do require surgery on rare occasions.

When to Seek Help

Women using Norplant should get medical attention if they experience any of the following problems: severe lower abdominal pain (a possible sign of ectopic pregnancy), heavy vaginal bleeding, arm pain, pus or bleeding at the insertion site, expulsion of an implant (when the implant comes out—very rare), jaundice, delayed menstrual period after a long interval of regular periods, migraine headaches or blurred vision.

Although pregnancy is rare among Norplant users, when it does occur, it is an ectopic pregnancy about 15 percent of the time. However, the rate of ectopic pregnancy has been only 1.3 per 1000 woman-years of Norplant use, which is much lower than the rate estimated for women in the United States who use no contraception (2.7 to 3.0 per 1000 woman-years).

Advantages

Norplant is highly effective, long lasting and easily reversible (assuming that removal is problem-free), doesn't interrupt lovemaking and enables women to avoid the negative effects of estrogen, which is found in all combination birth control pills. It also doesn't require a woman to do anything on a regular basis (like remember to take a pill). For some women, decreased menstrual bleeding is an advantage as well.

For women who do not want to have any more children, Norplant will offer an important alternative to sterilization.

Disadvantages

The complications and negative effects described above are, of course, possible disadvantages. Some African-American women who tend to form keloids (excessive growth of scar tissue on the skin) have expressed concern that Norplant may trigger even further keloid formation. This needs to be studied more. Also, Norplant does not provide any protection against STDs, including HIV infection.

Norplant's most serious disadvantage may be its provider dependence; that is, the method is not fully in the control of the woman who uses it, as is also true with the IUD and long-term injectable methods. Like the IUD, Norplant must be inserted and removed by a practitioner. As such, the method may be misused as a tool of social control over women.

In some developing countries, already there have been reports of women who sought and were unable to obtain removal of Norplant. Even when removal was not refused, there were cases in which personnel trained in the removal technique were simply not available. This underscores the importance of having an adequate system of family-planning or health care services in order to provide Norplant appropriately.

Although these two problems are far less likely to occur in the United States, misuse is possible in other ways. For example, a legislator in Kansas has proposed that mothers receiving welfare benefits be offered a payment of $500 for using Norplant. In California, a judge made Norplant use a condition of probation (an alternative to imprisonment) for a woman convicted of abusing her children. This decision, made without consideration of her medical status, was subsequently appealed. Such controversial or unethical uses of Norplant may well become a reality in this country, especially among poorer women and women of color, unless there is strong and outspoken op-

position to each and every proposal to misuse Norplant.

Responsibility

A woman bears the total responsibility for Norplant use. However, men can take responsibility for STD (including HIV) prevention by using condoms.

A woman must remember to remove Norplant after five years if she does not remove it sooner. Experience in other countries already demonstrates that some women will forget to have it removed. In our mobile society, it may be difficult for clinics and other providers to follow women for five years to remind them about removal if that should be necessary.

Each woman who uses Norplant should be given a card with the date of insertion and the date by which she should have the implants removed. She should keep this card with her medical records. Her practitioner should also note these dates on her medical records kept in the office or clinic.

DEPO-PROVERA AND OTHER INJECTABLE CONTRACEPTIVES

Depo-medroxy progesterone acetate (DMPA), better known as Depo-Provera or "the shot," is a long-acting synthetic hormone (progesterone) used as an injectable contraceptive in over ninety countries. It is manufactured and distributed by the Upjohn Company. It suppresses ovulation, at least to some extent, makes cervical mucus unable to support sperm survival and makes the lining of the uterus unsuitable for implantation. It is usually given as an injection every three months and is about as effective as the combination pill.

Although the FDA has refused for many years to approve DMPA for contraceptive use in the United States, the drug has been on the market for several other approved uses (for example, the treatment of uterine cancer). Because DMPA is available, some physicians have chosen to use it as a contraceptive. However, some do not follow informed consent procedures, so women may not understand fully what they are getting.*

Safety

According to current evidence, DMPA causes fewer major health problems than the Pill. However, women can experience serious problems

---

*The practice of prescribing drugs for *nonapproved* uses is legal, but physicians who do this are supposed to obtain signed consent forms demonstrating that the drug's unapproved status, as well as potential risks, are known to the woman.

with DMPA, including extreme weight gain, hair loss, severe depression, acne and very heavy periods, irregular periods or no periods at all.

In one ten-year study of fifty-two rhesus monkeys, two monkeys developed uterine cancer. Studies of women indicate that DMPA does not increase liver or ovarian cancer (it is protective against endometrial cancer). It may increase the risk of cervical cancer but does not increase the risk of breast cancer among women who have used DMPA for a long period of time and who were followed up to a decade after use was discontinued.[18]

Immediately after a DMPA injection, a woman has very high levels of the drug in her bloodstream and, if lactating, in her breast milk. Although we have little long-term evidence establishing the safety of DMPA for breast-feeding infants, Upjohn has at times marketed DMPA in some Third World countries as the "ideal contraceptive for lactating women."

Reversibility

Although most studies indicate that ovulation resumes within one year after discontinuing DMPA injections, there have not been enough studies to prove conclusively that DMPA did not contribute to long-term infertility in some cases.

The Controversy

Many women's health activists have opposed the widespread use of DMPA in the absence of more long-term studies. The National Women's Health Network played an active role in opposing the approval of DMPA in the United States as a contraceptive at a special Board of Inquiry hearing convened by the FDA in 1983.* At the same time, some family-planning providers believe that many women would choose DMPA over other contraceptives *even with full information about possible risks.* Although this is true, important concerns still remain to be addressed. The example of the Pill (also marketed prematurely) should warn us to be very careful with new hormonal contraceptives. Also, DMPA is different from other reversible contraceptives, because a woman can't change her mind after receiving a shot. Although we can stop using other methods immediately when we have problems, DMPA must remain in our system for at least several months until it is fully metabolized.

Quickly and easily administered, injections may be attractive to both providers and users.

*In mid-1984, this board recommended that DMPA be *denied* approval for contraceptive use. Upjohn subsequently withdrew its application for approval but then reapplied in 1992. As of mid-1992 approval is a real possibility.

However, for those of us who are not informed about DMPA and who are considered by providers as "ideal acceptors" for DMPA (this usually means we are poor white, black or Latin women or mentally retarded women who "cannot use other methods responsibly"), it may *not* be in our best interests to have DMPA widely available. Until we can be sure that true informed consent for *all* women will be the rule rather than the exception, misuse of DMPA and similar methods that a woman cannot discontinue by herself represent a serious threat to those women already most vulnerable to abuse.

PILLS FOR MEN

A pill for men could inhibit the production of sperm or prevent sperm from maturing and surviving. Compared with efforts directed at women, much less research is being done on contraceptive methods for men.[19] Many women have been lobbying for more research on male methods. It remains to be seen whether or not men would be willing to take a pill that exposed them to as many effects and potential risks as the Pill or IUD does to women. So far, there has not been any birth control pill developed for Western men, and there probably won't be for at least the next decade.

Researchers in the People's Republic of China have shown that gossypol (extracted from cottonseed) stops sperm production and changes sperm motility. However, China has abandoned this as a male method due to the toxicity of gossypol.

What if there were a pill or shot for men? Not all of us can absolutely trust our sex partners. As part of the active–passive, pursuer–pursued, predator–prey, male–female stereotypes that we act out in sex, men say many persuasive things to women to get us into bed. If the man lied about taking birth control pills, the woman would still be the one to get pregnant. Getting men to share the responsibility for birth control involves a lot more than finding methods for them to use (see Men and Birth Control, p. 260). For now, many of us prefer to keep the control in our own hands.

AFTER UNPROTECTED INTERCOURSE— THE MORNING-AFTER PILL

The morning-after pill is a series of very high doses of synthetic estrogens, progesterones or combination pills (Ovral) that must be started *within three days* of unprotected intercourse.

The FDA *has never approved* using DES or Ovral as morning-after pills.

The negative effects of morning-after pills containing estrogen are the same as those for combination birth control pills—nausea and vomiting, headache and breast tenderness. (Ovral seems to cause fewer of these effects, perhaps because of its lower dose of estrogen.) With DES, the nausea and vomiting may be severe.

Currently, practitioners recommend 200 milligrams of Ovral, a combination birth control pill (two fifty-milligram pills within seventy-two hours of unprotected intercourse and then two more Ovral pills twelve hours later). Ovral's failure rate ranges from 0.16 to 1.6 percent, partly because of the relatively low rate of pregnancy involved: about four out of a hundred women who have a single act of unprotected intercourse during a cycle conceive. For unprotected intercourse in midcycle, the rate is 15 to 25 percent.[20] *You should be examined* before taking a morning-after pill. If you should not take combination birth control pills, you should not take a morning-after pill (see pp. 282–83). If warning signals of heart attack and stroke occur (see p. 282), *stop taking the pills immediately and see a health practitioner.*

The most common morning-after treatment used to be DES. *Because the long-range effects of even one-time use of DES on the user have not been adequately studied, you should consider DES only in an emergency if at all.* Because DES has been used widely as a morning-after pill for twenty years, some doctors and clinics (especially university health services) still prescribe it. Pills containing progestin alone have also been used twenty-four hours after each time a woman has intercourse, with a failure rate ranging from zero to 45.2 percent. Progestins may prevent fertilization by immobilizing sperm or prevent implantation by making the uterus unable to support the fertilized egg. Especially when used regularly, progestins can cause irregular bleeding. (For contraindications to taking progesterone, see p. 288.) For signs of heart attack and stroke, see p. 282.

If you have had unprotected intercourse, you may prefer not to take a morning-after pill. You may prefer to wait to see if you are pregnant and, if so, have an abortion. Although abortion is more expensive and more difficult emotionally, it may be safer in the long run (see section on DES in Chapter 24, pp. 583–86). If you take morning-after pills and get pregnant anyway, *you should seriously consider having an abortion because of the potential danger to your offspring.*

THE INTRAUTERINE DEVICE (IUD)

Centuries ago, when camel drivers in the Middle East started out on a long journey across the desert, they would insert pebbles into the uterus of a female camel to keep her from becoming pregnant on the trip. A foreign body in the uterus seems to prevent pregnancy most of the time. IUDs became popular contraceptives for women in the 1960s. In the United States, use of this birth control method has declined dramatically from as many as 10 percent of all U.S. women using contraception in the 1970s to less than 1 percent today. Worldwide, however, use of IUDs has increased and today about 85 million women use them, mostly in Third World countries. Unfortunately, poorer health and more limited access to medical care exacerbate the risks and complications of IUDs.

In the mid-1960s, the IUD seemed to be the perfect alternative to the Pill. It was almost as effective and didn't introduce synthetic hormones into women's bodies. Once the IUD was inserted, women couldn't forget to use it. It was an inconspicuous method: It couldn't be discovered by the wrong person. Because it requires minimal involvement on our part, it seemed especially "appropriate" for young or poor women (especially women of color) in the United States and Third World countries, whom population control advocates often view as uncooperative and irresponsible.

Like the Pill, IUDs were marketed before sufficient research had been done to demonstrate their effectiveness and safety over a long period of time. In some cases, such serious problems emerged that IUDs were removed from the market.

An extreme example is the Dalkon Shield, an IUD marketed from 1971 to 1975 and manufactured by the A. H. Robins Company. It was soon implicated in a high number of cases of PID and spontaneous septic abortions (miscarriages). In the United States, twenty women died as a result of Dalkon Shield–related septic abortions. In 1974, the Shield was taken off the U.S. market (although devices already sold were not recalled). It was still distributed abroad, however.

In 1981, and again in 1983, the National Women's Health Network filed a class-action lawsuit against A. H. Robins, seeking a worldwide recall of the Shield, then inside an estimated 50,000 women in the United States and 500,000 women in other countries. Although unsuccessful, the lawsuit provided an important means of educating the public about the Shield and about the need to hold corporations accountable for their defective products, not just in the United States, but internationally.

Currently, there are only two IUDs for sale in the United States, the TCu-380A (ParaGard) and the Progesterone T device (Progestasert). IUDs may be more satisfactory than other methods for women who are at low risk of STDs, who want effective long-term contraception and who do not plan to have children in the future. For some women, IUDs will be a better alternative to sterilization. The information below is about the TCu-

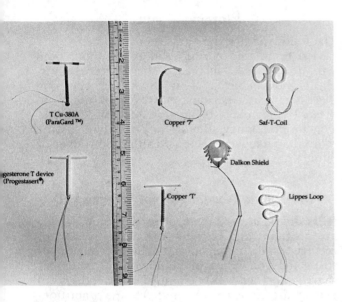

Different types of IUDs.

Jennifer S. Edwards
and Alice Steinhardt

380A and the Progesterone T device, unless another type is specifically mentioned.

Description

IUDs are small devices that fit inside the uterus. Some contain copper or synthetic progesterone; others are made of only white plastic. One or more strings are usually attached to IUDs. When the IUD is in place, these strings extend into the upper vagina. IUDs come in different sizes and shapes (see photo).

How It Works

No one is absolutely sure how the IUD works. The most widely accepted theory is that the IUD causes an inflammation or chronic low-grade infection in the uterus. This causes the body's defense system to produce higher numbers of white cells in the uterus. These cells may damage or destroy sperm or the egg and prevent them from joining; they may also hinder the buildup of the uterine lining, which must occur before implantation of a fertilized egg. (This does not preclude conception, however, and it allows the possibility of ectopic pregnancy [see p. 298], one problem associated with IUD use.) IUDs may also work by speeding up movement in the fallopian tube, causing the egg to arrive at the uterus too soon; by increasing the production of prostaglandins, which inhibit implantation; or by causing an implanted egg-sperm unit (blastocyst) to dislodge.[21]

Different Types of IUD

The TCu-380A (ParaGard) is a plastic IUD that has a thin copper wire wrapped around the vertical stem and a sleeve of copper on each "arm," with a clear or whitish string attached to it. Other IUDs containing copper are the Copper-7, the Shanghai V, the Multiload and various forms of Copper-Ts. Copper IUDs tend to increase bleeding during menstrual periods.

The Progesterone T device (Progestasert) is a plastic IUD containing synthetic progesterone and has a blue-black double string attached.* (See p. 288 for contraceptive effects of progesterone.) This IUD decreases bleeding during menstrual periods but has a higher rate of ectopic pregnancies than other IUDs.

All plastic IUDs are coated with barium so that they will be visible under X-ray (see Perforation, p. 297).

The Majzlin Spring, the Birnberg Bow and the Dalkon Shield have been removed from the market and should *not* be used because they are more strongly linked with perforation and infection.

Effectiveness

The IUD is considered a very effective form of birth control. Its typical failure rate is 3 percent.

Pregnancy rates for IUDs are lower among women over thirty.

For almost 100 percent effectiveness, use contraceptive cream, jelly or foam, or have your partner use a condom along with the IUD—all the time or when you know you are fertile (see Fertility Observation, p. 276). *It is a good idea to use a supplemental birth control method for at least the first three months after IUD insertion,* as that is the time when the IUD is most likely to be expelled and conception most likely to take place.

Expulsion

A major drawback of the IUD is its high expulsion rate. Our bodies have a natural tendency to expel foreign objects. Within one year of use, between 2 and 20 percent of women with IUDs will have expelled them, sometimes without knowing it has happened. These women could be vulnerable to pregnancy without their being aware of it. IUDs containing copper or progesterone seem to be expelled less frequently than the other IUDs.

---

*You can see the IUD string(s) if you use a speculum and a mirror to look at your cervix (see Chapter 12, "Anatomy and Physiology of Sexuality and Reproduction").

If your body is not going to tolerate the IUD, it will usually expel the device during the first three months after insertion. This happens most frequently during menstruation. Because you might not feel it coming out, check for it in the toilet and on your tampon or sanitary napkin. Be sure to feel the length of the string a few times each month, especially right after your period.

Signs of IUD expulsion include an unusual vaginal discharge, cramping or pain, spotting, a longer string or an ability to feel the IUD in your vagina or cervical os. When an IUD is being expelled, your male partner may feel pain or irritation during intercourse.

The longer your body retains the IUD, the better your chance of not expelling it.

Reversibility

The IUD can harm our fertility through pelvic inflammatory disease, perforation, embedding or ectopic pregnancy. These serious complications can cause impaired fertility or sterility and may lead to hysterectomy. Health practitioners should tell this to every woman who chooses an IUD as her form of birth control, especially to those of us who hope someday to have children.

If you don't have any of these problems during the time you use an IUD, your chance of becoming pregnant after it is removed is probably the same as it was before using the IUD (although there is some controversy on this).

Safety

Studies have documented serious negative effects suffered by IUD users. Some women have died from IUD complications; others have had serious injury (see below). IUDs increase a woman's chances of developing PID and subsequent infertility and are a poor choice for any woman at risk of developing an STD. In addition, IUDs offer no protection against STDs, including HIV.

How Long to Keep Your IUD

Copper devices must be replaced every four years, although some studies show that they are effective for at least five years. They probably lose some of their contraceptive quality after that, either because a corroded crust has formed over the device, prohibiting the copper from being released or, as some research suggests, because the copper has dissolved, presumably having been absorbed by the body. IUDs containing progesterone should be changed every year because the supply of progesterone in the device is used up after twelve months.

Warning Signals

The following are signs of serious problems: late period or missed period; abdominal pain; pain with intercourse; increased temperature, fever, chills; noticeable or foul discharge; spotting, bleeding, heavy periods, clots. *Report these immediately*, for they are signs of infection, perforation or pregnancy. Report *any* problem lasting more than a few cycles to a health practitioner or clinic.

Who Should Absolutely Not Use the IUD

IUDs should *absolutely not* be used by women who are pregnant and women with active, recent or recurrent pelvic infection, including known or suspected gonorrhea or chlamydia. (Remember that gonorrhea and chlamydia infections in women are often *asymptomatic*.) Some practitioners also recommend that the IUD should absolutely not be used by women who have acute cervicitis or nonspecific vaginitis until these conditions are controlled.

Who Is Strongly Advised Not to Use the IUD

Women with the following situations or conditions are *strongly advised not* to use IUDs: women for whom pregnancy in the future is a high-priority goal, abnormal Pap smears, irregular or abnormal pelvic bleeding, acute cervicitis, difficult access to emergency treatment, disorders of blood or impaired coagulation, endometritis, exposure to DES *in utero* (DES daughter) *if* it results in an alteration of the shape of the uterus or fallopian tubes, gynecological malignancy, history of ectopic pregnancy, an abortion within the past three months that was followed by infection, impaired response to infection (in women with diabetes or taking steroids), multiple sexual partners or a partner who has multiple sexual partners (because of risk of an STD), sickle cell anemia, inability to check IUD string or identify warning signals (including some women with spinal cord injury or multiple sclerosis), history of severe fainting or severe vasovagal reaction. Women at risk of exposure to HIV are also strongly advised not to use the IUD (see Chapter 15, "AIDS, HIV Infection and Women").

Who Should Probably Not Use the IUD

Women with the following situations or conditions *should probably not* use the IUD: anemia, bicornate uterus, cervical stenosis, endometrial polyps, endometriosis, leiomyomata, past history of fainting, severe menstrual cramps or bleeding, small uterus, valvular heart disease. Women who have a copper allergy or Wilson's disease (a rare inherited disorder of copper excretion) should probably not use *copper* IUDs.

Complications and Negative Effects

Infections

Recent analyses show that PID (see p. 588) is twice as likely to occur in women using IUDs than in women using *no* contraception; PID is two to nine times more likely to occur in women using IUDs than in women using *other methods* of birth control. Because PID most commonly occurs in the first month after an IUD is inserted, some practitioners recommend short-term use of antibiotics at the time of insertion to prevent infection.[22] (Some practitioners think that the string dangling from the IUD into the vagina can act as a ladder for germs to climb into the uterus.) Women who have an STD while using an IUD are at high risk for developing PID. PID will not go away by itself. It can lead to tremendous pain, future ectopic pregnancy, sterility and even death (see PID for symptoms and treatment, pp. 588–92).

Another form of infection that may occur is an infected miscarriage, called a *septic abortion*. Women who become pregnant with an IUD in place are more susceptible to septic abortion, especially during the second trimester. In extreme cases, this can cause death to the woman as well as the fetus and in most cases leads to hospitalization. That is why most doctors recommend having the IUD removed if you become pregnant.

Excessive Bleeding and Cramping

A common problem for women with IUDs is increased menstrual bleeding, sometimes excessive, and painful cramping and/or backache. Some women experience longer periods and bleeding or spotting and/or cramping between periods, too.

Usually these symptoms are more intense during the first three to six months after the IUD is inserted. Approximately 15 percent of IUD users have the IUD removed within one year because of bleeding and cramping.

The Lippes Loop and Saf-T-Coil increase blood loss by about 75 to 100 percent each cycle, and the copper-containing IUDs increase it by 20 to 50 percent. Heavier menstrual flow may make you anemic. Although the Progestasert decreases menstrual flow, women using it may experience spotting or light bleeding between periods. Because many menstruating women are marginally anemic anyway, it is a good idea to have a blood test before you get an IUD and at each follow-up appointment. Eat plenty of iron-rich foods.

Embedding

This is a problem (much less common than the above) where the lining of the uterus begins to grow around the IUD. If an IUD becomes partially embedded in the uterine wall, the device will usually still be effective. But embedded IUDs can cause more pain during removal. In some cases, you may need a dilation and curettage to get it out (see p. 358). In several cases we know of, women had hysterectomies because of embedded IUDs, a devastating blow for anyone who wants to have a child.

Check the string carefully at least once a month. A shorter string may indicate an embedded IUD, and you should have it checked by a health worker, who may remove it to avoid further complications, such as perforation. You can have the IUD replaced, or you may want to choose another method of contraception.

Perforation

Although rare, one of the most serious complications of IUD use is perforation of the uterine wall. This can happen partially, with part of the IUD pushing through the wall and part staying in the uterus; or it can happen completely, with the entire IUD pushing out of the uterus into the abdominal cavity. In the latter case, the IUD can migrate to other organs and become embedded in them, sometimes causing medical emergencies. Perforation occurs or begins to occur most frequently during insertion, due primarily to a practitioner's poor technique. It happens less often when a uterine sound has been taken, so always insist on this procedure (see p. 429).

Unfortunately, there are usually no symptoms accompanying perforation. The first sign may be a shorter string or no string at all during your monthly check (a good reason to check the string more than once a month). If this happens, be sure to see a health worker immediately. You should also use another form of birth control, because if the IUD has left the uterus, you are no longer being protected against pregnancy. In fact, some women only become aware of perforation after finding out they are pregnant.

Missing String

Because a missing string can mean either expulsion or perforation, there is no way of knowing what has happened unless you see the IUD come out. Otherwise there are several procedures available for trying to locate it. A medical practitioner can probe your uterus with a uterine sound or a biopsy instrument. If sounding fails to locate the IUD, an X-ray or ultrasound (see p. 429) may work. If the IUD is still in the uterus s/he can then try to pull the string down to remove the

IUD. This may involve dilating the cervix, which can be painful.

If no IUD can be located, this probably means it was expelled. If you are pregnant and elect not to have an abortion you should not have an X-ray. Ultrasound may be used instead, although this procedure can be expensive, and as yet no one knows the long-range effects, if any, of ultrasound on developing fetuses.

If the IUD is located outside the uterus, it should be removed, because it increases your chances of developing internal scar tissue. Copper and progestin are particularly damaging. Also, the IUD may prevent other organs from performing their functions properly or may puncture or strangle organs in the abdominal cavity, such as the bowel.

Recovery of an IUD that is not in the uterus and not expelled requires surgery. This can often be done in the outpatient services of your hospital or clinic. A laparoscopy operation is performed in this case (see p. 567). If the IUD is not accessible by laparoscopy, more extensive surgery may be required.

Pregnancy

If your period is late and you have an IUD, have a pregnancy test. If you know you are pregnant and you have an IUD in place, you should have the IUD removed *whether or not* you wish to continue the pregnancy. If you do *not* have it removed, your chances of miscarriage are about 50 percent, and during the second trimester your chances are ten times greater than normal. The miscarriage could become infected. If you *do* have the IUD removed, your chances of miscarrying are about 25 percent.

If you carry a pregnancy close to term with an IUD in place, there may be a higher likelihood of a premature or low-birth-weight baby or still-birth.[23]

Ectopic Pregnancy

If you get pregnant with an IUD in place, there is a 5 percent chance of ectopic pregnancy. Women who conceive with the Progestasert are six to ten times more likely to have an ectopic pregnancy than women using a copper IUD. *An ectopic pregnancy is a serious problem* that can cause hemorrhage and lead to infection, sterility and sometimes death. Frequently it is misdiagnosed, so IUD users should be aware of possible symptoms of ectopic pregnancy (see p. 508 for more information).

Other Possible Effects

The copper in the TCu-380A and other IUDs containing copper may produce an allergic skin reaction, and there is some question as to how it might affect a developing fetus.

There is no evidence that the IUD can cause cancer, but it has not been studied long enough to know the long-term effects of either the material it's made of (polyethylene) or the material some IUDs contain (progestin and barium).

How to Get an IUD

Because of the risk of perforation, a well-trained person must insert the IUD. Choose a practitioner who has experience with IUDs and find out in advance which device s/he uses. If s/he doesn't insert IUDs or the kind of IUD you want, go to someone else.

You must have a full medical, pelvic and breast examination, including a Pap smear, pregnancy test and tests for STDs before being given the IUD. This is very important, because if you have an STD or if you are pregnant, you should not use the IUD. That means at least two visits, because it takes a few days to receive results from the Pap smear and the STD cultures. You should, by law, be given an informed consent form to sign at this time (see Our Rights as Patients, p. 682).

The practitioner should do a sounding of the uterus to measure its depth and position. An IUD can be put into a tipped uterus.

Insertion takes place through the os (the opening in the cervix), which is in diameter about the size of a thin straw. Just before insertion, the IUD is straightened out in a plastic tube like a straw. The practitioner gently puts the tube into the vagina and up into the uterus through the cervix (see illustration). Then s/he pushes the IUD through the tube and it springs back into shape within the uterus. The practitioner removes the tube and the IUD stays in the uterus, with its string dangling

The insertion of Copper T 380A   The Population Council

into the vagina. Make sure that you understand how to check the string.

The process can hurt, sometimes a lot, because the inserter stretches the os open and the device irritates the uterus. You may have cramps during the insertion and for the rest of the day, especially if you have never given birth. Bring a friend with you if you can, someone who can accompany you home after the appointment. You might want to have a local anesthetic or take a mild painkiller, or you can pant quickly or relax and take deep breaths.

When to Get an IUD

This is controversial. Many advise inserting the IUD during or just after your period. The os is slightly opened at that time, so insertion may be less painful. Also, the fact that you are having your period probably means you aren't pregnant (although sometimes women have one or even two scant periods during pregnancy). Some suspect there may be a greater chance of incurring infection during menstruation, however, and avoid inserting IUDs at that time. Practitioners also used to think that IUDs should be inserted right after abortion. However, now many practitioners are afraid of infection or other complications at that time. Similarly, in the past few years, practitioners have changed their views about insertion of IUDs after childbirth; they now believe that IUDs can be safely inserted immediately after childbirth if a woman has had a normal labor and delivery, her uterus is firm and the bleeding has subsided. However, there is a higher rate of expulsion at this time.

Consequently, the best time for insertion may be between periods and at least six weeks after childbirth or abortion.

Checking Your IUD

At first you'll want to check your IUD string before intercourse (you may want to ask your partner to do it) and after each period. After three months or so, once or twice a month is enough.

You can try to feel the string with your finger or look for it during a cervical self-exam using a speculum (see pp. 564–65). To check with your finger, squat, bringing your bottom down near your heels to shorten the length of your vagina and reach into your vagina with your longest (clean) finger. The bathtub or shower is a good place, or bear down while you are sitting on the toilet. You may be confused by the folds in your vagina, but when you reach your cervix you will know it, as it is harder and firmer than anything else you'll touch. Find the dimple in your cervix;

this is the entrance to your uterus, and the strings of the IUD should be sticking out a little way. Some days your uterus may be tipped in such a way that you can't reach the cervix or find the hole; try again the next day. If you cannot find the strings for a few days or if they are much longer or shorter, or if you feel a bit of plastic protruding, call your health practitioner or clinic.

Advantages

You don't have to worry about forgetting to take a pill, checking your signs of fertility or using a barrier method at the time of intercourse.

Checking the string a few times each month encourages you to get to know your vagina and cervix and to feel comfortable about touching your genitals.

If you have an IUD containing progesterone, you will probably have less bleeding during your menstrual periods.

Disadvantages

Most of the disadvantages in terms of pain and risk have been described already. Note particularly the likelihood of long-term infertility due to PID. IUDs offer no protection against STDs, including HIV.

Responsibility

The woman sees a practitioner for insertion, three months later for a checkup and at least once a year afterward. She experiences the insertion and any negative effects. The woman or her partner must check the string periodically.

Cost

An initial examination with screening and blood tests costs about $100. A second visit, including purchase and insertion of the IUD, costs from $220 at a clinic (for the two visits, the total cost is $320) to $300 at a private doctor's office (total $400).

New IUD Design

Researchers are always designing new products to improve the effectiveness and reduce the problems of IUDs. View *all* new IUDs cautiously, because experience has shown that many of their long-term negative effects will show up only after they're put on the market. Some new designs we've heard about include variations of the copper-bearing and progesterone-releasing IUDs, IUDs made out of a copper-silver combination, IUDs made without rigid frames and a device that ttaches to the uterine wall to produce "reversible terilization."

The IUD as Postcoital (Morning-After) Birth Control

Because the IUD may inhibit the implantation of a fertilized egg, it has been used as a postcoital contraceptive. So far only the copper IUDs have been used in this way on a few women, but they have proven successful at preventing pregnancy within one to five days after conception occurs.

Of course, women who should not use the IUD for birth control (see p. 296) should not use it postcoitally either.

WITHDRAWAL (COITUS INTERRUPTUS, "TAKING CARE" OR "PULLING OUT")

Worldwide, this is the most universally used of all methods, a folk method passed on from one generation to the next. Withdrawal involves removing the penis from the vagina just before ejaculation so that the sperm is deposited outside the vagina and away from the lips of the vagina as well.

Withdrawal is not very effective because the drops of fluid that come out of the penis right after it becomes erect can contain enough sperm to cause pregnancy. Also, the man cannot always get out in time to avoid contact with the vagina *and* vaginal lips (sperm can move all the way from the vaginal lips up into the fallopian tubes). Multiple acts of intercourse in a short period of time increase the likelihood of failure, because more sperm are mixed in with the lubricating fluid. It is not possible to give reliable failure rates for withdrawal because so few studies have been done. However, based on this small number, researchers estimate that withdrawal has a lowest expected failure rate of 4 percent but a typical failure rate of 18 percent.

Withdrawal has a number of drawbacks in addition to its high failure rate. The man must keep in control and therefore cannot relax. When used over a long period, it may lead to premature ejaculation by the male. Withdrawal can also be uncomfortable for the woman: The man may have to withdraw before she reaches orgasm, interrupting the flow of her sexual response; also, a part of her is wondering whether he's going to withdraw in time, so that she, too, cannot entirely relax. Some couples who have used withdrawal for a long time have been able to work out these problems. Finally, withdrawal does not protect you against STDs, including HIV infection.

NONMETHODS

Douching

Some women douche with water or other special solutions immediately after intercourse in an attempt to remove semen from the vagina before sperm enter the uterus.

Douching does not work. Sperm move fast, and some will reach your uterus before you've reached the bathroom; and the douche, which is liquid squirted into your vagina under pressure, will push some sperm up into your uterus even as it is washing others away.

Douching is the least effective of all methods, and it puts the burden exclusively on the woman, who must hop up to the bathroom immediately. Don't use it!

Avoidance of Orgasm by the Woman

Some people think that in order to conceive, a woman must have an orgasm. This is false. One of the major differences between men and women in reproduction is that a man must have an erection and ejaculation to cause a pregnancy, whereas a woman can conceive without any sexual arousal.

Breastfeeding

Although occasionally breastfeeding on demand with no supplementary food for the baby may prevent ovulation for some women, you should not count on this.

Astrological Birth Control

This doesn't work.

STERILIZATION

Since 1973, the use of sterilization as a permanent* method of contraception has increased rapidly. Today it is the most frequently used method of birth control among married couples in the United States. Sterilization is a *virtually 100 percent* effective form of birth control, available for both women and men. In women, the fallopian tubes are cut and/or blocked so the egg and sperm cannot meet. This is called *tubal ligation*. In men, the vas deferens is cut and/or blocked so sperm cannot mix with seminal fluid. This is called *vasectomy*. In some developing countries, population

---

*Although there have been some successful attempts at reversing both vasectomies and tubal ligations, *the operation should be considered permanent and not reversible.*

control advocates are promoting sterilization as the best form of birth control. As one advocate put it: "Sterilization is the most cost-effective method of birth control, considering the number of years of protection it provides."[24] However, many women are choosing this procedure without adequate information about the possible risks and consequences involved, or under coercive circumstances.*

Choosing to be sterilized is a major step. Studies have shown that nearly one-third of the women who were sterilized at one point in their lives regretted this decision later on, particularly if they were under thirty years old when sterilized. Some women turn to sterilization in desperation because there is no suitable form of contraception for them. (Nothing else points out so clearly our need for better temporary methods of birth control.) Many feel they have no other choice: "The lack of employment opportunities, education, day care, decent housing, adequate medical care; safe, effective contraception and access to abortion all create an atmosphere of subtle coercion."[25]

For some women, however, the choice to be sterilized is a positive wish to avoid pregnancy forever. Some have already had children; others decide they never want children.

Under whatever circumstances sterilization is chosen, the decision usually brings up deep feelings, as this thirty-six-year-old mother of two described to us:

The week before my sterilization I was very nervous, irritable and jumpy. I'd yell at my husband. I tried to pull out of myself all my fears about having an operation: I would die, there'd be a mistake, I'd be out of control, I'd get the wrong anesthetic; and fears about this particular operation: My husband would think that I wasn't a real woman anymore, he'd leave me for a fertile woman, I'd get all dried up and wrinkled. I felt angry at my husband for not wanting to deal with his feelings of loss of manhood by having a vasectomy (though that was a little irrational on my part, for his vasectomy couldn't give me my sexual freedom if I wanted to make love with another man).

Now, almost two years later, I am glad I made the choice I did. I feel much freer when I make love. . . .

Since 1974, women have revealed and studies have documented a terrible pattern of sterilization abuse. Victims of sterilization abuse are usually poor or black, Puerto Rican, Chicana or Native American, often with little or no undertanding of

English.* Sometimes physicians consider women mentally unfit.† Physicians pressure women into giving consent during labor or childbirth; welfare officials threaten the loss of benefits if women refuse; no one informs women that the operation is permanent. Black women in the South are all too familiar with the "Mississippi appendectomy," in which the fallopian tubes are tied or the uterus is removed without them knowing it. Sometimes sterilizations are done primarily for the purpose of training residents or interns. Of the million hysterectomies done each year, perhaps one out of five is done for sterilization only, with no legitimate medical reason. Hysterectomy, a major surgical procedure, is unnecessary for sterilization purposes. The risk of death or complication from a hysterectomy is ten to one hundred times greater than from a tubal ligation (see Hysterectomy and Oophorectomy, p. 598). Especially if women are poor, public and private programs make it easier to get sterilization services than abortions or prenatal care and financial assistance so that we can have healthy children; or they refuse to perform abortions until women agree to be sterilized. In recent years legislators in at least ten states have proposed compulsory sterilization for all women on welfare. (No such measure has yet passed.) Occasionally physicians refuse to sterilize fully informed white middle-class women with no children who request this procedure. Sterilization and its abuses are experienced differently by different groups of women.

Sterilization abuse also occurs internationally.

---

*Sterilization abuse is not a new development. Beginning in the nineteenth century, people known as *eugenicists* tried to popularize the idea that social problems such as crime and poverty could be eliminated by preventing certain "unfit" people from having children. The eugenics movement, which has proponents even today, argued that criminals, "imbeciles," blacks and immigrants would produce more "inferior" people like themselves if allowed to reproduce. Eugenicists urged the passage of laws empowering the State to sterilize such individuals against their will. These eugenics laws were passed in thirty-seven states and still remain on the books in some.

†A major investigation and report, produced only after great pressure from people such as Connie Uri, a Native American physician, found that large numbers of women living on Indian reservations had been sterilized without consent by government-sponsored programs. (See the U.S. General Accounting Office Report to Hon. James G. Abourezk, B164031 [5], November 1976.) At a major teaching hospital in Los Angeles, a resident went to the local newspapers to expose cases of sterilization abuse involving many poor Chicana women. (See "A Health Research Group Study on Surgical Sterilization: Present Abuses and Proposed Regulations," Health Research Group, 1973).

GAO reports (single copy) are free. Write to U.S. GAO, Distribution Section, Room 1518, 401 G Street NW, Washington, DC 20548. Indicate the report number and date. Health Research Group reports are available from HRG, 2000 P Street NW, Washington, DC 20036.

---

*Most (but not all) documented cases of coerced sterilization in the U.S. involve women. Here we focus on the experiences of women.

See Chapter 27, "Developing an International Awareness," for U.S. government participation.

Feminists, health activists and others joined together to expose sterilization abuse and to organize against it in hospitals, communities, courts and legislatures. In 1975, responding to this pressure, New York City became the first city in this country to produce guidelines. On March 9, 1979, federal sterilization regulations went into effect. The most important requirements of the federal regulations include

- Obtaining voluntary informed consent using a mandatory, standardized consent form in a person's preferred language.
- Prohibiting overt or implicit threat of loss of welfare or Medicaid benefits if someone doesn't consent.
- Explaining alternative methods of birth control and the risks, side effects and irreversibility of sterilization, orally and in writing, also in a person's language.
- Waiting at least thirty days after a person signs the consent form before sterilization (except for premature delivery and emergency abdominal surgery).
- Prohibiting obtaining consent while someone is in labor, before or after an abortion or while the person is under the influence of alcohol or other drugs.
- Prohibiting hysterectomies for sterilization in federally funded programs.
- Imposing a moratorium on federally funded sterilizations of people under twenty-one who have been declared legally incompetent or are involuntarily institutionalized.
- Auditing sterilization programs in the ten states where most federally funded sterilizations are performed.[26]

The government does not monitor or enforce these regulations, and often doctors and hospitals ignore them. In some places, however, they have reduced the amount of sterilization abuse. If you are considering sterilization, make sure that the clinic or hospital performing it complies with these regulations. If you suspect that it doesn't, contact your local women's health group or one of the following organizations:

- American Civil Liberties Union
  Reproductive Freedom Project
    132 West 43rd Street
    New York, NY 10036
- National Black Women's Health Project
    1237 Ralph David Abernathy Blvd., S. E.
    Atlanta, GA 30310
- National Latina Health Organization/Organización Nacional de la Salud de la Mujer Latina
    P.O. Box 7567
    Oakland, CA 94601

- National Women's Health Network
  1325 G Street NW
  Washington, DC 20005
- Native American Women's Health Education Resource Center
  P.O. Box 572
  Lake Andes, SD 57356

Tubal Ligation

Female sterilization is effective immediately. It can be done under general, spinal or local anesthesia, and women usually go home the same day.

Laparoscopy, or "Band-Aid" surgery, is the most common surgical technique for sterilization in the United States. Although a laparoscopy can be done under local, general or spinal anesthesia, usually local anesthesia with a light sedative is adequate. The actual procedure takes about thirty minutes and involves making a small incision in a woman's belly button and inflating her belly with gas (carbon dioxide or nitrous oxide) so the fallopian tubes can be more easily seen. The woman is tilted back, head down, allowing her intestines to move away from her fallopian tubes. The tubes are moved into view by inserting a clamp (tenaculum) onto the cervix and an instrument (sound or intrauterine cannula) through the vagina and then manipulating the uterus and tubes. Next, her belly is inflated with gas to make the tubes visible. A laparoscope (a thin tube containing a viewing instrument and a light) is inserted through the incision to view the tubes. An instrument to block the tubes is introduced through the laparoscope or through a second tiny incision below the belly button. The tubes can be blocked by burning (electrocoagulation or cautery) or cutting them, clipping them shut or applying rings to them. The incisions are sewn closed (see illustration). Afterward, some women feel pain in their shoulders from the gas.

The *minilaparotomy*, or minilap, involves making a small incision just above a woman's pubic bone, moving the tubes into view with a tenaculum and ultrasound (see above), pulling the fallopian tubes up through the incision and blocking them (usually by tying and cutting them). The incision is sewn shut. Women seem to have more cramping and pain afterward than with a laparoscopy, sometimes lasting a few days.

Laparoscopy and minilaparotomy have a failure rate of about 0.2 percent.

Tubal ligations can also be performed through a woman's vagina (*colpotomy* or *culdoscopy*) or cervix (*hysteroscopy*, an experimental procedure). Sterilization by *laparotomy* involves major surgery (see Chapter 24, p. 567).

Sterilization probably does not affect a woman's hormone secretions, ovaries, uterus or vagina. Her menstrual cycle continues but may become

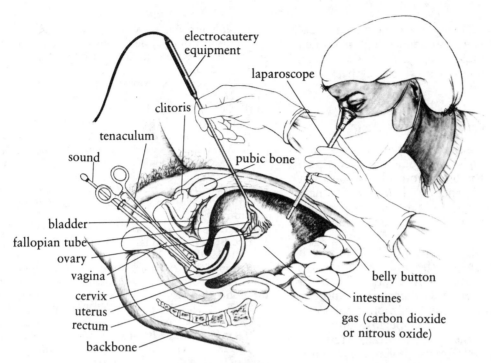

electrocautery
equipment

laparoscope

clitoris

tenaculum

sound

pubic bone

bladder

fallopian tube

ovary

vagina

cervix

uterus

rectum

backbone

belly button

intestines

gas (carbon dioxide
or nitrous oxide)

A tubal ligation (side view).   Christine Bondante

irregular. An egg ripens and is released from an ovary every month but stops partway down the tube and is reabsorbed by her body.

Complications and Negative Effects

Whenever surgery involving an anesthetic is performed, certain complications are possible. Major complications happen relatively rarely and depend a great deal on the skill and experience of the practitioner performing the sterilization. Cardiac irregularity, cardiac arrest, infection, internal bleeding and perforation of a major blood vessel are a few of the potential hazards.

Laparoscopic techniques may involve specific problems such as internal burn injuries or punctures to other organs or tissue, skin burns, puncturing of the intestine, perforation of the uterus and carbon dioxide embolism (which may cause immediate death).

Some women experience a post-laparoscopic syndrome including heavy irregular bleeding and increased menstrual pain, which may create the need for repeated dilation and curettages or, in some cases, complete hysterectomies.

Reversibility

No woman should undergo sterilization with the hope that the procedure can be reversed. If you think there is any chance you may want to have children someday, use a reversible form of birth control.

Nonetheless, recent advances in microsurgery have increased the possibility of tubal reconstruc-

tion, called *reanastomosis*. It is major surgery, requiring extreme skill on the part of the surgeon, highly specialized and expensive equipment and a woman in good health. The operation can cost $10–15,000 or more. This means that only women with substantial resources will be able to have plastic surgery to repair the tube(s), and even then success is not guaranteed.*

Before undergoing this operation, a woman and her partner should be tested for fertility potential. Also, the woman should have a laparoscopic examination to determine if her tubes are too damaged to be repaired. Cauterization tends to destroy a significant amount of the tube. Clips and rings seem to destroy much less of the tube but still make reversal highly unlikely.

New Techniques in Female Sterilization

Possible new techniques involve injecting substances into the fallopian tubes, inserting pellets or plugs, modifying surgical procedures and using

---

*A possible form of sterilization abuse may develop along these lines: Technology for sterilization reversal will improve greatly, due to a combination of physicians' recognition that many women do want reversal, scientific fascination with new surgical techniques and population establishment preference for sterilization as the most cost-effective form of birth control (see p. 301). The improved reversal techniques will lead to a popular misunderstanding that *all* women can count on reversal when and if they want it. Yet due to economic inequalities and racism, reversal will *not* be available to poor women and women of color in this country and around the world.

new types of clips or rings. We have heard of experiments using methylcyanoacrylate, also known as Krazy Glue or Superglue; and silicone plugs. The negative and long-term effects of these substances are unknown.

Male Sterilization—Vasectomy

Male sterilization is a much simpler process than female sterilization. Usually done in a doctor's office or in a clinic, the operation takes about half an hour. The practitioner applies a local anesthetic (such as Novocaine), makes one or two small incisions in the scrotum, locates the two vasa deferentia (singular: vas deferens, tubes that carry sperm from the testes to the penis), removes a piece of each and ties off the ends. Men are not sterile immediately, because sperm are already in the vasa deferentia. For this reason, use another method of birth control for two months or until the man has had two negative sperm counts.

Vasectomy leaves the man's genital system basically unchanged. His sexual hormones remain operative, and there is no noticeable difference in his ejaculate because sperm make up only a small part of the semen. Some men, although they know these facts, are still anxious about what a vasectomy will do to their sexual performance. Talking with someone who has had a vasectomy can help allay such anxieties.

In some men, antibodies to their own sperm can be found after a vasectomy. Some research suggests that these antibodies may lead to certain diseases of the immune system, yet many fully fertile men also have such antibodies, and so far this suggestion is without support.

Men who have a vasectomy may have an increased risk of prostate cancer.[27] A 1980 report indicating that vasectomy may induce atherosclerosis (hardening of the arteries) has not been supported by other studies.[28]

Experimental operations have placed plastic plugs or injectable chemicals into the tube to plug it up temporarily so that if the man later wants to have a child he can have the plug taken out. These methods appear to be reversible but not quite as effective as vasectomy. Researchers are also exploring ways to produce temporary sterility by increasing the temperature of a man's testicles through hot, shallow baths or ultrasound.[29]

Vasectomy should be considered irreversible.

NOTES

Note: Space limits mean that we can print only some of the documentation for points made in this chapter. Additional documentation is on file at the Boston Women's Health Book Collective office.

1. Malcolm Potts, "Why the World Is Not Getting the Contraception It Needs," *People*, Vol. 8, No. 4 (1981), p. 28. Published by the International Planned Parenthood Federation.

2. Dr. Frederick Robbins, quoted in Barbara Seaman. *The Doctor's Case Against the Pill*, rev. ed. New York: Dell, 1979, p. 11.

3. Dr. Frederick Robbins, quoted in Barbara Seaman, *The Doctor's Case Against the Pill*.

4. Willard Cates and Katherine M. Stone. "Family Planning: The Responsibility to Prevent Pregnancy and Reproductive Tract Infections," in A. Germain et al., eds., *Reproductive Tract Infections: Global Impact and Priorities for Women's Reproductive Health*. New York: Plenum, 1992.

5. James Trussell et al. "Contraceptive Failure in the United States: An Update," *Studies in Family Planning*, Vol. 21 (1990), pp. 51–54.

6. Linda E. Atkinson, Richard Lincoln and Jacqueline Darroch Forrest. "Worldwide Trends in Funding for Contraceptive Research and Evaluation," *Family Planning Perspectives*, Vol. 17 (1985), pp. 196–207.

7. Ortho Pharmaceutical Corporation. *Report on the 1991 Ortho Annual Birth Control Study*, Raritan, NJ: Ortho Pharmaceutical Corp, 1991. According to one survey conducted annually by Ortho Pharmaceuticals for the last twenty-four years, in 1983, 9 percent of women reported using condoms as their method of contraception as compared to 15 percent in 1991. (Among unmarried women condom use was 19 percent.)

8. H. Jick et al. "Vaginal Spermicides and Congenital Disorders," *Journal of the American Medical Association*, Vol. 245 (1981), pp. 1329–32.

9. S. Shapiro et al. "Birth Defects in Relation to Vaginal Spermicides," *Journal of the American Medical Association*, Vol. 247, No. 17 (1982), pp. 2381–84. J. L. Mils et al. "Are Spermicides Teratogenic?" *Journal of the American Medical Association*, Vol. 248, No. 17 (November 5, 1982), p. 2148.

10. J. Schwartz et al. *Connections: Nutrition, Contraception, Women, Eating*. Boston: Boston Family Planning Project, 1982.

11. A. Rosenfield. "Modern Contraception: A 1989 Update," *Annual Review of Public Health*, Vol. 10 (1989), pp. 385–401. R. Hatcher et al. *Contraceptive Technology 1990–1992*, 15th rev. ed. New York: Irvington, 1990.

12. D. L. Mishell, Jr. "Contraception," *New England Journal of Medicine*, Vol. 320 (March 23, 1989), pp. 777–87.

13. E. A. Holly. "Cutaneous Melanoma and Oral Contraceptives: A Review of Case-Control and Cohort Studies," *Recent Results in Cancer Research*, Vol. 102 (1986), pp. 108–17.

14. National Women's Health Network. "The Latest Studies in Breast Cancer and Oral Contraceptives," *The Network News* Vol. 14, No. 2 (March/April 1989), p. 4. Available from NWHN, 1325 G Street NW, Washington, DC 20005.

15. S. Harlap, K. Kost and J. D. Forrest. *Preventing Pregnancy, Protecting Health: A New Look at Birth Control Choices in the United States*. New York/Washington, DC: The Alan Guttmacher Institute, 1991. A. Fugh-Berman. "Should Women Over Forty Take the Pill?" *The Network News*, Vol. 14, No. 7 (January/February 1990), p. 4.

16. R. Hatcher et al. *Contraceptive Technology 1990–1992*, pp. 238–39.

17. R. Hatcher et al. *Contraceptive Technology 1990–1992*, pp. 266–67. D. R. Mishell, Jr. "Contraception," p. 782.

18. WHO Collaborative Study of Neoplasia and Steroid Contraceptives. "Breast Cancer and Depot-Medroxyprogesterone Acetate: A Multinational Study," *The Lancet*, Vol. 338 (October 5, 1991), p. 833. "Depot-Medroxyprogesterone Acetate (DMPA) and Cancer: Memorandum from a WHO Meeting," *Bulletin WHO*, Vol. 64 (1986), p. 375. There does appear to be a small increase in the risk of breast cancer in women within a few years after starting the drug. This could be due to better detection of breast cancer, to a speeding up of the growth of existing tumors or to causing new tumors.

19. Linda E. Atkinson, Richard Lincoln and Jacqueline Darroch Forrest. "Worldwide Trends in Funding for Contraceptive Research and Evaluation."

20. R. Hatcher et al. *Contraceptive Technology 1990–1992*, pp. 424–425.

21. K. Treiman and L. Liskin. "IUDs—A New Look," *Population Reports*, Series B, No. 5 (March 1988). Available from Population Information Programs, Johns Hopkins University, 624 North Broadway, Baltimore, MD 21205. Multiple copies are $2 each; free to developing countries.

22. Willard Cates and Katherine M. Stone. "Reproductive Tract Infections and Contraceptive Use/Safety."

23. K. Treiman and L. Liskin. "IUDs—A New Look."

24. Pourbe Bhiwandiwala. "New Approaches to Female Sterilization," *People*, Vol. 8, No. 4 (1981), p. 14.

25. Rahemah Amur et al. "Sterilization Rights Abuses and Remedies," *A Sourcebook for the 11th National Women and the Law Conference*, Spring 1980.

26. R. P. Petchesky. "Reproduction, Ethics and Public Policy: The Federal Sterilization Regulations," *Hastings Center Report*, Vol. 9, No. 5 (October 1979), pp. 29–41. Copies of the regulation are available from Marilyn L. Martin, Hubert Humphrey Building, Room 722-H, 200 Independence Avenue SW, Washington, DC 20201.

27. C. Mettlin, N. Natarajan and R. Huben. "Vasectomy and Prostate Cancer Risk," *American Journal of Epidemiology*, Vol. 132, No. 6 (1990), pp. 1056–61. L. Rosenberg et al. "Vasectomy and the Risk of Prostate Cancer," *American Journal of Epidemiology*, Vol. 132, No. 6 (1990), pp. 1051–55 (discussion, pp. 1062–65).

28. H. B. Petersen, D. H. Huber and A. M. Belker. "Vasectomy: An Appraisal for the Obstetrician Gynecologist," *Obstetrics and Gynecology*, Vol. 76, No. 3 (1990), pp. 568–72.

29. E. A. Lissner. "Latex and Hormones Aside. . . ." *WomenWise* (Spring 1991). Available from the Boston Women's Health Book Collective, Box 192, West Somerville, MA 02144.

RESOURCES

General

American Civil Liberties Union/Reproductive Freedom Project, 132 West 43rd Street, New York, NY 10036. Publishes *Reproductive Rights Update*.

Davis, Angela. "Racism, Birth Control and Reproductive Rights," in M. G. Fried, ed., *From Abortion to Reproductive Freedom: Transforming a Movement*. Boston: South End Press, 1990.

Gordon, Linda. *Woman's Body, Woman's Right: A Social History of Birth Control in America*, rev. ed. New York: Penguin Books, 1990.

Hartmann, Betsy. *Reproductive Rights and Wrongs: The Global Politics of Population Control and Contraceptive Choice*. New York: Harper & Row, 1987.

Hatcher, Robert, et al. *Contraceptive Technology, 1990–1992*, 15th rev. ed. New York: Irvington, 1990. A comprehensive handbook on birth control methods.

Luker, Kristin. *Taking Chances: Abortion and the Decision Not to Contracept*. Berkeley: University of California Press, 1975. A study of the complicated reasons why some women have sexual intercourse without using birth control, even when contraceptives are available.

Mintzes, Barbara, and Anita Hardon. *A Question of Control: Women's Perspectives on the Development and Use of Contraceptive Technologies*. Amsterdam, Netherlands: Women's Health Action Foundation, 1992.

Seaman, Barbara, and Gideon Seaman. *Women and the Crisis in Sex Hormones*. New York: Bantam Books, 1978 (paper). An excellent resource on the Pill, IUD, barrier methods, etc.

Todd, Alexandra Dundas. *Intimate Adversaries: Cultural Conflict Between Doctors and Women Patients*. Philadelphia: University of Pennsylvania Press, 1989.

Trussell, James, and Kathryn Kost. "Contraceptive Failure in the United States: A Critical Review of the Literature," *Studies in Family Planning*, Vol. 18 (September/October 1987), pp. 237–83.

Yanoshik, Kim, and Judy Norsigian, "Contraception, Control, and Choice: International Perspectives," in K. S. Ratcliff, ed., *Healing Technology: Feminist Perspectives*. Ann Arbor: University of Michigan Press, 1989.

Barrier Methods

Bruce, Judith, and S. Bruce Shearer. "Contraceptives and Developing Countries: The Role of Barrier Methods." 1983. A public-issues paper available from The Population Council, 1 Dag Hammarskjold Plaza, New York, NY 10017.

Chalker, Rebecca. *The Complete Cervical Cap Guide*. New York: Harper & Row, 1987. This is an excellent resource, not only for its clear and concise information about the cap, but about birth control more generally.

Concord Feminist Health Center, 38 South Main Street, Concord, NH 03301. Information packet on the cervical cap, $7.50.

"FDA Approves Vaginal Sponge as a Contraceptive Device," *Contraceptive Technology Update*, Vol. 4, No. 5 (May 1983).

Jick, H., et al. "Vaginal Spermicides and Congenital Disorders," *Journal of the American Medical Association*, Vol. 245 (1981), pp. 1329–32.

Lane, M. E. "Successful Use of the Diaphragm and Jelly by a Young Population: Report of a Clinical Study," *Family Planning Perspectives*, Vol. 8 (1976), pp. 81–86.

Liskin, L., et al. "Condoms—Now More than Ever," *Population Reports*, Series H, No. 8 (September 1990).

Available from Population Information Programs, Johns Hopkins University, 624 North Broadway, Baltimore, MD 21205.

McIntyre, S. L., and J. E. Higgins. "Parity and Use-Effectiveness with the Contraceptive Sponge," *American Journal of Obstetrics and Gynecology*, Vol. 155, No. 4 (1986), pp. 796–801.

Shapiro, S., et al. "Birth Defects in Relation to Vaginal Spermicides," *Journal of the American Medical Association*, Vol. 247, No. 17 (May 7, 1982), pp. 2381–84.

Tatum, Howard J., and Elizabeth B. Connell-Tatum. "Barrier Contraception: A Comprehensive Review," *Fertility and Sterility*, Vol. 36, No. 1 (July 1981), pp. 1–12.

Trussell, James, et al. "Contraceptive Failure in the United States: An Update," *Studies in Family Planning*, Vol. 21, No. 1 (January/February 1990), pp. 51–54.

World Health Organization. *Barrier Contraceptives and Spermicides*. Geneva, Switzerland: WHO, 1987.

Natural Birth Control

Note: These are some of the publications or resources currently available. Please understand that they are **not** meant to take the place of a group in which these skills are shared on a women-to-woman basis. We do not recommend that you use the information for contraception until you have participated in such a group.

Bell, Susan, et al. "Reclaiming Reproductive Control: A Feminist Approach to Fertility Consciousness," *Science for the People*, Vol. 12, No. 1 (1980), pp. 6–9, 30–35. Available from Science for the People, 897 Main Street, Cambridge, MA 02139.

Billings, Evelyn, and Ann Westmore. *The Billings Method*. New York: Random House, 1980. A popularized introduction to the ovulation method.

Cooper, Suzannah. *The Ovulation Method Charting Booklet*, 2nd ed. 1985. Three years of mucus/BBT charts with guidelines, $6.50. Available from Fertility Awareness Services, Box 986, Corvallis, OR 97339.

Doyle, Suzannah Cooper. "FA: Reclaiming Reproductive Control," *WomenWise*, Vol. 14, No. 2 (Summer 1991), p. 6.

———. *A Fertility Awareness Self-Instruction Course*. 1989. $45 (includes follow-up counseling). Available from Fertility Awareness Services, Box 986, Corvallis, OR 97339.

Guay, Terrie. *The Personal Fertility Guide*, 2nd rev. ed. New York: Beaufort Books, 1986.

Guren, Denise S., and Nealy Gillette. *The Ovulation Method—Cycles of Fertility*. Bellingham, WA: Ovulation Method Teachers Association. 1983. $4.70. Available from Denise Guren, 2908 Cottonwood, Bellingham, WA 98225.

Kass-Annese, Barbara, and Hal Danzer. *The Fertility Awareness Workbook*. 1986. $9.25. Available from Printed Matter, P.O. Box 15246, Atlanta, GA 30333.

Kippley, John, and Sheila Kippley. *The Art of Natural Family Planning*, 2nd ed. 1979. $8.20. Available from Couple to Couple League, P.O. Box 11084, Cincinnati, Ohio 45211.

Pfeiffer, Regina Asaph, and Katherine Whitlock. *Fertility Awareness*. Englewood Cliffs, NJ: Prentice Hall, 1984.

Trussell, James, and Laurence Grummer-Strawn. "Contraceptive Failure of the Ovulation Method of Periodic Abstinence," *Family Planning Perspectives*, Vol. 22, No. 2 (1990), pp. 65–75.

Wilson, Mercedes Arzu. *Love and Fertility*. Mandeville, LA: BBE Publishing, 1986. $16.00. Available from Family of the Americas Foundation, P.O. Box 219, Mandeville, LA 70448.

Winstein, Merryl. *Your Fertility Signals: How to Read Them to Achieve or Avoid Pregnancy*. 1988. $11.95. Available from Smooth Stone Press, P.O. Box 19875, St. Louis, MO 63144.

The Pill and Other Hormones

American Academy of Pediatrics, Committee on Drugs. "Breast Feeding and Contraception," *Pediatrics*, Vol. 68, No. 1 (July 1981), pp. 138–40.

Goldbaum, G. M., et al. "The Relative Impact of Smoking and Oral Contraceptive Use on Women in the United States," *Journal of the American Medical Association*, Vol. 258 (1987), pp. 1339–42.

Kay, Clifford R. "Breast Cancer and the Pill—A Further Report from the Royal College of General Practitioners OC Study," *British Journal of Cancer*, Vol. 58 (1988), pp. 675–80.

Kent, Ann. "Thirty Years on the Pill," *London Times* (March 22, 1990), p. 19.

Linn, Shai, et al. "Delay in Conception for Former 'Pill' Users," *Journal of the American Medical Association*, Vol. 247, No. 5 (1982), pp. 629–32.

Miller, Donald, et al. "Breast Cancer Before Age 45 and Oral Contraceptive Use: New Findings," *American Journal of Epidemiology*, Vol. 129, No. 2 (1989), pp. 269–80.

Minkin, S. "Nine Thai Women Had Cancer . . . None of Them Took Depo-Provera: Therefore Depo-Provera Is Safe. This Is Science?" *Mother Jones* (November 1981), pp. 34ff.

Mintz, M. "Annals of Commerce: Selling the Pill," *Washington Post* (February 8, 1976).

O'Malley, Becky. "Who Says Oral Contraceptives Are Safe?" *The Nation* (February 14, 1981).

Schwartz, J., et al. *Connections: Nutrition, Contraception, Women, Eating*. 1982. Available from Boston Family Planning Project, Department of Health and Hospitals, 818 Harrison Avenue, Boston, MA 02118.

Seaman, Barbara. *The Doctor's Case Against the Pill*. New York: Dell, 1979.

Stadel, Bruce. "Oral Contraceptives and Premenopausal Breast Cancer in Nulliparous Women," *Contraception*, Vol. 38, No. 3 (1988), pp. 287–99.

Stolley, Paul D., Brian L. Strom and Philip E. Sartwell. "Oral Contraceptives and Vascular Disease," *Epidemiologic Reviews*, Vol. 11 (1989), pp. 241–43.

"Triphasics and Ovarian Cysts: No Relationship?" *Contraceptive Technology Update*, Vol. 8 (August 1988), pp. 89–92.

IUD

Bevia, Maria, and Gordon Myron. "Common Complications from IUDs," *Resident and Staff Physician* (June 1976).

Cates, W. "The Intrauterine Device and Deaths from Spontaneous Abortion," *New England Journal of Medicine*, Vol. 295 (1976), p. 1155.

Foreman, Harry, et al. "Intrauterine Device Usage and Fetal Loss," *Obstetrics and Gynecology*, Vol. 58, No. 6 (1981), pp. 667–77.

Geyelin, Milo. "Dalkon Shield Trust Hailed as Innovative, Stirs a Lot of Discord," *Wall Street Journal* (June 3, 1991), pp. 1, 5.

"IUDs: An Appropriate Contraceptive for Many Women," *Population Reports*, Series B, No. 4 (July 1982). Available from Population Information Programs, Johns Hopkins Univerity, 624 North Broadway, Baltimore, MD 21205.

Kaufman, D. W., et al. "Intrauterine Contraceptive Device Use and Pelvic Inflammatory Disease," *American Journal of Obstetrics and Gynecology*, Vol. 136 (1980), pp. 159–62.

Mintz, Morton. *At Any Cost: Corporate Greed, Women, and the Dalkon Shield.* New York: Pantheon, 1985.

Treiman, K., and L. Liskin. "IUDs—A New Look." *Population Reports*, Series H., No. 5 (March 1988). Available from Population Information Programs, Johns Hopkins University, 624 North Broadway, Baltimore, MD 21205.

Sterilization

Gratton, N. Marcil. "Sterilization Regret Among Women in Metropolitan Montreal," *Family Planning Perspectives*, Vol. 20, No. 5 (1988), pp. 222–27.

Lissner, E. A. "Latex and Hormones Aside. . . ." *WomenWise* (Spring 1991), pp. 5, 8–10. Available from Elaine Lissner, P.O. Box 4208, Stanford, CA 94309.

Petchesky, Rosalind Pollack. *Abortion and Woman's Choice: The State, Sexuality, and Reproductive Freedom*, rev. ed. Boston: Northeastern University Press, 1990.

Winston, R. M. L. "Why 103 Women Asked for Reversal of Sterilization," *British Medical Journal* (July 30, 1977), pp. 305–7.

14

Sexually Transmitted Diseases

BY MARY CROWE, WITH
JUDY NORSIGIAN

With special thanks to Hilde
Armour, William McCormick,
Esther Rome, Pam White and Paul
Wiesner.

*This chapter in previous editions was
called "Venereal Disease" and was
written by Esther Rome and Fran
Ansley.*

*1992 Update by Judy Norsigian,
Michelle Topal and the American
Social Health Association with help
from Katherine M. Stone.*

Many people are surprised to learn that sexually transmitted disease (STD) is one of the most common kinds of infection going around today. Every year more than 12 million Americans get an STD, which is passed from person to person primarily through sexual contact. Until recently these infections were called venereal disease, or VD, a term many people associate with gonorrhea and syphilis. Actually, there have been more than twenty STDs identified; many are at epidemic levels in this country. In addition to the diseases themselves, which can range from mild to life-threatening, there is the possibility of complications for women that can impair their fertility.

Many of us still believe that "nice" girls don't get STD. When we do, we are labeled "promiscuous" if we are single or "unfaithful" if we are in a monogamous relationship. Worst of all, we may not get help when we are sick and need it most. As long as our society continues to look upon STDs as punishment for people who have casual sex, the problem will be hard to talk about, much less eradicate.*

No woman should be ashamed of having sexual feelings or choosing to be (or not to be) sexually active. But it is important to keep our sexual relationships healthy. That means learning how to prevent STDs, which are infections, before they happen, as well as how to get cured after the fact, whenever this is possible. We can help prevent the spread of infection without giving up our sex lives.

Because STD is hard to talk about, it can be difficult to find the information we need. Sometimes it seems easier to avoid the issue and forget about prevention, especially when our sexual partners are noncooperative or even hostile to the idea of "safer sex" (see Chapter 15). But the recent epidemic of AIDS and human immunodeficiency virus (HIV) infection (see Chapter 15) has raised public awareness about the need to practice prevention to avoid getting a deadly virus for which there is no cure. More of us now are willing to talk about using condoms—our primary means of STD prevention—although many people still don't. Changing our attitudes and behavior remains a major challenge of the 1990s.

STD has so many negative overtones. Even when we feel comfortable talking about sex we may not want anyone to know that we might have an STD.

---

*In Western culture this goes back a long way. Even before sexual nature was understood, syphilis and gonorrhea were considered just punishment for blasphemy.

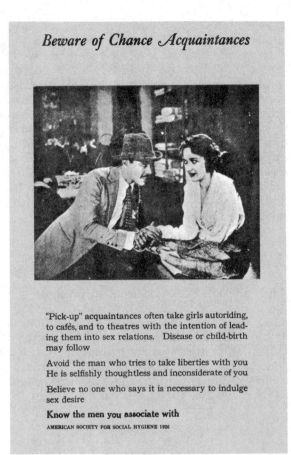

Beware of Chance Acquaintances

"Pick-up" acquaintances often take girls autoriding, to cafès, and to theatres with the intention of leading them into sex relations. Disease or child-birth may follow

Avoid the man who tries to take liberties with you He is selfishly thoughtless and inconsiderate of you

Believe no one who says it is necessary to indulge sex desire

Know the men you associate with

AMERICAN SOCIETY FOR SOCIAL HYGIENE 1926

Unknown

I've been so upset these last few days. My husband told me he'd slept with someone else and might have gotten an STD. I didn't know what to do. How could I call up my regular doctor and expose myself? If I asked any of my friends what to do, they would be mortified. I saw an ad yesterday for an STD hot line, and after a lot of hesitation I called. It was a relief to get information without anyone knowing who I was.

Having an STD can affect the way we feel about ourselves, our sexuality and our relationships. We may feel victimized, angry or depressed and even blame ourselves unfairly.

If one person in a supposedly monogamous couple gets an STD, it often serves as a dramatic focus for any problems the couple might have.

My husband and I, our toddler and sixteen-year-old baby-sitter went to the country at the end of the summer. When we returned home I started having a vaginal itch. Then I noticed my husband was itching, too. I asked him if he had slept with anyone else recently. He admitted to me he had slept with the baby-sitter. Otherwise he would never have told me.

Even when we feel comfortable about facing these issues, getting an STD usually means trouble. We will have to spend time and money for medical care; we will need to tell our sex partners so they can be treated too; and we will have our own feelings to deal with. Friends, counselors, therapists or a self-help group can all help when we have an STD.

WHAT ARE STDS?

STD is a term used to describe any disease acquired primarily through sexual contact. These can be caused by bacteria, viruses, tiny insects or parasites.

THE MOST COMMON STDS	
Chlamydia	Bacterial vaginosis (also
Gonorrhea	called hemophilus)
Human papillomavirus	HIV infection/AIDS
infection (e.g., genital	Syphilis
warts)	Pediculosis pedis (Crabs)
Genital herpes	Scabies
Nongonococcal urethri-	Chancroid
tis (NGU)	Hepatitis B
Trichomoniasis	

HOW STDS ARE SPREAD

The organisms (bugs, germs) that cause these diseases (except for crabs and scabies) generally enter the body through the mucous membranes—the warm, moist surfaces of the vagina, urethra, anus and mouth. Thus you can catch an STD through intimate contact with someone who already has the infection, especially during oral, anal or genital sex. When your partner has more than one STD you can become infected with all you are exposed to; gonorrhea and chlamydia are often transmitted together.

The stories about how you can get STDs from toilet seats, doorknobs or other objects are not true except under certain extremely rare conditions.* Nor can you catch STDs from heavy lifting, straining or being dirty. Animals don't transmit STDs to humans. Organisms that cause most STDs live best in a warm, moist environment like the linings of the genitals or throat. Outside the body most die in less than a minute or two.

*The inanimate object would need to have on it fresh, wet contaminated body fluid. See individual diseases for an explanation of when this could occur.

HOW LIKELY AM I TO GET STD?

Statistically, if you are young (between fifteen and twenty-four), are sexually active with more than one partner and live in an urban setting you are at highest risk for STD. Your chances of getting an individual infection will also depend on your ability to practice effective prevention. Basically, however, if you are heterosexual and have sexual contact with a man who has an STD, your chances of catching the infection are good. For example, after just one exposure to gonorrhea you have an 80 percent chance of catching the disease.

If you are lesbian, you are much less likely to get an STD because most STDs are not easily spread between women. It is possible to transmit herpes during kissing, oral–genital sex or through skin contact between an open sore and broken skin. It is also theoretically possible, though almost unheard of, to transmit gonorrhea to the throat during oral sex. If you have sex with both men and women, your chances of getting STD are the same as for heterosexuals. For more information, contact the American Social Health Association (ASHA) (see Resources).

BIRTH CONTROL AND STDS

While the Pill does not seem to promote gonorrhea, studies show that women using the Pill are more susceptible to chlamydial infections and possibly to HIV infection as well (see Chapter 15).

Barrier methods of contraception (latex condom, diaphragm, cervical cap, contraceptive sponge and spermicide) do offer protection against STDs, while the Pill, the IUD, and Norplant do not provide any protection.

HOW BIG IS THE PROBLEM?

Statistics show that the incidence of nearly every STD is on the rise. Of the ones we will be discussing in detail in this chapter, only gonorrhea has remained relatively stable (still at an epidemic level), thanks to massive federal programs for screening and control. Syphilis, considered under control in the late 1970s, is now increasing rapidly, especially among women, while the more newly recognized STDs, chlamydia and herpes, are growing so fast that they are called the "new epidemics." The incidence of genital warts is rising fast, particularly among women.

Chlamydial infections are now the primary preventable cause of sterility in women. Unfortunately, many clinics and physicians still do not provide diagnostic testing for this disease.

WHY PREVENTION?

1. Most literature on STDs stresses treatment and cure, which is not at all an effective way of controlling and reducing these diseases in this country. Because so many women (and quite a few men) have no symptoms, we can unknowingly start a chain of infection, which affects many people. We can stop this chain if each of us uses pro-

---

BRIEF SUMMARY

1. STDs are very common. If you are sexually active in anything but a totally monogamous relationship with someone who does not have an STD, you have a good chance of getting an STD.

2. The best way to deal with an STD is to avoid getting it in the first place. Use preventive methods wherever possible. The male and female condoms currently offer the best available protection, but the diaphragm, cervical cap, contraceptive sponge and chemical spermicides provide some protection, too.

3. If you think there is the slightest possibility you have an STD, get medical attention as soon as you can. In the meantime, try to figure out if the person you had sex with thinks s/he has been exposed to an STD.

4. Don't have sex until you have been tested or are sure you are cured (check with your practitioner).

5. If you do have an STD, inform all your recent partners personally or through an anonymous letter.

6. Before accepting treatment, make sure you understand what you are taking and for how long, the side effects and any follow-up tests or treatment required. Don't be embarrassed about asking questions. It's your life, not theirs.

7. Remember, if you are cured you can get the same STD again. Also, having one STD doesn't prevent you from getting any others.

To find out where you can get more information on symptoms, testing and treatment, see the Resources section at the end of this chapter; call the hot lines listed there.

The following methods are medically effective against STD in laboratory or clinical tests. No method is 100 percent effective, but using any of them should greatly reduce your chances of catching an STD.

1. Latex condoms (rubbers) used during vaginal, oral and anal intercourse are the best method of prevention we have so far. The man must put on the condom before his penis touches your vulva, mouth or anus.

2. Use the new female condom. This could be especially useful for women whose male partners can't or won't use a condom.

3. Use vaginal spermicides (contraceptive foams, creams and jellies).* You can purchase these in a drugstore without a prescription and use them with or without a diaphragm or condom. For maximum protection, use them with a diaphragm. When using with a condom, put an applicatorful of spermicide inside the vagina before sexual intercourse. If you take the Pill or have an IUD, it is wise to use spermicides, too.

4. Use a diaphragm (preferably with spermicide) to protect against STD that primarily affects the cervix (as with gonorrhea and chlamydia). Some researchers have found that women who use diaphragms have a lower incidence of chlamydial infection than those who use other forms of birth control.

5. Washing genitals before and right after sex is of questionable use for women. It is important for men to wash their testicles and penis, particularly after anal sex and before going on to vaginal or oral sex. Douching in most cases does not prevent STD, as it washes away normal vaginal secretions that help our bodies fight off infection and may even push infections higher up in your reproductive system.

6. We do not recommend morning-after antibiotic use. Taken just before or within nine hours after exposure to an infected person, these antibiotic pills contain enough drug *to prevent* these diseases, but *not enough to cure* an established infection. This method has serious drawbacks. Each time we use an antibiotic, we increase our chances of becoming allergic to that particular family of antibiotic, and then we cannot use that antibiotic for another illness for which it may be the most effective treatment. Also, if you take antibiotics frequently or in less than the optimal dosage, you may encourage the development of resistant strains of gonorrhea. *We do not recommend this method.*

7. There are also barrier methods that can be used for mouth-to-vagina or mouth-to-anus contact. These have not been scientifically tested or approved, but some people now place household plastic wrap over the area before contact and then discard it after one-time use.

---

*The creams, foams and jellies listed here have been shown in the laboratory to kill organisms that cause gonorrhea, syphilis, trichomoniasis, candidiasis, chlamydia, HIV, and the herpes virus. In actual use, they have been shown to be effective only against chlamydia and gonorrhea. These products have not been tested for use in anal sex and therefore may not be recommended. Some people may be allergic to one of the products. If you or your lover gets an itching or burning after using one, switch to another brand.

---

tection in addition to seeking a cure when we know we're infected.

2. By using prevention, we can protect ourselves from the serious STD complications, such as pelvic inflammatory disease (PID) and infertility, and our children from diseases of the newborn.

3. It takes a lot out of our bodies to be sick. It is also stressful to take the large doses of antibiotics required to cure some of the STDs. (For this reason, the so-called morning-after shot of antibiotics to prevent STD should not be used.)

4. Herpes and genital warts have no known cure at this time, but using latex condoms, contraceptive creams, jellies and foams *may* reduce their spread.

5. There is no cure for AIDS at this time, so prevention of HIV infection has to be a top priority (see Chapter 15).

HOW TO PREVENT STD

We can protect ourselves from catching STD in a number of ways. Some involve common sense. Talk to your lover about STD before having sex. Ask if s/he has been exposed to an STD. This is especially important if you are pregnant! Look carefully at your body and your lover's, checking for bad smell, unusual discharge, sores, bumps, itching or redness. If you think you or your partner may have an infection, don't touch the sores or have sex.

It's one thing to talk about "being responsible about STD" and a much harder thing to do it at the moment. It's just plain hard to say to someone I am feeling very erotic with, "Oh, yes, before we go any further, can we have a conversation about STD?" It is hard to imagine murmuring into someone's ear at a time of passion, "Would you mind slipping on this condom just in case one of us has an STD?" Yet it seems awkward to bring it up any sooner if it's not clear between us that we want to make love.

For some ideas on how to talk about sex more comfortably with a lover, see Chapter 11, "Sexuality."

TREATMENT—CONVENTIONAL VS. ALTERNATIVE AND SELF-HELP

In most cases, treatments for STDs caused by bacteria involve high doses of antibiotics, which kill the bacteria. Antibiotics are not effective against viral infections like herpes. Some people are allergic to penicillin or related drugs, while others suffer unwanted side effects from other antibiotics. Sometimes antibiotics just don't work. (For information on antibiotics, see pp. 315, 316, 322.) Most herbalists do not recommend treating serious infections like gonorrhea, chlamydia or syphilis with natural remedies—at least without first trying antibiotics.

No matter what treatment you use, remember, *curing STD does not provide immunity against future infection.*

SOCIAL PROBLEMS

Medical Care and the Morality Issue

The social stigma attached to STD often affects the quality of medical care more than we would like to think.

1. Until recently, medical schools virtually ignored STDs. As a result, physicians who received training prior to the past few years may not know much about diagnosing and treating STDs, especially when there are no symptoms, or symptoms characteristic of other infections. Though physicians and medical-care workers in clinics that regularly treat STD probably have the most up-to-date information, they are rarely informed about preventive methods (such as condoms or vaginal contraceptives).

2. Many medical-care providers consider STD an appropriate punishment for "immoral" sex. This is particularly true when they are dealing with women, because we are more readily labeled promiscuous than men. It is even more true for poor women and women of color than for white middle-class women. Too often, this attitude affects the quality of medical care provided.

3. Instead of blaming patients for the spread of STD, the medical profession must examine the reasons for their own poor record of adequate screening, diagnosis, treatment, reporting and follow-up of patients with STD. Make sure that your nurse-practitioner, doctor or other practitioner diagnoses and treats STDs according to the recommendations of the Centers for Disease Control (CDC). Because untreated STDs can have such serious consequences, prevention and early treatment must become priorities.

People at all levels of responsibility, too moralistic or too ashamed about sex, have slowed down research into improved methods of prevention and curtailed the spread of information about available methods of prevention and cure.

With the advent of widespread birth control, which reduced the fear of pregnancy, fear of STD became the last deterrent to sex outside of marriage. Yet information and access to contraceptive devices that help prevent STD may be difficult to get, especially for teenagers.

Money and Politics

The treatment of STDs and their complications such as PID costs over $3 billion a year. Funding for STD research, clinical training, screening programs and public education remains inadequate.

For the past few years, several members of Congress—especially those who are part of the Congressional Caucus for Women's Issues—have advocated the passage of the Infertility Prevention Act. This bill would authorize the CDC to give $50 million to family planning and other community clinics to offer outreach and counseling to women on the prevention and control of chlamydia and gonorrhea, screen women for these diseases and provide treatment to women and their partners. It would also fund public information and education programs. Public support for initiatives like this at both the local and national levels will be critical in the coming years.

Changes We Can Make Now

Although some medical professionals maintain that the only solution for our current STD epidemic is to develop a preventive vaccine, others believe that we can and should attempt to contain the diseases now.

It is possible to reverse the trend toward an increased incidence of gonorrhea. Several European countries and China have done so by educating the people about prevention, symptoms, testing and treatment. Sweden, by promoting the condom, has reduced the incidence of STDs without restricting sexual activity.

In order to use the tools we have now, we need to change the attitude that STD is a punishment for "immoral" sex. We must initiate more effective public education programs without moral overtones in our schools and communities. There are some nonjudgmental films, pamphlets and brochures (see Resources), though few deal with preventive measures women can use. We can distribute them in public places such as libraries, schools, movie houses, social centers and health facilities; we can talk with friends, parents and children to make sure they have as much accurate information as possible. We can support women's centers as they work for more complete sex and health education. When our society accepts sexuality it will be more likely to encourage STD prevention.

Practitioners must learn more about STDs. Self-testing kits have been developed and should be made available. More paramedics and lay health workers should be involved in running community screening programs to make tests, screening and treatment available to all economic and social groups. We can ask for routine screening tests for STD when we go for medical care; medical workers will be more apt to include tests automatically if a large number of clients request them.

SEXUALLY TRANSMITTED DISEASES— SYMPTOMS AND TREATMENT*

Gonorrhea

Gonorrhea is caused by the gonococcus, a bacterium shaped like a coffee bean, which works its way gradually along the warm, moist passageways of the genital and urinary organs and affects the cervix, urethra and anus. You can transmit this disease to another person through genital, genital–oral (which exposes the throat) and genital–anal sex. You can get a gonorrhea infection in your eye when you touch it with a hand that is moist with infected discharge. A mother can pass it to her baby during birth. Rarely, very young children can contract gonorrhea by using towels contaminated with fresh discharge. More frequently, children with gonorrhea are found to have been sexually abused. Gonorrhea has also been transmitted to women through semen used for donor insemination.

The disease is more likely to persist and spread in women than in men. Untreated gonorrhea can lead to serious and painful infection of the pelvic area, PID, which can lead to sterility.

*For more information about tests, drugs and how STDs affect men than we can include in this chapter, see *A Book About Sexually Transmitted Diseases*, by Donna Cherniak, Montreal Health Press, P.O. Box 1000, Station La Cité, Montreal, Quebec H2W 2N1, Canada, 1983, and contact the ASHA (see Resources).

A less common complication is proctitis, inflammation of the rectum. If the eyes become infected by gonococcal discharge (gonococcal conjunctivitis), blindness can result. Disseminated gonococcal infection, rare but serious, occurs when bacteria travel through the bloodstream, causing infection of the heart valves or arthritic meningitis. Gonorrhea can be treated and cured with antibiotics at any stage to prevent further damage, but damage already done usually cannot be repaired.

Remember, it is important to use preventive measures, because a woman often does not have early symptoms. By the time pain prompts her to see a doctor, the infection has usually spread considerably. A woman who has had a hysterectomy can be infected in the cervix (if it is left), the anus, urethra or throat.

Symptoms

Although women have gonorrhea most often without any symptoms, 80 percent don't notice symptoms because of their mildness, or confuse them with other conditions. Symptoms usually appear anywhere from two days to three weeks after exposure. The cervix is the most common site of infection. In cervical gonorrhea, a discharge develops that is caused by an irritant released by the gonococci when they die. If you examine yourself with a speculum you may see a thick discharge, redness and small bumps or signs of erosion on the cervix. You may at first attribute symptoms to other routine gynecological problems or to the use of birth control methods like the Pill. The urethra may also become infected, possibly causing painful urination and burning. As the infection spreads, it can affect the Skene's (on each side of the urinary opening) and Bartholin's glands. If the disease spreads to the uterus and fallopian tubes, you may have pain on one or both sides of your lower abdomen, vomiting, fever and/or irregular menstrual periods. The more severe the infection, the more severe the pain and other symptoms are likely to be. These symptoms may indicate PID.

Gonorrhea can also be spread from a man's penis to a woman's throat (pharyngeal gonorrhea). You may have no symptoms, or your throat may be sore or your glands swollen.

One to 3 percent of women with gonorrhea develop disseminated gonococcal infection (DGI). Symptoms of DGI include a rash, chills, fever, pain in the joints and tendons of wrists and fingers. As the disease progresses, you may have sores on the hands, fingers, feet and toes.

Men's Symptoms

A man will usually have a thick milky discharge from his penis and feel pain or burning when he urinates. Some men have no symptoms. Gonor-

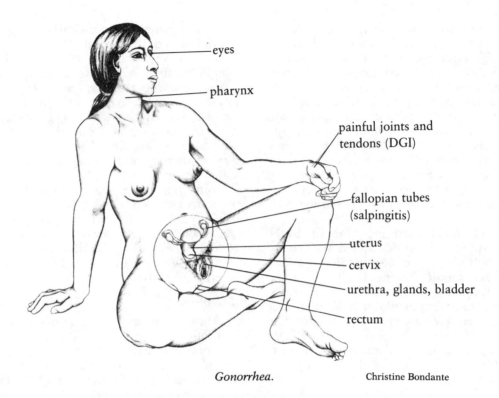

eyes

pharynx

painful joints and
tendons (DGI)

fallopian tubes
(salpingitis)

uterus

cervix

urethra, glands, bladder

rectum

Gonorrhea.   Christine Bondante

rhea in a man is often confused with nongono-coccal urethritis (NGU), which also produces a discharge and requires a different drug for cure. If you have had sex with a man who has a discharge from his penis, get him to go for a test right away. His discharge can be tested and diagnosed the same day. If he does not have gonorrhea or NGU, then you will not have to take unnecessary medication.

Testing and Diagnosis

It is important to be tested before taking medication, because a test done while treatment is being given is not accurate.

Don't douche right before a test, because you can wash away the accessible bacteria, giving a false negative test result. The gram stain and the culture are two standard tests for gonorrhea in current use. A woman can have them done during a pelvic examination or a throat exam. The widely used gram stain is very accurate for symptomatic men but only 50 percent accurate for women and asymptomatic men. In this test a smear of the discharge is placed on a slide, stained with a dye and examined for gonorrhea bacteria under a microscope. If your regular male partner's test is positive, you may want to be treated at the same time regardless of the test results.

The culture test (more reliable, but it takes longer) involves taking a swab of the discharge, rolling it onto a special culture plate and incu-bating it under special laboratory conditions for sixteen to forty-eight hours to let the gonorrhea bacteria multiply. Even the culture test can be inaccurate, primarily because it is difficult to maintain specimens in good condition during transportation to the lab. Test accuracy also depends greatly on which sites are chosen for testing. If you have the most commonly affected sites (cervix and anal canal) cultured, there is about a 90 percent chance of finding any existing infection. (Many women with gonorrhea also have tricho-moniasis and/or chlamydia.) The swab from the cervix is the best single test, about 88 to 93 percent accurate. Many women with infected cervices also have infection in the anal canal. If you have had a hysterectomy, ask for a urethral culture, too. If you have had oral–genital sex, ask for a gonococ-cal throat culture. Ask what kind of medium is used for culturing. Thayer-Martin or Transgrow are best.

Often women will have both tests, the gram smear for initial screening and the culture test to confirm the diagnosis. If the smear is negative but you have definitely been exposed to gonorrhea, you may want to be treated anyway while waiting for the results of the culture to come back.

Although these tests are not completely reliable, they are the most widely available in physicians' offices and clinics. If you have any doubts as to how accurate the results of your test were, try to have someone else do one or come back again within a week or two, the sooner the better.

Other Tests

The Food and Drug Administration (FDA) has recently licensed two new tests for gonorrhea. The *ELISA technique* (trade name, Gonozyme) detects antigens to the gonorrhea bacteria in cervical, anal or urethral specimens. This test can be performed in one or two hours, but the technology is more complicated and much more expensive than that of the culture test. Currently, medical practitioners still prefer the culture test when they have a good laboratory nearby to do it.

There are several FDA-licensed rapid gonorrhea tests. These tests can be performed in thirty minutes to several hours. While considered accurate, they may give a positive test when you are not infected (false positive) or a negative test when you are infected (false negative). These are not as reliable as the culture tests.

Treatment

Many physicians prescribe medication before the culture test is back or diagnosis is certain for three reasons: Tests are not always accurate; the physician is not sure you will come back; and the sooner the gonorrhea is treated, the easier it is to cure. Ask about medication for your partner.

On the other hand, some places refuse to treat you, even when you are certain of infection, until a positive diagnosis is made. One argument in favor of waiting for test results is that you should not take antibiotics unnecessarily.

An IUD may make cure more difficult because it helps spread infection and increases the chances of getting PID. Have your IUD removed before treatment.

The CDC recommend one dose of ceftriaxone as the preferred initial treatment for gonorrhea. Because chlamydia frequently coexists with gonorrhea, the CDC also recommend ongoing treatment with doxycycline (seven days) to treat the chlamydia. However, if it is possible to test for chlamydia (see p. 316), you should do this first in order to avoid possibly unnecessary use of antibiotics. Doxycycline is preferable over tetracycline only because the latter must be taken four times a day, while doxycycline is taken only twice a day. Neither should be used by a pregnant woman, who should take erythromycin instead (this is less effective but safer).

Follow-up

With ceftriaxone, a follow-up culture to test for cure is not necessary.

Gonorrhea and Pregnancy

Pregnant women should receive at least one routine gonorrhea culture during pregnancy. A pregnant woman with untreated gonorrhea can infect her baby as it passes through her birth canal. In the past, many babies went blind due to gonococcal conjunctivitis. All states now require the eyes of newborns to be treated with silver nitrate or other antibiotic drops in order to prevent this disease, even when the mother is sure she does not have gonorrhea and knows the treatment is unnecessary.

Chlamydia and Ureaplasma

Chlamydia, caused by the bacterium *Chlamydia trachomatis*, is the most common bacterial STD in the United States today. Chlamydia can cause very serious problems for women, including urethral infection, cervicitis (inflammation of the cervix), PID and infertility as well as dangerous complications during pregnancy and birth (see below). In men it can cause NGU, an inflammation of the urethra. This organism can also cause proctitis (inflammation of the rectum). Anal chlamydia has been found in sexually abused children.

Chlamydia is transmitted during vaginal or anal sex with someone who has the infection. It can also be passed by a hand moistened with infected secretions to the eye and from mother to baby during delivery. It is possible but unlikely to pass chlamydia to the throat if you perform oral sex on an infected man.

NGU can also be caused by *Ureaplasma urealyticum* (also called *T-Myocoplasma*), which is also a sexually transmitted bacterium. It has been found in the genital tracts of many apparently healthy people who have no symptoms of infection. While ureaplasma causes up to one-quarter of the cases of NGU in men,* it is currently not known what role ureaplasma plays with cervicitis or PID in women.† Some researchers believe it can cause pregnancy complications (see below).‡

Symptoms

Four-fifths of women with chlamydia have no symptoms. The most common symptom among women is increased vaginal discharge, which usually develops seven to fourteen days after exposure to the chlamydia bacterium. Painful urination, unusual vaginal bleeding, bleeding after sex and low abdominal pain are other signs. The cervix may or may not appear inflamed upon examination. If you have no symptoms, you must rely on your

---

*Fifty percent of cases of NGU are caused by chlamydia, 25 percent by ureaplasma and 25 percent by as yet unidentified organisms.
†Continued research needs to be done.
‡A related organism, *Mycolasma hominis*, may also be associated with infections leading to PID and, according to some researchers, infertility and/or premature birth.

fallopian tubes (chlamydial PID)

cervix
(chlamydia)

uterus
(chlamydial PID)

urethra

rectum

*Chlamydia. Chlamydia can also be transmitted to the
eyes via the hands.*   Christine Bondante

partner to tell you if he has symptoms or has been
diagnosed for NGU. You may want to get regular
chlamydia screening if you are sexually active.

Men's Symptoms

Men will usually have a burning sensation upon
urination and a urethral discharge that appears
one to three weeks after exposure. Symptoms may
be similar to those of gonorrhea but are usually
milder. The incubation period is also generally
longer—at least seven days. About 10 percent of
men have no symptoms, even though they can still
transmit the disease. Frequently only one member
of a couple will have symptoms, while the other
carries the infection. Both partners must be
treated to prevent passing the disease back and
forth.

Some practitioners are not aware enough of the
dangers of chlamydia. In addition, because chlamydial infection is so easy to confuse with gonorrhea and other diseases, practitioners often
misdiagnose it. They also overlook women's
symptoms or attribute them to other causes.

*It started out as cystitis. A few months later I started
having fever, chills and a lot of pain in my lower
abdomen. The doctor never said anything about the
possibility of chlamydia or PID. Instead they did
tests for gonorrhea, which were negative. After six
months of being really sick, they gave me ampicillin,
which didn't help. They kept saying, "There's nothing wrong with you. You must be having emotional
problems." After nine months I had a good case of
PID, which they called "a little pelvic infection." It
wasn't until my husband came down with symptoms
of NGU that they took me seriously and treated us
both with the right drugs.*

Remember, the usual treatment for gonorrhea
is *not* effective against these organisms. If you

think you have been exposed to NGU, wait for the
results of a test before accepting treatment for
gonorrhea.

Testing and Diagnosis

At present tests for chlamydia are *widely* available, although tests for ureaplasma are not. In
most cases, if you or your partner has a discharge,
you will be tested for gonorrhea, and if that is
negative, the practitioner will diagnose NGU/MPC
(mucopurulent cervicitis) by elimination. Incubation of the disease is also a clue. NGU takes
longer to show up than gonorrhea, although the
time period can vary, depending on whether chlamydia, mycoplasma, a combination of the two or
other bacteria are causing the infection. When the
organism causing the NGU is determined, the diagnosis will no longer be NGU. The person will
then be diagnosed with whatever was found and
treated for that organism. The CDC maintain that
a urethral smear is the only accurate test. Tests
for ureaplasma involve taking a swab from the
cervix and culturing the specimen, and are performed at large medical centers and some public
health laboratories. Nonculture tests for chlamydia (such as the monoclonal antibody test) are less
expensive, more rapid and now more widely available than culture tests. They are somewhat less
reliable but offer a valuable aid to diagnosis. For
information on where to get tested, call your public health department. The blood tests presently
available for chlamydia are currently considered
too impractical for widespread use.

Treatment

Tetracycline has been the standard treatment
for chlamydia and ureaplasma infections. The
CDC now recommend doxycycline as the treatment of choice, because it only has to be taken
twice a day instead of four times a day, as with
tetracycline. Erythromycin is often prescribed
when tetracycline or doxycycline cannot be given,
such as during pregnancy. Many of the other antibiotics commonly used for STD infections, including penicillin, are not effective. People with
chlamydial eye infections are treated with local
antibacterial agents, such as chlortetracycline.

Take all the medication prescribed, or the infection may come back at a later date, cause more
trouble and be harder to get rid of. Usually it
clears up within three weeks. If not, go back to the
practitioner, who will prescribe a different antibiotic or a longer treatment time. Regular sexual
partners should take tetracycline or doxycycline
whether or not they have symptoms. Because 10
percent of ureaplasma is resistant to tetracycline,
some practitioners recommend a follow-up culture one to four weeks after treatment.

316

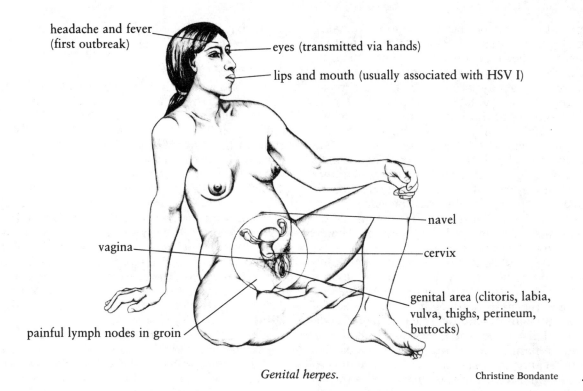

headache and fever (first outbreak)

eyes (transmitted via hands)

lips and mouth (usually associated with HSV I)

navel

vagina

cervix

genital area (clitoris, labia, vulva, thighs, perineum, buttocks)

painful lymph nodes in groin

Genital herpes.   Christine Bondante

Before taking any antibiotics, check with your doctor about possible undesirable effects. Pregnant women should not take tetracycline or doxycycline. Avoid alcohol until the infection is cured, as it may irritate the urethra. Have no sexual contact until you and your partner are cured. If you seem to keep having recurrent episodes of chlamydia and antibiotics have not cleared up the infection, you may have another bacterial infection or possibly a stubborn case of PID.

Chlamydia, Ureaplasma and Pregnancy

Studies indicate that 8 to 10 percent of all pregnant women may be infected with chlamydia, which, if untreated, can then be transmitted to the baby during birth. Infected babies may develop conjunctivitis or pneumonia. Chlamydia has also been linked to miscarriage, ectopic pregnancy, premature delivery and postpartum infections. Because of these risks, testing for chlamydia may soon be recommended for all pregnant women.

Because ureaplasma has also been strongly implicated as a cause of infertility, miscarriage and premature birth, some researchers feel that any woman with a history of infertility or ectopic pregnancies should be tested for ureaplasma or other mycoplasmas as well.

Herpes

Herpes (from the Greek word meaning "to creep") is caused by the herpes simplex virus, a tiny primitive organism studied considerably in recent years. The virus enters the body through the skin and mucous membranes of the mouth and genitals and travels along the nerve endings to the base of the spine, where it sets up permanent residence, feeding off nutrients produced by the body cells. There are two types of herpes simplex (HSV) viruses. Type I (HSV I) usually is characterized by cold sores or fever blisters on the lips, face and mouth, while Type II (HSV II) most often involves sores in the genital area. While HSV I is usually found above the waist and HSV II below, there is some crossover, primarily due to the increase in oral–genital sex. In this chapter we will be concerned with genital herpes.

You can get herpes by direct skin-to-skin contact during vaginal, anal or oral sex with someone who has an active infection. It may also be possible to spread it from mouth to genitals (or eyes) via the fingers. Although the disease is most contagious from the time the skin reddens until the sores crust over, herpes can be transmitted when no symptoms are present. Most transmission occurs when people are asymptomatic.

Symptoms

Symptoms usually occur two to twenty days after infection, although most people may not have symptoms or may not be aware of them until much later. An outbreak of herpes usually begins with a tingling or itching sensation of the skin in the genital area. This is called the *prodromal* period and may occur several hours to several days before the sores erupt, or it may not occur at all.

You may also experience burning sensations, pains in your legs, buttocks or genitals and/or a feeling of pressure in the area. Sores then appear, starting as one or more red bumps and changing to watery blisters within a day or two. Blisters are most likely to occur on the labia majora and minora, clitoris, vaginal opening, perineum and occasionally on the vaginal wall, buttocks, thighs, anus and navel. Women can also have sores on their cervix, which usually cause no discernible symptoms. Many women have sores on both the vulva and cervix during a first infection. Within a few days, the blisters rupture, leaving shallow ulcers that may ooze, weep or bleed. Usually after three or four days a scab forms and the sores heal themselves without treatment.

While the sores are active, you may find it painful to urinate, and you may have a dull ache or a sharp burning pain in your entire genital area. Sometimes the pain radiates into the legs. You may also have an urge to urinate frequently and/or a vaginal discharge. You may also have vulvitis (a painful inflammation of the vulva). During the first outbreak, you may also experience fever, headache and swelling of the lymph nodes in the groin. The initial outbreak is usually the most painful and takes the longest time to heal (two to three weeks).

Men's Symptoms

Men may experience pain in the testicles during the prodromal period, followed by sores that usually appear on the head and shaft of the penis but can also appear on the scrotum, perineum, buttocks, anus and thighs. Men can also have sores without knowing it, usually because they are hidden inside the urethra. There may also be a watery discharge from the urethra.

Recurrences

Some people never experience a second outbreak of herpes, but most people (75 percent) do, usually within three to twelve months of the initial episode and usually in the same area of the body. Recurrent episodes are usually milder, last from three days to two weeks and usually do not involve the cervix. They often seem to be triggered by stress, illness, trauma to the skin, menstruation or pregnancy. Most people find that the number of yearly recurrences decreases with time. Recurrent herpes is associated with lowered resistance, as are infections such as trichomoniasis, bladder infections, venereal warts, yeast infections and vaginitis. Poor diet and drugs that weaken the immune system (such as caffeine, speed, birth control pills and diet pills) may also make you more susceptible to recurrences. People who are deficient in B vitamins or who are unusually tense seem to get more frequent recurrences. Studies show that HSV II in the genital area is much more likely to recur than HSV I.

Testing and Diagnosis

You and your practitioner can usually diagnose herpes by sight when the sores are present, although herpes is occasionally confused with chancroid, syphilis or venereal warts. Several lab tests confirm the diagnosis or indicate the presence of herpes even when no sores are active.

The Tzanck Test

This test is similar to a Pap smear. A scraping is taken from the edge of an active sore, smeared on a slide sprayed with a cell fixative and sent to a lab for evaluation. A fairly accurate method of diagnosis, it can be used for both men and women, and is inexpensive (three to fifteen dollars). It cannot differentiate between HSV I and HSV II.

Viral Culture

A viral tissue culture can be taken using living cells to grow the virus. This test has an advantage in that it can distinguish between HSV I and HSV II, but it is expensive and few laboratories or doctors are equipped to perform it. The test is more accurate than the smear and should be done when the sores *first* appear. This is considered the most accurate method.

Other Tests

You can get a blood test to measure the level of herpes antibodies in the blood. (Once you have been exposed to the virus, your body manufactures antibodies to fight off the infection.) For this test, two ampules of blood are drawn, one during the initial attack and the second, two to four weeks later. If you have herpes, the second sample will show a much higher antibody level. (It takes about two weeks to build antibodies.) This test is only effective when performed during the initial infection of herpes in persons who do not have oral herpes (because this test cannot distinguish HSV I from HSV II). Because most people are asymptomatic with their first herpes infection, this test is not generally helpful.

Newer blood tests may soon be available.

Treatment

At present there is no medical cure for herpes, although researchers are investigating vaccines, antiviral therapy and immune-system stimulants. In the meantime, keep sores clean and dry. If they are very painful, you may want to get a prescription for xylocaine cream or ethyl chloride. If you are having an outbreak of genital herpes, your practitioner may prescribe an antiviral drug called acyclovir (trade name, Zovirax). For the first (primary) outbreak, acyclovir can be used topically to help with healing. For recurrent outbreaks acyclovir can be taken orally or at the onset of symptoms. Taken daily, it may help reduce the number of recurrences and the length of outbreaks. Taken at the onset of symptoms, it can reduce pain and how long the outbreak may last. Acyclovir is not considered a cure, however.

Some evidence suggests that early application of topical 15 percent idoxuridine (IDU) in dimethyl sulfoxide (DMSO) reduces the severity of lesions on the labia and shortens the healing time.* Homeopathic treatments have also been helpful (see Chapter 5).

Self-Help and Alternative Treatment

When sores first appear, take warm sitz baths with baking soda three to five times a day. In between, keep sores clean and dry. A hair dryer helps to dry sores. Sores heal faster when exposed to air, so wear cotton underpants or none at all. If it hurts to urinate, do it in the shower or bathtub or spray water over genitals while urinating (using any plastic squeeze bottle). When sores break, apply drying agents, such as hydrogen peroxide or Dom Burrows, which is available in drugstores. For pain relief, take acetaminophen (e.g., Tylenol) or aspirin.

Many women have found the following alternative treatments very helpful for herpes. They may or may not work for you. Because some of the products mentioned below must be purchased at a health food store, they may be expensive. We suggest that you pick one or two. Remember, all are most effective when combined with good nutrition and rest. (If you are pregnant, don't take medicinal teas or high doses of vitamin C without consulting your practitioner.)

1. Echinacea is a blood-purifying plant. Capsules made from it are available at health food stores. Take two capsules every three hours, make a tincture and apply (one teaspoon every two hours for three to four days), or make a soothing tea (four cups a day).

2. Take 2,000 milligrams of vitamin C. Vitamin E applied to sores may help.

3. Chlorophyll (in powder form) and wheatgrass are good antiviral herbs. Drink them with warm water. Also, eating blue-green algae (3,000 milligrams daily) may be helpful.

4. Lysine is an amino acid that many women find very effective in suppressing early symptoms. If you stop using it, symptoms may reappear. Take 750 to 1,000 milligrams a day until sores have disappeared. Thereafter take 500 milligrams a day. Lysine seems to work by counteracting the effects of argenine (a substance found in foods such as nuts—especially peanuts—chocolate and cola), which may stimulate herpes. During any herpes episode it is wise to avoid argenine-rich foods.

5. Take five to sixty milligrams of zinc daily.

6. Grape skins may be antiviral. Some women recommend eating red grapes.

7. Acupuncture treatments administered at the first signs of an attack sometimes prevent recurrences. Fingertip stimulation of acupressure points in the feet may also prevent outbreaks (three thumbs forward of the ankle bulge, along the line between the ankle bulge and little toe.)

For Symptomatic Relief

1. Make compresses out of tea made with cloves, use black tea bags soaked in water (tannic acid is an anesthetic) or take sitz baths with uva-ursi (also known as kinnikinnick or bearberry).

2. Apply vitamin E oil, A and D ointment, baking soda or cornstarch to the sores. (Some people believe that keeping the sores moist may make them feel better but last longer.)

3. Make poultices using pulverized calcium tablets, powdered slippery elm, goldenseal, myrrh, comfrey root or cold milk. Make a paste using any of these and apply to the sores. After applying, keep the paste moistened with warm water.

4. Aloe vera gel soothes and helps to dry out sores and promote healing.

Herpes and Pregnancy

Studies show that women with herpes have an increased risk of miscarriage and premature delivery. Equally important, when a mother is shedding virus at the time of delivery, herpes can be transmitted to the baby during passage through the birth canal, causing brain damage, blindness and death in 60 to 70 percent of cases. Scary as this sounds, it is important to know that this is rare, occurring only in one out of every 5,000 normal births. The risk is much higher when mothers have a primary (first) outbreak at the time of delivery; when they have sores, their babies have at least a 50 percent chance of contracting herpes during a vaginal birth. For a mother with recurrent sores, the risk goes down to less than 4 percent because she has passed antibodies on to the baby through the amniotic fluid and the baby's blood.

Pregnant women who don't have herpes should avoid unprotected sex during the last six weeks with partners who have herpes. If you are pregnant and have recurrent herpes, tell your physician or midwife. If you have prodromal symptoms or active sores at the time of delivery, you will usually have a cesarean section within four to six hours of the time the waters break. After birth, take care not to infect the infant.

---

*Contact the ASHA (see Resources) and get *The Helper* to follow the development of new treatments for herpes lesions.

Herpes and Cancer

Many researchers believed once that women with genital herpes had a greater risk than others of getting cervical cancer. This belief is no longer widely held. Nonetheless if you have herpes, it is advisable to get a Pap smear every year. It is possible that the factors that make us susceptible to herpes are similar to those that make us susceptible to cancer.

Prevention

Efforts to develop a vaccine against herpes have been unsuccessful so far. Researchers continue to pursue the possibility of a genetically engineered vaccine. Because there is no cure for herpes, it seems especially worthwhile to protect yourself from getting it. That does *not* mean that you should never have sex with someone who has the virus in a latent stage; it simply means using your common sense in evaluating the risk and taking simple precautions when possible. About 30 million Americans are infected, but only one-quarter to one-third of these know they are. The following suggestions (along with the general methods outlined on p. 311) may also reduce your chances of getting herpes.

1. You will be less susceptible to herpes when you are in good health, eating well and have ways of dealing with stress in your life (such as yoga, deep breathing, meditation—whatever works for you).

2. Avoid sex with someone who has active sores.

3. If your partner has herpes, it may be a good idea to take the precautions listed on p. 311, even if no symptoms are present. This is because herpes can be shed and transmitted without any symptoms.

4. Because herpes can be spread by skin contact from one part of the body to another, try to avoid touching an open sore. Wash your hands after examining yourself or touching the genital area. Always wash your hands before inserting contact lenses.

Protecting Others (If You Have Herpes)

1. If you have active sores, do not have sex. Consider using condoms when no sores are present (in between outbreaks).

2. Do not donate blood during an initial outbreak.

3. Males should not donate sperm during an active outbreak of herpes.

Preventing Recurrences

1. Herpes attacks seem to be triggered by stress. If possible, figure out what precipitated your attacks and try to eliminate or reduce tension in your life.

2. Limit the use of stimulants such as coffee, tea, colas and chocolate.

3. Increase your intake of vitamins A, B and C and pantothenic acid as well as zinc, iron and calcium to help prevent recurrences.

4. Avoid foods that have a lot of argenine (such as nuts, chocolate, cola, rice and cottonseed meal). Instead, eat foods high in lysine: potatoes, meats, milk, brewer's yeast, fish, liver and eggs.

5. If your outbreaks are very severe or frequent, consider taking oral acyclovir daily. This is expensive but does prevent outbreaks. Discuss the possibility with your practitioner.

Living with Herpes

Accepting herpes as a permanent part of your life may be difficult. You may feel shocked when you discover you have herpes and then frantically search for a cure. You may feel isolated, lonely and angry, especially toward the person who gave you the infection. You may become anxious about staying in long-term relationships, having children or getting cervical cancer. Not everybody experiences herpes in these ways, nor do these responses necessarily last forever.

After the first big episode of herpes, I felt distant from my body. When we began lovemaking again, I had a hard time having orgasms or trusting the rhythm of my responses. I shed some tears over that. I felt my body had been invaded. My body feels riddled with it; I'm somehow contaminated. And there is always that lingering anxiety: Is my baby okay? It's unjust that the birth of my child may be affected.

If you are in a close relationship with someone who doesn't have herpes, it can affect you both in subtle ways.

Sometimes it bullies both of us. When my lover feels she has to protect me from stress because I'm about to get herpes, she doesn't always ask for attention, time or comfort when she needs them.

How much herpes affects your relationships can depend a lot on how much you trust each other and how comfortable you feel about sharing your concerns.

The way we experience herpes may have a lot to do with our attitude about disease. For example, people who see herpes as a symptom of stress, illness or other problems rather than as a medical disaster seem to have a much easier time finding their own ways of coping with it.

Herpes is an inconvenience and a pain, but it's something you learn to live with. I think of it as an im-

balance. *Because I know it's related to stress, I keep myself in as good physical condition as possible and try not to get too upset about it.*

The one good thing I can say about herpes is that it keeps me honest in taking care of myself. When I feel my vulva start to tingle and ache, it's immediately a reminder to me to slow down. I take long, hot baths. I try to think relaxing, releasing thoughts and send healing, calming energy to that area. Sometimes I meditate.

Humor is the best way of coping with herpes. There is so much serious, scary stuff about it. You've got to recognize that it's just one of the bad tricks people have to live with.

Herpes may be easier to cope with if you feel comfortable enough to talk about it openly. Some people manage to talk themselves out of recurrences.

What turns out to be really useful is when my family and I talk about the viruses. We say things like, "They don't want to come down now. It's much cozier up by the spinal cord where they are. The weather is pretty bad out here and everyone's too busy to pay them much attention." I think what it probably does is calm me and ease whatever is bothering me. Who knows? Maybe they hear! All I know is that sometimes after I get the warning aches we sit at dinner having those discussions about how my little herpes viruses should stay where they are, and they don't come!

The Herpes Resource Center (HRC), an organization run by the ASHA, provides support, information and self-help groups for people with herpes. It also publishes an informative quarterly journal, *The Helper,* and operates The National Herpes Hot Line: (919) 361-8488. (See Resources.)

Syphilis

Syphilis is caused by a small spiral-shaped bacterium called a spirochete. You can get syphilis through sexual or skin contact with someone who is in an infectious (primary or secondary and possibly the beginning of the latent) stage when symptoms are present (see below). A pregnant woman with syphilis can also pass the disease to her unborn child.

Syphilis spreads via open sores or rashes containing bacteria that can penetrate the mucous membranes of the genitals, mouth and anus as well as broken skin on other parts of the body.

Symptoms

Once the bacteria have entered the body, the disease may go through four stages—depending upon when a person is treated.

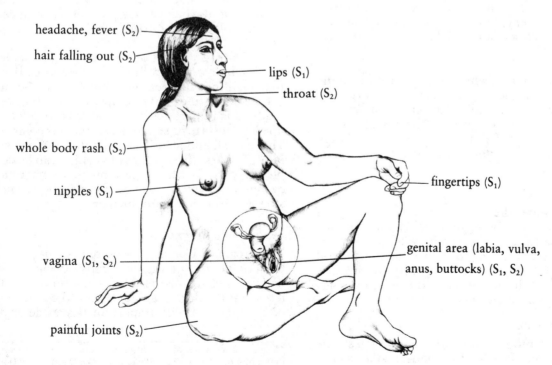

headache, fever (S₂)
hair falling out (S₂)
lips (S₁)
throat (S₂)
whole body rash (S₂)
fingertips (S₁)
nipples (S₁)
vagina (S₁, S₂)
genital area (labia, vulva, anus, buttocks) (S₁, S₂)
painful joints (S₂)

Syphilis. S₁, primary stage: chancre; S₂, secondary stage: red, sore area; rash.

Christine Bondante

Primary

The first sign is usually a painless sore called a *chancre* (pronounced "shanker"), which may look like a pimple, a blister or an open sore and shows up from nine to ninety days after the bacteria enter the body. The sore usually appears on the genitals at or near the place where the bacteria entered the body. However, it may appear on the fingertips, lips, breast, anus or mouth. Sometimes the chancre never develops or is hidden inside the vagina or folds of the labia, giving no evidence of the disease. Only about 10 percent of women who get these chancres notice them. If you examine yourself regularly with a speculum, you are more likely to see one if it develops. At the primary stage, the chancre is very infectious. The preventive methods outlined on p. 311 work only if the physical barrier covers the infectious sore. With or without treatment, the sore will heal, usually in one to five weeks, but the bacteria, still in the body, increase and spread.

Secondary

The next stage occurs anywhere from one week to six months later. By this time the bacteria have spread all through the body. This stage usually lasts weeks or months, but symptoms can come and go for several years. They may include a rash (over the entire body or just on the palms of the hands and soles of the feet); a sore in the mouth; swollen, painful joints or aching bones; a sore throat; a mild fever or headache (all flu symptoms). You may lose some hair or discover a raised area around the genitals and anus. During the secondary stage, syphilis can be spread through mucus patches or condylomalata, the raised areas.

Latent

During this stage, which may last ten to twenty years, there are no outward signs. However, the bacteria may be invading the inner organs, including the heart and brain. The disease is not infectious after the first few years of the latent stage (when no symptoms of second stage are present).

Late

In this stage the serious effects of the latent stage appear. Depending on which organs the bacteria have attacked, a person may develop serious heart disease, crippling, blindness and/or mental incapacity. With our present ability to diagnose and treat syphilis, no one should reach this stage. Syphilis in this stage is not infectious.

Men's Symptoms

Men's symptoms are similar to women's. The most common place for the chancre to appear is on the penis and scrotum. It may be hidden in the folds under the foreskin, under the scrotum or where the penis meets the rest of the body. In the primary stages, men are more likely than women to develop swollen lymph nodes in the groin.

Diagnosis and Treatment

Syphilis can be diagnosed and treated at any time. However, because syphilis used to be much less common, medical care workers may confuse early symptoms with several other STDs, including chancroid, herpes and lymphogranuloma venereum (LGV).

Early in the primary stages a practitioner can look for subtle symptoms like swollen lymph glands around the groin and examine some of the discharge from the chancre, if one has developed, under a microscope (a dark-field test). Do not put any kind of medication, cream or ointment on the sore until a doctor examines it. (The syphilis bacteria on the surface are likely to be killed, making the test less accurate.) Spirochetes will be in the bloodstream one or two weeks after the chancre has formed. Two blood tests are used to diagnose syphilis. One is a screening test called the *VDRL* or *RPR*. The second (*FTA-ABS* or *MHA-Tp*) confirms it. If you suspect that you have been exposed to syphilis and have been recently treated for gonorrhea with medication other than penicillin, you should have four tests one month apart to cover the possible incubation period. (Some drugs used to treat gonorrhea do not cure syphilis.) Remember, incubation can be as long as ninety days.* If you are sexually active with more than one partner or if your sexual partner is, request a syphilis blood test during regular health checkups.

Penicillin by injection or a substitute such as doxycycline or tetracycline pills for those allergic to penicillin is the treatment for syphilis. Because people sometimes have relapses or mistakes are made, it is important to have at least two follow-up blood tests to be sure the treatment is complete. The tests should be done six months and one year later. The first three stages of syphilis can be completely cured with no permanent damage, and even in late syphilis the destructive effects can be stopped from going any further.

Syphilis and Pregnancy

A pregnant woman with syphilis can pass the bacteria on to her fetus, especially during the first few years of the disease. The bacteria attack the fetus just as they do an adult, and the child may be born dead or with important tissues deformed

---

*A good description of the different blood tests used can be found in *A Book About Sexually Transmitted Diseases*, by Donna Cherniak.

or diseased. But if the mother gets her syphilis treated before the sixteenth week of pregnancy, the fetus will probably not be affected. (Even after the fetus has gotten syphilis, penicillin will stop the disease, although it cannot repair damage already done.) Every pregnant woman should get a blood test for syphilis as soon as she knows she is pregnant, again before she delivers and anytime she thinks she may have been exposed. If she has the disease, she can be treated for it before she gives it to her fetus.

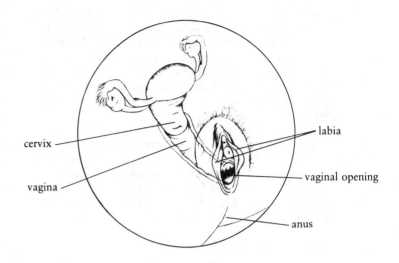

Genital Warts and Human Papillomavirus Infections*

Genital warts are caused by the human papillomavirus (HPV), similar to the type that causes common skin warts. Over twenty types of HPV cause invisible infections, warts or flat lesions in the genital area. HPV usually spreads during sexual intercourse with an infected partner. HPV infections may now be the most common STD in the United States. Some HPV-caused lesions on the cervix are associated with an increased risk of cervical cancer. Unfortunately, these invisible cervical lesions are not easily detected by either the health care practitioner or the woman with the infection.

Symptoms of genital warts usually appear from three weeks to eight months after exposure. During the presymptomatic period (as well as while they are present), warts are the most contagious, so it is advisable for your male partners to use condoms if any of you has been exposed to the virus. The visible genital warts look like regular warts, starting as small, painless, hard spots that often appear on the bottom of the vaginal opening. Warts also occur on the labia, vulva, inside the vagina, on the cervix or around the anus, where they can be mistaken for hemorrhoids. Warmth and moisture encourage the growth of warts, which often develop a cauliflowerlike appearance as they grow larger. Cervical lesions, though more prevalent than the visible warts, cannot be seen by the naked eye and have no symptoms.

Men's Symptoms

Warts occur on the head of the penis (often under the foreskin), on the shaft of the penis or occasionally on the scrotum. Using a condom can help prevent the spread of warts.

Diagnosis and Treatment

Diagnosis of warts is usually made by direct eye exam. An abnormal Pap smear may indicate the presence of HPV, and a colposcopy is usually

done to find the warts or flat lesions. If lesions are found, a biopsy may be done to diagnose HPV and to check unusual cell changes. If you have cervical warts or lesions, get a Pap smear every six months for early detection of unusual cell changes.

There are several treatments for warts.

1. Practitioners most often prescribe podophyllin solution. Apply it to the warts and wash it off two to four hours later to avoid chemical burns. Protect the surrounding skin with petroleum jelly (e.g., Vaseline). Sometimes several treatments are necessary, and they are not always successful. A safer self-treatment is also now available by prescription—podofilox.

2. Trichloracetic acid (TCA) is currently used by only a small percentage of practitioners but appears to be better than podophyllin in several respects. It is usually equally effective. The strength of TCA is more easily controlled; it works on first contact with the skin and then stops in about five minutes, reducing the danger of scarring. It does not seem to provoke severe reactions as podophyllin occasionally does. Some doctors use TCA during pregnancy, although no studies have been done to verify its safety at that time.

3. Cryotherapy (dry ice treatment) or acid can freeze or burn off small warts. This hurts briefly and sometimes causes scarring. You may want a local anesthetic.

4. You can apply 5-fluorouracil cream. It may cause irritation and discomfort.

5. Surgery or electrodesiccation (using an electric current to destroy tissue) becomes necessary for very large warts that fail to respond to other treatments. This procedure requires an anesthetic. If you have a cardiac pacemaker, the electric current may disturb it, so be sure to tell your practitioner.

6. Recent studies suggest that laser beams ap-

*See Who Is at Risk of CIN or Cervical Cancer, p. 573.

plied to warts are an effective treatment that does not affect normal tissue or cause scarring. Some practitioners recommend it particularly for HPV infections of the cervix (warts and other lesions). Local or general anesthesia may be necessary, depending on the number and size of the warts. Only physicians specially trained to do laser therapy should perform this treatment.

No matter what treatment you get, it is important to remove all warts, even those inside the vagina and on the cervix, to keep the virus from spreading. Sexual partners also should be treated. Removal of warts may not successfully get rid of all of the HPV. Therefore, warts may return and need additional treatment.

Genital Warts and Pregnancy

Warts tend to grow larger during pregnancy, probably due to the increasing levels of progesterone. If the warts are located on the vaginal wall and become very large or numerous, the vagina may become less elastic, making delivery difficult. Do *not* use podophyllin to remove warts, as it is absorbed by the skin and can cause birth defects or fetal death. ASHA maintains a program of support services for those infected with HPV (see Resources).

Other Sexually Transmitted Diseases

There are many more STDs than we can cover in this chapter. See Chapter 24, which deals with common medical and health problems, for information on common infections that can be transmitted nonsexually as well as sexually. Hepatitis B and STDs that are rare or tend to affect men more than women (such as chancroid, lymphogranuloma venereum, granuloma inguinale and intestinal STDs) are discussed in *A Book About Sexually Transmitted Diseases* by Donna Cherniak.

What to Do if You Think You Have an STD

Get a diagnosis as early as possible. Most STDs are easy to cure, though it can be difficult to wade through the medical system to get care. Women who think they may have an STD have several choices when it comes to medical treatment. Some of the advantages and disadvantages of each are listed below.

Private Physicians, Gynecology Clinics and Hospital Emergency Rooms (Varying Fees)

Many private doctors' offices, gyn clinics and hospital emergency rooms lack the equipment necessary to do a routine gonorrhea culture, much less test for chlamydia or herpes. In addition, many practitioners in these places tend not to test

> See Chapter 15 for a full discussion of HIV, AIDS and women. The ASHA, an excellent source of information on all STDs, operates several hot lines (see Resources) including the National AIDS Hot Line (800) 342-AIDS. Call them if you have any specific questions or would like further informational literature.

readily enough if a patient is white and middle-class.

The first time I asked a gynecologist for a routine gonorrhea culture, he smiled with a comradely look in his eye. "But I'm sure no man you'd be involved with would have gonorrhea."

On the other hand, they may be overly suspicious about the possibility of STD in patients who are black and poor.

Public Health Clinics (Usually Free or of Nominal Cost)

Public health departments run STD clinics throughout the country (sometimes located in hospitals), which are called "L" or "skin" clinics. Because they deal with STD on a daily basis, most clinics have personnel experienced in diagnosing STDs and good diagnostic equipment for major diseases. They also offer the services of a public health adviser who answers questions about STD. Most of the clinics do not test for hepatitis or the intestinal STDs, and some of the smaller ones may only be equipped to deal with gonorrhea, syphilis and common complications like PID.

Women who use public health clinics on a regular basis sometimes say they feel a definite stigma attached to them (as opposed to the experiences of patients at a hospital or neighborhood or private clinic).

Everyone looks at you when you're sitting in the Health Department clinic as if you're dirty or something. Then there are so many people reading your file: secretary, nurse, doctor. It's like they all know about you. It's very embarrassing.

Because clinics tend to be overcrowded, you may have a long wait before being seen by a hurried doctor or health care worker who may not take the time to answer your questions. The quality of service varies, of course, from clinic to clinic. To find the public health facility nearest to you, call the National STD Hot Line: (800) 227-8922.

Feminist Health Centers

Women's health centers often offer the most sympathetic care for women with STD. If they lack the necessary diagnostic equipment for your STD, they will refer you to a sympathetic doctor or clinic. For a list of feminist health clinics, write to us (the Boston Women's Health Book Collective) at Box 192, West Somerville, MA 02144, or write to the National Women's Health Network, 1325 G Street NW, Washington, DC 20005.

Going for Treatment

Before going to a physician or clinic, it's a good idea to call ahead to get an idea of services offered and charges. Tests are often free, but there may be a fee for the visit. If you are a minor and don't want your parents notified or sent the bill, ask about the policy on this.

If you are a minor, you can receive examination and treatment without your parents' permission in every state. The law, however, does not *prevent* the physician from telling your parents. You may want to ask your practitioner what her/his policy is before going for services.

Wherever you decide to go for care, you have a right to courteous and thorough treatment. Expect to have a medical history taken and a pelvic exam. The practitioner should explain any test, treatment and negative side effects. Before leaving, know what your follow-up care will be. If your doctor or medical care worker is too busy to answer your questions, ask to speak to someone else. It's always a good idea to take someone with you. Don't leave before your questions are answered. Even then, however, you may still feel uncertain about your treatment. Sometimes tests are not accurate; sometimes treatments don't work. That can mean more medical visits, time and money. Treatment can be painful—two big shots in the buttocks for syphilis, for example. But the alternative—not getting treatment—is worse.

STDs and the Law

State law requires that physicians and clinics report all cases of gonorrhea and syphilis to the state or local health officer. Chancroid, granuloma inguinale and lymphogranuloma venereum are also reportable in most states. Chlamydia is reportable in some states.

If you have gonorrhea or syphilis, a social worker may interview you and ask for names of your contacts (people you may have caught the disease from or given it to). Usually contacts are notified anonymously—your name is not mentioned. If you do not wish to give names of contacts, say you will contact them yourself. Then it is your responsibility to contact each person you've had sex with and ask them to seek treatment. Remember, you may be saving their fertility or even their lives.

RESOURCES

Books and Articles

American Social Health Association. "Can Alternative Medicine Work?" *The Helper* (Winter 1991).

Bell, Ruth, et al. *Changing Bodies, Changing Lives: A Book for Teens on Sex and Relationships.* New York: Random House, 1988, rev. ed. An *Our Bodies, Ourselves* for teens.

Cherniak, Donna. *A Book About Sexually Transmitted Diseases.* 1983. Available from Montreal Health Press, P.O. Box 1000, Station La Cité, Montreal, Quebec H2W 2N1, Canada. Also available in French: *Les Maladies Transmises Sexuellement.* Best single publication on STD, some on prevention.

Rosebury, Theodore. *Microbes and Morals: The Strange Story of Venereal Disease.* New York: Viking Press, 1971; Ballantine Books, 1973 (paper). An excellent historical look at STD, including examination of origin and spread.

Santa Cruz Women's Health Center. *Herpes.* 1986. Available from Santa Cruz Women's Health Center, 250 Locust Street, Santa Cruz, CA 95060. This is a comprehensive eighteen-page booklet on prevention, symptoms, traditional and nontraditional treatment of herpes.

World Health Organization (WHO) Study Group. *Management of Patients with Sexually Transmitted Diseases.* Technical Report Series, No. 810. 1991. Available from WHO, Distribution and Sales, 1211 Geneva 27, Switzerland. Publication Order No. 1100810.

Organizations

American Social Health Association (ASHA)
P.O. Box 13827
Research Triangle Park, NC 27709.

An excellent resource, which operates hot lines and publishes numerous materials. ASHA's National Herpes Resource Center publishes a special herpes newsletter. Single copies of ASHA's many publications, including the following, are available for free:

"Some Questions and Answers about NGU"
"Protect Yourself and Your Baby from Sexually Transmitted Disease (STD)"
"Some Questions and Answers about Chlamydia"
"Some Questions and Answers about PID"
"Herpes: Questions and Answers"
"Some Questions and Answers: HPV and Genital Warts"

Write or call (919) 361-8400 and ask for the Distribution Department.

Centers for Disease Control
Division of STD/HIV Prevention
Atlanta, GA 30333

Planned Parenthood
   Your local office is listed in the white and yellow pages of your phone book.

Public Health Department
STD Division (state level)
   Your local office is listed in your phone book.

National Herpes Hot Line
   (919) 361-8488
      Open Monday through Friday, 9:00 A.M. to 7:00 P.M., EST.

National HIV and AIDS Information Service
   (800) 342-2437
      Open twenty-four hours.

National HIV and AIDS SIDA Line
   (800) 344-7432
      For Spanish speakers. Open 8:00 A.M. to 2:00 A.M., EST.

National HIV and AIDS TTY Line
   (800) 243-7889
      For people who have hearing impairments. Open Monday through Friday, 10:00 A.M. to 10:00 P.M., EST.

National Sexually Transmitted Disease (STD) Hot Line
   (800) 227-8922
      Open Monday through Friday, 8:00 A.M. to 11:00 P.M., EST.

15

AIDS, HIV Infection and Women

EDITED BY MARY IDE, WITH
WENDY SANFORD AND AMY
ALPERN

Contributors: Amy Alpern, Marion
Banzhaf, Laurie Cotter of ACT/UP
New York, Risa Denenberg, Liz
Galst, Jenny Keller, Vicky Legion
and Chicago Women and AIDS
Project, Patricia O. Loftman, MS,
CNM (*Women of Color*), Janet L.
Mitchell, MD, MPH (*Women of
Color*), Jamie Penney and Lindsey
Rosen

Special thanks to Deborah Cotton

OVERVIEW ON WOMEN AND HIV/AIDS

Women—particularly women of color—are the invisible faces of AIDS in the United States, and the fastest-growing HIV positive (HIV+) group. Of the staggering 1 to 1½ million people in the United States who had been infected with the HIV virus as of September 1991, an estimated 300,000 to 400,000 of these were believed to be women and 19,796 women had been diagnosed with AIDS. Approximately 50 percent of the women were African-American and 20 percent were Latina; most were poor. More than half of the HIV+ U.S. women today became infected through sharing HIV-contaminated needles in intravenous (IV) drug use. At the same time, heterosexual transmission is increasing at an alarming rate, and women are nearly *eighteen times more likely to be infected by a male sexual partner than vice versa.* Figures are very low for woman-to-woman transmission, but this may be due to lack of studies on lesbian/bisexual sex. Women who are diagnosed with AIDS *tend to die twice as quickly as men with the same diagnosis,* and 63 percent will die of HIV complications without ever having been officially diagnosed as having AIDS. Women are by far the most frequent caregivers, often unpaid, for men, women and children who have HIV or AIDS.

Thus AIDS powerfully affects our lives as women. Yet in every aspect of the public response to AIDS, from research to drug trials, from health provider attitudes to insurance and disability practices, women's experience with HIV and AIDS has too often been overlooked. This chapter offers basic HIV and AIDS information for women. We encourage you to consult other sources listed in the Resources.

It is important to consider the wider world context of AIDS. Some 10 million people are infected with HIV worldwide, about a third of them women, and most of them in developing countries. Nearly all have been infected through heterosexual sex. In the world, then, as it is increasingly in the United States, AIDS is a disease of women and children, of people of color and of the poor. The politics of this, worldwide, are hauntingly similar to the politics of the AIDS epidemic in the United States, where the people who get AIDS most frequently and who suffer most from lack of treatment are not the ones who control the resources for research and treatment.

The Politics of Women's Later HIV/AIDS Diagnosis and Earlier Death

Why do women tend to die twice as quickly as men after being diagnosed with AIDS or so frequently die of HIV complications even before an

THE LANGUAGE OF HIV DISEASE: A GLOSSARY

AIDS: The abbreviation for *a*cquired *i*mmune *d*eficiency *s*yndrome. AIDS is a viral syndrome (a group of diseases) that weakens our immune system. A suppressed immune system weakens our body's ability to fight against various deadly infections and malignancies. To date, there is no cure for AIDS.

ANTIBODY: A special protein that is created by our body's immune system and used to fight specific agents that cause infection. In the case of HIV infection, however, the infecting virus is not destroyed by the antibody.

ASYMPTOMATIC: This means that a person has the HIV infection but shows no signs or symptoms. It is possible to infect others even if you are asymptomatic.

HIGH-RISK or UNSAFE BEHAVIOR: Specific sexual or drug-related activities that increase our chances of contracting or transmitting HIV. High-risk behaviors are those that allow the blood, semen or vaginal fluid of one person to contact the blood or mucous membranes (in the eyes, mouth, vagina, rectum) of another person. The two most high-risk activities are having sex without using protection and the sharing of intravenous (IV) needles in drug use.

HIV: The abbreviation for *h*uman *i*mmunodeficiency *v*irus. HIV is a slow-acting virus that is believed to be the main cause of AIDS. Although the term is often used interchangably with the term *AIDS*, it is not yet proven that everyone who is infected with HIV will develop AIDS.

HIV POSITIVE (HIV+)/HIV INFECTED/SEROPOSITIVE: This describes a person who is infected with HIV.

IMMUNE SYSTEM: The immune system protects the body from infection. In this system, specialized cells and proteins in the blood and other bodily fluids work together to eliminate disease-producing agents and other toxic foreign substances.

IMMUNOSUPPRESSION: Immuno-suppression is the term indicating that the immune system has been weakened, whether in response to HIV infection or other factors.

OPPORTUNISTIC INFECTIONS: Infections that take the opportunity to attack people whose immune system has been weakened, as in the case of AIDS. The most common opportunistic infections associated with AIDS in men and women are: *Pneumocystis carinii* pneumonia (PCP), cytomegalovirus (CMV), mycobacterium avium intracellulare (MAI) and toxoplasmosis. Common gynecological problems that *may* become opportunistic infections for HIV+ women are: PID, human papillomavirus (HPV), yeast infections, genital herpes and chronic vaginitis.

PERSON WITH AIDS (PWA): PWA is a positive term for someone who has AIDS. Using PWA helps avoid negative and judgmental terms such as AIDS victim, innocent victim or AIDS carrier.

SAFER SEX: Safer sex refers to practices that offer protection from HIV transmission during a sexual encounter. This means always using barriers that guard against the transmission of bodily fluids, which can carry HIV. Protective barriers include condoms (best combined with spermicide), plastic wrap or dental dams for oral sex, latex gloves or finger cots. Bodily fluids of an infected person that can transmit HIV include semen, blood (including menstrual blood), genital secretions and breast milk.

SEROCONVERSION: When a person's blood changes from having no HIV antibodies (seronegative) to having HIV antibodies (seropositive). This usually, but not always, happens within six months of exposure.

T CELL (also called CD$_4$ CELL): A type of white blood cell (lymphocyte) that is vital to the proper functioning of the immune system. T cells, or CD$_4$ cells, are the target of HIV. The virus encodes itself into the genetic information of the CD$_4$ cell/T cell and later can use the machinery of the cell to create new viral particles. The body's immune system is destroyed, because CD$_4$ cells are the central control cells of that system. Because HIV tends to reduce the number of T4 cells, this count is used as a marker of the severity of the HIV infection.

Source: Adapted with permission from ACT UP/New York Women and AIDS Book Group, *Women, AIDS, and Activism*, Boston: South End Press, 1990; and Peg Byron, "HIV the National Scandal," *Ms.*, Vol. 1, No. 4 January/February 1991, p. 133.

AIDS diagnosis? The answer lies in the persisting inequities of sex, race and class in our country. Sexism within the health-care system often renders women invisible with regard to AIDS. Instead of being viewed as persons who need health care, HIV+ women are often seen primarily as infectors of men and children. There is more public focus on prostitutes who may infect their clients and mothers who may infect their babies than there is on prevention and treatment for women. Family responsibilities are expected to—and often do—take precedence over our seeking health care for ourselves, so that many women delay seeking care long after experiencing symptoms of HIV infection. Because women tend to make less money than men, and often as single parents have financial responsibility for more family members, we have fewer financial resources with which to care for ourselves. Racism seriously affects the quality of health care options available to women of color in general and particularly to those who are HIV+. Racism and class discrimination also contribute to conditions in communities of color, which foster drug use, while impeding access to drug treatment programs.

Even HIV+ women who are able to make it to a doctor or a clinic may find our symptoms dismissed as not HIV related. The tendency in sectors of the medical world to discount women's complaints becomes compounded by the still widespread belief that this is a men's disease. Women reporting HIV symptoms like weight loss, headaches or fatigue may be told that these are stress related, not HIV related. Or we may report gynecological symptoms, which, because of insufficient research and inadequate definition, have taken a long time to be accepted as HIV or AIDS related.

The Centers for Disease Control's (CDC's) definition of AIDS, extensively used throughout the United States, defines a case of AIDS as an illness characterized by one or more indicator diseases in conjunction with laboratory evidence of HIV infection. For years the indicator diseases cited left out a woman's first HIV-related symptoms, which are often gynecological, such as recurrent vaginal candida (yeast); also omitted were some of women's opportunistic infections—a significant omission, although most women who die of AIDS die of the same infections that men do. As a result of this inadequate CDC definition, the total number of U.S. AIDS cases has been undercounted, women have frequently been misdiagnosed or undiagnosed for HIV (often dying before receiving treatment) and crucial research into women and HIV/AIDS has been delayed. Even worse, because so many public and private agencies rely on the CDC definition, women with HIV or AIDS who are ill but not officially diagnosed

HIV-positive peer counselors receive "Sister Care Awards" for volunteer service to the D.C. Women's Council on AIDS. Both women are now deceased.

D.C. Women's Council on Aids

have been denied access to treatment, services, insurance and disability benefits, drug trials and housing—that is, life itself.

Under pressure from AIDS activists and the National Commission on AIDS in the winter of 1991 to 1992, the CDC withdrew a new definition of AIDS that still did not include indicator diseases that often affect women. As of this printing, a more adequate definition has been put into effect. This demonstrates the tremendous importance of activism, much of it on the part of the gay and lesbian community, in moving a government that has been shockingly slow to respond to AIDS. The AIDS crisis became a crisis only because the U.S. government moved so slowly in the early 1980s to put money into research, treatment and, above all, education about how to prevent the spread of HIV. Thousands of men and women have died unnecessarily as a result. The reasons for this tragic delay are clear: prejudice against those whom AIDS hit first—gay men, then drug users, poor people, people of color. The media feeds this prejudice by referring to those who have contracted AIDS through blood transfusions as "innocent victims"—as though anyone who gets it through sex or drug use is "guilty." The only guilty party here is a public that withheld its resources while the virus spread.

It will continue to take persistent pressure from activists to achieve progress in combatting HIV and AIDS. To participate, we encourage you to contact one of the organizations listed in the Resources.

Women of Color

No matter how you look at the numbers, women of color are at higher risk of becoming infected with HIV than white women. The impact of substance abuse in women, long ignored, must be ad-

HIV-positive Latina AIDS activist Liz Ramos at an annual fund-raising walk in Boston   Ellen Shub

meaningful employment opportunities, substandard housing, high levels of violence and inadequate health care. All of these factors, when present in our society, contribute to the AIDS epidemic.

Of equal importance is the hierarchical placement of women in society, the role of women in communities of color and the role of women in the subculture of illicit drug use. What emerges is a picture of women who still maintain very traditional roles by defining ourselves in terms of our significant other and our ability to produce children. Women of color place our priorities second with the focus shifting to our children, significant others or family. Because of the myriad insensitivities of health and medical institutions, women are suspicious and enter them with great trepidation. As a result, women often neglect our own health and seek health and medical care only in moments of crisis and often at the most advanced stages of illness. HIV disease is no exception.

Although preventive messages and education proliferate, women hear them intellectually but ignore them emotionally because acting on these messages might mean being abandoned and isolated by our partners—a risk not balanced in favor of behavior considered safe.

Women in Prison

According to Susan Rosenberg, a political prisoner in the Marianna, Florida's women's maximum security prison,

Women in prison who are HIV positive or who have full blown AIDS are the front line of this crisis. We live isolated, enclosed and in a particular form of hell.

Women in prison contend with living conditions that are most often unhealthy and a health care system that is dramatically inadequate. Sisterhood and empowerment have become motivating concepts for women in prison to advocate for their own health needs and to build self-help programs. All AIDS activists are urged to support incarcerated women who are HIV positive in their demands for decent health care, participation in clinical trials with neutral group monitoring (that is, with no prison staff present), compassionate release for women who are ill and community participation within AIDS education in prisons.

Sex Workers

For women who support themselves by working in the sex industry, AIDS raises familiar issues. The public (media, police, courts) tends to blame prostitutes, not their male clients, for the buying and selling of sex. In the same way, prostitutes

dressed. Fifty percent of women infected with HIV list their own IV drug use as a risk factor and 20 percent report having a sexual relationship with a known male IV drug user. Substance abuse is consequently the most significant contributing factor for women of color who are HIV infected.

Substance abuse has been a major factor in the destruction of communities of color for decades. Its existence and destruction has been allowed to continue unabated because it had minimal effect on the larger white community and, in fact, provides economic support for segments of that community.

The high incidence of substance abuse can be traced directly to racism and its impact on communities through poverty, lack of educational and have been accused of spreading AIDS when, in fact, a woman sex worker is *eighteen times* more likely to contract the disease from a male client than she is to give it to him. While bearing the blame for men's choice not to protect themselves, women sex workers have built on years of experience in using condoms as protection from STDs and provide some of the most successful examples of women making changes to safer practices. Some have perfected a technique of getting a condom onto a client's penis without his knowing it; it involves starting out with the condom in your mouth and slipping it on while sucking, which may be a useful technique for any women whose partners resist using condoms or for couples trying to make condom use smoother or sexier. ("Try it on a banana first," counsels the excellent safer sex pamphlet *Making It*.)*

A sex worker's ability to protect herself from HIV is like every woman's: It depends on her

power in the relationship. More affluent sex workers are often freer to set the terms of the sexual encounter, although poor women who work on the street may not have the power to insist that their client use a condom, or condoms may simply be too expensive. Thus sex workers in poorer countries, and in poorer sections of the sex industry in the United States, are the ones who are most vulnerable to AIDS. Again, AIDS and poverty are cruelly linked. Power issues follow sex workers into their private relationships: Some who use condoms in sex for pay do not protect themselves with a lover; some may want sex with a lover to feel different, others may find it harder to set their own terms when it's not a business proposition.[1]

Around the world, women in the sex industry are organizing to improve their situation, with AIDS prevention as one focus. Dutch sex workers have designed a sticker saying, "I do it (with a condom)," to put up in the toilets of bars and discos, and in their own windows, to alert clients. The Prostitutes' Collective of Victoria, Australia, has launched a "Hello, sailor" education campaign for visiting servicemen.[2]

Making It: A Woman's Guide to Sex in the Age of AIDS by Cindy Patton and Janis Kelly (Ithaca, NY: Firebrand Books, 1987).

HOW HIV IS TRANSMITTED

It is a myth that only certain high-risk groups of people are at risk for infection with HIV (the virus that causes AIDS). This is not true. It is our *actions* that put us at risk for HIV, not what group we may belong to. Three conditions must be met for HIV to pass from one person to another.

1. *The virus must be present.* This means that one person must be HIV+. Gay sex, anal sex or using IV drugs do not themselves create infection. HIV is transmitted between people through the sharing of bodily fluids in which the virus is found. The virus can be transmitted through sexual activities including penile–vaginal intercourse, oral sex, anal sex, fisting, finger fucking, rimming and sharing uncleaned sex toys, such as dildos and vibrators. HIV can be transmitted through sharing needles that contain blood, including "works" for IV drugs (heroin, cocaine, speed) or needles that are shared and used for tatooing or body piercing.

2. *The virus must be present in sufficient quantity.* Blood, semen and vaginal and cervical secretions carry the highest concentrations of the virus, although saliva, tears and urine carry minuscule amounts or no HIV. Studies have shown that sufficient quantities of the virus can be present in male pre-cum, the clear liquid found on the penis before eja-

culation. Deep kissing is low risk, although theoretically could be risky if both people had bleeding gums or sores, allowing for blood-to-blood transmission. Sweat does not contain the virus, nor does vomit. HIV cannot be transmitted by insects, through food preparation, drinking out of the same glass, handshakes or toilet seats.

3. *The virus penetrates through the skin and into the body.* This is done through tiny tears or sores in the mucous membranes in the mouth, vagina or rectum; cuts in the skin or directly into the blood via a needle. Recent studies suggest that the virus may also penetrate intact membranes in the vagina. For information on possible infection of the fetus during pregnancy, see Reproductive Rights—HIV and Pregnancy (pp. 336–37).

HIV transmission can take place without our knowing that we or our sexual or drug partners are infected. The virus can live in a person's blood for ten years without causing any noticeable symptoms, so it's possible not to know for ten years, yet still be spreading the disease. This is what makes it so dangerous, why testing is so important and why it makes sense always to protect ourselves from HIV transmission. For information about prevention, see pp. 337–39.

Laws have been passed in many states requiring mandatory HIV testing of sex workers who are arrested, with no similar move towards testing their clients. The sexism is blatant. Sex workers ask for protection and decent health care, rather than harassment and mandatory testing.

Lesbians and HIV

Lesbians have been told we're a low risk group, yet defining risk in terms of groups rather than behavior is fatal.

There is a myth that lesbians are at low risk for contracting HIV, yet how often do we consider whether our activities are risky? Lesbians are not a homogeneous group with predictable behaviors, but rather live a variety of life-styles and engage in a vast range of sexual behaviors. Some lesbians, for example, sleep with men (as many as 45 percent, reports a 1987 Kinsey Institute study), some lesbians use IV drugs, some lesbians sell sex. And, just like heterosexual men and women, we don't always tell each other what we have been doing.

The number of cases of woman-to-woman transmission appears to be small at the present time, but bias on the part of the medical community may be responsible for these low numbers. For example, the CDC has not studied the issue of woman-to-woman transmission. The fact is, we don't know how many lesbians have AIDS, much less how many are HIV+. Given the possibility of women-to-women transmission of STDs such as chlamydia, herpes, or genital warts, it seems quite plausible that HIV could be transmitted as well.

Because HIV can be found in vaginal fluid and blood, including menstrual blood, there are many ways that a woman having sex with an HIV-infected woman lover could become infected. She could go down on her lover (have oral sex) without a barrier, especially when her lover has her period or has a yeast infection, and the virus could enter her circulation through small cuts in her mouth. She could get the virus on her fingers and put them in her mouth, her own vagina or her anus. She could penetrate her lover with a dildo and then use it herself, placing HIV inside her own vagina. She could be infected through cuts on her own fingers while penetrating her lover's vagina or anus with her fingers or hand. To protect ourselves and our lovers, we have to do more than know about safer sex, we have to use it (see Safer Sex Guidelines, p. 338).

WOMEN'S SYMPTOMS

Karen has chronic vaginitis, probably a yeast infection. After nearly a year of repeated treatments, her doctor continues to prescribe the same medication. Even though she tells the doctor the medication does not work, he keeps prescribing the same thing.

Denitra has a class II pap smear. She also has contracted veneral warts, which the clinic tells her is a sign of HPV (human papillomavirus). She has cryosurgery for her abnormal pap smear and is told later she is fine. She returns the next year and is shocked to find out her Pap smear indicates cancerous cells.

Marguerita is hospitalized for pelvic inflammatory disease. Her doctor does not understand why she is not responding to standard antibiotic treatment.

Early symptoms of HIV that can appear in both men and women in the asymptomatic phase of infection include weight loss, fatigue, swollen glands and the appearance of skin conditions, such as seborrheic dermatitis. During the symptomatic phase of the illness, symptoms will vary from bronchial infections to sores in the mouth, or thrush. There may be fevers, night sweats, a loss of appetite, trouble swallowing, headaches and diarrhea.

Some gynecological conditions can be indicative of HIV infection and may even be a woman's first symptom of HIV or AIDS. Most women with a well-functioning immune system will recover with standard treatment for a gynecological condition, but a woman who is HIV+ may require more intensive treatment or may develop a more rapid progression of infection. The gynecological

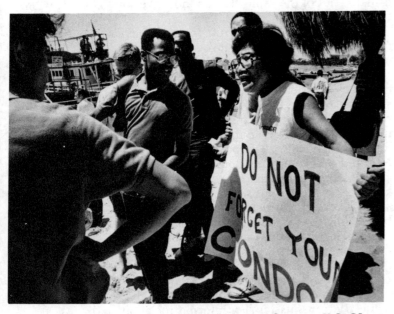

A nurse-midwife teaching about safer sex to U.S. GIs on Pataya, an island which the military has used for "R and R."
S. Asabe

conditions that can be *signs of HIV infection* are: (1) recurrent vaginal candida (yeast), which can precede the presence of oral thrush (a common opportunistic infection in men and women); (2) chronic pelvic inflammatory disease (PID); and (3) severe, extensive genital herpes.

There are also gynecological conditions that can be *risk factors for HIV infection*—that is, that may make us more likely to be infected by HIV if we are exposed to it.

1. A woman who has any sexually transmitted disease (STD) and is also exposed to HIV is probably at a higher risk for becoming HIV infected. Genital herpes, chancroid and syphilis (all genital ulcer diseases) offer easy passage for HIV by creating a more direct link to the bloodstream. Untreated STDs increase the likelihood of HIV transmission up to one hundred times.

2. Vaginal irritation due to yeast (candida), trichomonas or bacterial vaginosis can cause microlacerations or increased numbers of white blood cells, which increase a woman's risk for HIV transmission if exposed to the virus.

Human papillomavirus (HPV) is the virus that causes veneral warts (condyloma). Although it is not known conclusively whether HIV+ women are more likely to be infected with HPV or vice versa, it is known that women who have sex at an early age and who have had many partners are at high risk for both these viral infections. In all women, HPV has been linked to cervical cancer. Because HPV causes cell changes that can lead to cancer, it is recommended that HIV+ women receive a Pap smear at least every six months. Because some studies have shown Pap smears to miss abnormal cervical cells in women with HIV infection, some experts advise HIV+ women to have a colposcopy with biopsy (a microscopic examination of the cervical cells).

If you have an extensive history of gynecologic infections, you might want to consider getting tested for HIV.

Coping with Your Test Results

Even if you test negative for HIV (and have not risked infection in the past six months), you may find your relief and gratitude mixed with other feelings. You may ask, Why not me? as you watch friends suffer from the disease. Or you may find, as some people do, that it is difficult at first to keep practicing safer sex or using clean needles. A support group, counselor or good friend may help you find your balance.

If you test positive for HIV, remember that this does not mean you have or will ever get AIDS. It is a time to take particularly good care of your health if you can—such as eating better, resting more and protecting yourself from other STDs.

There are treatments like AZT, which, when started early, may make a difference in whether you develop AIDS or not. Thus finding health care is a crucial step; so is negotiating whatever insurance or disability benefits might be available to you. Finding emotional support is important, too: Without support you may feel too frightened to act or too angry to proceed. Seek out groups in your community for women who are HIV+; in groups you can give and get support, share ideas and learn. You can read, too, about other women's experiences; one resource is a Washington, DC-based newsletter, *The Positive Woman* (see Resources).

TREATMENTS

Medical Treatments

An ugly thing about the U.S. health care system is that we are likely to receive better care for HIV and AIDS if we are white and/or affluent and worse if we are women of color or poor. There are some highly dedicated health providers at every level of the system, but those in poorer facilities are working against immense obstacles to provide the care they believe is adequate. Even nonmedical factors have an impact: As simple a thing as child care can make the difference in whether a mother who is HIV+ can come for treatment. What follows is what should be the basic, minimal standard of care for all people with HIV or AIDS. An AIDS hot line or agency may be able to help you find the best care possible in your area (see Resources).

The best health care would mean frequent visits for physical exams and laboratory tests. A minimal standard of care for all people with AIDS includes the following:

1. *CD_4 cell monitoring.* The disease progress should be monitored frequently, using laboratory tests, or "markers," to provide a basis of planning for medical treatment. The primary marker in HIV disease is the CD_4-cell (known also as the T-cell) count. Medical providers need to understand that the meaning and applicability of these tests for women, pregnant women and all people of color may differ from the interpretation and suitability for white men.

2. *Vaccinations.* Vaccinations should be brought up to date.

3. *Prophylactic therapies.* Medical treatment can include initiating antiviral medications currently in use, such as AZT or DDI. Using medications prophylactically (for prevention) against PCP is essential. Prophylaxis for other opportunistic infections should be considered. Doctors treating people with HIV illness must have current knowledge of all available AIDS treatments

HIV TESTING

Finding out that you are HIV+ is life changing and traumatic; finding that you are not HIV+ is challenging in its own way. It makes sense to think through the decision carefully and to get as much support as you can while you do so. Check to see if there are support groups or counselors in your area for help with testing decisions, and/or look for a testing site where good counseling is provided.

What Is the HIV Antibody Test?
It is a blood test for antibodies to HIV, which is the virus believed to cause AIDS. When a person is infected with HIV, the body's immune system produces antibodies in an attempt to fight HIV. A small sample of blood, usually drawn from your arm, will detect the presence of these antibodies. The test is often inaccurately called an "AIDS test," but it does not tell you if you have AIDS.

What Are Reasons to Take the Test?
1. You want to know if you are infected so that you can consider getting medical help (including early intervention therapies), enrolling in drug trials or taking nonbiomedical treatments.
2. Knowing your antibody status will help keep you from having unsafe sex and/or sharing needles.
3. You are thinking about having a baby or breastfeeding your baby.

4. You would feel less stress if you knew for certain whether you are infected.

What Are Reasons Not to Take the Test?
1. You have never been at risk for HIV infection.
2. You do not feel able to deal with the strong feelings that might come up if you knew your test results (such as feeling like you would kill yourself), and you practice safer sex anyway.
3. You are being pressured by a health provider or other advisor to have the test in a setting where the results will not be anonymous (see below).

When Should the Test Be Taken?
Take the test a minimum of two to six months after your last possible exposure to HIV. Ninety-eight percent of people show antibodies within two months of exposure.

Where Should the Test Be Taken?
Antibody testing is available in many hospitals, clinics and doctor's offices, but it is important to choose carefully where to have it done. Some test settings offer confidentiality only; others offer anonymous testing. An anonymous test is done by code number, not by name, so that your name remains unknown throughout the process. In confidential testing, your test result will be recorded in

---

and their side effects, including how specific drugs will affect a woman's reproductive tract.

Support for your emotional well-being is important, as is nutritional advice and the assistance of a social worker. Finally, HIV+ women often have chronic vaginitis, pelvic infections, vaginal and cervical diseases, as well as bacterial lung infections. Unless these underlying problems are adequately treated, even the standard care regimen may fail to improve the health or extend the life of women clients.

If there are new drugs being tested for AIDS treatment, you may want to try them. Access to approved experimental therapies should be considered as part of your medical treatment plan. To keep current on new antiviral and other medications, we suggest that you contact the National Institutes of Health (NIH call them at (800) TRIALS A) for the latest in treatment protocols,

including clinical drug trials. A clinical drug trial tests new treatments on humans in an effort to prove drug safety, efficacy and appropriate dose levels. Participating in a drug trial is one way to benefit from the newest research and to receive free medicine and medical attention. It involves risks, too, but many PWAs prefer the risk of taking a new drug that might help to the near-certainty of suffering without it. However, many AIDS-related drug trials, including those under the direction of the NIH, have at least passively discriminated against women's participation. Many drug trials have been satisfied with simply studying males and have made no special efforts, such as providing child care or transportation, to include women; some, especially with drugs that may harm a developing fetus, require proof of sterilization or a pregnancy test before a woman can enter the program. Frustrated by the slow rate of your confidential medical record. Be aware that medical records are easily accessible to anyone in your health care setting and that courts and insurance companies can get access to medical records in certain situations. Your results could be used to prevent you from getting health insurance or proper care for other health problems. For this reason, many people prefer anonymous testing. Contact your local department of public health or AIDS agency to find the anonymous test sites nearest you.

In most cases, testing for HIV is voluntary. Mandatory testing is required for the military and for U.S. residency by noncitizens. Some prisoners and sex workers have also faced mandatory testing. Most AIDS activists regard mandatory testing as not only unjustly invasive, but a diversion of money that could be spent for AIDS education and treatment. For your own information, you might want to get an anonymous test if you know you will be in a circumstance where testing is mandatory.

What About the Test Results?

A positive result means that you have been infected with HIV and have developed antibodies to the virus. (Unlike antibodies to many other viruses, antibodies to HIV do not make you immune to the virus.) Being HIV+

does not necessarily mean that you now have AIDS or that you will develop AIDS in the future. It does mean that you can infect someone else with HIV if you exchange bodily fluids. False-positive results are rare, that is, your test results say that you are HIV+, when you are not. A negative result means you have not developed antibodies to the virus and in most cases means you are not infected with HIV. However, *a negative result does not always mean you are virus-free*. The immune system is likely to take three weeks to six months to produce antibodies after HIV infection and in some cases longer. If you were infected recently, the test may not detect it. A follow-up test four to eight weeks later is advisable. In rare cases, people may never produce antibodies and will consistently test negative although they are infected with HIV. An indeterminate result means that the presence or absence of antibodies to HIV cannot be confirmed in the blood sample taken, sometimes due to recent infection. You should have another test in four to eight weeks. Most people with indeterminate results are not really infected with HIV.

Source: Excerpted from "The HIV Antibody Test" pamphlet by the San Francisco AIDS Foundation, available at local AIDS agencies or from your local Department of Public Health, and "Anonymous HIV Antibody Testing" pamphlet by the Fenway Community Health Center. For copies, call (617) 267-0900.

FDA approval, some PWAs have found their own access to experimental drugs via AIDS activist organizations and an informal network.

Nonbiomedical Treatments

Alternative treatments, used in conjunction with more common, allopathic medical treatments like drugs, may reduce the severity of symptoms associated with HIV disease, as well as bolster the immune system, although there is no documented proof of their efficacy. The use of Chinese medicine—both acupuncture and Chinese herbs—may sometimes improve CD_4-cell counts and immune system functioning and abate some drug side effects and symptoms, such as night sweats, nausea, diarrhea and neuropathies (lack of feeling in the extremities). Many HIV+ persons who utilize Chinese medicine report feeling more in control

of their lives and better able to cope with their disease.

A number of mind/body medicine practices have helped to improve immune system functioning and enhance a person's sense of quality of life. Such practices include visualization, relaxation, physical exercise and cognitive therapy. Chiropractors and consumers have reported that chiropractic treatments may halt the progress of symptoms such as neuropathies and headaches. Chiropractic care can reduce stress and muscle tension and be a successful treatment for insomnia.

People with HIV infection usually become physically depleted from the disease and from some of the drugs used in treating it. Nutritional therapies, such as vitamins and supplements and high-calorie and low-sugar diets, may increase physical energy and create an improved sense of well-being. Meals should be varied and nutritious, food thoroughly cleaned and well prepared; avoid raw meat, raw fish and shellfish, raw milk and non-pasteurized cheese. HIV+ persons with cats, especially kittens, should not clean the litterbox (or should do so with gloves) to prevent toxoplasmosis, an opportunistic infection.

If you have health insurance, check with your insurance company to see if it will cover alternative treatments. You can also contact local AIDS service organizations, hospitals and clinics: Some provide nonbiomedical therapies regardless of an individual's ability to pay.

Whatever combination of medical and nonbiomedical treatments we may use, there is currently no cure for HIV infection and AIDS. As one PWA said of the struggle with one symptom after another, "having AIDS is like continually having to put out brush fires in my body."

REPRODUCTIVE RIGHTS—HIV AND PREGNANCY

Public policy in response to AIDS has greatly threatened the reproductive lives and choices of HIV+ women. An HIV+ woman's right to decide whether to continue or terminate her pregnancy is in serious jeopardy. She faces heightened discrimination, being viewed not as a potentially sick person in her own right but as a source of contagion, a "vector of transmission" to the "innocent victim" she carries in her body. Some AIDS policymakers in legal and medical programs actively discourage all HIV+ women from becoming pregnant and encourage pregnant HIV+ women to terminate their pregnancies. Yet the medical evidence regarding the effects of pregnancy on the health of HIV+ women and the rates, methods and risk factors for transmission to the fetus are inadequate and inconclusive.

Current research suggests that a pregnancy will not accelerate HIV disease, bring on symptoms or complicate pregnancy for a woman who is asymptomatic or shows no signs of sickness. However, pregnancy in women with advanced stages of HIV disease does appear to worsen symptoms.

It is possible for HIV to pass from a pregnant women to her fetus. Studies have shown that anywhere from 7 to 40 percent of the babies born to HIV+ women will develop HIV infection. Thus at least 60 percent, or three-fifths, of babies born to HIV+ women will remain infection-free. We do not know for sure how HIV passes from a woman to her fetus during pregnancy and/or during delivery. We do know that a woman is most likely to transmit the HIV virus to the fetus either immediately after she is infected or during childbirth. There is also some risk of transmission

through breastfeeding. A low CD_4-cell count (below 300), anemia, inflammation of the placenta, the presence of other infections and advanced AIDS in a woman may each increase the risk of transmission to the fetus and affect a woman's health and the progress of her pregnancy.

Every infant born to an HIV+ woman will have its mother's antibodies in its blood and may test positive for HIV for a period of time even if it is not infected. Because the current standard antibody test cannot distinguish between the mother's and the infant's antibodies, it has been necessary to wait a few months to determine whether the infant is infected. New tests have been developed that can determine HIV infection in infants as young as three to six months, and researchers are seeking tests that can reliably detect infection in a fetus. But testing is a complex issue. Some policymakers advocate routine testing of all newborns for HIV as a means of assessing the percentage of reproductive-age women who are infected with HIV. Those concerned with women's rights strenuously oppose any testing that is done without the informed consent of the mother. They argue persuasively that the time and money involved in widespread testing could better be spent on prevention, education and treatment of HIV disease.

Ironically, if you are HIV+ and pregnant and wish to terminate your pregnancy, you may find that abortion clinics will refuse to take you. This reflects some health-care providers' ignorance and fear regarding HIV transmission or what activists call AIDSphobia. You may face the untenable situation of being counseled to have an abortion yet being unable to find one—another serious restriction of your reproductive choices.

Advocates are fighting to preserve the reproductive rights of HIV+ women, whether we choose to become pregnant and to carry a pregnancy to term or to terminate it. These rights include access to nondiscriminatory health care and informed, up-to-date medical information and procedures. Even with support, the decision about motherhood is often a tough one; a question mentioned by many women is whether there is a dependable person in their life who would care for their child, should they themselves die of AIDS.

If you are considering artificial insemination, you need to know that donor insemination can be a source of HIV transmission. Today, sperm banks routinely test all donors for HIV and other STDs. They may freeze semen for at least two months to ensure that the donor did not produce the specimen while in the window period, when he may be infectious, but not yet testing positive. As a matter of protection, women who do not go through a sperm bank but seek a donor informally should insist that the donor be willing to frankly discuss his risk behaviors, to have one or more HIV tests and to practice safer sex during the period of at least two months before and during the insemination.

PROTECTING OURSELVES FROM HIV

HIV can live in the blood for at least ten years without creating symptoms. If we have unprotected sex or share needles with someone today, we expose ourselves to everyone s/he has exchanged bodily fluids with in the past decade. Even if we are in monogamous long-term relationships, our lovers may be bisexual and not telling us or using drugs and not telling us. Or they may have been infected by something they did long before they met us. The only answer is to act as though one or both partners is HIV+ and to use protection. There are barriers that are *known* to stop HIV transmission. Yet many of us are not protecting ourselves, or we do it sometimes and not others.

Why aren't we building safer sex into our lives? Here are a few reasons that women have mentioned.

1. *Our own attitudes.*

Who me??? I'm not a gay man or a junkie, so I'm safe. . . . I have good taste in men . . . or women. . . . I can tell who's infected. . . . If he had HIV he'd have oily hair and broken skin. . . . I love him so much, he'd never do anything to hurt me. . . . If I bring a condom, he'll think I'm a sleaze. . . . I want sex to be romantic. . . . I'm afraid he'll refuse . . . or get mad.

With thoughts like this, who's going to pull a condom or a roll of plastic wrap out of her pocketbook? As one woman said,

That condom seems to pour cold water on the romance by saying, "OK, to be brutally honest, we've both slept with other people." The condom seems like a statement of distrust: You could give me a disease, you could kill me.

Or you may want to have a baby, which means you don't want to use a condom or any birth control method.

2. *Our partner's attitudes.* Some men complain that condoms ruin sex. Some are afraid that they won't keep an erection while putting on a condom. Or they think it's not really sex without penetration and insist on intercourse even if there's no protection. If they are used to being in charge sexually, they may resent a woman initiating safer sex. They may feel accused of sleeping around. A lesbian lover may believe there's no HIV risk for lesbians. A sex worker's client may refuse to pay

for protected sex. Or there are cultural reasons. A woman's group from Chicago wrote

If you're poor and Latina, sexuality is one area over which men still feel like they have some control in their lives. If the women bring home the safer sex message we may become lightning rods for the frustration and anger the men feel as a result of racism, unemployment and poverty. The educational strategy has to be developed by the community itself.

Whatever the reason, our suggesting safer sex can provoke a response we didn't look for.

Ann's partner poked a pencil through the six condoms she brought home from the clinic, snarling, "I'll show you what I think of this shit."

The choice may seem to be unsafe sex or no sex.

A lot of these guys would rather dump you than use a condom.

3. *Other factors.* Expense and availability of safer sex supplies is a big factor for many women. One large Chicago clinic serving eight housing projects receives a state allotment of less than one-fifth of a condom per client each month. Teenage women often find themselves in a bind. A few high-school clinics distribute condoms, but conservative groups in many areas of the country have fought against AIDS education and condom distribution in the schools.

So we are up against a lot when it comes to protecting ourselves from HIV. What seems to make a difference is women helping each other. From the pioneering ACE prison-based peer education project (see Resources) to a group of women friends around a kitchen table getting down to basics about safer sex, we can help each other protect ourselves—and we have to.

Here are some things that different women have found effective: Read everything you can about condom use and practice putting one on a banana; practice with your friends what you are going to say with a partner; talk with your partner about how to make using condoms or plastic wrap (for oral sex on a woman) sexy; put the condom on together, put it on with your mouth; explore lovemaking that doesn't include penetration—more women have orgasm that way, anyway (see Chapter 11, "Sexuality"); if a man refuses to use a condom and overpowers you into having intercourse, at least get some spermicide into your vagina, or use a female condom (see p. 268); if he cares about having a family, try telling him that you don't want to get an infection that will hurt his ability to have children with you. Don't fool yourself: Challenge the myths. Remember that you can't tell by looking at someone if s/he is infected, love does not protect you from HIV, having only one sex partner doesn't protect you, having him pull his penis out before coming doesn't protect you, having penis–vagina intercourse instead of anal sex doesn't protect you, birth control pills and diaphragms protect you from pregnancy but not from HIV. (HIV can get through the wall of the vagina anywhere and so a diaphragm is not an adequate barrier.)

For women, safer sex is about power. Power in terms of feeling valuable, feeling worthwhile, having a high enough self-esteem to want to protect ourselves. Power in our relationships: being able to hold our ground and persuade a sex partner to use protection. Power in our pocketbooks: being able to support ourselves and our children if we leave a partner who endangers us by not using protection. Power in our friendships to support us in protecting ourselves. The power of feeling proud of our sexuality. There is the power, too, of speaking openly about sex, even when it is hard to talk about. Finally, our power to protect ourselves is weakened by drugs and alcohol; if we are addicted, the power we need depends on access to affordable treatment. All women deserve the power to keep ourselves and our loved ones healthy.

Safer Sex Guidelines

The idea behind safer sex boils down to four things:

1. You need to think and talk about HIV prevention long before having sex.

2. You should know that safer sex can be fun, imaginative and intimate.

3. Use barriers to protect yourself from potentially infected blood, semen or vaginal fluids.

4. Avoid drugs and alcohol that could get in the way of applying each of the first three.

Here is a listing of risky sexual activities and ways to enjoy them without getting infected with HIV. These methods are effective only if the condom or other barrier is in place **before** sexual contact. Please see Chapters 13 and 14 on birth control and STDs for more on spermicides and how to use a condom.

- *Penis–vagina intercourse.* For the best protection, the man uses a latex (not lambskin) condom, lubricated to avoid tearing, and the woman uses a vaginal spermicide containing nonoxynol-9, which has been shown to kill HIV in laboratory studies. The spermicide foam or gel should coat your entire vagina. (Read the package to make sure the spermicide concentration is greater than 9 percent.) Contraceptive sponges containing spermicide and suppositories are not

thought to be effective against HIV. Some women find some spermicides irritating to the vagina; you can try different brands. Some condoms contain a spermicide in the lubricant. If you use a lubricant, choose one that is water based, such as K-Y Jelly, Astroglide or Probe. Do not use oil-based lubricants like Vaseline, butter or Crisco, which will damage condoms within minutes.

The female condom is a promising new alternative that gives more control to us as women (see p. 268).

- *Oral sex on a man.* Oral sex is especially risky if the man ejaculates in your mouth, but even the pre-cum (drops of fluid that come out of the penis before he comes) can contain HIV. To protect yourself, use unlubricated latex condoms as soon as he is erect and a new one each time.

- *Oral sex on a woman.* Protection means using regular or microwaveable plastic wrap, but this does involve a small risk of suffocation. Be sure to cover both the labia and the anus. (Dental dams were initially suggested for this purpose, but they are small and thick and harder to get.) Use special care if the women has her period or a vaginal infection, as both can transmit HIV.

- *Penis–anus intercourse.* This is a high-risk activity, due to the fragile nature of the tissue in the rectum, which tears easily and thus can let HIV directly into the bloodstream. Many women choose to avoid anal intercourse entirely for this reason. If you do have anal sex, the man should use a latex condom with a water-based lubricant; he could use two condoms at once.

- *Fisting and finger play.* Fisting (putting a hand or fist into the rectum or vagina) or finger play (playing with the vagina or labia or touching your partner's anus) are risky because the internal tissue can be easily bruised or torn. HIV can travel into the bloodstream from cuts on your fingers or vice versa. For protection, use latex surgical or veterinary gloves (or finger cots for finger play) and change with each use.

- *Rimming* (mouth–anus contact). Rimming can spread disease carried in feces and saliva. For protection, use plastic wrap or dental dams.

- *Water sports* (sex partners urinate on each other). Wear goggles for this to protect your eyes, and avoid any broken skin or cuts.

- *Dildos/sex toys/vibrators.* These offer sexual enjoyment without the dangers of having semen entering your body, but if shared, they can transmit HIV from one partner to the other. Use a dildo with a condom and do not share dildos without putting on a new condom. Do not share sex toys and vibrators. Clean dildos and sex toys with hydrogen peroxide or bleach after each use.

- *Less risky activities.* Less risky activities include kissing (except deep kissing where there are un-

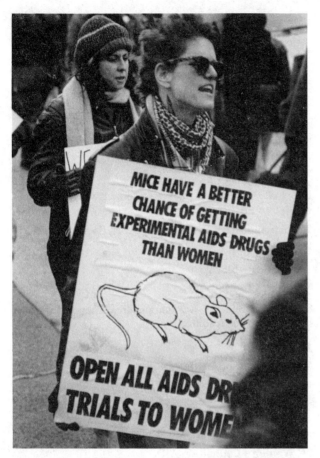

New York ACT UP demonstration at New York University Medical Center.   Miriam Lefkowitz

usual cuts in the mouth or gum disease), hugging, rubbing, hand jobs, mutual masturbation (avoid ejaculation on your skin if there are small cuts or sores), fantasizing and massage.

Safer Sex Supplies

Condoms (for men and, soon, for women), lubricants and spermicides are available from most drug stores, health clinics and sex boutiques. Plastic wrap is available in any grocery store. For latex gloves and finger cots, check with a local hospital, health clinic or sex boutique. Sex boutiques and other specialty stores carry dildos, sex toys and vibrators.* Planned Parenthood or STD clinics and some high schools supply free supplies of condoms.

HIV-Safe IV Needle Use

Sharing needles in IV drug use is the easiest way to get HIV from an infected person. One manual on protection advises:

*See Eve's Garden or Good Vibrations in Chapter 11's Resources.

If you want to use drugs as a regular part of your life, think about changing to a non-IV drug and finding the lowest-risk options. Drug centers can be useful in helping you evaluate your drug use. If you decide to continue using IV drugs, always clean your works before you shoot up. Take a small bottle of bleach. Draw bleach into your needle and squirt it out (three times) to kill the AIDS virus. Now draw up some clean water and squirt it out (three times) to get out the bleach. Make sure your cooker has been rinsed in bleach, too. Use fresh cotton each time you strain your liquid. In an emergency, rubbing alcohol, vodka or wine can also be used, but they are not as good as bleach.[3]

NOTES

1. H. Ward et al. "HIV Risk Behavior and STD Incidence in London Prostitutes," in *Abstracts of the VIth International Conference on AIDS, San Francisco, June, 1990*, FC 738. Quoted in *Triple Jeopardy: Women and AIDS*. London: The Panos Institute, 1991.

2. *Triple Jeopardy: Women and AIDS*. London: The Panos Institute, 1991.

3. Cindy Patton and Janis Kelly. *Making It: A Woman's Guide to Sex in the Age of AIDS*. Ithaca, NY: Firebrand Books, 1987, p. 11.

RESOURCES

Books and Articles

ACT UP/New York Women and AIDS Book Group. *Women, AIDS and Activism*. Boston: South End Press, 1990. Essays on the health and policy issues of concern to women affected in any way by HIV and AIDS.

Chicago Women's AIDS Project. *Girls Night Out: A Safer Sex Workshop for Women: Manual for Peer Leaders*. Available from the Chicago Women's AIDS Project, 5249 North Kenmore, Chicago, IL 60640, (312) 271-2242.

Cole, Rebecca, and Sally Cooper. "Lesbian Exclusion in HIV/AIDS Education: Ten Years of Low-Risk Identity and High-Risk Behavior," *SIECUS Report*, Vol. 19, No. 2 (December 1990/January 1991), pp. 18–23. This entire issue focuses exclusively on women and HIV/AIDS.

McCormack, Thomas P. *The AIDS Benefits Handbook*. New Haven, CT: Yale University Press, 1990.

Panos Institute. *Triple Jeopardy: Women and AIDS*. London: The Panos Institute, 1991.

Patton, Cindy, and Janis Kelly. *Making It: A Woman's Guide to Sex in the Age of AIDS*. Ithaca, NY: Firebrand Books, 1987. In Spanish and English. Good, frank discussion of the relative riskiness of specific sexual behaviors. Illustrated with cartoons by Alison Bechdel.

Peavey, Fran. *A Shallow Pool of Time*. Philadelphia: New Society Publishers, 1990. A first-person account by an HIV+ woman, activist, writer and comedian.

Reides, Ines, and Patricia Ruppelt. *AIDS: The Women*.

San Francisco: Cleis Press, 1988. Moving first-person accounts by women affected by HIV and AIDS.

The Positive Woman: A Newsletter by, for, and About the HIV Positive Woman.
P.O. Box 34372
Washington DC 20043-4372
(202) 898-0372
An excellent bimonthly newsletter for HIV+ women.

University of Massachusetts—Boston. *Searching for Women: A Literature Review on Women, HIV, and AIDS in the United States.* Boston: Law Center, College of Public and Community Service, University of Massachusetts, and the Multicultural AIDS Coalition, 1992.

Organizations

National

ACT UP (AIDS Coalition to Unleash Power)
135 West 29th Street, Suite 10
New York, NY 10001
(212) 564-2437
AIDS activist organization.

National AIDS Hot Line
(800) 342-AIDS
Spanish: (800) 344-7432
TTY: (800) 243-7889
Information, education and national and local referral. English language line is open twenty-four hours a day, 365 days a year; Spanish line is open seven days a week from 8:00 A.M. to 2:00 A.M., EST; TTY line is open Monday through Friday, 10:00 A.M. to 10:00 P.M., EST.

Northeast

AIDS Project
22 Monument Square, 5th Floor
Portland, ME 04101
(207) 774-6877
Support groups; hot line; HIV testing/counseling; meals program; case management.

AIDS Project New Haven
P.O. Box 636
254 College Street, Suite 200
New Haven, CT 06510
(203) 624-0947.
Buddy program; case management; massage clinic; meal delivery; support groups; counseling; hot line; education.

Blacks Educating Blacks About Sexual Health Issues (BEBASHI)
1528 Walnut Street, Suite 200
Philadelphia, PA 19102
(215) 546-4140
Sexuality workshops; HIV testing/counseling; support groups; community-based training for AIDS education; peer education; substance use recovery; referral.

Boston Women's AIDS Information Project
464 Massachusetts Avenue
Boston, MA 02118
(617) 859-8689.

Community-based training and education for women of color.

Health Education Resource Organization (HERO)
101 West Read, Suite 825
Baltimore, MD 21201
Hotline: (301) 945-AIDS
Counseling; support groups; legal assistance; advocacy; buddy program; financial assistance; referral.

New Jersey Women and AIDS Network
5 Elm Row, Suite 112
New Brunswick, NJ 08901
(908) 846-4462
Information and advocacy for women with HIV infection and AIDS.

Women and AIDS Resource Network (WARN)
55 Johnson Street, Suite 303
General Building
P.O. Box 020525
Brooklyn, NY 11202
(718) 596-6007
Counseling; referral; workshops for women with AIDS; resources for lesbians.

Southeast

AIDS Services of Austin
P.O. Box 4874
Austin, TX 78765
(512) 451-2273
Spanish: (512) 472-2001
Counseling; advocacy; educational materials; referral.

DC Women's Council on AIDS
Sistercare Support Network
725 8th Street
Washington, DC 20003
(202) 544-8255
Peer counseling; support groups; practical support; safer sex education; risk reduction education.

Health Crisis Network
1351 NW 20th Street
Miami, FL 33142
(305) 326-8833
Referral; counseling; support groups; Spanish and Creole; individual and group counseling for substance users.

NO/AIDS Task Force
1407 Decatur Street
New Orleans, LA 70116
(504) 945-4000
Counseling; educational information; referral.

Sisterlove Women's AIDS Project
1132 West Peachtree Street, Room 111
Atlanta, GA 30309
(404) 872-0600
Safer sex education; advocacy; workshops; women of color.

Women's Health Project
Nelson Tebedo Clinic
P.O. Box 190712
Dallas, TX 75219
(214) 521-5124

Comprehensive nurse-run project devoted to the health needs of women, particularly those involving HIV/AIDS, lesbian issues and breast health.

Midwest

Aliveness Project
730 East 38th Street
Minneapolis, MN 55407
(612) 822-7946
Women's support group; meals; drop-in center; clothing; library; massage therapy; acupuncture; chiropractic.

Chicago Women's AIDS Project
5249 North Kenmore
Chicago, IL 60640
(312) 271-2242
Support groups; referral; case management; safer sex education; peer education; child care and family services; buddy program; financial assistance; speakers bureau.

Community Health Awareness Group
3028 East Grand Boulevard
Detroit, MI 48202
(313) 872-2424
Community-based program for African-American and Latin communities; counseling; support groups; HIV and TB testing referral; bleach distribution; home visits; food and clothing bank.

Native American Women's Health Education Resource Center
P.O. Box 572
Lake Andes, SD 57356
(605) 487-7072
Reservation-based women's health resource center; HIV testing/counseling; safer sex education; financial assistance; culturally specific health education; advocacy.

Simon House
16260 Dexter Avenue
Detroit, MI 48221
(313) 863-1400
Emergency and transitional housing for women and their children, whether HIV infected or not; hospice; parenting classes; nutrition classes; referral; advocacy.

St. Louis Efforts for AIDS
5622 Delmar Boulevard, Suite 104E
St. Louis, MO 63112
(314) 367-8400
Support groups; buddy program; referral; educational materials; case management; outreach programs for women, lesbians and gay men, people of color and campuses; newsletter.

Topeka AIDS Project
P.O. Box 4726
Topeka, KS 66604
(913) 232-3100
Advocacy; case management; clinical services; referral; counseling; self-help; substance use recovery; support groups for people with AIDS (PWAs) and people living with AIDS (PLWAs); financial assistance;

buddy program; safer sex education; home health care; child care.

West

Cascade AIDS Project
408 SW Second Avenue, Room 412
Portland, OR 97204
(503) 223-5907
Support groups; counseling; educational materials; free legal advice; emergency financial aid; hotline; community health nurse.

Chemical Dependency Center for Women
1507 21st Street, Suite 100
Sacramento, CA 95814
(916) 448-2951
Counseling; street outreach; prison outreach; education.

Colorado AIDS Project
1576 Sherman Street
Denver, CO 80203
(303) 837-0166
Toll-free outside Denver: (800) 333-2437
Counseling; referral; emergency financial assistance; buddy program; support groups.

People of Color Against AIDS Network
1200 South Jackson, Suite 25
Seattle, WA 98144
(206) 322-7061
Prevention, outreach and educational materials.

Prevention Point Research Group
San Francisco, CA
(415) 861-6710
Street outreach; needle exchange; AIDS education

PROTOTYPES—W.A.R.N. (Women and AIDS Risk Network)
5601 West Slauson Avenue, Suite 200
Culver City, CA 90230
(213) 641-7795
AIDS prevention education and information; referral; court referral for sex workers; support groups; outreach; case management.

San Francisco AIDS Foundation
25 Van Ness Street, Suite 660
San Francisco, CA 94102
(415) 864-4376
Hot line: (800) 863-AIDS
Food bank; emergency housing; education programs and materials.

Women's AIDS Network
25 Van Ness Street, Suite 660
San Francisco, CA 94102
(415) 864-4589
Women's caucus of the San Francisco AIDS Foundation; education; information.

Legal Resources

AIDS Law Project, Gay and Lesbian Advocates and Defenders
P.O. Box 218
Boston, MA 02112
(617) 426-1350

Legal advocacy on issues of discrimination, confidentiality and access to health and medical care.

American Civil Liberties Union AIDS Project
132 West 43rd Street
New York, NY 10036
(212) 944-9800, ext. 545
Litigation and educational materials.

Lesbians' Resources

Gay and Lesbian Adolescent Social Services (GLASS)
8235 Santa Monica Boulevard, Suite 214
West Hollywood, CA 90046
(213) 656-5005
Counseling; housing; education; medical referral.

National Gay and Lesbian Health Foundation
1638 R Street NW, Suite 2
Washington, DC 20009
(202) 797-3708
Health care advocacy; publishes directory of lesbian/
gay health services in United States; sponsors national conferences on lesbian/gay health issues.

National Gay and Lesbian Task Force
1517 U Street NW
Washington, DC 20009
(202) 332-6483
Advocacy; activism; referral.

Whitman-Walker Clinic
1407 S Street NW
Washington, DC 20009
(202) 797-3500
An innovative workshop for the lesbian community on sexuality, safer sex and communication.

Teens' Resources

Adolescent AIDS Program
Montefiore Medical Center
111 East 210th Street
Bronx, NY 10467
(212) 920-2179
HIV testing/counseling; clinical services; support groups; case management; referral; safer sex education.

Hetrick-Martin Institute
401 West Street
New York, NY 10014
(212) 633-8920
TTY: (212) 633-8926
Support groups; counseling; social activities.

Teens and AIDS Hotline
(800) 234-TEEN
Nationwide referral service.

Treatment Resources

AIDS Treatment Data Network
259 West 30th Street
New York, NY 10001
(212) 268-4196
Information on research and treatment; educational materials; access to AIDS-related clinical drug trials; peer education and counseling.

Fenway Community Health Center
7 Haviland Street
Boston, MA 02115
(617) 267-0900
HIV testing/counseling; outpatient medical care; gynecological services; substance use treatment and counseling; acupuncture detox; nutrition information; massage; holistic therapy.

Project Inform
1965 Market Street
San Francisco, CA 94103
(800) 822-7422
Nationwide referral to treatment centers and information.

Whitman-Walker Clinic
1407 S Street NW
Washington, DC 20009
(202) 797-3500
Case management; clinical services; HIV testing/counseling; referral; safer sex education; support groups; hotline; buddy program; financial assistance; legal services; substance use recovery.

Prison Resources

AIDS Counseling and Education (ACE)
Bedford Hills Correctional Facility
287 Harris Road
Bedford Hills, NY 10507
(914) 241-3100, ext. 260
Nationwide model for peer education for prisons, created by women prisoners for women prisoners; peer counseling; education groups; peer support; health advocacy; inmate and worker education; workshops for general public.

National Prison Project
1616 P Street NW
Washington, DC 20036
(202) 331-0500
Information; studies; referral.

Social Justice for Women
MCI Framingham Women and AIDS Project
108 Lincoln Street, 6th Floor
Boston, MA 02111
(617) 482-0717
Monitors medical care, treatment and aftercare services for HIV positive women at MCI Framingham; group education programs; individual counseling.

16

If You Think You Are Pregnant: Finding Out and Deciding What To Do

BY JANE PINCUS AND
JILL WOLHANDLER

Some of us want to have a child and, within a matter of months or years, become pregnant.

Some of us become pregnant unexpectedly or when we don't want or can't have a child.

There are several ways of finding out whether you are pregnant. It is best to find out early. If you want to have a baby, you can take extra good care of yourself. If you decide not to continue the pregnancy, you can get an early abortion, the easiest and safest kind. *If you suspect pregnancy but haven't yet had a test, don't assume you definitely are pregnant. Use birth control if you have intercourse and don't want to be pregnant.*

Usual signs of early pregnancy (one to two weeks after conception) are (1) missing a period; (2) a period with less bleeding or fewer days than usual; (3) swelling, tenderness or tingling in your breasts (about two weeks after conception); (4) frequent urination; (5) fatigue; (6) nausea or vomiting (morning sickness); (7) feeling bloated or crampy; (8) increased or decreased appetite; (9) changes in digestion (constipation or heartburn); (10) mood changes. Keep in mind that some women become pregnant and are not aware of it for the first few months. Signs of pregnancy vary from woman to woman and pregnancy to pregnancy.

WHERE TO GET A PREGNANCY TEST

Pregnancy tests are available through many clinics and medical practitioners (doctors, midwives, nurse-practitioners, physicians' assistants). In many places family-planning organizations (Planned Parenthood, for example), women's health centers and abortion clinics offer the most frequently used pregnancy testing services. The yellow pages may also list labs that do pregnancy testing. You can buy a kit in a drugstore and do a test yourself at home (see below). In some places you may have to call a doctor or hospital to get a test.

You may be able to get a free test, but be aware that free services may be offered as a way to promote something else. For example, groups like Birthright advertise free pregnancy testing and counseling and offer help with problem pregnancies. These groups give out antiabortion propaganda, hoping to frighten you and convince you not to consider abortion even if you do not want to have a baby.

Wherever you go, the person who tells you the result of your test may make assumptions that do not apply to you: s/he may tell you about abortion but not about prenatal care and having a baby; tell your husband, boyfriend or parents without your permission; act as if you are in a crisis situation and feeling terrible; or congratulate you on the "happy news." Remember that it's your body and your choice. You may feel not at all the way anyone else expects you to feel.

KINDS OF PREGNANCY TESTS

All urine and blood tests react with a hormone called human chorionic gonadotropin (HCG), which is secreted into a pregnant woman's blood by the developing placenta. HCG shows up in the urine, through which it is excreted. *Urine slide tests* are the fastest, easiest and least expensive pregnancy tests. A drop of urine is mixed with the test serum on a slide; after two minutes the presence or absence of little clumps in the mixture indicates whether there is HCG in the urine. These tests are accurate for most women at about twenty-seven days after conception (when a period is about thirteen days late). In a *urine tube test* the urine is mixed with purified human HCG in a test tube. After one to two hours the cells sink to the bottom of the tube in a doughnut pattern if there is enough HCG for a positive test. These tests are generally accurate a few days earlier in pregnancy than the slide tests. Recently, new and more expensive urine tests have been developed that may be accurate as early as fourteen days after conception.

To collect a good urine sample use a *very clean, dry jar.* Do not use an old medicine container or shampoo bottle, because traces of chemicals or soap can contaminate the sample. Especially if it is early in the pregnancy, take the sample when you first wake up in the morning, because your urine is more concentrated then. A small amount (several tablespoons) is sufficient for the test. Cover the urine and keep it refrigerated. It is best not to use aspirin or marijuana the day before you take the sample, because they can interfere with the test.

Pregnancy test results can be positive, negative or inconclusive. A positive result almost always means pregnancy. A false positive—that is, a positive result when a woman is not actually pregnant—is rare. False positives can be caused by an error in reading the test, drugs (marijuana, methadone, Aldomet, large amounts of aspirin, synthetic hormones like birth control pills, some tranquilizers and other drugs that affect the nervous system), protein or blood in the urine, soap or other substances in the container, hormone changes of menopause* or certain tumors or other rare medical conditions.

A negative test may mean that you are not pregnant, but false negatives are fairly common. Often, it is too early in your pregnancy for the test to measure the small amount of HCG in your urine. Later, the amount of HCG starts to decrease after a couple of months; by four to five months the HCG level may be so low that a test may give a false negative. Other reasons for false negatives are (1) the urine became too warm; (2) the urine was not concentrated enough; (3) there was contamination from the jar or from certain medications; (4) it is an unhealthy pregnancy that may miscarry; (5) it is an ectopic pregnancy (pregnancy outside the uterus); (6) there has been a mistake in doing the test. A health worker can help you evaluate your chances of a false negative and discuss why your period may be late if you are not pregnant. If you suspect that you are pregnant even though a test is negative, have a pelvic exam and/or repeat the urine test. Don't just keep waiting for your period.

In two weeks I had three pregnancy tests; all of them were inconclusive, according to the lab reports I got. By the time I was given a blood test which established my pregnancy as real rather than imagined, I felt angry at the medical establishment for disbelieving me.

Home Pregnancy Tests

Some women appreciate the option of a home pregnancy test because it gives privacy, convenience and control over the experience. However, other women feel isolated doing a home test. The test itself is not hard to do, but home tests may give false results more often than lab tests. The instructions do not include enough information to evaluate whether the result is accurate, so you may need additional information.

Blood Tests

Two kinds of blood tests—radioimmunoassays (RIAs), which test for the beta subunit of HCG, and radioreceptorassays (RRAs)—are more sensitive than slide or tube tests. They can detect low levels of HCG in the blood even before the first missed period. (HCG appears earlier in the blood than in urine.) Blood tests may be needed to detect

---

*All the tests except the beta subunit tests cross-react with luteinizing hormone (LH) (see p. 256). For this reason, premature menopause and actual menopause can give false positives. Also, it is possible, though very rare, that a test at the LH surge at ovulation could give a false positive.

an ectopic pregnancy or missed abortion. The RIA test is accurate seven to twelve days after conception, whereas the RRA test, called Biocept-G, is accurate fourteen to seventeen days after conception. Like all tests, they sometimes give false results.

Pills and Injections

If the doctor suggests injections or pills to see whether they will bring on your period, *do not agree.* This procedure, sometimes called a *hormone withdrawal test,* is *not* an accurate test for pregnancy, and it is dangerous. The drugs used are synthetic hormones (usually progestin) that can cause negative effects in a woman who takes them and birth defects if she is pregnant and decides to have the baby. Though the FDA issued warnings against this procedure in 1973 and withdrew approval in 1975, a 1976 survey showed that doctors were still using it.*

Pelvic Exam

To check on the results of a pregnancy test or to find out how far along your pregnancy is, have a pelvic exam at around six weeks after your last menstrual period (six weeks LMP). If you are pregnant, (1) you, your doctor, midwife or other practitioner will feel that the tip of your cervix (neck of the uterus) has become softened; (2) your cervix may change from a pale pink to a bluish color because of increased blood circulation (you can see it yourself if you have a speculum and mirror); (3) your uterus feels softer to the person examining you; and (4) the size and shape of the uterus change.

Some women just know they are pregnant. Some of us feel we know the *moment* we become pregnant. Perhaps one sign—a missed period, tender breasts—tunes us in to the fact that our bodies feel different.

With my first child I missed a period and my breasts hurt. With Jesse, I knew the moment I conceived him. There's no way of pinning that down, no way of explaining how I felt. I just knew.

Now you know you are pregnant. If you are going to have the baby, see Part IV, Childbearing. If you plan to have an abortion, turn to Chapter 17, "Abortion." In either case, you may want to consider the information below.

---

*See *Biology of Women* by Ethel Sloane, New York: John Wiley & Sons, 1980, p. 264.

IF YOU'RE NOT SURE WHAT YOU'RE GOING TO DO

Think through the various possibilities and what they would mean to you. You may be able to decide what to do very quickly; you may think you know what you are going to do, but after more thought and talking about it, you may change your mind; you may be torn for a long time and find it incredibly difficult to make a decision. You are not required to talk to anyone in order to decide, but talking with people you think will be supportive can be immensely helpful. You may or may not want to include family members or the man involved. Talking may make you closer than before, or you may not get support when you most want or expect it. Often others have such strong feelings about your pregnancy that they are not helpful and may even upset you.

Whatever choice you make, it should be *yours* and no one else's. Other people (family, friends, lover) *may* help you figure out what you want, but sometimes it is wisest to talk to them *after* you have made your decision. *You should not have to justify your decision to anyone, but if you don't make any decision, you are in fact deciding to have a baby, without realizing that it is a decision.*

Counseling from experienced professional people in your own community is probably the most helpful, but choosing the right help can be extremely difficult, recently made much worse by legal pressure on many family-planning clinics to avoid any mention of abortion (see p. 361). *There are "abortion" centers whose only purpose is to frighten you and prevent abortion and "adoption" agencies whose main purpose is to get your baby away from you* (see below).

Having and Rearing Children

Get some idea about what it's like to raise children; observe and talk to mothers, fathers, children you know. Offer to take care of friends' children. If you are married or living with someone, think about how having a baby will change your life together. If you are single, think about how you would support and care for a child; where you would live; who, if anyone, you would live with. If you already have children, what will a new child mean to you and to them? Always keep in mind that we all need help at different times to bring up our children.

Abortion

For many women abortion is a positive choice. Having an abortion can be much less traumatic physically and emotionally than having an unwanted child. The safest and easiest time to have

345

an abortion is within the first three months (first trimester) of the pregnancy.

This is the first time I really told people because it was such a big thing for me. There are so many women who've had abortions. These women have made these choices, too—so nothing's wrong with me. . . . When you are willing to talk about it, it makes another feel she can talk to you.

I was the mother of three little boys. Being a mother and having children has always been very important to me, and this made the decision that much more difficult. Loving children as I do, I also knew that having the baby and then giving it up for adoption would not be an option for me.

Before I made the decision to have the abortion, I cried a lot. I would wake up around four-thirty in the morning and think about what to do, and cry. I'm sure experiencing the loss of a potential child was part of it.

My lover was opposed to having the child (as a team) and I didn't want another child without his help, so I decided on abortion. I was not happy with this because I wanted the child and was in love with the father.

I knew that abortions were legal, but that's all. I was afraid to mention it to my doctor. I thought he'd accuse me of being evil. (He didn't.) I also thought I'd be in terrible pain. The hospital had a program explaining the procedure the day before to the whole group of us. It was very helpful.

I get so bitter hearing people piously stating how those poor babies have a right to live and there are lots of people who want babies and can't have them. A baby isn't just produced and given away and that's that. You're talking about a part of the woman's body. That baby is part of her, and to expect her to give it up after going through a pregnancy is really ridiculous. I know many women could, but many couldn't. I couldn't have. I know that without my abortion I would have gone through nine months of hell, dealing with my boyfriend, my parents, my friends, my job, my financial situation, my health, my whole future and then thinking about the baby, its future, would I keep it or not, how to support it, and so on—one headache after another. At that time in my life, I don't think I could have handled it all. I couldn't even handle it now, and I'm better off now than I was a year ago.

Increasingly, younger women are vulnerable to right-wing or fundamentalist religious values and propaganda being disseminated in the wider society, believing even in peer groups that "good girls" don't use birth control and don't have abortions. Some also come to regret their abortions or feel silently guilty about them. From this pressure to carry a pregnancy to term you may become vulnerable to other pressures—to keep your baby or give it away (see below).

Adoption and Foster Care

Be sure to see pp. 347–49 for more about adoption.

Explore the adoption alternatives and services available to you. Find out about your legal rights from your *own* lawyer, a legal aid office, or an informed women's group, but not from anyone who will benefit or profit from your decision, such as a lawyer or social worker suggested by an adoption agency. Adoption agencies are geared primarily to performing adoptions rather than serving the needs of a woman with an unwanted child, although some claim to do both. All rights and laws vary from state to state. Some states allow only agencies to arrange adoptions while others allow private placement arranged by a lawyer, physician or the woman who is pregnant or has had the child. Never sign any papers until you are *absolutely sure* of your decision. In some states there is a grace period even after you sign during which you can change your mind.

The yellow pages ads of phone directories prey on vulnerable and unsuspecting pregnant teens, inviting them to come to another city, all expenses paid, to have their babies in privacy and surrender them secretly. Many of these newer self-described "adoption" agencies, which have sprung up in many states, gloss over the line between financial support to isolated and frightened unwed mothers and "baby selling," forbidden by law in most states. Many lawyers have gone into the business of private adoptions, some more unscrupulous than the agencies. A "black market" exists for healthy white infants and even for overseas children, which only comes to public attention periodically when a particularly outrageous case is discovered. Meanwhile, impatient infertile couples now openly seek out desperate pregnant young women directly through advertising, often moving to states where they can escape agency scrutiny. Some thoughtful professional leaders are becoming alarmed and outraged by this rapidly rising trend (see box on p. 350).

Many women have joined together recently to talk about what it meant to them to give their children up for adoption many years ago. Whether or not they felt they had done so of their own free will, whether or not they felt that it had been the right decision for them at the time, they all agree that giving your child up for adoption doesn't mean that you aren't a mother anymore; you will always be the child's birth parent.

ADOPTION ABUSE

by Carole Anderson and Lee Campbell, with Mary Anne Cohen. Reprinted from *Women-Wise*, Vol. 5, No. 3, Fall 1983.

You may never have heard the term birthmothers before, but we are the mothers who have surrendered children to adoption. We have joined together to form a national, non-profit group called Concerned United Birthparents, Inc. (CUB). We are the living proof of why all feminists must oppose legislation that now threatens to destroy the gains made for women in the past few years.

Most people assume that mothers who surrender their babies to adoption do so because they don't want their children. Or they assume that mothers choose adoption as a means of providing more for their children than they could offer. In our view, these assumptions are dangerously simplistic.

In a male-dominated society, a woman's expression of sexuality is permitted only within strict bounds. Traditionally, only when she is married is sexual activity considered legitimate; indeed, it is expected at a husband's whim as his right.

For thousands of years men have sought to control women's sexuality and fertility. Out-of-wedlock pregnancies have historically merited harsh punishment. In some cultures, that punishment is even death. An unmarried pregnant woman is still considered, in some Moslem countries, to be such a stain on the family's honor that it can be cleansed only through the woman's death, and the murderer is rarely prosecuted.

America's preferred punishment appears more civilized. We favor removal of the evidence: before birth, in maternity homes, segregated educational programs, or away at Aunt Sally's; after birth, by adoption. When these preferences are ignored, we mount subtle but effective campaigns to condemn the perpetrators. We sympathize with infertility among married couples in the same breath that we bemoan the so-called "unwed teenage pregnancy epidemic," as though the issues are related. We proclaim that "adoption builds families" without reference to the female-headed families adoption has separated, as though they never existed. We begrudge the subsidies that help economically deficient single-parent families to remain together, while we uncomplainingly subsidize foster care and adoption.

Most younger single mothers have little knowledge of rights. They are accustomed to following the advice of parents, teachers, and other authority figures. Frightened, vulnerable, and economically dependent, mothers whose parents are not supportive are easy prey to the social workers, attorneys, and doctors who arrange adoptions and collect placement fees of as much as $30,000 for healthy white infants.

Most CUB members surrendered children at a time when they were unaware of financial help that would have enabled them to keep their children, or when such help did not exist. Most encountered social workers who failed to give information about alternatives that could have aided mothers to keep their families together. Children of single parents, it was said, would be ridiculed at school as bastards, or grow up to be homosexual because they lacked a father image, or would live in poverty forever because no decent man would marry their mother. Through the 1960's most schools expelled pregnant students, thus denying them a chance to graduate. And day care opportunities were rare even if a mother could find a job that would support her and her child. Denied education, denied jobs and denied any knowledge of financial assistance, few had any option but to surrender their children.

The loss of a child to adoption is a unique and unnatural one. Unlike death, which is final, adoption creates a loss that is renewed daily, as each day is a new day of trying to live without the surrendered child whose life continues separately. It is a limbo loss, in which there are constant questions but no answers. Is my child well or ill? Happy or miserable? Alive or dead?

For ten years I tied up all my emotional energy in trying to pretend it never happened, and I almost believed it. I had to stay emotionally detached to survive. I was afraid to face all this pain, but I was numbing myself to everything else in life, too.

Part of me died. I feel empty inside, I'm afraid to make decisions about anything, and I can't

continued

trust anyone. I was told so many lies. I can't let anyone get close to me, especially men, and I cringe if a man touches me.

When I was eighteen I believed what the social worker said about adoptive couples. That they were screened so they were totally perfect parents who had everything my child needed, and I had nothing. Now I know adoptive parents are the same as everyone else. They're not perfect. I feel cheated. Why did I have to compete with other people for the right to raise my own child?

Forcing me to surrender my child was an ultimate act of rape. I wish that when they were through with me, they had put a bullet in my head so I wouldn't have to live in such anguish.

When a mother surrenders her child, she is allowed no options in the terms of that surrender. She has no right to participate in selecting who will raise her child, to know anything about her child's adoptive parents, to know anything about her child's health or welfare. She has no right to choose whether or not she wishes to be anonymous to the adoptive parents or to her child, even after her child is an adult. She has no right to legal counsel, no right to be informed of alternatives, no right to copies of information about her. She has no right to her child's original birth certificate, nor to the falsified version that will later be substituted to state that the adoptive parents gave birth. She has no right to know the legal process involved in adoption. She even has no right to receive a copy of the surrender document that separates her child from her.

Social workers defend this process by claiming that adoption is a positive choice for a young woman with an unplanned pregnancy since it permits the mother to correct her mistake. They insist that the mother's pain is temporary, and that she will be able to begin a new life. That same child who was described as a burden to the mother is transformed into a blessing for a married couple able to pay a placement fee.

Many adoptive mothers, too, have sought to keep birthmothers in the role of brood mares. While some adoptive mothers have joined in CUB's efforts, others loudly proclaim that they alone are really mothers, that birthmothers do not deserve to know of their children's welfare, that God gave the child to adoptive parents, or that birthmothers should be grateful to adoptive parents for having saved their children from the stigma of illegitimacy. These adoptive parents demand that birthmothers respect adoptive parents' efforts, while they ignore birthmothers' sacrifices.

These women, too, are victims. Many have reported feelings of inadequacy and insecurity as a result of their inability to bear children of their own. Made by our society to feel their value as women depended on their ability to bear children, some feel they have to adopt babies and act as if they had borne them. The final proof of motherhood—the child's birth certificate—is permanently sealed, and a false one issued to reinforce the idea that birth alone confers motherhood.

Feminists have been slow to recognize adoption's exploitation of their sisters. Perhaps one reason is that women have been not only the victims of adoption abuse but also its chief perpetrators and beneficiaries. Just as it is women like Phyllis Schlafly who have led efforts to defeat the Equal Rights Amendment and advances for women's rights, it is women

They use yourself against you—your fears, insecurity, guilt! You give all your power away. You don't see it happening overtly, so you're never at the point where you'll run out the door with the baby. I can't believe I signed that paper. I thought I was doing the best thing: I didn't want her to be taunted and marked for life. For years afterward I couldn't remember anything about how I gave her up. I heard about one woman who forgot she even had a baby.

When I hear people say that adoption is the option women should choose instead of abortion, I get a *knot in my stomach and all my memories come back. Adoption may be an option for some people, but it wasn't a good answer for me.*

Foster care is a way of having someone else raise your child temporarily. If your relatives take care of your child, you avoid the necessity of going through an agency. When you go through an agency, you are giving up control of your baby, and your future wishes may not be respected.

who have fought to continue adoption abuse.

Reflecting the changes brought about by the women's movement, in the recent past single mothers have succumbed less frequently to adoption abuse. But know these things: Although only 3 percent of mothers under twenty now choose adoption, 43 percent of 125 cities with a population of 100,000 or more offer adoption services. The clientele being served today are infertile couples who, unwilling to adopt the many older or special-needs children who are available, wait in frustration on ever-lengthening lists for healthy, white infants. Joining agency workers' and infertile couples' demand for adoptable babies are anti-choice proponents who blithely tout adoption as the answer to abortion. . . .

Unless we exert the same effort in this area of reproductive rights as we do in others, single-parent families will be unnecessarily separated by adoption in the same manner they have always been. Adoption is especially susceptible to exploitation because there are no laws granting rights to birthmothers, no system of accountability for agency workers, and no recognition among lay people of the conflict of interest that inevitably arises when counselling centers and maternity homes double as adoption agencies.

Despite claims by the New Right to the contrary, adoption as it is traditionally practiced is not the panacea for all of society's ills. The unnecessary separation of mothers and children is a cruel, but regrettably usual, punishment that can last a lifetime.

A lifetime of suffering is too much to demand for any woman's expression of her sexuality. Even if contraception is obtainable, no fertile woman is ever safe from the possibility of unintended pregnancy, since there is no method that is 100% reliable. Even abstinence has its failures since rape exists.

We birthmothers are openly fighting for the rights of the young women of the future who may be threatened with our fate. Our lives are testimony to the devastating effects of the oppression of women that is our mutual foe. Help us, and let us help you, in our common cause. We are your mothers, your daughters, your sisters, perhaps even yourselves.

Lee Campbell is the founder of CUB (Concerned United Birthparents), a national support and advocacy group (see Resources). Lee and Carole Anderson are both former CUB presidents. Mary Anne Cohen is an original CUB member, a poet and a leader in Origins, a New Jersey–based support group.

Editor's note: Currently our federal government, responding to presidents and wealthy right-wing political supporters, has provided funds for expensive Department of Health & Human Services TV ads, often run late at night, openly promoting adoption as the government-sponsored answer to unwanted pregnancy. Several state welfare programs have attempted to force pregnant teens to live at home with parents rather than try to make it on their own. All of these programs are dangerous to prospective single mothers and single-parent families, attempting to impose an official governmental view of morality on all women, especially those who are most impressionable and least powerful. They attempt to punish the "immoral" by forcing them to give birth and then depriving them of their children through adoption as the only or first-choice option.

APPENDIX: ADOPTEES' LEGAL STATUS

An estimated 40 million people in the United States are affected by the institution of adoption, directly or through close relatives. In most states, however, the legal status of an adoptee is different from all other persons, no matter how old the adoptee is. Usually, the original birth certificate is sealed permanently and a new falsified certificate is issued by the state as if the adoptive parents had given birth to the child. Originally designed exclusively to protect the privacy of adoptive parents, the practice is now defended as protecting the adoptee from the stigma of illegitimacy and the birth mothers' stigma as "unwed mothers." The result is that in most states today when you surrender a child to adoption, that child is to be barred *forever* from knowing his/her original family origins, and you are to be barred *forever* from finding out about his/her new identity or welfare.

Although the law in some states allows adoptees to petition the court to open the sealed record for a "good purpose" (usually medical information), judges often refuse. Agencies' response to returning adult adoptees and birth parents seeking information is very mixed and varies from

IT'S TIME FOR SWEEPING CHANGE

by Annette Baran and Rueben Pannor.
Excerpted and edited from *AAC Decree*, No. 4,
June 1990.

What have we, in the adoption-reform movement, really been doing during the last two decades? It seems to us that, if we take off our blinders, we must admit that we have been co-opted into supporting a system that causes pain and lifelong suffering to the parties involved.... Each year that we delay, thousands of new adoptees, adoptive parents and birth parents join the long list of the afflicted.... We have always maintained that adoptive placement is the last resort, to be considered only when all other options have been thoroughly explored. However, our practice has never reflected this concept. Indeed, we are now embarked on a world of "How to" books, video tapes and seminars to teach couples methods and ruses of locating and convincing pregnant women to give up their babies. We are a heavy presence in the high school classroom, and the advertising columns luring vulnerable and economically deprived pregnant teenagers.... What have we done to underwrite and support keeping babies and helping the family stay together? Where in the world of adoption reform have we heard any emphasis on prevention and education and contraception? Knowing the agony and lifelong pain that would result from an unplanned pregnancy and subsequent relinquishment, why have we not made prevention a major issue? This issue has been clouded by religious dogma and politicized to obscure the real problems.... We offer the following issues for serious consideration.

Relinquishment of children to a new set of parents, as a final irrevocable act, severing all rights of the birth parents, must be discontinued. Open adoption, which we helped pioneer, is not a solution to the problems inherent in adoption. Without enforcement, open adoption is an unenforceable agreement at the whim of the adoptive parents. Instead, a form of guardianship adoption would be in the best interests of all concerned, with special benefits for the adoptee. It decreases the abandonment/ rejection issue and permits the child to know that the birthparents cared but could not raise him [sic].... The struggle to open records and address the wrongs of the past must continue. However, simultaneously and with equal emphasis, we must begin to look at the future and address the need for sweeping change. Do we have the courage to address the issues that will truly eliminate the problems we have struggled with for so many years?

Annette Baran, M.S.W., and Rueben Pannor, M.S.W., are professional leaders in adoption social work and coauthors of numerous books and articles.

state to state, some also involved in falsifying or concealing information and outright lying. Most adult adoptees remain in a sort of permanent "chattel" relationship to the state: The state possesses crucial information about them that it will not reveal, even to their adoptive parents and certainly not to birth mothers (even though they also may need it for the sake of later children). Adoptee-organized registries and search/support groups have tried to fill that vacuum, not always successfully. State-sponsored registry legislation has also been largely a failure, in some cases even creating new barriers by requiring signed legal releases from birth fathers as well as birth mothers—a clear perversion of the intent.

Professionals and legislators who claim adoptees' falsified legal status also protects birth mothers, supposedly promised confidentiality and anonymity at the time of surrender, are simply ignorant of history and common practice. Most birth mothers claim this guarantee of legal protection was never explained or even offered; most signed and surrendered, as one mother said, "without even a receipt." Certainly they never wanted anonymity from their own children, which is very different from public disclosure. It is clear that only opening the sealed state records can bring justice to the adult adoptee and to the birth parents.

Each year thousands more infants are legally surrendered and become adoptees in the system of closed adoption. The adoption reform movement's state-by-state campaign to open sealed records is slowly gaining momentum across the United States, led largely by adoptees, birth parents and a few enlightened professionals and adoptive parents. Meanwhile, older adoptees age and even die still wishing to learn the secrets of their unique identity. Birth mothers also wait for change, most silently, many going to their graves without even a scrap of information about the child—often their only child—they surrendered long ago.

RESOURCES*

Books

Aigner, H. *Adoption in America: Coming of Age.* Greenbrae, CA: Paradigm Press, 1986.

Arms, S. *A Hand Full of Hope: The Promise of Open Adoption.* Berkeley, CA: Celestial Arts, 1989.

Baker, N. *Babyselling: The Scandal of Black Market Adoption.* New York: Vanguard Press, 1978. A classic book.

Baran, A., et al. *Lethal Secrets: The Shocking Consequences and Unsolved Problems of Artificial Insemination.* New York: Warner Books, 1989.

Gediman, J., and L. Brown. *Birthbond: Reunions Between Birthparents and Adoptees: What Happens After.* Far Hills, NJ: New Horizon Press, 1989.

Gilligan, C. *In a Different Voice.* Cambridge, MA: Harvard University Press, 1982.

Kirk, H. D. *Adoptive Kinship: A Modern Institution in Need of Reform.* Port Angeles, WA: Ben Simon Publishers, 1985.

Krementz, J. *How It Feels to Be Adopted.* New York: Knopf, 1982.

Lifton, B. J. *Lost and Found: The Adoption Experience.* New York: Harper & Row, 1988.

Riben, M. *The Dark Side of Adoption.* New York: Harlo Press, 1988.

Silber, K., and P. Dorner. *Children of Open Adoption.* San Antonio, TX: Corona Publications, 1990.

Silverman, P. *Helping Women Cope with Grief.* Sage Human Services, No. 25. Beverly Hills, CA: Sage Publications, 1981.

Simon, R. J., and H. Alstein. *Transracial Adoptees and Their Families: A Study of Identity and Commitment.* New York: Praeger, 1987.

Sorosky, A., A. Baran and R. Pannor. *The Adoption Triangle: The Sealed or Opened Records: How They Affect Adoptees, Birthparents and Adoptive Parents,* 2nd ed. San Antonio, TX: Corona Publications, 1989.

Triseliotis, J. *In Search of Origins.* Boston: Beacon Press, 1973. A classic book.

Winkler, R., and D. Brown. *Clinical Practice in Adoption.* Elmsford, NY: Pergamon Press, 1988.

Articles

Anderson, R. "The Nature of Adoptee Search: Adventure, Cure, or Growth" (Practice Forum), *Child Welfare,* Vol. 68, No. 6 (November/December 1989).

———. "Why Adoptees Search: Motives and More," *Child Welfare,* Vol. 67, No. 1 (January/February 1988).

Baran, A., and R. Pannor. "It's Time for Sweeping Change" (Commentary), *AAC Decree* (American Adoption Congress), Vol. 4 (Summer 1990), p. 5. See box, p. 350.

Deykin, E., et al. "The Post-Adoption Experience of Surrendering Parents," *The American Journal of Orthopsychiatry,* Vol. 54, (January 1984), pp. 271–80.

Griffin, K. "The Open Adoption Option" (Family), *IN HEALTH* (January 1992), pp. 24–27.

Klerman, L. "Adoption: A Public Health Perspective" (Editorial), *American Journal of Public Health,* Vol. 73 (1983), p. 10.

Silverman, P., et al. "Reunions between Adoptees and Birth Parents: The Birth Parents' Experience," *Social Work,* Vol. 33, No. 6 (November/December 1988), pp. 523–28.

Simpson, M., et al. "Adoptees in Search of Their Past: Policy Induced Strain on Adoptive Families and Birth Parents," *Family Relations* (1981), pp. 427–34.

Periodicals

Adoption Therapist
Hope Cottage Adoption Center
4209 McKinney Avenue, Suite 200
Dallas, TX 75205

Chain of Life
Janine Baer
P.O. Box 8081
Berkeley, CA 94707
This newsletter offers feminist, gay and lesbian perspectives.

Reader's Guide to Adoption-Related Literature
William L. Gage
2300 Ocean Avenue
Brooklyn, NY 11229
The guide is updated periodically.

Reunions
Edith Wagner
P.O. Box 11727
Milwaukee, WI 53211-1727

Organizations

Adoption Circle: Choices, Education, Search, Support (*ACCESS*)
401 East 74th Street, Suite 17D
New York, NY 10021

Adoption Connection, *Happenings*
O'Shea Building, Room 6
11 Peabody Square
Peabody, MA 01960

ALMA (Adoptees Liberty Movement Association)
P.O. Box 154
Washington Bridge Station
New York, NY 10033
This organization offers a databank service. There are local chapters.

American Adoption Congress, *Decree*
1000 Connecticut Avenue NW, Suite 9
Washington, DC 20036
The hotline telephone number is (505) 296-2198. There are local chapters.

Child Welfare League of America, *Adoption Report*
440 First Street NW
Washington, DC 20001

---

*Please also see the Resources for Chapter 17, "Abortion."

CUB (Concerned United Birthparents)
  2000 Walker Street
  Des Moines, IA 50317
This organization offers an extensive list of publications. There are local branches.

Donor's Offspring (Children of donor insemination)
Candace Turner
  P.O. Box 37
  Sarcoxie, MO 64862

International Soundex Reunion Registry (ISSR)
  P.O. Box 2312
  Carson City, NV 89702
This organization offers the best adoption registry.

National Adoption Information Clearinghouse
  1400 I Street NW, Suite 1275
  Washington, DC 20005

Orphan Voyage
  Cedaredge, CO 81413
Adoptee support and a clearinghouse service are offered.

OURS (International Adoptions/Monthly Magazine)
  3307 Highway 100 North, Suite 203
  Minneapolis, MN 55422

PACER (Post Adoption Center for Research and Education)
  2255 Ynacio Valley Road, Suite L
  Walnut Creek, CA 94598
This organization offers regional adoptee support and resources.

PACT (Pre- and Post Adoption Consulting Team): COMPACT
The Family Center
  385 Highland Avenue
  Somerville, MA 02144

Parenting Resources, Inc. (multiresource)
  250 El Camino Real
  Tustin, CA 92680

Tri-Adoption Library
  P.O. Box 638
  Westminster, CA 92683
Write to them for referrals and publication lists.

17

Abortion

Physical and emotional aspects of abortion by JILL WOLHANDLER, with RUTH WEBER *Abortion history and politics* by TRUDE BENNETT, with JILL WOLHANDLER and DANA GALLAGHER

With special thanks to Vickie Alexander, Diane Balser, Terry Courtney, Margie Fine, Linda Gordon, Debra Krassner, Jane Pincus, Meredith Tax, and members of the Reproductive Rights Action Group at Brooklyn College.

This chapter in previous editions was written by Carol Driscoll, Nancy P. Hawley, Elizabeth McGee, Pamela Berger and Wendy Sanford.

1992 Update by Marlene Gerber-Fried, with Judy Norsigian. Special thanks to Sarah Buttenweiser, Concord Feminist Health Center, Helen Caulton, Liz Hill, Ana Ortiz, Stephanie Poggi, Loretta Ross, Kira Sarpard, Jill Wolhandler and Susan Yanow.

Women have always used abortion as a means of fertility control. Unless we ourselves can decide whether and when to have children, it is difficult for us to control our lives or participate fully in society. Legal, safe and affordable abortions help to give us that control.

Women of various ages, races, religions, economic and marital status and sexual preference choose to have abortions for many reasons. We may become pregnant because of inadequate birth control methods, information and access. Since no birth control method is 100 percent effective, abortion is a necessary backup when birth control fails. We may be pregnant, want a child and not be able to afford it or decide that even a planned pregnancy is a mistake after our economic or personal circumstances change. We may find out through amniocentesis that our fetus has a serious genetic disability. We may become pregnant because of rape, incest or other kinds of sexual coercion so common in our society. Little or nonexistent sex education leaves young women particularly vulnerable to sexual pressures.

Deciding whether to have a baby or an abortion is always a serious choice. You have to decide what you believe is responsible, moral and best for yourself and the important people in your life, depending on your needs, resources, commitments and hopes. We believe that compulsory pregnancy and forced motherhood are morally wrong.

For women who may experience a spiritual quandary about taking away the potential for human life, some spiritual teachers have sug-

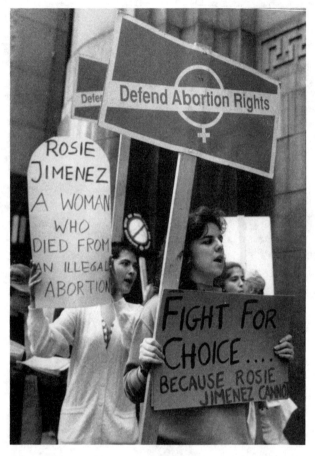

Ellen Shub

gested that we make this difficult choice based upon what will cause the least suffering for all of those involved.

The fact that I was able, for so many reasons, to choose to have an abortion has made an enormous difference in my life since then. Other decisions that I've made (where to live, to go back to school, to come out as a lesbian, what kinds of work to do) might all have been different if abortion hadn't been available to me in the past . . . I feel so strongly that those options should be open to other women. Of course, this means not just abortion but child care, decent incomes and housing and education, struggling with racism and more. But I know from my own experience what is involved for a woman to decide on an abortion and follow it through. Knowing that afterwards my feelings weren't as simple as I'd expected just makes it clearer for me that no one else has any right to interfere with a woman doing what she needs to do, according to her own wisdom and judgment.

As black women we have never been able to say clearly that we support abortion because being able to control our reproduction directly affects the qual-

ity of our lives and, in some cases, whether we even have lives. It is very hard for women to say that when the deal goes down, we choose ourselves.

I was sixteen, pregnant and couldn't tell my parents. It's not that they would hurt me or anything like that—but I didn't want to hurt them. Because I wasn't getting my parents permission, I had to go in front of a judge. I felt like a criminal. I was scared that he would say no. My lawyer helped a lot, but it was still so hard to do. It made me angry, too. This judge doesn't even know me. Even though he let me do what I wanted to do—have an abortion—I'm still mad about the judge. The abortion itself was fine. I feel good that I was able to do all of this.

Opponents of abortion tell us that no woman ever wants to have an abortion, that abortion is always traumatic, but sometimes women are forced by economic necessity or psychological desperation to have them. When I was young and unwillingly pregnant and afraid I wouldn't find an illegal abortion in time, that was traumatic. My desperation consisted of not wanting to be a mother at that time. I did want to be sexually active. Having an abortion produced great relief, the end of my trauma.

It seemed like a punishment. I used birth control and got pregnant anyway. I no longer trusted my diaphragm, my lover, my body. My guilt about being pregnant turned into anger when I learned that no method of birth control is 100 percent effective! I took all the precautions and still needed an abortion. At the clinic, so many women had similar experiences.

Deciding to have an abortion wasn't a difficult decision or a big deal. From the way everyone I told reacted, though, I started wondering if something was wrong with me for not being upset.

MEDICAL TECHNIQUES FOR ABORTION

When you are considering an abortion or choosing where to have an abortion, you have a right and a need to know the procedures used at each stage of pregnancy, the risks and possible complications and the cost.

In pregnancy, a tiny ball of cells attaches itself to the lining of the uterus about one week after conception. A mass of tissue called the *placenta* develops in the uterine lining to nourish the *embryo.* By the end of the second month, the embryo, now called a *fetus,* is surrounded by a protective fluid-filled sac, the *amniotic sac.* At about twenty weeks the woman begins to feel the fetus move. Sometime between the twenty-fourth and twenty-eighth weeks the fetus reaches the point where it may live outside the mother for at least a short while under intensive hospital care.

354

Procedure	Techniques	Weeks LMP	Where Performed	Common Anesthesia (see p. 360)
1. Preemptive abortion Endometrial aspiration Menstrual regulation (See section on menstrual extraction)	Suction	4–6	Clinic MD office	None (Local)*
2. Early uterine evacuation (EUE)	Suction	6–8	Clinic MD office	None Local
3. Vacuum aspiration	Dilation, suction, sometimes curettage	6–14	Clinic MD office (Hospital)*	None Local (General)*
4. Dilation and curettage (D and C)	Dilation, curettage	6–16	(Clinic)* (MD office)* Hospital	(Local)* General
5. Dilation and evacuation (D and E)	Dilation, suction, curettage, use of forceps	12—upper limit varies from 16–24	(Clinic)* MD office Hospital	(Local)* General
6. Induction abortion Instillation procedure Saline abortion Prostaglandin abortion	Injection of liquid through the abdomen into amniotic sac; uterine contractions (labor) expel the fetus and placenta	16–24	Hospital	Local for the injection and painkillers for the labor and delivery
7. Prostaglandin suppositories (rarely used)	Drug inserted into the vagina to cause labor and miscarriage	13–?	Hospital	Painkillers for labor and delivery
8. Hysterotomy	Uterus is cut open	16–24 or later if woman's life in danger	Hospital	General

*Parentheses mean "less common."
LMP: last normal menstrual period.
Dilation: enlarging the cervical opening by stretching it with tapered instruments called dilators, or with laminaria (see p. 358). Many medical technicians use the word "dilatation" to mean the same thing.
Suction: drawing out the contents of the uterus through a narrow tube attached to a gentle vacuum source.
Curettage: scraping the inside of the uterus with a metal loop, called a curette, to loosen and remove tissue.
Forceps: grasping instruments used to remove tissue.
Amniotic sac: sac of fluid surrounding the fetus.
Prostaglandin: hormonelike substance that causes uterine contractions.
Saline: salt water.

Procedure	Complications
1. Preemptive abortion Endometrial aspiration Menstrual regulation	Infection Retained tissue (incomplete abortion)
2. Early uterine evacuation (EUE)	Perforation Hemorrhage
3. Vacuum aspiration	Continuing pregnancy (missed abortion)
4. Dilation and curettage	Cervical tear Reaction to anesthesia or other drugs
5. Dilation and evacuation	Postabortal syndrome (blood in uterus)
6. Induction abortion	Infection, retained tissue, hemorrhage, cervical tear, drug reaction, others (see p. 359)
7. Prostaglandin suppositories	Often unsuccessful, severe gastrointestinal side effects
8. Hysterotomy	Risks of major surgery (see p. 359)

HOW PREGNANT ARE YOU?

The length of a pregnancy is usually counted from the first day of the last normal menstrual period (LMP) and not from the day of conception (fertilization). LMP dating is inaccurate and misleading. It can make you think that you are two weeks further along in the pregnancy than you really are. It assumes that every woman not only has a twenty-eight-day cycle but ovulates exactly two weeks after her period began. (Nobody has a regular cycle *all* the time.) The *first trimester* is the first thirteen weeks; the *second trimester* is the fourteenth through twenty-fourth weeks LMP; twenty-five weeks LMP and later is the *third trimester*. Abortion is safer, easier and less expensive in the first trimester. It may be difficult to find a facility that provides second-trimester abortions, and impossible to get a third-trimester abortion unless your life is endangered by your pregnancy.

The first day of the last menstrual period is the most common way to date a pregnancy, but you must consider whether that period was normal for you. If it came at an unexpected time or was lighter than usual, conception may have happened *before* that bleeding.

If you chart your body changes with a fertility awareness method (see p. 276), you will have a written record of ovulation and will be able to recognize pregnancy quite early on. If you do cervical self-examination, you may notice that your cervix has changed color and become bluish-purple, which happens early in pregnancy.

Signs of pregnancy can help confirm the date of conception (see p. 343).

An experienced health worker or medical practitioner can estimate the length of a pregnancy by feeling the size of the uterus during a pelvic exam. This is usually accurate within a two-week range. Ultrasound, another method for determining the length of a pregnancy, also has a two-week margin of error. The practitioner doing the abortion makes the final decision about how far advanced the pregnancy is and whether s/he is willing to perform the abortion. If the practitioner refuses to do the abortion, you may have to find someone else. Statistically, abortion risks increase as the pregnancy progresses and the uterus becomes larger and softer.

In an abortion, the contents of the uterus (embryo or fetus, placenta and built-up lining of the uterus) are removed. Different methods are used, depending on how large the pregnancy tissue has grown, the training of the person performing the abortion, the approaches favored by the local medical community and the equipment available. The chart summarizes medical abortion procedures. The numbers in this section refer back to the chart. These procedures may not all be available in your area, or different names may be used for some of them. Ask for explanations of words and terms you don't understand.

During an aspiration abortion (1, 2 and 3 on the chart), the contents of the uterus are removed through a strawlike tube that is passed through the cervix into the uterus. The tube, called a *cannula*, is attached to a source of gentle suction—an electric or mechanical pump or a syringe—which draws out the tissue.

Aspiration is now the most common abortion technique. Of all the methods, it carries the least chance of complications and considerably less risk than pregnancy, labor and delivery. In fact, it is now the safest of all operations, safer than tonsillectomies or circumcisions. It only takes a short time (five to fifteen minutes).* Aspiration abortions are now available throughout the United States, though some women still have to travel many hours to get to an abortion facility. *This kind of abortion is the safest and least disruptive for a woman, both physically and emotionally. It can only be done during the first three months of pregnancy.*

1. An aspiration procedure before five to six weeks LMP, when pregnancy cannot yet be verified by a pelvic exam, is called *preemptive abortion*, *endometrial aspiration* or *menstrual regulation*. (Some people also call it *menstrual extraction*, but that term describes a different procedure and should not be used for this one. See p. 358.) A syringe is attached to the cannula to suction out the lining of the uterus, including the small amount of fetal and placental tissue if there is a pregnancy. Since a syringe rather than a motorized pump is used to create a vacuum, electricity is not needed.

No dilation (stretching of the cervical opening) is needed to insert a small (four to five millimeters) flexible plastic cannula into the uterus. Local anesthetic is rarely used, because there is no dilation

---

*First-trimester aspiration abortions can be done by trained practioners as easily and safely as by doctors. Unfortunately this is illegal in most states. In Vermont, women trained as physician assistants have performed one-third of the abortions for years, with an excellent safety record. However, antiabortion politicians have been trying to change Vermont laws to restrict the performance of abortions to MDs only. This would make abortions harder and more expensive to obtain, prevent women from turning to other skilled women for abortions and reinforce the power of doctors.

Cannulas
6-, 8-, 12-mm diameters

Robbie Pfeufer

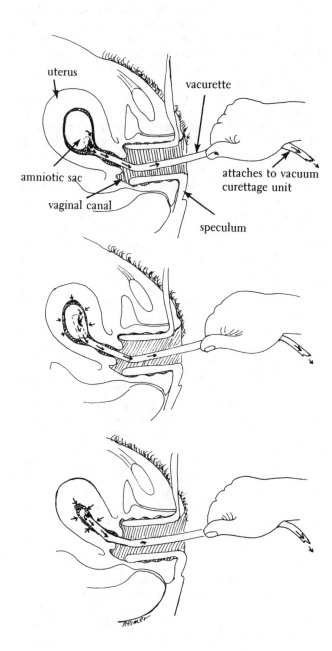

Vacuum suction abortion.　　Nina Reimer

and the procedure only take a few minutes. The same complications can occur as with an aspiration abortion performed a few weeks later, after pregnancy is confirmed. However, because only flexible instruments are used, there is less risk of perforating the uterus, and problems that might result from dilating the cervix are avoided. But there is slightly more chance that the practitioner may miss aborting the pregnancy, if there is one, since the fetal tissue is so minimal.

Some women want to remove a pregnancy as soon as possible or prefer not to know whether they actually are pregnant. However, having an abortion before you know for sure that you are pregnant does not necessarily mean that you won't have any feelings about pregnancy and abortion to deal with. One drawback is that you may indeed not be pregnant; there are many reasons for a period to be late, including anxiety about being pregnant! (If blood tests for very early pregnancy are available in your area, you can avoid an unnecessary procedure by confirming your pregnancy in this way.) Also, tests for the Rh blood type are not usually part of preemptive abortions and Rh-negative women are not usually offered Rhogam (see p. 363).

2. Abortions by *early uterine evacuation (EUE)*, done when a pelvic exam confirms pregnancy, use a technique similar to number 1, except that a five- to six-millimeter flexible cannula is used. Population control projects have exported this technique to many Third World countries because it is easy to train laypersons to do it and it does not require a motorized suction pump or much equipment.

3. During a *vacuum aspiration abortion*, the cervical opening is stretched (dilated) so that a larger cannula can be used. An electrically powered aspirator is the source of suction.

There are several variations of this method. For over a decade women have been working to create the safest, least physically traumatic vacuum aspiration techniques. A number of woman-owned and -controlled feminist health centers have trained practitioners to use minimal dilation and small flexible cannulas, which reduce the chance of tearing or perforating the uterus or cervix. (An eight-millimeter cannula can be used for abortions through eleven to twelve weeks LMP.) *Curettage*, or scraping the inside of the uterus with a metal loop called a *curette*, is not routinely necessary. Experiences at these clinics and others show that this approach is more comfortable for women than that of most conventionally trained abortionists, who use larger, rigid plastic or metal cannulas (which require more dilation) and a curette after the suction.*

---

*Doctors are trained to consider new information about medical procedures only if it comes from so-called medical authorities. They are not trained in give and take or in learning from health workers "below" them in the medical hierarchy or from women on whom they do the procedures.

4. *Dilation (dilatation) and curettage (D and C)* is a standard gynecological procedure used to treat conditions such as excessively heavy bleeding and to diagnose various uterine problems. It is usually done in a hospital under general anesthesia. Because medical students routinely learn D and C, this used to be the most common method for first-trimester abortions. Now it has been virtually replaced by the quicker, easier and safer aspiration techniques, which are usually done in clinics with local or no anesthesia. Some doctors will do a D and C for abortions from twelve to sixteen weeks.

5. *Dilation (dilatation) and evacuation (D and E)* is a newer method that combines D and C and vacuum aspiration techniques for abortions later than twelve weeks LMP. Because the fetal tissue is larger and the uterus is softer and easier to injure than in the first trimester, a D and E is more complicated and requires a high level of skill on the part of the person performing the abortion. An ultrasound examination (sonogram) may be required beforehand.

MENSTRUAL EXTRACTION

In the early 1970s self-help groups at the Feminist Women's Health Center in Los Angeles and elsewhere developed a technique using a small flexible plastic cannula to remove the lining of the uterus at about the time that the menstrual period is due. Women practiced on each other in order to develop safe instruments and techniques. Menstrual extraction is done on an experimental research basis by women in advanced self-help groups; it cannot be obtained at a medical facility. Menstrual extraction helps women avoid the discomfort of a menstrual period, provides information about menstruation and enables women to learn basic health care skills. A very early pregnancy, if present, would probably be removed along with the lining of the uterus. We need to do more research before we can know whether frequent extraction of the uterine lining creates any long-term or delayed health problems, although there is no evidence of any so far. Several aspects of the techniques developed for menstrual extraction have been incorporated into medical practice for early abortion with flexible cannulas. Menstrual extraction is a powerful example of medical research done by women on and for ourselves.

The cervix needs to be dilated more than with an earlier abortion so that larger instruments can be put into the uterus to remove the pregnancy. Often dilation is begun by placing one or more laminaria sticks into the cervical opening the day before the D and E. (This extra visit may be inconvenient for some women and difficult or even impossible for others.) Laminaria is a sterilized seaweed that absorbs moisture and expands, gradually stretching the cervix. Dilation taking place this way over a number of hours is probably safer and more comfortable than dilation done all at once at the time of the abortion, especially with later pregnancies. Some women feel pressure or cramping with laminaria in place. There is a small risk of infection, and occasionally laminaria itself starts to bring on a miscarriage.

The laminaria is removed at the time of the abortion. Dilators are used to enlarge the cervical opening further, if necessary. Then the doctor uses forceps, a curette and vacuum suction to loosen and remove the uterine lining, placental and fetal tissue. A drug (oxytocin) may be given to help the uterus contract, slowing down the bleeding that normally occurs.

6. In an *induction abortion*, the doctor injects (instills) an abortion-causing solution through the abdomen into the amniotic sac, which surrounds the fetus. (Before sixteen weeks LMP this sac is not large enough to be located accurately, so the induction procedure cannot be used until this time.) Hours later, contractions cause the cervix to dilate and the fetus and placenta to be expelled. A D and C is often performed after the abortion to remove any remaining tissue and to give doctors in training (residents) more chance to learn. A hospital stay of twelve to forty-eight hours is involved, which is expensive.

The first commonly used solution was hypertonic saline (salt) solution. In recent years use of prostaglandins has become widespread, as well as combinations of saline, prostaglandins, urea and/or other ingredients. For details and a comparison between saline and prostaglandin abortions, see p. 367. Induction abortions are often called *saline* or *prostaglandin abortions*, according to the abortion-causing solution used.

7. *Prostaglandin suppositories* placed in the vagina sometimes cause strong uterine contractions resulting in miscarriage. This is the newest, least-known abortion method. Many hospitals use prostaglandin suppositories only when a fetus has died and the woman isn't going into labor to expel it from her body. Nausea, vomiting, diarrhea, fever and failure to cause abortion are common problems.

8. In a *hysterotomy* the surgeon removes the fetus and placenta through an incision into the abdomen and uterus, like a small Cesarean section. The incidence of serious complications for this kind of major surgery is considerably higher than for other methods of abortion. You may need a hysterotomy when induction methods have been repeatedly unsuccessful or can't be used for medical reasons.

RISKS AND COMPLICATIONS

As with any medical procedure, there are possible risks and complications. The chance of a complication for a first-trimester abortion is about 1 percent. The later the abortion, the more chance of complications. Signs of a complication will generally appear within a few days after the abortion. Listed below are possible risks and complications of aspiration abortions, their symptoms and treatments. (See p. 367 for additional risks and complications of induction abortions.)

Infection

Infection is one of the more common complications. Even though sterile instruments and antiseptic are used, bacteria sometimes travel into the uterus. Signs of an infection are fever of 100.5 degrees Fahrenheit or higher, bad cramping and/or vaginal discharge with a foul odor. Treatment consists of antibiotics, usually tetracycline or ampicillin. It is important to have an exam after finishing the medication to make sure the infection is gone and there is no sign of retained tissue. Left untreated, an infection can cause serious illness, sterility or even death.

Retained Tissue

Since the practitioner can't actually see inside the uterus during the abortion, occasionally s/he leaves some tissue behind. Signs of retained tissue include very heavy bleeding, passage of large blood clots, strong cramps, bleeding for longer than three weeks or signs of pregnancy (for instance, sore breasts, nausea, tiredness) lasting more than a week. Tissue remaining inside the uterus is likely to become infected. Sometimes drugs (Methergine or Ergotrate) are given to stimulate the uterus to contract and push out the retained tissue. The other treatment is removing the tissue by an aspiration procedure similar to an aspiration abortion, but shorter or occasionally a D and C.

Perforation

Perforation of the uterus occurs if an instrument goes through its wall. There is more risk of perforation in a D and E than in a first-trimester abor-

tion. If a woman is awake, she is likely to feel a sharp pain or cramp. If perforation occurs, the medical staff will monitor pulse, blood pressure, cramping and bleeding very closely. The uterus is a very strong muscle and often heals quickly on its own. However, if there are any indications that a large blood vessel or another organ may have been injured, you will need hospitalization and possibly surgery. If the abortion has not been completed when the perforation occurs, it is usually finished in a hospital.

Hemorrhage

Uterine hemorrhage (excessive bleeding) during or after an abortion is more likely to occur in second-trimester abortions. Excessive bleeding can sometimes be a sign of retained tissue, perforation or failure of the uterus to contract. Drugs may be given to stimulate the contractions of the uterus, or an aspiration procedure may be done to slow down the bleeding. Check before you leave the clinic and inform the recovery room staff of the amount of bleeding.

Cervical Laceration (Tear)

There is more chance of the cervix being injured during a second-trimester abortion than an earlier abortion. A woman may not feel a tear when it happens, but the practitioner should inform her and record it in her medical record. A small tear heals without treatment. A more serious tear may require stitches, and there may be some bleeding from the tear.

Missed Abortion—Continued Pregnancy

In very rare instances, some tissue is removed and yet the woman remains pregnant. This is more likely early in pregnancy (less than four weeks after conception, six weeks LMP). All clinics should inspect the tissue removed from the uterus right after the abortion to be sure that all the pregnancy tissue has been removed. In cases of a multiple pregnancy, sometimes one pregnancy is removed but another remains (either in the same uterus, or, more rarely, in a double uterus). If this happens, signs of pregnancy are likely to continue. The abortion will have to be repeated in a week or so.

Postabortal Syndrome (Blood in the Uterus)

If the uterus doesn't contract properly or if a blood clot blocks the cervical opening and prevents blood from leaving the uterus, blood collects within it. As blood accumulates, pain, cramping and sometimes nausea increase. Sometimes you can push the clots out by deep massage directly over the uterus (pressing hard with your fingers just above the pubic bone). If this doesn't work, the clots need to be removed by reaspirating the uterus.

Possible Effect on Future Pregnancies

Having an abortion does not decrease the chances of having a healthy baby in the future. There is some indication that having several abortions may slightly increase chances of miscarriage or premature birth, but enough good research on this issue has not been done. (Dilating the cervix should be done as little and as gently as possible in order to minimize the chances of weakening it.)

ANESTHESIA

If you are going to have an abortion by a suction method, you may have the choice of using anesthesia (pain-reducing drugs). If you understand what your options are and how they may affect you, you can decide which type of anesthesia you prefer, or decide not to have any at all.

There are two basic types of anesthesia: *local*, which affects only the cervix, and *general*, which makes you unconscious ("asleep"). There is also a newer method that combines a local anesthetic with drugs that cause partial loss of consciousness. This is called *augment*.

Local anesthesia is injected into the cervix (neck of the uterus). It relaxes the cervical muscle, easing cramps that may occur when instruments such as dilators are passed through the cervix. Cramps caused by contractions of the uterus as it is emptied are not lessened by this method, however.

General anesthesia is usually given intravenously (injected into a vein in the arm). It causes unconsciousness; you won't see what's happening or feel pain but you may well hear what is being said. Augment anesthesia, such as narcotics or tranquilizers, is also given intravenously.

Any anesthetic drug has risks and complications, in addition to the risks of the abortion. With a local you may briefly experience ringing in your ears, tingling in your hands or feet or lightheadedness. Seizures or serious allergic reactions are rare. If you have general anesthesia you may feel groggy, nauseated and disoriented after you wake up; some people do not feel well even a couple of days later. You may wake up with cramps.* Rarely, a serious reaction may damage the liver or other organs. In addition, general anesthesia

*These cramps may not be different from cramping after an abortion with local or no anesthesia, but it can be much harder to deal with them when you are waking up mentally affected by the anesthetic drugs.

increases some of the risks of the abortion itself. For example, there is more bleeding because the uterine muscle is more relaxed. There is also a greater chance of a serious perforation because doctors, unfortunately, have been known to be less gentle with the instruments if the woman is asleep and cannot complain about unusual pain. The risks, negative effects and recovery from augment vary with the particular drugs used, but generally last several hours or less.

For a first-trimester abortion, general or augment anesthesia is not medically necessary. For a second-trimester D and E, which takes longer and may be more uncomfortable, these strong drugs are more commonly used. Some women, for their own reasons, choose not to be awake. Most women find the cramps quite bearable with a local or no anesthetic.

I felt real good about my decision not to be put to sleep for my abortion. I found out that I have the strength to face my fear of pain. My cramps were bad for a few minutes, but I concentrated on deep breathing and held my counselor's hand. Ten minutes later I felt fine and ready to go home.

With general or augment anesthesia you have little control over the abortion experience because you will most likely not be aware of what occurs during the procedure. Sometimes doctors or nurses will express hostility during those emotionally vulnerable minutes just before the drugs take effect and as they are wearing off.

During my last abortion . . . I was put to sleep. . . . I couldn't deal with being awake. . . . Before I went under, the doctor said to me, "This is your third abortion, isn't it? What birth control are you using?"

Unfortunately, it is hard to get evidence of how frequently this kind of emotional abuse occurs. Women are often either unconscious or partially conscious when it occurs, and any witnesses are medical personnel who find this kind of behavior acceptable or who will not risk their jobs and professional status by telling on other professionals.

Each woman's abortion experience is a unique one, within a known range of possibilities. No one can predict whether you will find the cramping painful or mild, or what the effects of anesthesia will be for you. Try to find out what drugs are used in the facility you go to. Information about drug effects and risks should be a part of your preparation for an abortion and will help you make the best choices if decisions are left up to you. Some facilities have a set way of doing things, and they may or may not respond to your requests.

Sometimes abortion facilities have their own reasons for using general or augment anesthesia for first-trimester abortions. A nurse-counselor at one abortion facility said:

Black and Hispanic women are all screamers. We try to give them general anesthesia so that they don't upset the other patients or the staff. Teenagers and Medicaid patients also should have a general.*

There can also be financial motives for encouraging women to accept general anesthesia. With the woman unconscious there is no need to be reassuring or gentle during the procedure, and the doctor can work faster, performing more abortions and making more money.

ABORTION FACILITIES

This section refers to legal abortions, although with the current political situation our right to legal abortions is in serious danger. How much choice you have about where your abortion takes place depends on where you live, how much money you have or what your insurance will cover, how old you are, how far along you are in your pregnancy and which referral sources are available to you.

Agencies That Can Help You Get an Abortion

Since abortion was legalized there have been a variety of responsible sources of information about where to get an abortion. However, because of a 1990 U.S. Supreme Court decision (Rust vs. Sullivan), some changes may occur. The Court upheld the gag rule prohibiting physicians and counselors who receive federal funds under Title X from providing information on and making referrals for abortion. This decision affects family planning and Planned Parenthood clinics. Although many clinics have not decided how to handle this situation, most will probably refuse the funds because of their commitment to providing full and accurate information and care to women. Congress has voted to overturn the gag rule, but President Bush has promised to veto the legislation, and it is not clear that there are enough votes to override his veto.

Some antiabortion groups masquerade as referral agencies and try to "persuade" women not to have abortions. These are often listed as "problem" or "crisis" pregnancy centers. If the gag rule

---

*This is an example of racist stereotyping as well as value judgment by a woman whose culture approves of quiet and forbids loud noises to express emotions. Why should all women of a certain race, culture, economic status or age automatically be subjected to the health risks of general anesthesia, while middle-class white women are given the choice of a local anesthetic?

stands, there will be more of these. If you're not getting the information you want, feel free to leave or hang up the phone. If you can, take someone you trust with you.

For reliable information, contact: abortion providers (may be listed in the yellow pages), gynecology clinics at non-Catholic hospitals, neighborhood health centers, family-planning clinics, women's centers and feminist health centers (listed in phone books, local newspapers and college campus directories). Planned Parenthood has offices in almost every state, providing referrals and, in some areas, operating abortion clinics. You can also get information from the National Abortion Federation Hotline, (800) 772-9100; the National Women's Health Network, (202) 347-1140 or the other national organizations listed in the Resources. They also have information about Medicaid funding and funds for low-income women seeking abortions.

What to Look for in Choosing a Facility

Most first-trimester abortions are done in free-standing clinics that are not part of hospitals. Abortions are also done in doctors' offices, hospital outpatient clinics, and in hospitals, sometimes with an overnight stay. *A hospital setting is not necessary for first-trimester abortions except when certain serious health conditions require hospital emergency facilities to be immediately available.* Second-trimester D and E abortions can also be performed safely in a properly equipped clinic or doctor's office. However, they are less available and you may have to travel to get one.

Legalization has meant safe facilities, but how we feel after an abortion can also be influenced by the quality of counseling and the treatment by the staff, which vary with the motivations of those who run or own a facility and with abortion politics. Antiabortion propaganda is pervasive in our society. Messages that abortion is wrong, that women who have abortions are selfish or irresponsible about sex and birth control, that abortion is murder and that abortion is an emotionally traumatic experience have created a climate in which abortion is cloaked in guilt, shame and fear. Even many supporters of abortion rights often portray abortion as a necessary evil. Unfortunately, some counselors and medical staff at clinics express these views. Unsupportive, insensitive treatment by clinic staff is especially problematic and can make an abortion unpleasant or worse. You are entitled to be treated with respect. A staff member at a feminist clinic says how it should and can be:

At our clinic counselors are trained to help each woman sort out her feelings. We do not invade any-

one's privacy if she tells us that her decision is clear, not coerced, and that she does not want to discuss her reasons or feelings. Women talk with each other, not just with the counselor. We provide very detailed and accurate information about the abortion procedure, A woman can have a friend stay with her during the abortion. When there is a decision to be made, the woman herself is an active participant.

I wish women could walk into any medical facility feeling that we deserve to be treated with respect and demanding it when it isn't there. We should stop feeling grateful every time we are not overtly abused.

Racial and cultural barriers also shape our experience.

Just because they give you a white woman to talk to don't mean you got counseled. She was nice; she gave me good information. I'm explaining to her how I feel about this whole thing. She tells me that she thinks that I'm not ready to have an abortion and she's going to send me home. Well, I hit the roof! "You're going to send me home? Do you know how hard it is to get here?" She didn't understand what I was saying to her. I was saying, "Yeah, if I had a baby I could deal with it. I have to deal with anything that comes up. This is how my life has been, how my mother's life, all the people I knows life has been. You deal with whatever shit happens. But if I had a choice, I would prefer not to have this baby. And since I do have this choice, this is what I want to do." . . .

. . . I think that a lot of the problem was she was white and I was black. She didn't understand what it meant to me, a black woman, and I guess to black women, period, to have a baby.

An African-American counselor says,

I am the only woman of color working at the clinic. It is important for me to be there for women of color who come to have abortions, otherwise all they see are white faces. I became a counselor because I knew I could make a difference—I wanted to help all women.

WHAT YOU NEED TO KNOW

Whether you have to search to find one abortion service or you can choose among several facilities, ask questions beforehand. Not only must you get an idea of what to expect, but you can also prepare yourself to negotiate for options that may not be part of the standard procedures.

1. Cost? Must the fee be paid all at once? Will Medicaid or health insurance cover any of it? Is everything included or may there be additional charges (for example, for a Pap smear or for Rhogam)?

2. Are there age requirements or special consent requirements? Do I have to tell my parents or husband, get their consent and/or bring proof of age?

3. How long should I expect to be at the facility? Will everything be done in one visit?

4. Will child care be provided for my child(ren)?

5. What do I need to bring with me?

6. Is there anything in my medical history that would interfere with my getting an abortion at that facility?

7. Can I bring someone else with me? Can s/he stay with me throughout the counseling and the abortion procedure if that's what I want?

8. Will there be a counselor or nurse with me to provide information and support before, during and after the abortion?

9. Will there be staff people who speak my native language? If not, will the facility provide an interpreter?

10. Can the facility accommodate any special needs I have (for example, wheelchair accessibility)?

11. What type of abortion procedure will be done?

12. What anesthesia and other medications are available? What choices do I have?

13. Will the facility be responsible for routine follow-up? For treating complications? What type of backup services are available in case of emergency?

14. Will a breast exam, Pap smear and gonorrhea culture be done?

15. Will birth control be available if I want it?

16. Are abortions performed if women are HIV positive?

17. Could there be antiabortionists picketing or blocking me from entering the clinic? If so, what arrangements are there to deal with this?

Ask about *anything* that concerns you. Often the way the staff answers questions indicates their attitude toward women coming for abortions. Trust your feelings about the way you are treated on the phone as well as in person.

The antiabortion movement has made abortion and family planning clinics, their clients and personnel targets for harassment and violence. It is not uncommon for there to be antiabortionists demonstrating outside clinics or trying to prevent you from entering. When making your appointment, ask about protesters and what procedures the clinic has for handling them. Many have escorts who will meet you outside and accompany you for your appointment. Some clinics have alternate entrances to avoid protesters. Often there will be abortion rights advocates at the clinic to support and protect women going to the clinic.

Many women feel upset and angry at having to deal with protesters at clinics. Some want to confront them, others prefer to avoid or ignore them. We believe that antichoice protests at abortion clinics constitute harassment—no one but you has the right to decide whether you will have an abortion. No one has the right to try and interfere with that decision.

TO ANTIABORTIONISTS

Do you know me.
Have we met.

Surely you must know me
because here you are today.

Today you seek to help me make a decision
reserved for myself—and a personal few.

Today you tell me I am wrong and
you seek to decide my fate.

Surely you must know me.

Were you there as I struggled to raise my children
Perhaps I missed you along the way.

Do you know the doors closed in my face
I have forced open

Although your face is not known to me
Surely you must know me.

YOU SAY WE'VE NEVER MET!

How then do you dare with a smug indignant
*   face*
intrude on my personal choice.

How dare you lay your body
in my path.

I will walk over you
I will crawl under you

My choice will be mine, because now—
*   it's quite clear—YOU DON'T KNOW ME AT*
*   ALL!*

HELEN R. CAULTON

HAVING A VACUUM ASPIRATION ABORTION

The large majority of abortions currently done in the United States are first-trimester vacuum aspiration procedures in an outpatient clinic. Clinics vary a great deal, and your experience may be very different from another woman's, even at the same clinic.

Medical Preliminaries

After arriving at the clinic, you will fill out a medical history form. A health worker will draw blood to check for the Rh factor* and for anemia, do another pregnancy test and check your pulse, blood pressure and temperature (vital signs).

Counseling

Most clinics provide individual and/or group counseling. The counselor explains the abortion procedure and what to expect afterward. She may also talk about birth control options. The counseling session is a time for you to ask questions and express any fears or concerns, especially about the pregnancy or the abortion. Being in a group provides an opportunity to talk with other women who are having abortions. Discussing your experiences together can help you feel clearer, stronger and less alone.

The two rooms where the abortions were done opened onto the porch where the six of us were waiting. One girl from the group, who had said she never had a pelvic examination in her life, was just coming out of the abortion room. She had just had her abortion and looked okay. That was comforting. A seventeen-year-old girl came in. She was very scared. I held her hand and comforted her. I hadn't had my abortion yet and was scared, too (although I'd had one operation, two children and a D and C with a spinal). Something amazing happened when I held her hand. Any fear I'd had disappeared as if it were drawn out of me. We were all such different women who for varying reasons were having the identical physical thing done to us.

*Blood is either Rh positive or Rh negative. When an Rh-negative woman carries an Rh-positive fetus, antibodies against the Rh factor can build up in her blood. The most likely time for this to happen is at the end of the pregnancy, whether by abortion, miscarriage or birth. In a later pregnancy these antibodies can react against an Rh-positive fetus, causing serious harm and even endangering its survival. An injection of a blood derivative (one brand name is Rhogam) within seventy-two hours after the end of every pregnancy usually prevents antibody formation. If you need Rhogam, it should be given before you leave the clinic.

Lynn Vera

The Abortion

The counselor will take you to the exam room after you go to the bathroom. Before the abortion itself, the practitioner performs a bimanual exam to feel the size and position of your uterus, confirming the stage of pregnancy. S/he needs this information to decide how large a cannula to use and the angle at which to insert instruments safely. If you've never had a pelvic exam, tell your counselor. Whether this is your first exam or you have had others, make sure that the practitioner goes slowly, is gentle, explains what is happening and allows you to have some control over the procedure.

Next, the practitioner inserts a speculum into your vagina, separating the vaginal walls to see the cervix. You may feel pressure, but this should not hurt. Have the practitioner readjust the speculum if it pinches. A chlamydia and gonorrhea culture may be taken, and a Pap smear if you haven't had one recently.

The practitioner thoroughly wipes your vagina with antiseptic solution to help prevent infection. If you are having a local anesthetic, it is injected into the cervix. Since the cervix has very few nerve endings, you may not feel this at all, or it may feel like a pinch or pressure. Next, a tenaculum is attached to the cervix to keep the cervix steady. You may feel a pinch, cramp or nothing at all. Some practitioners then measure the inside of the uterus with a thin rod called a *sound*; others believe that this is not necessary. Sounding may cause a short cramp. The cervical opening is gradually stretched by inserting and removing dilators of increasingly larger sizes. You will probably feel some kind of cramping, perhaps similar to mild

or stronger menstrual cramps. Two to eight dilators may be used. Dilating usually takes less than two minutes.

A sterile strawlike tube is inserted through the cervix into the uterus. Cannulas are made in different diameters, from the size of a small drinking straw to the size of a large pen (five to twelve millimeters). The later the pregnancy, the larger the cannula needed to remove it. Tubing connects the cannula to a bottle. The *aspirator*, a motorized suction machine, creates a vacuum in the bottle. As the cannula is moved along the uterine walls, gentle suction draws pregnancy tissue out through the cannula and tubing into the bottle. The aspiration usually takes no more than a few minutes, depending on how many weeks pregnant you are.

Forceps may also be used to remove tissue. Some practitioners insert a curette and scrape the inside of the uterus to check that it is completely empty. Others think that this additional step is unnecessary. It causes extra bleeding, increases the risk of perforation, lengthens the abortion and causes discomfort or pain.

As the uterus is emptied, it starts to contract to its nonpregnant size. These contractions can range from hardly noticeable to painful cramps—each woman is different. Breathing deeply and in a regular pattern, especially with the help of a counselor or friend, can help you to relax your body, "riding through" the cramps. It is also important to keep your stomach muscles as relaxed as possible and not to move around. Cramps should

1	2	3	4	5	6	7	8	9	10

1: speculum   6 and 7: flexible plastic cannulas
2: tenaculum   8: rigid plastic cannula
3: sound   9: curette
4 and 5: dilators   10: forceps   Lynn Vera

lessen immediately after the cannula is removed or within the next ten minutes or so.

After the Abortion

After wiping out your vagina and checking for bleeding, the practitioner will remove the speculum. Then you can move into a more comfortable room to sit or lie down for a while. You may feel weak, tired, crampy or nauseous for a while, or you may be ready to get up immediately. Before you leave, a counselor should explain aftercare instructions (what to expect and watch for). Your vital signs, cramping and bleeding should be checked before you leave.

The abortion itself was very uncomfortable, like having an IUD put in but more intense. It didn't last long and the doctor was good.

I received no counseling of any kind from the doctor. There was, however, a beautiful, middle-aged nurse there who explained the whole procedure carefully and stayed with me. I especially appreciated her because while I was not particularly frightened of the abortion itself, I was, and still am, terrified of doctors and hospitals.

The abortion itself was amazingly quick and painless (considering the propaganda to the contrary). I spent an hour lying down to recover. I remember being elated—it was over and it had been so simple!

It hurt so much. It was incredible. The people at the clinic were really sweet and helpful but they should have told me how much it was going to hurt. What hurt the most was that I could feel when they were scraping around inside. I've talked to a lot of girls who said the same thing happened to them when they were really far along. That's why it pays to have an abortion as early as possible.

I experienced some pain with the procedure but mostly it was just a series of new sensations. I had never been so aware of my uterus.

When I found out I was pregnant I was numb, unfeeling. This scared and confused me. I had never blocked my feelings so totally or unconsciously before. I wonder now if that's why the abortion itself was so physically painful.

SECOND-TRIMESTER ABORTIONS

Very often, women choose second-trimester abortions because they were unable to get the money together in time to have first-trimester abortions. Ironically, a later abortion is an additional financial drain: It costs more, requires more time off from work and may involve extra expenses for travel to an appropriate facility. Other reasons for second-trimester abortions may include errors in pregnancy detection: false-negative pregnancy tests or inaccurate uterine sizing by medical practitioners. Women who were pregnant when they started taking birth control pills or who were not told that it is possible to get pregnant with an IUD in place sometimes do not even suspect pregnancy for several months. Some states now require women under eighteen to get parental consent or a court order, which can result in delays of weeks or even months. Occasionally a woman (especially a teenager) may not admit the possibility of pregnancy. Because she lacks support, money or information, she may feel afraid, overwhelmed and unprepared to deal with pregnancy, so she denies it, hoping it will somehow go away on its own. Given these all-too-common situations, a woman may come to the experience of a later abortion already emotionally exhausted.

A large percentage of women who are forced to seek second-trimester abortions are young, poor or women of color. They bear the brunt of attitudes that "blame the victim." A woman may be treated as though she is stupid and/or irresponsible and deserves to be "punished" by an unsupportive atmosphere and a painful experience.

Most doctors and hospitals choose not to perform second-trimester abortions. Someone from Planned Parenthood told us, "Many doctors wish the problem would go away." In February 1975, a Boston jury convicted Dr. Kenneth Edelin of manslaughter for performing a routine hysterotomy on a woman whose pregnancy was between twenty and twenty-eight weeks LMP. Though the Boston jury's decision was reversed in a higher court and Dr. Edelin was acquitted of the charge, hospitals around the country (never enthusiastic about late abortions in the first place) have reacted by closing down their second-trimester abortion services or by bringing in costly equipment to try to keep alive fetuses that show signs of life when expelled (costs to be passed on to the woman).

The Advantages of the D and E Procedure

The D and E has several advantages over the induced-miscarriage procedures more commonly used for abortions in the second three months of pregnancy. Not only is the D and E safer, but it is physically and emotionally easier for a woman than an induction abortion, where she goes through labor and delivery of a fetus, often while in a hospital room by herself. D and E is much quicker (ten to forty-five minutes, compared to many hours with an overnight stay in a hospital for induction abortion), and complications are less likely, although more studies are needed. D and E can be done in a properly equipped doctor's office or clinic with local anesthetic and perhaps also a tranquilizer, although most are still done in hospitals using general anesthesia. A few doctors are doing the D and E procedures through twenty-four weeks LMP with good results, although a limit of sixteen, eighteen or twenty weeks is more common.

The biggest problem with D and E, however, is that it is not widely available. There are not enough people yet trained to do D and E procedures, especially in the eighteen- to twenty-four-week LMP range. Many doctors dislike the idea of removing a second-trimester fetus by performing a D and E. They would rather provide induction abortions, which do not require their presence after the injection. (The woman and the nursing staff are left to deal with the aborted fetus.) Unfortunately, not enough doctors are willing to accept the personal strain of doing D and E's. We need more doctors who place greater priority on the fact that *a D and E is both safer and less upsetting for women.*

In some places a D and E costs more than an induction abortion. Or a D and E may be available to women who can afford private gynecologists or to women who can afford to travel to another state but not to women who must get their medical care from local government-funded clinics and teaching hospitals. This kind of unconscionable discrimination means that women who have less money are forced to accept an induction procedure, which involves more pain, more time and more chance of health complications.

Having a Second-Trimester Instillation Abortion

Choosing a Facility

Having an induction abortion from sixteen to twenty-four weeks of pregnancy is a more difficult experience than a first-trimester abortion or a second-trimester D and E abortion. There may be hours of uncomfortable labor as the uterus contracts to open the cervix and expel the fetus. The complication and mortality rates, though no higher than for full-term pregnancy and delivery, are higher than for earlier abortions or D and E by a skilled doctor. Emotionally, too, it can be a hard experience, even when you are very sure you do not want to have a baby. The pain and/or discomfort, the length of time, the similarity of the experience to delivery of a baby, an intimidating or unsupportive hospital atmosphere and the influence of a very vocal part of society that says that later abortions are "bad"—these factors can make induction abortion upsetting.

EFFECTIVENESS AND COMPLICATIONS OF ABORTIONS PERFORMED AT THIRTEEN WEEKS' GESTATION BY D AND E, SALINE AND PROSTAGLANDIN F_2a*

Outcomes	Intraamniotic Instillation		
	D and E	Saline	PGF₂a†
Effectiveness			
Success rate	99.90%	97.60%	92.50%
Induction-abortion time (hours)	0.50	29.20	24.80
Specific complication‡			
Incomplete abortion	9.90	28.27	36.10
Hemorrhage	0.71	1.86	5.80
Transfusion	0.19	0.96	1.53
Cervical laceration or fistula	1.16	0.55	0.64
Convulsions	0.02	0.08	0.32
Uterine perforation	0.32	0.05	0.16
Any complication	5.83	37.45	53.26

This table appears in Robert A. Hatcher et al., *Contraceptive Technology*, New York: Irvington Publications, 1982, p. 178.

*Source: W. Cates, D. A. Grimes, K. Schulz, H.W. Ory and C.W. Tyler, "World Health Organization Studies of prostaglandin versus saline as abortifacients," *Obstet Gynecol* 52.493, October 1978.

†Data derived from the Joint Program for the Study of Abortion under the auspices of the Centers for Disease Control.

‡Complications per 100 procedures.

ABORTION, AMNIOCENTESIS AND DISABILTY

We believe that the availability of amniocentesis (see p. 430) with the option for abortion if serious genetic defects are found should not conflict with our commitment to build a better world for people with disabilities. The disability rights movement has pointed out the danger in equating the presence of a genetic defect with the notion of a life not worth living. A woman should have the right to bear a child with a disability and not be punished by lack of support for that choice. All of us can reach out and create networks of information so that a woman confronting the diagnosis of Down's syndrome or any other serious disability in her fetus can meet other parents and children living with these conditions, and learn realistically about the quality, cost and availability of the services that make such lives better.

Pay attention to both emotional and physical needs when choosing a facility. (Unfortunately, it may be difficult to find *any* medical facility near you where second-trimester abortions are performed.) Doctors usually do induction abortions in general hospitals where the quality of care and degree of personal attention vary greatly. A few small hospitals and clinics specializing in abortion try to make late abortion as comfortable as possible. Some hospitals have a separate second-trimester abortion unit with counseling and special staff. They avoid insensitive treatment such as placing abortion patients in rooms with women who are having babies. In any hospital you may be left alone a lot, not told clearly what is being done to you, not offered enough pain medication (if you want it). Unfortunately, if you do not have the time and money to travel for an abortion, you may have to accept whatever kind of care you can find. Talk with the doctor beforehand, as well as the hospital, about the type of care you want to receive. Try to bring a friend who can give you support and help see that your needs are respected and responded to.

A Comparison of Saline and Prostaglandin Abortions

In an induction abortion the practitioner injects a miscarriage-causing solution through the abdomen into the amniotic sac and uterine contractions expel the fetus. The two most commonly used solutions are a saline (salt) solution, which usually causes fetal death followed by uterine contractions, or the prostaglandin F_2a, which causes labor contractions. Sometimes urea or saline is added to a prostaglandin solution. In some hospitals you will have a choice of methods if you are firm about requesting it. Also, refer back to the table of complications on p. 355.

Saline solution has a lower complication rate, a lower rate of incomplete abortion and consequent D and C and a lower chance of having to repeat the injection. The disadvantages of saline include a longer wait before labor begins and a slight risk of serious emergency, such as shock, and possibly death if careless instillation allows salt to enter a blood vessel. Liver or kidney problems, heart failure, high blood pressure and sickle cell anemia are medical reasons not to have a saline abortion.

The prostaglandin F_2a works more quickly and does not have the same risk of serious emergency carried by saline. However, it has more negative effects, including nausea, vomiting and diarrhea; a higher rate of failure of the first instillation and a higher rate of excessive bleeding and retained placenta (requiring immediate D and C). The labor contractions are usually faster, sharper and more painful, and there is a risk of the cervix tearing.

(Use of laminaria to stretch the cervix before contractions begin may reduce this risk.) In very rare cases the fetus is expelled with signs of life and does not expire until shortly afterward. Medical reasons to avoid prostaglandin are a history of convulsions, epilepsy and asthma.

Preliminaries

Read the box (p. 362) for suggestions of questions to ask when you set up an appointment. Plan to be at the hospital overnight. If you are having an out-of-town abortion, make sure before you go that you have the name and phone number of a doctor or clinic at home to call in case of questions or complications after the abortion.

The same tests and examinations are necessary as for suction abortion. In taking your medical history, the medical staff should check for conditions that would contraindicate use of saline or prostaglandin methods. If you are going to have a prostaglandin abortion, the hospital may ask you to come in the day before for insertion of laminaria.

The Procedure

Instillation

The doctor cleans your abdomen, numbs a small area below your navel with a local anesthetic and then inserts a needle through the skin into your uterus. This may sound scary, but you will probably feel only a slight cramp when the needle enters your uterus. For saline, some amniotic fluid is removed. The miscarriage-inducing solution is slowly injected into the amniotic sac. You may experience pressure or a bloated feeling. If you are having saline and feel waves of heat, dizziness, backache, extreme dryness or thirst, tell the doctor right away; this may indicate that the salt is entering a blood vessel, which is dangerous.

Waiting

It will take hours before the labor contractions begin, from eight to twenty-four or more with saline and less with prostaglandin. Medication can relieve nausea and diarrhea caused by prostaglandin. If labor contractions don't begin within the expected time, oxytocin may be given to stimulate contractions. This carries a risk of rupture of the uterus if contractions are too strong. Sometimes the instillation is done a second time.

Contractions

At first contractions will probably feel like mild cramps. Later you may feel a lot of pressure in the rectal area and then a gushing of liquid from the vagina—this is the breaking of the amniotic sac (bag of waters). Each woman's labor is different in terms of how long it takes and how it feels.

When prostaglandin or oxytocin is used, contractions are quicker and sharper than with saline.

As a rule the contractions are not as strong as those of full-term labor and delivery, but they can be painful. Relaxation, deep breathing or panting can help make the later contractions easier to tolerate. Sitting or squatting may be the most comfortable, though hospital staff may want you to lie down. Support and comfort from a friend can help, too. No general anesthesia is given, but tranquilizers and pain medication should be offered if they won't slow down the labor.

Expulsion

Eventually the contractions will expel the fetus and, within an hour, the placenta.

Recovery

You will probably stay in the hospital for some hours after the abortion. If all of the placenta was not expelled, you may need an aspiration procedure or a D and C to remove the retained tissue. Aftercare is the same as for a suction abortion.

AFTER AN ABORTION

Aftercare

Women have a variety of experiences after an abortion. Most of us feel fine and do not have any problems, but some feel tired or have cramps for several days. Bleeding ranges from none at all to two to three weeks of light to moderate flow, which may stop and then start again. Signs of pregnancy may last up to a week. Some women experience a variety of changes four to seven days after an abortion because of the drop in hormone levels that happens at this time. Because of the drop in hormone levels, bleeding, cramping, breast soreness and/or feelings of depression may increase or appear if they have not been present.

Here is a list of ways to take care of yourself after an abortion:

1. Try to follow what your body needs—rest for a day or so if you feel tired. (If you can't rest because you have no one to help take care of your children or you have to go to work to keep from losing your job, you may recover more slowly.) Avoid heavy lifting or strenuous exercise in the next few days, as it may increase your bleeding. Drinking alcohol may also have this effect. Sometimes Ergotrate or Methergine (drugs that stimulate the uterus to contract) is prescribed on the theory that it may keep bleeding to a minimum and help expel any tissue retained in the uterus.

2. To help prevent infection, don't put anything into your vagina. This will avoid introducing germs that may travel up into your uterus before it has had a chance to heal completely. Don't use tampons, douche or have intercourse for two to three weeks.* It is okay to take tub baths or swim, unless you are bleeding.

3. Watch for signs of complications. If you have fever of 100.5 degrees Fahrenheit or higher, severe cramping or pain, foul-smelling vaginal discharge, vomiting, fainting, excessive bleeding (soaking an entire pad in an hour or less or passing quarter-sized clots) or signs of pregnancy that last longer than a week, report this to the clinic or doctor immediately. If you often get high on alcohol or drugs during this time, you may not be alert enough to pay attention to these warning signals. Remember that complications are rare, but they do happen to some of us. It is not your fault if you have a complication. If a complication is not taken care of as soon as possible, it might turn into a serious situation, so don't ignore possible warning signs. Often a call to the clinic will reassure you that what is happening to you is not a complication after all, but within a range of normal experience.

After the abortion, I had retained tissue. I needed a reaspiration [basically, a second abortion] to prevent an infection and remove the remaining tissue. Although the national rate of complications is very low, I was enraged to be a statistic. I had decided to terminate my pregnancy, but I didn't expect another abortion one week later. I didn't have any choice but to see it through and get my body back to normal.

4. Often the place where you had the abortion is the best source of information and medical advice or care in case of a possible complication. Call them if anything is bothering you, even if you cannot go back there for care. If you need follow-up medical attention, try to consult people who are experienced in treating women who have had legal abortions. Stay away from hospitals, clinics and practitioners who believe in forced motherhood and are against abortion. They may try to make you feel that you "deserve" the complication as "punishment" for having had an abortion, and they may not be well informed about proper treatment for postabortion problems.

5. It is important to get a checkup in two to three weeks. A pelvic exam gives information about the small possibility of retained tissue or infection that may not be causing any symptoms yet. Also, you can get any routine gynecological care that was not done at the time of the abortion.

---

*You may have been given antibiotics (usually tetracycline or ampicillin). Some people think that this cuts down the chance of developing infection; others think you should never take unnecessary antibiotics. They may also mask signs of infection. If you do decide to take antibiotics, be sure to take them according to directions.

This is often a good time to discuss birth control, which may have been difficult to talk about at the time of the abortion. A feminist health center should offer you a chance to learn more about your body, including breast and cervical self-examination techniques. You may also be asked to talk about what's been happening since your abortion—both body changes and feelings. It can be especially helpful to talk with other women who have had abortions recently. Most of us are reassured by having questions discussed and learning that our experiences have happened to other women, too. If you are one of the few women who has a continuing problem or complication, you need good information and medical help until the problem is over.

6. Your next period will probably start four to six weeks after your abortion. If you do not get your period in six weeks, contact your health care provider. *You can get pregnant immediately after an abortion, even before your next period, so you need to use reliable birth control if you have intercourse and don't want another pregnancy.* You may say and believe, "I'll never have intercourse again, so I don't need birth control." And although there are many wonderful ways of making love without intercourse (see Chapter 11, "Sexuality"), you may later change your mind. *One thing that you have in common with all women having abortions is that you know you can get pregnant.* If you weren't sure before, you know beyond any doubt that you need to use birth control if you have intercourse again and do not want to become pregnant.

Choosing a birth control method is a very individual matter (see Chapter 13, "Birth Control"). Some facilities will encourage you to use certain methods, especially pills, which you can start taking the day of a first-trimester abortion. If you do this, you will be protected after the first cycle of pills, four weeks later. However, the hormonelike drugs of the pills affect your whole body and can cause changes that are similar to signs of pregnancy, which could be confusing right after an abortion. It is probably not a good idea to have an IUD inserted at the time of an abortion, because of greater risks of infection and perforation. Also, the IUD effects of cramping and bleeding may mask the symptoms of an abortion-related infection. A diaphragm or cervical cap can be fitted or refitted at the postabortion checkup. You can start a natural birth control class after an abortion or obtain foam and condoms from a drugstore without a prescription. If the clinic or practitioner encourages you to use "the Shot" (Depo-Provera) or be sterilized, be sure to find out about the risks and the other methods that are more likely to allow you to become pregnant later if you want to. (See Chapter 13 for discussion of the reversibility of various methods of birth control.)

Feelings after an Abortion

There is no single way in which women experience abortion—positive, negative, or mixed feelings are all natural. Women often feel new strength in having made and carried out an important, often difficult decision.

I feel proud of myself that I made the choice to have an abortion and finish college. I never made a decision before that said I was the most important person. Choosing abortion is about empowerment. It's about making a choice in favor of myself and my own future. It was giving myself a vote of confidence.

My unwanted pregnancy and my abortion led me to explore and gain a full understanding of my fertility cycle and my body. This knowledge has helped me feel whole. I have always been prochoice, but now I feel able to face antichoice propaganda with the power of my own personal experience. I feel good that I can use my experience to help my sisters, my women friends and, possibly someday, my daughter.

I am a fifteen-year-old Latina woman. When I got pregnant I couldn't tell my mother. In my family my pregnancy would be considered a disgrace and an insult to the family. I would have to leave the house. My boyfriend thought I should have an abortion and so did I. I didn't really feel that I had a choice. We did not have the time or money to bring a child into this world. I know what I did was right. I also know that after the abortion I wept tears of sadness and tears of satisfaction.

I felt huge relief. I knew from the moment I found out I was pregnant that having an abortion was the right thing for me. I felt the same way after the abortion and ready to move on with my life.

The escorts took me and my boyfriend through the crowd. The demonstrators held pictures of bloody fetuses and yelled at me not to murder my baby. The whole thing really stirred me up. After the abortion I was so angry. Who do they think they are trying to tell me what to do?

My friends supported me in my decision. They talked about it with me and came to the clinic, too. I was a little tired for a day or so afterward but that's all.

Sometimes women feel guilty about having an abortion. This is not surprising because our society still doesn't particularly accept the choice of abortion. So much emphasis is put on motherhood and fetal rights that many people act as though a fetus were more important than a woman.

The antiabortion movement, playing on women's fears, has portrayed abortion as a traumatic and dangerous procedure. They talk about "post-abortion" syndrome, claiming long-term psychological effects on women and harm to future fertility. These claims are not true. Legal abortion does not hinder fertility; dangerous illegal abortions do. Severe depression after an abortion is extremely rare. In fact, most women experience relief. At the same time, some women experience sadness or a sense of loss, especially if they were unable to work through feelings before the abortion. We can support each other by breaking the silence and isolation surrounding abortion.

I had an abortion in 1970, yet I find it difficult to write about abortion. I have escorted friends to get abortions, yet I find it difficult to talk with them about abortion. They felt they needed to be secretive about their experience. They did not hear voices validating their decision, so they questioned their choice. It is not easy for black women to talk about abortion. It is not easy for black women to have abortions. But we have spoken silently with our actions, having abortions at twice the rate of white women . . . and without community support because of the conspiracy of silence surrounding abortion. A silent community cannot support sisters doing what they need and choose to do.

We need to start telling our stories about how illegal abortion killed our mothers and how legal abortion saved our lives. We have to talk to each other as black women, sister to sister.

Being able to talk about your feelings with a sympathetic and objective friend, relative, counselor or group is the most important thing you can do to help you feel better, resolve difficulties and move on.

My conflicts about the abortion were resolved about a year and a half later, when I found the courage to speak of it in a women's group. The calmness and caring the other women shared with me, as well as some of their own experiences with abortion, helped me resolve my own feelings.

Some of us may have negative feelings about sex, or intercourse in particular, for a while after the abortion. On the other hand, some of us had a chance to choose a reliable method of birth control for the first time after the abortion and are more relaxed about sex. Sometimes the abortion provokes other changes. Relationships may end. The whole experience may strengthen a relationship or enable us to make other positive changes in our lives.

If you would like help from someone with special training, the facility where you had the abortion or any of the groups listed earlier in this chapter can refer you to someone to talk with—social worker, counselor, clergyperson. There are also a few postabortion support groups run by prochoice women. If there is none near you, consider a women's support group, a therapy group or individual therapy.

Some of us may have other ways besides talking to resolve difficult feelings: yelling, crying, prayer, music, meditation, art, athletics or other physical activity. Some of us block our feelings rather than feel them, joke about them, put them away to deal with later or take pride in getting through something on our own without expressing our feelings. We must respect the different ways women deal with feelings.

We may also be angry and bitter if we had to have an abortion because we did not have the resources—decent jobs, child care, education, food—to raise a child. We may be angry that Medicaid did not pay for the abortion and we had to spend money needed for food, rent and clothes.

Taking away Medicaid funding says to poor women, "you don't deserve this." With Medicaid abortion, poor women had a little bit of control. They don't seem to get it—for poor women, abortion is a matter of survival. If I have this one more child, it etches away my margin of survival.

Some of us choose to translate our feelings into action: do political work to keep abortion legal, work for improvements in abortion services, demand child care and jobs, fight against restrictions that prevent Medicaid or insurance from paying for abortions, educate our daughters about sex, help a friend who is dealing with an unwanted pregnancy.

I started doing counseling a short while after my first illegal abortion. Someone would call me to find out where to get an abortion. I would automatically ask them to come to my home and would spend time talking about it.

When I was fifteen and pregnant, abortion was illegal. I was denied any choice—I had a baby that I gave up for adoption. This experience has been a driving force in my life. I became an ob-gyn; I do abortions because I am totally committed to making sure that other women have the options that I didn't have.

HISTORY AND POLITICS OF ABORTION

Anthropological studies show abortion to be widespread in ancient and preindustrial societies throughout the world, throughout history. In the

Western world, before Christianity, Greeks and Romans considered abortion acceptable during the early stages of pregnancy.

Over several centuries and in different cultures there is a rich history of women helping each other to abort. Until the late 1800s women healers in western Europe and the United States provided abortions and trained other women to do so, without legal prohibitions.

In other parts of the world today skilled women abortionists still practice, despite the expansion of institutionalized medicine. In Thailand, Malaysia and the Philippines, for example, village abortionists continue their traditional technique of abortion by massage.

From its beginnings Christianity considered all abortion sinful, although the Church had—and has—no fixed position on when the fetus becomes a person.* In the earliest centuries abortion was clearly considered a sin against the Church's sexual codes—not a sin of "killing." American and English common law dating back to the thirteenth century tolerated abortion up until "quickening," the moment at about twenty weeks when a pregnant woman first feels the fetus move.

The State didn't prohibit abortion until the nineteenth century, nor did the Catholic Church lead in this new repression. Britain first passed antiabortion laws in 1803, which then became stricter throughout the century. The United States followed, as individual states began to outlaw abortion at any stage of pregnancy. By 1880 most abortions were illegal in the United States, except those "necessary to save the life of the woman." But the tradition of women's right to early abortion was rooted in American society by then; abortionists continued to practice openly with public support, and juries refused to convict them.

When in 1869 Pope Pius IV declared all women having abortions to be subject to excommunication, whatever the duration of the pregnancy, the Catholic Church assumed its crusading role against abortion.

Abortion suddenly became a crime and a sin for a number of reasons. A trend of humanitarian reform in the mid-nineteenth century broadened liberal support for criminalization of abortion, because it was at that time a dangerous procedure done with crude methods, few antiseptics and high mortality rates. But this alone cannot explain the attack on abortion. For instance, other risky surgical techniques were considered necessary for people's health and welfare and were not prohib-

ited. "Protecting" women from the dangers of abortion was actually meant to control them and restrict them to their traditional childbearing role. Antiabortion legislation was part of an antifeminist backlash to the growing movements for suffrage, voluntary motherhood and other women's rights in the nineteenth century. The prevailing public prudery and antisexual moralism condemned feminism and considered sex for pleasure evil, with pregnancy as punishment.* At the same time male doctors were tightening their control over the medical profession. Doctors considered midwives, who attended births and performed abortions as part of their regular practice, a threat to their own economic and social power. The medical establishment actively took up the antiabortion cause in the second half of the nineteenth century as part of its effort to eliminate midwives.

Finally, many countries were concerned about declining populations in the nineteenth century. Developing industries and expanding territories in the United States needed workers and farmers. With the declining birth rate among whites in the late 1800s, the U.S. government and the eugenics movement urged white, native-born women to reproduce, and warned against the danger of "race suicide."† Budding industrial capitalism relied on women to be unpaid household workers, low-paid menial workers, reproducers and socializers of the next generation of workers. Without legal abortion, women found it more difficult to resist the limitations of these roles.

Then, as now, making abortion illegal neither eliminated the need for abortion nor prevented its practice. In the 1890s, doctors estimated that there were two million abortions a year in the United States. A recent study in New York City showed that over 45 percent of women who had legal abortions would have tried to get them even if they had been illegal.

Women who are determined not to carry an unwanted pregnancy have always found some way to try to abort. Lacking better alternatives, all too often they have resorted to dangerous, sometimes deadly methods, such as inserting knitting needles or coat hangers into the vagina and uterus, douching with dangerous solutions like lye and swal-

---

*In the thirteenth century, the Church favored the notion that male fetuses got a soul (became a person) at 40 days gestation, whereas female fetuses got a soul at 80 days. Abortion was still prohibited at all stages.

*Anthony Comstock, fanatical secretary of the New York Society for the Prevention of Vice, was responsible for legislation in 1873 that banned "obscene" materials from the U.S. mail—including anything to do with contraception or abortion. Also see Linda Gordon's *Woman's Body, Woman's Right*, rev. ed., New York: Penguin Books, 1990.
†"Race purity must be maintained, we must have more native white births." (Teddy Roosevelt, 1905, quoted in Angela Davis, *Race, Sex and Class*, Chapter 12, footnote 13, in Melvin Steinfeld, *Our Racist Presidents*. San Ramon, CA: Consensus Publishers, 1972, p. 212).

lowing strong drugs or chemicals. The coat hanger has become a symbol of the desperation of millions of women who have risked death to end a pregnancy. When these attempts harmed them, it was hard for them to obtain medical treatment; when these methods failed, women still had to find an abortionist.

Illegal Abortion

Many of us do not know what it was like to need an abortion before legalization. Women who could afford to pay skilled doctors or go to another country had the safest and easiest abortions. Most women found it difficult if not impossible to arrange and pay for medical abortions.

With one exception the doctors whom I asked for an abortion treated me with contempt, their attitudes ranging from hostile to insulting. One said to me, "You tramps like to break the rules, but when you get caught you all come crawling for help in the same way."

The secret world of illegal abortion was frightening and expensive. Although there were skilled and dedicated laywomen and doctors who performed safe, illegal abortions, most illegal abortionists, doctors and those who claimed to be doctors cared only about being well rewarded for their trouble. In the 1960s abortionists often turned women away if they could not pay $1,000 or more in cash. Some male abortionists insisted on having sexual relations before the abortion.

Abortionists emphasized speed and their own protection. They often didn't use anesthesia because it took too long for women to recover, and they wanted women out of the office as quickly as possible. Some abortionists were rough and sadistic. Almost no one explained what was happening, discussed birth control techniques or took adequate precautions against hemorrhage or infection.

Typically, the abortionist would forbid the woman to contact him or her again. Often she wouldn't know his or her real name. If a complication occurred, harassment by the law was a frightening possibility. The need for secrecy created isolation for women having abortions and those providing them.

The woman who did my abortion did not charge very much. No one in our neighborhood had much money, and finding a "doctor" to do an abortion was impossible. After I got home, I developed a high fever. I was so sick I was delirious with the pain and fever. My mother took me to the emergency ward. The doctors asked her who had done the abortion. When she didn't tell them, they refused to treat me. They said that they would let me die if she didn't tell them the name and address of the abortionist. Frightened, she gave them a false name and address and then they started treatment for me. When the police went to arrest the abortionist and found out that my mother had given false information, they went to my house and arrested my husband. They kept him in jail for several days until he agreed to give the information they wanted. The police took him with them to the woman's house to be sure he had told the truth. He called out to her in Spanish to warn her that the police were there, but they made him be quiet. Even though I almost died, I felt that the woman had done the best she could and had been trying to help me when I was desperate and had nowhere else to turn. It would have been impossible for me to have another child then. I hope other women will never have to go through what I experienced—to be treated like a criminal even when you need immediate medical care.

In the 1950s about a million illegal abortions a year were performed in the United States, and over a thousand women died each year as a result. Women came into emergency wards only to die of widespread abdominal infections, victims of botched or unsanitary abortions. Many women who recovered from such infections found themselves sterile or chronically and painfully ill. The enormous emotional stress often lasted a long time.

Poor women and women of color ran the great-

Woman dead on motel room floor. Her death was due to an air embolism suffered during an illegal abortion.
Files of Dr. Milton Halpern, former medical examiner, New York City

est risks with illegal abortions. In 1969, 75 percent of the women who died from abortions (most of them illegal) were women of color. Ninety percent of all legal abortions in that year were performed on white private patients.

Attempts to Make Illegal Abortion Less Dangerous

Many communities had informal networks of people who knew where women could obtain an abortion. In the 1960s, clergy groups and feminist groups set up their own referral services to help women find safer illegal abortions. Some groups found that they needed to learn more about women's bodies and about abortion techniques in order to evaluate abortionists and help women avoid dangerous procedures. As they learned, they began to seek and create better, safer alternatives. In Chicago a group of women formed the Jane Collective, which provided safe, effective and supportive illegal abortions. When they discovered that one of the skilled abortionists they used was not a doctor, Jane women realized that they could learn to perform the abortions with adequate training, and they did. Over a four-year period the Jane Collective was able to help over 11,000 women get illegal first- and second-trimester abortions with a safety record comparable to legal abortions done in medical facilities. They also reduced the cost to fifty dollars and never turned any women away because of inability to pay the fee. In this way, they put many of Chicago's expensive and unsafe illegal abortionists out of business.

Groups like the Jane Collective and other less well-known women's groups demonstrated that determined and dedicated laywomen with no formal medical training can, with careful instruction and practice, perform abortions competently and humanely. Because what they were doing was illegal, they had to set up security measures to protect the identities and safety of those involved. They could not discuss their role in providing abortions over the phone or in writing. Nor could they speak publicly about what they were doing, to encourage other women and help them in similar work. A common rule was not to tell any person, *no matter how close a friend*, any information about abortion activities that she did not need to know, because this could make her an accessory to the "crime" as well as a potential source of danger to the safety of the group. Complicated arrangements protected the anonymity of women providing the abortions and the locations where they were performed. Instruments and supplies had to be obtained, stored and transported in secrecy. If a woman had a complication during or after her abortion, or when she wanted a routine postabortion follow-up, she needed to know where to go for help and what information to give to the medical personnel to get care while protecting security. And, most impressive of all, these groups of women insisted that all these arrangements include emotional support, reassurance and kindness.

Despite the existence of groups like the Jane Collective most women having to seek an illegal abortion endured substantial risk and trauma. It is crucial that we keep abortion safe, legal and accessible, so that abortion will never have to go underground again.

Some women have written about learning how to do nonmedical abortions and claim to have had good results with alternatives, especially one to four weeks after conception. Yet information about many nonmedical abortion techniques, especially herbal ones, is incomplete, vague or even inaccurate. While attempting to induce an early abortion with acupuncture, acupressure or vitamin C may not be successful, it is not likely to involve serious risks. Taking herbal preparations, however, may be dangerous, sometimes even deadly, when women do not have extensive knowledge of herbs and cannot recognize signs of complications. In 1978 the Centers for Disease Control reported three cases of pennyroyal oil poisoning from unsuccessful attempts to induce abortions. One of the women died. Pennyroyal is a potent herb listed in many books and articles as an abortion-causing substance (abortifacient) without clear instructions about safe dosages, dangers of overdose and differences between the oil and a tea brewed from the leaves.

There has been a revival of interest in menstrual extraction, a simple technique that uses mild suction to remove a woman's period within a few days of when it is due. Over the past two decades women in small self-help groups have learned the procedure by practicing upon one another, over an extended period (see Resources). Now, with the possibility that abortion could once again become illegal in the United States, some women want to learn menstrual extraction in order to be able to help other women whose periods are a day or two late and who suspect they may be pregnant.

The Push for Legal Abortion

In the 1960s, inspired by the civil rights and antiwar movements, we began to fight more actively for our rights as women. The fast-growing women's movement took the taboo subject of abortion to the public. Rage, pain and fear burst out in demonstrations and speakouts, as women burdened by years of secrecy got up in front of strangers to talk about their illegal abortions. We marched and rallied and lobbied for abortion on demand. Civil-liberties groups and liberal clergy supported us.

Reform came gradually. A few states liberalized abortion laws, allowing women abortions in certain circumstances (e.g., pregnancy resulting from rape or incest, being under fifteen years of age) but leaving the decision up to doctors and hospitals. Costs were still high and few women actually benefited.

In 1970 New York State went further with a law that allowed abortion on demand through the twenty-fourth week from the last menstrual period if it was done in a medical facility by a doctor. A few other states passed similar laws. Women who could afford it flocked to the few places where abortions were legal. Feminist networks offered support, loans and referrals and fought to keep prices down. But for every woman who managed to get to New York, many others lived in isolated communities and had limited financial resources. Without money or mobility, these women could not be helped as easily. Illegal abortion was still common. The fight continued; a number of cases before the Supreme Court urged repeal of all restrictive state laws.

On January 22, 1973, the U.S. Supreme Court, in the famous Roe vs. Wade decision, stated that the "right of privacy . . . founded in the Fourteenth Amendment's concept of personal liberty . . . is broad enough to encompass a woman's decision whether or not to terminate her pregnancy." The Court held that through the end of the first trimester of pregnancy, it is only a pregnant woman and her doctor who have the legal right to make the decision about an abortion. States can restrict second-trimester abortions only in the interest of the woman's safety. Protection of a "viable fetus" (able to survive outside the womb) is allowed only during the third trimester. If a pregnant woman's life or health is endangered, she cannot be forced to continue the pregnancy.

Though Roe vs. Wade left a lot of power in doctors' hands, it was an important victory for us. Although the decision did not guarantee that women would be able to get abortions when they wanted to, legalization and the growing consciousness of women's needs brought better, safer abortion services. Severe infections, fever and hemorrhaging from illegal or self-induced abortions became a thing of the past. Women health workers improved abortion techniques. Some commercial clinics hired feminist abortion activists to do counseling. Local women's groups set up public referral services and women in some areas organized women-controlled nonprofit abortion facilities. These efforts have turned out to be just the beginning of a longer struggle to preserve legal abortion and to make it accessible to all women.

We have learned that legalization, though essential, is not enough. Laws and their enforcement vary, depending on who is in power. A strong movement needs to maintain constant public pressure.

In 1978, Italy passed a law giving women the right to free first-trimester abortions. The law requires a doctor's approval, a waiting period and parental consent for women under eighteen. Abortions can only be performed in public hospitals where anyone involved, from administrators to surgeons to anesthesiologists, can claim "conscientious objector" status and refuse to participate. In this Catholic country where the Church exerts a lot of pressure, 72 percent of Italian doctors became objectors within a year and refused to perform legal abortions. Some of these same doctors, however, continued to perform illegal abortions outside of hospitals, collecting high fees from women who could not obtain legal abortions.

Passage of the law was just the beginning of the fight for Italian feminists. They had to keep demanding abortions from clinics and hospitals. In 1978 they occupied and operated the abortion clinic in the Policlinico, Rome's largest hospital, whose director had promised to provide abortions and then changed his mind. After three months (and three police attacks), the women were finally ousted.

The hospital occupation helped consolidate the Italian prochoice movement. When a measure came up to repeal legal abortion in May 1981, it was defeated two to one. This was an impressive victory in a Catholic country with wealthy and powerful antiabortion forces.

Services After Legalization

Although legalization greatly lowered the cost of abortion, it still left millions of women in the United States, especially women of color and young, rural and/or poor women, without access to safe, affordable abortions. State regulations and funding have varied widely and second-trimester abortions are costly. Even when federal Medicaid funds paid for abortions, fewer than 20 percent of all public county and city hospitals actually provided them. This meant that about 40 percent of American women never benefited from liberalized abortion laws.

During the late 1970s and early 1980s, feminist health centers around the country provided low-cost abortions that emphasized quality of care and maintained political involvement in the reproductive rights movement. Competition from other local abortion providers, harassment by the IRS, and a profit-oriented economy made their survival difficult. By the early 1990s, only twenty to thirty of these centers remained.

RU-486 plus Prostaglandin: An Early Abortifacient

RU-486 (mifepristone) is a steroid drug that, when combined with a prostaglandin, is an effective early abortifacient (abortion-causing substance). Also called the *abortion pill* or the *French pill* (because its first widespread use has been in France), RU-486 has generated substantial controversy and media attention during the late 1980s and early 1990s.

How Does RU-486 Work?

By blocking the normal action of progesterone in the uterus, RU-486 can prevent implantation of a fertilized egg in the uterus or can bring on menses even if implantation already has taken place. This "antiprogesterone" drug is most effective when used within nine weeks of the last menstrual period and when followed forty-eight hours after ingestion by a dose of prostaglandin, either by suppository, by injection or orally. The prostaglandin increases uterine contractions and enhances the effectiveness of RU-486.

Is RU-486 plus Prostaglandin Safe and Effective?

RU-486 plus prostaglandin has been tested in over a dozen countries, mostly on a small scale. Most information comes from France, however, where over 100,000 women had used the drugs as of late 1991 and where one-third of all abortions are now done using this method. So far, RU-486 plus prostaglandin appears relatively safe in the short term. There are common negative effects, however, such as abdominal cramps (sometimes severe), dizziness, diarrhea and vomiting. In addition, about one woman in a thousand will experience bleeding sufficient to require a transfusion. (This is about twice as frequent as hemorrhage after vacuum suction abortion.) Long-term follow-up of women using these drugs is essential to determine long-term effects, if any.

RU-486 plus prostaglandin is successful 96 percent of the time when used within nine weeks of a woman's last menstrual period. When it fails, a suction abortion or D and C is necessary. If a pregnancy should continue after administering RU-486 plus prostaglandin, the effects on the growing fetus are unknown. It is possible that RU-486, as a steroid, might cause birth defects, so women should be aware of this. There are, however, several known cases where a woman took RU-486, did not subsequently take the prostaglandin and went on to have a baby that appeared normal in all respects.

RU-486 can be used alone, with lower success rates, as has been demonstrated in studies in Los Angeles and elsewhere.

The Experience of French Women

Several women's health activists, including representatives of the Feminist Women's Health Centers, visited France in the spring of 1989. Their trip report indicates a favorable response to this early abortion method. When women compared RU-486 plus prostaglandin to a surgical abortion, they overwhelmingly preferred the former. (However, it is important to note that first-trimester surgical abortions in France—and in most of Europe—are still performed under general anesthesia, so women there understandably view surgical abortion as more invasive and stressful.) Also, because most women developed strong contractions quite soon after receiving the prostaglandin, they chose to remain in the clinics, in the company of other women, to wait for the abortion to take place there. In some cases, women stayed overnight rather than go home, in order to avoid being alone when the uterine contents, including the embryo, came out.

Potential Advantages of RU-486 plus Prostaglandin in the United States

Because RU-486 can be administered in a doctor's office as well as in a clinical setting, women seeking early abortions may more easily avoid the antiabortion picketers and harassment so common at many abortion clinics in the United States. Possibly, more physicians and other practitioners will be willing to offer RU-486 plus prostaglandin, because they, too, would be able to avoid such harassment. Remember, however, that later first-trimester abortions will always be needed and that the problem of clinic harassment will remain whether or not RU-486 is licensed in the United States.

For women who are aware of their unwanted pregnancies in the earliest stages, RU-486 plus prostaglandin offers the option to end their pregnancies as soon as possible. It also offers a drug alternative to women with a strong aversion to inserting any instruments into their uterus. Possibly, greater media attention to this method will educate more women about the first signs of pregnancy and thus expand the number of women who could choose a very early abortion.

Potential Disadvantages of RU-486 plus Prostaglandin in the United States

An abortion with RU-486 plus prostaglandin takes considerably more time than a first-trimester vacuum suction abortion. It also involves at least one extra visit to a clinic or doctor's office (to receive the prostaglandin). A "combined" pill—one that would contain both RU-486 and prostaglandin in delayed-released form—is theoretically possible, but no drug company yet admits to working on such a formulation.

Long-term effects of RU-486 plus prostaglandin are unknown at this time.

RU-486 plus Prostaglandin in Developing-Country Settings

Women in so-called developing countries have expressed great interest in RU-486, especially in settings where abortion is illegal and maternal mortality rates due to illegal abortion are high. On the one hand, they are concerned about the long-term effects of RU-486, the possible short-term problems that might appear with poor and malnourished women (something the French experience cannot address) and the unsafe situation for the women who will bleed seriously and not have access to blood transfusions. On the other hand, they acknowledge the current dangers of common practices, such as inserting unsterile objects and caustic solutions into the uterus. Even without proper medical backup, some women argue, use of RU-486 would provide a safer overall situation, because the risk of infection would be greatly reduced by avoiding use of unclean instruments in the uterus.

There is no question that women desperately need safe abortion procedures, especially in countries where abortion is illegal. In Brazil, for example, thousands of women have used an easily available oral prostaglandin—alone—to attempt an early self-abortion. Although unsuccessful much of the time, many women who fail with this approach then go to a hospital for treatment of their bleeding—usually a D and C—that completes the abortion.

Other Issues for Consideration

Because RU-486 has become so politically controversial and because many antiabortion groups have been opposing its use in the United States even for research purposes, it may be some time before RU-486 plus prostaglandin is approved for use as an abortifacient in the United States. Meanwhile, RU-486 is being studied for other potential uses, such as in the treatment of breast cancer, Cushing's syndrome and endometriosis.

If and when introduced into the United States, it is crucial that rigorous postmarketing surveillance of RU-486 plus prostaglandin be conducted to determine long-term effects, if any. (Ideally, this should take place in many countries.) Clinical trials involving women of different racial, cultural and socioeconomic backgrounds are also essential to demonstrate safety and efficacy for women of different backgrounds and with different health problems, such as malnutrition.

Should RU-486 become more widely available, suction and surgical abortion services must still be preserved for women who need or want them, especially in instances where a later abortion is required. Unfortunately, if current abortion clinics face substantial competition from other providers who choose to offer RU-486, it is possible that some of these clinics (including women-controlled health centers) will be forced to go out of business, thus limiting access to suction/surgical abortions.

RU-486 also has potential as an occasional menses inducer, to be taken several days before a woman's period is due. It could not be used regularly, however, because of its tendency to disrupt the menstrual cycle, making it difficult to know when the next menstrual period would be due. Similar drugs may offer more promise as a once-a-month menses inducer and need to be researched further. Such an approach to fertility control would not require a positive pregnancy test and could be used by women who suspect they might be pregnant but would rather not delay action.

Reproductive Freedom versus Population Control

While we see the fight for abortion rights in the context of defending the rights of all women to make their own decisions about reproduction, not all advocates of abortion rights share this understanding. Some view legal abortion and contraception as tools of population control, especially as ways of limiting Third World populations. As one black feminist activist has observed,

Too often arguments from within the prochoice movement have appealed to racist and genocidal notions about "overpopulation" by Third World people. Put this together with a racist history and the continuing virulence of racism in the United States and there is little question as to why blacks link abortion to genocide.

At the same time many black women are choosing to have abortions. Accessible abortion is essential for black women, but we must refuse to be used and abused by someone else's political agenda for our womb.

Rejecting population control perspectives means rejecting all efforts to coerce or otherwise influence women *to* have abortions at the same time that we resist attempts to prevent women from having abortions. Creating the conditions that enable women to have the children they want to have is a long-term goal of reproductive rights activists.

Low-income women, young women, and women of color in the United States and throughout the world have been the primary targets of the population control policies of the U.S. government and others whose goal is to limit the numbers of people they consider "undesirable." For example, although abortion has become increasingly less accessible, sterilization is all too available for women of color. The federal government stopped funding abortions in 1977, but it has continued to pay for sterilizations. During the 1970s, women health activists exposed various forms of sterilization abuse (see Sterilization) and emphasized the lack of real choice when sterilization is easily available while abortion is not.

Abortion itself can be a population control tool if certain groups of women are coerced into having them. For example, women with AIDS (overwhelmingly women of color) who are pregnant currently experience pressure to have an abortion. There is also concern that they will be targets of forced sterilization. (See Chapter 27, "Developing an International Awareness," for the international dimensions of population control.)

Eroding Abortion Rights: The Antiabortion Crusade Since Roe vs. Wade

When the Supreme Court legalized abortion in 1973, the antiabortion forces, led by the Catholic Church hierarchy, began a serious mobilization using a variety of political tactics including pastoral plans that map out organizing strategies to eliminate legal abortion, political lobbying, campaigning and picketing abortion clinics. These activities continue today. In 1990 the National Conference of Catholic Bishops hired a public relations firm and allocated $3 to $5 million to be spent over a three-year period to push its antiabortion position. And in 1991 the Vatican announced yet another antiabortion initiative.

The Church hierarchy does not truly represent the views of American Catholics on this issue nor the practice of Catholic women who have abortions at the same rate as the national average for all women.

Other religious groups, like the Mormons and some representatives of Jewish orthodoxy, have traditionally opposed abortion. In the 1980s, rapidly growing fundamentalist Christian groups, which overlap with the New Right and "right-to-

life" organizations, were among the most visible boosters of the antiabortion movement.

Antiabortion groups talk as if all truly religious and moral people disapprove of abortion. This is not true now and never has been. (For prochoice religious perspectives, write to RCAR—the Religious Coalition for Abortion Rights. See Resources.)

The long-range goal of the antiabortion movement is to outlaw abortion. Their short-range strategy has been to attack access to abortion, and they have had successes.

Their first victory, a major setback to abortion rights, came in July 1976 when Congress passed the Hyde Amendment banning Medicaid funding for abortion unless a woman's life was in danger. Following the federal government, many states stopped funding "medically unnecessary" abortions. The result was immediate in terms of harm and discrimination against poor women. In October 1977 Rosie Jiminez, a Texas woman, died from an illegal abortion in Mexico after Texas stopped funding Medicaid abortions.

It is impossible to count the number of women who have been harmed by the Hyde Amendment, but before Hyde, one-third of all abortions were Medicaid funded—260,000 women per year. Without state funding, poor women with unwanted pregnancies are forced to have babies, be sterilized or have abortions using money really needed for food, rent, clothing and other necessities.

Although a broad spectrum of groups fought against the Hyde Amendment, this attack on poor women was not made a priority by the prochoice movement. There was no mass mobilization and public outcry. When the Hyde Amendment was upheld by the Supreme Court in 1980 (Harris vs. McRae), this was the beginning of the erosion of constitutional protection for abortion rights. Since then, three other Supreme Court cases have dealt severe blows to abortion rights.

In Webster vs. Reproductive Health Services (1989), the Court upheld various provisions of a Missouri law restricting abortion including a preamble stating that "the life of each human being begins at conception," a provision enabling a state to prohibit "public facilities" and "public employees" from being used to perform or assist abortions not necessary to save the life of the pregnant woman and a requirement that a physician must conduct tests to determine fetal viability if a woman seeking an abortion appears to be at least twenty weeks pregnant. In the decision, several justices indicated a willingness to reconsider—and some were ready at that time to overturn—Roe vs. Wade and to consider further restrictions on abortion.

In Hodgson vs. Minnesota (1990), the Court upheld one of the strictest parental notification laws

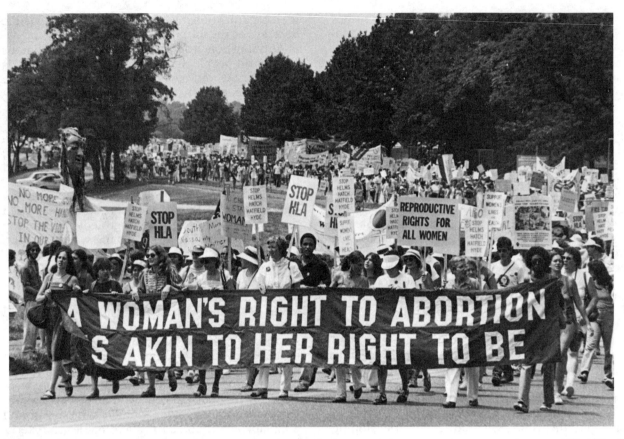

David Beach

in the country—two-parent notification, even if they have never lived with the young woman and do not have legal custody (the law does provide the alternative of a judicial hearing). The Court also upheld the constitutionality of imposing waiting periods after notification of both parents before the abortion can be performed.

In Rust vs. Sullivan (1991), the Court upheld the gag rule that prohibits counselors and physicians in federally funded family-planning clinics from providing information and making referrals about abortion. If a woman asks about abortion, she is to be told that it is not considered an appropriate method of family planning. The regulations require that all pregnant women be referred to prenatal care providers that promote the life and health of "mother and unborn child." They also require that clinics physically and financially separate their Title X programs from the provision of both abortion and abortion counseling and referral services.

As of this writing, abortion is still protected by the Constitution, but it seems only a matter of time until Roe vs. Wade, now gutted, will be completely overturned. The Supreme Court currently has a solid antiabortion majority.

The erosion of judicial support for legal abortion is even more serious because of the continu-

ous onslaught, especially since the Webster decision, of restrictive legislation at both the federal and state levels. Restrictions such as parental consent/notification laws (thirty-five states have such laws); denial of state funding (as of 1991 only thirteen states fund abortions); criminalization with penalties; reinstating spousal consent; and prohibitions against the use of public facilities and federal funds for abortion services, counseling or referrals, all make abortion less accessible and more difficult for increasing numbers of women.

Antiabortion forces have also used illegal and increasingly violent tactics in pursuit of their goals. During the 1980s, the antiabortion movement began routinely attacking abortion clinics. Over 80 percent of all abortion providers have been picketed and many have experienced other forms of harassment including bomb threats, blockades, invasions of facilities, property destruction, assault of staff and patients and death threats. Hundreds of clinics have been vandalized, bombed and burned. In the late 1980s a group called Operation Rescue initiated a strategy of civil disobedience by blockading clinic entrances and getting arrested. There have been thousands of arrests of antiabortionists nationwide as clinics have increasingly become political battlefields.

Taking Action

To the antiabortion movement and the New Right, abortion symbolizes women's independence and sexual freedom, the breakdown of the male-dominated family and women's bolder demands as workers and mothers. Their attacks on women's freedom are part of a backlash effort to turn back the gains of the women's, civil rights and gay and lesbian movements. In their unrealistic efforts to control sexuality, they have created an atmosphere that is volatile, irrational and sometimes violent, so that being vocally prochoice can be risky.

Yet the abortion rights movement is growing. The attacks on abortion have challenged us to mobilize our strength, expand our numbers and fight to regain and extend our rights. Activists have responded to Operation Rescue with physical defense of clinics and escorts for patients. In the aftermath of the Webster decision, existing organizations have grown and new ones have been created. All forms of political activism have intensified, including direct action, lobbying, demonstrations and political education.

More and more of us are coming together to express our rage, to share our visions for the future and to create a new movement that will fight for all of the rights all women need to make reproductive freedom a reality. We are transforming the prochoice movement. While we work for abortion rights, we also make the connections with opposition to sterilization abuse and racism, and de-

---

LANDMARK SUPREME COURT ABORTION DECISION IN 1992

In July of 1992, the United States Supreme Court issued a decision in a case entitled *Planned Parenthood v. Casey*. This decision sets the stage for the future of abortion rights in the United States for the next decade. In *Casey*, while a bare five-justice majority of the Supreme Court defended eloquently the importance of reproductive choice to women's privacy, bodily integrity and equality, seven out of nine justices emphatically rejected the Court's two-decade-long tradition of vigorously protecting women's access to abortion services from the most restrictive government regulations.

The Pennsylvania statute at issue in *Casey* required that a physician provide women seeking abortions with counseling biased in favor of childbirth. After this counseling, the statute required a 24-hour wait before the abortion. The statute also mandated spousal and parental notification. The Supreme Court upheld all of Pennsylvania's requirements—although most were found to be burdensome and medically unnecessary—with the sole exception of spousal notification. Spousal notice was struck down as unconstitutional because five justices considered the requirement "unduly burdensome," particularly with regard to women in violent abusive or otherwise dysfunctional marriages.

But two frightening themes in the Court's analysis should fill women with great foreboding. First, the Court sanctioned the view that government may regulate the health care of pregnant women to protect fetal life from the moment of conception so long as it does not "unduly burden" access to an abortion. Second, the Court showed little concern for the severe impact of state restrictions on abortion in the context of poverty. For example, the 24-hour waiting period can require extra travel, lodging and child care costs beyond the financial means of poorer women. For these women, such extra costs can turn a burden into a veritable ban on access to abortion.

The immediate consequence of the Court's decision in *Casey* will be a massive onslaught of state regulatory measures designed to create obstacles to women's access to reproductive choice with no underlying medical rationale. These restrictions will have the cumulative effect of reducing, if not denying, the availability of abortion services to an ever-increasing underclass of women; abandoning norms of neutrality and informed consent in reproductive health care; and diminishing the rights and equality of pregnant women generally.

The decision promises grave uncertainty about the future of reproductive liberty. We are one justice away from the complete loss of any constitutional protection for abortion and we have already lost *Roe's* promise that states cannot regulate abortion services out of existence. Ultimately, the decision confirms the necessity of a strong reproductive rights movement dedicated to a congressional "Freedom of Choice Act" and, finally, to the restoration of the vitality of *Roe v. Wade*.

By: Rachael N. Pine, The Center for Reproductive Law & Policy, 120 Wall Street, New York, NY (212-514-5534) (a feminist legal organization dedicated to the protection of women's reproductive freedoms throughout the world).

AFRICAN-AMERICAN WOMEN FOR REPRODUCTIVE FREEDOM

Choice is the essence of freedom. It's what we African-Americans have struggled for all these years. The right to choose where we would sit on a bus. The right to vote. The right for each of us to select our own paths, to dream and reach for our dreams. The right to choose how we would or would not live our lives.

This freedom—to choose and to exercise our choices—is what we've fought and died for. Brought here in chains, worked like mules, bred like beasts, whipped one day, sold the next—244 years we were held in bondage. Somebody said that we were less than human and not fit for freedom. Somebody said we were like children and could not be trusted to think for ourselves. Somebody owned our flesh and decided if and when and with whom and how our bodies were to be used. Somebody said that black women could be raped, held in concubinage, forced to bear children year in and year out, but often not raise them. Oh, yes, we have known how painful it is to be without choice in this land.

Those of us who remember the bad old days when Jim Crow rules and segregation were the way of things know the hardships and indignities we faced. We were free, but few or none were our choices. Somebody said where we could live and couldn't, where we could work, what schools we could go to, where we could eat, how we could travel. Somebody prevented us from voting. Somebody said we could be paid less than other workers. Somebody burned crosses, harassed and terrorized us in order to keep us down.

Now once again somebody is trying to say that we can't handle the freedom of choice. Only this time they're saying African-American women can't think for themselves and, therefore, can't be allowed to make serious decisions. Somebody's saying that we should not have the freedom to take charge of our personal lives and protect our health, that we only have limited rights over our bodies. Somebody's once again forcing women to acts of desperation, because somebody's saying that if women have unintended pregnancies, it's too bad, but they must pay the price.

Somebody's saying that we must have babies whether we choose to or not. Doesn't matter what we say, doesn't matter how we feel. Some say that abortion under any circumstance is wrong, others say that rape and incest and danger to the life of the woman are the only exceptions. Doesn't matter that nobody's saying who decides if it was rape or incest, if a woman's word is good enough, if she must go into court and prove it. Doesn't matter that she may not be able to take care of a baby, that the problem also affects girls barely out of adolescence, that our children are having children. Doesn't matter if you're poor and pregnant—go on welfare or walk away.

What does matter is that we know abortions will still be done, legal or not. We know the consequences when women are forced to make choices without protection—the coat hangers and knitting needles that punctured the wombs of women forced to seek back-alley abortions on kitchen tables at the hands of butchers. The women who died screaming in agony, awash in their own blood. The women who were made sterile. All the women who endured the pain of makeshift surgery with no anesthetics and risked fatal infection.

We understand why African-American women risked their lives then and why they seek safe legal abortion now. It's been a matter of survival. Hunger and homelessness. Inadequate housing and income to properly provide for themselves and their children. Family instability. Rape. Incest. Abuse. Too young, too old, too sick, too tired. Emotional, physical, mental, economic, social—the reasons for not carrying a pregnancy to term are endless and varied, personal, urgent and private. And for all these pressing reasons, African-American women once again will be among the first forced to risk their lives if abortion is made illegal.

There have always been those who have stood in the way of our exercising our rights, who tried to restrict our choices. There probably always will be. But we who have been oppressed should not be swayed in our opposition to tyranny of any kind, especially attempts to take away our reproductive freedom. You may believe abortion is wrong. We respect your belief and we will do all in our power to protect that choice for you. You may decide that abortion is not an option you would choose. Reproductive freedom guarantees your right not to. All that we ask is that no one deny another human being the right to make her own choice. That no one condemn her to exercising her choices in ways that endanger her health, her life. And that no one prevent others from creating safe, affordable, legal conditions to accommodate women, whatever the choices they make. Reproductive freedom gives each of us the right to make our own choices and guarantees us a safe, legal, affordable support system. It's the right to choose.

We are still an embattled people beset with life-and-death issues. Black America is under siege. Drugs, the scourge of our community, are wiping out one, two, three generations. We are killing ourselves and each other. Rape and other unspeakable acts of violence are becoming sickeningly commonplace. Babies linger on death's door, at risk at birth: born addicted to crack and cocaine, born underweight and undernourished, born AIDS infected. An ever-growing number of our children are being abandoned, being mentally, physically, spiritually abused. Homelessness, hunger, unemployment run rife. Poverty grows. Our people cry out in desperation, anger and need.

Meanwhile, those somebodies who claim they're "prolife" aren't moved to help the living. They're not out there fighting to break the stranglehold of drugs and violence in our communities, trying to save our children or moving to provide infant and maternal nutri-

tion and health programs. Eradicating poverty isn't on their agenda. No—somebody's too busy picketing, vandalizing and sometimes bombing family-planning clinics, harassing women and denying funds to poor women seeking abortions.

So when somebody denouncing abortion claims that they're "prolife," remind them of an old saying that our grandmothers often used: "It's not important what people say, it's what they do." And remember who we are, remember our history, our continuing struggle for freedom. Remember to tell them that we remember!

Byllye Avery (National Black Women's Health Project)
Rev. Willie Barrow (Operation Push)
Donna Brazile (Housing Now)
Shirley Chisholm (National Political Congress of Black Women)
Representative Cardiss Collins (U.S. Congress)
Romona Edelin (National Urban Coalition)
Jacqui Gates (National Association of Negro Business and Professional Women's Clubs, Inc.)
Marcia Ann Gillespie (*Ms. Magazine*)
Dorothy Height (National Council of Negro Women)
Jewel Jackson McCabe (National Coalition of 100 Black Women)
Julianne Malveaux (San Francisco Black Leadership Forum)
Eleanor Holmes Norton (Georgetown University Law School)
C. Delores Tucker (DNC Black Caucus)
Patricia Tyson (Religious Coalition for Abortion Rights)
Maxine Waters (Black Women's Forum)
Faye Wattleton (Planned Parenthood Federation of America)

Note: Organizations for identification purposes only.

mands for welfare rights, disability rights, gay and lesbian liberation, economic rights, child care and health care.

These changes are the most exciting aspects of the past few years. We have participated in international days of protest and gatherings that build solidarity and communication among women all over the world. Within the United States, new organizations representing and led by women of color have become prominent in the abortion rights struggle. And these trends have pushed the prochoice movement to see abortion rights in the broader context of women's health and freedom. All of us who believe that safe abortions contribute to the preservation of human life must be active in the political battle for accessible legal abortions as part of the struggle for reproductive freedom for all women.

RESOURCES

Organizations

American Civil Liberties Union (ACLU)
Reproductive Freedom Project
   132 W. 43rd Street
   New York, NY 10036
   (212) 944-9800
Involved in litigation relevant to abortion rights, publishes a number of pamphlets and the bi-monthly *Reproductive Rights Update.*

Boston Reproductive Rights Network (R2N2)
   P.O. Box 686
   Jamaica Plain, MA 02130
A feminist, grassroots, activist organization working on a broad range of reproductive rights and women's health issues. Publishes a quarterly newsletter.

Catholics for a Free Choice (CFFC)
   1436 U Street NW, Suite 301
   Washington, DC 20009
   (202) 638-1706
A national educational organization that supports the right to family planning and abortion.

The Committee to Defend Reproductive Rights (CDRR)
   25 Taylor Street, Suite 704
   San Francisco, CA 94102
   (415) 441-4434
Grassroots, feminist, membership organization. Does public speaking and community education on a wide variety of reproductive rights and health access issues. Publishes a newsletter and fact sheets.

Civil Liberties and Public Policy Program
   Hampshire College
   Amherst, MA 01002
   (413) 549-4600, ext 645
A resource for campus and community reproductive rights organizing. Publishes a newsletter, puts on an annual reproductive rights conference and distributes videos.

The Federation of Feminist Women's Health Centers
   3701 Folsom Boulevard, Suite A
   Sacramento, CA 95816
   (916) 737-0260
A nonprofit association of women's health projects that provides health services to women, including abortion, well-women care and birth control. They distribute a video, *No Going Back,* about menstrual extraction.

The Fund for the Feminist Majority
   1600 Wilson Boulevard, Suite 704
   Arlington, VA 22209
   (703) 522-2214
An advocacy and research group that aims to get women into positions of leadership throughout society and to promote a national feminist agenda. The Feminist Majority Foundation (186 South St., Boston, MA 02111, [617] 695-9688) is the research and education arm of the Fund.

International Women's Health Coalition
   24 East 21st Street
   New York, NY 10010
   (212) 979-8500
A private, nonprofit organization dedicated to improving women's reproductive health in less industrialized countries. It supports health care projects, policy-oriented field research and public education.

Native American Women's Health Education Resource Center
   P.O. Box 572
   Lake Andes, SD 57356
   (605) 487-7072
Has organized a Native American reproductive rights coalition.

The National Abortion Federation (NAF)
   1436 U Street NW
   Washington, DC 20009
   (202) 667-5881
An association of abortion providers, individuals and organizations working in reproductive health and abortion rights. NAF distributes informational publications and has a toll-free hotline which gives referrals for abortion services and funding. HOTLINE: (800) 772-9100, M-F, 9:30–5:30 E.S.T. In Canada, (800) 424-2280.

The National Abortion Rights Action League (NARAL)
   1101 14th Street NW, 5th Floor
   Washington, DC 20005
   (202) 408-4600
Works to elect prochoice officials to all levels of government and to protect the right to choose in the legislatures, the courts and at the clinics. It has a Campus Organizing Project which assists young activists.

The National Black Women's Health Project (NBWHP)
   1237 Ralph David Abernathy Drive SW
   Atlanta, GA 30310
   (404) 758-9590
Public Policy/Education office: 1133 15th St., NW. Suite 550, Washington, D.C. 20005, (202) 835-0117 (or 0118). A self-help and advocacy organization addressing vital health issues facing Black women and

their families. Activities and resources include: self-help chapters, networking, national and regional conferences, the newsletter *VITAL SIGNS* and the film *On Becoming a Woman*.

The National Latina Health Organization (NLHO)
P.O. Box 7567
Oakland, CA 94601
(415) 534-1362
Promotes self-help methods and self-empowerment processes. Latinas for Reproductive Choice, part of NLHO, takes public stands on reproductive issues and is involved in education and advocacy work in order to include Latinas in the national reproductive rights debate.

The National Organization for Women (NOW)
Action Center
1000 16th Street NW, Suite 700
Washington, DC 20036
(202) 331-0066
A top priority is keeping abortion and birth control safe and legal. NOW works on obtaining grassroots support and lobbying on state and national levels.

The National Women's Health Network (NWHN)
1325 G Street NW
Washington, DC 20005
(202) 347-1140
Works for abortion rights as one of many women's health issues. Maintains national communications about antiabortion legislation, RU-486, and harassment of feminist abortion providers.

The Religious Coalition for Abortion Rights (RCAR)
100 Maryland Avenue NE, Suite 307
Washington, DC 20002
(202) 543-7032
An ecumenical coalition of thirty-six religious denominations and organizations. Has many publications on positions of religious organizations with regard to abortion rights.

The Reproductive Health Technologies Project
1601 Connecticut Avenue NW, Suite 801
Washington, DC 20009
Promotes public education and dialogue about RU-486 and other contraceptive/abortifacient drugs.

Students Organizing Students (SOS)
1600 Broadway, Suite 404
New York, NY 10019
A national group organizing students on high school and college campuses in the fight for reproductive freedom.

Women of All Red Nations (WARN)
4511 North Hermitage
Chicago, IL 60640
An American Indian women's group whose purpose is the empowerment of Indian women. Primary issues include: promoting Indian women's health and reproductive rights; fighting against violence against women; supporting Indian treaty rights; and stopping spiritual and cultural exploitation.

The Women of Color Partnership Program (WOCPP) of RCAR (see address above) works on reproductive rights issues and reproductive health care concerns from the unique perspectives of women of color. It publishes a newsletter, *Common Ground—Different Planes*.

Books

Baehr, Ninia. *Abortion Without Apology: A Radical History for the 1990's*. Boston: South End Press, 1990.

Bonavoglia, Angela. *The Choices We Made*. New York: Random House, 1991.

Cohen, Sherrill, and Nadine Taub, eds. *Reproductive Laws for the 1990s*. Clifton, NJ: Humana Press, 1989.

David, Henry P., and Zdenek Matejeek. *Born Unwanted: Developmental Effects of Denied Abortion*. New York: Springer, 1988.

Davis, Susan E., ed. *Women Under Attack—Victories, Backlash and the Fight for Reproductive Freedom*. Boston: South End Press, 1988 (originally published by CARASA, Committee for Abortion Rights and Against Sterilization Abuse, New York).

Dworkin, Andrea. *Right Wing Women*. New York: Putnam, 1983.

Faux, Marian. *Roe v. Wade: The Untold Story of the Landmark Supreme Court Decision that Made Abortion Legal*. New York: New American Library, 1988.

———. *Crusaders: Voices from the Abortion Front*. New York: Birch Lane Press, Carol Publishing Group, 1990.

Federation of Feminist Women's Health Centers. *A New View of A Woman's Body*. New York: Simon & Schuster, 1981.

Ferraro, Barbara, and Patricia Hussey with Jane O'Reilly. *No Turning Back: Two Nuns Battle with the Vatican over Women's Right to Choose*. New York: Poseidon Press, 1990.

Francome, Colin. *Abortion Freedom: A Worldwide Movement*. London: George Allen and Unwin, 1984.

Frankfort, Ellen, with Frances Kissling. *Rosie, the Investigation of a Wrongful Death*. New York: Dial Press, 1978.

Fried, Marlene Gerber. *From Abortion to Reproductive Freedom: Transforming a Movement*. Boston: South End Press, 1990.

Gage, Suzanne. *When Birth Control Fails: How to Abort Ourselves Safely*. Hollywood, CA: Speculum Press, 1979.

Garfield, Jay L., and Patricia Hennessey. *Abortion: Moral and Legal Perspectives*. Amherst: University of Massachusetts Press, 1984.

Ginsburg, Faye D. *Contested Lives: The Abortion Debate in an American Community*. Berkeley: University of California Press, 1989.

Gordon, Linda. *Woman's Body, Woman's Right: Birth Control in America*, rev. ed. New York: Penguin, 1990.

Harrison, Beverly Wildung. *Our Right to Choose: Toward a New Ethic of Abortion*. Boston: Beacon Press, 1983.

Hartmann, Betsy. *Reproductive Rights and Wrongs: The Global Politics of Population Control and Contraceptive Choice*. New York: Harper & Row, 1987.

Hartmann, Betsy, and Hilary Standing. *The Poverty of Population Control*. London: Bangladesh International Action Group, Third World Publications, 1989.

Lader, Lawrence. *Abortion*. Boston: Beacon Press, 1966.

———. *Abortion II.* Boston: Beacon Press, 1973.

———. *RU 486: The Pill That Could End the Abortion Wars and Why American Women Don't Have It.* Reading, MA: Addison-Wesley, 1991.

Luker, Kristin. *Abortion and the Politics of Motherhood.* Berkeley: University of California Press, 1984.

McDonnell, Kathleen. *Not an Easy Choice: A Feminist Re-examines Abortion.* Boston: South End Press, 1984.

Melton, Gary B., ed. *Adolescent Abortion: Psychological and Legal Issues.* Lincoln: University of Nebraska Press, 1986.

Merton, Andrew. *Enemies of Choice: The Right to Life Movement and Its Threat to Abortion.* Boston: Beacon Press, 1981.

Messer, Ellen, and Kathryn E. May. *Back Rooms: An Oral History of the Illegal Abortion Era.* New York: Simon & Schuster, 1988.

National Women's Health Network. *Abortion Then and Now: Creative Responses to Restricted Access.* Washington, DC: National Women's Health Network, 1990.

Petchesky, Rosalind Pollack. *Abortion and Woman's Choice: The State, Sexuality, and Reproductive Freedom,* rev. ed. Evanston, IL: Northeastern University Press, 1990.

Radl, Shirley L. *Over Our Live Bodies: Preserving Choice in America.* Dallas: Steve Davis Publishing, 1989.

Raymond, Janice et al. *RU-486: Misconceptions, Myths and Morals.* Cambridge, MA: Institute on Women and Technology (Department of Urban Studies and Planning, MIT), 1991. (Cottingham, Jane, and Paul Van Look. "RU-486: Misconceptions, myths and morals: A critique," June 1992. Available for $2.00 from the Boston Women's Health Book Collective, Box 192, West Somerville, MA 02144.)

Rodman, Hyman, Betty Sarvis and Joy Bonar. *The Abortion Question.* New York: Columbia University Press, 1987.

Rothman, Barbara Katz. *The Tentative Pregnancy: Prenatal Diagnosis and the Future of Motherhood.* New York: Penguin, 1987.

Schulder, Diane, and Florynce Kennedy. *Abortion Rap.* New York: McGraw-Hill, 1971.

Tribe, Laurence. *Abortion: The Clash of Absolutes.* New York: W. W. Norton, 1990.

White, Evelyn C., ed. *The Black Women's Health Book: Speaking For Ourselves.* Seattle, WA: Seal Press, 1990.

Articles

Bart, Pauline. "Seizing the Means of Reproduction: An Illegal Feminist Abortion Collective—How and Why It Worked." Available for $2.00 from Boston Women's Health Book Collective, Box 192, West Somerville, MA 02144.

Binion, Gayle. "Webster v. Reproductive Health Services: Devaluing the Right to Choose," *Women & Politics,* Vol. 11, No. 2 (1991).

Centers for Disease Control. "Abortion Surveillance." CDC, Public Health Service, U.S. Dept. of Health and Human Services, Bureau of Epidemiology, Family Planning Evaluation Division, Atlanta, GA 30333. Free.

Gallagher, Janet. "Prenatal Invasions and Interventions: What's Wrong with Fetal Rights." *Harvard Women's Law Journal,* Vol. 10 (Spring 1987), pp. 9–58.

Henshaw, S.K. "Induced Abortion: A World Review, 1990," *International Family Planning Perspectives* (March/April 1990).

Henshaw, S.K., Lisa M. Koonin and Jack C. Smith. "Characteristics of U.S. Women Having Abortions, 1987," *Family Planning Perspectives,* Vol. 23, No. 2 (March/April 1991).

Jacobson, Jodi L. "Global Politics of Abortion," Washington, DC: Worldwatch Institute (1990).

Mertus, Julie A. "Fake Abortion Clinics: The Threat to Reproductive Self-Determination," *Women & Health,* Vol. 16, No. 1 (1990).

Nsiah-Jefferson, Laurie. "Reproductive Laws, Women of Color, and Low-Income Women," in Sherrill Cohen and Nadine Taub, eds., *Reproductive Laws for the 1990s.* Clifton, NJ: Humana Press, 1989, pp. 23–67.

Paltrow, Lynn M. "Amicus Brief: Richard Thornburgh v. American College of Obstetricians and Gynecologists," *Women's Rights Law Reporter,* Vol. 9, No. 1 (Winter 1986).

Petchesky, Rosalind Pollack. "Foetal Images: The Power of Visual Culture in the Politics of Reproduction," in Michelle Stanworth, ed., *Reproductive Technologies: Gender, Motherhood and Medicine.* Minneapolis: University of Minnesota Press, 1987.

Relkin, Ellen, and Sudi Solomon. "Using State Constitutions to Expand Public Funding for Abortions: Throwing Away the Carrot with the Stick," *Women's Rights Law Reporter,* Vol. 9, No. 1 (Winter 1986).

Roberts, Dorothy E. "The Future of Reproductive Choice for Poor Women and Women of Color," *Women's Rights Law Reporter,* Vol. 12, No. 2 (Summer 1990).

Rogers, James, Robert Boruch, George Stoms and Dorothy DeMoya. "Impact of the Minnesota Parental Notification Law on Abortion and Birth," *American Journal of Public Health,* Vol. 81, No. 3 (March 1991).

Stearns, Nancy. "Roe v. Wade: Our Struggle Continues," *Berkeley Women's Law Journal,* Vol. 4 (1988–1989).

Villarosa, Linda. "Our Bodies, Their Laws," *Essence,* Vol. 20, No. 6 (October 1989), pp. 24–26.

Periodicals

Family Planning Perspectives
   Published bimonthly
The Alan Guttmacher Institute
   111 Fifth Avenue
   New York, NY 10003

Special Publications

Women's Global Network for Reproductive Rights. "Maternal Mortality and Morbidity: A Call to Women for Action," WGNRR, N2 Voorburgwal 32, 1012 R2 Amsterdam, The Netherlands. May 28,1990.

"No Way Out: Young, Pregnant, and Trapped by the

Law," ACLU Reproductive Freedom Project, 132 W. 43rd Street, New York, NY 10036, 1991.

"Protecting Access to Health Care for Women: A Guide to Legal Strategies to Prohibit Violence and Interference at Clinics," NOW Legal Defense and Education Fund, 99 Hudson Street, New York, NY 10013, 1991.

"Protecting Young Women's Right to Abortion: A Guide to Parental Notification and Consent Laws," NOW Legal Defense and Education Fund, 99 Hudson Street, New York, NY 10013, 1990.

"Reproductive Rights: The Global Fight," *Connexions: An International Women's Quarterly*, No. 31, 4228 Telegraph Avenue, Oakland, CA 94609.

"Shattering the Dreams of Young Women: The Tragic Consequences of Parental Involvement Laws," ACLU Reproductive Freedom Project, 132 W. 43rd Street, New York, NY 10036.

Audiovisual Materials

Abortion Denied: Shattering Young Women's Lives, 1990, color, a video about the devastating effect of parental consent/notification laws. Available from The Feminist Majority Foundation, 1600 Wilson Boulevard, Arlington, VA 22209.

Abortion for Survival, 1989, color, video showing the availability of birth control and abortion as basic rights for women's survival, not only in the United States but internationally. A major criticism of it is that family planning in the Third World is discussed in terms of population control and not women's control. Comes with fact-filled booklet. Available from The Feminist Majority Foundation, 1600 Wilson Boulevard, Arlington, VA 22209.

Abortion: Stories from North and South, a 16-mm 1984 color film/video. A documentary that attempts a historical and cross-cultural view of abortion. Segments filmed in Ireland, Japan, Thailand, Peru, Colombia and Canada. The film is quite powerful, however, important criticisms have been raised: international family-planning programs are presented uncritically. Available from Cinema Guild, 1697 Broadway, New York, NY 10019.

Back-Alley Detroit: Abortion Before Roe v. Wade, 1992, 45-minute color video by Daniel Friedman and Sharon Grimberg. Using interviews and archival footage, this excellent historical documentary depicts the full range of women's experiences, exposes the underworld that criminalization of abortion created and tells the stories of those who defied abortion laws. A must. Available from Filmmakers Library, 124 East 40th Street, New York, NY 10016.

Casting the First Stone: Portraits of Women and Men on Both Sides of the Abortion Controversy, 1-hour 1991 video. Tells the story of six women and spans three decades. Available from Women Make Movies, 225 Lafayette Street, Suite 207, New York, NY 10012.

Holy Terror, a 16-mm 1986 color film/video. A documentary presenting the rise of antiabortion efforts of the religious New Right. Although it predates Operation Rescue, it is still the best film about the antiabortion movement. Available from Cinema Guild, 1697 Broadway, New York, NY 10019.

In Defense of Roe, a 35-minute 1989 color video. Speakers place the abortion rights struggle in the context of health care needs and perspectives of poor women and women of color and emphasize coalition building as a priority in the agenda for reproductive freedom. Available from the ACLU Reproductive Freedom Project, 132 W. 43rd Street, New York, NY 10036.

No Going Back. This 1988 video presents menstrual extraction as an abortion method that can be used by women in self-help health groups. Women's health activists disagree about the safety of this procedure. Available from the Federation of Feminist Women's Health Centers, 1043 University Avenue, No. 169, San Diego, CA 92103, (619) 298-0967.

On Becoming A Woman, a 1989 color video about mothers and daughters working to communicate honestly with each other. Full of candid, emotional conversations about menstruation, sexuality, birth control, teen pregnancy and relationships. Available from National Black Women's Health Project, 1237 Ralph Abernathy Drive, SW, Atlanta, GA 30310.

Our Right to Abortion, a 1987 color video combining footage of the 1986 "March for Women's Lives" and interviews with longtime activists. It does not deal with the experiences of poor women and women of color. Available from Women Make Movies, 225 Lafayette Street, Suite 207, New York, NY 10012.

Silent No More, a 1989 color video. Four white women talk about their illegal abortions. This was made during a speak out at Hampshire College. Available from Civil Liberties and Public Policy Program, Hampshire College, Amherst, MA 01002.

Speaking Out for Reproductive Freedom, a 1991 color video. Twenty speakers from the United States and the Third World talking on a wide range of issues. Available from Civil Liberties and Public Policy Program, Hampshire College, Amherst, MA 01002.

With a Vengeance, a 40-minute black-and-white 16-mm film/video. Explores the history of the struggle for abortion rights since the 1960s, reflecting the wider history of the women's liberation movement. Available from Women Make Movies, 225 Lafayette Street, Suite 207, New York, NY 10012.

You're What? A Story of Teenage Pregnancy, a 1986 color video. A docudrama portraying a fifteen-year-old faced with an unplanned pregnancy in a state with parental consent laws for abortion. Available from Boston Women's Health Book Collective, Box 192, W. Somerville, MA 02144.

18

New Reproductive Technologies

By Ruth Hubbard, with
Wendy Sanford

With special thanks to Gena Corea.

*1992 Update by Diane Clapp, with
Judy Norsigian.*

From *in vitro* fertilization and sex preselection to embryo transfer, scientists and physicians are working hard on new technologies that could drastically change women's relationship to childbearing. These technologies raise a dilemma for those of us who are writing and consulting on this book. On the one hand, we know that some technologies have helped or have the potential to help women who badly want biological children and would otherwise be unable to have them. We want to support a woman's right to choose to have children and by the means she sees best. We know also that certain technologies can help parents avoid passing on hereditary diseases to their children.

Yet we have serious questions. The technologies involve a degree of invasiveness and medical manipulation of women's bodies, which alarms us. Most of the money that goes into developing these technologies would be better spent on preventive measures and basic health care services for all women. What's more, white, professional, affluent men make up the overwhelming number of the scientists who research these technologies, the physicians who apply them, the legislators who approve and fund the research and the drug company directors who translate them into products to be advertised, sold and profited from. Despite claims that these technologies are to "serve"

women, our experience with the use of other medical technologies has taught us to be suspicious; physicians and hospitals now virtually force birthing technologies on us, and sterilization has been outrageously misused against poor women and women of color. Most doctors offering even something as technically simple as donor insemination have so far restricted their services to married women. We can reasonably predict that those in control of the technologies of the future will show a continued resistance to sharing them with women in nontraditional relationships, particularly lesbians.

We have questions, too, about the long-range goals of this research. One source lists as the final goal of reproductive engineering "the ultimate manufacture of a human being to exact specifications." Who will decide these specifications? Our guess is that without a major political revolution it won't be women, and it especially won't be women of color or women who are poor. Will these new reproductive technologies truly serve us? Or, in a society where women have less power than men, will they be a means of further controlling our freedom to make choices about our bodies?

We are also critical of the way the society measures our worth as women by our fertility. We are made to feel inadequate or unwomanly if we can't bear children "of our own." The mother of the first test-tube baby expressed the guilt she had felt:

"I'm not a normal woman," I told John. . . . "I wouldn't even blame you now if you went off with someone else." . . . It wasn't John's fault. He could have as many children as he liked with another woman. A whole football team. . . .[1]

Wanting a baby and not being able to have one can be intensely painful. But society heaps an extra load of guilt on us. Is this one of the reasons why some of us are so willing to go through all kinds of time-consuming, painful and at times degrading tests and medical manipulations to have a child? Even the less invasive infertility techniques expose a very private corner of our lives and open us to endless questions and advice from relatives, friends and physicians, who may also recommend surgery, drugs or other risky and invasive procedures. Our male partner may share our sense of violation as he ejaculates on command, so his semen can be examined and his sperm counted.

There is no inner recess of me left unexplored, unprobed, unmolested. It occurs to me when I have sex that what used to be beautiful and very private is now degraded and terribly public. I bring my [menstrual cycle] charts to the doctor like a child bringing home a report card. Tell me, did I do well? Did I ovulate? Did I have sex at the right times as you instructed me?[2]

It would be a lot better if we felt less pressured to produce our "own" children and could express our needs to love, nurture and be loved by becoming close to children of neighbors, friends or relatives, by adopting children who need parents or by becoming foster parents. At present, adoption and foster parenting involve personal and legal problems that many of us aren't willing or able to take on. And yet the biotechnical solutions aren't easy, either.

We must judge the value of the reproductive technologies in the context of the social, political and economic setting in which they are produced and used. We must look at who owns them and who profits from them, whether they give professionals more power over us or whether they increase the power and self-sufficiency of those of us who use them. We must assess their dollar cost and judge how easily ordinary people can have access to them. We must also recognize that researchers may be seeking the fame and funding that come from achieving scientific breakthroughs and triumphs rather than working for the well-being of women.

In this chapter we have tried to help inform women considering the use of these technologies, while at the same time raising the strong doubts we hold.

DONOR INSEMINATION (DI)

This is the simplest, least invasive and most widely used of the technologies we are considering. It doesn't require professional help, and we can do it at home.

To use DI on your own, you should have no fertility problems and your menstrual cycle should be fairly regular. Then you begin by charting your basal temperature and mucus consistency for a few months (see "Fertility Observation," p. 276) so that you know when you are likely to ovulate. You must also find a fertile man who is willing to donate sperm. You can do this yourself or, if you want anonymity, through a friend. When you know from past cycles that you are about to ovulate, the sperm donor must masturbate into a clean (preferably boiled, *but cooled*) jar. Within an hour after ejaculation, you suck the semen into a needleless hypodermic syringe (some women use an eye dropper or a turkey baster), gently insert the syringe into your vagina while lying flat on your back with your rear up on a pillow and empty the syringe into your vagina to deposit the semen as close to your cervix as possible. Then continue lying down comfortably for about ten minutes, so that as little sperm as possible leaks out of your vagina.

It's a good idea to repeat this with fresh sperm samples in two or three days, during and after the time you ovulate. Most women become pregnant after trying DI during three to five cycles. If you aren't pregnant after having tried it five or six months, you may want to consult a fertility clinic to check on your and your donor's fertility.

This kind of DI is often called *artificial insemination by donor*. At present, probably more than 30,000 babies a year are conceived by DI in the United States by women whose husbands either have fertility problems or are at risk of passing on a serious hereditary disease, as well as by women who are single or part of a lesbian couple. Some married couples are occasionally advised to use the husband's sperm for DI. This is useful when there are structural or psychological barriers to sexual intercourse. In addition, if the husband provides normal motile sperm, but not enough, he may be advised to collect the first few drops of the ejaculate separately from the rest. Since the first portion contains most of the active sperm, that's what you use for donor insemination.

The American Fertility Society has issued guidelines indicating that only frozen, not fresh, semen be used when doing DI. They suggest that the donor have an HIV test for the AIDS virus, that the sperm be frozen and held until he is tested again in three months and only if that test is negative should the frozen, stored semen be used. It takes longer to get pregnant with frozen semen because sperm movement is decreased after freezing. Often, an average of eight to ten cycles is needed before a pregnancy occurs. Many clinics now are improving pregnancy rates by (1) doing intrauterine insemination with the frozen sperm, (2) inseminating twice at midcycle and (3) adding ovulatory enhancement drugs like human menopausal gonadotropin (HMG) (Pergonal) or clomiphene to trigger more eggs to be released, thereby increasing the likelihood of conception.

When a procedure is this simple, why do some of us take on the expense and other drawbacks of involving physicians and lawyers? For one thing, when a physician does the insemination, it is easier to provide anonymity for both donor and recipient (see below). Ideally, the donor also would be properly screened for possible health problems although in fact most physicians ask prospective donors only a few questions about their health and family histories for various diseases.* Indeed, since donors usually receive $25 to $40 per ejaculate, some men may conceal health problems in order to be eligible. A survey of physicians' practices shows that most of them don't offer you more protection than you could provide yourself.

Physicians do have access to sperm banks that store frozen sperm, so that you don't need a donor on call to produce sperm when you ovulate. Unfortunately, however, using frozen sperm usually costs you more time and money. (At about $70 per insemination, DI through a physician costs about $140 a month at two inseminations per cycle and $200 to $300 if frozen semen is used.)

Mutual anonymity between you and the man who donates the sperm may be important for both of you and can forestall legal and emotional complications. Problems have arisen when a man who gave his sperm had a change of feelings later and sued for visitation or wanted to give the child his surname. Single and lesbian women especially have to guard against this kind of harassment. The sperm donor, too, may need protection, because a court may later assert a donor's responsibility for child support.†

There are also arguments against anonymity. Many unmarried women, both heterosexual and lesbian, want the donor to be a friend who will possibly be involved in the child's life. Also, just as adopted children are making increasing efforts to locate their biological parents, some children conceived by DI may be disturbed and angry if they cannot find out who their biological fathers are. Also, health problems may arise that may make us or our children want to have access to the biological father's medical history.

As you think about the entire situation, as well as about other alternatives such as adoption or structuring your life without a child, you may want to talk with others who have used DI or with an infertility counseling or educational group such as Resolve, Inc. (see Resources). The procedure isn't right for everybody and raises different questions for different people.

Some married women have said that they felt as though they were committing adultery. (The Roman Catholic and Orthodox Jewish religions do consider DI adultery.) A partner may not feel as involved in the pregnancy or parenthood as you had hoped, because the baby isn't his or her biological child. If you value genetic continuity and family resemblances highly, then DI is not for you. Think about what you will tell close friends and family, and—most important—what you will tell your child. Many parents in the past have kept DI a secret, perhaps to protect the man from the embarrassment of having people know he is infertile. (Fertility and sexual potency—particularly in the sense of the ability to achieve erection and ejaculation—are very often mistakenly linked and overvalued.) Don't assume from the start that you must be secretive or, conversely, tell all.

Some people feel more comfortable with a carefully worded consent form, signed by all parties—the woman who plans to be inseminated, her partner (if she has one), the sperm donor and preferably also his partner (if he has one). Such a contract can spell out future financial obligations and visitation rights for the donor (if he is to have any) and for partners in case of separation or divorce. However, courts don't have to honor such a contract if they decide that some other arrangement would be in the child's best interest. What's more, some lawyers think that it is a mistake for the recipient or donor of sperm to sign anything, since a signature could be construed as an admission of paternity that could be used against either of them in later litigation.*

Under proper circumstances, DI may be right. Two lesbian partners, who plan to raise children together, told about the bond it created between

---

*There is preliminary evidence that more women are contracting pelvic inflammatory disease as a result of DI (see p. 588).
†The legal status of DI differs in different states and is sometimes unclear. Some states have considered children conceived by DI to be "illegitimate"; others acknowledge paternity of the social father. The legal ground is shifting as DI becomes more widespread, so it is a good idea to be aware of the situation in your state.

---

*An excellent resource for anyone choosing DI is *Lesbians Choosing Motherhood: Legal Implications of Donor Insemination and Co-Parenting* edited by Maria Gil de la Madrid. (See Resources.)

them for the one to help the other with her insemination. Another woman, more ambivalent, said:

Our daughter is really extraordinary—enormous energy, very strong-willed and totally different-looking from either of us. I am reminded constantly that her father was a stranger.

And one wrote:

My husband and I had more than our share of doubts right up until the moment of our daughter's birth. When we saw our baby girl, all our doubts disappeared.

SURROGATE MOTHERHOOD

Surrogate motherhood (more appropriately called *contract motherhood*) is extremely controversial. As it is most often practiced in the United States, one woman—the so-called surrogate—contracts with a man to be inseminated with his sperm and to bear a child that she will turn over to him at birth. Typically, the man is married and his wife adopts the baby. The surrogate is paid her expenses and a fee (usually around $10,000). Also, a mediating agency and/or lawyer gets fees ranging from $10,000 to $25,000. As of 1990, there have been about 4,000 such births in this country.

There are also *gestational surrogacy* arrangements in which the contracting woman has no genetic relationship to the child. The eggs and sperm of the contracting couple are brought together in a laboratory and the resulting embryo then implanted in the surrogate. As of 1990, there were eighty such births.

Surrogacy appeals to some heterosexual couples in which the woman cannot get pregnant or carry a fetus to term, whereas her partner produces normal amounts of active sperm. It also affords possibilities for gay male couples, lesbians, single heterosexual women or men—any people who want to parent their own biological children but for a variety of reasons are not in a position to do so.

As you may imagine, this enterprise raises a host of social, legal and financial questions. Our strongest concern is that this option puts pressure on some of us to "rent out" our bodies for most of a year as a way to earn money. Can we really contract to give up a child before we become pregnant and be sure that we'll be able to live with the decision once the baby is born? Aren't the issues currently being raised by birthmothers who have given up children for adoption likely to surface for surrogate mothers?

Some surrogate mothers have in fact changed their minds and wanted to keep the child. Some succeeded in doing so, whereas others didn't, sometimes after painful legal battles. The question of whether or not such contracts signed beforehand should be legally binding after birth is now being debated in many state legislatures.

It is also far from obvious what the couple's obligations should be if they separate or change their minds during the pregnancy. And what if the baby they contracted for is born with an unanticipated health problem? Can they go back on the contract? And must the biological mother then care for it, or does a judge decide whose child it is?

The economics are also complicated. Some surrogate mothers have asked to be paid only for their expenses, saying that they want to give the child as a gift to women who cannot bear children. For others it is a way to earn money. One surrogate mother said, "It's a business endeavor that satisfies monetary needs and emotional needs." But what is a fair price? Even a $10,000 fee provides a contract mother with only $1.57 per hour.

Concerned about the issues of enforcing contracts, the fine line between "gestational services" and the actual "purchasing" of a child and the potential problems for children of surrogacy arrangements, the National Women's Health Network issued this statement in 1987:

1. *Commercial surrogacy arrangements are contrary to public policy and existing laws, disregard the value of human life, exploit women, and should be prohibited by law.*

2. *Laws against commercial surrogacy arrangements should be directed against any party to such an arrangement including, but not limited to, the man and/or woman who seek to purchase a child, the woman who carries and/or gives birth to the child, the agency or attorneys who are paid for the transaction, the physician or medical center which is paid for the medical testing and procedures, and any other brokers to the arrangement.*

3. *All surrogacy contracts or agreements should be unenforceable, because no woman should be forced to give up a child based on a surrender signed prior to conception or birth. The gestational mother—the woman who gives birth to the child—is, and should continue to be recognized as, the mother for all legal purposes. Furthermore, surrogacy contracts violate existing laws and public policy.*

Other feminists disagree, arguing that paid surrogacy enhances choices for all parties involved. The books by Andrews and Field (see Resources) offer a much fuller discussion of this controversy.

ASSISTED REPRODUCTIVE TECHNOLOGIES

In vitro fertilization (IVF) is a biologically and technically complicated procedure that is still experimental in many respects.

It is intended primarily for women whose ovaries and uterus appear to function normally, but whose fallopian tubes are blocked or don't function properly so the egg cannot get to the uterus.

Every year 20,000 couples undergo IVF in this country, resulting in 2,000 babies born as of 1990. Though IVF costs between $8,000 and $10,000, plus the medical expenses associated with pregnancy and birth, many women still seek to be screened to determine whether IVF might help them.

In vitro is Latin for "in glass." In IVF, the technical feat is to extract a ripe egg from the ovary, fertilize it with sperm in a glass dish and get the embryo back into the womb. The first successful IVF and subsequent implantation was achieved in England in November 1977 and resulted in the birth of Louise Brown.

Different physicians and clinics are developing their own modifications, but the procedure involves these steps:

1. To trigger the development of "good follicles," women are given combinations of various hormones including an LhRh agonist (for example, Lupron), HMG (Pergonal), clomiphene citrate and HCG. Ultrasound monitoring of the follicles and frequent blood tests to check hormone levels are required. (About 10–20 percent of women entering IVF programs are canceled at this point because of poor follicle development.

2. At a precise time, the eggs are retrieved from the ovary using ultrasound-guided needle aspiration. While a woman is under light sedation, a thin needle is inserted into the vagina and through the vaginal wall in order to remove the mature egg(s) from the ovarian follicles. Local anesthesia is often used to numb the upper vaginal wall. The eggs are then mixed with sperm.

3. If fertilization takes place, the embryos are transplanted to the uterus when they reach the four- to eight-cell stage. In order to increase implantation rates many programs put two to eight embryos into a woman's uterus. Any additional embryos can be frozen if the couple has designated this beforehand. (The frozen embryos can be thawed and used later if the initial IVF cycle fails. About 50 percent of frozen embryos survive the thawing process, and 10 percent result in pregnancy.)

4. Twelve to fourteen days after the embryo transfer, a pregnancy test can be done. If the test is positive, progesterone shots are continued for up to twelve weeks. Only 10 to 15 percent of women undergoing IVF get to this point.

IVF is an expensive and rigorous experience. If you choose to undergo IVF, it is important to select a clinic that is getting good pregnancy results. Ask what the clinical pregnancy rate is per embryo transfer for women of your age and with your diagnosis. For example, a twenty-year-old woman with tubal damage has a much higher chance of success than a forty-year-old woman with endometriosis. Don't be fooled by distorted reports of success rates. As Dr. Richard Marrs, director of the Institute of Reproductive Medicine at Good Samaritan Hospital in Los Angeles, has said, "Regulation needs to take place because there is a lot of exploitation that's going on."[3] You can contact Resolve (see Chapter 22's Resources) for more specific information on specific IVF clinics.

It is also important to know the risks involved with IVF. The ectopic (tubal) pregnancy rate is about 7 percent, miscarriage rates are as high as 22 to 24 percent, some women have side effects from the hormonal treatments and there is an increased chance of multiple pregnancies (which are riskier than single pregnancies). Twins occur in one of every three IVF pregnancies, triplets in one out of every ten. Clomiphene citrate and HMG are also suspected risk factors for ovarian cancer. Good studies are still needed to determine the true risks of taking these drugs.[4]

Several other techniques have resulted from IVF. In *gamete intrafallopian transfer* (GIFT), the egg is "harvested" by ultrasound-guided needle aspiration (as in IVF). Egg and sperm are mixed during a laparoscopy and put back in the fallopian tube. GIFT has a higher success rate than IVF, but it does not document fertilization. *Zygote intrafallopian transfer* (ZIFT) involves the laparascopic "harvesting" of egg and sperm, their fertilization outside a woman's body and then placement of the embryo (at an early stage of cell division) in the fallopian tubes. ZIFT has a 30 percent success rate in some studies. *Micromanipulation* of the egg (making a small opening in the outer membrane of the egg wall) is another technique used to increase fertilization rates.

Donor egg IVF has become an option for women with premature ovarian failure (early menopause) or who have diseases or disabilities that may be genetically transferred. In these cases, either a woman or her clinic finds another woman willing to donate her eggs. This donor will have the same ovulation induction hormone treatment as any woman undergoing IVF, but once her eggs are retrieved and fertilized, any resulting embryos will be placed in the uterus of the woman seeking to become pregnant. There is a 30 to 40 percent pregnancy rate for women with premature ovarian failure using this option. They are, of course, not genetically related to the fetuses they carry as a result of donor egg IVF.

Most physicians who use IVF believe that the risks are negligible. They argue that if an egg or embryo is damaged, it simply won't develop. But we don't know whether that's true until thousands of babies conceived *in vitro* have had a chance to grow up. This is why some critics of IVF, as of other reproductive technologies, have said that in this procedure, women and their babies become guinea pigs.

And what of the ethical, legal and emotional issues? A procedure that requires this much technical expertise is completely under professional control. We and our partners will never have much say about where or how we want it done. Because the pregnancies are so precious (emotionally, technically and economically), couples are under pressure to manage the prenatal period and birth just as the physicians order. Many women who have IVF are having cesareans.*

All these techniques raise profound questions too numerous to explore here. What does it mean, for example, to force multiple embryos into our uteruses and to strive for pregnancies when our natural reproductive cycles have ceased? Our dreams for a pregnancy and a biologically related child may be strong, but we must consider carefully all the costs to our health and well-being.

SEX PRESELECTION

Some couples try to choose the sex of their child for medical reasons, because certain inherited diseases—for example, hemophilia and a type of muscular dystrophy—are much more likely to affect boys than girls. But some people just feel strongly that they want to have a child only if they can be sure it will be the gender they "prefer."

Techniques for choosing the sex of a child before conception depend on the fact that a child's sex is determined by the father. The reason is as follows. All our cells contain forty-six chromosomes, which come in twenty-three pairs. We get one member of each pair from our mother, the other from our father. One of the twenty-three pairs determines sex. They are the *sex chromosomes*, called X and Y. Women have two X chromosomes; men have one X and one Y. Mature eggs and sperm contain only one member of each chromosome pair and therefore only one sex chromosome. Since a woman has only X chromosomes, all her eggs contain an X. Since a man is XY, about half his sperm cells contain an X chromosome and half a Y. If an egg (which is always X) is fertilized by a sperm that contains an X, the child will be a girl (XX); if it is fertilized by a sperm that contains a Y, the child will be a boy (XY).

Methods of sex preselection try to favor the X-

As thousands of women try to enroll in IVF programs, we must question why it is that many of us gladly accept painful medical interventions and unknown health risks in order to bear a child. We must look at the socialization we undergo as women that makes childbearing seem more important than our own health and well-being. We mustn't feel pressured by the fact that this technology now is available. *There is nothing wrong with us as women if we decide not to become involved with complicated, expensive and experimental procedures whose risks cannot be known with certainty for a long time.*

Clearly the procedure is sufficiently expensive, complex and of such uncertain outcome that it can serve relatively few of us. Despite great promises that, with more experience, IVF clinics would improve their success rates, the fact is that success rates remain about the same as we begin the 1990s.[5] Meanwhile, many of us will risk invasive exploratory procedures and repeated attempts at IVF only to end up disappointed. In some cases this happens because the medical profession emphasizes high-technology "solutions" to preventable problems instead of stressing simple preventive measures that could benefit many more of us. Many of us who end up wanting IVF would not need it if we had known earlier about possible *preventable* long-term effects of untreated or mistreated pelvic inflammatory and sexually transmitted diseases, and about risks from IUDs.

---

or the Y-bearing sperm, but none is very effective. They rely on observations that Y-bearing sperm tend to swim faster and would be more easily damaged by the acidic environment of the vagina than X-bearing sperm, whereas X-bearing sperm appear to live longer and be more sensitive to the alkalinity in the cervix, uterus and fallopian tubes.

One recommendation is that to improve the likelihood of conceiving a girl, you should have intercourse thirty-six to forty-eight hours before ovulation and, for a boy, try delaying intercourse until two to twenty-four hours before you ovulate (see Fertility Observation, p. 276). Confusingly, other researchers have come up with the opposite recommendation: that intercourse a few days before ovulation weights chances in favor of boys,

---

*Cesareans always give doctors more control over the birth without necessarily improving birth outcomes. Many physicians prefer to do cesareans with "precious pregnancies," regardless of how the woman wishes to give birth. Some women who require IVF also have medical complications that may make a cesarean necessary.

intercourse at the time of ovulation very slightly in favor of girls.

Another recommended technique makes use mainly of the differences in the sensitivities of X and Y sperm to acid and alkali. Proponents suggest that to load the dice in favor of a girl, you use a mildly acidic douche (two tablespoons of white vinegar in a quart of lukewarm water) before intercourse, allow only shallow penetration of the penis (so that the sperm must spend a longer time in the acidic environment of the vagina), be in a face-to-face position and avoid orgasm, which increases the alkalinity of the vagina. If you prefer a boy, you use an alkaline douche (two tablespoons of baking soda in a quart of water) and reverse the other conditions. Neither method guarantees success, but they may improve chances.

Obviously these methods deal only in probabilities. If your genetic history is such that a male child would have a fifty-fifty chance of inheriting a disease you want to avoid, you may want to be more certain. In that case, you can have a physician determine the fetus's sex after you are pregnant, so that you can have a choice of having an abortion if it is male or be more prepared for coping with the disease both emotionally and practically should you decide to continue the pregnancy. Increasing numbers of sex-linked diseases can now be diagnosed in the fetus, so that you don't need to consider abortion unless prenatal tests show that the fetus you are carrying has the disease* (see p. 428 for a discussion of prenatal diagnosis).

In the United States, fetal sex usually is determined by amniocentesis, which cannot be done until about the fourteenth week of pregnancy. Since it takes another three or four weeks to complete the chromosomal analysis, if you decide to abort, it means a second-trimester abortion—more painful, risky and psychologically difficult than early abortion.

Abortion for reasons of sex selection has become a focal point of the antiabortion movement, which has attempted to manipulate qualms about this practice into opposition to all abortions. Exaggerating the incidence of sex selection abortions, they claim this is further evidence of the callousness and selfishness of those who advocate choice.

Feminists in other countries such as India have protested sex selection for different reasons. Where there has been strong cultural pressure to bear male children, women have used amniocen-

tesis plus abortion to avoid giving birth to female children. In India, for example, the situation is so serious that the usual sex ratio has been reversed, resulting in a significant demographic imbalance in favor of men. Indian feminists have called for an end to the widespread use of amniocentesis and chorionic villus tests for sex selection. Although this practice is now illegal in places, it continues in a country where female infanticide is still practiced. Furthermore, the death rate for girls and women is higher than that of boys and men at every stage of their lives, because females have less access to resources, including food and medical care.

Studies have shown an almost universal preference for males, especially as first-born children. Because of this, population control advocates have supported sex selection as a way of limiting population growth. They argue that people often have more children than they really want because they keep trying for a boy. Preselecting will therefore lead to fewer children born, and if fewer girls are born, there will be fewer women bearing children in the next generation.

Among feminists there is disagreement about how best to oppose this practice and change the conditions that give rise to it. In both China and India, women's groups are engaged in public education and other political campaigns to change the societal values and attitudes toward women that are the root causes for this destruction of female fetuses. Although some advocate banning the tests, arguing that they do not offer real choices, others distrust government intervention and believe that women must ultimately make their own decisions. Some oppose sex selection, seeing it as part of a growing trend to create "made to order" children. Still others see the effort to police sex selection as part of the effort to control and criminalize the behavior of pregnant women.

Although we may disagree about the morality of sex preselection or what to do about it, we must recognize the different realities in women's lives and the importance of supporting each woman's right to make her own reproductive decisions.

CONCLUSION

In conclusion, many of us in the collective would not advise using any of these technologies except DI, unless we are fully aware of the physical, emotional and financial burdens often involved. Although some of us know from personal experience the strong desire many women feel to have a biological child, these techniques involve so much social and medical manipulation of women and of our reproductive systems that we think the risks and costs are too high.

---

*A group of women advising us on living with a physical disability expressed a concern about the pressure to have an abortion in cases of predicted disability, as each one was glad herself to be alive. If this society were less demanding of physical "perfection" and more helpful to parents and children with special needs, women might worry less about having a child with special health problems.

NOTES

1. Lesley and John Brown with Sue Freeman. *Our Miracle Called Louise.* London: Magnum Books, 1979, p. 83.

2. Barbara Eck Menning. "The Emotional Needs of Infertile Couples," *Fertility and Sterility*, Vol. 34, No. 4 (October 1980), pp. 313–9.

3. Richard Marrs. *ObGyn News*, Vol. 23, No. 14 (July 15–31, 1988).

4. Patricia A. St. Clair Stephenson. "The risks associated with ovulation induction," *Iatrogenics*, Vol. 1, 1991, pp. 7–16.

5. Medical Research International and Society for Assisted Reproductive Technology (SART). "In vitro fertilization-embryo transfer (IVF-ET) in the United States: 1990 results from the IVF-ET Registry," *Fertility and Sterility*, Vol. 57, No. 1 (January 1992), pp. 15–24. Data collection for this article was supported by a contract from Serono Laboratories, Inc., which markets fertility drugs.

RESOURCES

Books

Andrews, Lori. *Between Strangers: Surrogate Mothers, Expectant Fathers and Brave New Babies.* New York: Harper & Row, 1989.

Arditti, Rita, et al., eds. *Test Tube Women: What Future for Motherhood?* Boston: Routledge and Kegan Paul, 1985.

Baruch, Elaine Hoffman, et al., eds. *Embryos, Ethics and Women's Rights: Exploring the New Reproductive Technologies.* New York: Harrington Park Press, 1988.

Birke, Lynda, Susan Himmelweit and Gail Vines. *Tomorrow's Child: Reproductive Technologies in the '90's.* London: Virago Press, 1990.

Cohen, Sherrill, and Nadine Taub, eds. *Reproductive Law for the 1990's.* Clifton, NJ: Humana Press, 1989.

Corea, Gena. *The Mother Machine: Reproductive Technology from Artificial Insemination to Artificial Wombs.* New York: Harper & Row, 1985.

de la Madrid, Maria Gil. *Lesbians Choosing Motherhood: Legal Implications for Donor Insemination and Co-Parenting*, 2nd ed. San Francisco: National Center for Lesbian Rights, 1991.

Field, Martha A. *Surrogate Motherhood: The Legal and Human Issues.* Cambridge, MA: Harvard University Press, 1988.

Klein, Renate D. *Infertility: Women Speak Out about Their Experiences of Reproductive Medicine.* Boston: Pandora Press, 1989.

Noble, Elizabeth. *Having Your Baby by Donor Insemination: A Complete Resource Guide.* Boston: Houghton Mifflin, 1987.

Rothman, Barbara Katz. *The Tentative Pregnancy: Prenatal Diagnosis and the Future of Motherhood.* New York: Penguin, 1986.

———. *Recreating Motherhood: Ideology and Technology in a Patriarchal Society.* New York: W.W. Norton, 1989.

Saffron, L. *Getting Pregnant Our Own Way: A Guide to Alternative Insemination.* 1986. Available from Women's Health Information Centre, 52 Featherstone St., London, EC1, United Kingdom.

Spallone, Patricia. *Beyond Conception.* New York: Bergin & Garvey, 1989.

Spallone, Patricia, and Deborah Lynn Steinberg, eds. *Made To Order: The Myth of Reproductive and Genetic Progress.* New York: Pergamon Press, 1987.

Stanworth, Michelle. *Reproductive Technologies: Gender, Motherhood and Medicine.* Minneapolis: University of Minnesota Press, 1987.

Articles

American Fertility Society. "Ethical Considerations of the New Reproductive Technologies," *Fertility and Sterility*, Vol. 46, No. 3 (Supplement 1, 1986).

Pollitt, Katha. "When Is a Mother Not a Mother?" *The Nation* (December 31, 1990), pp. 825, 840–46.

Sandelowski, Margarete. "Compelled to Try: The Never-Enough Quality of Conceptive Technology," *Medical Anthropology Quarterly*, New Series, Vol. 5, No. 1 (March 1991).

Souer, M., R. Paulson and R. Lobo. "A Preliminary Report on Oocyte Donation Extending Reproductive Potential for Women Over 40," *New England Journal of Medicine*, Vol. 323, No. 17 (October 25, 1990), pp. 1157–60.

Periodicals

Reproductive and Genetic Engineering: Journal of International Feminist Analysis. Pergamon Press.

PART IV

Childbearing

Introduction

By Jane Pincus
and Judy Luce,
with Norma Swenson

*This introduction in previous
editions was written by Jane Pincus
and Robbie Pfeufer.*

Having a child involves the whole of a woman's social, physical, sexual and spiritual being. When you bear children, you have great strengths and capabilities—flexibility, determination, humor, endurance and inner knowledge about what feels best for you.

You also have great needs. Women have the right to have these needs met. Our society has the responsibility to provide the resources necessary for women to have healthy pregnancies and births. You have a right to love; sufficient resources, financial security and the support of friends and family; a safe environment; adequate food, rest and exercise; a skilled, wise, trusted practitioner who respects you, a comfortable and safe place of birth and continuity of care; confidence in your ability to give birth and the knowledge that people are interested in you and care about you as well as your baby.

During labor you need food and drink to keep up your strength, people around you who have confidence in you and patience with the natural unfolding of your labor. You need people to provide physical and emotional support, help you relax and sustain and guide you and freedom to move around and adopt comfortable labor positions.

After the birth, you need to be in surroundings that enable you to be with your baby whenever you want. You may need help if you are breast-feeding and a helping hand during the following days and weeks so that you can be sure your family is well cared for. You continue to need plenty of good food and rest. With your first child, you need support and encouragement in learning to be a mother. You need appropriate medical resources reasonably nearby in case of emergency. You need control over your fertility so that you can plan your pregnancies.

Woman-centered birth places women at the heart of the childbearing experience. It affirms that pregnancy and birth are normal, healthy life events. It values our strengths and our perceptions of our own needs, paying careful attention to the language we use and the life experiences we have had. It involves the use of a whole range of midwifery skills on the part of birth attendants.

In this country we could create a maternity system that would revolve around women, babies and families. If we were a more humane society, we would. We know enough about childbearing to give women confidence, banish ignorance and minimize fear. We have enough food. We could develop a network of midwives to attend the majority of births. Women would have their babies wherever and however they want, assured of skilled assistance. Physicians would provide med-

Peter Simon

The prevalent system makes it difficult to choose alternatives such as midwives, freestanding birth centers and home births. Most physicians pay little attention to the overwhelming evidence in lay and scientific literature that alternatives to conventional obstetrics are better and safer for most women and babies. Moreover, they often actively harass and persecute alternative practitioners and settings at every opportunity.

Because obstetrics is big business, changes come about only when middle-class white women act as "consumers," threaten to go elsewhere when dissatisfied and as citizen-activists work to effect changes in policy. Institutions make cosmetic changes when economically threatened, with a lot of strings attached: Hospitals build birthing rooms—but women must meet a long list of conditions in order to use them; fathers are "allowed" to be present at birth—but it is not always considered their right; commercial birthing chairs are installed—but they restrict women to only one labor position; nurse-midwives invited into some hospitals must perform a delicate balancing act so as not to encounter resistance or lose their jobs, meeting excessively restrictive protocols for "normal" birth.

These token modifications offer an illusion of choice, but they do not represent fundamental change. The power relationships between women and doctors remain unequal. The underlying denigrating beliefs about women's bodies and childbirth have not changed. Medical training is as narrow, shortsighted and technology-bound as ever. The average cesarean rate is 24 percent, and higher in some hospitals. Low-income women in cities and rural areas are not getting the compassionate community-based preventive care they so desperately need, and their babies are dying. The U.S. infant mortality rate is rising once again. Increasingly high medical fees for maternity care are bankrupting Medicaid and burdening average families. Many childbirth educators who genuinely want to change the system end up compromising their insights and convictions so as not to antagonize the powers that be. Many midwives also have to compromise their beliefs and practice in order to continue to be able to attend women.

Pregnant women are more frightened than ever. For a few short years in the late 1960s and early 1970s when so many of us learned about the joys and benefits of natural childbirth, we expanded our awareness of what childbirth could be like. Optimistically we believed that we could give birth the way we wanted as long as we informed practitioners about our desires. Naively we believed that we could change obstetrics. But the last decade has seen obstetrical power and practice more firmly entrenched than ever, with the proliferation of pregnancy tests and childbirth

ical backup when needed in the name of public health and community responsibility. National health insurance would guarantee care for everyone. Generous family leave and day-care policies and programs would provide job security and enable us to stay home with our new babies.

If we were able to bring about the essentials of the environment described above, most births would be natural and most babies would be fine. Instead, our obstetrical system, part of a larger medical-industrial complex, trains its physicians to consider childbearing as a potentially life-threatening situation. Women internalize this view. It focuses upon the risks and pathology of childbirth, viewing labor and birth as dangerous, unbearably painful processes, if not illnesses, to be "managed" only in hospital settings with routine use of a wide array of drugs and technologies. It ignores or suppresses the sexual, social and spiritual dimensions of childbearing. It may punish pregnant women when they do not behave in expected ways. It too often neglects or abandons women who do not meet particular income criteria. Indifferent to the circumstances of our lives, it offers medical solutions to problems caused by social and economic ills and concentrates on the most costly kinds of medical surveillance and rescue in times of crisis, upholding social and economic inequality. It pits mother against child, treating women merely as vessels for their babies. Women who have limited resources not only have to struggle with general health problems but have to confront the built-in race and class biases of the system.

technologies—their risks often undisclosed and their benefits to most women and babies unproven. Because of this increase, most women have become more vulnerable than ever to the idea that childbearing is inevitably risky and dangerous. We are overly scared that something will go wrong and often made to feel guilty and selfish when we question invasive, experimental procedures. Wanting to feel in control, or simply giving in, we become persuaded, then compelled to look beyond ourselves to blood tests, monthly ultrasound photographs and amniocentesis reports for confirmation that things are all right. Sometimes we can pick and choose among the procedures offered to find the one that makes us feel at ease and do without the rest. But the deceptively simple question, "Don't you care about your baby?" leads most women to believe that a barrage of procedures is absolutely necessary. Because they exist, they become the norm. After all, isn't everyone having them done? Thus we consent to a process of medicalization that has the ultimate effect of making us mistrust our own feelings and intuitions, our healthy bodies, our deepest selves. Said

one woman, "I feel so overwhelmed—I am consumed with deciding what tests to have. I can hardly enjoy being pregnant or cherish the changes in my body."

The technocratic orientation of each succeeding generation erodes our wealth of accumulated knowledge of childbearing and drives it undergound. Let's bring that knowledge to light and preserve it. Let's challenge the medical takeover of our bodies and souls. Let's celebrate pregnancy, birth and motherhood as natural, satisfying and strengthening events of life and honor the women who are bringing babies into this world.

*I sit here on the porch as if in a deep sleep, waiting for this unknown child. I keep hearing this far flight of strange birds going on in the mysterious air about me. How can it be explained? . . . Suddenly everything becomes alive . . . like an anemone opening itself, disclosing itself, and the very stones themselves break open like bread.**

---

*Meridel Le Sueur, "Annuciation," in *Ripening* (Old Westbury, NY: Feminist Press, 1982), p. 128.

19

Pregnancy

By Jane Pincus, with
Norma Swenson

With special thanks to Jenny
Fleming, Linda Holmes, Bebe Poor
and Becky Sarah.
*This chapter in previous editions was
written by Ruth Bell and Jane
Pincus.*

*1992 Update by Jane Pincus, with
Judy Luce, Linda Holmes, Robin
Blatt, Judi Rogers and Norma
Swenson.*

PRENATAL CARE: PREPARATION FOR PREGNANCY, LABOR AND BIRTH

Prenatal care is the care you give yourself, as well as the care you receive from friends and family. We no longer believe that it is enough just to "see the doctor regularly" or "leave it all to the doctor." When you visit your practitioner (midwife or doctor) every month and then every week, s/he is simply monitoring the care you give yourself.* When you have conditions that require watching or medical attention, you especially need to care for yourself to keep in top shape and minimize complications. Caring for yourself means that your good mothering has already begun.

Eating Well

Also read Chapter 2, "Food."

It is essential to eat well during pregnancy. Even when you are trying to get pregnant you can begin to change and improve your eating habits. Think of it as eating for yourself, for when you are healthy, most likely your baby will be healthy too.

By eating well:

- You expand your blood volume to meet the increased demands pregnancy makes on your body. Blood bathes and washes over the placenta where the exchange of oxygen and nutrients takes place.
- You help make sure that your uterus and all other tissues grow and increase in elasticity, that your baby grows to its full genetic potential and weighs as much as it should.
- Healthy birth weight, which can vary, and placental "sufficiency" increase the likelihood that labor and birth will be uncomplicated. Eating well lowers the risk of complications such as infections, anemia and toxemia in the mother and prematurity, low birth weight, stillbirth, brain damage and retardation in the baby.
- Your body stores the fats and fluids you will need when you begin to breastfeed. You will need to continue to eat and drink a lot of healthy foods and fluids after your baby is born.

Don't deprive yourself to feed other family members. You may be eligible for the WIC (Women, Infants and Children) program, a supplemental food program sponsored by the government. Designed for pregnant and lactating women, it provides milk, fruit, cereal, juice,

---

*In some places, women conduct part of their own prenatal exams (test their urine, take their own blood pressure and keep their own charts). See Maternity Center Association's self-help list (MCA address in Resources in Chapter 20, "Childbirth").

AS FOR WEIGHT GAIN, DON'T FIXATE ON A MAXIMUM NUMBER OF POUNDS. EVERY WOMAN'S METABOLISM IS DIFFERENT. IF YOU EAT WELL AND NUTRITIOUSLY, YOUR WEIGHT WILL TAKE CARE OF ITSELF. PREGNANCY IS NOT THE TIME TO DIET.

A SUGGESTED DAILY DIET FOR PREGNANCY

1. Two to four protein servings of meat, fish, poultry, cheese, tofu (soybean curd), eggs or nut-grain-bean-dairy combinations (see p. 37). If you do not drink one quart of milk a day, add additional protein foods.
2. A quart of milk (whole, skim, buttermilk) or milk equivalents (cheese, yogurt, cottage cheese). Use dry milk powder when cooking other foods. If you are allergic to dairy products, take calcium lactate. Seaweed, sesame seeds, butter, molasses and shellfish contain calcium; some tofu is also made with calcium lactate.
3. A serving of fresh, leafy green vegetables—spinach; dark, loose-leaf lettuce; broccoli; cabbage; Swiss chard; kale; collard; mustard or beet greens; alfalfa sprouts.
4. One or two vitamin C–rich foods—whole potato, grapefruit, orange, melon, green pepper, cabbage, strawberries, fruit, orange juice.
5. A yellow or orange vegetable or fruit.
6. Four to five slices of whole-grain bread, pancakes, tortillas, cornbread, or a serving of whole-grain cereal or pasta. Use wheat germ and brewers' yeast to fortify other foods.
7. Butter, fortified margarine, vegetable oil.
8. Salt to taste. (Avoid foods and drinks with needless sodium.)
9. Six to eight glasses of liquid—fruit and vegetable juices, water and herb teas. Avoid sugar-sweetened juices and colas.
10. For snacks, dried fruits, nuts, pumpkin and sunflower seeds, popcorn.

---

cheese and eggs. Contact a public prenatal clinic, your local health department or your public health nurses to find out how you can join. If you are on public assistance, a physician may request a higher food allowance from welfare for you.*

You may not be able to eat large meals, especially during early pregnancy if you are nauseous or toward the end when your uterus takes up so much room. Instead, eat smaller amounts more often. Eat regularly. Don't go for long stretches of time without food.

Special Food Needs During Pregnancy

Pregnancy increases your need for *calories and protein*. Your protein needs double. Almost all foods contain some protein. You'll also need to eat a wide *variety* of foods, as other nutrients are scattered around in different foods.

Folic Acid

Folic acid is found in green leafy vegetables. It is essential for protein synthesis in early pregnancy and also for the formation of blood and new cells. Your baby needs folic acid to grow. Symptoms of folic acid deficiency are anemia and fatigue (anemias may also have other causes). Your body doesn't store folic acid, so if you are anemic, daily supplements are necessary.

If you have taken birth control pills and are now pregnant, you may have depleted your supply of vitamins B_6 and B_{12} and folic acid and may need supplements. If you are planning to get pregnant, take folic acid supplements before pregnancy. It can reduce the incidence of spina bifida by 70 percent.

Iron

Iron is obtained from prune juice, dried fruits, legumes, blackstrap molasses, lean meat, liver, egg yolk and cooking food in iron pots and pans. It is a main component of hemoglobin, which, composed of complex molecules of protein and iron, carries oxygen to your baby and your cells. The baby also draws on your iron reserve to store iron in its liver to last for the duration of his/her milk diet after birth. You'll also need oxygen (supplied by hemoglobin) during labor for your uterus; the baby's brain cells need oxygen, too. If you eat a well-balanced, iron-rich diet, your system may contain enough iron. If not, you'll require a supplement; ask for ferrous gluconate or ferrous fumarate rather than ferrous sulfate, which tends to take vitamins out of your system. Organic iron, a

---

*For more information, contact the Children's Foundation, Suite 800, 1426 New York Avenue NW, Washington, DC 20005, (202) 347-3300, and/or your public health nurse.

natural form of iron, is available in health food stores.

Calcium

Similarly, your need for calcium increases during pregnancy and lactation.

Fluids

Fluids aid the circulation of blood and body fluids and the distribution of mineral salts and stimulate the digestion and assimilation of foods. Drink eight to ten glasses of fluids a day. Use care in drinking caffeine. Colas—*all* of them—have too much caffeine.

Weight-Gain Restriction, Salt-Free Diets, Diuretics and Diet Pills

Physicians in previous decades (and perhaps some older practitioners today) restricted weight gain and salt intake during pregnancy. They also gave women dangerous diet pills (amphetamines) and diuretics (which eliminate liquids from the body). They did so because they believed that such precautions would prevent the condition called *toxemia*, or, as it is called today, *preeclampsia*. They were mistaken. Pregnant women must be well nourished and gain weight. A reasonable amount of salt is fine, and some swelling of hands and feet (edema) is normal. By enjoying the food you eat and eating in a balanced way, you are caring well for yourself and your baby.

Practitioners, the Medical System and Nutrition

Midwives, nurse-practitioners and family practitioners emphasize eating well much more than the vast majority of obstetricians do. Medical training includes little or nothing about the science of applied nutrition. Many obstetricians consider eating well barely worthy of mention beyond the admonition to "eat a balanced diet." They are taught that they can "rescue" women and babies through technology, drugs and operations when problems arise during pregnancy, labor and birth.

Substances and Procedures to Avoid

Drugs*

Commonplace substances such as coffee, tea and over-the-counter medications like aspirin are drugs. They contain many chemicals that have

---

*Drug research gives us conflicting results because it is difficult to do scientific studies using human beings. Drug dosage can be controlled in animal studies, but as animals metabolize drugs differently from humans, results cannot be directly applied. Also, not all fetuses will be affected by the same dosage.

been investigated as possible agents causing birth defects. In the United States a pregnant women ingests, on the average, seven or eight different drugs during her pregnancy.

Most of the drugs we take during pregnancy will cross the placenta. Fetuses are extremely susceptible to drugs, especially during the first three months when vital organs are forming. We can classify direct effects of substances on pregnancy and the fetus into three different types: *teratogenic* (causing birth defects), *toxic* (having a more severe pharmacological effect on the fetus) and *addictive* (causing dependence). Although only a handful of drugs have been shown to be teratogenic, there is much we don't know about possible subtle or long-range effects of many drugs and environmental agents. Therefore, take as few drugs as possible during pregnancy. Sometimes you have to weigh the risks of an illness versus known or unknown risks of the drug in question. For example, if you have a high fever during the first months of pregnancy, your best course of action may be to take Tylenol to reduce the fever, because prolonged high fever can be teratogenic. If you have a serious condition such as diabetes or hypertension, you may need to take prescribed drugs to control the disorder, since your illness can affect the baby's development. If you are bothered by more common disorders such as headaches, nausea or constipation, first try nonmedical remedies. If they don't work, consult your practitioner before taking *any* medication, prescription or nonprescription.

It is not possible to state a level of *alcohol* regarded as safe during pregnancy. An occasional glass of wine or beer should not cause you anxiety, but you would be wise to limit your drinking to little or nothing. *Caffeine* is a common drug found in coffee, tea, chocolate and over-the-counter drugs. Present evidence, though limited, indicates that moderate amounts of coffee (three cups a day) seem to present no special risks. *Smoking*, on the other hand, has consistently been shown to have detrimental effects on fetuses. Heavy smokers (more than fifteen cigarettes a day) have a higher rate of miscarriage, stillbirths, premature and low-birth-weight babies. If you can't stop smoking altogether, then reduce the number of cigarettes you smoke and eat well.

X-Rays

Avoid them or delay them until after you have given birth. From a practical standpoint, there is no threshold for a safe level of fetal radiation exposure.[1] In some places they are being replaced by ultrasound. Avoid X-rays to assess the size of your pelvis (pelvimetry). They are dangerous, inaccurate and increase your chance of having a cesarean.

MATERNITY CARE IN A LARGER CONTEXT

Society can make it difficult for us to take good care of ourselves: "While our health is undeniably assaulted by natural forces frequently beyond our control, all too often the enemies of our physical and emotional well-being are social and political" (Angela Y. Davis, "Sick and Tired of Being Sick and Tired: The Politics of Black Women's Health," in *The Black Women's Health Book*, Seattle, WA: Seal Press, 1990, p. 19). Whenever economic, educational, social and political constraints limit people's access to good food, there are accompanying stresses which debilitate childbearing women. (Murray Enkin et al., *Effective Care in Pregnancy and Childbirth*, Oxford: Oxford University Press, 1989, p. 20.)

It is intolerable that in this wealthy democratic country we do not treat access to good health care as a fundamental human right. Every woman, man and child should be well fed, clothed, housed and protected socially and economically. Instead, physicians and hospitals spend millions of dollars on facilities, research and monitoring equipment for "high-risk" women and low-birth-weight babies. Our money could be better spent educating women and preventing the conditions that lead to serious health problems.

The United States currently ranks twenty-second among nations in its infant mortality rate (*Medical World News*, June 11, 1990, p. 46). The most recently available national infant mortality rates, from 1989, are, white babies, 7.9 per thousand; Hispanic babies, 8.5 per thousand; and black babies, 18.6 per thousand (National Center for Health Statistics, "Advance Report of Final Mortality Statistics, 1989," Vol. 40, No. 8, Supplement 2, January 2, 1992). In some areas the discrepancy is much higher (from 24 per thousand and up). These numbers do not take into account institutional misreporting and underreporting of infant mortality data.

A 1989 Harvard Medical School Dean's report states that infant deaths are caused by

the relatively poor health status of poor women; inadequate provision of prenatal care services; the growing social systems based on insurance coverage; inadequate mechanisms for providing community-based care to high-risk infants after they leave the hospital and most fundamental, the dramatic increase in the numbers of children being born into poverty, as this can always overwhelm what medical science can provide.

Jane Hodgson's review (*JAMA*, June 13, 1990, p. 3090) of Margaret Boone's book *Capital Crime: Black Infant Mortality in America* (Newbury Park, CA: Sage, 1989) contains a description of the intensive care units at Columbia Hospital for Women in Washington, DC, where tiny babies are born "incompletely formed, to be attached to electronic monitors and infusions . . . the survivors too frequently develop blindness, hearing loss, infections and permanent handicaps."

California's Native American infant mortality has been higher than in any other reported ethnic group except blacks. In December 1979, 38 percent of all pregnancies at the Pine Ridge Sioux reservation in South Dakota resulted in miscarriage before the fifth month or excessive hemorrhage, and 60 to 70 percent of the children suffered breathing problems. A study indicated that the reservation water contained pollutants and radioactive materials (Winona LaDuke, "They Always Came Back," *Sinister Wisdom* Vol. 22/23, 1979).

Physical Activity and Exercise

See also Chapter 4, "Women in Motion."

Physical activity and exercise are essential when you are pregnant. Throughout pregnancy, women swim, run, walk briskly, dance and do yoga. Use common sense when exercising. Make sure you can still speak comfortably; then you'll know you're not overdoing. If what you are doing makes you feel good, then continue.

In her book *Essential Exercises for the Childbearing Year*, Elizabeth Noble describes many exercises in detail. You can practice labor positions, such as squatting, which can increase your pelvic opening by 30 percent. See Sheila Kitzinger's book *The Experience of Childbirth* (listed in Resources) for a lot of good ideas about breathing and relaxation.

In many places, health care is not available. In Georgia, for instance, 79 out of 152 counties have no obstetrical practitioners, and 58 percent of the state's obstetricians will not offer prenatal care to uninsured women (Gail Vernon and Zuri Jordan, "Home Birth: A Matter of Choice," *Vital Signs*, October 1991, p. 15).

Many women of color and low-income women avoid available prenatal care because health professionals and institutional bureaucratic procedures humiliate them and offer little they perceive as valuable. It is not unusual to have to make nine different trips in six weeks to several different locations just to begin prenatal care and receive Medicaid eligibility ("Death by Red Tape," *New York Times*, May 19, 1991, p. 16). Difficult, sometimes tragic experiences are not uncommon:

Pregnant Black women, uninsured and without the means to pay hospital entrance fees, have been known to give birth in parking lots outside the hospitals that have refused them entrance. . . . Because so many programs designed to ameliorate the conditions of poor people . . . have been abolished or cut back in recent years, accessibility to health services has become a pressing problem (Angela Y. Davis, The Black Women's Health Book, *p. 19).*

Evelyn C. White, introducing *The Black Women's Health Book*, protests the racism that cripples the medical establishment: "Black women have had enough of the statistics that tell us that the life expectancy for whites is 75.3 years compared with 69.4 for blacks; that 52 percent of the women with AIDS are black; that more than 50 percent of black women live in a state of emotional distress . . ." (p. xv). Low-income white women are little better off as economic conditions worsen and services are cut.

Infant mortality is not a health problem . . . [it] is a social problem with health consequences . . . the solution is not primarily medical but environmental, social and educational (Marsden Wagner, "Infant Mortality in Europe: Implications for the United States," Journal of Public Health Policy *[Winter 1988], p. 473).*

Once women in poor health do arrive at the hospital, they receive the crisis-oriented interventive care that many of us have been criticizing as inappropriate for *all* childbearing women. Technology as a last resort may indeed be lifesaving for some women and babies. But it will never replace the compassionate, preventive community-based care we all need, nor does it make up for the lack of an equitable social and health care system. Many countries in Europe make provisions for caring for *all* pregnant women; we can and we should look to them for appropriate and effective models of care.

Women are getting together to help themselves. The National Black Women's Health Project has ninety-six self-help groups in twenty-two states. They are setting up community centers to do health screening and referral for pregnant women and hook them up with the social services they need. These centers will offer computerized learning programs and individualized tutorial programs, work with community members to develop job-related skills and continue holding self-help group meetings. "We hope this will be a model program that can be duplicated anywhere. . . . Our time is coming"; (Byllye Y. Avery, *The Black Women's Health Book*, p. 10; see also Chapter 26, "Organizing for Change: U.S.A.)

Putting Yourself at Ease During Pregnancy

Explore your own and your partner's greatest hopes and deepest fears about pregnancy and birth, about becoming parents. Picture what you want the birth to be like. Learn about the baby growing within you, about what happens during childbirth. Practice relaxation skills, read books. Create a community around you by finding a variety of people—your partner, friends young and old—to advise and encourage you. If you don't know any other women who are pregnant, put up a sign at the market or laundromat. *Women were never meant to go through childbearing alone.*

Childbirth Classes

Many women have met other pregnant women and learned about pregnancy and birth by attending childbirth classes.

You may or may not have a choice of classes

ELEVATOR (KEGEL) EXERCISES

It is simple to do Kegel exercises—contracting your pelvic-floor muscles. They help you prepare for childbirth.

A good way to locate the pelvic floor muscles is to spread your legs apart and to start and stop the flow of urine—your ability to do this is one indication of how strong your muscles are. Another method is to try tightening around a man's erect penis during intercourse (this will feel very pleasant to him and can help to enhance your pleasure, too). Or use one or two of your fingers.

Begin exercising these muscles by contracting hard for a second and then releasing completely. Repeat this ten times in a row to make up one group of exercises (this takes about twenty seconds). In a month's time, try to work up to twenty groups during one day (about seven minutes total). You can do this at any time—while sitting in a car or bus, while talking on the telephone, or even as a wake-up exercise. Some of us have noticed improved muscle tone (and occasionally increased pleasure during sex) in only several weeks. For more detailed instruction on Kegel exercises, consult your local childbirth group.

where you live. In large cities there is a wide range: private classes taught by nurses, midwives or physicians; hospital-based classes; prepaid health-plan classes and community-based classes taught by childbirth education organizations, Bradley and Lamaze method advocates, home birth groups and independent teachers. If no classes exist, *you can create your own* with the assistance of a layperson or professional who knows about childbearing and with the help of groups already active.*

Community-based classes are likely to be smaller and more personal than hospital classes and much richer in content. You may meet people going to different kinds of birthplaces as clients of a variety of midwives and physicians. You get a better idea of the possible choices. You may make friends who will enjoy trading child care and providing mutual parenting support for years to come.

Home birth classes can often give you the most positive and complete information about normal labor and birth; people planning other kinds of birth attend them also. They touch on a wide range of concerns—the physiology of labor and birth; visualization of the process (you imagine yourself giving birth); relaxation techniques; the importance of someone (other than hospital staff) to assist you and be your advocate; the practice of supported positions during labor; discussions of fantasies and feelings; risks of routine drugs and interventions and their occasional benefits; what it's like to breastfeed, to be parents. Couples visit with their new babies to describe their own experiences and answer questions. Films are shown.

It was the first time I'd ever seen anything be born. Hearing people talk, hearing the sounds, made it real. I see that it's a lot of work; people are working hard to make the birth happen. A person can go through all that and be fine!

Those sounds she made were upsetting. I wanted her to stop. They were so intimate, sexual. I could be making those sounds.

Every class we got to know each other better. During breaks we'd talk about our dreams, problems, questions, over apples, tea and crackers. After our babies were born we continued to meet every month for two years.

Most hospital classes tend to focus on labor and delivery and prepare you to accept hospital "management" of birth, presenting their procedures and techniques as if they were a normal and inevitable part of childbirth. Occasionally in hospitals you will find instructors strongly dedicated to your having the best possible experience.

If your hospital class doesn't suit you, change to another if you can, or take more than one kind.

The hospital class was useful in preparing couples for the emotional aspects of childbearing. . . . There were twenty people. The teacher told us about her own experiences. She stressed taking care of yourself afterwards and gave support in being assertive with hospital personnel. In the Lamaze class, the teacher was more distant but gave better information, role-played us through difficult situations. Classes were indispensable in getting Joel involved.

Women with Physical Disabilities

Many women with physical disabilities can give birth to healthy children. If you are considering

---

*To find out what's available in your area, ask public health nurses, other nurses, midwives and physicians you like. Contact your local childbirth organization: ICEA (International Childbirth Education Association), NAPSAC (InterNational Association of Parents and Professionals for Safe Alternatives in Childbirth), VBAC (Vaginal Birth After Cesarean), CPM (Cesarean Prevention Movement) or your local women's center.

Jim Harrison/Stock Boston

motherhood, you have many of the same concerns as most women. You'll want to consider how pregnancy will affect your life and to establish a community of support. More specifically, you will explore how motherhood will affect your immediate and long-term health and determine as well as you can your individual requirements. You may need to coordinate your care by bringing together your practitioner and disability specialist, if you have one; and make sure that if you go to a hospital the staff is appropriately informed and prepared to meet your needs. Also think ahead on how you can adapt child-care paraphernalia to your circumstances.

Judy Rogers and Molleen Matsamura's *Mother-to-Be: A Guide to Pregnancy and Birth for Women with Disabilities* (New York: Demos, 1992) contains interviews with thirty-six mothers who have a variety of disabilities, from mild to severe. They all encourage disabled women to consider having children. Most found that pregnancy had not been as uncomfortable or difficult as expected, and some felt better than usual during pregnancy. All of them stressed the importance of being well informed especially because they sometimes faced more risks than able-bodied women. Ann Finger's *Past Due: A Story of Disability, Pregnancy and Birth* (Seattle, WA: Seal Press, 1990) is a complex personal account emerging from her own experiences with childbearing and the women with disabilities movement. Also read Susan Browne, Debra Connors and Nancy Stern's *With the Power of Each Breath: A Disabled Woman's Anthology* (San Francisco: Cleis Press, 1985).

Childbirth preparation has become equated in the popular mind with the Lamaze method (psychoprophylaxis, "prepared" or "natural" childbirth), which teaches women how to breathe and relax in specified ways during labor and birth. In the 1960s, prepared childbirth advocates did fight for women to be awake and conscious during birth—an important advance, since during the previous forty years they had been drugged to the point of unconsciousness. Yet critics of the method point out that it fits all too well with the American way of birth, coexisting with *all* forms of intervention. We are led to believe that we are having "natural" births when in fact we are lying in bed, horizontal, motionless; our labors are accelerated by Pitocin; we are shaved, hooked to monitors, cut (episiotomy) and sometimes partially drugged. Mentally active—concentrating on breathing, panting away like machines—but physically inactive, we are not "in control" but doubly controlled by the interventions and by the breathing method itself. In the words of a labor attendant and childbirth preparation teacher:

I've seen women told to "do your breathing" as they were objecting to painful exams and procedures.

From a conversation with a midwife:

Teach women how to breathe? Why, we know how to breathe, honey—we've been doing it all our lives!

Limits to Choice

The alternatives or choices available in childbirth may not address parents' . . . concerns about maternity care adequately because the choices offered are limited, and because parents are not really free to choose. Obstetric care is organized in ways that limit choices, being a hierarchical system dominated by an engineering model of birth, in which caregivers contact parents very briefly and are themselves interchangeable, where efficiency is paramount, and where the technology that has been adopted is confining rather than freeing.[2]

In certain areas of the country where women have been working to expand birthing alternatives, you may be able to choose both practitioner and birthplace—from family practitioners and obstetricians to nurse- and independent midwives, from freestanding birth centers to home births backed up by hospitals, to hospital birthing rooms and the usual labor and delivery rooms.

However, your town or the city nearest you may have only one clinic, one hospital and one physician, or a group of physicians who have the same ideology. Economic pressures may reduce your options—the local maternity clinic has been closed down for lack of funding, the prepaid health plan you belong to limits your choices because of its stringent rules, you can only afford to use the public hospital clinic and birthing facilities, your insurance coverage restricts you to one type of care. Also, practitioner and place are usually linked: Most physicians will not attend you at home and most independent midwives cannot or will not attend you in hospitals. Laws in most states limit nurse-midwives to attending women in hospitals or birthing centers, though some states permit them to attend home births. The greatest range of choices is available mostly in a narrow, concentrated band in suburbs and edges of cities. Women in rural areas and inner-city areas have little if any real choice of attendant or place of birth. Most inner-city women are forced into clinics to be cared for by ob/gyn residents in training. In these situations, the best you and your partner can do is to be as informed and assertive as possible, and seek out supportive nurses.

Your choices are also limited by the fact that the medical establishment is just that—a *medical* system. Some books and childbirth classes generate a liberal-type illusion that it's possible to make nonmedical choices within that system. It may be possible—up to a certain point. But once in the hospital, despite books, classes, "best doctor in town" and even written statements sent beforehand to hospital administrators and nursing staff, you often have very limited control over the environment. Chance and luck play huge roles in what happens during labor: A wonderful, encouraging nurse may be on duty, or there may be a nurse who knows practically nothing about normal labor and doesn't respect your wishes. Your physician, whom you trust, may be busy with another birth or on vacation, and a doctor you've never seen before thinks your ideas absurd and does things his own way, at your expense. In addition, the presence of drugs and equipment nearby and personnel trained and eager to use them alters your choices if you don't have enough support when labor becomes intense.

If you do have real choices where you live, ask yourself, What is most important? Where and with whom will you feel most secure? You are the only one who can decide. Each situation is unique; your priorities may be different from another woman's. Also, each region has its own history of obstetrical and midwifery practice to take into account. Your choices may not always be clear and simple. In many cases, no absolute answers exist. Once you make a decision, you can remain flexible in case you want to or have to change your mind.

TYPES OF PRACTITIONERS

A nurse-midwife:

When women go to practitioners for checkups, they should walk out from every visit feeling ten feet tall! . . . Every site of care and style of care, no matter who gives it, ought not only to give surveillance but should educate and empower, should enhance every woman's feeling of her ability to do what she's doing well.

Physicians

See pp. 673–76.

Every good-sized community has physicians.

Obstetricians/gynecologists, trained primarily as surgeons, see women for brief periodic checkups, are usually in and out during labor and often arrive just before delivery. Often they practice in groups and may control childbirth practices in one hospital or throughout a whole region. They do not usually practice in rural areas. In most suburban and metropolitan areas only ob/gyns have delivery room privileges in hospitals; in teaching hospitals and medical centers all MDs will be ob/gyns or ob/gyn residents in training. Though most obstetricians are not trained to deal with *normal* labors (see p. 439, Physicians' Obstetrical Training Contributes to the Climate of Doubt), their surgical skills are invaluable in real emergencies. Their prenatal care is often seriously inadequate.

From a conversation among pregnant women:

a. I really didn't think much of the doctors at the clinic. They were very impersonal and . . . it's a real mill. . . . They want you out of there in 20 minutes.
b. So do private obstetricians. They want you out of there in 10.
c. Mine didn't even know my name *through the whole pregnancy.*[3]

When I go for checkups at the health plan office, nurses check my weight, urine and blood pressure. The doctor listens to my baby's heartbeat. They never ask me how I am feeling, what I eat, if I get enough exercise and rest or if I have any questions or problems.

Family practitioners (MDs and DOs, or osteopaths) and *general practitioners* (almost extinct) are "primary care" physicians trained in family medicine, which means that they can give basic, comprehensive care to any person of any age. They are more likely to see you as a whole person and to know other family members. Most of them have a fair amount of obstetrics experience and some specialize in obstetrics. They have delivery room privileges in most community hospitals.

The family practitioners and obstetricians who have our interests at heart listen to what we want, teach us a lot, learn from us and alter their practices as they learn.

A family practitioner:

In my relationship with families I get as much as I give. I see people doing marvelous jobs: During labor and birth they are autonomous, assertive, really pleased with themselves. To be part of their birth experiences is exciting for me in turn. My presence helps them to feel safe having babies at home.

A male family practitioner:

When I attend women in labor I am as much my woman-self as I can be. Sometimes I know when they are fully dilated, for my own stomach feels crampy. I've asked the midwives about this and they say it happens to them, too.

A mother:

When I was ready to give birth the nurse said, "Push with your mouth shut." But I thought to myself (it wasn't exactly thinking), "That's not the best way for the baby to get oxygen." I wanted to groan, so I groaned deep, loud primal groans and pushed my daughter out. My doctor was amazed. He'd never heard such sounds before. They worked so well he said he would suggest them to other women.

In a hospital birthing room:

Dr. E. checked me out during my pregnancy because I had a particular medical problem. (Otherwise the midwives he works with would have seen me.) Though he stayed with me during labor, Bonnie, my labor coach, acted as midwife, suggesting what to do, applying hot compresses. Dr. E. showed her a lot of respect, the respect she deserved to have. It tickled me to overhear him say to the medical student present, "Now, here's birth with dignity! I certainly don't need to be here."

Such physicians are rare.* Many of them are either scorned or harassed by their colleagues.

---

*See Michel Odent's *Birth Reborn* and S. Sagov et al., *Home Birth: A Practitioner's Guide to Birth Outside the Hospital*, for informed descriptions of attitudes toward childbirth and how medically trained people can change their attitudes. (Both listed in Resources in Chapter 20, "Childbirth.")

Midwives

Women have cared for childbearing women for centuries. In many communities they were recognized as "wisewomen" and consulted about issues other than childbearing—illness, abortion and child health.

In the United States today there are two main types of midwives—*certified nurse-midwives* and *independent midwives*. They often share similar philosophies about childbearing, although their education and training differ.

At the heart of midwifery lies the belief that the passage through the birth canal is a healthy experience for mother and baby. The midwife believes in the ability of a woman's body to move toward health, to compensate for irregularities and to overcome pain. She sees birth as an expression of spirit in a physical act [and] believes that the baby benefits from this creative expression and actually likes being born.[4]

In the words of a nurse-midwife working in a hospital:

I want to be where women are. I want to be where women want to be. I am fascinated to watch them be powerful. I see them emerge from their birth experiences and make changes in their own lives.

When midwives are free to practice as they want, they offer us continuous care during pregnancy, labor and birth and after the baby is born.
Midwives, *at their best,*

- Pay attention to the woman in her family context, to family dynamics. They help expectant and new parents sort out their feelings and deal with practicalities.

Suzanne Arms

- Bring to their work a strong combination of practicality and spirituality. They are concerned with the woman's well-being and satisfaction as well as with the safety of mother and baby.
- Encourage women to take charge of their care, to believe they are equal to the responsibility, to feel in control of their experience.
- Are knowledgeable about normal pregnancy, labor and birth.
- Respect the process of birth, trust the unique course of each labor, patiently watch it unfold, sustain and guide you, encourage you to find comfortable, efficient labor positions and help you ease the baby out.
- Bring you through difficult moments, sometimes turning what looks like a complicated labor into a normal one.
- Recognize complications that require a doctor's attention and call upon doctors for help when necessary.

[A midwife's] skills, besides medical techniques, include elusive abilities to intuit, evoke and channel. Her hands are among her most precious tools.[5]

For me, Janet, my nurse-midwife, meant the support I'd hoped for; for instance, coming to our apartment for my actually fairly short labor. When I thought I was really not holding up under the stress she'd say, "That was pretty intense," verifying that it was okay to be "falling apart" and that I was doing great. We ended up going to the hospital birthing room when I was pretty far along—unpleasant having to move, but it certainly kept my labor going. For me, even the pushing hurt, but again I felt such confidence that everything was going well. . . . After Jackie was born, I felt only Janet understood what I'd been through and what I was going through.

Certified Nurse-Midwives (CNMs)

More and more communities and hospitals have CNMs, nurses educated in graduate programs as specialists in normal pregnancy and birth and in well-woman care. They follow an organized program of study designed to meet present standards for knowledge, skill and judgment. Graduates are evaluated and certified after passing examinations, and each state licenses nurse-midwives to practice under its own regulations.

CNMs work in their own private practices, in private physician practices, freestanding birth centers, hospitals, health departments and sometimes homes. They *always* practice in conjunction with physicians, referring women who have problem pregnancies to them and calling upon them in situations and emergencies which require medical care, advice and/or surgical attention.

CNMs in the United States got their start in the 1920s, when nurses associated with the Frontier Nursing Service and Maternity Center Association began attending poor women in Appalachia and New York City. CNMs worked in and out of hospitals for the next fifty to sixty years. The American College of Obstetricians and Gynecologists (ACOG) waited until 1971 to recognize the profession officially. Nurse-midwives have been instrumental in creating out-of-hospital birth centers and in-hospital alternative maternity care programs in response to parents' complaints about conventional hospital care. They often attend poor women when physicians will not and fight along with clinic patients for simple changes in obstetrical routines.

It is a victory for us to enable clinic women to labor upright. . . . Otherwise they'd be flat on their backs the whole time.

Despite this excellent record, and although nurse-midwives are in increasingly high demand (most women attended by nurse-midwives prefer them to physicians), there are simply not enough of them, for the following reasons: Too few training programs exist that are acceptable to women who would choose to be midwives; for a number of years many state laws restricted or prohibited nurse-midwifery practice (rarely the case now); nurse-midwifery is a collaborative profession and nurse-midwives may find it difficult to find physicians to work with. While some physicians appreciate the quality care nurse-midwives offer, many others, especially obstetricians, consider nurse-midwifery an economic threat as well as a challenge to their competence as clinicians. As a result they may either refuse to develop the necessary cooperative relationship, attempt to prevent other physicians from doing so or punish them when they do. Also, the increasingly technological approach to birth makes it difficult to adopt a midwifery approach.

Nurse-midwives are now covered by most insurance policies. However, against all the evidence of successful midwifery practice, the malpractice rates for some obstetricians practicing with midwives are increasing.

The American College of Nurse-Midwives (ACNM) and the Midwives Alliance of North America (MANA) are now working together to try to create "direct-entry" programs for professional midwives.

MIDWIFERY CARE IS . . . PRIMARY CARE, IS SAFE, ENHANCES ACCESS, MEETS NEEDS OF VIRTUALLY ALL CHILDBEARING WOMEN, INVOLVES JUDICIOUS USE OF TECHNOLOGY, IS ASSOCIATED WITH A HIGHLY FAVORABLE LIABILITY RECORD, IS WELL-RECEIVED BY CHILDBEARING WOMEN, AND IS HIGHLY COST-EFFECTIVE.[6]

Independent Midwives

Over the past twenty years, a new group of independent midwives has come into being. They are rooted in their communities and attend women who choose to give birth at home and seek out their assistance. They acquire their skills through apprenticeship with other midwives and (sometimes) supportive physicians and through reading and study. Other women combine apprenticeship with attendance at one or several of the midwifery schools that have emerged over the past ten years in Texas, Washington, New Mexico, Colorado and Massachusetts. They become specialists in normal pregnancy, labor and birth.

Increasingly, they are the most skilled, knowledgeable and competent birth attendants in their community. They know their limits, screen pregnant women for risks and encourage them to obtain physician backup when needed. They know how to recognize labor complications, and they call for assistance when necessary.

What's unique about having the community midwife is that when I see the mother at her home and help her I'm going to see her again—we go to the same foodstore and . . . we know the same people, so there's that continuity. . . . A midwife doesn't just catch babies. A midwife is an educator as well. . . . What I see as the most powerful aspect of

---

In this set-up that man has to do away with the midwives, God is yet on his throne. . . . So don't you worry about Alabama doing away with the midwives. God is in Alabama—unh-hunh—and in other places, too.

Miss Annie Lee James, midwife
Louisville, Alabama

Miss James and many other southern granny midwives believe in keeping the faith. In fact, many of these women can trace their faithkeeping heritage to great-grandmothers who were midwives during slave times. These traditional midwives say God gave midwives their work and the powers of the supernatural will always be present to guide them.

As recently as 1950, the majority of all black babies born in the South were attended by granny midwives, primarily older, self-educated black women. Today, however, granny midwives' hands provide care for less than 1 percent of childbearing mothers. White granny midwives practicing mostly in Appalachian areas and Hispanic grannies in the southeastern United States have also been legally eradicated or forced underground.

Besides their profound sense of spirituality, granny midwives were particularly sensitive in understanding their clients' emotional, social and psychological needs. Midwives, for example, often waited on generations of the same family. ("Waited on" is an expression used by traditional southern midwives to describe their childbirth attendant activities.) Other aspects of their community roles as midwives included counselor for baby ills, advisor for women's health problems, household support person for postpartum mothers, adviser on gynecological problems, community her-

bologist and general healer. Midwives who maintained culturally based expressions around the birth event were also recognized as ritual specialists.

As for actual midwifery practices, these midwives were precursors to the current wave of birthing alternatives. Traditional grannies kept their mammas stirring, as they say, during labor. These women were masters of various massage techniques that they applied during pregnancy and birth. Many grannies assisted mothers in using the traditional birthing positions taught to them by their mothers or the community's elder midwives; midwives recognized the wisdom of stooping, kneeling or squatting to make birthing much easier. Most of these traditions are African and are still alive in African culture today. Many granny midwives remain proud of their knowledge of the use of various teas as purgatives, labor stimulants and muscle relaxants.

Although traditional granny midwife practices no longer flourish, they are being increasingly recognized. Newly published oral histories and other historical records are linking today's midwife with her midwife roots. Contemporary midwives are finding that the traditional midwife was skilled both in assisting normal childbirth and in attending more complicated births such as twins, triplets and breeches. Now, various organizations, including the Midwives' Association of North America (MANA), the Black Women's Health Project and the Childbearers of African Descent (CPAD), are embracing the granny midwife. The granny midwife's stories are valuable to all women working to sustain the midwife-attended homebirth tradition.

—Linda Holmes

[the Traditional Childbearing Group] is that we teach Black empowerment . . . we want you to know that you're somebody. . . . You have to love yourself, you have to love your unborn baby and that your baby's being born Black. It already has something against it. You're all it's got and you have to get yourself empowered to keep this baby alive, so that he or she can make and be the great spirit that's meant to be. . . . Go back to our history. Start with someone in your family who knows the power of your family line. You have to honor yourself and be proud so that you can maintain your pregnancy and do it with dignity by taking care of yourself. You can read. You can eat right. . . . Things you can control, let's start with that and then we can challenge the system.[7]

In somewhat the same way that nurse-midwives are meeting standards and offering peer support, so women in the best independent midwifery communities keep in constant communication about their work.

Midwives are actively engaged in developing and maintaining communication with the medical community so that women will have the best possible care. They also try to educate physicians, nurses and medical personnel about the competency of midwives and the benefits and limits of midwifery care.

Although midwives are often the best practitioners for childbearing women, they differ in personality and practice. You'll want to interview a midwife as you would a physician, looking for competence, flexibility and empathy. You'll want to communicate your needs and desires and see if her commitments and her life-style will enable her to give you the care you want. Some certified nurse-midwives have a more medicalized approach than others, especially when they work in hospitals rather than in freestanding birth centers or in homes. Some independent midwives are able to keep a clearer vision of what normal childbirth is like than can women working in more medicalized settings. Independent midwives can differ greatly in levels of experience and the manner in which they acquire their skills. Be sure to inquire.

Choosing a Practitioner

Check out the options where you live. Get names of practitioners from people you know and trust; from local childbirth groups, childbirth teachers, women's health groups, the American College of Nurse-Midwives, MCA, NAPSAC, ICEA or the BWHBC (see Resources in Chapter 20, "Childbirth," and see Appendix, pp. 425–26).

Once you know what choices are available, look around. Be as clear as you can about the kind of pregnancy, birth and portpartum experience you want. Ask other women who have had babies recently, "What happened?" Then visit practitioners

or phone them, and ask them about their beliefs and practices. Some will treat you well and welcome your questions. Some physicians may be resentful, even hostile, at your efforts to evaluate them, because they aren't used to it. Persist—you have a right to make an informed choice.

As you speak with practitioners, state your preferences. Ask questions clearly and tactfully; aim to communicate well from the start. Ask for equally clear and specific answers. Bring someone with you, preferably the person who will share pregnancy, birth and child care with you, for company and support, and to help you remember what you want to ask. Trust your own instincts. If you think that the practitioner resists or resents your

---

SAFETY

We all want to be "safe." None of us wants to risk our own or our children's lives. From childhood we are taught that hospitals are the place to go when we are injured, when our lives are in danger. These beliefs extend to childbirth. It is true that maternal mortality rates in hospitals are good. They improved most dramatically in the 1940s when antibiotics were introduced. But pregnancy and birth are not illnesses. Hospitals are not necessarily the best places to have babies. It is difficult for many women to hear negative statistics and facts about hospital care. We are taught to believe that infant or maternal deaths in the hospital are unavoidable, whereas if they happen during a home birth they could have been prevented. Marjorie Tew, a medical research statistician who set out to prove the safety of hospital birth, found the opposite: that increased hospitalization for birth was *not* responsible for decreased maternal and infant mortality (see *Safer Childbirth*, in Resources), as obstetricians have been taught and would have us believe. Instead, safety depends mainly on the mother's good health and the skill and vigilance of her birth attendants.

It may be true that we are "safest" where we feel the most comfortable. It is also true that many people use the concept of "safety" as a form of intimidation, which prevents some women from seeking alternatives that would be more compatible with their values and beliefs. Think about what the people in your life and you yourself mean by "safety."

questions, it should not have to be your task at this time to educate him or her, though if you live in an area of limited choice you may have to. Especially important: If, during the course of your relationship with your practitioner, you feel dissatisfied with answers to your questions, or demeaned, then consider changing if possible.

It can be hard even to think of switching. Often you feel unaccountably loyal even to a person who makes you uncomfortable, hurts you in some way, or whom you actively dislike. More emotional than usual during pregnancy, you may hesitate to make such a big change, especially if you are feeling unsure of yourself. Ask your partner and friends to help you. Once you decide, you may find it easy and strengthening to choose someone else. It is never too late to switch.

I was in labor for two days at the hospital. My labor wasn't progressing fast enough for my doctor. He was angry at me because I refused to have it speeded up by Pitocin. I knew I was doing fine. Finally the hospital decided I wasn't in labor (at five centimeters' dilation!). My doctor sent me home. As soon as I got home my labor picked up and became so intense I knew I was about to give birth. My husband rushed me to another hospital (I was afraid to return to the first—no way!) and I had the baby then and there, attended by the very surprised nurse-midwife on duty!

HOSPITAL BIRTH

Also see Chapter 20, "Childbirth."

When you choose a practitioner or a clinic, you are usually choosing a hospital, too. Most hospitals find it easier to treat all women the same way. Hospital routines may or may not coincide with those of your practitioner. Learn what you can. (See Appendix for questions to ask.) Take a tour early so that the surroundings become familiar. Ask questions. Talk with the nurses, too, if you can. Some nurses encourage women to have as natural births as possible.

Deciding

Actually, if there were a birth center nearby, I'd have my baby there. But since there isn't, and since I'm completely healthy, I don't want to go to a hospital and be made to feel unhealthy. We're having a home birth with a very fine midwife. The more I learn, the more I'm sure that's what I want.

I chose the hospital because I wanted the whole experience to be separate from the rest of my life, and I felt safest there.

It would freak out our landlords if we gave birth in our apartment. I don't feel at home there anyway, and have no special attachment to it. I'm also a little nervous. So we're planning to use the hospital birthing room. Our doctor is a family practitioner.

I had my first two children in a hospital. Both were good experiences, but after having a home birth I know what a truly good experience is. I felt rested, healthy, ready to have a baby. My husband was as involved, eager and interested as he could be. I wanted to have the least intervention possible. My friends were all around me. It's incredible to think about doing the hardest, most concentrated intense work you will ever do in your life in an unfamiliar place—the most intimate experience and you are sharing it with strangers. Here I was in my own bed, my own clothes, in an atmosphere so familiar.

Another factor against home birth was having to deal with such "stuff." It was complicated-sounding getting everything set up—backups, et cetera. And I didn't really want to deal with all the people who would be appalled, the explaining we'd have to do. Everyone (like my mother) was satisfied with the idea of a nurse-midwife. I could say, "Oh, yes, the doctors are there if needed"; "It's in a medical facility"; et cetera.

I was aware of the home birth movement, but for me I couldn't do it comfortably. If anything happened, I'd never forgive myself. My parents would never forgive me. But I know childbirth is a fairly normal process so I didn't want to go to the Boston crisis centers. I wanted a labor coach because I wanted to stay home as long as possible during labor. So I chose Dr. M. and the birthing room of the small hospital he worked at.

Hospital Birthing Rooms

Many hospitals offer birthing rooms, sometimes called *alternative birth centers, not* to be confused with freestanding birth centers. The mere existence of a birthing room does not guarantee you a more autonomous labor and delivery. If someone else has gone into labor ahead of you, it may not even be available. In some places birthing-room regulations are so stringent that you must meet rigid criteria to be "eligible." Then, when you are "allowed" to use it, the moment your labor deviates from a mythical "norm" you may be transferred to a conventional labor room. You may feel you have to prove yourself, an added stress that can make you tense and slow your labor. Only when hospital staff and administration respect the noninterventionist policy behind a birthing room is it a *real* alternative. A midwife describing the birthing room at her local hospital:

It's a really casual place. I went over and sat on the rug. [The] woman and her husband were dancing together . . . they were cheek to cheek . . . just lost in their own worlds. After a while he opened his eyes . . . and gave me this incredible smile. He said, "Oh, this is the prom we never had." It was as if we were watching a ballet of lovers. She would pull herself away from him and . . . undulate and wriggle and boogie . . . and he'd come to her and massage her. . . . When the woman would look at us—you know how they're so far out there, they need a tether—she'd look, and all we had to do was smile and nod our heads . . . then, all of a sudden she said, "Oh damn! unnh! I'm pushing already! I was having such a great time!"[8]

FREESTANDING BIRTH CENTERS

Freestanding birth centers are homelike primary care centers with access to specialist consultation and hospital acute care services as needed. Although nurse-midwives operate or staff 80 percent of the 135 centers in the United States, obstetricians and family physicians who support a more natural approach to birth are increasingly interested in them. The birth center philosophy is simple—that pregnancy and birth are normal until proven otherwise. Programs focus upon safe and sensitive care, promoting family health and enhancing your confidence in your body and your ability to give birth and nurture your newborn. Practitioners encourage families to become involved and participate in the program of care and the celebration of a new life.

A study of almost 12,000 women in freestanding birth centers published in the *New England Journal of Medicine* concluded that "birth centers offer a savings in cost and minimize the rate of cesarean section" and that "few innovations in health care promise lower cost, greater availability and a high degree of satisfaction with a comparable degree of safety."[9] The cesarean section rate in the National Birth Center Study was 4.4 percent* compared to 24 percent nationally. The National Association of Childbearing Centers' annual surveys of charges consistently report a savings of 30 to 50 percent over in-hospital care for normal birth. Most insurers, including CHAMPUS and Medicaid, pay for birth center services. This American innovation is receiving increasing international attention as the world struggles to provide affordable, continued quality care to all

women and childbearing families. Look for centers licensed by the state and/or accredited by the Commission for Accreditation of Freestanding Birth Centers. Call the NACC (in Chapter 20's Resources) for the birth center nearest you.

A midwife describes the Childbearing Center of Morris Heights, in the Bronx, New York:

[This center] is just one small model of what women in a community can do when they are given access to resources, to education and to policy. . . . I feel that [we have] an ideal program for teen-agers because they really feel nurtured. We've done a lot of four-month parenting programs that a percentage of the girls go through which really helps in trying to have them feel competent. . . . We held grandmother brunches . . . to try to reach the older women in the community . . . and we tried to explain about the kind of care we considered the highest quality because it combined the best of midwifery tradition with access to modern health care. It was, in fact, a process of reeducating and ourselves being educated as to the needs of the people with whom we were working. . . . We have [community] women . . . fully participating in the running of the birthing center.[10]

HOME BIRTH

Home birth offers you the chance to labor and give birth in familiar surroundings and to choose your own attendants. You may want to invite family and friends to share the wonder of birth and welcome the new baby. At home you can engage in a whole range of pleasurable activities that make you happy and make labor bearable. Home provides the opportunity to have a birth that is not interfered with. The rhythm of your labor will be respected and your unique needs addressed. Birth is a family event, and there will be no disruption of family bonds. After the birth you can relax, eat the food you like, be cared for and get to know your baby without institutional interference, pressures and expectations. You have all the time in the world.

If you are physically and emotionally healthy, eating well, getting exercise; if your pregnancy progresses normally; if you are supported and encouraged by family and friends, then you may be reasonably certain that things will go well and that your labor will be successful and your baby will be healthy. Remember that prenatal care is the care we give ourselves in pregnancy. Midwifery care is oriented toward health promotion and prevention of complications. A few insurance policies will reimburse independent midwives for home birth service.

In this country if you choose to give birth at home, you are swimming against the cultural

---

*Hospital "birth centers" have higher rates.

stream and you will have to take a great deal of initiative and responsibility in planning for the birth. There is institutional opposition to home birth. Women who plan to give birth at home are often denied prenatal care or backup emergency care by local obstetricians who are openly hostile and say, "We can't afford the risk." Most physicians oppose home birth outright. They may frighten you with horrible tales of what might happen without discussing ways of making home birth safe. They may not be able to prescreen adequately for risks or provide emergency backups. They will ignore excellent statistics from Europe and our own Kentucky Frontier Nursing Service. Behind this smoke screen lie other, sometimes unspoken, factors: Home births are inconvenient for physicians; it is frightening for them to be away from all their hospital equipment; it is psychologically threatening for them to be the invited guest in your home, where you set the tone and they are not in complete control. Fear of malpractice suits and peer condemnation are added issues.

Most complications of childbirth can be handled without difficulty by a practitioner experienced in normal births at home (see Midwives, p. 409). There is almost always enough time to get more specialized help. Birth is not risk-free anywhere. The times when hospital care unexpectedly becomes instantaneously necessary are rare.* A matched, controlled study comparing the outcomes of 1,046 home births to 1,046 hospital births, found no significant differences in maternal or infant mortality or morbidity.[11]

While hospital emergency rooms are required by law to accept anyone who appears for emergency care, both parents and birth attendants feel more comfortable knowing that they have made arrangements in advance for such an emergency transfer in case it becomes necessary.

Birth attendants have different criteria for transferring a birth to the hospital. Their decisions may vary depending on the nature of the problem, their experience, the equipment available, their agreements with supporting physicians and the nature of the backup facility as well as its distance from the birth and the women they are attending.

It was a really beautiful thing to do—not only to be freed from the atmosphere and personnel of the hos-

pital (and who knows what it means for a newborn to see wood walls and carpeted floor, to smell real human smells, to feel wool and cotton and flannel clothes instead of starchy, white, deodorized . . .) but also to know that my body and her body knew what to do, and probably did it better than any doctors could. She was crying before the push that sent her into the world had faded and was wide awake from the start.

THE PREGNANCY ITSELF

During your pregnancy, several processes are going on at once: You are going through physical changes and emotional changes and your fetus is growing within you. Your pregnancy will have much in common with other women's. Yet it is yours, and unique (and each pregnancy you go through will differ from the others). In talking to mothers and to women who are pregnant at the same time you are, you will discover that there's no one right way to be pregnant.

Many changes take place in your body as the fetus develops in you. Some of these changes are just changes. Some can be uncomfortable at times. You may feel many changes and discomforts, few or none at all. You'll want to know what they are, why they occur, when they are likely to occur. Eating well and exercising reduce or eliminate many discomforts. Some minor discomforts, if ne-

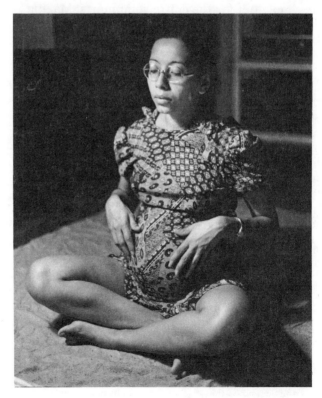

George Malave/Stock Boston

---

*In 1982 ACOG and the obstetrical establishment circulated throughout the media raw and undifferentiated statistics from several state health departments that purport to show that there is a higher risk of death when babies are born at home. These statistics represent unplanned, premature, precipitous home births. ACOG hired expensive public relations experts to mislead the public and their colleagues in other specialties. What these figures actually show is what happens when women are denied adequate medical care by physicians and welfare bureaucrats.

glected, can lead to major complications. And you should know that in every pregnancy there's a possibility of miscarriage (though the likelihood decreases with the passing months), so that if it happens to you, you won't be totally unprepared.

Your feelings will vary tremendously according to how you feel about having children; your previous pregnancies and/or abortion experiences, if any; how you feel about your own childhood, your parents or the people who reared you; whether or not you are with a partner—and if you are, how you feel about him or her.

At each stage you may feel conflicts as well as harmonies. Sometimes you'll feel positive, sometimes negative. You'll have doubts and fears. It's important to know that these doubts and fears occur during a "good'" pregnancy, too, for your body has been taken over by a process out of your control. You can come to terms with that takeover actively and consciously by knowing what's happening to your body, by identifying your specific feelings (especially the negative ones, because they are the most difficult to deal with) and also by learning what the fetus looks like as it grows. Its growth is dramatic and exciting (see p. 420 for more on feelings).

Our society tends to treat pregnancy as a solitary, clinical experience. Many nonindustrialized societies have invested it with religious significance, respect it as an altered physical and psychic state and celebrate it as significant not only for the couple but for the entire community. Making and deepening bonds with people who make you feel special can be an important source of strength.

Due Date

The length of a normal pregnancy can vary from 240 to 300 days. It's good to know approximately when your due date will be, but don't get fixated on a particular day. Only 5 percent of women give birth on their projected due date! (Some practitioners advise rounding it off to the nearest month!)* Since there are so many changes and

---

*If you and your obstetrician disagree seriously about the conception date, this can affect your baby's well-being. For example, if your obstetrician thinks the baby is "postmature," s/he may advise induction. If you are right and s/he is wrong, the birth may be premature. If your doctor thinks you are *less* pregnant than you are, you may give birth before anyone is prepared for it.

We have talked with dozens of women whose doctors refused to believe that they knew when their babies were conceived and thus approximately when they were due. Some had problems as a result. *Don't let the due date tyrannize you.*

Nowadays, obstetricians tend to dismiss their judgment and yours and rely on ultrasound to assess fetal maturity. Unfortunately, some doctors recommend *monthly* ultrasound pictures and depend on these rather than on physical exams. This is not sound medical practice.

feelings to talk about, it's more convenient to talk within the framework of trimesters.

First Trimester (First Twelve Weeks)

Testing During Pregnancy
See Appendix pp. 427–32.
A proliferation of newly developed tests and technology obliges us to make choices and decisions undreamed of twenty years ago. Many of these tests are too often overused. Occasionally, some are useful.

Physical Changes
You may have none, some or many of the following early signs of pregnancy. If you have had regular periods, you will probably notice that you have missed a period. However, some women do bleed for the first two or three months even when they are pregnant, but bleeding is usually short and there's scant blood. Also, about seven days or so after conception, the *blastocyst*, the tiny group of cells that becomes the embryo, attaches itself to the uterine wall, and you may have slight vaginal spotting, called *implantation bleeding*, while new blood vessels are being formed. *Be sure to get a pregnancy test* (see pp. 343–44), or do one for yourself at home.

You may have to urinate more often because of increased hormonal changes; pituitary hormones affect the *adrenals*, glands that change the water balance in your body, so you retain more body water. Also, your enlarging uterus presses against your bladder.

Your breasts will probably swell. They may tingle, throb or hurt. Your milk glands begin to develop. Because of an increased blood supply to your breasts, veins become more prominent. Your nipples and the area around them (areola) may darken and become broader.

You may feel nauseated, mildly or enough to vomit, partly because your system is changing. One theory is that the higher level of estrogen accumulates even in the cells of the stomach and causes irritation as acids tend to accumulate. The rapid expansion of the uterus may be involved. If you feel nauseated, eat lightly throughout the day rather than taking large meals. Eat food high in protein. Munching crackers or dry toast slowly before you get up in the morning can help a lot. Avoid greasy, spiced food. Don't fast, and at least drink juice. Take vitamin B_6 and other B vitamins. Apricot nectar helps some women. Powdered ginger in capsules or as a tea can help too.

You may feel constantly tired.

You may have increased vaginal secretions, either clear and nonirritating or white, yellow, foamy or itchy. The chemical makeup as well as the amount of your vaginal fluids is changing. If you are very uncomfortable or if such a condition persists, see your practitioner.

The joints between your pelvic bones widen and become more movable about the tenth or eleventh week. Occasionally the separating bones come together and pinch the sciatic nerve, which runs from your buttocks down through the back of your legs; this can cause pain.

Your bowel movements may become irregular, in part because the heightened amount of progesterone relaxes smooth muscles; therefore, your bowels may not function as efficiently as they did. Also, if you are resting more often, your decreased activity may cause some constipation. Eat foods high in fiber content and/or simply add bran to other foods. Eat salads and fresh fruits frequently and drink fruit juices.

During the first ten weeks you'll feel relatively few body changes. All those above are fairly common and not too annoying, though nausea and tiredness can wipe some women out.

Early pregnancy surprised me. I was expecting to feel very different and instead was feeling things I'd felt before. It was like premenstrual tension. I was a little nauseous. But it's amazing—once I realized I was pregnant the symptoms were tolerable, because they are not signs of sickness but of a life growing.

I felt at the same time more vulnerable and more powerful than ever.

Prenatal Exams

Obstetricians and clinics usually set up a fairly cursory routine examination schedule. Midwives and family practitioners will see you as regularly, but most likely will spend much more time with you.

During your first visit the practitioner will take a complete medical, reproductive and family history, including menstrual history, previous births, pregnancies, operations, abortions, illnesses, drugs taken, family illnesses such as high blood pressure or heart disease. Bring any medical records that you have and describe as completely as you can what's happened to you physically in the past. You should have a general physical exam and then an exam for pregnancy, which includes a breast examination to see if there are changes in your glands and a pelvic exam, which shows the position and consistency of your uterus, the condition of your ovaries and fallopian tubes and the consistency and color of your cervix. You will give blood to determine your blood type and the presence or absence of the Rh factor and to provide blood for a blood count and hemoglobin analysis.

You'll probably have tests for rubella* and possibly for toxoplasmosis (a disease resulting from cat feces or raw meat that causes retardation in newborns). You may also get other tests and cultures for STDs. (See Chapter 14, "Sexually Transmitted Diseases," for a description of the effects of untreated STDs on newborns.) The urinalysis will check for protein and glucose in the urine and a urine culture will reveal any urinary tract infections.† Your weight and blood pressure will be checked and you may have a Pap smear. If you have a history of diabetes and a specific risk factor (large babies, family history of diabetes, previous history of stillbirths), you will want to check your blood sugar level and get nutritional counseling.

Some practitioners ask you to chart what you eat over a three-day period and then discuss it with you. Ask for complete information about the purposes as well as the results of all tests. You have choices about whatever is done.

Your next visits will be monthly. The heartbeat and position of your baby will be checked, as well as your urine, weight and blood pressure. If you or your partner has a history of herpes, be aware of outbreaks and use condoms during lovemaking. Seek out ways to minimize outbreaks by eating well and minimizing stress.

At the beginning of your eighth month you'll probably see the practitioner every two weeks.

During the ninth month you'll see him or her once a week. It's best at this time to keep internal exams down to a minimum to prevent infection.

At the other extreme of exam scheduling, many rural and inner-city women never see a nurse or doctor until it's time to deliver. Conditions in some hospitals and clinics are so bad—crowded,

---

*If you are not immune to German measles (rubella), try to avoid exposure. When you have it, you may have a rash, tenderness of the lymph nodes in the back of your neck and possibly mild joint pains. If you are exposed in the first 16 weeks of pregnancy and if you get the disease, chances are high that the fetus will have problems. At this point you will have to make a decision about whether or not to continue your pregnancy. A blood test will tell you if you have or have had rubella.
†When you are pregnant you become more susceptible to urinary tract infections (UTIs) because the hormone progesterone relaxes smooth (involuntary) muscle and the collecting area in the kidneys and the tube connecting the kidneys to the bladder becomes larger. Urine tends to stagnate there, aggravating any latent infection. Signs of infection are increased urination, pain and/or a burning sensation. More extreme signs are back pain, chills and fever, bloody urine.
To prevent UTIs, it helps to drink fairly large quantities of fluids throughout pregnancy, especially acidic juices. You can make your own cranberry juice by boiling cranberries in water, straining and adding honey. Or add the juice of one whole lemon or lime to a half-gallon of water, keep it cold and drink three to four glasses a day. Also empty your bladder completely and frequently. Acupuncture may help, too.
In the first trimester of pregnancy your infection should be treated with sulfa drugs if juices and frequent urination don't work.

long waits, careless medical people, lack of respect for women and families—that women become discouraged and don't want to come for appointments.

What I hated most about City Hospital was the "cattle run." There was always a mad rush for the elevator immediately before clinic was about to begin. When we arrived every patient was assigned a number. We waited, seated in rows on long, hard benches. The bathroom stank. The rooms were dirty, drab and overheated. The medical staff were often overworked and overwhelmed; the nurses and doctors were impersonal. I rarely saw the same doctor twice. Another concern was, why didn't I ever see any women doctors or physicians of color?

Your Feelings About Yourself and Your Pregnancy

At the beginning of a first pregnancy or of any pregnancy, there are many variations in feeling, from delirious joy to deep depression.

Some Positive Feelings

You may feel an increased sensuality, a kind of sexual opening out toward the world, heightened perceptions, a feeling of being in love. A lot of new energy. A feeling of being really special, fertile, potent, creative. Expectation. Great excitement. Impatience. Harmony. Peace.

It gave me a sense that I was actually a woman. I had never felt sexy before. I went through a lot of changes. It was a very sexual thing. I felt very voluptuous.

It meant I could get pregnant finally after a lot of trying, that I could do something I wanted to do. It meant going into a new stage of life. I felt filled up.

Some Questions

What's going to happen to me? How will being pregnant change me? Will I be able to cope well? Can I physically handle birth? Will I miscarry? How long can I keep my job? Who am I? What image can I form of who I want to be? What is my baby going to be like? What about my partner?

Some Negative Feelings

Shock. I'm losing my individuality. I'm not the same anymore. I'm a pregnant woman; I'm in this new category and I don't want to be. I don't want to be a vessel, a carrier. I won't matter to people now, only my baby will. I can't feel anything for this thing growing in me. I can't feel any love. I'm scared. I'm tired. I feel sick. I wish I weren't pregnant. I'm not ready. I don't understand motherhood.

Negative feelings are natural. When you deal with them and don't avoid or ignore them, you'll be better prepared to handle them close to the birth and afterward. Also, miraculously they usually change a lot from one trimester to the next, most often in a positive direction.

Sometimes it seemed like I had gotten pregnant on a whim—and it was a hell of a responsibility to take on a whim. Sometimes I was overwhelmed by what I'd done. A lot of that came from realizing that I had chosen to have the baby without the support of a man. I was scared up until the third trimester that I wasn't going to make it.

Some of you will be too busy to think often about your pregnancy. Others will have more leisure. Some of you will be interested in your pregnancies in different degrees, your awareness switched inward at different times.

When I first felt her move, I knew there was life inside me. But I didn't realize I was having a baby until my doctors literally pulled her out of me upside down and she sneezed, and then she lay next to me and I felt her tiny breath on my fingers.

Maybe the last three weeks I started looking at other babies.

At the beginning of pregnancy it's sometimes a relief not to think about it, and you can even forget it if you want to. At some point during pregnancy you may wish you could escape from the inevitability of what is happening to you.

Growth of the Fetus

You can't feel the changes going on inside you. Both the placental systems and the complicated systems of your fetus are deveoping on a miniature scale. See *A Child Is Born* for wonderful photographs.

Pregnancy and AIDS

(See Chapter 15, "AIDS, HIV Infection and Women.")

Second Trimester
(Thirteenth to Twenty-Sixth Week)

Physical Changes

At about the fourth month the fetus begins to take up much more space. Your waist becomes thicker, your clothes no longer fit you, your womb begins to swell below your waist and, around the fourth or fifth month, you can begin to feel light movements ("quickening"). The fetus has been moving for months, but it's only now that you can feel it. Often you will feel it first just before you fall asleep.

You are probably gaining weight now. Eat as well as you can.

Your circulatory system has been changing and

WOMAN IN 16TH WEEK
OF PREGNANCY

Nina Reimer

your total blood volume increasing, as your bone marrow produces more blood corpuscles and you drink and retain more liquid. Your heart is changing position and increasing slightly in size.

In some women the area around the nipple, the areola, becomes very dark due to hormonal changes. The line from the navel to the pubic region gets dark, too, and sometimes pigment in the face becomes dark, making a kind of mask. The mask goes away after pregnancy. Usually the increased color around your nipples and in the line on your abdomen will not go away after the pregnancy, but it may fade.

Some women salivate more. You may sweat more, which helps to eliminate waste material from your body. Sometimes you'll get cramps in your legs and feet when you wake up, perhaps because of disturbed circulation. Calcium relieves these cramps, or drink raspberry leaf tea at bedtime. Just relax—the cramps will go away. Keep your feet elevated and warm, or pull your toes toward your knees.

Your uterus is changing, too. It's growing. Its weight increases twenty times, and the greater part of this weight is gained before the twentieth week.

As your abdomen grows larger the skin over it will stretch and lines may appear, pink or reddish streaks. Your skin may become dry; add oil to your bath and rub your skin with oil.

By midpregnancy your breasts, stimulated by hormones, are functionally complete for nursing purposes. After about the nineteenth week a thin amber or yellow substance called *colostrum* may come out of your nipples; there's no milk yet. Your breasts are probably larger and heavier than before. If you are planning to breastfeed, it's a good idea to begin gently massaging your nipples. If your nipples are inverted (turned in), pull them out gently several times a day by putting your thumbs on each side of them, pressing down into the breasts and away from the nipple. Wash your breasts daily with mild soap or clean water. It's also a good idea to wear a supportive bra, as your breasts can begin to feel very heavy.

Your bowels and your entire digestive system may move more slowly. Indigestion and constipation can occur. You may have heartburn because of too much acid in your stomach. Again, a good diet and regular exercise ease these situations. Eat frequent small meals if possible. Avoid greasy foods and coffee. Drink a lot of fluids and increase bran and fiber. Avoid taking strong, oily laxatives or laxatives containing sodium, such as baking soda or Alka-Seltzer. Papaya pills (available at health food stores) may be helpful.

As a result of pressure of pelvic organs, veins in your rectum (hemorrhoidal veins) may become dilated and sometimes painful. To prevent hemorrhoids you can practice rectal exercises, which resemble elevator exercises (see p. 406) except that you contract your rectal muscles instead. When you go to the bathroom, prop your feet up on a stool. Eat a lot of roughage. If you have hemorrhoids, lie down with your rectum high and apply ice packs or heat. Tucks pads and Preparation H are okay. Or take warm baths and apply Vaseline. Vitamin E oil may help. Eat fewer spices. Continue to exercise.

Varicose veins are veins in your legs that have become enlarged and can hurt. Because of pressure, the veins and blood vessels that carry blood from your legs to your heart aren't working as smoothly as before. A tendency to varicose veins can be hereditary. Many women find it very helpful to wear support stockings a half-size larger than their ordinary stockings. And lots of rest, with legs elevated, is good, alternated with walking or mild exercise.

Many women have nosebleeds because of the increased volume of blood and nasal congestion or perhaps because of increased hormone levels. (It's also possible to have "sympathetic" nosebleeds during periods.) A little Vaseline in each nostril may stop the bleeding.

Edema (Water Retention)

Your feet, ankles, fingers, hands and even your face may swell somewhat. When you are eating well, including adequate protein intake, edema is normal and no cause for worry, especially during the last half of pregnancy. Pregnancy hormones manufactured by the placenta, principally estrogens, cause connective tissue throughout your body to retain extra fluid, which benefits you and your baby. It serves as backup for the expanded blood volume needed to nourish the placenta, protects you from going into shock if you lose blood and assures you an adequate milk flow during early breastfeeding. With twins, edema will increase as will your weight gain. Normal edema is associated with healthy infants—higher birth weight and lower infant mortality.[12]

If you are uncomfortable, try to lie down with your feet raised several times a day. Exercise helps squeeze water from the tissue spaces in your blood vessels. Cut down on refined carbohydrates. Rest.

Preeclampsia

After the twenty-fourth week of pregnancy, some women develop a combination of high blood pressure, edema and protein in the urine. While these conditions can occur separately and sometimes all together for many reasons, they may also be symptoms of preeclampsia. Check with your practitioner. S/he should observe your blood pressure on at least two occasions a minimum of six hours apart and check the amount of albumin (a protein) in the urine. Toward the third trimester of pregnancy, if you develop very high blood pressure, a large amount of protein in your urine with a decrease in the amount of urine, a severe continuous headache or swelling of your face or fingers, you may have severe preeclampsia. These conditions can develop in just a few hours, and unless you have them checked immediately, eclampsia—convulsions and coma—may occur. Some mild conditions can be treated at home after medical evaluations; others and all serious preeclamptic conditions *must* be treated in the hospital; your life and the baby's are at stake.

The incidence of preeclampsia in pregnancy may be lessened by good prenatal care.

Clothing

Wear loose, comfortable clothing, warm in winter and cool in summer. Many women modify their own pants by piecing in an elastic stretch panel in the front. Simple unbelted smocks are useful as dresses. Large men's shirts are useful, too. Maternity clothes in stores are often expensive. Ask your friends for any clothes they may have.

Get as much rest as you possibly can. If you are very busy, try to set aside segments of time for total relaxation, even if it's only fifteen minutes at a time.

Your Feelings About Yourself

How will you feel about your changing body?

I was excited and delighted. I really got into eating well, caring for myself, getting enough sleep. I liked walking through the streets and having people notice my pregnancy.

But many of us watch ourselves growing outward so quickly with mixed emotions.

I don't like being pregnant. I feel like a big toad. I'm a dancer, used to being slim, and I can't believe what I look like from the side. I avoid mirrors.

Your Feelings About Your Baby

The first movements you feel your baby make can be amazing.

I was lying on my stomach and felt . . . something, like someone lightly touching my deep insides. Then I just sat very still and for an alive moment felt the hugeness of having something living growing in me. Then I said, "No, it's not possible, it's too early yet," and then I started to cry. . . . That one moment was my first body awareness of another living thing inside me.

And after the first movement—in the fourth or fifth month—you may wait days for another sign of quickening.* Then the movements will become frequent and familiar. The baby begins to feel real. You can feel from the outside the hard shape of your uterus.

Last night its kicking made me dizzy and gave me a terrible feeling of solitude. I wanted to tell it, "Stop, stop, stop, let me alone." I want to lie still and whole and all single, catch my breath. But I have no control over this new part of my being, and this lack of control scares me. I feel as if I were rushing downhill at such a great speed that I'd never be able to stop.

Sitting on a rock overlooking the domesite, trees growing right out of the rock. They cling and flourish on nothing. Images of the growing life inside me, also coming from nothing, getting nutrition from my body the way the tree does from the rock. . . . Occasionally I give it warmth, mostly when it moves. The more it moves, the more I like it. I also resent it an awful lot; I feel big, ugly and uncomfortable, and in spite of Len's protestations, I feel alone.

Even during the most positive pregnancies you may have moments, hours and days of depression, anxiety and confusion. These depressions may be connected to submerged anxieties you have in relation to your own childhood, doubts you have

---

*Even if you aren't sure when you conceived your baby, you can be almost certain that quickening occurs between the eighteenth and twentieth weeks of your first pregnancy, earlier in subsequent pregnancies.

about your own identity, economic problems, having too many children already and problems in your relationship with your partner.

It seems that my feelings about my pregnancy, my body, the coming of the baby, were inextricably wound into my feelings, problems, hopes and fears for our relationship. . . . It's hard to separate which feelings were a result of my unhappiness about us (a lot of the bad feelings about my body arose because Bob showed very little interest in my enlarged, changing body), which ones were my own negative feelings about having a less functional body (I wanted to keep working and active, but my body was so cumbersome that I was always worn out and tired) and which ones were just moods caused by pregnancy.

We have general fears, too; there is fear of the unknown, especially if it's a first pregnancy. No matter how much we do know about the physiological changes in our bodies, there's something incomprehensible about the beginnings of life. And by becoming pregnant we open ourselves to changes and complications. We become much more aware of being vulnerable.

I remember feeling overwhelmed by sad things I saw, and was overwhelmed by things that could happen to innocence. I'd wake in the night and think people were going to come in and take things, take the baby from me. I was beginning to be out of control, I was terribly afraid of chance. I've always been afraid of irrationality, of fate.

You may have vivid unsettling dreams.

For two nights now my falling asleep has given rise to that old childhood dream-image of falling down a deep, dark, square hole ever diminishing in size.

I'm in a hospital in a room all alone, a cold room. The nurse gives me a shot; I have my baby and I don't feel a thing. I look up and see my baby floating in a beaker, alive. I can't go to her; I'm sad and frustrated.

The baby starts coming out of my belly. I have to hold it in. My skin is transparent.

We fear that our babies will be born with a disability. While most babies are born healthy, between 3 and 4 percent of babies are born with diseases and 1 percent with physical malformations. Some women have dreams, fantasies and nightmares about flaws and physical disabilities. These are normal and universal.

When I was about six months pregnant and Dick was starting school again, I was home alone, isolated for days at a time. My nightmares and day-

dreams started around then, really terrible fears of the baby being deformed. All my life I've always been the good girl. I knew I wasn't really good. I knew I had bad thoughts, but I was never allowed to express them. So I thought that my baby's deformities would be the living proof of the ugliness and badness in me.

We fear our own death, the child's death.

In fact, some women miscarry and some babies die. While it's difficult, threatening and sad to think of, it happens. Though it's very hard and not usually useful to try to prepare for death, it helps to know what has happened to some women, so that if we or our friends experience such loss, we can in some way be acquainted with the event. This knowledge is a kind of preparation. It's vitally important to be able to reach out to friends when tragic things happen to them, and to help ease their feelings of isolation. It also helps us to know that we can and need to ask for help if such a thing happens to us.

I went into the hospital for the birth of my first child. . . . The child's lungs became infected and he died two days later. I never saw him. When I began to return to myself I found that despite all those times I had told myself that nothing could really happen, I had nothing but an empty belly. I don't know if we should be warned ahead of time to worry needlessly about something that happens to a very few women, but as one of those women, I definitely need to feel some sense of sharing with others in the same position—not to cry over what happened but to work out how to face other people. That's the hardest part—nobody wants to deal with death, especially when your friends are at the childbearing age themselves and can't help being afraid of you for what you stand for. I found that my friends wanted me to pretend nothing had happened—even that there had

Vaughn Sills

421

been no pregnancy. I don't think it was just my particular friends—it's natural to want to avoid those things. And so my fantastic pregnancy, in which a lot of things went on in my head and body that helped me to change and get myself together, had to be buried. Even now, after a year, I can see their pain and fear for me as I start into my eighth month of pregnancy with my second child. I have to be the one who keeps them calm, and I especially must assure everyone that this one will be okay.

You may also feel guilty about being afraid. Doesn't it mean that as a mother you will be weak and inadequate? The myth is that you can't allow yourself these depressions because you are supposed to be strong, mature, maternal, accepting, loving all the time.

Your feelings are legitimate. You must feel free to know them, to express them and to be strengthened by them.

Men's Feelings About You and Your Pregnancy

How will the man you are involved with respond to you? That depends on how you feel about yourself, on the relationship between you, on how he feels about himself and about fatherhood and what he sees his part to be in your pregnancy. It's best when he is as involved as possible. Enjoy your pregnancy together, prepare and learn together. He may feel close and attracted to you and fascinated by your growing body. Or for reasons having to do with his own upbringing and particular problems, he may feel upset, confused and threatened by all your changes and by what's to come. His feelings may vary enormously.

Sometimes I thought you were very beautiful and your belly was beautiful. And sometimes you looked like a ridiculous pregnant insect. Your navel bulging out looked strange.

If you are having problems, see if you can talk together about your feelings. Talk can also lead you to question the conventional ideas of beauty we are all exposed to. It's possible that he won't be able to talk about or to cope at all with the changes and responsibilities that your pregnancy implies. He may be jealous or resentful. Some men seek out women other than the pregnant women they are living with, whether they're married or unmarried. Others, although not actually leaving you, may withdraw from you emotionally at this crucial time.

Being Lesbian and Pregnant

More and more lesbians are choosing to have babies together through artificial insemination*

---

*See Chapter 18, "New Reproductive Technologies," for information on artificial insemination.

or intercourse and to create families. You will have most of the same joys and anxieties as heterosexual couples do. In many places, practitioners, clinics and birth centers will accept you as a couple when you go for prenatal care; other people may be prejudiced and punitive. Depending on the situation, you may not want to come out to your practitioner (or you may end up changing practitioners). But sometimes when you do, it can have a positive effect.

I had requested early in pregnancy to have Mary with me during labor and birth. I asked the hospital, wrote them a letter, and was told it had to go to the Board. They kept giving me the runaround. Meanwhile I was developing a good relationship with my obstetrician. At the beginning he had negative value judgments about me. As he got to know and like me, everything changed. He went to bat for me, got permission for Mary to be with me. I was also told afterward that he had spoken to the obstetrical staff to prepare them for our being there together. He told them that if any of them had negative feelings about lesbianism, they should not be there when we were. The result was that everyone at my labor and birth was extremely supportive.

Making Love During Pregnancy

You may have many different feelings about making love during pregnancy. Your moods and desires will shift.

I wanted to make love more than ever.

I remember feeling very sexy. We were trying all these different positions. Now that we were having a baby, I felt a lot looser, a lot freer. I used to feel uptight about sex for its own sake, but when I was pregnant I felt a lot freer.

I felt very ambivalent about making love. I had miscarried several times. I wanted to make love and I was scared to make love. As a single woman it was hard to find men who found me attractive with my belly so big. I had no sexual contact at all during the last two months.

You may feel more open, giving and sensuous than ever before (some women have orgasms or multiple orgasms for the first time). You may turn inward. With each month, each trimester, you may feel different. You may be afraid that making love will hurt the baby. It won't.

You can use pregnancy as a time to experiment with many different ways of loving, from touching and sensual massage to exploring a whole range of lovemaking positions. At the end of pregnancy, the man-on-top position is the most uncomfortable of all for women. Try propping yourself up on pillows, you on top, both of you relaxed side by side like two spoons fitting into each other, mutual masturbation or anything you want to think up that feels sensual and satisfying.

You can use pregnancy as a time to learn what your genitals look like and how to contract and release pelvic-floor muscles (see Kegel exercises, p. 406). Experiencing orgasms during masturbation and lovemaking is pleasurable and good for you. Lovemaking brings you closer to your partner and can prepare you for the giving, taking, opening up and deep relaxation of labor. Childbearing can be a vivid expression of your sexuality.

After making love your uterine contractions may continue. You can feel your uterus tighten, then relax. But lovemaking can bring on labor toward the end of pregnancy *only if you are ready to begin your labor.* Some researchers believe that prostaglandins concentrated in semen can cause uterine contractions but have found no conclusive link.

You probably should not have *intercourse* if you have vaginal or abdominal pain, if you have any uterine bleeding, if your membranes have ruptured (then there *is* danger of infection), if you think that miscarriage may occur. If your partner works in an environment where toxics may concentrate in sperm, he should wear a condom (see p. 109). If either you or your partner have open herpes sores, avoid any contact with the sores.

Third Trimester (Twenty-Seventh to Thirty-Eighth Week)

Physical Changes

Your uterus is becoming very large. It feels hard when you touch it.

I remember my friends' surprise when they put their hands on my belly to feel it. They expected it to be soft and somehow jellylike and were amazed at its hardness and bulk.

It's a strong muscular container. You can feel and see the movements of your baby from the outside now, too, as it changes position, turns somersaults, hiccups. Sometimes it puts pressure on your bladder, which makes you feel that you need to urinate even when you don't and which can hurt a little, or sometimes a lot, for very brief periods. Sometimes toward the end of pregnancy it presses on the nerves at the top of your legs, which can be painful, too.

Your baby will be lying in a particular position, sometimes head down, back to your front, sometimes crossways. It moves around often. Your practitioner can help you discover which position the baby is in.

Sometimes your baby lies still. It's known that babies sleep *in utero.* If you don't feel movement for three to four days and you're anxious about it, call your practitioner if you can and ask whether s/he thinks it's a good idea to check the fetal heartbeat. Usually these are periods of rest for the baby and can last several days.

You will feel your uterus tighten every now and then. These painless contractions (called *Braxton-Hicks contractions*) are believed to strengthen uterine muscles, preparing them for eventual labor.

It becomes increasingly uncomfortable for you to lie on your stomach. You may experience shortness of breath. There's pressure on your lungs from your uterus, and your diaphragm may be moved up as much as an inch. Even so, because your thoracic (chest) cage widens, you breathe in more air when you are pregnant than when you are not. Sometimes when you lie down you may not be able to breathe well for a moment. Prop yourself up with pillows or turn on your side, and the pressure on your diaphragm will be lessened.

The peak load on your heart occurs in about the thirtieth week. After that the heart usually doesn't have to work so hard until delivery.

You are still gaining weight. If you have hemorrhoids or varicose veins, try to avoid standing up for long periods of time, and when you sit or lie down, be sure your feet are raised.

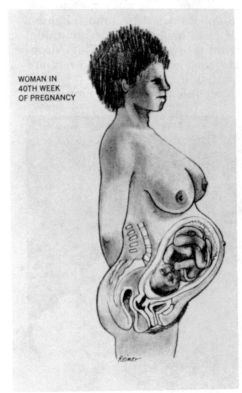

WOMAN IN 40TH WEEK OF PREGNANCY

Nina Reimer

423

Your stomach is pushed up by your uterus and flattened. Indigestion becomes more common. If you have heartburn, sleep with your head and shoulders raised. Eat small amounts. Don't take mineral oil—it causes you to excrete necessary vitamins.

If you have insomnia or trouble sleeping because the baby's movements make you uncomfortable, take walks and hot baths. Drink warm milk or raspberry tea. Avoid sleeping pills. Brisk exercise during the day will help you sleep better.

I think there is a reason for this nonsleeping: there's work getting done. That restlessness needs to happen. Your energy builds up for the coming crisis. I remember pacing around my house at midnight, burning with energy, finally finding the tiny sandals my first child had worn as a toddler. I carefully cleaned and polished them for the new baby. Then I slept fine.

Your navel will probably be pushed out.

Since your body has become heavier, you'll tend to walk differently for balance, often leaning back to counteract a heavier front. This can cause backaches, for which there are exercises. Your pelvic joints are also much more separated.

At about four to two weeks before birth, and sometimes as early as the seventh month, the baby's head settles into your pelvis. This is called "lightening" or "dropping." It takes pressure off your stomach. Some women do feel much lighter. And if you have been having trouble breathing, pressure is now off your diaphragm. This "dropping" can cause constipation; your bowels are more obstructed than they were.

As for water retention, an average pregnant woman retains from 6.5 to 13 pints of liquid, half of this in the last ten weeks. Swollen ankles are common.

Your Feelings About Yourself and Your Pregnancy

I had a feeling of being at the end, of nothing else being terrifically important.

I thought it would never end. I was enormous. I couldn't bend over and wash my feet. And it was incredibly hot.

At the end I started to feel it was too long. Dick took pictures of me during the eighth month. I saw my face as faraway and sad.

I had insomnia. I couldn't get comfortable. I couldn't sleep, he'd kick so much.

The relationship of mother carrying child is most beautiful and simplest.
  I pity a baby who must come out of the womb.

I wonder what it looks like. How fantastic that it only has to travel one-and-a-half feet down to get born.

My kid is dancing under my heart.

Ed Pincus

POSTURES TO TURN A BREECH BABY

Begin after the thirtieth week of pregnancy for up to four weeks before birth or until version (turning, a shift in position) takes place, whichever happens first.

1. Lie on your back on a hard surface with the pelvis raised by pillows to a level nine to twelve inches above the head. Stomach should be empty. (This posture corrected breech to head-first position of baby for 89 percent of patients in one study.) Lying head-down on a collapsed ironing board with one end propped on a couch or chair is sometimes more comfortable than the pillow position. Practice twice a day for ten minutes each time.

2. Knee–chest position: Kneeling on all fours, fold your arms and place your head on them, keeping your knees about eighteen inches apart and your back straight. Bladder should be empty. If you do this posture with your head at the edge of your bed, a book can be placed on the floor below and it is possible to read comfortably. Practice twice a day for ten minutes each time.

Fairly confidently and calmly awaiting the baby— quite set on a home delivery. Doctor said Thursday I was already dilated two-and-a-half centimeters, so it must be getting close. Getting a bit anxious, listening to every Braxton-Hicks contraction, awaiting with hope—and fear, too—its change into the real thing.

I feel exultant and tired and rich inside. My belly is large, and last night the baby beat around inside it like a wild tempest. I thought the time had come and was panicked and nauseated, then very excited. I woke Ed up. Then at five I fell asleep. Meanwhile I move in slow motion and wait.

APPENDIX

Questions for Practitioners Who Work in Hospitals

These questions are purposely broad and vague. You can use them to lead into a more detailed interview once you have read these chapters and other books.

What is your philosophy of childbirth? What kind of prenatal care do you offer? What kind of childbirth preparation do you favor? Do you consider good nutrition and exercise important and can you help me with them? Do you recommend childbirth preparation classes? What kind? What kind of tests do you do during pregnancy and just before birth? Will you be easy to reach if I need you?

How many births have you attended? Where? Where has your training been? How do you usually conduct labor and birth? Do you stay with women throughout labor or appear at the end of labor? Do you approve of labor coaches? Of family, friends, children being present? What percentage of your clients walk around during labor? Eat or drink during labor? Labor in positions of their choice? Have no drugs at all? Have no episiotomy? Hold their babies and breastfeed right away? Under what circumstances and what percentage of the time do you use drugs and interventions: IVs? Amniotomy? Electronic monitors? Pitocin to start or speed up labor? Episiotomy? Forceps? Cesareans? Who backs you up if you can't be present at prenatal visits or at labor and birth? Do they share your beliefs? Can you give me the names of some women who have used your services? What is your overall fee for prenatal care and a vaginal delivery? For a cesarean? If I've had a cesarean, do you encourage trial labor and vaginal delivery?

How often will I see you after my baby is born?

Two important points: (1) Be sure to compare what the practitioner says with hospital rules and anesthesia department requirements, which may

David Alexander

be different. (2) No matter what your physician says, the attitudes and practices of nurses attending you during labor can influence or determine what happens.

Questions for Nurse-Midwives Who Give Care in Private Offices, Clinics or Hospitals

Very much like the above questions. Add: Will I need to make contact with someone other than you? What percentage of your clients require physician care? Under what circumstances do you call in the doctor to assist you? If I am transferred to physician care in an emergency, will you still be able to be with me?

Questions for Nurse-Midwives and Physicians Who Work in Freestanding Birth Centers

Most of the same questions as above. Add: What are your requirements for birth center admission? What are your screening protocols? What percentage of your clients have been "risked out" prior to labor? Why? What are backup arrangements? What are your protocols for hospital admission? When do you advise women to go into the hospital?

Questions for Midwives Who Attend at Home

What is your philosophy of birth? Of prenatal care? Do you offer comprehensive care, including laboratory work, either on your own or in connection with a facility, interpreting urine, blood, diagnostic tests? Can I do these tests myself? Do you provide nutritional counseling? How often do you visit before and after the birth? What kind of childbirth preparation do you favor? Do you recommend classes? What kind?

What has your training been? Whom have you trained with? Are you in communication with other midwives in your area? How many births have you attended? How many births have you been responsible for?

What medical/hospital backup do you have? What have your experiences been?

How do you conduct labor and delivery? When do you check the baby's heartbeat, my blood pressure and pulse, dilation, baby's position and descent?

How do you define complications? How do you handle complications? Under what conditions would I see a physician or go to the hospital?

How do you reduce or prevent perineal tearing? What about repair? How do you define newborn distress? Handle it? Do you know how to do mouth-to-mouth resuscitation on newborns? Do you make postpartum visits? When? For how long a period of time? Who is your backup? Does s/he share your beliefs? Can I meet her/him? Can you give me the names of some women you have assisted? What do you charge?

Questions for Hospitals*

May I preregister, or will I have to fill out forms when I arrive in labor? Do you have a birthing room? What are the criteria? What percentage of women use it? What percentage of doctors use it?

What procedures are routine here? Do you remove personal belongings? Do preps (shave pubic hair)? Give enemas? Do you have a place for women in early labor—a special room or a lounge? May my partner/relatives/friends/labor coach be with me during labor and delivery? May my child(ren) be present? Do you routinely require IVs and fetal monitors? May I walk around during labor? Take showers or baths? May we take photos? May I stay in the labor room for the whole time instead of going to the delivery room?

If it's a teaching hospital, how will that affect me? (In some teaching hospitals women are approached during labor and asked if they will take part in studies; in others, they may undergo certain procedures unnecessarily for the sake of a study, without being told.)

What is the cesarean rate at your hospital, both for primary and repeat cesareans? Have there been nursery staph infections during the past year?

Can my partner and coach be with me in the delivery and recovery rooms if I have to have a cesarean? Can my partner hold the baby right afterward?

May I hold my baby immediately after delivery and nurse her/him? May we stay together in privacy after the delivery? Are mothers and babies separated after delivery? For how long? Why?

Do you have rooming-in? What kind: Complete? Modified? What hours? Can my baby feed on demand? Do you have experienced advice available for breastfeeding mothers?

What are visiting hours? May my partner and family visit whenever they want? Can I decide the length of time I want to stay? Do you have early discharge? What is your exact policy?

You can write a letter to your practitioner, hospital administrator and head of nursing staff stating your preferences and priorities concerning labor and birth. Bring a copy with you when you go to the hospital to have your baby. Your wishes and desires may be honored. Decide what your bottom line is—what you absolutely *won't* give up.

Testing Before or During Pregnancy

Sickle Cell Trait and Sickle Cell Anemia

One in twelve black people in the United States carries only a single gene for sickle cell anemia and consequently has sickle cell *trait*. This is a benign condition that rarely has any effect and that most people don't know they have. The sickle cell gene developed thousands of years ago in people who lived in Africa and in countries around the Mediterranean Sea, apparently because having sickle cell trait helped protect them from malaria. However, if you have sickle cell trait and your partner does, too, each of your children will have one chance in four of having sickle cell anemia.

About 1 in 165 black people is born with the inherited disease of *sickle cell anemia*. Symptoms can include poor physical development, jaundice, weakness, abdominal pains, lowered resistance to

---

*If hospitals really met women's needs, we wouldn't have to ask all these questions!

infections, bouts of swelling and pain in muscles and joints. The red blood cells, shaped like a farmer's sickle, don't live as long as normal cells and are destroyed at a faster rate, so movement of oxygen is reduced. The clinical picture is variable. Some people who have severe anemia during childhood may find the symptoms becoming milder as they grow older. For others, the anemia is tiring at times but tolerable, or it can be extremely painful. In order to have the disease, you must inherit a *pair* of genes for sickle cell, one from each parent.

If you are black and if you are planning a pregnancy with someone of similar background, you may want to be tested for sickle cell trait. The blood test is simple and you can have the results in thirty minutes. Then, if your test is positive, your partner may want to be tested, too.

If you have the trait and your partner doesn't, then your children have a fifty-fifty chance of having the trait. If one of you has sickle cell anemia and the other has neither sickle cell anemia nor the trait, all your children will have the trait and therefore have no problems. If you both have the trait, every time you have a child, s/he will have one chance in four of having completely normal blood, one chance in two of having the trait and one chance in four of having sickle cell anemia. If one of you has the trait and the other has sickle cell anemia, each child will have a fifty-fifty chance of having sickle cell anemia.

Ideally, your test for sickle cell trait or anemia should be part of a program that will do several things for you. It will inform you as soon as possible of test results and keep them absolutely confidential. If you and your partner both have the trait, it will provide counseling if you want it as you decide about having children. If you have sickle cell anemia, it will identify which form you have, as some are not as troublesome as others. It will help you learn about the problems and risks of going through a pregnancy; some of your symptoms may be intensified by pregnancy (circulatory problems may become worse; you may be more tired or depressed than usual and more prone to miscarriage). Finally, a good program will provide counseling and support services to you and your family if your child or your partner has sickle cell anemia and you need these services.

To locate a sickle cell program in your area, check with your local hospital, neighborhood health clinic or department of health.

Tay-Sachs Disease

Tay-Sachs disease is another genetic disease, rare in the general population (one in 100,000) but much more common in Jews of eastern European origin (1 in 3,600 births) and in French-Canadians. It results from the deficiency of an enzyme (hex-osaminidase A) involved in the metabolism of some of the fatty substances essential for the nervous system's proper functioning. Infants with Tay-Sachs disease are born seemingly normal, but early in infancy their development slows down and paralysis, blindness, severe behavioral changes and disorders of the nervous system follow. It is always fatal, usually by age three or four.

If you are a Jew of eastern European descent or French Canadian and plan to have a baby, you and your partner can be tested for the trait. If you both have it, your baby has one chance in four of having Tay-Sachs disease. In 1970 a relatively simple test became available to detect carriers of the trait (the test determines the concentration of hexosaminidase A in the blood). It is also possible to detect affected fetuses *in utero* through amniocentesis (see below).

Rh Factor in Blood

The Rh factor is a substance in the blood. At least 86 percent of us have this substance coating our red blood cells; we are called Rh positive (Rh+). Those of us who don't have it are Rh negative (Rh−).

If someone with Rh− blood receives transfusions of blood containing the Rh+ factor, the Rh− blood gradually builds up antibodies that defend the blood from the hostile Rh factor, causing some red cells to be broken down and their products spread through the body.

This same process can occur during pregnancy, because a certain amount of blood is transferred between you and your fetus through the placenta, though each circulatory system remains fairly separate. Most of the change goes from the mother to the fetus. At birth, however, because of the separation of the placenta from the uterus, there can be a much larger spillover, and a quantity of the baby's blood can be absorbed by the mother. This mixing does not occur often. If you have Rh− blood, are pregnant for the first time and have not had a transfusion containing Rh+ blood, your first child will probably be all right. But at birth you can absorb your baby's Rh+ blood, causing your own blood to react and begin developing antibodies. These antibodies will be present in your blood during your next pregnancy. They can get into the bloodstream of your second child as it grows and attack and destroy some of its red cells. As a result, the baby may be stillborn, severely anemic or retarded.

Thus every Rh− woman should have her blood checked regularly, beginning early in pregnancy. If you are Rh−, pay careful attention to the following:

1. The father's Rh factor should be checked. If he is also Rh−, all your offspring will be Rh− and there's no need for further checking. If he's

Rh +, it should be determined whether he has both Rh + and Rh − genes, in which case the fetus will be Rh + only 50 percent of the time. If the man has only Rh + genes, the fetus will always be Rh +.

2. You should know whether you have had previous blood transfusions. It's possible (though rare now that people are aware of the Rh factor) for a woman with Rh − blood to have received Rh + blood in a transfusion, and thus to have already developed antibodies.

3. You should have your own blood tested for Rh sensitization (the presence of antibodies) during your pregnancy.

4. A fetal amniotic fluid sample can be taken during amniocentesis to see whether the blood cells of the fetus are being altered. If the bilirubin level in the fluid is high, it indicates that the fetus is affected, and a blood transfusion may be given to the baby *in utero*.

Rhogam

A drug called Rhogam has been developed that prevents you from producing antibodies. *For Rhogam to be effective, you must get it within seventy-two hours after a miscarriage from the second month on and after every abortion or pregnancy.* In some states you can get free Rhogam shots. Check with your health department.

What can be done if the blood of the fetus is being invaded by maternal antibodies? There are now techniques for exchanging invaded fetal blood for healthy blood while the fetus is still in the uterus, and for exchanging the baby's blood after it is born. Check with your practitioner about the risks and benefits of these techniques. Ask for names of other Rh − women and find out from them what their experiences were. Thanks to Rhogam and these new techniques, most Rh incompatibles are now born healthy.

Testing During Pregnancy*

Deciding

Prenatal genetic testing during pregnancy may pose numerous dilemmas for many women. Over the past decade, new genetic tests have been introduced into the prenatal care "market" by both nonprofit and commercial genetic laboratories. Many of these medical and surgical tests are now

---

*For more discussion, see "Can Aborting Imperfect Children Be Immoral?" by Adrienne Asch, in Nancy K. Rhoden and John D. Arras, eds., *Ethical Issues in Modern Medicine*, 3rd ed., Palo Alto, CA: Mayfield, 1989. Also see Robin J.R. Blatt's *Prenatal Tests: What They Are, Their Benefits and Risks, and How to Decide Whether to Have Them or Not*, New York: Vintage Books, 1988, and her forthcoming *Prenatal Genetic Testing: A Guide for Pregnant Women and Couples* (tentative title), South Hadley, MA: Bergin & Garvey.

---

routinely performed upon women during pregnancy to provide information, with varying degrees of accuracy, without adequate information about them or sufficient investigation of their safety. The Human Genome Project (see p. 694) will generate and confront women with even more new tests. Because so many of these tests are being developed, patented and marketed, you are likely to be persuaded to undergo them not for your own good or the good of your baby, but to enable physicians to acquire experience in performing them and to assess the results; that is, you may be included in ongoing studies. *You have the right to refuse any test.*

Testing may be reasonable when we anticipate that a fetus may be "at risk" for a particular health problem. There may be advantages to knowing beforehand if there are certain problems with the fetus. For example, it enables women and their families to prepare during pregnancy and birth for the special needs of the new baby or for putting a newborn up for adoption. Sometimes experimental fetal surgery techniques are available for certain conditions. In addition, based on test results, some women may decide not to continue the pregnancy (see p. 366).

Having a child always involves unknowns and even with the available testing, many problems cannot be detected. Often we come to believe, in our technological, medicalized culture, that the newly developed prenatal tests magically "prevent" disease and disability and that we are irresponsible when we decide not to have them. Though tests may be appropriate in specific instances, it is not reasonable for them to be done routinely—they may not always be safe for us or our babies, they further medicalize the pregnancy experience and they can cause unnecessary anxiety. Unfortunately, often their very existence pressures us into having them done.

My son was born fourteen years ago. In the past three years I had an abortion and a miscarriage. Once again I became pregnant. Though I had planned to have an amniocentesis done that last pregnancy, the miscarriage changed my mind: When the medical center sent out an informational pamphlet about amniocentesis which said that there was a 1.5 percent chance of miscarriage or fetal damage,* and after Steven and I had done a lot of reading, I realized that if I had to go through another loss I'd be a basket case. So I decided not to have it done.

Then came the enormous pressure: Here I was, thirty-eight. My doctor urged me; so did my father, my husband's parents; my sister had had one and

---

*If you are at a place that presents this high a risk, go elsewhere if you can.

so had all my friends, without questioning. I even knew abstractly that I'd rather have a miscarriage than a Down's syndrome baby.

For three weeks I was a wreck. Then one of my friends asked me, "What would be the worst *thing?" I said, "The worst thing would be if the baby were healthy and amniocentesis caused a miscarriage."*

That did it: no amniocentesis. I'd really made the decision. We lived with it fine.

And Sarah is wonderful and healthy.

There is no easy answer.

You are much more likely to be subjected to a barrage of tests if your practitioner is a technologically oriented obstetrician or if you are planning to have your baby in a large teaching hospital. Midwives are much less likely to suggest that any of these tests be performed routinely, and many strongly believe that they are not necessary and that they lead to medicalization of pregnancy.

Physicians will frequently offer or perform ultrasound, alpha-fetoprotein (AFP) screening and amniocentesis. Though some of them are concerned about our babies' welfare, others may be simply protecting themselves, "doing everything possible" in case something goes wrong. It can be overwhelming.

My doctor insisted I should have amniocentesis and downplayed any risks. "Well, when are you going to do it?" he kept asking. Finally, during one checkup, he got me when I was feeling very vulnerable. Yet even when I got up on the table to have it done, I hadn't really made up my mind about it.

It is important to think about why we have these tests, to learn about the procedures, not to feel pressured and to be comfortable with the decisions we make.

I was thirty-seven, healthy, had had two children and was pregnant again after seventeen years. I just knew I didn't want a needle poking into my womb.

I am planning a home birth and thought long and hard about amniocentesis. You have to use technology selectively. I finally decided to have it done— that if there was something wrong, I owed it to my family to find out. I wanted to have the chance to decide about continuing the pregnancy. After it was over, what a relief! We don't have the results yet, but I'm not at all wondering or worried!

Several prenatal tests can provide specific information about the condition of the fetus: *ultrasound* or *sonography* (UTS), *amniocentesis* and *AFP screening* are the three most common procedures. With these tests, doctors can identify certain fetal disabilities such as spina bifida, Down

syndrome, cystic fibrosis and some types of muscular dystrophy.

Ultrasound and AFP screening (a blood test) are simple medical procedures (although a positive AFP test can lead to a further series of tests, including ultrasound and amniocentesis). Amniocentesis is a more difficult, time-consuming and costly procedure and carries a small (less than 1 percent) risk of miscarriage or infection.

The tests were once intended for women who have reason to be concerned about the health of their fetus, because they have already given birth to a child with a disability, because a particular disability runs in their or their partner's family or because they have some other reason to believe their children to be at risk for a particular disability. They are now presented to almost all pregnant women. For approximately 95 percent of women who are tested, the results are negative. However, a negative result on a particular test does not guarantee that the baby does not have some other problems, though it's unlikely. Many conditions cannot yet be tested for.

When considering each test, here are some questions to ask:

- What is the nature of the disability for which the test is being done? Where can I get more information from people who have this disability?
- What medical facility is best for the particular test I'm considering? Which practitioner is best?
- What will I learn from the test? How accurate is it?
- What are the risks to me and my baby if I take the test?
- How long do I have to wait to learn the results?
- What options do I have if the test yields positive results?

Be sure that you want and need the test in question. Talk it over with your physician, especially if s/he performs tests routinely. Ask to talk with a genetic counselor. Be sure you understand what is happening and why. If you have any doubts, get a second opinion. Talk with other women who have had the test.

Ultrasound

Ultrasound may now be used throughout pregnancy, although the place, if any, for routine ultrasound has not been convincingly established. It uses intermittent high-frequency sound waves to create pictures of the body's inner organs by recording their echoes, much as sonar measures shapes in the water. The procedure is done either vaginally or abdominally. With vaginal ultrasound (which is new) the *transducer*, or probe, is inserted into the vagina. Some women feel more comfortable inserting it on their own. With abdominal ultrasound, a technician or physician runs the transducer back and forth over your abdomen, and a computer translates the resulting echoes into pictures on a video screen. When performed by a capable technician, ultrasound can be valuable. Most doctors consider it to be safe, *yet we don't know enough about its long-term effects and must question its routine use, especially during early pregnancy.*

Amniocentesis (Amnio or Tap)

This is an invasive procedure that can be used to reveal chromosomal conditions and certain metabolic and biochemical disorders in the fetus. It can also be used for certain DNA tests such as cystic fibrosis or sickle cell conditions. It is standard medical practice for physicians to offer it to women thirty-five years and older, because older women have an increased chance of having babies with Down syndrome (trisomy 21—a form of mental retardation), and now it is increasingly being offered earlier and earlier. Age thirty-five was originally set as the cutoff because at this age the likelihood of having a baby with a chromosome condition is about the same as or greater than the risk that the test will injure the fetus or induce a miscarriage. The risk to the fetus is estimated to be one loss in 400 amniocentesis procedures at large city hospitals specializing in prenatal testing. In places where the staff is not well trained and has much less experience with performing the test, the risk is higher. Down syndrome is the most common chromosome abnormality found by amniocentesis and has an incidence of approximately 1 in 400 births for women aged thirty-five. The risk increases with age and reaches 1 in 100 at age forty.*

Physicians bring up amniocentesis when you are close to age thirty-five because of recent lawsuits in which parents who have had a child with Down syndrome have sued doctors who have not warned them and told them about amniocentesis. Many doctors recommend it by age thirty-eight. Some physicians will not accept women in their forties as clients if they refuse amniocentesis. If your obstetrician has suggested amniocentesis because of your age or a genetic condition in your family, your decision to have the test or not depends on many personal considerations, such as your family situation, your feelings about medical procedures and risks, your feelings concerning abortion and the way you feel about the possibility of having a child with a disability.

Disabilities differ a lot in their severity. Getting to know children with disabilities and/or their parents can often help you to acquaint yourself with what the situation would mean to you and your partner. Different people feel very differently about this matter, and it is important that you not feel pressured into a decision you won't be comfortable with.

You may choose to have amniocentesis even if you would not have an abortion.

When I became unexpectedly pregnant at forty-three, my doctor told me about amniocentesis, but I told him that because of my religion I wouldn't consider having an abortion no matter what the results of the test. He then suggested I consider having the test just to find out the condition of the baby—that probably we would be reassured that it was all right. I talked it over with my husband and he thought this idea made sense. It was very upsetting when we first learned the baby had Down's, but this didn't change our original feelings. Learning the baby's condition early made all the difference. I attended a clinic which helps parents care for children with Down's and talked with many parents. As well as preparing ourselves, my husband and I were able to help our three teenage children know what to expect. We all picked out the baby's name together and the children are waiting for him to come home so they can help take care of him.

It is also important to discuss your and your partner's family's medical history and ethnic background with your physician, since amniocentesis can also test for approximately eighty rare disorders, among them Tay-Sachs disease and sickle cell anemia, though the latter can be done only in a few specialized centers. Tests other than routine chromosome analysis and AFP screening for neural tube defects (see p. 431) will be performed only if your physician indicates that they are necessary, because they are costly and time-consuming. Ordinarily you would not consider any of them unless you had special reasons to believe that your baby was at risk.

The procedure: A physician performs amniocentesis on an outpatient basis in a hospital or his or her office, under the continuous guidance of a competent technician to check the location of the fetus and the placenta. Some physicians use a local anesthetic to numb the skin, others don't. The physician then inserts a long, thin needle through your abdominal wall into the womb and draws off approximately four teaspoons of fluid into a syringe. On rare occasions s/he may have to try a second time to get enough fluid. You may have some or all of the following sensations during the procedure: pricking or stinging of your skin, cramping when the needle enters the uterus and pressure when the fluid is withdrawn. These reactions are normal and don't mean that anything

---

*Increased paternal age may contribute to Down syndrome. Amniocentesis, of course, permits diagnosis in either case.

is amiss, but they should diminish and disappear within a day. If they don't, call your physician.

Whereas some women find the procedure easy, others find it an unpleasant, upsetting experience.

I was nervous. But my obstetrician met us in the waiting room and told me that discomfort is unusual. First they showed it on the ultrasound screen and then made a pen mark on my stomach where the needle was to go in. The whole procedure turned out to be completely painless. My doctor talked his way through: "Now I'm going to do. . . . Now you'll feel. . . ." It was reassuring. Then he told me to take it easy for a day. After, we spoke to a genetics counselor and asked a lot of questions. She told us as much as we wanted to know and showed us "pictures" of imperfect chromosomes which cause birth defects. It was abstract but it hit home. It helped that nothing had gone wrong during the procedure. We didn't worry at all about what the results would be.

I hadn't been anxious about the procedure but looking back I'm glad my husband decided to come. No one had prepared me for how important it was to have someone there holding your hand and being supportive. The doctor couldn't get the needle in the right place and kept moving it around for a long time. This really hurt and I was upset and anxious. Finally he took the needle out and tried again. The second time there was no problem but I was quite distraught by that time. The staff and doctors were wonderful but I wish I had talked beforehand to someone who had gone through the experience.

The procedure itself wasn't bad. My husband went with me. I found it kind of creepy thinking of that long needle so I didn't look. It took longer than I thought. Having my own doctor there made a difference; I would have been more nervous in a clinic in somebody else's hands. Afterwards, however, I had bad cramps and was in great pain. I found it traumatic to hear (from the counselor) about all the genetic disabilities that could not be picked up and why the test might have to be done again. The cramps did go away but I stayed in bed for two days because I had lost a baby a few years before and was afraid of miscarriage. When it became clear that things were all right I felt better.

The correct use of ultrasound and proper needle size are important. When hospitals use improper techniques, risks to the fetus increase. You may want to consider traveling to a hospital other than the one near you if the facilities are better and the personnel more experienced. Find out who specializes in the procedure and the number of amniocentesis procedures they do. Talk to other women who have had amniocentesis.

The sample of amniotic fluid contains some of the baby's cells and fluids. The cells are cultured and a photograph is made of their chromosomes. You may receive a picture of the chromosomes (karyotype) if you wish. Some people choose not to see it, since you can tell the sex of the baby from the chromosomes. Others prefer to know their baby's sex before it is born.

Amniocentesis is traditionally performed between sixteen and eighteen weeks of pregnancy. However, there are experimental protocols assessing its use and safety as early as twelve weeks.

Maternal Serum Tests (AFP Tests) for Neural Tube Disorders

Approximately 2 in 1,000 infants in the United States are born each year with a neural tube disorder (NTD). In this disorder, the developing neural tube, which forms the brain, spinal cord and spinal column, does not close over completely. The disorder, which usually leaves an open lesion, can occur anywhere along the neural tube. If the tube remains open at the top, the baby will be born with only a rudimentary brain and open skull. This condition, called *anencephaly*, is always fatal. If the opening is along the backbone, its severity will depend on several factors: whether the lesion is covered with skin, whether nerve tissue protrudes from the defect, and the size and location of the lesion. This condition is known as *spina bifida* or *meningeomyelocele*. Children with open lesions can have severe medical problems, such as mental retardation, lack of bladder or bowel control, some degree of paralysis, requiring extensive medical and surgical procedures. However, many forms of spina bifida are much less disabling, and people with the condition lead rich, full lives.* Unfortunately, the AFP test gives no indication of the severity of the problem, although ultrasound can help with the diagnosis in some cases.

During the last decade, researchers discovered that the amount of AFP was higher for women who carried an affected fetus. Elevated levels may indicate women who have a higher than "normal" chance of carrying a fetus with an NTD and may indicate when further testing ought to be considered. The AFP test can diagnose about 85 percent of fetuses with an open lesion. About 10 percent of fetuses with NTDs have lesions covered with skin. They are not detectable and usually less serious.

Although the blood test itself is routine and easy to do, the results are difficult to interpret for the following reasons:

1. The amount of AFP varies during pregnancy.

---

*Contact the Spina Bifida Association of America, 343 South Dearborn, No. 317, Chicago, IL 60604, (312) 663-1562, for more information.

Therefore it is important to know when you became pregnant. An ultrasound may help find out how old the fetus is.

2. The blood test may give false positives. An increased amount of AFP may occur for reasons other than NTDs in 5 percent of the tests. Multiple births, certain rare disorders and an incorrect estimate of fetal age can result in false positives. Lower levels may be due to incorrect pregnancy dating.

Because of the many false positives, further tests are done on women who have a high AFP reading. These include a second blood test or just ultrasound to check the fetus's age. Women with low levels are usually sent for ultrasound. When the reason for the higher level cannot be determined, a woman will have amniocentesis. Each step increases the accuracy with which the relatively few cases are diagnosed.

Medical and laypeople have raised questions about routine AFP screening, which subjects numbers of women to tests when so few will actually have any problems and will have to wait so long for results. Inadequate counseling, lack of cultural and linguistically appropriate information and the procedures themselves can cause extreme stress.

If you decide to have an AFP blood test, keep in mind that other tests, such as UTS or amniocentesis, may be necessary to determine whether or not the fetus has a given condition. If you are having amniocentesis anyway, the AFP blood test is unnecessary since the AFP level in the amniotic fluid will be measured.

Researchers do not know what factors can produce NTDs and believe them to be brought on by a combination of genetic and other unknown factors. One study found that supplementary vitamins around the time of conception and for the first month of pregnancy may help prevent the disorder.[13] This should not be interpreted as meaning that megavitamins are useful to women who eat a complete diet. Most of the vitamin research has been done with women whose diets are poor and lacking in certain essentials.

Chorionic Villus Sampling (CVS)

This new and still experimental test provides earlier results for pregnant women than amniocentesis. An early surgical test that removes from the uterus a piece of the chorion, the outer tissue of the sac surrounding the fetus, it is used to identify chromosome and biochemical conditions, such as Tay-Sachs disease, inherited conditions and the fetus's sex. It cannot identify neural tube conditions. *The safety, accuracy and long-term effects of CVS are still unknown.* The preferable time to have it done is between nine and twelve weeks. It can be performed in an outpatient clinic or a doctor's office by an experienced obstetrician who has had thorough training and experience in performing it. A diagnostic ultrasound must always be performed just before. It can be done vaginally or abdominally. *Ultrasound-guided aspiration* is the technique most commonly done in the United States. The physician inserts a catheter through your vagina and cervix into the chorionic villi (fingerlike projections of tissue that eventually form the placenta), and then a small amount of villi is cut with a fine forceps or aspirated via suction. The abdominal technique, like amniocentesis, involves inserting a needle through the abdomen into the center of the chorion.

The chorionic tissue does not necessarily reflect the genetic status of the fetus. Some risks are infection for the mother, bleeding, harm to the fetus such as limb deficiencies, cervical lacerations and miscarriage.

Percutaneous Umbilical Blood Sampling Test (PUBS)

PUBS is one of the newest experimental methods of fetal blood sampling. Fetal blood is obtained by guiding a needle through the abdomen and uterus into the umbilical vein. It can be used to test for many of the same genetic conditions as amniocentesis but can generate results in as few as three days. It is only offered under very special conditions. It is now being performed between eighteen and thirty-six weeks of pregnancy.

Testing Before Birth (Antepartum Fetal Testing)*

Another set of tests exists, originally designed as screening and diagnostic tools for women with health problems (diabetes, heart or kidney disease or excessively high blood pressure) or for women who have had a previous problem, such as stillbirth. These tests are also performed when a woman or her practitioner thinks that a baby is overdue—usually after forty-two weeks of pregnancy—or that a fetus still in the uterus has stopped growing (IUGR, intrauterine growth retardation), for the placenta can reach a point where it no longer functions at its peak. The goal of these tests is to discover whether the baby is healthy enough to remain in the uterus. While sometimes successful in reassuring worried

---

For further reading, see Judith Lumley, "Antepartum Fetal Heart Rate Tests and Induction of Labor," in Diony Young, ed., *Women and Health: Obstetrical Intervention and Technology in the 1980s*, Vol. 7, Nos. 3/4 (New York: Hawthorne Books, Inc., 1983), pp. 9–28; also Adrian Grant and Patrick Mohide, "Screening and Diagnostic Tests in Antenatal Care," in Murray Enkin and Iain Chalmers, eds., *Effectiveness and Satisfaction in Antenatal Care* (Philadelphia: J. B. Lippincott, 1982), pp. 22–59.

women and practitioners, and sometimes leading to a truly lifesaving cesarean (as in the case of preeclampsia), these tests, like the tests previously discussed, do not *guarantee* a healthy baby. In addition, researchers have not performed enough randomized clinical trials to prove that testing and knowing the results actually do reduce perinatal death. The tests have high false-positive rates and medical people disagree as to which results constitute "normalcy" and which mean danger. Despite such cautions, many doctors have begun performing biophysical and biochemical tests routinely on healthy women toward the very end of their pregnancies. This practice does reassure some women, and because some tests are performed in the hospital, can serve to acquaint women with the birthplace and practitioners there, if the hospital is small enough. But tests also cost more money; further medicalize pregnancy; worry many women excessively, causing them to mistrust their bodies and their health; and sometimes lead to unnecessary medical induction of labor or to further (unnecessary) interventions.

You can check your baby's movements. When you see your practitioner s/he will listen with a stethoscope or doptone to the baby's heartbeat after each of several movements to determine whether the heart tones speed up (accelerate) after each movement, an indicator of good health.

Keep in mind that women experience a lot of variation as their babies move around. Some babies are more active than others, and most babies alternate between periods of activity and periods of rest. Your own perception of the baby's movements may vary greatly depending on what you are doing.

Non-Stress Test

This test may also be performed, based on the idea that when a healthy baby moves in the uterus, its heart rate will speed up with each movement. The test takes twenty to forty minutes and is usually performed in a hospital maternity ward or wherever an external fetal monitor is available. Go for the test at a time when you know your baby is "awake." The nurse determines fetal heart rate by hooking you up to the fetal monitor as you lie on your left side or sit up. The baby moves either by itself or when you push or your practitioner pushes at it. (Drinking a glass or two of orange juice very often makes the baby move, according to one maternity nurse we know.) The test is "reactive" if fetal heart tones accelerate fifteen beats above baseline (120 to 160 beats a minute) twice or three times within twenty minutes. However, practitioners don't all have the same standards as to what a normal response should be, or they may misinterpret their findings. Negative results—a "nonreactive" baby—don't necessarily mean that the baby is in danger. This test is almost always performed before the contraction stress test.

Contraction Stress Test

This test takes two forms. The first, less interventive than the second, simply consists of *nipple stimulation*, causing you to secrete oxytocin, which leads to uterine contractions. You are lying on your left side or sitting up, hooked up to an external fetal monitor. You stimulate your nipples with your fingers, a warm or dry washcloth or a breast pump. Contractions begin within twenty to forty minutes, and usually much sooner. You should have three moderate contractions within ten minutes, each lasting around forty-five seconds. The monitor records the fetal heart's response to each contraction. The aim of this test is to determine your baby's condition by seeing how the placenta responds to the stress of a contraction. If nipple stimulation doesn't succeed in bringing on contractions, then you will have the oxytocin challenge test (OCT), in which a small amount of Pitocin (synthetic oxytocin) is introduced via an intravenous drip. Once contractions begin the fetal heart tones are checked. The OCT has a high false-positive rate with results sometimes difficult to interpret and different observers giving different readings. Its risks lie in the fact that it is an unnatural intervention. It can lead to artificial induction of an entire labor, to cesareans and to hospital-caused (iatrogenic) prematurity—a baby simply may not be ready to be born.

Use your own judgment in relation to these tests. Their very existence and availability may mean that you will be more likely to use them, that you will be pressured into using them. It is most important that you feel as calm as possible toward the end of your pregnancy. The tests may or may not contribute to your peace of mind. You may not want to have any done at all, especially when you are feeling fine.

NOTES

1. M. Enkin, M.J.N.C. Keirse and I. Chambers. *A Guide to Effective Care in Pregnancy and Childbirth.* Oxford: Oxford University Press, 1989, pp. 67–9.

2. M.P.M. Richards. "The Trouble with 'Choice' in Childbirth," *Birth: Issues in Perinatal Care and Education*, Vol. 9, No. 4 (Winter 1982), p. 253.

3. Jo Ann Bromberg. "Having a Baby: A Story Essay," in *Childbirth: Alternatives to Medical Control*, Shelly Romalis, ed. Austin: University of Texas Press, 1981, p. 40.

4. Peggy Spindell. "Midwives and Physicians: Making Home Birth Work Together," Chapter 3 in *A Prac-*

titioner's Guide to Birth Outside the Hospital, S. Sagov et al., eds. Rockville, MD: Aspen Systems Corp., 1983.

5. Elizabeth Davis. *Heart and Hands: A Midwife's Guide to Pregnancy and Birth*. Berkeley, CA: Celestial Arts, 1987, p. 4.

6. Summary, *Childbearing Policy Within a National Health Program: An Evolving Consensus for New Directions*. Available from Jane Pincus, Box 72, Roxbury, VT 05669. $5.00.

7. Shafia Monroe, midwife, interviewed in *Sojourner* (March 1991), p. 2H.

8. Candace Whitredge, interviewed in *The Birth Gazette*, Vol. 5, No. 3 (Spring 1989), p. 8.

9. Judith P. Rooks, Norman L. Weatherby, Eunice K. M. Ernst, Susan Stapleton, David Rosen and Allan Rosenfield, "Outcomes of Care in Birth Centers: The National Birth Center Study," *New England Journal of Medicine*, 321.26 (December 28, 1989), pp. 1804–11.

10. Jennifer Dohrn, inerviewed in *The Birth Gazette*, Vol. 7, No. 4 (Fall 1991), p. 16.

11. Lewis E. Mehl. "The Outcome of Home Delivery: Research in the United States," in Sheila Kitzinger and John A. Davis, eds., *The Place of Birth*. New York: Oxford University Press, 1978, pp. 93–117.

12. Leon Chesley. "Toxemia," in F. Gary Cunningham, *Williams Obstetrics*. Norwalk, CT: Appleton & Lange, 1989. This is the most widely used ob/gyn textbook.

13. *The Genetic Resource*, Vol. 6, No. 1 (1991), p. 61.

RESOURCES

Books and Pamphlets

Davis-Floyd, Robbie E. "Birth as an American Rite of Passage," in Karen L. Michaelson, ed., *Childbirth in America: Anthropological Perspectives*. South Hadley, MA: Bergin & Garvey, 1988, pp. 153–72. Shows how typical obstetrical routines incorporate the fundamental values of our broader culture, making the premises of the technological model of birth appear to be true so that the birthing woman perceives her experience in those terms only.

Martin, Emily. "Medical Metaphors of Women's Bodies: Birth, Resistance, Race and Class," and "The Creation of New Birth Imagery," in *The Woman in the Body: A Cultural Analysis of Reproduction*, Boston: Beacon Press, 1989. The author argues that medical texts depict birth through industrial production metaphors, with the uterus as the machine and the woman as laborer, under the efficient and coercive management of physicians. She interviews women and shows how their views agree or disagree with this model.

Oakley, Ann. *Telling the Truth About Jerusalem*, New York: Basil Blackwell, 1986. A collection of essays that include reflections on the way ultrasound has transformed social relations between physicians, pregnant women and their babies; the meaning of motherhood and the way it has been shaped by the medical paradigm; and the significance of social support in pregnancy.

Pfeufer-Kahn, Robbie. "Taking Our Maternal Bodies Back," in Joyce Antler and Sari Knopp Biklen, eds., *Changing Education: Women as Radicals and Conservators*, Albany: State University of New York, 1990. An essay about successive versions of *Our Bodies, Ourselves*.

Pincus, Jane. "Advice Books for Childbearing Women: Choice or Coercion?" Available from the author at P.O. Box 72, Roxbury, VT 05669. A critical examination of modern childbirth books. Most of them offer women seriously conflicting messages about pregnancy and birth, undermining women's strength and confidence and forcing them into a medical mindset.

Women's Institute for Childbearing Policy. "Midwifery Education in the United States: A Compilation of Selected Resources." Available from Judith Dickson Luce, 30 Park Street, Barre, VT 05641. $5 for syllabus/bibliography; $45 for syllabus/bibliography and copies of the more than sixty cross-disciplinary documents listed. (Make checks payable to WICP.)

20

Childbirth

BY JANE PINCUS, WITH
NORMA SWENSON

With special thanks to Jenny
Fleming, Judy Luce and Becky
Sarah.

*This chapter in previous editions was
called "Prepared Childbirth" and was
written by Ruth Bell and Nancy P.
Hawley.*

*1992 Update by Jane Pincus, with
Judy Luce and Gail Sullivan.*

CLIMATE OF CONFIDENCE

To birthing . . . we bring our histories, our relationships, our rituals . . . needs and values that relate to intimacy, sexuality, the quality and style of family life and community, and our deepest beliefs about life, birth and death. . . . [1]

When you believe in your basic health and strength, in your ability to give birth in your own way, trusting yourself and the people around you to provide guidance and support, when your practitioners believe in you, bringing to the birth of your baby their cumulative experience of seeing many normal births and healthy babies, then you and they together create a climate of confidence.

I had a long, drawn out labor. Each person there got a chance to rest. They switched on and off being with me. I'd take hot showers. I could do what I wanted. I was standing most of the time and walking around. I was so pleased not to be in bed. They encouraged me to eat; I did drink some tea. Finally they convinced me to lie down and I got a little sleep.

Labor was painful. Pain isn't an adequate word. I was bowled over by the intensity of the physical experience. I remember thinking as labor got heavy, women are fantastic, they get pregnant over and over again and are strong enough; people go through this all the time. Nobody could have prepared me for it in words.

I could imagine myself understanding how I'd take drugs if someone urged them on me in a hospital. But here, because everyone was saying, "Everything is fine," it was easy to keep going.

Finally it was dragging on. Laura (my midwife) said, "You and Lewis run around the back yard." We did. We tromped around. Every time I had a contraction I leaned against the pear tree. Then I ran up and down the stairs a few times. Labor became more intense.

Laura called Peter (the doctor). He came over, sat in a corner and read a magazine, saying, "This could take up to two hours. Don't worry, you have plenty of time."

Then came the best time of all. Pushing wasn't at all painful. Mary was holding the mirror; each time I pushed I could see the effects. Laura: "Try breathing—blow out from really deep inside you. Let your cheeks puff out." It worked. I started squatting, then sitting up with Lewis behind me. My final delivery position was on my side, one leg up on Laura's shoulder. With every single push I could see Emma coming out, bigger and bigger. After every push Laura would massage my perineum. The little—no, the big—head came out. She was cooing. It was the sweetest thing I ever heard. Laura said to Lewis and me, "Reach down and pull out your baby." It was a big surprise to us! We did! We pulled her out! I brought her to my breast. We were enthralled. The afterbirth came out with no problem. Laura showed it to us.

The whole experience changed my life. It taught me how deeply physical life is, and connected me much more with my body. I'd learned a refined kind of Catholicism where nothing was earthy, nothing was said aloud. But there's nothing subtle about being pregnant and having a baby!

Another woman and her husband created their own climate of confidence when they had their second baby in a large, busy city hospital where they were more or less left to themselves.

Labor really began at twelve-thirty A.M. on Monday. At two A.M. we went to the hospital. At two P.M. the next day I was working harder but still four centimeters dilated. The obstetrician wanted to give me morphine, saying, "This has gone on too long for a second labor. I'll put you to sleep for five hours and you'll wake up in active labor." Jack and I looked at

Suzanne Arms

each other and said, "This guy's really hot to trot." But we knew that when the baby's ready to be born, it will be born. We said we'd decide at three P.M. At three P.M. I was five centimeters dilated. Nurses were changing shifts. Though they were wonderful there were never many of them around. I was sitting up all the time. Jack and I used a lot of imagery. He helped me to breathe into the pain. We imagined wind and waves. I made sure the sensation would go down and through my cervix, and pictured my cervix opening, pictured myself being born. That helped a lot. Looking at Jack was best, or burying my face in his neck, or closing my eyes and going inside. If he hadn't been there, forget it. We were so concentrated on what we were doing. We knew it was our experience. He knew exactly what to do. He never left me.

At three-thirty they said they were thinking of breaking my bag of waters, but because of the change in shifts, they never got around to do it. Then my waters broke by themselves and labor got harder. I knew it was toward the end. I felt pressure against my pubic bone, which was relieved by counterpressure and singing. Singing was exactly what I needed to do with this one. All of a sudden I needed to push. "Don't push," they said. "I can't not," I said. They took me to the delivery room. I delivered my baby quickly. It was intense. I did my share of yelling. Her head came through while the doctor was still getting dressed, so I had no episiotomy. I made the doctor show me the placenta. My baby nursed in the recovery room, just as I had dreamed about it last summer.

And a midwife states:

All efforts are made to see birth as a continuum. I tell people who have prepared for home birth, who begin labor at home and then end up at the hospital, "Who you are never changes: your planning, ideals, values, beliefs, principles never change just because you end up in the hospital, or with a cesarean. You are stronger than you would have been because you've gone through all those decisions and made the choices you did."

These women who give birth confident in their own birthing powers, at home, in birth centers and in hospitals, show us that giving birth can be richer than we ever imagined. They speak of excitement, doubt, determination, effort, learning about themselves; of momentary lapses and pulling themselves together; of hard work and giving in; of contentment, amazement, ecstasy and exaltation. They listen to their bodies, remain open to their attendants' encouragement to relax and renew themselves. Their experiences make it vividly clear what birth can be and, in contrast, to what extent the purely medical view of birth focuses primarily upon fears: fears of pain, fears that something will go wrong.

CLIMATE OF DOUBT

How did this focus upon the most negative aspects of birthing come about? In fact, the climate of doubt has been in the making a long time. To begin with, obstetrics in the United States began as a surgical specialty practiced by males.

Brief History

More drugs and technologies are now used in "normal" births in America than anywhere else in the world. This reflects in part the desire to master, conquer and control nature that was present among the colonists from the beginning.[2]

The present system was born in and shaped by the competition between male and female healers.[3]

In colonial, preindustrial America, midwives and community women attended childbearing women with excellent results. Sometimes—rarely, when all else failed—they called upon barber-surgeons: "Small wonder that the men who were called by midwives to assist in births regarded birth as deadly and dangerous. They lacked the midwives' experience of hundreds of routine births that required no assistance."[4] *Man-midwives*, as they were called at first, used forceps and hooks, as few women would or did. A formal training period was deemed necessary, and obstetrics became the first specialty to be taught in medical schools in the United States in the eighteenth century.

Many of our own and our doctors' present attitudes originated during the nineteenth century.* Male doctors gradually gained control of childbirth among the upper and middle classes, a control that represented political and economic triumph rather than scientific necessity. They deliberately, systematically excluded women from medical training.[5] "Doctors feared, not without reason, that if women were admitted to the profession, women patients would prefer physicians of their own sex, especially for childbirth."[6]

Although in the 1830s and 1840s a strong grassroots popular health movement campaigned against medical elitism and many kinds of healing sects flourished, and although the medical "regulars"—upper- and middle-class men—had

nothing to recommend them over lay practitioners—"they still couldn't claim to have any uniquely effective methods or special body of knowledge"[7]—the regulars won out through political influence.

Around the same time, doctors performed cruel experimental surgery upon many women, especially black slaves and poor women, in the name of science[8] (an experimentation that continues in gynecology and obstetrics to this day[9]). Out of this early experimentation grew "cures" for gynecological conditions, many of which were actually created by barbarous childbirth practices (although this was not recognized at the time). These skills increased gynecologists' powers enormously, since the promise of cures and even of prevention lay with them.

The Victorian era saw gynecologists and obstetricians gain even more control over women. Middle- and upper-class women, admiring education and science and able to afford doctors' fees, changed their allegiance from midwives to scientifically trained doctors, men of their own class. Some of these doctors eventually became advisers in all sorts of personal matters and went so far as to become judges of their moral conduct (a role that continues to this day). These women were rarely physically active. Meanwhile working-class women continued to work day and night in factories and fields, their pregnancies and births attended by local midwives. Physicians continued to look upon midwives both as economic threats and threats to the masculine, medical order they were in the process of establishing.* They waged a virulent campaign against midwives, stereotyping them as ignorant, dirty and irresponsible. Physicians deliberately lied about midwifery outcomes to convince legislators that states should outlaw it, when in fact midwives often had safety records superior to those of physicians.[10] In addition, though most people of that time believed that birth was usually a healthy, natural process:

Obstetricians campaigned to reverse that belief. They set out to make mothers "fear" the dangers of pregnancy and childbirth, and think of "no precaution as excessive"; and then to comfort them with the assertion of their right to the care of the only ones who could provide it, the professional obstetricians.[11]

As medical boards and state legislators systematically suppressed midwifery, women had to

---

*To understand more fully the origins of these attitudes, see G. J. Barker-Benfield, *The Horrors of the Half-Known Life*, for a fascinating and informative description of the U.S. male mentality in the nineteenth century. Also read Barbara Ehrenreich and Deirdre English, *For Her Own Good*, and *Witches, Midwives and Nurses*; and Richard and Dorothy Wertz's *Lying-In: A History of Childbirth in America*; and all the writings of Robbie E. Davis-Floyd (see Pregnancy and Childbirth Resources).

*"It is at present impossible to secure cases sufficient for the proper training in obstetrics, since 75% of a material otherwise available for clinic purposes is utilized in providing a livelihood for midwives." (Dr. Charles E. Zeigler, quoted in Barbara Ehrenreich and Deirdre English, *For Her Own Good*, p. 95.)

move out of their homes into hospitals to give birth, which did not prove to be safer or better for them and their babies.[12] In 1900, 5 percent of babies in the United States were born in hospitals; by 1935, 75 percent; and by the late 1960s, 95 percent.[13] By giving birth in hospitals women took the last step toward total dependence on the man-made obstetrical system, which became a de facto monopoly. Our struggle to escape this monopoly continues to this day.

Some Attitudes That Create and Sustain a Climate of Doubt

Taking their own bodies as the norm, most doctors see women's bodies as abnormal. Influential obstetricians in this country have come up with some striking descriptions of labor and birth, among them Joseph B. DeLee, who in 1920 compared labor to a crushing door and birth to falling on a pitchfork, the handle driving through the perineum:

In both cases, the cause of the damage, the fall on the pitchfork and the crushing of the door, is pathogenic, that is disease provoking, and anything pathogenic is pathologic and abnormal.[14]

The well-known author of *Birth Without Violence*, Dr. Frederick Leboyer, says:

One day, the baby finds itself a prisoner... the prison comes to life... begins, like some octopus, to hug and crush... stifle... assault... the prison has gone berserk... with its heart bursting, the infant sinks into this hell... the mother... she is driving the baby out. At the same time she is holding it in, preventing its passage. It is she who is the enemy. She who stands between the child and life. Only one of them can prevail. It is mortal combat... not satisfied with crushing, the monster... twists it in a refinement of cruelty.[15]

The orthodoxy reflects an anxious view of birth... as a treacherous course mined with sudden, unexpected disasters requiring the medical equivalent of a military alert.[16]

These ideas and others less dramatic but equally negative underlie and shape many routine obstetrical practices. The practices then reinforce our fears that our bodies won't work right and something will go wrong. They cause new doubts, disrupt the physiology of labor, distort our experiences or completely prevent them from taking place normally. Attitudes themselves—our own and our practitioners'—affect the course of labor—slowing it down, speeding it up—as much

as any drug or mechanical intervention.* When we accept medical descriptions of what we should feel, do and take during labor and birth we allow our powers to be diminished and tamed.

Institutions Contribute to the Climate of Doubt

During the 1950s and 1960s, operations research techniques used to expedite the manufacture of various forms of weaponry in WW II were applied to developing more effective obstetrical suites. ... Priorities were formulated to facilitate the efficient processing of as many women as possible rather than to allow for an adjustable tempo for each individual birth. The factory approach was soon incorporated into textbooks on hospital design: "The conveyer belt concept has its use in analyzing our problems. It emphasizes the repeated transference of a mother (as in motor-car assembly) from place to place, and also that unequal time periods at any station can render the process uneconomical."[17]

Hospitals reduce labor and birth to a medical, debilitating event. As healthy, strong women with good energy, we enter these places for sick people and our strength is systematically depleted. Often we are put into wheelchairs. Our personal effects are taken away. We are cut off from our friends and the people closest to us, isolated among strangers and made dependent and anonymous. Medical personnel desex and infantalize us when they give us enemas and shave us. We are not allowed food and drink, which weakens us, slows labor down and endangers our health. We are hooked up to IVs, which immobilize us: "You don't want to get exhausted, do you?" We are given epidurals: "It will get worse before it gets better (and you won't be able to handle it)." As one nurse-midwife said, regretfully, "The most natural aspects of birth—sexuality, blood, sweat, shit, movement and sounds—have no place here." We are assaulted by assumptions about our inability to give birth without intervention (at times even by the best intentions of hospital staff wanting to "do something useful"). Each "stage" of labor must take place within a given amount of time.

"Continuity of care," one of medicine's own standards for quality care, does not exist. We see

---

*Ann Oakley's *Subject Women* (New York: Schocken Books, 1980) has an excellent discussion of women's attitudes about themselves and professionals' attitudes toward them. Diana Scully's *Men Who Control Women's Health* describes obstetrical residents' attitudes toward the women they see in hospitals. Gayle Peterson, in *Birthing Normally*, details some of the ways in which *our* beliefs and attitudes can affect pregnancy and labor.

many people and have to cope with different personalities, which is neither easy nor particularly good for us. During pregnancy, one doctor or series of doctors checks us out, often hastily and impersonally. During labor in the hospital all kinds of strangers—anesthesiologists, nurses, nursing students, residents, medical students and lab technicians—walk in and out of the room. Some nurses do all they can, but there are not enough of them.

The nurses came and went and didn't stay. My husband did fine, but I was a crab. He couldn't relieve my backache from back labor. One nurse gave me good massages—she knew just where to press—but she was so busy that she had to leave all the time. That upset me.

We also may have no one at all with us for periods of time. *Few cultures leave laboring women so alone.* The doctor, appearing briefly or just at the end of labor, may be someone we have never seen before. When the baby is born, we often have a new set of nurses and an unfamiliar pediatrician. In large hospitals a doctor who specializes in newborns (neonatologist) may appear as well.

This "care" distracts us, causes insecurity and confusion at a time when we should be relaxed, comfortable, focused on ourselves and our babies.

Isolation and immobility during labor increase pain, which increases tension and fear, which brings on more pain. In such surroundings, women end up "needing" pain relief, and obstetricians, anesthesiologists, researchers, and drug companies hasten to provide it in abundant variety.

Physicians' Obstetrical Training Contributes to the Climate of Doubt

Men and women trained in medical schools, clinics and hospitals rarely, if ever, see a normal spontaneous labor and birth. To most students, childbirth means a woman lying on her back during labor, her bag of waters broken artificially, labor "accelerated" by Pitocin, often hooked up to a fetal monitor, drugged or anesthetized, feet in stirrups for delivery in the lithotomy position, given an episiotomy, with a possibility of forceps or perhaps a cesarean section.

As a result, physicians don't know how to relate to a fully conscious, unanesthetized woman. They don't sit through labor from beginning to end to learn how or what a woman feels, to become acquainted with the rhythm of her labor, the positions she chooses and the sounds she makes, to monitor the baby's descent, encourage her and simply to do nothing at times—"mastering the art of inactivity," as one childbirth educator said.

My first home birth, in a trailer in Maryland, was also the first time I had ever been alone with a woman throughout her whole labor. It took hours. There were no nurses, no shifts, no system to shield me from how long having a baby really takes. I remember opening my obstetrics book, examining the course of labor charted on the page and feeling reassured, for the hours of labor were no longer than the hours of the curve.[18]

Nor do medical students learn "hands-on" skills so important to laboring women—massage, physical support, perineal massage. In sum, they do not learn midwifery skills. Most find it boring and undramatic to sit through a labor. Even when they want to, they don't have enough time. Instead, they learn to use mechanical interventions of all kinds routinely to speed up labor, unaware of just how invasive and even dangerous these interventions can be (see pp. 454–59). Also, since obstetrics is a surgical specialty, they must meet a quota for procedures performed, practicing their craft not because women need certain procedures done, but because students need experience. Many of them learn to manipulate us into accepting and submitting to interventions "for our own good" and "for the safety of the baby," strongly suggesting that if we don't agree to undergo certain procedures, we do not care about the baby. They also learn that unless they use or have close at hand every available tool and instrument, they may be sued for malpractice at some point in their future career. Drugs and intervention used routinely in the name of safety become instruments of control and debilitation.

After such training it is no wonder that physicians genuinely believe that we cannot and should not give birth without medical interventions and hospital assistance.

Women Internalize the Medical Model

Childbearing has always involved a perfectly natural fear of something going wrong, of the unknown, of pain and the risk of death. We can never be completely certain of the outcome wherever and however we give birth. Medical attitudes and practices encourge, indeed thrive on these fears. One mother says:

It is as if our confidence is a large, bright piece of fabric. When little pinprick holes of fear and doubt appear, the medical mentality makes them larger and larger until the once beautiful cloth is nothing but gaping holes.

When we are isolated and have no experienced, empathetic women around us to answer questions, listen to us and help us keep feeling positive;

when we put our faith only in doctors who don't believe in our ability to give birth; when we depend, as they do, only on their medical techniques—then we reinforce their belief that we can't do without them. TV, with its images of groaning women giving birth draped in white sheets, and women's magazines repeat the message:

The single factor most responsible for recent advances in helping mothers and infants through the prenatal period (defined as from conception through the first month of the infant's life) is sophisticated technology. It allows physicians to closely monitor fetal development through pregnancy and labor. If the pregnancy is developing entirely normally and if the delivery is totally uncomplicated, the full weight of this technology need not be brought to bear, although it sometimes is.[19] [Emphasis ours.]

Millions of women read articles like this one, which sets up an impossible "model" of pregnancy and labor while suggesting that almost no one will have one. Such propaganda subtly demoralizes us, making us believe that technology must be inevitable. In absorbing the medical model of childbearing we allow our fears of what might go wrong to win over our knowledge that *all* living is risk, that life is to be lived fully with reasonable care rather than with unreasonable caution.

Childbearing is *your* experience—you, not anyone else, are having your child. If you want to give birth in a climate of confidence, you must know it is possible, create it, seek it out, surround yourself during pregnancy with friends and practitioners who feel positive about childbirth. You must know how pervasive the climate of doubt is these days so that you can recognize it in its many forms. Many experienced independent and nurse-midwives; a few physicians, especially family practitioners; some nurses and special labor attendants can help you have the childbirth you want, either in your home, in freestanding birth centers or sometimes even in hospitals.

LABOR

Your body prepares for labor. During labor, uterine muscles gradually stretch the cervix open for the baby to come out, and the muscles also push the baby down into the vagina so it can be born.

Throughout your pregnancy you have been having contractions—called *Braxton-Hicks contractions*—as uterine muscles tighten, then loosen, exercising the uterus and preparing it to work efficiently during labor. Toward the end of pregnancy you may feel these contractions pulling and stretching more intensely and frequently; occa-

sionally they are uncomfortable. Your cervix is softening, ripening.

Both effacement (thinning and drawing up of the cervix) and dilation (opening of the cervix) can occur before you *feel* your labor beginning. Some women remain slightly dilated for weeks before labor begins. Others go into labor *before* dilation starts and have their babies a few hours later.

When you feel stronger contractions, more like menstrual cramps, you may think you are beginning early labor (and sometimes you are). Called "false labor" by the medical profession, these contractions play an important role in initial dilation and effacement. It's as if your uterus were warming up for labor. These contractions usually stop after a while, though they can last for hours. When you feel them, get up and walk around, and see if they continue or if the intervals between contractions become longer or shorter.

What Causes Labor?

We know a lot about labor, but we don't know exactly what causes it to begin. We do know that the physical and emotional readiness of mother and baby is the factor that produces changes in the mother's hormonal levels. Prostaglandins ripen or soften the cervix, and oxytocin causes regular rhythmic contractions that dilate the cervix. The baby's position as well as your emotional state and physical positions can also affect labor. What is important for you to realize is that each labor has its own unique rhythm with periods of intense activity, plateau periods and rest periods, depending upon and reflecting your circumstances as you go through labor.

Some First Signs of Labor

Some body signals let you know that labor may be approaching. Warm-up contractions may become more intense and frequent. You may have diarrhea for a few days or on the day labor begins, your body's way of emptying itself so that labor is less obstructed. You may feel an extraordinary burst of energy and want to cook, clean house, organize—a kind of nesting instinct. You may suddenly want to do nothing.

Bloody Show

As your cervix begins to stretch open, the small mucus plug that seals it comes out, not usually in one piece but as pink mucus, "bloody show," blood-tinged from the broken capillaries formerly attaching it to the cervix. Many women never have a "show." Others have it all through early and active labor.

Dana Sibley

Waters Breaking

As your baby's head presses down against the membranes containing amniotic fluid, they may break. (Most often they break during labor. Rarely, they remain intact until after the baby is born.) Your "waters" may rush out or, more commonly, just trickle out, usually clear and odorless, or milky. Some women think they are wetting their pants. Check color and smell. If you can't stop it by holding it back, it is probably amniotic fluid. *No matter how much fluid comes out, your body replaces it every few hours. There is no such thing as a "dry birth."* After your membranes break, labor will probably begin within twelve to twenty-four hours, though some women trickle for a few days or even weeks. Practitioners disagree about what should be done after your waters break. Physicians are more likely to say that you should come

right to the hospital to prevent infection. Some of them routinely induce labor after twenty-four hours if you haven't started on your own. Midwives and birth attendants are more likely to tell you to relax, that labor will begin soon.

Even if you are planning to give birth in the hospital, consider staying at home; there's usually *less* chance of your getting an infection at home in your customary environment. *Don't* take baths, put anything into your vagina (no internal pelvic exams) or have sexual intercourse. Stay clean. Drink a lot of fluids. Take your temperature regularly, twice a day or more. After twenty-four hours, another thing you can do is to get a white-blood-cell count every day to make sure there's no infection. Your practitioner may want to check your baby's heartbeat periodically.

If your waters broke suddenly, you may want

your practitioner to check externally that the baby's head fits right into your pelvis so that the umbilical cord hasn't slipped in front of the baby's head (which happens sometimes if the baby is in breech position or presenting "high"). Also, if you notice any brown or green staining, let your practitioner know, as it means that meconium (the tarry substance in your baby's bowels) has been squeezed out—common but occasionally an indication of fetal stress or distress.

Contractions (One of the Most Common Signs of Labor)

Your uterus will begin to contract regularly and/or strongly after a while. At first it may feel like gas pains, menstrual cramps, backache, a pulling and stretching in your pubic region. In early labor, contractions may be as regular as clockwork—perhaps ten minutes apart—or they may be irregular, inconsistent, widely spaced. If you begin labor during the daytime, go about your daily routine, especially if this is your first baby, when labors usually take longer. More often, labor begins at night when you are relaxed. It's a good idea to get some more sleep if you can.

At five A.M. I felt period cramps, was really excited. They weren't particularly painful. I knew something was happening! I waited for other signs. Had "bloody show." Beryl, my birth attendant, examined me. I was fully effaced and not dilated at all. Rick and I thought about what we wanted to do with the day. I baked a birthday cake, we took naps, had a quiet day together. I ate lightly all day, had spaghetti for dinner. We went to sleep; I woke up at eleven-thirty P.M. truly in labor.

An unplanned home birth:

I was probably in labor all day and didn't realize it. I went to take a shower, to wash my hair and shave my legs to be presentable. Lo and behold, my son was born then and there. The three of us went to the hospital, my head covered with shampoo.

Some women know when they are about to go into labor, and some can make it happen.

My body felt different the night before, as if I'd become lighter and the baby had shifted position.

I went into labor with my second child very consciously because I needed to. I don't believe in trying to control a process like labor, but it was wonderful to know I could invite it/allow it to start. My blood pressure had been climbing the last weeks of the pregnancy because of overwork and extreme stress. The midwife said to me firmly, "Just have the baby," so I went home to try. I thought about it, we made love, I let go of the reasons why it wasn't a good day, and

in two hours my water broke with mild contractions starting up soon.

I know a midwife who covers the delivery service for only twelve hours a week at a large city hospital. She has delivered four babies for this one woman with whom she has a deep rapport. The woman has managed to time all four labors to fit into the midwife's twelve-hour segments, which shift around from week to week.

Early Labor

In early labor, walking around, taking long walks, taking long baths or making love if your waters haven't broken, lovemaking without intercourse if your waters have broken, showering, hugging, kissing, stroking your nipples or having them sucked all can stimulate your contractions and relax you. (Says one nurse: "Pizza, beer and orgasms—our favorite induction!")

When we went for a walk it was fun running into friends: "What are you doing up? I thought you were in labor." It was fun changing people's image of a woman in labor.

We went to the movies because our apartment was small, and it was too cold out to take a walk. I don't remember much of the film.

We made love while I was in labor. We went to bed and had a wonderful time. I was happy to be giving—to him and to myself—and not just concentrating on contractions.

When you rest or go to bed, contractions may slow down and that's fine. Alternate moving around with brief naps. Stay rested.

Women should stay at home until contractions are frequent and strong. *The longer you stay out of the hospital, the less likely you are to have labor interventions.* Some women prefer to go and settle in before contractions become so strong that walking and riding in a car are uncomfortable. (Afterward, some wish they had never gone to the hospital, others that they had left home sooner.)

Active Labor

When labor really gets going, contractions are strong and rhythmic. You feel them building like a wave, pulling and tightening first in one place, then expanding throughout your uterus, into your back or your groin, and then lessening. In between you can rest, sleep, stay still, walk, talk. *Make sure to empty your bladder regularly.* Relaxing deeply *between* contractions gives you energy for each new one. Relaxing deeply during them helps reduce pain sensation.

Contractions when most intense felt like a belt around my lower back and abdomen. Most of the feeling was in my lower back. Contractions had a curve: strong at the beginning and then slowing down. You get to know them. What surprised me was that you're in two worlds. You have to concentrate on them when they happen, but when they stop, you're just regular. I've never felt so lucid, so clear, as in between contractions.

Language was really important, and I didn't like the word "contraction." . . . I found that when I was having my babies that if I thought "contraction" it meant making something tight. It's true the uterine muscles are contracting, but if everything's working right, at the same time the cervix is expanding. It's much more useful to think of the expansion. . . .[20]

You adapt to labor. The hardest part comes early sometimes. Then you accept that it's really happening, it's a baby, it hurts—no abstractions. Later it can get easier, though contractions may be much stronger.

There is a lot else going on besides the pain in the belly. I felt my nose and teeth going numb, rather as from drinking too much wine. I also saw the colors in the kitchen getting brighter and stronger. I'm not into mystical things, or thinking about auras, but yes, labor is a kind of high if you flow with it, and a room full of loving people does produce energy . . . gives you strength.[21]

Some Ideas for Maintaining Your Identity While Coping with Hospital Routines

- Go in with your partner and/or birth attendant. It's better to be with someone familiar, never necessary or helpful to be separated. It helps if

Ann McQueen/Stock Boston

Suzanne Arms

you bring two support people—one to help you physically during labor and one to troubleshoot in case you have problems getting what you want.
- If they bring you a wheelchair and you feel comfortable standing and walking, ignore it. Take advantage of it if you want to. There is no medical reason for you to use it.
- You can wear your own clothes. If you wear the hospital johnny, take two, and use one as a robe. Bring soft, stretchy socks, preferably knee socks. Hospital rooms are often air-conditioned.

Procedures You Will Encounter

- If you haven't preregistered, you may be asked to sign a patient consent form. It states that you always have the right to informed consent, to say no and to know the risks and advantages of all drugs and procedures. It may also ask you for an "ether permit"—your agreement to be anesthetized in an emergency. You can withdraw your consent at any time.*

---

*Be sure you don't automatically sign a circumcision consent form. If you are a Jehovah's Witness, you need to sign a specific form for yourself and baby to refuse blood products. Signing a form does *not* prevent you from taking legal action in the future should that become necessary.

LABOR

Midwifery Approach to Labor

Midwives describe labor as a continuous process that includes the birth of the baby and the delivery of the afterbirth (placenta). Midwives and other sensitive practitioners know that each labor has its own rhythm and takes its own time. They will not set arbitrary limits for the length of each phase, but will use approaches and techniques to facilitate labor at certain points. This attitude respects and makes possible an experience women describe as being timeless. Some women open up in a steady, gradual way. For others, the process is marked by plateaus and rest periods. Some women slip their babies out, while others take a much longer time helping their babies work their way through the pelvis. Midwives recognize that it is just as important for the mother to deliver the placenta as to deliver the baby. Medically defined "stages" (see below) refer only to the medically perceived relationship of the baby to the woman's body and not at all to labor as women experience it.

Medical Approach to Labor

Medical tradition divides labor into three stages: (1) the time it takes to become fully effaced and dilated; (2) pushing the baby out; and (3) expelling the placenta. Most physicians and hospital personnel set strict time limits in which they expect each of these stages to take place (Friedman's curve), and most physicians are aggressive in their approach to the delivery of the placenta. These limits vary from one practitioner and place to another. Some hospitals may wait twenty-four hours before "accelerating" labor with Pitocin; others wait only twelve hours or even less or do a section for "failure to progress." Most physicians do not like "second-stage" labor to last more than one or two hours.*

---

*Often this is because if you have received anesthesia, it has a depressant effect on the baby.

- A nurse or resident will ask you some questions about your pregnancy and labor. A lab technician will probably take a blood sample, just in case it becomes necessary to match your blood. Hospital staff may listen to the fetal heartbeat with a fetoscope or doptone or see if the fetal heart remains steady during and after contractions. Since the doptone is a form of ultrasound, you may want to ask for a regular fetoscope instead. (Some nurses have never been trained to use regular fetoscopes, however.)
- During all these procedures you can stand or sit. You don't need to get into bed or lie down, though you may be urged or expected to. (You will need to lie down for a fetoscope but not for a doptone.) A mother who labored and gave birth two times lying flat on her back observed:

I've often thought that the best thing a woman can do for herself when she gets into the hospital is to stay upright, standing, sitting, kneeling, squatting. That way she remains active, in control.

- In some hospitals the nurses may want to do a "test strip," using the external fetal monitor to check the course of the baby's heartbeats during a series of contractions. They will ask you to lie still for twenty minutes to an hour. Remember

that when you lie down, your contractions change. If you are in early labor, they may slow down and even stop altogether. They may become more uncomfortable, making you tense up, which affects their efficacy. Ask for a human monitor instead! If the nurses aren't around and you have a birth attendant who knows how to listen to the fetal heartbeat, she can check the fetal heart rate.
- You will probably have an internal exam to check dilation. In some hospitals nurses do them, in others, residents or doctors.

One resident must have been magic. He was a small, silent young man. I didn't feel his exams at all.

I'd brought tapes and music, was walking and dancing. We'd created a wonderful mood. Then the resident came in and blew it. He examined me internally, causing more pain than ever in my life.

- You have the right to turn away residents, to say, "I want my own doctor." Often in teaching hospitals, residents are the only doctors you get, and several of them may want to look at you. You have the right to say no.
- You can refuse to participate in teaching programs. You can always refuse any procedure

from anyone even in life-threatening situations.* Your partner and/or birth attendant can advocate for you.

- Nurses will be your most constant medical attendants if you have no midwife or labor coach. Let them know what you want. Many nurses are encouraging and helpful.

I was in labor for thirty-six hours altogether, most of them in the hospital. One nurse stayed in the room with me the whole time, sleeping in the other bed, keeping people from coming in. She'd tell them, "This is my patient; I'm in charge!" She helped me to have a beautiful vaginal delivery. Without her I would not have done it.

If you have a bad rapport with one nurse, ask for another. It's not always easy to do so (or possible to get another), but it's worth a try.

- If, during any of the procedures mentioned above, you are having a contraction, let the people around you know. They may not be aware of it. Hold up your hand, tell them. Your partner can tell them. They should stop what they are doing and wait. You should not be distracted. Focus on what you want and need. This is your labor and your birth.

Achieving Full Dilation and Effacement (Sometimes Called Transition)

A range of signs indicates that you are becoming fully open and getting ready for the baby to actually be born. You may have a powerful "opening up" feeling, contractions may come rapidly or be more intense than before. The more relaxed you are at this time, the better you'll feel. You may need others especially now to help you breathe deeply and focus your energies, to hold you, encourage you.

You may be very vocal during contractions and doze or be very still in between. Or you may be inward and concentrated throughout. Many women choose one particular position at this time—kneeling, on hands and knees, on their side in bed. This time has been associated with nausea, shaking, trembling of thighs and legs, chills and irritability, though these things can happen at the beginning of labor and be absent at this time. Some women are comforted by the incredible intensity, even by their own irritability, because they know it means that they are close to the end of this part of labor.

*Sometimes the staff proceeds anyway. The hospital is usually protected against any legal action in the future, on the grounds that they acted to save your life.

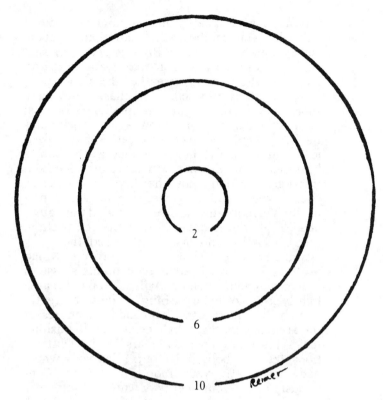

Cervical dilation in centimeters, shown actual size.
Nina Reimer

When you reach full dilation labor often slows down, with contractions farther apart, as if your body were taking a rest. Often women will want to just rest and will experience no urge to bear down, a phase that can last for a brief period or up to two hours. Or contractions may come so close together they feel like one long one. Or you may scarcely have time to take a breath before your enormous uncontrollable "pushing" contractions begin.

The Baby Moves Down Through Your Vagina

Some women suddenly feel an amazing urge to bear down. For some women this is a great relief because they feel in control. For other women, depending on the baby's position, it can be a very painful part of labor. Some women never feel that strong urge to push, as they move the baby down with contractions that feel no different from labor.

Women who attend childbirth preparation classes are often taught to practice pushing by taking huge, deep breaths, holding them and bearing down as hard as they can. Yet strenuous active pushing doesn't necessarily get the baby out faster.[22] In fact, it can lead to the baby's being deprived of oxygen.[23]

Your uterus contracts involuntarily and will push the baby out itself most of the time if not interfered with. *Feel* it pushing and bear down only when you feel the urge. If your mouth is open, your vagina will be open. Breathe deeply or sigh between contractions. You may want to grunt, moan, howl or simply "breathe" the baby out.*

Today many physicians emphasize having a short second stage (typically two hours or less) without evidence to prove that a longer one hurts the baby.† This phase of labor can, in fact, take a few minutes or five hours, as long as the baby's heartbeat is fine. When you relax between contractions and don't push hard, you don't get as tired as you would if you were pushing. Your perineum has more time to stretch around the baby's head as it moves down during the contraction, then back a little, down during the next, then back again. It can be a slow, gradual process, which protects the baby's head and the mother's tissues. Sometimes your attendant will ask you to breathe lightly so as not to be pushing at all as s/he gently stretches or massages with oil and hot compresses the area around the baby's head. Gentle pushing means fewer or no perineal tears. During contractions, let your belly bulge out; relax your whole body, especially your mouth and jaws. Consciously direct your energy downward, outward.

---

*See Sheila Kitzinger's books, Rahima Baldwin's *Special Delivery* and Elizabeth Davis's *Heart and Hands*, for more detailed descriptions of this phase of labor.
†Roberto Caldeyro-Barcia, a well-known South American ob/gyn, says that fetal lack of oxygen (hypoxia) has been a "reason" to push the baby out quickly and thus have a short second stage, when in fact it's the sustained pushing that can cause hypoxia in the first place. Physicians often feel hysteria at the idea of the baby "trapped" in the "birth canal" and rush to pull it out. Nurses also contribute to the rushed atmosphere by calling MDs in too soon. Since they're all there they say, "Let's get her delivered," especially when they are very busy.

I was holding back. This thought raced into my mind and out the other side: If I push hard enough, I'm going to become a mother. Ann said, "Next time you have a contraction, push a little bit; think open; *you'll feel better." Amazing—I could feel her coming down; it did feel better.*

You can be in any position to let the baby come out. When you are on hands and knees or squatting with knees apart, your pelvis is at its widest. You may feel most comfortable kneeling or on the toilet at first, then go to kneel on the bed or sit, or lie on your side with one leg up on an attendant's shoulder.

THE LITHOTOMY POSITION—LYING ON YOUR BACK WITH YOUR FEET UP IN STIRRUPS—IS THE WORST, MOST INEFFECTIVE AND MOST DANGEROUS POSITION FOR LABOR. IT IS USED IN MOST HOSPITALS FOR THE CONVENIENCE OF THE DOCTOR.

Suzanne Arms

Jim Harrison/Stock Boston

Pushing was the strangest and in some ways the nicest sensation I've ever had. I could actually feel the shape of the baby, feel myself sitting on the head as it moved down . . . the thought of moving, especially from a good, comfortable, well supported seated position, to flat-out on a bed seemed ridiculous. So there I was on my rocking chair, with my feet up on two little kitchen chairs, with Hersch on one side and the doctor on the other . . . it was like moving a grand piano across a room: that hard, but that satisfying.[24]

BIRTH

Your baby's head will be born first, unless the baby is in breech position (see p. 452). You must usually wait for the baby to rotate a quarter-turn in order for the rest of it to be born—shoulders, one at a time, then body. During this time your attendant may ask you to keep in eye contact and to blow gently and to reach down and touch the baby's head, then breathe the baby out. S/he will check to see if the cord is around your baby's neck and perhaps also to suction mucus from its nose and mouth.

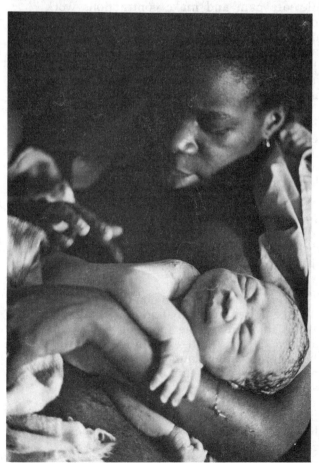

Suzanne Arms

Within a few minutes, the baby was coming. I knelt on the bed, leaning forward against Thomas. It was a wonderful position, very solid and stable, yet my hands were free to reach down and feel her head. My older daughter was ready with a blanket to wrap the baby, and I will never forget the feeling of the little body sliding out and into my hands just as the sun came up. It's a great moment—the baby is there, it doesn't hurt anymore, both in the same instant. The room was full of light.

I got to shouting, "That's enough, that's enough." "My hemorrhoids hurt," I got to blubbering. Marya said, "Run some water; take a bath." It felt good to have all that water sloshing around. Nothing was happening on the bed; it seemed so much easier in the water. Everything I needed was there at the time. I said, "I feel kind of open!" Then I saw my son float out. It was great. He was so peaceful and calm. His eyes were open under the water.

I felt godlike—a miracle worker. It was the best moment of my life. I felt my baby's head, then saw his face—I got to cut his cord and put him to my breast. I felt like I did the impossible. I couldn't believe he was finally out into the light. I felt holy.

RIGHT AFTER

If your baby breathes as soon as the head is completely out, s/he may be born looking pink. Otherwise s/he will look very still and bluish until breathing becomes regular and sustained. Not all newborns cry. Some cry for a moment, then stop. They may just breathe, blink and look around or snuffle.

Right after birth, hold your baby close. S/he's your own; s/he belongs next to you. Cover her/him with blankets for warmth and hold her/him naked against your breasts and belly in order that s/he may touch your skin, smell you, feel you, hear you, look at you and your partner. You'll want to caress, touch, talk to her/him. Enjoy this slow time. If you are exhausted, your partner can hold the baby against you or close to him/herself.

So much has been written about this moment. It is important to recognize birth as the continuation of a process that began with conception. The connection is already an intimate one. Newborns recognize their mother's scent, their parents' voices and familiar sounds. We want hospitals to respect how crucial it is for us, our partners and children to continue to be close to our babies at this time. The further attachment of babies to mothers after birth, called *bonding* (as if babies and mothers had not been connected for months) cannot be created or forced just by going through the motions. As Sheila Kitzinger said in

CREATING A NURTURING BIRTH ENVIRONMENT

Surroundings. When you feel comfortable and safe, with familiar people around you, you are better able to relax. Women give birth at home to be in familiar territory where they are free to be themselves. Out-of-hospital birth centers are usually like homes; you can cook your own food, use the living room, spend time with your children and friends. If you go to the hospital, bring "home" along with you—favorite clothes, photographs, pictures, beloved objects, a rug or blanket, records or tapes for music.

People you feel comfortable with. It is important that the presence of others, their touch, advice and actions give you comfort and strength and make you happy and confident and that they feel comfortable with you.

The pain was like a hurricane shaking me apart. I yelled a lot and walked around and took showers. I remember looking at Paul and thinking, What are you so happy about? This is terrible. Yet I know that the grin on his face sustained me. I needed his touch and his joy, and I needed—very differently—the midwife's words and knowledge and reassurance.

Choose support people who can understand what you want and don't want without having their feelings hurt. Too many and/or the wrong people (sometimes even your partner) can hinder labor by being too solicitous, too anxious, too noisy, too bossy.

Breathing. Whether or not you've practiced breathing beforehand, deep breathing can help you to relax. Imagine your breath carrying oxygen to every part of your body. Breathe in whatever way is comfortable. Loosen your jaw. Open your mouth and throat. Smile. Laugh.

I found my own way of breathing. I knew I had to relax into the tenseness.

Some women may use the breathing they've practiced and become too controlled, too tense. Combine breathing with different positions, with sounds.

I was with a woman doing rigid strong labor breathing she had learned in a childbirth class. She was tight, exhausted. I said, "You don't have to do that." "What will I do?" "Just see what happens." She began to relax. When she let go trying to keep her control, her energy started to flow. Over the next few hours she started doing little sighs which became moans at the end. On the floor, kneeling, she breathed into her husband's lap and rocked her pelvis. He started to breathe and rock with her.

Endorphins. You may feel exhilarated during labor, mellow and peaceful between contractions, especially when your labor is progressing naturally and uninterruptedly. Your body is producing its own substances for pain relief, called *endorphins*, which have a morphinelike effect. (High levels have been found in the placentas of animals and humans after birth.[25]) Tension and fear cause you to secrete adrenaline, which tenses you up, slows your labor and makes it more painful. This inhibits the secretion of endorphins. By relaxing, you enable endorphins to flow again. If labor is painful, don't blame yourself. Deep relaxation can be difficult, even in an ideal environment.

Change position and move around. Positions in which your spine is upright, as when you are walking or rocking, can help you relax, alleviate pain and make contractions work more effectively. Being on hands and knees also helps, especially when you have back labor. You can rock back and forth, dance slowly and rhythmically and move in ways you'd never dream you'd move! Many women find sitting on the toilet most comfortable.

Food and drink. When you drink and eat—light foods at the beginning of labor, juices, tea with honey, juice popsicles as it becomes more intense—you keep up your strength and blood sugar level. You don't become dehydrated and you are better able to handle contractions. Drink, and remember to pee often.

Birth is a time of great energy: No one should be expected to run a marathon or swim the English channel if she had been deprived of sustenance and was unable to continue to nourish herself from time to time.[26]

Emotions. Some women don't want or need to make noise, but many find that expressing strong emotions of the moment—anger, exaltation, fear, pain—groaning, grunting, shouting, moaning, laughing, singing, chanting—can loosen them up. During second-stage labor as you breathe or push the baby out, you'll probably be making sounds along with the pushing. Low sounds seem to work better than high-pitched ones—more of a *downward* feel to them, say some midwives.

Water is wonderful. Baths and showers can relax and soothe us during labor. Some women stay in the shower for hours. When tub water is shallow, someone can pour warm water over your belly during contractions. (One midwife says, "It's better than Pitocin for getting contractions going!") When the water is deep, your uterus will be lifted up and away from your body, which can reduce the intensity of labor, especially back labor. Lying mostly underwater, leaning against supports, you can float slightly and relax deeply.

Help: physical support, touch, massage and holding. Ask your partner, friend, birth attendant or nurse to help you when you squat, stand or kneel; to lean against you; hold you under your arms; let you hang from his/her shoulders; hold you however you want to be held.

"Drink in" touch and massage. Human companionship and/or contact can make you feel at ease, sustained and loved. Your partner or attendant may know exactly what to do without being asked. Or s/he may not. If the touch doesn't feel right, ask until something feels better. Some women do not want to be touched at all.

I asked my two friends to massage deeply and hard, putting a lot of pressure on my lower back muscles to counter all that force. I liked feeling their hands supporting my belly at the same time.

Imagining. In South India, birth attendants place a flower near the laboring woman; as its petals unfold, her cervix opens. Opening is a ceremony, a celebration.

Imagine being in a place you love the best, where you are most happy. Imagine you are a flower opening, light exploding. Open your mind to images. Imagine your baby hugged by your uterus, pushing down, ready to be born in its own way, opening you. Say to yourself, "I feel my baby moving down my pelvis, I feel my muscles letting go; my cervix is stretching, opening, opening MORE—open . . . open . . . OPEN."

Advice for your attendants, family and friends. Pay attention. Observe. Be quiet, present, in tune. Focus your attention on her. Be joyful, encouraging, positive, uplifting. Move slowly, breathe slowly, stay calm. Don't communicate anxiety or fear. Leave the room if you feel uncomfortable. Don't expect her to be stoic. Don't expect her to tell you politely what she wants. Sometimes she may not want you to touch her at all. If she tells you to go away, don't take it personally. It's just labor. Don't feel sorry for her. Yes, it hurts, but show your belief in her strength. Or she may say, "I can't stand this anymore." Tell her she can. She is. Change what's happening. Make it better. Maybe a walk, a shower, a bath, a change of position will make her feel better. Keep her focused on the present. If she is losing her concentration, help her focus. Hold her, sing, chant, laugh, moan, rock with her. Just before the baby is born, at the most intense time, she may need touch, eye contact. Breathe along with her. Hold hot compresses against her perineum; she can relax into the heat. Or let her lean against/on you.*

---

*Special thanks to Becky Sarah!

Vaughn Sills

one of her talks, "Some hospitals act as if it is a special glue that can be sprayed on and will take in five minutes. After that they think it's too late." One mother fighting separation from her baby was told, "You're bonded to her now, so what's the problem?"

And if for some reason the first moments after birth don't turn out the way you want, you will have many ways of becoming attached to your baby and her/him to you. Bonding in humans is an ongoing process.

Right after the birth, practitioners evaluate your baby's well-being. Their conclusions are often expressed in the one- and five-minute Apgar score (from one to ten). Most infants score between seven and ten. Your attendant will have oxygen and suctioning equipment at hand in case the baby needs help breathing. Gentle suctioning of the nose and throat is done if needed. The baby will be wet-looking, covered with a waxy substance called *vernix* and usually not very bloody. Her/his head may be oddly shaped temporarily, having been molded during its passage through your vagina.

The first few hours of life are a time of heightened awareness for your baby. That is why you need peace, quiet and no interruptions. Your baby will nurse (s/he has been sucking in the womb before birth). Some babies know exactly what to do right away. Babies born to unsedated and/or unanesthetized mothers often have strong sucking reflexes. Others take time to learn. If you have received drugs, your baby may not be able to nurse until they wear off. It is good to let your baby suckle even if you don't plan to breastfeed, for when babies first nurse, they receive important antibodies and nutrients from your colostrum. If the baby doesn't seem to want to nurse right away, or if hospital staff objects, remember that *you are in charge and can make it happen.** Sucking is important for you, too. It stimulates oxytocin, which makes your uterus contract to expel the placenta and stay contracted afterward. It also slows down any bleeding.

You are still connected to your baby by the umbilical cord, attached to the placenta inside you. Physicians in hospitals used to cut the cord as soon as the baby breathed or cried; many still do. But now many practitioners wait five or ten minutes until the cord has stopped pulsating. Then they clamp the cord, cutting it a few inches from the navel. Often, one's partner cuts the cord. In a week

or so, the bit of cord left on the baby's navel dries up and falls off.

DELIVERY OF THE PLACENTA

After a certain interval—five to thirty minutes or longer—the cord lengthens, you may feel a contraction, have a rush of blood and expel the placenta. Contractions usually come sooner when you are sitting up or squatting and the baby is suckling. It is extremely important to have the placenta totally out, which completes the birth cycle. Until this happens, blood vessels remain open and women are especially vulnerable to infection and hemorrhage. Once the entire placenta is born, blood vessels close down. Your uterus clamps down and begins to shrink. Breastfeeding helps this process. If all else is normal, it's reasonable to wait, watchfully. Often, the best way to ensure that there will be no problems is to let things happen. Usually the placenta comes out by itself, helped along by your baby suckling or by someone else sucking on your nipples. If the placenta doesn't come out, your attendant may give you a shot of Pitocin, pull gently on the cord (controlled traction) or extract it manually (if, for example, there is hemorrhage, and it must come out quickly). If you are at home and have problems at this point, you may have to go to the hospital.

THE FIRST FEW HOURS AFTER THE BABY IS BORN

Mother and Baby

It is best if your baby stays with you and your partner for as long as you want after birth. Parents and child sleep and wake together, get to know each other, and the baby nurses whenever s/he wants.

Although parents and baby stay together at home, in freestanding birth centers and some hospital rooms, it is more difficult in most hospitals. (Definitely make your wishes known beforehand.) *There is no medical reason to separate healthy mothers and babies after birth. It is your right to keep your baby with you; s/he belongs to you.* Babies with minor and even major health problems benefit from being close to their parents; they also may need medical observation at the same time.

The First Hour or Two

Practitioners will do a complete physical exam of your baby. It is not necessary that they do it right away (unless there is an obvious problem). In the hospital ask to have it done in your presence so

---

*It is important for you to have discussed breastfeeding with your practitioner (and your pediatrician, if possible) in advance and to have made sure that you can reach her/him after the baby is born, so that any hospital orders preventing you from being with your baby can be changed.

that you can see exactly what is happening and ask any questions you may have.

Silver Nitrate Drops and Vitamin K

In all hospitals it will be recommended that babies' eyes be treated with a substance that can prevent gonococcal infection. Traditionally, silver nitrate was used, but now erythromycin is offered.* Parents can sign a waiver and refuse the treatment. The gonococcal bacteria, if left untreated, can lead to blindness (see Chapter 14, "Sexually Transmitted Diseases"). Home birth attendants leave the decision up to parents as to whether or not they want the baby to receive drops. If you refuse the treatment, pay close attention to your baby's eyes during the first week or so to make sure that they remain clear and don't look infected. If they do become runny and/or swollen, with lashes stuck together, your baby must get medical care.

Pediatricians recommend that babies receive vitamin K injections after birth to prevent a rare (1 in 2,000) disorder known as hemorrhagic disease of the newborn (when the blood doesn't have enough clotting factor). Twenty-five years ago these injections became mandatory in hospitals to counteract the anticlotting effects of many drugs, which sometimes caused jaundice. In out-of-hospital births, most attendants will not use vitamin K unless there has been trauma. Vitamin K injections may or may not be given. If it has been a traumatic birth with excessive head-molding, vitamin K is necessary. You can give vitamin K orally to the baby, but it's not clear that it works as well, and it tastes bad. Ask your practitioner about silver nitrate and vitamin K. You have a legal right to refuse both treatments.

Where You Are After You Give Birth Affects How You Feel

The comfort of being at home cannot be overestimated, being in my own bed afterward, familiar cracks in the ceiling, my family all around.

After a normal delivery in a freestanding birthing center, most women go home within twelve to twenty-four hours. The usual stay in a hospital is four hours to three days or three to five days after a cesarean. If you want to leave soon after the birth, make arrangements with your practitioner and the hospital.

We had planned a home birth but, because of an unexpectedly long labor, wound up delivering in the hospital instead. Our disappointment, however, was tempered by our doctor's promise that if everything went okay, we could return home right after the birth. Megan was born that day at noon, and by five P.M. I was back at home taking a much needed shower, while Peter and my mother and his parents prepared supper and admired the baby. Then we all sat down to a celebration birthday supper, complete with cake and champagne and Megan in the middle of the table in her basket. By nine P.M. Peter and I were asleep in bed with Megan snuggled between us. The next day, the midwife came, checked me and the baby and answered my barrage of questions. Later in the day, friends came bringing food and baby presents. I remember those days as among the happiest in my life.

You may want to stay in the hospital a few days, especially if you have other children at home or no household help.

I have five kids at home. I look on this as my only vacation this year!

Some hospitals have *rooming in*, where your baby stays with you all the time; they may have *modified rooming in*, where your baby stays with you whenever you want, or just during the day, and then goes back to the central nursery whenever you are tired or at night. Often, mothers who keep their babies with them are more rested than mothers whose babies stay in the nursery. But many hospitals still separate mothers and babies routinely, sometimes for twelve to twenty-four hours at first and then most of the time except for feedings; nurses place babies in warming cribs, take them to central nurseries and bring them to mothers for feedings every four hours. Most newborns and mothers find it difficult to adapt to hospital routines. In addition to the stress of being in a strange, sterile environment, hospital rules can interfere with the natural process of recovery and with getting to know your baby.

I had my first baby in the hospital. For the next four days I hardly slept. My roommate was nice, but she liked the TV on all the time. Then there were the nurses who came in every couple of hours to take my temperature or give me a laxative or scold me for nursing "too long" on one side. During visiting hours and at night, they took the baby to the nursery, and I would fantasize that she was the one I heard crying. I felt tense and depressed most of the time.

There are good reasons for going home as soon as possible. Babies in hospital nurseries are at sig-

---

*Most states have a law requiring silver nitrate; some physicians and hospitals may feel they cannot administer antibiotic alternatives without changes in the law.

LESS USUAL PRESENTATIONS

In the previous description of labor, we have assumed the baby's position in the uterus to be the most common—*left occipito anterior* (LOA). This means that the baby is head down in the uterus, lying on its left side, with the occiput, or back part of the skull, toward the mother's front. It is the most efficient way for a baby to slip past the pubic bone and into the birth canal.

Another position is head first but faced the opposite way, with the baby's face toward the mother's front. This is called *posterior presentation*. It can mean a longer labor, since the baby may try to turn around during labor in order to be born in the more favorable way, facing the mother's back. With a posterior baby, you may experience labor pains in your back. Feel free to take labor positions most comfortable for you.

Some babies present buttocks down or feet (footling) or hands first. They are in *breech* position, which can mean a long back labor. Sometimes you can turn a breech baby around yourself from the thirtieth week of pregnancy on (see p. 424). They may turn themselves during labor or may not turn at all. A *skilled* practitioner may be able to turn them from the

outside (external cephalic version).* If your practitioner has delivered many breech babies successfully and if your pelvis is big enough and the baby small enough, you'll be able to birth her/him vaginally. *Squat: It widens your pelvic outlet significantly!* A danger in breech birth is that after the baby is delivered the head will be trapped, and the baby will try to breathe and will suffocate. Knowledgeable practitioners wrap the baby's emerging body in warm blankets to keep cold air from shocking her/him into taking a breathful of mucus; they also insert a finger into the woman's vagina, clearing a passageway for air. Footling breeches are usually delivered by cesarean (unless they are the second of twins, when the cervix has opened wide enough). These days most obstetricians in training rarely if ever learn the necessary skills to perform external cephalic versions or to help deliver breech babies vaginally; they perform cesareans instead.

Some babies lie horizontally (*transverse lie*) and their heads never engage. They must be born by cesarean.

---

*See Brigitte Jordan, "External Cephalic Version," *Women and Health*, Vol. 7, Nos. 3/4 (Fall/Winter 1982), pp. 83–102, for a historical, cross-cultural and physiological description of this procedure.

nificant risk for infection.* There's an advantage to immediate hands-on practice in taking care of your baby, especially if it's your first.

SOME SIGNS OF ABNORMAL LABOR AND DELIVERY

If complications should arise during labor, your body will usually give you some warnings. It is, of course, of vital importance that you be aware of them and tell your practitioner. When you are awake and not medicated, you will have a much

clearer sense of what is going on. Also, some complications are set into motion by anesthesia.

Here are a few signals that should warn you to notify your practitioner immediately.

Continuous and Severe Lower Abdominal Pain, Often Accompanied by Uterine Tenderness

This is different from the pain of normal labor contractions, which comes on with increasing intensity and then gradually disappears completely until the next contraction—a pain that comes and goes.

An Abnormal Presentation or Prolapse of Cord, Placenta or Extremity

If any of these occurs, an experienced practitioner must decide if a cesarean is required. Prolapsed cord (when the cord falls into the vagina and there is the danger that it might be compressed, thereby cutting off oxygen to the baby) and placenta

---

*Central nurseries used to be considered sanctuaries where babies were kept safe from infections, chilling, mucus problems and overexhaustion from medicated or operative deliveries. Yet in large nurseries, infants receive intermittent and often impersonal care, a poor substitute for mothering. some nurseries breed *Staphylococcus aureus*, *Streptococcus* and *Salmonella* (which cause *nonsocomial* infections—infections acquired in a hospital). These clearly *iatrogenic*—hospital-caused—illnesses can be serious, sometimes resulting in infant death.[27]

previa (placenta first instead of baby first) generally call for a cesarean section.*

Excessive Vaginal Bleeding

There are a number of reasons for this, such as cervical laceration, placenta abruptio (when the placenta suddenly becomes detached from the uterus) or delivery before the cervix is fully dilated. It is normal, however, to have a bloody mucus discharge just before complete dilation, especially when the cervix is opening up very quickly.

Abnormally Slow Dilation of the Cervix

When contractions are severe and the cervix is still not dilating regularly, then the ineffective contractions may be creating undue stress on the fetus, the mother or both. This is a particularly hard condition to diagnose, since pain is subjective and many labors last much longer than others. This is part of the dystocia category discussed in Cesarean Section (p. 459). Many midwifery techniques can change this type of labor. However, sometimes even then there will be little or no cervical dilation.

Abnormality in Fetal Heartbeat

This condition is a sign that the baby may be in trouble. Fetal heartbeat should be checked regularly throughout labor.

Any Adverse Change in Condition of Mother or Baby

If the pattern of heartbeat and/or blood pressure changes, if the woman develops a fever or if some other difficulty arises, it is essential that an experienced doctor or midwife be present to interpret the signs.

PREMATURE LABOR AND DELIVERY

A premature baby is one who is born during or before the thirty-seventh week of pregnancy. Until recently a baby of five and a half pounds or less was considered premature, but now doctors are more concerned with the maturity and functional development of the baby than with her or his birth weight.

We know little about the cause of prematurity in nearly half the cases. Poor health, inadequate nutrition, stress and heavy smoking all increase one's chances of having a premature delivery.* Some specific causes of premature labor are infectious diseases (such as syphilis), toxemia of pregnancy, diabetes, thyroid disturbances, fetal abnormalities, placental abnormalities (placenta previa, placenta abruptio, etc.) and multiple pregnancies—twins or triplets. Some of these problems can be avoided through adequate nutrition and health care. Statistics show that low-income women and young teenagers receive poorer and less prenatal care and are more likely to deliver prematurely than middle-class women.

Premature labor proceeds like normal, full-term labor. It may be a little slower owing to weaker contractions or more rapid because the baby is smaller. *Premature babies are extremely susceptible to the dangerous effects of the drugs used during labor,* so if you are prepared to handle labor without drugs you will be doing your baby a great service.

The smaller and more feeble the baby, the more s/he needs immediate care. In the United States, most premature babies are placed in oxygen-, temperature- and humidity-controlled incubators, kept in intensive care nurseries and protected from every possible source of infection, since they are very susceptible and infection is common in hospitals. Increasingly, mothers are spending more time with their babies in these nurseries, some of which are set up for parents, others not. Be assertive about staying with your baby as much as possible—your presence, your voice, your touch, your love will help her/him thrive. Some doctors are exploring the advantages of keeping older or larger premature babies in incubators close to their mothers' bedsides, so that mothers can take them out to cuddle and hold close.† These babies grow and develop much more quickly than those who are left more to themselves in incubators. Mothers turn out to be the most watchful attendants, and if anything seems to be going wrong, they quickly signal nurses or doctors.

It is best to feed your baby breast milk.[29] The antibodies in colostrum fight the very infections to which the premature baby can succumb. You can pump your own milk with an electric or hand

*Michel Odent, in *Birth Reborn*, discusses the possibility of vaginal birth if only a bit of the placenta covers the cervical opening.

*Seventy percent of deaths of newborn babies in the United States are due to low birth weight. This is a tragedy, since we can prevent much prematurity by good nutrition, competent prenatal medical care and adequate birth control for those who may be unable to carry a fetus to term (e.g., young teenagers whose bodies are not yet developed enough).[28]
†Michel Odent, at his clinic in Pithiviers, France, is one. See *Birth Reborn*. Also see Robert B. Berg, " 'Early' Discharge of Low-Birth-Weight Infants," *Journal of the American Medical Association*, Vol. 210, No. 10 (December 8, 1969), pp. 1892–96.

breast pump (some hospitals have them handy) if your baby must stay in an incubator, and feed it to her/him (see p. 479 for more).

You may not be prepared yet for delivery and motherhood; you feel uncertain and anxious, constantly worried about your baby. Find people with whom you and your partner can talk. All hospital staff should be aware of your feelings, encourage you to spend as much time with your baby as you want, explain the reasons for all hospital procedures and answer all your questions as completely as possible.*

OBSTETRICAL ROUTINES, PROCEDURES AND DRUGS

The mechanism of labor is both powerful and delicately balanced. Each part and process has a function in helping the baby be born well. Our attendants must respect the process and not interrupt it, hinder it or speed it up (unless absolutely necessary). Contractions massage the baby to squeeze excess fluid out of its lungs, amniotic fluid equalizes pressure and cushions the baby's head, membranes hold the waters in, the perineum has a chance to stretch slowly. Like any other animal, we need a calm environment for labor to proceed at its own pace, and we tense up when we are afraid, causing labor to slow down. Like elephants and dolphins, we labor best with empathetic females like ourselves nearby.

Occasionally things go wrong and medical intervention becomes necessary. Most obstetrical drugs and hospital procedures have never been scientifically proven beneficial for healthy mothers and infants.[30] Most of the time medical obstetrics interferes with our bodies in outrageous ways, as if male doctors over the course of the past century had sat down and systematically figured out how to interrupt each natural step of the labor process, one by one.† It is a credit to our basic health and resilience that, despite such assaults, we and our babies emerge so healthy. It is sad that so many of us expect intervention as the norm and rely on it for safety and pain relief when it is not always safe and we can deal with pain in so many other ways. It makes no sense for us to accept routine tampering with our bodies, our strengths and the safety of our children. It is useful to learn about obstetrical routines so that we use medical resources during labor only when we really need them.*

Drugs and Interventions in a Hospital Birth

Like a snowball rolling down the hill, as one unphysiological practice is employed . . . another frequently becomes necessary to counteract some of the disadvantages, large or small, inherent in the previous procedure.[31]

If you are planning a hospital birth, find out what procedures and drugs are in common use there and the choices you will be able (allowed) to make. Discuss your preferences beforehand, write them down and send copies to your physician or midwife, to the hospital and to the head of nursing.

Once you arrive at the hospital, you have a right to know the names and risks of anything done or given to you, and to refuse them (see Our Rights as Patients, p. 682).

"Prepping" (Shaving Pubic Hair)†

This used to be done routinely. It is totally unnecessary. It is just one part of the male medical ritual of depolluting, purifying women.[33] (We heard one doctor say, "I like my women clean.") Prepping desexes us, makes us look like little girls again. Doctors believe that pubic hair contains germs and prepping decreases the risk of infection. In fact, prepping *increases* the risk of infection, when surface skin cells are scraped off and sometimes razors nick skin. As hair grows back, it is itchy and uncomfortable.

Many hospitals have eliminated this practice or offer it as an option.

Enemas

Enemas used to be routine, but most hospitals don't give them anymore. They are not necessary. Women often have a natural diarrhea before labor begins or during labor. You can request an enema if you think it will make you feel better or if feces in your rectum seems to be holding up your labor. Often enemas stimulate labor. But if you are in

---

*See Sherri Nance, *Premature Babies: A Handbook for Parents*, for a sensitive discussion about all aspects of prematurity.
†Michel Odent, throughout *Birth Reborn*, speaks of modern obstetric practice as "the systematic elimination of the mother from the childbearing process." Sally Inch's *Birthrights* gives a detailed description of the effects of drugs and interventions. Doris Haire wrote *The Cultural Warping of Childbirth* out of a concern that obstetrical practices and drugs are causing retardation, brain dysfunction and learning disabilities in our children.

---

*See *Home Birth: A Practitioner's Guide to Birth Outside the Hospital*, by Sagov et al., for discussions of the ways in which women in labor, their partners and practitioners mutually decide about whether or not to use interventions and drugs, balancing medical necessity with personal values.
†Two British studies conclude that routine prepping and enemas constitute "unjustified assaults" on women, and that there is no evidence of benefit.[32]

active labor already, it can make your contractions stronger and more uncomfortable, which in turn may make you ask for drugs, thereby setting off the chain of procedures related to their use. One reason given for administering enemas is to prevent contamination of the perineum by feces. Yet enemas result in watery feces, which may be less "clean" than natural diarrhea.

Making Women Lie Down

This increases the length of labor and the risk of distress to the baby while decreasing the strength and efficiency of contractions.[34] When you lie down you press in your inferior vena cava (a major vein), which decreases blood flow and oxygen supply to the fetus. Since it is often more uncomfortable to lie still than to be upright and/ or moving around, you may become tense, which can slow labor even more and make you feel more pain. At this point you may ask for drugs or your labor may "need" medical intervention, when in fact what you *really* need is a change of position, movement, a shower or bath to relax you, and loving, holding, touching.

Rupturing the Amniotic Sac (Membrane)— Amniotomy

Some physicians routinely rupture membranes early in labor, or if they think your labor isn't progressing fast enough, by puncturing the sac through your cervix with a small hook. It doesn't hurt; you can feel the waters rushing out. The baby's head then moves down to press aginst your cervix, perhaps releasing more oxytocin and thereby causing stronger contractions. Early amniotomy, more convenient for the doctor, does not usually benefit baby or mother.[35] The stronger contractions can place pressure on the placenta or umbilical cord as the baby pushes against it; if the cord is wrapped around the baby's neck or is very short, it can also be affected by such pressure, which may cut off the flow of blood, which contains oxygen. In addition, the baby's body and head are no longer cushioned by amniotic fluid. Stronger contractions may be more difficult for you to handle; you are also more prone to infection. The medical answer: possibly drugs to weaken (counteract) strong contractions or Pitocin to speed up labor because of the risk of infection; fetal monitors to check the baby's heartbeat; and occasionally cesareans because these interventions have endangered your baby's life.

Sometimes when a woman is dilated about eight centimeters and the baby's head has descended far enough, a practitioner may rupture the membranes to speed labor. If your practitioner suspects fetal distress, s/he may rupture the membranes to check the amniotic fluid for the presence of meconium (not a completely reliable indicator).

(Some practitioners use an amnioscope, a rod with a light and mirror on it, to "see" the color of the fluid without having to rupture the membranes, a less invasive procedure.)

Intravenous Solution (IV)

Many hospitals set up an IV for every woman early in labor. A nurse will introduce a hollow tube into a vein in your hand or arm and affix it with adhesive tape so that fluids can flow (be infused) into your bloodstream. The IV is used "just in case" something goes wrong and emergency anesthesia becomes necessary or to prevent hypotension (lowered blood pressure) from epidural anesthesia; to nourish you with a glucose solution and prevent you from becoming depleted and dehydrated when you are not allowed to eat or drink during labor; to introduce oxytocin (now almost routine in many teaching hospitals in order to speed up labor); to teach students about IVs.

IVs should not be used in normal labors; instead you should be able to drink fruit juices, water, honeyed teas. They *are* useful, however, when you can't keep anything down and vomit a lot (rare) or when you have become extremely dehydrated.

IVs make it difficult for you to move around (immobility can slow down your labor). They can be uncomfortable and make you feel awkward and passive. They may make you anxious. If you must have an IV, ask the nurses to put it securely into the arm or hand you use the least. Ask for an IV pole so you can continue to move around. Ask someone to push it. You must be sure to urinate often, at least once an hour or more, as fluids accumulate and a full bladder can hinder your baby's descent. Be as active as you can. You can even take a shower with an IV.

Elective Induction and Acceleration of Labor

When labor does not begin within a given amount of time or moves "too slowly" (each physician and hospital has a particular policy), many physicians will induce or accelerate ("augment") it. When there is no reason for induction other than the physician's or the woman's convenience, it is known as "elective induction." In 1978, the FDA came out against the practice of elective induction by Pitocin (see below), yet often physicians get around this ban by performing amniotomy to start labor or by "stripping" the membranes.

The first step in induced or accelerated labor involves artificial rupture of the membranes with attendant risks (see above). Sometimes the physician will "strip" rather than rupture the membranes: During an internal examination in the hospital or even during a routine office visit, if s/he feels the baby is "ready," s/he uses a finger to separate the amnion (bag of waters) from the uterine wall. No one knows exactly why this causes labor to begin. When obstetricians strip the membranes, they often do it without informed consent. It is an unnecessary, invasive and risky procedure, for if there is an unrecognized placenta previa (a placenta nearer to the cervix than the baby is), the placenta could be stripped away from the uterus, with harmful and possibly catastrophic effect to the baby, or if the baby is not ready, a premature birth may result.

To start or speed up labor, physicians have used a drug called Pitocin, or "Pit," to substitute for oxytocin, a hormone present in natural labor. It is obligatory to administer Pitocin through an intravenous drip with a pump because then the dosage can be controlled. Control is essential because Pitocin can cause very strong contractions, creating potential dangers for both the baby and the woman.

Prostaglandins are now being used in hospitals to induce and augment labor by ripening the cervix. A gel is inserted into your vagina either directly or via a diaphragm. Sometimes it begins to work in as little as an hour or two, but more often you will wait for six to twelve hours before being rechecked. Sometimes prostaglandins cause contractions to begin. If too much is used, your uterus could be overstimulated. Sometimes it causes nausea.

Induction and acceleration involve considerable risks. Many physicians' estimates of fetal maturity are off by three to seven weeks.[36] Without knowing the baby's age, we can't know if s/he is ready to endure the stresses of labor and delivery and extrauterine life. Some induced babies born too soon have hyaline membrane disease (immaturity of the lungs) and respiratory disease syndrome. Pitocin may cause jaundice in the newborn. Induction is sometimes begun before a woman's cervix is ready ("ripe")—before a certain amount of dilation and effacement—so that her uterus doesn't respond strongly enough to Pitocin and the baby must be born by cesarean. Artificially provoked uterine contractions can be much more violent and prolonged than natural ones, and they may interfere with blood flow to the uterus and placenta, causing fetal distress. Such contractions also can cause uterine rupture and hypertension. Even with the smallest dose, some women have prolonged contractions that close up the cervix. Most women experience these unnatural contractions as more painful than natural ones because they don't follow a wavelike course but reach high intensity instantly and remain intense for a long period. If you are unprepared (and even when you are prepared), you may become discouraged by the pain and rely upon an epidural, with its accompanying risks, to reduce pain.

Induction or acceleration may be appropriate when there is some question about the baby's survival and/or when the mother has toxemia, hemolytic disease (Rh factor) or maternal diabetes. Yet these complications are now usually regarded as indications for a cesarean section, since the use of Pitocin may further compromise the baby.

If you are being induced, or if the physician is accelerating your labor, make sure of four things.

1. Be as certain as possible that your baby is mature enough to be born.

2. Nurses and physicians must start you with the *smallest* dose of Pitocin. There's no way beforehand to gauge the sensitivity of your uterus to Pitocin.

3. You must have expert medical assistance; the baby's heart must be constantly monitored.

4. You must have good labor support, someone near you to help you to relax and to breathe.

My doctor decided to induce my labor.

At the hospital I got some injections of what I thought was Pitocin. My labor was very intense and unexpectedly short—four hours. My daughter had to be delivered by forceps because her heartbeat was slowing down and I couldn't push her out quickly enough. I was told her life had been endangered because my contractions were too strong and the placenta had separated from the uterine wall too early. My doctors were heroes! They had saved her life.

Three years later, seven months pregnant, I asked my doctor a casual question about my first labor and delivery. He began reading my record to me.

Amazed, I said, "That's not my labor. That's someone else's record."

It turns out that the Pitocin stimulated my labor too strongly so that indeed it wasn't natural and was dangerous, and then they gave me Demerol to slow everything down. My strong contractions made the placenta separate early. I'm sure that the Demerol slowed my daughter's heartbeat and oxygen intake. It also explains why she was so sleepy the first three days and didn't immediately nurse.

Now I know my doctors were responsible for the dangers to my daughter's life—if not completely, at least in great part. Induction complicated my labor and delivery.

Fetal Monitors

Fetal monitors are machines that electronically record the baby's heart rate during labor. There are two basic kinds of monitors: external (noninvasive) and internal (invasive). The most accurate external monitor is applied by temporarily sticking gummy electrodes onto the laboring woman's abdomen. The electrodes pick up and record the fetal heartbeat. In addition, two straps, about two to three inches wide, are placed around the woman's abdomen. The upper belt holds the tocody-

Sam Sweezy/Stock Boston

namometer, which records the existence and the duration of the uterine contractions. The lower strap holds an ultrasonic transducer (ultrasound), which monitors and records the fetal heart rate.

Internal fetal monitors are used in most hospitals.* Electrodes connected to wires within a plastic tube are introduced into the woman's vagina and attached directly to the baby's presenting part (usually the scalp) by means of metal clips or screws. (No one has bothered to find out if this causes pain to the baby; it certainly seems as if it must!) The wires coming out of the vagina are held in place by an elastic strap around the woman's thigh. These electrodes measure the baby's heartbeat. The woman's contractions are measured either by a catheter designed for that purpose, introduced into her uterus through her vagina, or by the external tocodynamometer strap described above. A printout shows the baby's heartbeat, which is also audible. The woman will probably have a blood pressure cuff and often an IV.

Though the monitor may be useful in some truly high-risk situations and necessary when labor is induced or accelerated or the woman anesthetized, it entails many discomforts and risks to women and babies.[37]

1. Ultrasound has never been proven safe.

2. The straps and the pressure of the transducer may be uncomfortable.

3. Ironically, fetal stress picked up by the monitor may be a product of invasive hospital routines/

procedures, including the monitor itself. Since women with a monitor cannot move around much, if at all, labor may slow down or stop.

4. Machines get old and break down. They often interpret normal signs as pathological or indicate normality when something is really wrong. The machine may lose the baby's heartbeat when s/he moves, or the electrode may slip out of the baby's scalp.

5. Hospital personnel tend to pay *less* attention to women with monitors. Also, partners and attendants may direct their attention and support away from the woman and pay attention mainly to the machine.

6. Hospital personnel may interpret machine data incorrectly. Incomplete understanding of the range and fluctuation in fetal heart rate during and between contractions has led to unnecessary forceps and, these days, unnecessary cesarean deliveries.

7. Women and babies run a greater risk of infection with the internal monitor. Infection frequently occurs when the uterine catheter is used. The baby's scalp may bleed because of the way the screw has been attached. Postdelivery rashes are common where the electrode was attached (85 percent in one study), and scalp abscess is not uncommon (20 percent).

8. Monitoring has contributed to the recent rise in cesareans, an added risk for mother and baby.

Routine use of fetal monitors has not significantly decreased the newborn death rate nor the number of brain-damaged children. Several randomized controlled clinical trials demonstrated that the use of fetal monitoring, as compared with supervision of labor by nurses with stethoscopes, did not improve Apgar scores or decrease neonatal mortality. David Banta recommends that electronic fetal monitoring "should be limited to specific high-risk groups as part of carefully designed evaluative trials of efficacy,"[38] and Havercamp and Orleans add that fetal blood scalp sampling should be used along with electronic fetal monitor to avoid false positive diagnoses of fetal distress.[39] This procedure, in fact, is the *only* way to verify distress recorded by the monitor; it analyzes the acidity of the baby's blood. Not all hospitals that use fetal monitors have the capability to interpret blood acidity ranges. In addition, "the technique is difficult, awkward, uncomfortable for women and technically difficult even with considerable experience."[40] It involves another puncture in the baby's scalp.

K. Kirkwood Shy et al., in the *New England Journal of Medicine*, described a six-year study of the fetal monitoring of 189 premature babies that showed that fetal monitors fail to improve neurological development.[41] Monitors may also cause higher rates of cerebral palsy.[42]

---

*A monitor becomes *essential* if a woman has epidural anesthesia. Because it is known that fetal distress gradually begins to increase as the epidural is used, mandatory use of the monitor is the only responsible way to employ this type of anesthesia. Not incidentally, the "two-hour limit" for second-stage labor also arose from the combined use of the epidural and monitor, since it is at about two hours at most that fetal distress begins to show almost routinely. Given the combined risks of the monitor and the epidural, this "option" for women must be questioned seriously.

Two new developments are the *intrauterine pressure catheter* and the *fetal acoustic stimulator*. The intrauterine pressure catheter is inserted vaginally into the uterus between the baby and the uterine wall. It is used to determine the intensity of contractions if a woman has received Pitocin ("been pitted") and her labor is not progressing. In fetal acoustic stimulation, an instrument, used abdominally, emits sound waves to shock and "wake" a baby up. It creates a sudden, marked rise in the heart rate of a healthy baby. It is clear that the efficacy and safety of these procedures have not been adequately assessed.

Episiotomy

Episiotomy is the most frequently performed obstetric operation in the West. It is one of the most intense and dramatic ways in which the territory of women's bodies is appropriated, the only operation performed on the body of a healthy woman without her consent. It represents obstetrical power: Babies can't get out unless they are cut out. It prevents women from experiencing birth as a sexual event, and is a form of ritual genital mutilation.[43]

An episiotomy is an incision through skin and muscles in the perineum, the area between the vagina and the anus, to enlarge the opening through which the baby will pass. The procedure is necessary only in rare cases of fetal distress, when the baby must come out quickly and the woman's tissues just won't stretch any more.

Most doctors are taught that episiotomies will prevent perineal tears extending to the anus (third-degree lacerations); that they prevent damage to the baby's head; that they keep the pelvic floor from becoming too stretched; and guard against uterine prolapse, cystocele and rectocele (when the uterus falls into the vagina, when the bladder or rectum protrude into or through the vaginal walls). Yet the available data reveal that episiotomy doesn't accomplish the above goals.[44]

There is no justification for routine episiotomy,* yet many physicians continue to perform it. They rarely learn those midwifery techniques that can prevent or minimize tearing. For instance, in most births you will have little if any tearing when you are upright, sitting or squatting to breathe or push your baby out, resting between contractions; when your practitioner helps you to control your pushing, open up and relax; when s/he carefully massages, softens and supports your perineum using warm oils and wet compresses.

Some physicians believe that they are performing a service to the woman's partner.

I saw my doctor at the checkup six weeks after my baby was born. Full of male pride, he told me during my pelvic exam. "I did a beautiful job sewing you up. You're as tight as a virgin; your husband should thank me."

Many women find intercourse extremely painful after being stitched up too tightly. Stitches are often itchy and extremely painful for several weeks as they heal. Some women are allergic to the stitches; others have had stitches that didn't dissolve. While there are no studies to prove it, many women report permanently impaired sexual sensation after episiotomies.[45]

You have a legal right to refuse episiotomy.

Vacuum Extractors and Forceps

These days vacuum extractors are used before or in place of forceps to help the woman push the baby out and to rotate the baby. They have a small suction cup that fits onto the baby's presenting head. They are used to help speed the pushing part of labor if there is fetal distress, if the umbilical cord is tightly wrapped around the baby's neck or if the cord prolapses or to shorten what physicians consider a long "second stage" of labor. The vacuum extractor is also used with epidurals, because you can't feel pushing sensations. Sometimes after the extractor is used, the babies are born with bumps on their heads, which usually disappear in twelve to twenty-four hours. And sometimes a kind of blood blister (cephalohematoma) develops, which can become infected. Vacuum extractors are much safer for mother and baby than forceps, and they enable you to be active in birthing your baby. These days, younger physicians are taught to use vacuum extractors rather than forceps.

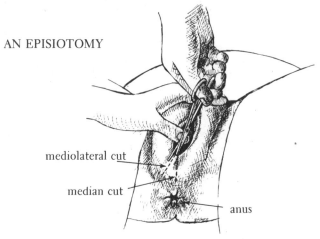

AN EPISIOTOMY

mediolateral cut

median cut

anus

Nina Reimer

---

*When a woman is in the lithotomy position (on her back with legs raised) she literally has to push uphill, against gravity, thus putting enormous strain on her perineum and "necessitating" an episiotomy. Once she sits up, or squats, that strain is lessened.

Forceps may still be used in certain cases and by older physicians. They resemble hinged salad tongs, except that the blades are longer and curved to fit the shape of the baby's head. The doctor introduces each blade into your vagina separately and places them on the sides of the baby's head, usually over the ear but sometimes at the temples. Then s/he attaches the two blades together outside. In previous years (and perhaps even now) doctors used them even in uncomplicated labors to shorten the pushing phase, which they believed to be exhausting to the mother and possibly dangerous to the baby. Yet this phase of labor takes its own time and normally goes from a half-hour to three, five or more hours. *Unless there is some indication that the baby is having trouble getting out, doctors have no medical reason for introducing forceps.* Forceps have caused serious damage. Midwifery techniques should be tried first.

Today cesarean sections are replacing forceps in most situations—one reason for the spectacular rise in cesarean sections. You may choose to have a cesarean rather than a forceps delivery; on the other hand, you may prefer forceps to a cesarean operation.

Cesarean Section

Cesarean section appears to be a sometimes useful and needed technique presently utilized in an undocumented, unclarified and uncontrolled manner.[46]

Cesarean sections are life-saving operations when women have certain problems before or during labor—severe preeclampsia, serious diabetes, transverse lie of the baby, failure of the baby to descend at all, cord prolapse, placenta previa, baby much too large, active herpes lesions, sudden unexplained fetal distress.

She had been head down for three months before the birth but somehow she turned, put her foot through the amniotic sac, tore off the placenta and the uterus collapsed. My contractions were very painful and came every three minutes. Then I started bleeding. We watched her heart rate go down on the monitor. The doctor said a cesarean was necessary. They tried a spinal three times; it didn't take. My husband was going through hell; he couldn't do anything. Finally I was given general anesthesia. I came to three hours later. I'd lost a lot of blood.

Afterwards every day I asked the doctors and nurses if there was anything I could have done to make it less traumatic, more normal. I got the facts. There was nothing I could have done. I kept reliving it, asking my husband lots of questions like a child. The hospital people were wonderful.

Not having seen her born really hurts. They gave

A cesarean birth.   Vaughn Sills

her to my husband to hold right after. It took me three days to unwrap her and look at her naked and see that she was really all right.

It was so quick and different than we'd planned. So much happens in such a short time; there's no time to process it. I wish there had been some way to prepare for it. It was good that it was done; it saved my life and hers.

Please let women know that in regard to cesareans there is a "gray area" between the life-or-death emergency situation and the absolutely unnecessary operation. In my case, I had been in extremely painful labor for hours and hours, with back-to-back long-lasting contractions (unexpected because my first labor had been intense, but short and manageable). David held me, massaged me; I walked, stood, squatted, took baths. Now, I'm no martyr, but I think I could have stood it if there had been any progress, but there was very little. Most discouraging, the baby's head wasn't engaged. After nine hours I said to my doctor, "I need a cesarean." Not one to jump into a C-section, he didn't want to do it right away. Finally, I had an epidural. When it took effect, I could smile again. We waited a while longer—no progress. When he finally did the cesarean, he was amazed by the size of my baby. She was a giant! I know that some people believe that women can birth just about any size baby vaginally. Perhaps I would have been able to do so, too, if I had done other things and been willing to labor for twenty-four more hours. Maybe not. I wonder whether the intense pain wasn't my body's way of telling me that vaginal birth was impossible this time. I am glad I made the choice I did.

Cesareans must be performed in hospitals with proper drugs and anesthesia techniques, antibiotics and blood transfusion equipment. Nurses will shave your pubic hair and insert a catheter into your urethra to empty your bladder. If you are awake for the operation, nurses may place a screen below your shoulders so that you don't see, though sometimes you can look in a mirror. They will wash you down with an antiseptic solution. You'll have either regional (spinal or epidural) or general anesthesia. With general anesthesia you should receive as small a dose as possible (epidural doses will be greater than for labor-pain relief). When your abdomen has become numb or when you are unconscious, the physician makes a small horizontal cut in your abdominal wall, low down near the line of your pubic hair. (Sometimes a vertical cut will be necessary to get the baby out quickly.) The physician then cuts horizontally through the uterine muscle and eases the baby out. The baby's nose and mouth will be suctioned with a mucus catheter. When s/he is breathing well, you or your partner can hold her/him. The physician then removes the placenta and sews you up, layer by layer.

Almost every woman needs to believe that her cesarean was necessary. However, in response to the tremendous increase in cesareans over the past decade, two major investigatory studies suggest that 33 to 75 percent of cesareans were *not* necessary, having been performed as a result of current medical procedures and attitudes alone.[47]

With Deb, my first baby, around the time of my due date my doctor told me that he'd had a dream about me which worried him: that the baby was okay now, but the head would be too big to fit through my pelvis and there would be trouble. He wanted to do a cesarean right away. I made him wait two weeks; I didn't think he was giving me half a chance. But I was not allowed to go into labor, and he did his cesarean. Three years later, after a smooth labor at home with a midwife attending, I gave birth to Emily, whose head was much bigger than Deb's had been.

A childbirth educator from C/SEC (see Resources) tells a more typical story:

A woman phoned me today. She had given birth to her first child eight weeks ago. After being in labor for only four hours she had dilated from four to nine centimeters. Suddenly they transported her to the delivery room, and yelled at her to push even though she didn't feel the urge to push and told them so. But they pressured her and, half-sitting up, holding her legs (a typical Lamaze position), she pushed for twenty-six minutes—she has it on record. At the end of that time her cervix was swollen—of course it swells when you push like that—and they told her that she wouldn't be able to deliver vaginally. Within

fifteen minutes she'd had a cesarean. Reason given: "Failure to progress."

The above-mentioned studies conclude that cesareans, being major operations, carry two to four times greater risk of death than vaginal deliveries.* They cause postoperative infections in 33 percent of women. They frequently cause respiratory distress problems in both premature and full-term babies and psychological damage to the mother, if not to the family unit as a whole. In addition, anesthesia exposures during cesareans may leave large numbers of babies with delayed motor development and other neurological defects.

What is happening, and why? In 1968, the average cesarean rate was 5 percent. In 1987 the national average had risen to 25 percent. Factors responsible for the increase—some statistically measurable, others not—include

1. *Physicians' practice of defensive medicine.* The most common cause of cesareans today is not fetal distress or maternal distress but obstetrician distress.[48] Physicians think that if they do a cesar-

---

*Studies of maternal mortality are continuing at the CDC (Centers for Disease Control).

A vaginal birth after cesarean.   Suzanne Arms ean and a baby is born "less than perfect," they have covered themselves legally. In fact, more suits have been instigated for malpractice associated with cesarean surgery than for failure to perform it.

2. *"Once a cesarean, always a cesarean."* This dictum accounts for 30 percent of all cesareans. Repeat cesareans are elective surgery, not obligatory. *In fact, many women—perhaps the majority—can have vaginal births after cesarean (VBACs).* They need information, encouragement, self-confidence and support to do so.[49] A woman who had two VBACs tells this story:

One day in the supermarket I started to talk with a woman who was looking at my youngest child with such longing. She said, "I so much want to have more kids, but I had a cesarean and I'll never go through that again." There was such pain in her eyes. I said, "I'm here to tell you that you don't have to!" and told her my story. You could see that she started to light up; then she sort of flickered out. "But my doctor said women who have cesareans can't deliver vaginally." She agreed to find out why she'd had it in the first place. At least she now had some hope. No one had ever allowed her to hope before.

Most often the condition that makes a cesarean necessary in one birth, if it was necessary at all, won't exist in the next. Physicians claim uterine rupture is a risk,* but ruptures occur so rarely that women must weigh this fact against the many known risks of abdominal surgery. VBACs are far safer in most cases. ACOG's March 1982 pronouncement that women who meet certain criteria can have "trial" labors will enable only a few women to have vaginal births after cesareans, as long as the medical climate remains negative.†

3. *Obstetrical training.* Physicians and residents are not trained in normal obstetrics, and now don't even learn skills such as external cephalic version (gently turning breech babies around) or delivering breeches vaginally. In addition, at the same time that the birth rate has come down, obstetrics/gynecology is growing as a surgical specialty; new residents need training and have to perform a certain number of procedures in order to meet a quota.

4. *Belief that cesareans mean "better babies."* In-

fant mortality and morbidity rates *have* declined in recent years, but not primarily because of obstetrical intervention. In fact, cesarean-section babies are often distressed. The existence of neonatal intensive care units has been largely responsible for keeping alive low-birth-weight and premature babies who otherwise would have died.

5. *Changing indications for cesarean sections.* Women's bodies haven't changed, but physicians' eagerness to perform cesareans has led them to expand the meaning of the word *dystocia*. Physicians tell women that their pelvis is too small (cephalopelvic disproportion) or their labor is too slow (failure to progress in labor),[50] and call both *dystocia*, when in fact if women could labor naturally, moving around and squatting, they could deliver normally in most cases. Dystocia has been called a "wastebasket" term. It accounts for 43 percent of all cesareans and 30 percent of the increase in cesarean sections from 1970 to 1978.

Now that physicians are less experienced in delivering them, the number of cesarean deliveries for *breech* babies continues to increase and now accounts for 12 percent of the cesarean rate. Cesareans can mean healthier babies for very large or very small breech babies but, in general, many more breech babies could be delivered vaginally just as safely if practitioners learned how to do it and encouraged women to squat for delivery. Cesareans are also replacing forceps deliveries.

6. *Economic incentives.* Cesareans are more lucrative for obstetricians, anesthesiologists and hospitals.

7. *Obstetrical practice and technology.* Fetal monitors, induction, oxytocin challenge tests, epidurals, amniotomies and women laboring on their backs all cause problems that then necessitate intervention, which leads to cesareans.

8. *Physician attitudes.* Underlying these factors, physician attitudes, while not statistically measurable, point up why cesareans are so dear to the medical heart. This discussion was heard among a compendium of doctors:

What's so great about delivery from below? . . . You don't want the baby squeezed out like toothpaste in a tube? . . . You might say we're helping women to do what nature hasn't evolved her to do for herself.

By and large, I think American obstetrics has become so preoccupied with apparatus and with possible fetal injury that the mothers are increasingly being considered solely vehicles. In many cases small and uncertain gain for the infant is being purchased at the price of a small but grave risk to the mother.[51]

Several organizations have sprung up over the past decade, two among them being Cesarean/Support, Education and Concern (C/SEC) and the

---

*Ruptures occurred (rarely) in the past when incisions made vertically in the upper half of the uterus didn't heal properly, and when modern surgical techniques and emergency medicines were not available to minimize risks.
†Conditions: The mother must have the shorter horizontal scar; the baby must be properly positioned, head down; the baby must be no more than eight pounds, eight ounces; the pregnancy must have been completely normal; the mother's condition must be monitored.

Cesarean Prevention Movement (CPM). C/SEC aims to inform women and families about cesareans and to humanize medical attitudes and policies. CPM grew out of C/SEC. Its founders, all of whom had had cesareans, realized that their cesareans had been medically unnecessary and that in the future most of them could labor naturally and deliver vaginally. These convictions were reinforced by the experiences of hundreds of women who contacted them. As a result, CPM's goals are to educate women and practitioners in order to decrease the number of women having a first (primary) cesarean and to increase the number of women having VBACs. Both organizations have brought about positive changes in hospital cesarean practices, both advocate VBACs and have positively affected women's attitudes about themselves and their capabilities. Throughout the country, women are forming or joining VBAC classes, in which they talk about their previous experiences, fears and hopes and learn concrete ways of preparing physically and emotionally for the births of their next babies. They learn how to prevent unnecessary cesareans (see the box Creating a Nurturing Birth Environment, pp. 448–49, and Cohen and Estner's book *Silent Knife*).

Drugs

Every single drug given to the mother during labor crosses the placenta and reaches her baby, some in greater amounts and with greater rapidity than others. If the baby is premature, smaller than average or in poor health, the consequences can be particularly dangerous. Even a normal baby can suffer from the effects of maternal medication.

No drug has been proven safe for mothers and babies. Most obstetric drugs used routinely for labor and delivery have not been approved for that purpose by the FDA, and thus they assume the status of experimental drugs.[52]

Some infants whose mothers received analgesia and anesthesia during labor and delivery have had retarded muscular, visual and neural development in the first four weeks of life.[53] This doesn't mean all babies will be so affected, nor will the babies affected be permanently retarded in development; but four weeks is a long time in the life of a newborn infant.

Anesthetized mothers often feel quite separate from their newborns:

I was really doped up when my baby was delivered and barely got to see that she was alive before she was whisked away to the nursery. When I finally woke up and she was able to be brought to me, I remember thinking, Is this really my baby? Do I really want to take her home with me? It took me a while to feel connected to her.

We mothers sometimes suffer more from the aftereffects of the drugs used in our labor than we might have from the labor itself. The problem is compounded because along with each drug often come two or three other procedures designed by the hospital to reduce, as much as possible, the risk of the medication used.

Analgesics decrease our overall perception of pain, and *anesthesia* removes our sensation of pain altogether by creating loss of consciousness, "sleep" or a temporary loss of feeling in the specific area affected. Although drug development and administration is being refined and improved, and many of the old, seriously dangerous drugs and procedures are disappearing, keep in mind that in hospitals where older physicians practice, some of these drugs may still be administered.

Analgesia: Tranquilizers and Narcotics

As soon as labor becomes intense, you may be offered a tranquilizer or a narcotic "to take the edge off your contractions." Tranquilizers (Vistaril, Phenergan) are given primarily for anxiety; they are not painkillers. They can relax you in early labor or if you are very tired. But once you have established a good pattern of labor, they can make you feel out of control, sharply reducing your ability to cope with your contractions. You may find yourself falling asleep until a contraction reaches its peak and then wake, panic and actually experience more pain than you would have without the drug. Tranquilizers may have a depressant effect on the newborn. For instance, Valium (diazepam) reduces a newborn's body temperature, muscle tone and ability to suckle. Other tranquillizers may cause labor to slow down or even cease altogether.[54]

Barbiturates (Nembutal, Seconal), derivatives of barbituric acid, should no longer be used for obstetrical purposes. Used to promote sleep, they are dangerous to the fetus, seriously depressing fetal respiration and responsiveness.* (They used to be given in combination with scopolamine, called *twilight sleep*, an amnesiac and a hallucinogen, which had the nightmare effect of making women become physically violent during labor, talk uninhibitedly or go into a stupor. Women felt the sensations but "forgot" what happened and later felt they had lived through some kind of torture.)

Narcotics can provide relief from pain but make babies less able to suck. They may be sleepy, dopey and not responsive to their environment. Even

---

*T. Berry Brazelton determined that barbiturates taken by the woman lodge in the baby's midbrain for up to a week after delivery.[55]

small amounts of Demerol (meperidine) affect your baby's responsiveness. Narcotics can affect you, too, causing drowsiness and nausea.

Most women receiving analgesics are instructed not to walk around during labor as they may become dizzy or faint.

General Anesthetic Agents Inhaled by the Mother

Inhalation gases used to be administered during labor with each contraction. The point was to breathe in the right amount of the vapor just in time to have it working during the peak of the contractions. These drugs slow down labor, serve as depressants to the newborn's responsiveness and have potentially fatal complications if too much is inhaled. *Nitrous oxide* can delay for *months* the development of the baby's motor skills—attempts to sit, stand and move around. Penthrane (methoxyflurane) can be self-administered with a hand-held inhalator.

Anesthesia

General anesthesia puts the woman completely to sleep. It should never be used during labor because it slows it down and has a severely depressant effect on the baby. Furthermore, injudicious use of general anesthesia for delivery can lead to the woman's (and sometimes the baby's) death.

Physicians who want their patients to be totally unaware of the obstetrical procedures used during the last minutes of labor will often give them general anesthesia. Sometimes it is used during a cesarean section. But physicians are using it less than in previous years because of the risks involved and because newer technology has been developed.

If the physician decides s/he wants a numbing effect only during delivery to perform an episiotomy or to use forceps, s/he may give the mother a *regional anesthesia*, a *pudendal block*.* The pudendal block anesthetizes only the vulva, or external female organs, by injections of novocaine. Even this relatively minor anesthetic can cause a "persistent decrease in oxygen saturation in the newborn during the first 30 minutes of postpartum observation."[56]

Another form of anesthesia, the *paracervical block*, is in use.† Many anesthesiologists consider it dangerous to both fetus and mother. Complications such as convulsions and severe hypotension are common, and it has led to a significant

number of fetal deaths. Because the anesthetic is injected into the area around the cervix, there is the possibility that it will accidentally be injected into the presenting part of the baby. Moreover, the injection site is very close to the main artery of the uterus, which increases the chance of its being absorbed rapidly by the placenta and depressing the fetus.

Spinal anesthesia has been used just during delivery to anesthetize the entire birth area (from belly to toes). The anesthesiologist injects spinals, or subarachnoid blocks, into the subarachnoid space around the spinal column. Spinals totally stop labor, all motor functions and our urge to bear down, so instead of our pushing the baby out, the obstetrician must use forceps. Aftereffects may include headache (usually the result of an overly large needle, which causes spinal fluid to leak, though this problem is rare now), stiff neck and backache. Misadministration of the spinal has resulted in failure of heart and lung function and even death. Spinals can and should be avoided, except when necessary for an emergency delivery.

If everything has gone normally and no drugs have been administered up until this point, the actual delivery is the worst time to give anesthesia. In fact, the perineum usually becomes numb at delivery—a natural anesthesia. And, if you have learned how to "breathe" or push your baby out in a comfortable position, you are able to experience fully the satisfaction of delivery without an anesthetic to cut off sensation and make your recovery that much more difficult.

Two forms of *continuous regional anesthesia* are given to the woman during active labor and continuously readministered until delivery. They require the services of a trained anesthesiologist, not available twenty-four hours a day in most hospitals.

For most of us, the end of active labor, from eight centimeters to ten centimeters of dilation, is intense. During this time you may feel like or be pressured into taking some medication "to tide you over." But *transition* is for the great majority of women the shortest part of labor. So when you consider anesthesia, you need to weigh the possible risks and aftereffects of the technique against your ability to cope. This anesthesia will persist in almost every case as you push the baby out, eliminating sensations of giving birth. It may in fact prolong your labor, requiring further intervention.

---

*Pudendal block anesthesia is named for the pudendum, or external female genitalia. *Pudendum* in Latin means "that of which one ought to be ashamed." Obviously we can't imagine a more inappropriate name!

†It is used mainly by obstetricians rather than anesthesiologists. The only possible excuse for its continuance is the unavailability of better anesthesia technology and of better-

trained anesthesiologists. The FDA Subcommittee on Anesthetic and Life Support Drugs considered placing warnings on the drug bupivacaine and then declined to do so. If this is the procedure presented to you, consider trying to find another physician or another hospital. (Some Lamaze programs actually encourage the use of this procedure because the physicians who "accept" Lamaze use it.)

The *caudal* requires an injection into the sacral canal at the base of the back. For a continuous caudal (given from about eight centimeters of dilation), a catheter is introduced into the lower back and the anesthetic is injected into the catheter in measured doses. A caudal requires a significantly larger dose of anesthetic than does either a spinal or an epidural (explained below), and it therefore carries a greater risk to both mother and baby. Furthermore, the failure rate for caudals is higher than for epidurals, owing to the greater chance of improper needle placement. Maternal hypotension (sudden drop in blood pressure)* and subsequent lack of oxygen to the baby is a potential problem that the anesthesiologist must carefully guard against.

Epidural anesthesia can be administered to laboring women at any time, but it should be started no earlier than four centimeters of dilation and no later than nine. Many obstetricians, anesthesiologists and women as well would have us believe that the epidural is the answer to our labor problems. Increasingly, as older types of pain relief are found to be hazardous, *to choose a hospital birth is to choose the epidural.*

Epidurals can be useful when a woman has serious respiratory disease as the drug involved reduces the work the lungs have to do. It may make it easier for a diabetic woman, for it reduces the demands on her metabolism. It can slow down precipitate labor and also moderate a premature urge to push, as with a footling breech. It is used increasingly in cesarean operations instead of general anesthesia.

Epidurals have been assumed to be safer than caudals for mother and baby because a different type of anesthesia is used. However, like caudals, they can cause maternal hypotension. Transverse arrest (the baby's getting stuck in a sideways position in the uterus) is another possible complication of epidurals, as they can cause the uterine muscles to relax too much.

Behavioral changes in newborns whose mothers received epidural anesthesia include decreased rooting activity (a basic food-searching survival technique) and muscular floppiness.[57] Esther Conway and Yvonne Brackbill also found negative behavior changes after continuous regional anesthesia, but they concluded that the effects on the baby were less than those suffered by babies whose mothers had received high doses of labor medication or general anesthesia.[58]

Epidurals are administered like a continuous caudal through a tiny catheter placed in the back by a needle. An injection is made in the middle of the woman's back and the catheter moved into her epidural space (not into the spinal column), the space around the base of the spinal cord. The anesthetic is dripped in, in measured doses. An experienced anesthesiologist must administer the anesthetic, because a mistake in placement can lead to serious consequences for the mother—in the extreme, paralysis or death.

When administered properly, epidurals will eliminate the sensations of labor in most cases and, unlike the standard spinal, numb only the area immediately around the perineum and lower uterus, belly to knees. However, when you choose epidurals you also invite a number of interlocking procedures, most of which increase the risks of the method. (These procedures are done for caudals, too.) These include

1. *An intravenous hydrating solution attached to one arm.*

2. *Blood pressure gauging.* Your blood pressure will probably be checked every fifteen to thirty minutes, because a drop in blood pressure is common and can have serious effects on the fetus as well as on the mother. You will probably have to wear a blood pressure cuff continuously on the other arm.

3. *Artificial rupture of the membranes (bag of waters).* If your membranes have not already ruptured by themselves, your doctor will probably rupture them before you are given an epidural or caudal. This is done to make sure that the baby's head is firmly positioned in the birth outlet and to prepare for the attachment of an internal fetal monitor.

4. *Pitocin.* Some doctors give Pitocin to women receiving continuous regional anesthesia to start again or speed up contractions stopped or slowed down by the anesthetic. Ruptured membranes plus Pitocin create very strong uterine contractions that *must* be monitored, since the baby is at risk of distress; you cannot feel their strength, and your uterus might rupture.[59] Some hospitals now measure the dosage by machine so that this is much less likely to happen.

5. *An external or internal fetal monitor, with all its attendant risks.* It is essential during continuous anesthesia (caudal or epidural) to check the baby's heart rate, because fetal distress rises with the length of time the anesthesia is administered.

6. *A catheter.* The sensation that you have to urinate diminishes, so you may need a catheter.

7. *Much higher (three to four times) incidence of*

---

*If the woman becomes hypotensive, she should turn (or be turned) on her side immediately to take pressure off the *inferior vena cava,* the major source of blood returning to the heart. Hypotension can be contained or prevented in most cases by this maneuver and by the generous use of an intravenous solution started well in advance. Some effects of hypotension on the mother may be shocklike symptoms, altered pulse rate, nausea and vomiting. Its effects on the fetus are slowed heart rate, decreased flow of blood through the placenta and insufficient oxygen intake. These effects tend to show up immediately.

vacuum extractor or forceps delivery. As the urge for and coordination of pushing are decreased, many babies remain in an occiput, transverse or posterior position. The mother can't push her baby out and ends up "needing" forceps.

8. *A cesarean section.* With epidurals there is a higher cesarean rate. Because the monitor is used almost routinely these days and the epidural is usually administered early in labor, it is difficult to separate the influence of the epidural from the monitor in increasing the cesarean-section rate. "Failure to progress in labor," the prime indication for cesarean sections, is often the direct iatrogenic result of a labor slowed down by epidural anesthesia.

AFTERWARD

Your baby is born. You have done all in your power to give her/him the healthiest and safest birth possible. You may feel delighted with the labor and birth—high, fulfilled, ecstatic and immensely close to your partner and your baby.

Birth is a powerful event. We relive the births of our children many times over during the following days, weeks and months, thinking and talking about them, feeling them in our heart. This reenactment is a natural and sometimes essential means of understanding what has happened. When we have experienced birth in the setting of our choice, with no or few complications, we relive the event in a clear, happy way. But when unexpected complications and medical interventions alter the experience, we may have conflicting feelings—joy *and* disappointment, confidence *and* a sense of inadequacy. We may feel confusion and less satisfaction.

Knowledge alone cannot enable us to find a language adequate and powerful enough either to express our wonder and sense of accomplishment or our frustration, anger and outrage. Memories of negative experiences can haunt us. Unhappiness may be right on the surface, easily accessible, taking the form of grief, anger, of having been violated. We may think, *I* didn't have my baby; the system had it for me. Or we may bury our strongest emotions, denying how terrible the experience was because to admit it would bring us to the edge of such deep anger that we don't know how to handle it or whom to blame. We excuse and defend physicians and institutions, describing bad experiences as good ones. We become defensive: "Yes, others don't need these unnecessary, even barbaric procedures, but in my case it was necessary." We apologize for being selfish and wanting something different: "It doesn't matter. After all, my baby is fine and that's all that counts. But why am I crying?" We feel ashamed of not having had that

"natural" birth we'd prepared for. Often other mothers make us feel badly, too, by subtly implying that we were at fault. Or we feel distant from the baby.

My next memory was waking up the next morning. "You have a beautiful daughter," they said. "Where is she? Give her to me. She's mine!" They brought her. I wasn't even glad to see her. I wasn't sure she was mine.

And worst of all, inappropriately, we blame ourselves—"My body just didn't work right"—instead of seeing clearly how the system undermines our knowledge and self-sufficiency; instead of saying to ourselves, as one author did, "Whatever the luck of the draw for your labor, be assured that you have done the best you could on that day for your baby."

If you were dissatisfied with your experience, it can be healing to reflect on it and come to terms with it. Question what happened, talk about it, send for your hospital records and check them against your memories of the event. Understand the choices you made and why you made them. Allow yourself to feel the deep range of your emotions. A good friend or an experienced counselor may help you to go through this process; perhaps a group of women might be more helpful.

After you explore your feelings and get your questions answered, you will then be able to move on, to think of doing things differently next time if you plan to have more children. Sometimes it takes many years to understand fully what happened, a process that can be difficult but enormously strengthening. For some of us, it has been the beginning of activist work to change childbearing conditions.

Even now, seventeen years after my daughter's birth, I am still learning how dangerous the medical techniques used were for her. I didn't know that my doctors, the "best in town," were as ignorant as I. As for "natural" maternal feelings, well, I just didn't have them. Move around during labor? I lay flat on my back, never dreaming another position was possible. Insist on keeping her with me after she was born? I held her for a moment, felt her breath on my hand and let them take her away. (Though I kept repeating over and over, like a song to the white walls of the recovery room, "I have a daughter! A daughter! A daughter!" and I felt like a child at Christmas who had been given a marvelous present.) Sometimes I blame myself, but not for long. My tears still turn to anger as they have for years; both fuel my determination to help other women find alternatives to conventional obstetrical care. When I am lucky enough to be present at the births of my friends' children, the simplicity and joy of these births affirm and vin-

dicate all of us who work toward loving and informed care for all childbearing women.

NOTES

1. Judith Dickson Luce. "Birthing Women and Midwife," in Helen B. Holmes, Betty Hoskins and Michael Gross, eds., *Birth Control and Controlling Birth: Women-Centered Perspectives.* Clifton, NJ: The Humana Press, 1980, p. 240.

2. Dorothy Wertz. "Man-Midwifery," in *Birth Control and Controlling Birth*, p. 147.

3. Barbara Ehrenreich and Deirdre English. *Witches, Midwives and Nurses.* Old Westbury, NY: The Feminist Press, 1973, p. 41.

4. Dorothy Wertz. "Man-Midwifery," p. 149.

5. Mary Roth Walsh. *Doctors Wanted—No Women Need Apply: Sexual Barriers in the Medical Profession 1835–1975.* New Haven: Yale University Press, 1977.

6. Dorothy Wertz. "Man-Midwifery," p. 153.

7. Barbara Ehrenreich and Deirdre English. *Witches, Midwives and Nurses*, p. 30.

8. G. J. Barker-Benfield. *The Horrors of the Half-Known Life: Male Attitudes Toward Women and Sexuality in 19th-Century America.* New York: Harper & Row, 1977.

9. Diana Scully. *Men Who Control Women's Health: The Miseducation of Obstetrician-Gynecologists.* Boston: Houghton-Mifflin, 1980. Michelle Harrison. *Women in Residence.* New York: Penguin Books, 1983. Gena Corea. *The Hidden Malpractice: How American Medicine Mistreats Women.* New York: Jove/HBJ, 1978.

10. Richard and Dorothy Wertz. *Lying-In: A History of Childbirth in America.* New York: Schocken Books, 1989, Chapter 7. Neal Devitt. "Hospital Birth vs. Home Birth: The Scientific Facts, Past and Present," Chapter 37. D. Stewart and L. Stewart, eds., *Compulsory Hospitalization: Freedom of Choice in Childbirth*, Vol. 2, Marble Hill, MO: NAPSAC Publications, 1979.

11. G. J. Barker-Benfield. *The Horrors of the Half-Known Life*, p. 63.

12. Neal Devitt. "Hospital Birth vs. Home Birth," pp. 487–92.

13. Neal Devitt. "Hospital Birth vs. Home Birth," pp. 493–94.

14. Joseph B. DeLee. "The Prophylactic Forceps Operation," *American Journal of Obstetrics and Gynecology*, Vol. 1 (1920), pp. 32–44.

15. Frederick Leboyer. *Birth Without Violence.* New York: Alfred Knopf, 1975, pp. 24–26.

16. Stanley Sagov et al. "The Issue of Safety," Chapter 2 in *Home Birth: A Practitioner's Guide to Birth Outside the Hospital*, Rockville, MD: Aspen Systems Corporation, 1983.

17. Roslynn Lindheim. "Birthing Centers and Hospices: Reclaiming Birth and Death," *American Review of Public Health*, Vol. 2 (1981), pp. 1–29.

18. Michelle Harrison. *Woman in Residence*, p. 17.

19. Ellen Switzer and Joan Kline. "Pregnancy and Childbirth 1982: New Options," *Family Circle Magazine* (March 16, 1982).

20. Ina May Gaskin. "Practicing Midwifery—A Talk by Ina May Gaskin," *Childbirth Alternative Quarterly* (Summer 1981), p. 4.

21. Barbara Katz Rothman. *In Labor: Women and Power in the Birthplace*, 2nd ed. New York: W. W. Norton, 1992, p. 290.

22. Constance Beynon. "The Normal Second Stage of Labor: A Plea for Reform in Its Conduct," *Journal of Obstetrics and Gynecology of the British Empire*, Vol. 64, No. 6 (December 1957), pp. 815–20.

23. Roberto Caldeyro-Barcia. "The Influence of Maternal Bearing-Down Effects During the Second Stage and Fetal Well-Being," *Birth and the Family Journal* (Spring 1979).

24. Barbara Katz Rothman. *In Labor*, p. 20.

25. C. D. Kimball, C. M. Chang, S. M. Huang and J. C. Houck. "Immunoreactive Endorphin Peptides and Prolactin in Umbilical Vein and Maternal Blood," *American Journal of Obstetrics and Gynecology*, Vol. 140, No. 2 (May 15, 1981), pp. 157–64. Michel Odent. "The Evolution of Obstetrics at Pithiviers," *Birth and the Family Journal*, Vol. 8, No. 1 (Spring 1981), pp. 7–15.

26. Nancy Wainer Cohen. *Birth, A Commentary.* Available from the Boston Women's Health Book Collective.

27. Ruth Lubic. "The Impact of Technology on Health Care—The Childbearing Center: A Case for Technology's Appropriate Use," *Journal of Nurse-Midwifery*, Vol. 24, No. 1 (January/February 1979), pp. 6–10.

28. National Institutes of Health, Department of Health and Welfare Publication No. 77-1079, 1977.

29. V. Crosse et al. "The Value of Human Milk Compared with Other Feeds for Premature Infants," discussed in Doris Haire and John Haire, *Implementing Family-Centered Maternity Care*, pp. v, 42–43, ICEA publication (see Resources).

30. "Obstetrical Practices in the United States," Washington, DC, April 17, 1978, 95th Congress, 2nd session, U.S. Senate, Committee on Human Resources. Washington, DC: U.S. Government Printing Office, 1978.

31. Doris Haire, *The Cultural Warping of Childbirth*, p. 32. Available from ICEA (see Resources).

32. M. L. Romney. "Predelivery Shaving: An Unjustified Assault?" *American Journal of Obstetrics and Gynecology*, Vol. 1 (1980), pp. 33–35. M. L. Romney and G. Gordon. "Is Your Enema Really Necessary?" *British Journal*, Vol. 282 (April 18, 1981), pp. 1269–71.

33. Ann Oakley. *Subject Women*, New York: Schocken Books, 1980.

34. Susan R. McKay. "Maternal Position During Labor and Birth: A Reassessment," *JOG Nursing* (September/October 1980), pp. 288–91.

35. S. Gabbe, B. Ettinger, R. Freeman and C. Martin. "Umbilical Cord Compression Associated with Amniotomy," *American Journal of Obstetrics and Gynecology* (October 1, 1976), pp. 353–55.

36. National Institutes of Health. *Cesarean Childbirth*, Publication No. 82-2067, October 1981, pp. 31–318.

37. "Antenatal Diagnosis," Bethesda, Maryland, 1979, National Institutes of Health Consensus Development Conference, NIH Publication No. 79-1973. A. D. Haverkamp, M. Orleans, S. Langendoerfer et al. "A controlled trial of the differential effects of intrapartum

fetal monitoring," *American Journal of Obstetrics and Gynecology*, Vol. 134 (1979), p. 399. A. D. Haverkamp, H. E. Thompson, J. G. McFee et al. "The Evaluation of Continuous Fetal Heart Rate Monitoring in High-Risk Pregnancy," *American Journal of Obstetrics and Gynecology*, Vol. 125 (1976), p. 310.

38. David Banta. "Risks and Benefits of EFM," in Holmes et al., *Birth Control and Controlling Birth*, p. 191.

39. Albert Havercamp and Miriam Orleans. "An Assessment of Electronic Fetal Monitoring," *Women and Health*, Vol. 7, Nos. 3/4 (1982), p. 132.

40. A. Havercamp and M. Orleans, "An Assessment of Electronic Fetal Monitoring," p. 119.

41. K. Kirkwood Shy et al. *New England Journal of Medicine* (March 1, 1990), pp. 588–93.

42. A. Grant et al. "Cerebral Palsy Among Children Born During the Dublin Randomized Trial of Intrapartum Monitoring," *Lancet* (November 25, 1989).

43. Sheila Kitzinger's talk at Boston College, Autumn 1981.

44. D. Banta and S. Thacker. "The Risks and Benefits of Episiotomy: A Review," *Birth*, Vol. 9, No. 1 (Spring 1982), pp. 25–30.

45. Sheila Kitzinger. *Episiotomy: Physical and Emotional Aspects* and *Some Women's Experiences of Episiotomy*, London: The National Childbirth Trust, 1981.

46. Helen Marieskind. *An Evaluation of Cesarean Section in the United States*, a report submitted to the Department of Health, Education and Welfare, June 1979, National Institutes of Health, Report of the Task Force, *Cesarean Childbirth*, NIH Publication No. 82-2067, October 1981, p. 25. Jeanne Guillemin, "Babies by Cesarean: Who Chooses, Who Controls?" The Hastings Center Report, Vol. 11, No. 3 (June 1981), pp. 15–18.

47. National Institutes of Health. *Cesarean Childbirth*. Helen Marieskind, *An Evaluation of Cesarean Section*.

48. Dr. Gerald Stober, quoted in Christopher Norwood, *At Highest Risk*. New York: Penguin Books, 1980, p. 227.

49. Nancy Wainer Cohen and Lois Estner. *Silent Knife: Cesarean Prevention and Vaginal Birth after Cesarean*, South Hadley, MA: J. F. Bergin, 1983. Elizabeth Shearer, "Education for Vaginal Birth after Cesarean," *Birth: Issues in Perinatal Care and Education*, Vol. 9, No. 1 (Spring 1982), pp. 31–34. Nancy Wainer Cohen, *Open Season: A Survival Guide for Natural Childbirth and VBAC in the 90's*, New York: Bergin & Garvey, 1991.

50. D. Neuhoff, M. Burke and R. Porreco. "Cesarean Birth for Failed Progress in Labor," *Obstetrics and Gynecology*, Vol. 73, No. 6 (June 1989), pp. 915–20.

51. Dr. I. Kaiser, quoted in Helen Marieskind, *An Evaluation of Cesarean Section*, pp. 114–15.

52. Doris Haire. "Research on Drugs Used in Pregnancy and Obstetrics," presented to the Subcommittee on Investigations and Oversights of the House Committee on Science and Technology, Washington, DC, July 30, 1981. Available from the Boston Women's Health Book Collective. "Use of Drugs for Unapproved Indications: Your Legal Responsibility," *FDA Drug Bulletin* (October 1972).

53. Doris Haire and John Haire. *Implementing Family-Centered Maternity Care*, pp. iii–10, in W. Bowes, Y. Brackbill, E. Conway and A. Steinschneider, *The Effects of Obstetrical Medication on Fetus and Infant*, Monograph of the Society of Research in Child Development, Vol. 35, No. 4 (1970). Control groups showed that this effect was directly related to the obstetrical medication used. Furthermore, R. Kron, M. Stein and K. Goddard show, in "Newborn Sucking Behavior Affected by Obstetrical Sedation" (*Pediatrics*, Vol. 37 (1966), pp. 1012–16), that newborn sucking behavior may be depressed for as long as four days after delivery by barbiturates used routinely on the laboring mother.

54. John J. Bonica. *Principles and Practice of Obstetric Analgesia and Anesthesia*, Vols. 1 and 2. Philadelphia: F. A. Davis Co., 1972, p. 268.

55. T. Berry Brazelton. "Effect of Maternal Medication on the Neonate and His Behavior," *Journal of Pediatrics*, Vol. 58, No. 4 (1961).

56. Doris Haire and John Haire. *Implementing Family-Centered Maternity Care*, pp. iii–13.

57. John Scanlon. "Obstetric Anesthesia as a Neonatal Risk Factor in Normal Labor and Delivery," *Clinics in Perinatology*, Vol. 1, No. 2 (September 1974), p. 479.

58. John Scanlon. "Obstetric Anesthesia as a Neonatal Risk Factor in Normal Labor and Delivery," p. 478.

59. E. Daw. "Oxytocin-Induced Rupture of the Primigravid Uterus," *Journal of Obstetrics and Gynecology of the British Empire*, Vol. 80 (April 1973), pp. 374–75. The uterus of a first-time mother ruptured due to excessive contractions caused by oxytocin and the rupture was not discovered until after the baby had died, since the strength of the contractions was masked by the epidural anesthesia and the fetal heart was monitored only intermittently.

RESOURCES

Each of these books contributes to an understanding of childbirth in America. Many are recent; others—some of the most useful—are out-of-print and (we hope) available in libraries.

General Books About Childbearing and Reproduction

Arditti, Rita, Renate Duelli Klein and Shelley Minden, eds. *Test Tube Women*. Boston: Pandora Press, Routledge and Kegan Paul, 1984. The articles in this book provide a strong feminist insight into new reproductive technologies and issues such as testing during pregnancy and *in vitro* fertilization.

Arms, Suzanne. *Immaculate Deception: A New Look at Women and Childbirth in America*. New York: Bantam Books, 1986. The first and still powerful systematic exposure of the abuse of technology and intervention in normal childbirth and of how women have lost their power over normal childbearing to male doctors. Angry, passionate. A beautiful tribute to midwives.

Armstrong, Penny, and Sheryl Feldman. *A Midwife's Story*. New York: Ballantine Books, 1986. Armstrong tells what she learned about the beauty of birth while assisting Amish women at home.

———. *A Wise Birth: Bringing Together the Best of Natural Childbirth with Modern Medicine.* New York: William Morrow, 1990. The authors ask crucial questions about childbirth as women in the United States experience it today. Rare, poetic descriptions of birth.

Barker-Benfield, G. J. *The Horrors of the Half-Known Life: Male Attitudes Toward Women and Sexuality in 19th-Century America.* New York: Harper & Row, 1977. Read this dense, witty description of the nineteenth-century medical and moral climate in America if you want to understand the origins of current male attitudes towards women.

Buss, Fran Leeper. *La Partera: Story of a Midwife.* Ann Arbor, MI: University of Michigan Press, 1980. Jesusita Aragon's story told in her own words—a midwife who has delivered 12,000 babies.

Chard, Timothy, and Martin Richards. *Benefits and Hazards of the New Obstetrics.* Philadelphia: J. B. Lippincott, 1977. Researchers and practitioners discuss the pros and cons of using medical technology for childbirth. These essays were gathered together in the 1970s when the use of technology was increasing in intensity in America and England. The issues raised remain valid today.

Cohen, Nancy Wainer. *Open Season: A Survival Guide for Natural Childbirth and VBAC in the 90's.* New York: Bergin & Garvey, 1991. This book continues where *Silent Knife* leaves off, angrily, passionately criticizing an obstetrical system that does not change.

Cohen, Nancy Wainer, and Lois Estner. *Silent Knife: Cesarean Prevention and Vaginal Birth After Cesarean.* South Hadley, MA: J. F. Bergin, 1983. Discusses in an upbeat way how to prevent cesareans, how to have a vaginal birth after cesarean and how to create positive attitudes toward childbearing. Well researched, contains women's poignant birth stories.

Davis-Floyd, Robbie. *Birth as an American Rite of Passage.* Berkeley: University of California Press, 1992. An anthropologist links interviews about birth to an analysis of obstetric procedures as rituals designed to convey the core values of American society to birthing women, values that center around science, technology and patriarchy.

DeVries, Raymond G. *Regulating Birth: Midwives, Medicine and the Law.* Philadelphia: Temple University Press, 1985. Explores the laws that regulate midwives and the history of those laws and emphasizes that control over women's health care must be returned to women.

Eakins, Pamela S., ed. *The American Way of Birth.* Philadelphia: Temple University Press, 1986. Chapters examine conflicts between childbearing women and the medical profession, cesarean birth, birth and social class, midwifery and much more.

Edwards, Margot, and Mary Waldorf. *Claiming Birth: History and Heroines of American Childbirth Reform.* Trumansburg, NY: The Crossing Press, 1984. This woman-centered book skillfully weaves together the life stories of many key women who worked for childbirth reform with a clear and critical assessment of the movement's successes and failures.

Ehrenreich, Barbara, and Deirdre English. *For Her Own Good: 150 Years of the Experts' Advice to Women.* New York: Anchor Books, 1979. No other book makes modern women's manipulation by succeeding generations of male experts so devastating. It exposes the unscientific basis of "scientific" expertise used to control women. Indispensable for an understanding of how women's role becomes defined in modern industrial society.

———. *Witches, Midwives and Nurses.* Old Westbury, NY: The Feminist Press, 1973. This powerful booklet gives a brief history of how male doctors seized control of healing and then of birthing.

Enkin, Murray, Marc J. N. C. Keirse and Iain Chambers. *A Guide to Effective Care in Pregnancy and Childbirth.* Oxford: Oxford University Press, 1989. An invaluable resource, a condensed version of a 1,500-page two-volume worldwide review of obstetrical studies and practices. It is being updated in database form every six months.

Haire, Doris. *The Cultural Warping of Childbirth.* Available from ICEA Bookcenter, PO Box 20048, Minneapolis, MN 55420. A classic pamphlet that reviews cross-cultural childbearing practices and soundly criticizes our own.

Harrison, Michelle. *Woman in Residence.* New York: Penguin Books, 1983. A look at what actually occurs in hospitals among doctors and medical students and residents as they give gynecological and obstetrical care to women, from the viewpoint of a caring, conscientious doctor.

Holmes, Helen B., Betty Hoskins and Michael Gross, eds. *Birth Control and Controlling Birth: Women-Centered Perspectives.* Clifton, NJ: The Humana Press, 1980. Roundtable discussions of papers presented at the Ethical Issues in Human Reproduction Technology: Analysis by Women (EIRTAW) Conference, held in Amherst, MA. Rich, lively reading, all issues still relevant today.

Inch, Sally. *Birthrights.* New York: Pantheon Books, 1984. Since its publication, this book, with its systematic description of the few advantages and the many disadvantages of current obstetrical practices and drugs, has been used as a reference by parents, educators and practitioners.

Jordan, Brigitte. *Birth in Four Cultures.* St. Albans, VT: Eden Press Women's Publications, 1980. An anthropologist compares U.S. birth customs with those of Sweden, Holland and the Yucatan. She points out that those practices we label as "scientific" are actually a variety of birthing rituals.

Kitzinger, Sheila, and John Davis, eds. *The Place of Birth.* New York: Oxford University Press, 1978. Reflects issues raised at meetings of British and some American health-care providers, including the safety of home vs. hospital birth, routine obstetrical intervention, fathers' participation, etc.

Leavitt, Judith Walzer. *Brought to Bed: Childbearing in America 1750–1950.* New York: Oxford University Press, 1986. Helps readers understand in detail the history of childbirth in America and the intricacies of women–physician interactions.

Logan, O., and K. Clark. *Motherwit: An Alabama Midwife's Story.* New York: E. P. Dutton, 1989.

Michaelson, Karen L., ed. *Childbirth in America: Anthropological Perspectives.* South Hadley, MA: Bergin & Garvey, 1988. Discussions about decision making during pregnancy, birthplace and birthstyle, and becoming parents. Useful articles.

Newland, Kathleen. *Worldwatch Paper 47, Infant Mortality and the Health of Societies*. December 1981. Available from Worldwatch Institute, 1776 Massachusetts Avenue NW, Washington, DC 20036. A summary of the relationship between a country's wealth and its infant mortality rate. It documents education of mothers as the most important factor in predicting healthy babies and stresses the need for a more humane distribution of resources.

Oakley, Ann. *The Captured Womb: A History of the Medical Care of Pregnant Women*. Oxford: Blackwell, 1984.

———. *Women Confined: Towards a Sociology of Childbirth*. New York: Schocken Books, 1980. Describes childbirth as a complex event of a woman's life and critiques the socialization of women and the medicalization of birth.

Pfeufer-Kahn, Robbie. *The Language of Birth: Representation, Power, and the Maternal Body*. Chicago: University of Chicago Press, 1993. Weaves together a description of attitudes toward birth in Western texts, the relationship between traditional and current protocols and practices, women's own stories and the author's own experience as a mother.

Rich, Adrienne. *Of Woman Born: Motherhood as Experience and Institution*. New York: W. W. Norton, 1976. The poet draws upon her personal life, history, research and literature to discuss many aspects of motherhood from a feminist viewpoint.

Rothman, Barbara Katz. *Encyclopedia of Childbearing*. Phoenix, AZ: Oryx Press, 1992. Rothman has drawn on the expertise of hundreds of knowledgeable women, compiling a wealth of knowledge about pregnancy and birth.

———. *In Labor: Women and Power in the Birthplace*, 2nd. ed. New York: W. W. Norton, 1992. Rothman combines her personal childbirth experiences with a critique of obstetrics in the United States today and compares the medical and midwifery models of birth.

———. *Recreating Motherhood: Ideology and Technology in a Patriarchal Society*. New York: W. W. Norton, 1989. A discussion of the ways in which patriarchy, technology and capitalism impinge upon women's procreative lives.

———. *The Tentative Pregnancy: Prenatal Diagnosis and the Future of Motherhood*. New York: Viking Press, 1986. An in-depth discussion of women's reactions to amniocentesis and its predictions.

Sagov, Stanley, Richard Feinbloom, Peggy Spindell and Archie Brodsky, eds. *Home Birth: A Practitioner's Guide to Birth Outside the Hospital*. Rockville, MD: Aspen Systems Corporation, 1983. A detailed, useful description of how this particular family practice group handles pregnancy, labor and birth. Sensitive discussions of the midwife–physician relationship and of home birth. An essential book for medical students, doctors and midwives. Also an enormously reassuring guide for parents.

Scully, Diana. *Men Who Control Women's Health: The Miseducation of Obstetrician-Gynecologists*. Boston: Houghton Mifflin, 1980. A fascinating, behind-the-scenes study of obstetrical training, including analyses of gynecology texts, observations of operating rooms and teaching hospital clinics and interviews with medical students. It brings out the inadequacy of residency training and how it often conflicts with women's needs.

Susie, Debra Anne. *In the Way of Our Grandmothers: A Cultural View of Twentieth-Century Midwifery in Florida*. Athens: University of Georgia Press, 1988. History of midwifery in Florida and conversations with Southern women who remember when midwifery evolved organically from women's needs and existed outside the realms of men.

Tew, Marjorie. *Safer Childbirth? A Critical History of Maternity Care*. London: Chapman & Hall, 1990. This important book contains statistical, biological and observational evidence that obstetric care has made a negative contribution to safer childbirth. It concludes that safety in childbirth depends primarily upon women's good health.

Wertz, Richard, and Dorothy Wertz. *Lying-In: A History of Childbirth in America*, rev. ed. New Haven: Yale University Press, 1989. The most complete social, legal and cultural history of childbirth in the United States up to and through the 1980s.

Books to Help You with Pregnancy and Childbirth

Ashford, Janet Isaacs, ed. *The Whole Birth Catalog*. Trumansburg, NY: The Crossing Press, 1983. Directory of groups, ideas and products, detailed description of books and journals. Fun to read. Gives an idea of women's childbearing culture.

Baldwin, Rahima. *Special Delivery: The Complete Guide to Informed Birth*, rev. ed. Millbrae, CA: Les Femmes Publishing, 1990. Positive discussion of pregnancy, labor and birth. Especially useful if you are planning a home birth.

Chester, Laura, ed. *Cradle and All: Women Writers on Pregnancy and Birth*. Boston: Faber & Faber, 1989. Essays, poems and excerpts from novels.

Davis, Elizabeth. *Heart and Hands: A Midwife's Guide to Pregnancy and Birth*, rev. ed. Berkeley, CA: Celestial Arts, 1987. About setting up a midwifery practice. It describes pregnancy, labor and birth from a midwife's point of view and is strong on emotional aspects of childbearing. Good practical information.

Dick-Read, Grantly. *Childbirth Without Fear*, rev. ed. New York: Harper & Row, 1987. The first book to speak of "natural childbirth." The author stresses education and relaxation rather than activity and breathing during childbirth and discusses the fear–tension–pain syndrome.

Gaskin, Ina May. *Spiritual Midwifery*, 3rd ed. Summertown, TN: The Book Publishing Co., 1990. Story upon story about childbirth from The Farm's midwifery service, followed by practical midwifery information. The Farm provides an excellent model for an alternative birthing practice.

Hazell, Lester. *Commonsense Childbirth*. New York: Berkley Medallion, 1976. Good reading. A complete, sensible approach to childbirth. The author has had four children and conveys what it feels like to lose a child. An excellent critique of childbirth problems caused by the medical profession and an encouraging view of home birth.

Hosken, Fran P. *The Universal Childbirth Picture Book*, illustrated by Marcia L. Williams, 6th ed. Lexington, MA: Women's International Network News, 1983. Used by community groups and hospitals throughout the world. Related charts and color slides. The pictures have been helpful to many women. Available in French, Spanish, Arabic, six Indian languages and many others.

Kitzinger, Sheila. *The Experience of Childbirth*. New York: Penguin, 1984. Psychological and physical aspects of childbearing discussed in an informative, empathetic, broadminded manner. One of Kitzinger's best.

Lang, Raven. *Birth Book*. Palo Alto, CA: Genesis Press, 1972. About home deliveries and confident, woman-centered birth. Moving personal descriptions of birth by mothers and fathers. Vivid photographs. Gives a good idea of what the home-birth movement of the 1970s was like.

Moskowitz, Richard. *Homeopathic Remedies for Pregnancy and Childbirth*. Berkeley, CA: North Atlantic Books, 1992. An excellent guide by a physician specializing in this area.

Nilssen, Lennart. *A Child Is Born*, rev. ed. New York: Delacorte Press, 1990. Astonishing photographs. Human reproduction from pregnancy through birth.

Odent, Michel. *Birth Reborn*. New York: Pantheon, 1984. Dr. Odent describes the evolution, practices and philosophy of his maternity clinic in Pithiviers, France, a gentle, calm birth environment in which women are encouraged to "listen to their bodies" during labor and birth, supported mainly by midwives. This book is a useful guide for practitioners who are trying to "demedicalize" their point of view.

Peterson, Gayle. *Birthing Normally: A Personal Growth Approach to Childbirth*. Berkeley, CA: Mindbody Press, 1984. How women's attitudes and emotions affect their pregnancies and births.

Steiger, Carolyn. *Becoming a Midwife*. Portland, OR: Hoogan House Publishing, 1987. Describes midwifery apprenticeship and practice in a broad, informative way. Useful for midwives and also for parents who want to learn about midwifery.

Young, Diony. *Changing Childbirth: Family Birth in the Hospital*. Rochester, NY: Childbirth Graphics Ltd., 1982. An optimistic, realistic book about every facet of birth in hospitals from family needs to obstetrical practices to strategies for implementing change.

Articles

Barkan, S., and M. Barkan. "Delayed Childbearing: No Evidence for Increased Risk of Low Birth Weight and Preterm Delivery," *American Journal of Epidemiology*, Vol. 125, No. 1 (1987), pp. 101–9. More evidence that infants of first-time mothers over thirty have no greater risk for these problems than those of younger women.

Breece, Connie, Ellen Israel and Laurie Friedman. "Closing of the Nurse-Midwifery Service at Boston City Hospital: What Were the Issues Involved," *Journal of Nurse-Midwifery*, Vol. 34, No. 1 (January/February 1989), pp. 41–44. How a successful midwifery practice was challenged and destroyed within a city hospital setting.

Chavkin, W. "Drug Addiction and Pregnancy: Policy Crossroads" (Public Health and the Law), *American Journal of Public Health*, Vol. 80, No. 4 (April 1990), pp. 483–87.

Davis-Floyd, Robbie E. "The Role of Obstetrical Rituals in the Resolution of Cultural Anomaly," *Social Science and Medicine*, Vol. 31, No. 2 (1990), pp. 175–89. Identifies eight "conceptual and procedural dilemmas presented to American society by the natural process of birth, and resolved by obstetrical rituals." For example, can the powerful female phenomenon of birth be made to support patriarchy?

———. "Obstetric Training as a Rite of Passage," *Medical Anthropology Quarterly*, Vol. 1, No. 3 (NS) (September 1987), pp. 288–318. Interviews with obstetricians and obstetrical residents. Examines how medical students are transformed into obstetricians.

Grant, A., et al. "Cerebral Palsy Among Children Born During the Dublin Randomized Trial of Intrapartum Monitoring," *The Lancet* (November 25, 1989) pp. 8674–80. Intensive internal electronic fetal monitoring during labor does not protect against cerebral palsy (all hospital births).

Guyer, B., et al. "Medicaid and Prenatal Care: Necessary but Not Sufficient" (Editorial), *Journal of the American Medical Association*, Vol. 264, No. 17 (November 7, 1990), pp. 2264–68. Prenatal care alone does not guarantee better outcomes.

Holland, Endesha Ida Mae. "Granny Midwives," *Ms.* magazine (June 1987). A readable history of granny midwives in the South.

Jordan, Brigitte. "Cosmo-political Obstetrics," *Social Science and Medicine*, Vol. 28, No. 9 (1989), pp. 925–44. Describes reasons for the failure of efforts to upgrade the skills of village traditional birth attendants in the Yucatan—the didactic mode of teaching is not appropriate in communities where people learn through apprenticeship. Brings to light the different ways in which people learn. Applicable to women and learning in the United States today.

Kennel, J., et al. "Continuous Emotional Support During Labor in a U.S. Hospital, A Randomized Controlled Trial" (Original Contributions), *JAMA*, Vol. 265, pp. 2197–2201. Support produced significant reductions in cesarean sections, forceps deliveries, as well as similar effects on use of epidural anesthesia, oxytocin use, prolonged infant hospitalization and maternal fever.

Luthy, D., et al. "A Randomized Trial of Electronic Fetal Monitoring in Preterm Labor," *Obstetrics and Gynecology*, May 1987. Reductions in perinatal mortality or morbidity through use of EFM was not demonstrated in this very rigorous study.

Mason, Jutta. "The Meaning of Birth Stories," *The Birth Gazette*, Vol. 3, No. 3 (Summer 1990), pp. 14–19. A wonderful discussion of how women's stories about birth surface when women give birth as they want, and disappear when obstetrical control intensifies.

Also a discussion of the pros and cons of licensing midwives.

Neuhoff, C., et al. "Cesarean Birth for Failed Progress in Labor," *Obstetrics and Gynecology*, Vol. 73, No. 6 (June 1989), pp. 915–20.

Rooks, J., et al. "Outcomes of Care in Birth Centers: The National Birth Center Study" (Special Article), *The New England Journal of Medicine*, Vol. 321 (December 28, 1989), pp. 1804–11. Free-standing birth centers [84] run by nurse-midwives are safe and acceptable alternatives to hospital births for many women, result in fewer cesarean sections.

Sakala, Carol. "Content of Care by Independent Midwives: Assistance with Pain in Labor and Birth," *Social Science and Medicine*, Vol. 26, No. 11, 1988, pp. 1141–1158. Independent midwives in Utah help women to mobilize and enhance their own resources in a variety of ways.

Shearer, B., and D. Young. "Leading OB's repudiate Standard Practices," *The Midwife Advocate* (Mass. Friends of Midwives), Vol. 4, Nos. 3/4 (Fall/Winter 1987/1988), p. 2. The top leadership in academic obstetrics and the inventor of fetal monitoring confess the failures of routines they helped establish.

Shy, K., et al. "Effects of Electronic Fetal Heart Rate Monitoring, Compared with Periodic Auscultation, on the Neurologic Development of Premature Infants," *New England Journal of Medicine*, Vol. 322, No. 9 (March 1, 1990), pp. 588–93. 93 premature births show Electronic Fetal Monitoring does not result in improved neurologic development for "premies."

Stafford, R. S. "The Impact of Nonclinical Factors on Repeat Cesarean Sections" (Original Contribution), *JAMA*, Vol. 265 (January 1991), pp. 59–63. 45,425 births showed reasons for repeat cesarean births were due more to nature of the hospital than to medical condition of fetus or mother.

Thorp, J. A., et al. "The Effects of Continuous Epidural Analgesia on Cesarean Section for Dystocia in Nulliparous Women," *American Journal of Obstetrics and Gynecology*, Vol. 161, No. 3, pp. 670–75. 711 births among matched women in rigorous study showed significant increases in cesarean sections when epidural anesthesia was used.

Treffers, J., et al. "Home Births and Minimal Medical Interventions" (Letter from Amsterdam), *JAMA*, Vol. 264, No. 17 (November 7, 1990), pp. 2203–4. Thorough review of Dutch system shows safety of home births and midwives.

Women's Institute for Childbearing Policy. "Childbearing Policy within a National Health Program: An Evolving Consensus for New Directions." A collaborative paper, coordinated by Carol Sakala, of WICP, the National Women's Health Network, the National Black Women's Health Project and the Boston Women's Health Book Collective. Available for $5 from Jane Pincus, Box 72, Roxbury, VT 05669. Calls for an approach to maternity care policy that combines women's health and public health perspectives and promotes midwives as the appropriate caregiver for childbearing women.

Periodicals

Birth: Issues in Prenatal Care and Education
Blackwell Scientific Publications
Three Cambridge Center, Suite 208
Cambridge, MA 02142

Cesarean Prevention Clarion
P.O. Box 152
Syracuse, NY 13210

Journal of Nurse-Midwifery
Elsevier Science Publishing Co., Inc.
655 Avenue of the Americas
New York, NY 10010

The Midwife Advocate
c/o MFOM
P.O. Box 3188
Boston, MA 02130

Mothering
P.O. Box 8410
Santa Fe, NM 87504

Midwifery Today
Box 2672-4
Eugene, OR 97402

The Birth Gazette
42, The Farm
Summertown, TN 38483

Women and Health
The Haworth Press
10 Alice Street
Binghamton, NY 13904-1580

Catalogs

Send away for these five catalogs and you will get an idea of just how many pamphlets, books, educational materials and videos are out there!

ICEA Bookmarks
ICEA Bookcenter
P.O. Box 20048
Minneapolis, MN 55420
(800) 624-4934
Fax: (612) 854-8772

Imprints
Birth and Life Bookstore
7001 Alonzo Avenue NW
P.O. Box 70625
Seattle, WA 98107-0625
(206) 789-4444

Cascade Birthing Supplies
P.O. Box 12203
Salem, OR 97309
Instruments and equipment for midwives as well as items and books for mothers and babies are offered.

Moonflower Birthing Supply
P.O. Box 128
Louisville, CO 80027
(800) 747-8996
Supplies midwifery equipment, and books are also offered.

Childbirth in History
Janet Isaacs Ashford
   327 North Glenmont Drive
   Solana Beach, CA 92075
Write for a brochure listing booklets and scripted slide shows with images and information concerning birth, midwifery, positions for labor, etc.

Organizations Concerned with Childbirth Education

American College of Nurse-Midwives
   1522 K Street NW, Suite 1120
   Washington, DC 20005
   (202) 347-5445
The professional organization for nurse-midwives in the United States. It administers national certification examinations, accredits nurse-midwifery educational programs, provides membership services, produces publications for its members and the public and holds an annual convention.

American Foundation for Maternal and Child Health, Inc.
   30 Beekman Place
   New York, NY 10022
Concerned with protection against abuses of drugs, interventions and obstetric procedures that could cause damage to the fetus, infant or child in later life.

Association for Childbirth at Home International (ACHI)
   P.O. Box 430
   Glendale, CA 91209
   (213) 667-0839
Founded in 1972. It trains childbirth educators, is developing midwifery training programs to comply with state laws throughout the United States and provides pamphlets and reprints.

Cesareans/Support, Education and Concern (C/SEC)
   22 Forest Road
   Framingham, MA 01701
   (508) 877-8266
C/SEC serves parents and professionals who want information and support in relation to cesarean childbirth, cesarean prevention and VBACs. It has been instrumental in humanizing cesareans.

Informed Homebirth, Inc.
   P.O. Box 3675
   Ann Arbor, MI 48106
It offers classes to prepare parents for home birth, prepares certification for childbirth assistants and childbirth educators and provides tapes for people planning a home birth. Sells books and videos.

International Association of Parents and Professionals for Safe Alternatives in Childbirth (NAPSAC)
   Route 1, Box 646
   Marble Hill, MO 63764
   (314) 238-2010
NAPSAC's goals are to promote education about the principles of natural childbirth; act as a forum facilitating cooperation among parents, childbirth educators and medical professionals; encourage and aid in the implementation of family-centered maternity care in hospitals; assist in the establishment of maternity and childbearing centers; help establish safe home birth programs; and provide educational opportunities to parents and parents-to-be that will enable them to assume more personal responsibility for pregnancy, childbearing, infant care and child-rearing. NAPSAC is openly antiabortion.

International Cesarean Awareness Network (formerly called the Cesarean Prevention Movement)
   P.O. Box 152
   Syracuse, NY 13210
   (315) 424-1942
It has as its goal the reduction of the primary cesarean rate and the increase of vaginal births after cesareans (VBACs). It puts out a feisty newspaper, the *Cesarean Prevention Clarion*.

International Childbirth Education Association (ICEA)
   P.O. Box 20048
   Minneapolis, MN 55240
   (612) 854-8660
ICEA is an interdisciplinary organization, founded in 1960, that represents a federation of groups and individuals, both parents and professionals, who share an interest in childbirth education and family-centered maternity care. There are regional chapters.

La Leche League International, Inc.
   Box 1209
   9616 Minneapolis Avenue
   Franklin Park, IL 60631
   (708) 455-7730
It provides all kinds of information and support about breastfeeding. There are chapters in many cities.

Maternity Center Association
   48 East 92nd Street
   New York, NY 10128
   (212) 369-7300
Founded in 1918, it began training public health nurses in midwifery in 1931. It established the MCA Childbearing Center in New York City in 1975, the country's first freestanding birth center. This organization offers excellent publications, such as the *Birth Atlas*, and conducts all sorts of classes, conferences and seminars. Its general director, Ruth Watson Lubic, has worked long and hard to improve maternity care.

Midwives Alliance of North America (MANA)
   P.O. Box 1121
   Bristol, VA 24203
   (615) 764-5561
MANA was created to expand communication and support among North American midwives; form an identifiable and cohesive organization representing the professional midwife on a regional, national and international basis; promote guidelines for the education and training of midwives and assist in development of midwifery educational programs; promote guidelines for basic competency of practicing midwives; promote midwifery as a quality health-care option for women and their families; promote research in the field of midwifery care; and establish channels for communication and cooperation between midwives and other professional and

nonprofessional groups concerned with the health of women and their families.

National Association of Childbearing Centers (NACC)
3123 Gottschall Road
Perkiomenville, PA 18074
(215) 234-8068
Begun in 1981. It is working on the public and policy levels in government, industry and the health professions. NACC is dedicated to developing closer ties within the rapidly growing national childbirth center movement and to promoting an understanding of the birth center concept. NACC constituents are operating birth centers, individuals and groups interested in establishing childbirth centers and consumers of maternity care.

Traditional Childbearing Group
P.O. Box 638
Boston, MA 02118
(617) 541-0086
Group of midwives of African descent offering home birth, childbirth classes, counseling about patients' rights and traditional healing approaches.

Traditional Midwife Center International
c/o Linda Holmes
64 Cambridge Street
East Orange, NJ 07018
A networking organization for individuals interested in collecting and preserving documents and artifacts pertaining to the practices of traditional Southern granny midwives of African descent.

21

Postpartum

BY DENNIE WOLF AND
MARY CROWE

With special thanks to
Robbie Pfeufer.

*This chapter in previous editions was
written by Paula Doress, Vilunya
Diskin, Esther Rome and Marty
Ruedi.*

*1992 Update of postpartum
depression and Resources by Alice
LoCicero.*

BECOMING A MOTHER

*The months after having a baby are a mix, a real
mix. Some days you love it. Imagine having the
chance and time to roll on the bed and drink in the
smell of a baby and find the tiny daily changes in a
body your body made. Other days you're on a bus
with a wet baby and a stroller that's rolling down
the aisle. You look at the neat, childless people in the
other seats and you feel messy, clumsy, alone and in
the way. I remember Mondays when I could barely
shuffle between my part-time job and the sitter's,
with the baby wailing in the car seat. Then Wednes-
day would roll around, she'd wake up laughing with
her arms out, we'd sail through the morning and I'd
come to work thinking, This isn't easy. But, God,
does it matter!*

Celebration and change surround the birth of a
baby. But the new life isn't just the baby's—it's
yours, too. Being a mother can bring deep pleasure, intimacy and skill.

But in this culture, at this time, motherhood
also challenges our well-being. As mothers, many
of us assume the role of the all-time giver, and
bury our own needs for adult company, nurturance, sexuality. Increasing numbers of us are
under the chronic stress that comes from balancing the roles of mother, worker and lover. We ne-

glect our own physical and mental health, even
those of us who wanted children and who have
the protection of enough income, help and closeness with friends or lovers. The strain is even
greater for low-income and single mothers and for
women who do not fit the motherhood ideal (like
lesbian women or women who do not want their
babies).

Motherhood can be a time of insight. Birth and
nursing give us a new respect for our bodies. Car-

Suzanne Arms

474

ing for, playing with and cuddling children, we discover new dimensions to loving. Many of us wake up, as never before, to the politics of being women and caregivers. As we move between homes and workplaces, our own lives teach us the changes in housing, health care, wages and work structures that families need. Hours spent caring for others make us more concerned about what sexism, racial prejudice and nuclear weapons mean for the future.

When we move into the first year of motherhood prepared and aware, we can wrestle with the issues and take hold of the possibilities. In this chapter we present the stories, wisdom and strategies of many new mothers: women who had difficult and easy postpartum experiences, women who became mothers alone or with partners, women with male and female partners, first- and many-time mothers, mothers who worked at home and mothers who chose or had to take on or continue outside work.*

THE POSTPARTUM EXPERIENCE

Many women describe three phases of postpartum experience. During the first days after delivery, we deal with the emotional and physical effects of having given birth. Over the next few months we learn what it means to be parents and adjust to life with a baby. Eventually, after daily life becomes more settled (usually in the second half of the postpartum year), we begin to face some of the long-term issues motherhood raises for us.

This doesn't mean, however, that you will experience postpartum in terms of defined phases or that postpartum ends when a year is up. You will probably have some of these feelings at various times and at various levels of intensity for years to come. Postpartum, like birth, is a very individual experience.

THE FIRST PHASE: TRANSITION TO PARENTHOOD

During the first few days postpartum we make the transition from pregnancy to motherhood. This is a time of enormous change; physically our bodies recover from birth and begin to nourish the baby; emotionally we may feel everything from exhilaration to exhaustion, uncertainty and sadness.

---

*In this chapter we have focused on the experience of birth-mothers and do not discuss adoptive mothers' or stepmothers' transition to motherhood. We believe that the experience of assuming the social role of motherhood is much the same for any woman who becomes a primary caretaker, regardless of the circumstances.

Our birth experience may also affect how we feel, as may our readiness to become mothers and whether or not we have support from partner, family and friends.

Feelings About the Birth

If the birth has gone well and the baby is healthy, you may feel incredibly high, tremendously relieved and proud of what you have just accomplished.

Even though I'd had a long and difficult labor, I felt ecstatic after the baby was born. I wanted to leap out of bed and run around the room to celebrate. Then, after a couple of hours, fatigue caught up with me and I began to feel utterly exhausted. Every muscle and bone ached. Still, I didn't mind somehow. It was a good kind of tiredness—the kind that comes when you've been pushed to the limits of your capabilities. Along with the weariness came new, quieter feelings of peace, happiness, tenderness for my baby and a connection to all womankind!

But you may have other feelings, too, especially if the birth did not live up to your expectations or if you encountered unexpected intervention or complications.

We had planned a birth with no intervention, and I had an emergency cesarean instead. Even though I was relieved that everything was okay and thrilled with my baby, I had the nagging sense that I had failed somehow. Later I got over feeling that it was my fault, but I still felt cheated out of the birth experience we had hoped and planned for. Sometimes I still can't help feeling a little jealous when I hear women talk about their wonderful birth experiences.

In the days following delivery you may think about the birth a lot, want to talk about it in detail and try to resolve your feelings about it. You may relive it over and over, perhaps fantasizing different outcomes for parts you feel ambivalent about (see p. 484 for more).

The Baby Blues: Early Postpartum Depression

Within a few days after birth, you may experience the *baby blues*. They can appear as anything from a fleeting sense of inexplicable sadness to a full-blown depression that temporarily incapacitates you. You may cry unexpectedly, feel worried about your lack of maternal feelings or frightened by the reality of the sudden responsibility thrust upon you. Many of us have vivid dreams and fantasies.

The birth of my baby was wonderful, but the next day I kept having the sense that something was miss-

ing, that I'd lost something in the process. Looking at my soft, flat belly, I finally realized what it was: I missed being pregnant. For days afterwards I found myself wanting to feel the baby kick. Even though I had a real, live baby to deal with, I felt hollow inside. It took a while to accept the fact that this baby was the same one I'd carried for so long.

Immediately after the birth of my baby I felt high and exhilarated. But that night I got sad. I cried all night long. During the next few days I lay on my bed thinking of how I would kill myself. I couldn't sleep at all. I tried to tell the nurses I was depressed and all they gave me were sleeping pills. I felt like I'd never feel anything again but this incredible despair. I had nightmares. The one I remember best is where I would be feeding the baby. I would fall asleep and the baby would fall off the bed and be killed. I don't know why I had these dreams and impulses. I have a happy marriage and it was a wanted pregnancy.

Almost everyone has these feelings to some extent; postpartum blues often appear just as your milk comes in. Hormonal changes may be at least partly responsible for sudden shifts in mood, and depression can be heightened by being physically run down, anemic or exhausted from being woken repeatedly at night.

Usually these feelings last only a day or two. If you are insecure about your ability to care for or relate to your baby, your confidence will grow as you get to know her/him better. In addition, talking with other mothers about fears and anxieties can help you feel less alone. With a caring partner, friends or family, the baby blues are less likely to occur and easier to handle.

When depression lasts more than a few days it is usually caused by a combination of social and physical factors. For a discussion of more serious postpartum depression, see p. 485.

Physical Changes After Birth: Taking Care of Ourselves

For me, physical recovery was no big deal. Because I had an easy birth and no episiotomy, I healed very fast and felt back to normal within a few days. The only thing that bothered me was sore nipples (for the first couple of days) and night sweats, which lasted about a week. Otherwise I felt terrific. Maybe I was just high from the birth, but I seemed to have a lot more energy then than I do now, several months later.

For at least two weeks after the birth I was very uncomfortable. In addition to feeling the episiotomy stitches, my whole pelvic area ached, and it hurt to stand for more than a few minutes. I couldn't sit for a week! Even after I got home, I found I couldn't do

anything. I hated the feeling of being helpless. Because I was in so much pain, I was very touchy and found it hard to respond to my husband or to the visitors who came to see me and the baby.

Our bodies undergo enormous changes after birth—a pregnancy in reverse. Your uterus will become firm, contracting often, reducing in size so that by the tenth day after delivery you will no longer be able to feel it above the pubic bone. Breastfeeding your baby speeds up this involution process by releasing the hormones you need to trigger uterine contractions and keep them going. (Sometimes milk not coming in can be a sign of retained placenta.) These postdelivery contractions of the uterus are often strong and may startle you, especially following a second or subsequent child, but they will ease within a few days. Drinking raspberry tea and resting with a heating pad on your belly will help.

In another dramatic change your blood volume is reduced by 30 percent during the first two weeks postpartum. Under any other conditions this loss would be felt as exhaustion, but many women are exhilarated instead.[1] If you feel very tired or weak, you may be anemic. Be sure to eat enough iron-rich foods and/or continue taking iron and vitamin supplements.

As the uterine tissue breaks down, it is expelled in a discharge called *lochia*, similar to a heavy menstrual flow, which usually lasts from two to four weeks after birth. If bleeding is unusually heavy or suddenly resumes after this time or if the lochia smells bad (a sign of infection), talk with your doctor or midwife. The immediate postpartum period is a time when infection can occur easily. Be on the lookout for signs—excessive bleeding, fever—that something might be wrong.

Many women find that after delivery, their pelvic floor and abdominal walls are very slack. Kegel exercises (see p. 406) immediately after birth, followed by gentle abdominal exercises and leg lifts, will help restore your muscle tone.

It may take a while for your bowels to start up and become regular. Drinking a lot of liquids keeps bowel movements soft and helps prevent urinary tract infections as well. Eat bran and stewed prunes. Relax and let your body take over. As long as you don't strain, you won't dislodge your recovering organs (a common fear), tear your stitches or aggravate hemorrhoids (varicose veins of the anus), which sometimes appear during pregnancy or the second stage of labor. If you have them, wipe with toilet paper soaked in water or witch hazel after each bowel movement, and take frequent sitz baths (one and a half inches of water with a strong brew of comfrey tea to promote healing).

During the first twenty-four hours after delivery, apply ice packs to the perineum, labia, anus, etc., to reduce swelling. After twenty-four hours, try warm sitz baths (see above). Some midwives recommend honey or vitamin E to heal stitches and tears; others prefer keeping the area dry and exposing it to infrared light for a few minutes at a time. Most also recommend waiting two weeks before taking tub baths (showers are fine, however).

As your tissues rid themselves of excess fluids stored up during pregnancy, you may drink, urinate and perspire more than usual. The sudden loss of estrogen can also cause night sweats, which may last for several weeks after birth. (These are similar to night sweats at menopause.) Some women also experience "hot flashes" during nursing, as their milk lets down.

When you nurse your baby from birth onward, without the hospital-enforced twelve-to-twenty-four-hour wait and according to the baby's demand for food, engorgement (painful swelling of breasts) will probably not occur. If you are not nursing regularly, your breasts may become markedly engorged when your milk first comes in, during the second or third day after delivery. Nursing frequently (to keep the breasts empty); applying heat in the form of hot showers, compresses or heating pad; and massaging the breasts (to promote circulation and letdown) should relieve engorgement quickly. Some women also recommend ice packs for pain. Whatever you do, don't stop nursing!

Some hospitals routinely give new mothers shots of DES or androgen (male hormone) to suppress their milk supply.* *We do not recommend these shots.* If you do plan to breastfeed, be sure to tell your practitioner and the hospital staff so they'll know *not* to give the shots. If you do not nurse your baby, binding your breasts tightly will ease discomfort when your milk comes in and will inhibit the supply. Before making the decision not to breastfeed, we hope you will consider the advantages carefully (see below).

After a normal delivery you will probably be out of bed within a few hours. Getting on your feet soon after birth means fewer bladder and bowel problems and a quicker recovery of energy. Getting up earlier can also reduce the hospital stay. Some hospitals, as well as birthing centers, now encourage the new mother to leave within twenty-four hours of a normal birth. This doesn't mean, however, that you should resume normal activities right away. It is very important to take care of yourself during these early days after birth. Resuming strenuous activity too soon can prolong the healing process and leave you feeling exhausted a week or two later. Even when you are feeling terrific, keep visitors to a minimum and let other people take care of household chores and any other children you may have. If you are alone at home, ask friends, relatives or neighbors to run errands and bring in meals. Your hospital may also provide homemaker services or social services. For at least six weeks, you should set aside extra time for rest and exercise.

Our friends set up a great system. Each night for the first week they would bring over a pot of something to eat. But they liked to stay and eat with us. We had to be their hosts! Finally, we asked them just to bring the food and let us eat by ourselves. We were too tired for company.

Recovery After a Cesarean Birth

If you had a cesarean birth, you may feel sick and weak for a day or so, as well as very sore around the incision. You will probably have an intravenous feeding tube (IV) and a catheter (to drain the bladder) for twenty-four to forty-eight hours. Many women find the catheter very uncomfortable, so ask if it can be removed earlier. Also ask that the IV be placed so that it doesn't interfere with nursing the baby. If you had general anesthesia during the operation, your lungs will have accumulated fluid that must be coughed up. The "hut" or "chest" breathing exercises you may have learned in childbirth classes can help you to do this without too much discomfort. Many women also experience gas pains and/or constipation. Eating light, easily digested foods for the first few days will help.

After a cesarean, you will be on your feet within a day. Walking may be painful, but it helps you to get your digestive system going and avoid blood clots in your legs (thrombosis). Within a few days you can begin exercises (see E. Noble, *Essential Exercises for the Childbearing Years*, listed in Resources) that speed healing and restore muscle tone, but you should avoid heavy lifting and strenuous exercise for at least six weeks.

Because you have had major surgery, you may be in the hospital for several days, so it's important that you feel cared for during your hospital stay. Ask for whatever makes you feel better, whether it's frequent visits from your partner, family and friends, food from home or a massage when you're feeling tired and sore. Some hospitals allow partners to stay overnight (you may have to provide your own sleeping bag on the floor).

---

*DES may soon be banned for this purpose. Even if you are given the shots to suppress your milk, you can nurse. Just put your baby to your breasts regularly and persistently, and the suckling will cause your milk to come in. However, the hormones will reach the baby. Mothers are also at risk from DES (breast cancer, thromboembolism) (see p. 585).

On the second day, I insisted on getting up and taking a shower. Washing my hair was a big step toward recuperation. It made me feel that I was taking charge of my body again. Exercising helped, too—I started stretching my legs and doing ankle rotations immediately.

When you are feeling well enough, have adequate help at home and feel uncomfortable in the hospital, ask if you can leave early. (Perhaps you could return as an outpatient to have your stitches removed.)

Feeding Your Baby

Most of us working on this book breastfed our babies because we wanted to and were proud that we could provide the best possible nourishment for our children. Even after returning to work, many of us found ways to continue breastfeeding. Both the advertising industry and hospitals continue to promote formula, even though research shows that breast milk is the best food for infants. Women who choose to breastfeed may have trouble finding information and support for their decision or be pressured by family or doctors into

George Malave/Stock Boston

stopping because they think that the baby isn't getting "enough" milk. Also, because our society tells us (in subtle and not so subtle ways) that breasts are sex symbols and bodies are sex objects, we may feel embarrassed or uncomfortable about using our breasts to feed our babies. We hear that nursing "spoils our figures" or ties us down so that we can't resume work or other activities. These myths serve to discourage women from making the choice to breastfeed.

Research shows that there are many good reasons to breastfeed and almost no reasons not to.[2] Human milk (unlike cow's milk) is ideally suited to a baby's needs. It provides exactly the right balance of nutrients, which adapt to your baby's changing requirements. Even babies who can tolerate no other food digest breast milk easily. In addition, breastfeeding helps to strenghten the infant's resistance to infection and disease, something no formula can do. Colostrum, the liquid in a new mother's breasts before the milk actually comes in, is especially high in antibodies that protect the tiny newborn against staphylococcus infections, polio virus, Coxsackie B virus, infant diarrhea and *Escherichia coli* infections, the very germs to which infants are usually most susceptible. Breastfeeding also gives our babies a natural immunity to almost all common childhood diseases for at least six months and often until we stop breastfeeding completely.*

In general, breastfed babies have fewer problems with allergies, constipation, indigestion, skin disorders and future tooth decay than bottle-fed babies. Breastfeeding is even thought to encourage better development of the dental arch, preventing the need for orthodonture later on.[3] For all these reasons, the American Academy of Pediatrics officially endorses breastfeeding as the preferred way of feeding babies.†

There are practical advantages, too. Formula must be prepared for each feeding in sterilized bottles. Breast milk is economical and always available at the right temperature, and there are no bottles to carry around! In addition, the milk supply adjusts to the baby's needs; the more the baby nurses, the more milk the breasts produce. As the baby weans, the milk supply tapers off.

Women who breastfeed tend to get back into shape earlier than those who don't. From right after birth, breastfeeding helps your body to expel

---

*Because of immunities in breast milk, some women delay having their babies inoculated against diseases until they stop breastfeeding. You might discuss this with your practitioner.
†There are serious disadvantages to formula use. An estimated 5,000 babies die annually in the United States due to formula abuse in some hospitals that actively promote its use, especially among poor women. Other health scandals in this country and abroad have involved deaths of babies who received contaminated or improperly mixed formula.

excess fluids and tissue. Because the body burns about 1,000 calories a day to produce breast milk, nursing mothers tend to lose weight gained during pregnancy gradually during the first few months postpartum.

Finally, breastfeeding can be relaxing and sensual, close and satisfying. Some women become sexually aroused and even have orgasms while breastfeeding. This is because oxytocin, the hormone that triggers orgasm (and labor), is also responsible for the letdown of milk when stimulated by the baby's suckling. The breastfeeding mother and her baby have an intimate and interdependent relationship; many women feel extraordinarily close to their babies while nursing.

If you decide to breastfeed your baby, it is a good idea to have access to advice from experienced, successful nursing mothers. The La Leche League provides just this kind of advice plus literature and support groups. Breastfeeding is a learned skill that takes determination and practice, especially since we don't grow up among a lot of women who do it. You can solve most breastfeeding problems with patience and the right kind of support.*

Some women choose formula so that others can feed their babies and because it is easy to tell exactly how much milk the baby is getting. Occasionally women who want to breastfeed have severe difficulties that lead them to switch to partial or complete bottlefeeding at some point. If you decide to bottlefeed for these or other reasons, be assured that you can still have a close relationship with your baby. Whether you feed babies by breast or bottle, they like to be held close and cuddled during feedings. This physical closeness is important to the baby's emotional health, for it satisfies her/his need for touching and sucking, which is especially strong in the early months.

Breastfeeding Under Special Circumstances

There is no reason why women who have had cesarean births cannot breastfeed their babies, though it may be a little more difficult getting started if the mother is uncomfortable after surgery and/or the baby is sleepy from drugs used during delivery. Some cesarean mothers choose not to take painkilling drugs after surgery that will pass through their milk to the baby.

Mothers of premature babies and twins usually can and should nurse their babies.* If your baby is too small and weak to suck, you can express milk to be fed to her/him via a tube until s/he is strong enough to nurse. Even if you are separated from your baby by a prolonged hospitalization, you can usually make arrangements to breastfeed part-time (see below).

With few exceptions, mothers with illnesses requiring medication can and should continue to nurse. If you are taking drugs that will pass through your milk to the baby, you and your practitioner can often make substitutions, lower the dosage or eliminate the drug. Make it clear to your practitioner that you want to continue to breastfeed your baby.

If for some reason you must stop breastfeeding (or choose not to initially), you may be able to reactivate your milk supply later by allowing your baby to suckle frequently. It may take some time for your milk to come in, and the process can be frustrating and difficult. Some determined women have resumed nursing weeks or even months after stopping completely. Occasionally, mothers of adopted children have even managed to breastfeed their babies successfully.

The La Leche League (see Resources) has documented examples of all the cases mentioned above and can provide invaluable information, advice, literature and encouragement through a difficult period.

Sharing Feelings

If you plan to return to work, want time for yourself or feel it's important for your partner or other members of the family to feed the baby, it is possible to establish a part-time breastfeeding arrangement, especially after the first couple of months. You can express milk (by hand or breast pump), chill or freeze it (if it is not used within a few hours) and leave it for others to give to the baby. Alternatively, you may be able to find another nursing mother who would be willing to nurse your baby while you are out.

If you must miss feedings on a regular basis, be sure to express milk at the appropriate feeding times to keep up your milk supply. Remember, breastfeeding is a matter of supply and demand. We know of airline stewardesses who express milk while they are traveling and breastfeed their babies on the days that they are home.

Some women find that expressing milk is a real inconvenience. Others have trouble expressing enough milk to keep up an adequate supply. In

---

*Some common problems include difficulty with letting down milk and maintaining an adequate milk supply when the baby grows quickly. If you do have problems, we recommend consulting nursing mothers or supportive groups (such as La Leche) rather than relying on pediatricians for advice. Few physicians are experienced and/or supportive enough of breastfeeding to be really helpful; many actively discourage women from breastfeeding if the slightest problem arises.

---

*Research shows that the milk of mothers of premature babies contains more protein than that of mothers with full-term babies. (La Leche information Sheet No. 13, December 1980, available from La Leche League International. See Resources for address.)

these cases, you may nurse only once or twice a day, giving your baby juice or formula in between, or switch entirely to bottlefeeding. The point is to reach a compromise that you feel good about for yourself and your baby.

Breastfeeding and Contraception

When you are totally breastfeeding your baby (i.e., no supplementary formula or solid food), your menstrual periods usually do not return for seven to fifteen months after birth, because the hormones that stimulate milk production also inhibit menstruation. Breastfeeding, however, is *not* a reliable form of contraception after four to five weeks postpartum. It is possible (though rare) to ovulate and conceive before getting a period. Once you have resumed menstruation, you are even more likely to become pregnant. In choosing a form of birth control, avoid the IUD because of increased risk of pelvic inflammatory disease. Recently, the American Academy of Pediatrics cautioned that extended use of combination pills may affect your milk supply and/or the length of time you are able to nurse.[4] We have serious reservations about oral contraceptives. Also, since steroids can get into the milk supply, there may be as yet undiscovered effects on the baby. (See Chapter 13, "Birth Control.")

Tips for Successful Breastfeeding

In order to establish and maintain a good milk supply, you must take care of yourself. This means eating high-protein foods (a pregnancy diet plus 300 to 500 calories). Be sure to include foods rich in vitamins B and C, iron and calcium.* If you have been taking prenatal supplements, keep taking them until your practitioner advises otherwise. Don't try to lose weight at this time. The ten or so extra pounds you retained after birth will help your body sustain milk production during the first few months. In addition, sudden weight loss can be harmful: If your body is forced to mobilize its fat supplies, your milk may contain higher amounts of some of the potentially hazardous chemicals found in our environment and food supplies.[5]

Be sure to drink plenty of fluids. A good rule of thumb is to drink a big glass of juice, milk or water every time you nurse. Keep one by your bedside at night, too.

Getting enough rest is *very* important. It is difficult for your body to produce increasing amounts of milk when you are tired and run-down. If you feel your milk supplies are inadequate, try to cut

down on outside activities and rest whenever possible. Some women also recommend supplemental brewers' yeast (which contains high amounts of B vitamins) or a glass or two of dark imported beer (which contains yeast). You can also drink teas made from blessed thistle, camomile, fennel or fenugreek seed thirty minutes before nursing.

Remember, whatever you eat or drink will be passed on to your baby via your milk. For this reason, it is wise to avoid caffeine and drugs* (including over-the-counter remedies). Also, don't take more than one or two alcoholic drinks.

Some Problems You May Encounter

Sore Nipples
Some women have sore nipples the first few days of breastfeeding. While hospitals often advise women to nurse only five minutes on each breast at four-hour intervals, many women find that nursing more frequently actually works better because the breasts don't become engorged (see below) and the baby sucks less vigorously at the nipple. If your nipples do become sore, exposing them to sunlight and air whenever possible will help, as will sparing applications of vitamin E oil, lanolin or calendula cream. Other ointments contain ingredients that could be toxic to the baby.

Engorgement
When your milk comes in on the second or third day, your breasts may feel full, heavy and painful to the touch. In some cases, they are so full you may have to express a little milk by hand before the baby can grasp the nipple. Frequent nursing on demand often prevents engorgement, but if it occurs, hot showers or hot compresses made with comfrey applied before nursing will usually remedy the situation within a day or so. By that time, your body will have adjusted its supply to the baby's demand for food.

Sore Breasts
If you have swelling, redness or a painful lump in one area of your breast, you may have a plugged duct, which can be caused by poor letdown, engorgement, infrequent nursing, tight clothing and/or stress and fatigue. Hot compresses, massaging the area and increased nursing will usually ease the discomfort. If the swelling is accompanied by fever and a tired, run-down, achy feeling (like flu), you probably have a breast infection (*mastitis*). In that case, contact your practitioner or midwife and make sure to get more rest. Some people recommend taking two to four capsules of echinacia

---

*Women who cannot drink milk because of a lactose intolerance can add lactase (a milk-digesting enzyme) to ordinary milk, making it digestible. This product is available in drugstores and goes under the trade name of Lact-Aid.

*Before taking any drugs, consult your practitioner as to whether they are safe for nursing mothers. Contact the La Leche League for a list of drugs to avoid while nursing.

root or putting garlic (a natural antibiotic) under the tongue overnight.[6] If the condition does not improve in twenty-four hours, you may need medication. Rarely, a breast infection develops into an abscess that may have to be surgically drained. In most cases, however, early treatment will prevent this.

THE SECOND PHASE: ADJUSTING TO LIFE WITH A BABY

During the first few months after birth we learn what it means to have a baby in our lives. Many women describe early postpartum as a period of fragmentation and disorganization.

During those early weeks I felt like I was disappearing. I seemed to exist only in terms of other people's needs. Sometimes I wasn't sure where the baby ended and I began. I felt that I had lost my old self and was too tired, physically and emotionally, to find her again. But I was also discovering a new part of myself that I hadn't known about before: unexpectedly intense feelings for my new baby, a resurgence of love for my mother, connection with other women. I went from despair to overwhelming feelings of tenderness, all within the space of an hour.

During this time we have to find ways of coping with the changes this upheaval brings about.

Fatigue

Of all the stresses associated with postpartum, fatigue is the one most mentioned by almost all parents. At some point most of us "crash" under the pressure of night after night of interrupted sleep—some for only a short while, others for months, especially when there are other children at home and/or little outside help.

For the first week after the birth I was flying. I seemed to have plenty of energy for everything—my new baby, my husband, even the constant stream of visitors who filled the house. Then, one day, it just caught up with me. Suddenly I could hardly get through the day with two or three naps. By nine A.M. I was exhausted. In addition, my perineum, which was nearly healed, suddenly began to ache and feel sore again. My body was clearly sending me a message. When I slowed down and began to take care of myself, I felt better, but I never did recapture that initial high of those days after the birth.

The first six months of my third baby's life are a blur to me. Constantly tired and irritable, I somehow got through each day, but it certainly was no fun for us

all. The older children (three and six) suffered from not getting enough attention. Because the baby was breastfeeding six times a day there was almost no time to take the kids out or even get through the daily housekeeping. I still feel spread thin most of the time.

Some physical discomforts also contribute to fatigue. Common ones that last two to three weeks after birth are sweating (especially at night), loss of appetite, thirst (due to loss of fluids and nursing) and constipation. If you continue to lose sleep, you build up a backlog of REM* sleep loss, which can lead to emotional and physical disturbances. Your partner may also suffer the effects of sleep deprivation.

Some women get enough REM sleep even though the baby disrupts their usual sleep pattern. However, if you sleep most soundly in your sixth or seventh hour of sleep, have someone else feed the baby during the night, early in the morning or in the late afternoon, so that once a day you can sleep for a longer stretch than the few hours between feedings. Keep housework to a minimum and ask for help with it and any other children you may have. If possible, nap whenever the baby naps.

Sexuality

Some of us have little or no interest in sex for a while after childbirth. Others resume sexual activity fairly quickly. We each need to set our own pace.

Low sexual interest can result from having your life shaken up, feeling exhausted, having to take care of your new baby, a mate and possibly other children. You may need to be nurtured and cared for, too.

All that first year, our old forms of go-to-it sexuality were just too much. I was too tired and I'd fall asleep in the first five minutes, leaving Jack frustrated, even angry. Other times I'd have the nursing and holding of the baby on my mind and intercourse seemed rough and crude. Also, I think that by the end of a day I had had a lot of skin-to-skin rubbing and touching and didn't feel sexually hungry at all. But Jack hadn't had much at all. The unevenness of it all was driving us nuts. After months and months of snarling, we just had to invent "middle ways" of being physical with one another. I think I picked it up from watching each of us with the baby—the nuzzling and snuggling that goes on with no expectation of orgasm, just affection.

---

*REM (rapid eye movements) are associated with dreaming, which occurs during the deepest phase of sleep, and is believed to be necessary for physical and psychological replenishment.

Low sexual interest can have physical causes. If you had an episiotomy or tear in the perineum during birth, the area may be sore for several weeks. Your vagina may feel dry, lacking its normal lubrication because of lowered estrogen levels (more common in nursing mothers). Penetration—by a finger, penis or dildo—may hurt, although other kinds of lovemaking that don't involve penetration may be just what you want.

If the vaginal area feels okay and the bleeding (lochia) has stopped, there is no medical risk in having intercourse with a male partner, or with a female partner, lovemaking that includes penetration. Masters and Johnson report that many women resume sexual intercourse within three weeks following delivery.[7] U.S. physicians advise no intercourse for six weeks to prevent infection; however, this rule originated in the days before antibiotics. If you sleep with one person regularly, you probably already share the same germs.

If penetration is uncomfortable and you still want it, use an unscented lubricant such as K-Y Jelly or a clear vegetable oil.* Be aware that some nursing mothers also experience painful cramps during and after intercourse.

If your partner is a man, you must use reliable birth control as soon as you are ready to have intercourse again, even if you haven't had a period. Your old diaphragm will not fit. You can use condoms with lots of foam or jelly until you get a new diaphragm fitted (see Breastfeeding and Contraception, p. 480, and Chapter 13, "Birth Control").

Learning How to Be Mothers

We may have grown up believing that because we are women, we are supposed to know how to care for a baby. Yet it is really experience that teaches us to be good mothers, including our own experiences babysitting or watching our mothers care for younger brothers and sisters. In the beginning we may be uneasy and afraid to trust our own good sense, especially with a first baby. Talking with other mothers about our feelings and fears can give us the confidence to try different things.

The first month was awful. I loved my baby but felt apprehensive about my ability to satisfy this totally dependent tiny creature. Every time she cried I could feel myself tense up and panic. What should I do? Can I make her stop—can I help her?

After the first month I got the hang of it, partly because I had such an easy child. She slept a lot, and when she was awake she was responsive—she'd look at me alertly and smile. Gradually my love for her overcame my panic. I relaxed, stopped thinking so much about my inadequacies and was just myself. It was pretty clear from her responses that I was doing something right.

I didn't know how to change a diaper any more than my husband did. In fact, I may have been more nervous about it, since I was "supposed" to know how. I learned to do it because I had to learn, and my husband learned, too.

Don't expect to love being a mother all the time. for instance, when your baby sleeps a lot, wakes up for feedings, smiles at you and goes back to sleep again, the baby business is a breeze. But when a baby is *colicky* (a catchword to describe baby discomfort, fussiness, crankiness) and cries sixteen hours out of twenty-four (that is not an exaggeration; one couple we know just went through forty-eight hours of constant wailing), your physical and mental powers may be stretched to their limits. There is nothing quite so jarring to the nerves as your own baby's cries. Watching the baby writhe in discomfort or pain fills a new parent with feelings of impotence, guilt and understandable anger. No amount of preparation can really equip you to withstand this calmly. But just realize that most babies are colicky for only a few hours each day—often in the late afternoon and evening—and usually outgrow it by around four months.

At around two weeks old she started crying from ten or eleven P.M. until six in the morning. We tried everything—walking, rocking, massage—but nothing seemed to help. Underneath I was sure it was my fault. One night, in desperation, Mark started dancing around the floor with her. I was so tired and they looked so funny that I started to laugh. Mark began to laugh, too, and the baby was so surprised that she stopped crying for a minute. It was enough to break the tension. After that, it seemed to get gradually better. I stopped blaming myself and realized that this was something she just had to go through, and all we could do was be there with her. After a few hard weeks she tapered off.

In many cases, colic is thought to be due to the immature digestive system of the baby.* Sometimes, however, an allergy to a protein in cow's milk is responsible. If you are breastfeeding, you can try to avoid dairy products for a week to see

---

*Avoid estrogen creams and/or pills recommended by some physicians, as the long-term effects of hormones on you and the baby are unknown.

*During the 1950s, colic was usually thought to be caused by maternal hostility to the baby. Some doctors still believe this. If your pediatrician questions your feelings about motherhood, switch to another topic. What you need is practical help, not psychoanalysis.

if it helps. Some vegetables (onions, garlic, cabbage, broccoli, cauliflower, brussels sprouts) and occasionally wheat can also cause gas pains in breastfed babies. It's a good idea to avoid any foods to which you are allergic, as the baby may also be sensitive to these substances. If you are bottlefeeding, you might try changing the formula.

You can try massaging your colicky baby's tummy, getting in a warm bath with her/him (heat often has a soothing effect) and offering weak solutions of camomile or spearmint tea. In very extreme cases, your practitioner may prescribe a drug (such as Donnatal) for your baby. Beyond that, the only advice we can offer is to have lots of people around to hold and walk the baby so you can get away for a period each day.

Whether your baby is easy or colicky, getting along with her/him may take some time and work.

Other Changes

Living with a new baby means changing our lives in many ways. We discover we are on twenty-four-hour call.

I was used to getting out of the house in five minutes when I wanted to go somewhere. Now it can take me an hour to get organized for even a simple expedition. By the time I've gathered up the diapers, blankets and rattles, fed and changed the baby and put her in the snuggly, sometimes it's almost too late to go. And if I ever want to go out alone, I've learned I need to start phoning babysitters a week in advance.

Many babies are unpredictable in their sleeping and eating habits for the first few weeks. Some breastfed babies continue to nurse frequently and wake at night for months. We may be overwhelmed by the constant demands of baby care and find it difficult to get on with the rest of our lives.

I had been told that most babies ate every three or four hours and slept the rest of the time. Not mine! She wanted to nurse every two hours and sometimes more often than that. Sometimes she would sleep for an hour, sometimes for fifteen minutes. I loved her, but I also felt consumed by her needs. It was hard to adjust to the fact that I couldn't get anything finished, whether it was an article I was reading or folding the laundry. At the end of the day I would realize I hadn't accomplished anything. Once I accepted the fact that I was not going to function at my old efficient rate (at least for a while) and stopped feeling guilty about what I wasn't getting done, I felt freer to enjoy the time I was spending with my baby.

Some of us are reluctant or resentful about giving up activities we used to take for granted; for others, it's a holiday if we can stay at home for a while. Though it may seem like forever when you are living it, this phase passes. Within a few months, when the baby is older and on a more predictable schedule, you'll have more flexibility.

Isolation

For many of us, life with a new baby means coping with the monotony and isolation of long hours spent alone with an infant. This is particularly true after the first weeks when you do not work outside the home, the excitement of the birth event has worn off, friends and family are no longer coming around to visit and your partner has returned to work. There may be day after day without adult company.

You can get very nutty from being alone at home. I get so that I invent errands. I go outside just to buy a loaf of bread, just to see people. I notice that the streets are full of people like me, mothers with babies in strollers or carriages. I stand behind them in line and see how they try to engage in a bit of conversation because they want someone to talk to, just like me.

It is only in Western, modernized cultures that women are expected to "go it alone" with children. In other cultures, postpartum mothers live among mothers, aunts, sisters and cousins and are able to draw on their time, interest and wisdom.[8] Many of us feel more connected with our own mothers after giving birth, but when we are geographically or psychologically separated, we may overlook them as an important source of help and affection.

In fact, research into postpartum depression suggests that one of the most important protections a woman can have is a network of social relations.

For single mothers especially, family and friends are, as one woman put it, "better than vitamins, more than money."

When Alison was still a baby, I was in pretty hard shape. I didn't have work; I'd dropped out of school. The man I was living with was having a real bout with drinking. It would have been worse if it hadn't been for one of my brothers. He'd come down to the cottage after high school in the afternoon. We'd just hang out together. He adored both of my kids. I think he really took the hard parts out of being a mother alone.

When Willie was just a few months old, I joined a playgroup with several other mothers in the area.

Nancy Hawley

While the group was formed to get the babies together, its real function was as a support group for the mothers. It was reassuring to hear that someone else's baby was colicky and had been up all night and trade information and suggestions as to what we could do. It was also a help to share some of my ambivalent feelings about motherhood and discover that I wasn't the only one. I came to look on the playgroup as an oasis in what was otherwise a somewhat lonely existence.

Maintaining our friendships with people who don't have children may mean taking the initiative.

Before we had a baby, we used to go to dinner a lot with some friends. For a couple of months after the baby they went on calling us on the spur of the moment. We couldn't get organized fast enough to find a sitter and go. They stopped calling. I missed them, so I called up and asked them to our house. Of course, the baby cried on and off, and they were put off. I could see what was happening, so I just said, "This isn't working. How about you call us way in advance, we'll be able to plan, and we can go."

There are other ways of avoiding isolation. Small babies are *very* portable, especially if you have a baby carrier (a frontpack or backpack) or stroller. As long as they are fed and changed regularly, babies make surprisingly good companions for almost any outing.

*After a week, I was going crazy being alone at home with the baby. So I borrowed a baby carrier and just took her everyplace with me. I learned how to nurse in public without being obtrusive and discovered she would sleep anywhere—in the carrier, on the floor of a friend's house, in a shopping cart, even in res-*taurants and movie theaters. Being mobile made me feel less confined and kept me in touch with the world.

Feelings During Postpartum

Once the full impact of living with a baby hits us, we may feel pride, elation, love, attachment, warmth—but many internal and conflicting feelings, thoughts and fears may also surface: I am supposed to be fulfilled because now I am a mother, but I feel ambivalent; I have to go back to work and fear losing touch with my baby; I have to be around all the time just to meet my baby's needs, so I don't have time for my other interests; I've lost my independence; I feel scared and inadequate—I need mothering myself.

After the baby was born, she became the focus of everyone's attention, and I was reduced to the role of caretaker. People would come up and say, "What a lovely baby," and never even look me in the eye. I was proud of my baby, but I felt a nonperson myself. I wanted to say, "I'm the one who cleans up the messes and gets up at night. Pay attention to me, too!"

We may feel angry at ourselves, our partner or our babies when we are particularly exhausted or isolated, or when we are not the perfect mothers we expected to be. Anger does not fit in with our fantasies about motherhood. Neither does grief, frustration, panic, jealousy. But they happen. Acknowledgment is the first step in dealing with our feelings.

I am a psychiatric nurse and therefore was aware of how angry thoughts about a baby postpartum are a normal part of the adjustment process. But I was unprepared for the enormous amount of anger I felt. I was angry about everything, it seemed. First, we had so carefully planned the conception (scientifically) of a baby girl, and I gave birth to a boy; then my sister-in-law, who had given birth six weeks before me, used the name I had reserved for my child for her baby. Then I realized how much my son resembled my father, who thirty years ago had rejected me. I also heavily identified with my oldest child about his displacement as kingpin. When I attempted to share child care with my husband, who worked at home, I found myself at the mercy of two schedules, the baby's and his. It wasn't until six months later that I knew that my anger was dissipating. It was a full two years before I felt myself again. During this time I had obsessive fantasies about hurting the baby, how fragile he was, how easily I could drop him, how maybe I would forget him and leave the house, et cetera. I hated myself for such thoughts, but they persisted. It wasn't until I finally accepted the fact that a "nice woman like me" could have such anger that the fantasies abated.

Postpartum Depression

The six or eight months after Peter was born were hard. My physical energy started to return when he slept through the night and more when he stopped needing a ten P.M. feeding. But my mental and emotional energy seemed to have disappeared for good. It was all I could do to get through a day. I took long naps and cried often. I got jealous about women my husband saw at work. I was out of touch about the me who had been an interesting, active and humorous person. Love him as I did, in some moods I resented Peter for even existing. To most people I pretended to be a "happy, young mother," but I was quite depressed. I didn't know about postpartum depression, so I blamed what I was feeling on my own failure to be a good mother. I think I also blamed my husband, as though he could have made me feel better. He was worried about his job and resentful that I was too low to give him any comfort. He accused me of having a child and now "not wanting one." (He didn't know about postpartum depression either.)

A lot of things contributed to my feeling better. I began admitting to friends how bad I was feeling; I began a cooperative playgroup with four other mothers. Most important, I went to a women's health group and learned that many women are depressed for several months after childbirth. All of a sudden I knew it wasn't my fault. I wasn't a bad person for what I was feeling.

In modern technological societies, most mothers experience periods (not just moments) of fear and depression. Almost a third suffer recurring depression. Up to two women out of each thousand experience depression that is deep and disabling enough to require hospitalization. Clearly we need information about postpartum depression in order to act to prevent it, to identify it, to cope with it in ways that will reduce its lasting effects.

Types of Postpartum Disorder

1. *The baby blues.* See page 475.
2. *Mild depression.* In this form of depression, bouts of feeling unable, lonely, guilty or frightened reappear and may make it difficult to eat, sleep, make love, work. The feelings may be provoked by a specific incident, such as your baby crying all night or a talk with a childless friend who seems so much more energetic and interesting. Depression may descend when you are run-down or under pressure (when you have guests or a job interview). Periods of depression last up to several

days or a week. However, rest, time away from the house and child care or talking with someone who knows what it is like to care for an infant can break through the depression (see Preventing and/or Coping with Depression).

3. *Postpartum psychosis.* If, in addition to the baby blues, you also are having extreme highs and/or lows of mood or are agitated, see and/or hear things that others don't, are confused, have odd or strange thoughts or fears or impulses to harm or even kill yourself and/or your baby or feel you are being "ordered" to do things you normally would not, you deserve to get help from an experienced practitioner right away. This rare condition is thought to be connected in some way to the massive hormonal changes that occur after childbirth, although no one yet knows why some mothers are more vulnerable to these changes than others. You may have periods of relative calm and clarity in your thinking, but the difficulties of postpartum psychosis often return suddenly after such periods, so be sure you get help.

4. *Postpartum panic disorder.* If you develop a panic disorder, you may feel as if an inner alarm system had been turned on; you will have sudden, extremely high anxiety and physical symptoms such as rapid heartbeat, sweaty palms or difficulty breathing. These attacks are extremely unpleasant. Because there are various treatments for panic disorders, you may want to discuss alternatives with your practitioner.

5. *Chronic or severe depression.* If you suffer a serious postpartum depression, the bouts of anxiety and helplessness are frequent and last over weeks, even months. Under these circumstances, activities as basic as cooking, dressing and caring for your child seem impossible. This kind of depression is disabling—women suffering from it cannot get out of bed or out of their homes. If you (or a woman you know) are suffering these feelings, it is very important to seek outside help from someone whom you trust—a family practitioner, a therapist, a spiritual healer.

What Causes Postpartum Depression?

Forty years ago most people believed that women who suffered more than the baby blues were mentally ill or unconsciously rejecting the normal responsibilities of motherhood. In fact, two different types of stress may be at the root of postpartum depression.[9]

Physical-stress theories say that the dramatic reduction in estrogen and progesterone in the postpartum period triggers depression.[10] They suggest that postpartum depression is similar to premenstrual depression and note that some women are more sensitive than others to these hormonal swings. The hormonal changes of the postbirth period are also apparently similar to what occurs when people are in other high-stress situations, such as combat.

Although these biochemical theories do shift the blame from the individual woman, their major drawback is the implication that postpartum depression can be completely cured chemically with the help of mood-altering drugs. (For risks of these drugs, see Chapter 3.) These drugs may treat the *symptoms* of depression temporarily and make a depressed woman feel better able to face the routines of child care, but they do not cure depressions that are caused or aggravated by nonchemical factors such as isolation, poverty or stress.

Other studies demonstrate that a woman's life situation can make her vulnerable to postpartum depression. In Ann Oakley's studies of postpartum mothers living in London, 98 of the 102 women interviewed experienced recurrent depression. Oakley pointed to the conditions that influence postpartum depression: (1) the amount a woman's partner participates in the process of having and caring for the child, (2) how realistic her picture of motherhood is, (3) whether she has and can hang on to interests outside of child care, (4) how much she can call on a network of friends and relations for help and advice, (5) whether she lives in housing that cuts her off from other adults and (6) whether she had little control over what happened during pregnancy and birth (see p. 465). Oakley's work confirms the findings of American research during the 1960s.[11] Apparently, whenever motherhood brings isolation and a loss of control, many of us get depressed.

New motherhood can bring a variety of losses, which we may mourn through depression. For more, see below, Losses in New Motherhood and Treatment for Postpartum Disorders.

Who Is Most Likely to Suffer from Depression?

Some women are only briefly depressed following a birth, but a few end up in hospitals. Why are some of us so much more vulnerable than others? There are a number of factors that predict who will be hardest hit by postpartum depression. You are more likely to be depressed (1) if you are having your first baby or you have been through the postpartum-depression experience before; (2) if moving and changes of lifestyle have created either geographic or emotional gaps between you and your family; (3) if your own family history includes the death of either of your parents when you were young, memories of desertion, sexual abuse, physical abuse or traumatic divorce that make you anxious about becoming a parent. Other factors affecting depression are (4) your own physical health; (5) your own mental health (it helps to have a history of being able to handle stress or knowing others who can) and (6) your partner's willingness to share the plea-

sures and responsibilities of child care.

One study found that 60 percent of women with a number of the situations described above developed mild or chronic depression.[12] If your history and circumstances put you at risk, you can act before your baby is born to make yourself less vulnerable. Reach out to friends or relatives who care about you. Lay the groundwork for sharing parenthood with your partner.

Preventing and/or Coping with Depression

Mothers who have been through postpartum depression themselves make the following suggestions:

- Find out if the hospital, birthing center, a nearby women's center, La Leche League or a church sponsors a discussion group for new parents. Try it. If it helps, make long-term child-care plans so that you can go on attending.
- Talk with a friend about what troubles you.
- Take time for yourself *each day*.
- Don't feel guilty about your feelings: They are not a sign of your inadequacy as a mother or as a partner.
- Go outdoors, with or without the baby, anytime the weather permits. Make an effort to talk with other adults you meet—parents with children, the mail carrier, neighbors.
- Whatever your share of the household tasks, do a little each day so that it does not defeat you by piling up. Better yet, do it with a friend, one day at her/his house, another day at yours.
- Locate another adult who can give you the "long view," someone who has raised children and who can tell you what it was like, what was hard, what made a difference. Houses and apartments everywhere are full of women who know a great deal about surviving and enjoying motherhood. They rarely talk about it because they think no one has any use for what they have learned.
- Take care of yourself. Find some kind of exercise you enjoy and do it as regularly as you can. Eat as nutritiously as possible. Pay attention to pleasure. Wear something you like in the middle of the day. At the store, buy one food you love to eat. Try learning something new.

If your mood still does not change, you may need outside help. Signs that indicate you need help:

- You have lost interest in doing anything on your own behalf or feel the baby would be better off without you.
- You have become dependent on alcohol or drugs.
- You have attempted suicide or fear that you will.
- You have abused your child/children.
- You and your partner have serious, constant difficulties coping with the changes brought by parenthood; these difficulties include long, in-

sulting arguments, physical abuse, affairs that threaten your ability to stay together, desertion.

- As a single person, you find yourself so desperate for affection that you become involved in a series of brief relationships that drain your energy and self-esteem without providing the affection or comfort you hoped for.

If you seek outside help, it is essential to find a counselor or therapist willing to look outside as well as within you to find the cause of your depression, one who won't simply prescribe drugs and send you away. In a culture like our own, which tends to devalue people who spend time caring for others, you may have to search for someone who will take your depression seriously. You also want a person who will help you learn to be assertive and constructive about making the changes in your life that may protect you from later depression. Do not hesitate to ask other women if they can recommend anyone. Ask for recommendations through parent groups, women's centers, a nurse practitioner or pediatrician you like. After getting this kind of private help, your first-hand knowledge of postpartum feelings can enable you to reach out to other mothers as an individual or as a part of community action (see p. 495).

Losses in New Motherhood That May Contribute to Postpartum Depression

If your baby was premature or ill, had to remain in the hospital after you were discharged or has ongoing health problems, depression may be a part of the process of your grieving. Allowing yourself to mourn the image of a robust newborn may be helpful. Social structures tend to reward new mothers for being strong and "in control," when open expression of pain, disappointment and sadness might, at times, be more helpful. Whether or not your baby has been ill, it may be helpful to allow yourself to mourn past losses that come to mind, such as past pregnancy losses through miscarriage or abortion or loss of your parents or loved ones. Also allow yourself to mourn losses associated with becoming a mother, such as loss of freedom and autonomy and loss of your pregnant state. If the birth itself did not measure up to your expectations, you may be grieving that loss as well. In the United States, most women giving birth are anesthetized, cut (either for cesarean section or episiotomy) or both. This is not the case in all parts of the world. Even in some other Western industrialized countries—those where midwives have a strong presence—rates of cesareans and episiotomies are far lower, and the results better, than ours. Many commentators feel that experiencing these interventions makes women vulnerable to depression following childbirth. As your baby grows, becomes more interested in others and in toys, becomes mobile and weans, you may also grieve the loss of the closeness you had with the baby as a newborn.

Examine your schedule and decide whether your expectations of yourself are realistic, given that you are going through major physical, psychological and social changes. Take care of your need for regular exercise. Cut down on unnecessary activities. Consult a nutritionist or read materials from La Leche League to be sure you are drinking and eating properly to support breastfeeding. Cut out or at least down on caffeine, alcohol and refined sugars. Be sure you are getting the nutrients you need, every day. If, after taking these steps, you find you are continuing to have difficulties, or that they are getting worse, an experienced practitioner may be needed.

Treatment for Postpartum Disorders

Baby blues requires no professional care; it resolves itself in a few hours or days. At the other end of the spectrum in severity, both postpartum psychosis and severe postpartum depression require immediate care from a knowledgeable and experienced practitioner. You may decide to seek help for mild or moderate depression or postpartum panic disorder as well, especially if taking care of your needs doesn't lead to improvement.

Many practitioners believe that medication and hospitalization are necessary in the treatment of postpartum psychosis and severe postpartum depression. This is due to the fact that, in these rare situations, there is risk to the well-being and even survival of mother and baby. Unfortunately, temporary weaning and separation of mother from baby are necessitated by these treatments, because there are currently few, if any, units in the United States that accept mothers and babies together. (This kind of unit has proved successful in England, but lack of awareness and sensitivity to the needs of mothers and babies have lead U.S. hospitals to allow cost and liability factors to dictate the types of care offered. Mutual support groups and women's groups should lobby hospitals to establish such units.) We can negotiate frequent, regular visits with our babies, with assistance and oversight by caregivers, during the short time when hospitalization is needed. Some very innovative, determined, energetic families, with considerable community support, may be able to arrange alternative forms of care for individual mothers. This should not be undertaken lightly, however. Ongoing therapy, monitoring and consultation by experienced and knowledgeable caregivers must be a necessary part of such an alternative plan.

Medication may also be recommended for moderate postpartum depression and panic disorder. Some medications do require weaning. Be sure to

Suzanne Arms

We are surviving. Just. Why don't they give Croix de Guerres to people who can go without more than two hours total daily sleep for five weeks? I thought babies ate at six-ten-two-six-ten-two—mine does. He also eats at five-seven-nine-eleven and four-eight-twelve. I am getting rather used to going around with my breasts hanging out. They are either drying from the last feed or getting ready for the next one. But the love—I never knew, never imagined that I would love him like this. This incredible feeling of boundless, endless love—a wish to protect his innocence from ever being hurt or wounded or scratched. And that awful, horrible, mad feeling in the first week that you'll never be able to keep anything so precious and so vulnerable alive.

THE THIRD PHASE: LONG-TERM ISSUES

The period between six and twelve months after birth is often a time when chaos, fatigue and uncertainty ebb away and a tide of confidence and energy washes in. This is partly because our babies begin to sleep through the night, eat solid food, take predictable naps in the morning and afternoon. But this return to normal also comes from our own practicing, experimenting and learning during that first chaotic half-year.

I was getting together all the stuff I needed to take Pablo out—you know, the blanket, the diapers, the toys. I did it very smoothly, thinking all the time about the different buses we had to take. "This is it," I said to myself. "Being a mother is under my skin, in my brain, part of the way I pick things up and put them down."

No matter how much smoother daily life becomes, parenthood alters practically all of our "old" ways.

Partnership: Jealousy, Sex Roles and Intimacy

When I think back on it, adding a baby was like sending our relationship through a wringer and planting a garden smack in its middle—both at once.

Throughout the first year, adult caresses or conversations often lose out to a cry from the crib. Our partner becomes less a lover or a companion than "the other babysitter." Earlier in this chapter, we talked about practical issues in sexuality and child care that come up during the first months. Some deeper or more complicated issues arise as the people in a couple relationship undergo a gradual shift to parenthood. This is not an easy transition. First, whether we have children at eighteen or thirty-eight, we have to balance being a parent with all the other concerns of our

talk it over with your practitioner if continuing to breastfeed is important to you. Perhaps dosages or choice of medication may be arranged to allow you to continue. Or perhaps you and your practitioner can collaborate on a plan that does not require medication. If you and your practitioner decide that the best treatment for you includes medication that necessitates weaning, you may wish to relactate and resume breastfeeding when your need for medication has passed. Discuss this with your caregiver and get help from La Leche League.

Competent practitioners will discuss their recommendations carefully, and be sure you have some part in the decision-making process. If a practitioner doesn't seem to be willing to take your preferences and wishes into account, you can state that you wish to consider other alternatives. This may be hard to do when you are experiencing significant confusion or depression. Partners, friends or family may help in this process. If the care offered by one practitioner doesn't seem adequate, there are the options of obtaining a second opinion or switching to a different practitioner.

Celebrating the Pleasures

I had heard about the negatives—the fatigue, the loneliness, loss of self. But nobody told me about the wonderful parts: holding my baby close to me, seeing her first smile, watching her grow and become more responsive day by day. How can I describe the way I felt when she stroked my breast while nursing or looked into my eyes or arched her eyebrows like an opera singer? This was the deepest connection I'd felt to anybody. Sometimes the intensity almost frightened me. For the first time I cared about somebody else more than myself, and I would do anything to nurture and protect her.

lives, whether it's finishing high school, finding work or caring for our own parents.

For both lesbian and heterosexual couples, one of the most difficult issues is jealousy, or competition for affection. Often there just isn't enough energy, time and affection for everyone.

When I nursed at night, the sight of me holding my full breast to this sleepy little baby used to drive Les nuts. When I'd get back into bed, he'd be wild to make love, fast and hard. It got to be quite a thing because I'd come back to bed feeling mild and sleepy. Les wanted to screw and I wanted to snuggle. We fought over it a lot until we realized we had to make time for some sex that was hard and fast and some that was cozy. A couple of months past the worst of it, we began to joke about "hard" and "soft" sex.

Second, we become parents in a culture that is riddled with strong, even irrational beliefs about men's and women's roles in child rearing. The belief that mothers do their part by caring for children while fathers do theirs by contributing income affects our own behavior and shapes the social institutions all around us.* It requires hard work and self-awareness for men and women in heterosexual couples to stay friends and lovers as they become parents.[13]

Parents who adopt conventional sex roles may be jealous when each of their daily lives contains completely different people, routines, tasks and rewards.

There I was at home, by choice and liking it, except for this. Every day there were hundreds of small things—great ones like the baby rolling over or playing while I worked. Terrible ones like him choking or falling out of the infant seat. All these things were big to me. But when Marty came home, he'd listen for a minute, then start winding his watch or sorting the mail. I got to feeling like a housekeeper and he seemed more and more to be the invited guest.

It's one of those "grass-is-greener" things—I envied, sometimes even hated Sam when he went out to work. I don't know what I was imagining—that he hung around talking, went out to lunch, did interesting things. One time he was watching me bathe Annie in the sink. He asked if he could do it—he stood there, soaping her back over and over like he couldn't get enough of it, and he talked about how he hated to leave us in the morning and how he

Mary rests while Joseph cares for baby.   Book of Hours
(French, 15th century), Walters Art Gallery, Baltimore, MD

worried he would be closed out, left looking in at what she and I had together.

TO MY HUSBAND
*I mothered you,
then weaned you,
so we could parent
together.
Children grow so tellingly.
And who will dare
share this startling
gut
tenderness
when my son (soon)
moves on beyond where I
can pull him on my lap
and smell his hair;
I've lost the smell of your
grown-up hair.
Will this parenting lose us
each other?*

We have to find ways of breaking through the barriers set up by jealousy, emotional fatigue and sex-role isolation. Many of us have found that our most powerful solution is to share the responsi-

---

*The process of becoming parents can bring out traditional sex-role behavior. In early motherhood, women tend to act more passive, to become more emotionally expressive and more responsive to the needs of others. In becoming fathers, some men feel they should assert their authority, control their emotions and act rationally.

bilities of parenthood more equally. To share parenthood, both partners have to contribute time, work and caring. In some arrangements, the adults split days at home fifty–fifty. In other situations, the one parent who does the most daily parenting asks her or his partner for limited but important commitments of time and interest that go beyond occasional "babysitting."

When Laurie was born I was bound and determined to do it all—be a full-time mother, a full-time, perfect housekeeper. I spent that first year rushing like a madwoman from one duty to the next. I ended up feeling either like the good mother and the wicked wife or the wicked mother and the perfect wife. When I had Peter, my second, I said, "Hey, these kids are ending up with a six-thirty sweetheart, not a father, and I'm tired and lonely. There are two parents here; why am I in this alone?" When I asked Mike to help, he started taking Thursday afternoons off—out of back-vacation time. I still had the kids most of the time, but the idea that he would do that made a big difference between us.

Realistically, not all partners can take time off. In that case, the one who is away most can do whatever *is* possible: bathe the baby in the evening, put the baby to bed, make dinner.*

Postpartum: The Second Time Around

For many of us, postpartum is a very different experience the second time around. Some aspects are much easier; having been through it all before, we know what to expect and are comfortable with many of the practical and emotional issues of child care and parenthood. At the same time, incorporating a second child into our existing family can be difficult and stressful, especially if our children are closely spaced and/or we lack a partner, family or friends to turn to for support and help.

I started having children in my late thirties so I wanted them close together. My second child was born seventeen months after the first. In some ways I enjoyed the whole experience more. As a second-time mother I was more relaxed and less anxious about every little thing, and my second baby was more easygoing than my first. But that first year was also very hard. I was exhausted just trying to take care of two babies in diapers. In addition, my oldest child was jealous and needed a lot of extra attention which I couldn't always give. Having two babies on different feeding and nap schedules made life chaotic

at times. I was much less mobile with two babies. Going to the grocery store could take all morning. What I found the hardest was having no time to myself. Someone always was wanting something. Unfortunately, my husband was not much help—his job required a lot of traveling and he was gone at least half of the time.

Now—a year and a half later—things are much easier. The kids go to family day care three days a week and I've been able to go back to work part-time and resume some of the interests and friendships that I had given up. I finally feel like my life, which was out of whack for so long, is beginning to have a rhythm again. I feel like a survivor. I'm proud of my kids and myself for having made it through.

THE HEALTH AND WELL-BEING OF MOTHERS

There are plenty of manuals on health care for infants. But almost nowhere is there a discussion of the health problems women encounter because they are mothers.

The Stress That Comes of Being a Mother

Caring for infants and young children is rewarding but *hard* work. If you have a child between one and three, you are doing something for or with that child about every five minutes, for as long as she or he is awake. While studies of stress have tended to ignore women at home with young children, research on factory workers shows that the result of routine work is fatigue, loss of concentration and appetite and eventual loss of self-esteem. In M. Howell's studies of child-care workers, she found that *six hours* marked the limit of an adult's patience and endurance when working closely with young children.[14] To avoid being worn down, we have to find ways of providing breaks, "recesses," even vacations. This is especially true for those of us who are on our own whether by choice, through separation from a partner or because our partners are uninvolved;* it is vital that women at home organize to provide breaks for each other through trading child-care hours, playgroups or sharing the cost of hiring a sitter.

Mothers experience a second type of stress. Everything from myths to current research has made us believe that a woman must always put her family's needs before her own.

---

*For a more detailed discussion of the issues and "how-tos" of shared parenting, see Chapter 6 of *Ourselves and Our Children* by the Boston Women's Health Book Collective (New York: Random House, 1978).

---

*Many married women who are entirely responsible for the daily care of children live lives similar to those of single women, though they may have more money. Women who have distant or uninvolved partners may benefit from talking to single mothers about how they cope.

Getting ready to leave in the morning is a good example. It doesn't only mean me getting breakfast. It means being sure that each of the kids has what they need: the oldest one needs lunch money, the middle one needs boxes for art class, the baby needs eardrops and the right blanket for day care. But it also means to me that everybody should go away feeling loved and safe and ready. If one of them cries, I get to work feeling sad and like I messed up.

Researchers have repeatedly found that almost twice as many women as men suffer recurrent or serious depression. Until recently this fact has been hard to explain, because men have been thought of as suffering higher levels of stress. Currently, we are coming to see that what men suffer are periods of high stress (e.g., job pressures, illness). What women, and especially mothers, experience is *chronic stress*, the continuing feeling that we must respond to what others ask of us, that we should, but rarely do, meet everyone's needs. All this may help make us vulnerable to depression during the postpartum months and throughout our years as mothers.

I have this dream that keeps coming back, since just a couple of months after my second baby was born. In it, I am caught in a wall, so that I am part of what is keeping the room from falling in on itself. In the room there are a a lot of people—mostly family—eating and drinking. I want to come out, but they can't or don't hear me. I want to leave the wall, but I am caught and it seems like I am invisible to them.

For as long as we nominate ourselves as what one mother called the "universal shock absorber," we are bound to fall short. We have to give some of the responsibility to others, whether through shared parenthood, community living or asking older children to pitch in.*

Who Cares for the Caregiver?

It usually feels right to be completely absorbed by a newborn baby. Once routines and basic skills are (more or less) in hand, however, it is essential to balance this preoccupation with an interest in caring for ourselves.

One day when I was leaning over to put Ben in the crib, I realized I had no idea what clothes I had on.

I stayed there with my eyes half closed, not looking, trying to figure it out. I couldn't. I tried to remember brushing my teeth and I couldn't. I knew what shoes I had on, only because I only wore one pair ever.

Research on maternal health is beginning to show that we look after the physical and mental health of our children but skimp on our own well-being.* We insist that our children sit down and eat a nutritious meal while we eat leftovers. We send children out to play, to get exercise, sunlight and fresh air, while we stay inside and clean the living room. After the stitches heal, past the six-week postpartum checkup, medical programs usually ignore maternal health in favor of children's.

We may well spend fifty additional years—or more—in the bodies that gave us the children we so carefully watch over. We have to stand back from the ideals of self-sacrifice and monitor our own health just as we do our children's: tooth for tooth, vitamin for vitamin.

Part of the difficulty lies with the medical system. The dollar and hour costs are high for young families. Moreover, the practice of separating pediatric from adult care means that one bus or car ride and waiting period accomplishes only individual, not family, care. We need medical facilities with practitioners for adults and children, lab facilities under the same roof, nutrition and mental-health workers available, staffed playrooms so that mothers can take their time during their appointments.

Modern Theories of Attachment: What Is the Cost to Mothers?

Anytime we leave our babies and feel a guilty, sinking sensation, we are responding to a cultural myth that states that any mother who loves her child would never leave that child if she had a choice. There is *no* question that children need the love and care adults can offer. Yet current beliefs about "the child's tie to his [sic] mother" cause many women to spend their child-rearing years leading lives that are narrower and guiltier than is healthy for any active adult.

Between 1930 and 1950 scientists observed how traumatic it was for infant monkeys to be reared without their mothers. Researchers began to ask the same sort of question about human infants and mothers: in the "natural laboratories" provided

---

*For a detailed discussion of the sources and effects of stress in low-income women, see *Families and Stress*, D. Belle, ed. (New York: Russell Sage Foundation, 1982). Women of all income levels can learn a great deal from this book about how the ongoing responsibilities of child care may affect their well-being.

*Studies by John Eckenrode and his colleagues at the Harvard School of Public Health indicate that mothers do sacrifice their health care in favor of seeing that children are taken care of. It appears that in the days following stressful situations, children make more visits to clinics but mothers' visits drop off.

Jim Harrison/Stock Boston

that challenge our options, we find the following:

1. The original research was done in very severe circumstances. Sharing care with a partner, a sitter or relative is simply not the same as wartime or hospital separation.

2. In many cultures older children, aunts, even grandfathers assume major caregiving roles. Children are not harmed by being lovingly cared for by more than one person or by a person who is not the mother. Many families in this culture provide loving environments for children while single mothers go about the business of working and living.

3. When it has mattered economically or strategically, white middle-class families, as well as the federal government, thought it fine for women to be separated from young children. When women joined the work force during World War II, the government built large day-care centers where children could even eat supper with their mothers, then spend the night.[16]

In light of these facts, if we can make decent child-care arrangements, we won't go to work, a night course or an exercise class feeling as if we had "abandoned" a child. When our children have problems, we will not automatically think, Oh, if only I had stayed at home.

Being Workers and Mothers

The real personal decisions and compromises involved in going to work while you have a baby at home are enough for any woman. Sometimes the baby is sick, some days she cries when you leave, other times you love her to bits. But the tangle of guilts and shouldn'ts and dangers that have come to surround making that decision has just got to be cut away.

For many of us the prospect of working when we have very young children is complicated both practically and emotionally. We have to find child care and juggle the double demands of home and workplace. We love and miss our children; we are afraid of being replaced in their affections; we want to know that other caregivers will care deeply, too.

These kinds of anxieties and questions are normal signs of caring. *However, the deep doubts and guilt that many of us feel in making and carrying out the decision to work are not a necessary part of being a working mother.* These doubts are our response to being raised as females in a culture that insists that nurturing, and especially child care, is "women's work." Since nearly 60 percent of women with children under school age are in the work force,[17] it is time to question the equation between motherhood and constant child care.

by World War II and hospitalizations, they observed children's mourning and depression when separated from their parents.[15] They reasoned that the fuss an eight- or nine-month-old makes when approached by strangers signals the appearance of a very special tie to a particular human caregiver, the mother. In the end, what emerged was a theory of attachment, which says that between six and nine months of age children become deeply attached to their mothers. After that time any prolonged or regular separation from the mother causes feelings of desertion that affect a child's ability to form relationships in later life.*

Pediatricians and conservative political groups have used these ideas to argue against mothers working outside the home, publicly funded day care, part-time jobs or schooling that would open up alternatives to women with young children. But when we look closely at these arguments

---

*Some positive results from this work should not be ignored. This research has convinced hospitals to let parents stay with sick children and prompted orphanages to seek adoption for children as early as possible.

CHILD CARE

For many of us the thought of child care brings up images of too many children in a crowded, messy room looked after by overworked, poorly paid women. Reliable, affordable, high-quality child care is hard to find.

There is a big difference between what child care in this country could be and what it has been forced to become because it lacks social support. The federal government has consistently refused to plan for or provide significant financial support to a national child-care program, giving as a major reason the desire to keep families "intact" and provide for the emotional needs of young children. The net result has been that, for the most part, it has been impossible to build the thoughtfully designed, well-equipped, well-staffed child-care centers that we need. Many centers become shoestring operations in living rooms, basements and YMCAs. Wages of about $11,500 a year for full-time work make it difficult to build a group of committed, experienced, skilled child-care workers.

Based on these circumstances, many of us fear that group child care will hurt our children, that they may be ignored, unloved, bored. Our fears trap us: "If I can't afford a private sitter, then I belong at home." Some women can afford this choice. Others must go on welfare, borrow money, become dependent on support payments. Yet dropping out of the job market for several years can have both economic and personal costs (loss of seniority, benefits, personal identity). In order to make our decisions, we have to shake off some myths about child care.

Myths About Child Care

- *Child care means institutional day care.* If you decide to work, you have some choices about the kinds of alternative-care arrangements to make. Depending on income and circumstances, you can call upon extended family, trade hours with other parents, form playgroups and parent cooperatives, use private or publicly funded day care.*
- *Group care for a young child can be harmful.* The experiences of other countries like China, Sweden and Israel demonstrate that children raised

Elizabeth Crews/Stock Boston

in group care situations grow into normal adults. Studies done in the United States clearly show that children who experience group care, even from infancy, are just as affectionate, bright and emotionally healthy as children who have been raised totally at home. In fact, children who spend time in day care may be more creative and indepedent than children who stay home.[18]
- *It is selfish for a woman to "sacrifice" her child so that she can work.* Contrary to the arguments of the political right, increasing numbers of us are not "choosing" to work. We are doing what we must to keep our families financially afloat. Only 29 percent of married women have partners with an income over $15,000 annually, while it costs about $27,000 a year to support a four-person family. Additionally, half of us—one out of every two women—will be separated from a partner while we still have the responsibility for child support.* Single women and lesbian couples have to face the fact that women earn only seventy-one cents where men would earn one dollar. Most women who have children on their own have no choice but to work or receive welfare.
- *Children are the losers when mothers work.* A great deal of child development research states that mothers who play with and talk to their babies have children who speak earlier, are more imaginative, seem brighter. This research makes us believe that we always ought to be on hand. It does matter that children's environments are interesting and that people care enough to help them practice skills, play, experiment. But that

---

*Because we do not have the space to discuss the advantages and disadvantages of the different types of day care here, we suggest that you talk with other parents about their experiences and/or consult one of the following resources: *Ourselves and Our Children* by the Boston Women's Health Book Collective (New York: Random House, 1978); *Family Day Care* by Alice Collins and Eunice Watson (Boston: Beacon Press, 1976); *The Penguin Book of Playgroups* by Joyce Lucas and Vivienne McKennell (New York: Penguin, 1974).

---

*Even though fathers are often legally responsible for contributing to child support, only 37.4 percent of mothers receive payments and only 68.3 percent of these receive the agreed-upon amount. (See "Child Support and Alimony: 1989," Bureau of the Census, No. 112, Series P60, No. 173.)

responsiveness can come from many different kinds of people. *Other* caregivers can give them experiences that we could never offer. For example, children who have additional caretakers learn to turn to other adults, to get along with other children (if they are being cared for in group situations), to understand more fully the many roles women take on. Instead of asking, What do children lose when mothers work? we must ask, What are the costs—to children, women and society—when women who want and need to work stay at home "for the sake of the children"?

Finding and Using Child Care

All mothers need to find child care sooner or later, whether it is for an afternoon off or for daily eight-to-six care. Here are some brief suggestions that may make this task more manageable. (See Resources for books and other material that can be of further help.)

Planning Ahead

To get a head start on child care, try to think during pregnancy what your child-care needs are most likely to be during the first year: Will you be looking for occasional babysitting, part-time care, full-time care? If you work, find out what your employer provides in terms of maternity leave. Talk with your employer about your plans for returning to work. Find out from your employer or other workers about maternity leave (will it cost you seniority, vacation days, benefits?), taking sick days when your baby is sick, exemptions for working parents (some factories will give parents preference among shifts).

Talk with other people you know who have babies. Ask them what their child-care needs were, how they met them, how they found good sitters, day-care centers or other forms of child care. Visit home child-care facilities: an infant day-care center; a local babysitter; a family day-care home. Talk to several people's favorite babysitters to find out what makes caring for someone else's child pleasant or difficult. These visits and conversations will give you a feel for the kind of child care you'll want to use.

Child-care arrangements will help, but they are not a substitute for working out the sharing of care with your partner, another family or friends. When children are sick, when your usual arrangements fall through, at night, on vacations, in emergencies, you will need people to help out.

When to Start Day Care and How Often to Use It

Some experienced parents suggest that you stay at home with your new baby for at least three or four months if you can. This will let you get back on your feet and permit you to get to know your infant (babies begin to be much more responsive to faces, voices, games about that time). If you can afford it, use child care at least occasionally before your baby is eight or nine months old, the age at which many infants become very frightened of strangers. Approach the task of finding child care with the understanding that children of different ages require different kinds of care. The quiet, calm care that was perfect for the first four months may be boring and frustrating for a child who is learning to walk.

There is the possibility of too much child care. Five days a week from seven A.M. to six P.M. is a long time for anyone to be away from home. We believe that children need private time with people they know and love. Part of planning child care is providing time for parent and child to be together. If your schedule demands you find care for such extended periods, plan times in the morning and evening when you can focus your attention and affection on your child. Alternatively, consider if a family member or friend can pick up your child early on some days.

Finding Quality Child Care

What each of us wants from child care varies, but there are some basics:

- Caregivers must be responsive to children, even when children are tired or cranky. They must care enough to notice when children are unhappy, sick or needing new activities. Children are growing human beings and need more than just watching.
- The physical space should not be overcrowded, dirty or chaotic. It should include areas for resting, quiet play, active play.
- The experience should have variety: indoor and outdoor time; rest periods and playtimes. Even small babies need this kind of variety to counteract monotony.
- Other children involved should be healthy, free of infectious diseases or behavior disorders that the caregiver or the other children cannot handle.
- You should be able to find out what goes on during child-care hours, should be free to observe and to talk with caregivers about things that concern you and them.
- The environment should be safe: no detergents within reach, no open doors to the street, no stairways without protective gates.

Beyond these basics, choosing child care is a matter of what you feel comfortable with, can find, can afford. But whatever situation you choose, you must trust the caregiver.

As much as you want the child care you choose to be perfect and trouble-free, it is a human arrangement and requires attention, planning, looking after. Get to know the person(s) taking care of your child. Tell her/him what you know about your child. Ask them what they notice. If you have a feeling that something is not right, look into it. Talk to the caregiver(s), observe, ask other parents. If you are still concerned that the care is less than what you want, get together with other parents to try and change the situation or find something else if you can. Try not to communicate your doubts to your child. Unless you have no choice, don't go for a stopgap situation just "to tide you over." Multiple changes are hard on children and on parents.

Returning to Work

Most of us make plans for returning to work while we are still pregnant. After a baby is born, we may feel different about work than we expected. Some of us won't be ready or interested in returning to work after the usual eight- to ten-week maternity leave; others may be restless long before our scheduled time at home is up.

I went back to work six weeks after my daughter was born. I remember the midwife saying to me, "You have your whole life to work; your baby will only be little for a short time. Why don't you just enjoy your stay at home with her for a while?" She even suggested talking with my employer, but I was afraid of losing my job. I think now that I was overaccommodating. I wish I had waited longer before going back. Every morning when we are struggling to get out of the house by eight, I think, Wouldn't it be wonderful to be able to stay home with my baby today? I really missed something by not waiting at least a few more weeks.

Designing Work Options

Given the limits of the job market, women have been inventive when faced with the demands of wage earning and child care. Some women have found jobs to do at home: computer programming, editing, catering, family day care, illustrating, typing. Some have also learned to use existing work structures, such as factory shifts, so that they can share child care with a partner. In some cases, women have found, created, talked employers into part-time jobs that permit them to keep a foot "in both worlds." Women have also helped in the design of newer options: *flex-time*, an arrangement that permits workers to come in quite early in the morning or much later in the day, as long as they work their assigned number of hours, and *job-sharing*, which occurs when two people, both interested in part-time employment, share a single position.[19]

Though all working mothers need these options, few of us currently have them. To get them and to help make them available to other mothers, we have to pursue them everywhere—in union elections, in new contracts, by lobbying the benefits office at corporations where we work and by personally requesting them from supervisors and employers.

INVENTING A DIFFERENT KIND OF MOTHERHOOD

There is nothing quite like the first year of being a mother to wake up to what it's like to be stuffed into a role or a way of being that's too small. Inside your head you know that you are different, bigger, stronger, wiser. On the outside, people look at you like you're another one of those stroller-pushers.

Having female reproductive organs need not and should not determine how we spend what could be some of the fullest years of our lives. To open up the possibility of combining motherhood and selfhood, nurturance and sexuality, working and child rearing, we need these changes in society:[20]

1. Timely help for pregnant women who do not have a working system of human support; who have been laid off from work; whose births may be problematic.

2. A new definition of prenatal classes that includes discussion of events past the birth, helping couples to think ahead to the role of divisions and separations that may occur postpartum or by helping single mothers to plan for child care.

3. Postpartum health care that includes the mother's (and father's) health as well as that of the baby. Women's groups coould form around postpartum issues (infant care, working, social stress, couple relations). Women should be encouraged to think about designing their days so that their own health care (exercise, sitting down to meals, rest) is a part of their routine. Local health clinics could offer group counseling, and six-week checkups for mothers would include more than routine checks of stitches, weight and so on.

4. A postpartum hotline staffed by both experienced mothers and new mothers could operate twenty-four hours a day and offer both the opportunity to obtain concrete woman-to-woman advice and suggestions about where to turn for help with more serious problems.

5. A government-subsidized service in which women would be paid to visit new mothers, teach the how-tos of baby care, discuss the difficult issues that arise in the postpartum weeks and months and help women to explore their immediate community in order to locate child care, other new mothers and other resources. At the very least, every well-baby clinic and doctor's office ought to have a bulletin board where these resources are listed.

6. Paid maternity and paternity leave for new parents, with full pay provided by all places of employment, as in Sweden and China; subsidized day care so that there are enough places for the families who want them and so that day-care workers can be paid decently and work shorter hours under the kinds of physical conditions that will permit them to be responsive and inventive caregivers.

7. Day care to be provided by *all* places of employment (as well as through at-large community centers) so that mothers can return to work if they want or need to. Employers must come to see this benefit as similar to offering health insurance and must cease arguing that it makes women more expensive to hire than men. Employment-based centers should encourage women to nurse and parents to eat meals with their children.

8. Awareness on the part of architects and planners that families with children have special needs that can and should be met: ramps so that we can ease strollers off sidewalks, parks with enclosed areas, common spaces with open carpeted areas where babies can play—maybe beside the washers and dryers in apartment basements.

9. Changes in the work structure so that part-time work becomes more widely available and better paid; tightening of the laws regarding equal pay for comparable work so that women's contributions to family incomes can be more substantial.

10. Paid consumer and citizen involvement by women in planning, monitoring and delivery of health care and community services, especially those that are meant to touch the lives of mothers and children, such as local clinics, public hospitals and mental-health facilities, park and recreation departments, housing authorities.

To see the problem as larger than ourselves helps.

One day I thought about all the mothers in all the households: apartment buildings, one- and two-family houses, farmhouses, mobile homes, rented rooms. I thought of us at home alone with our children. I thought how if we were all to come out from inside those walls and see how many of us there were, talk about all we knew and what we needed, we would see how large the problem was and we would take action.

Beyond imagining, we have to act. Now, as in the past, we have to offer each other what we need as mothers—child care, advice, time to talk. We

Jerry Berndt/Stock Boston

also have to work together in larger, more public groups to change the institutions and attitudes that often make parenthood difficult: whether it is an advertising industry with its one-dimensional portrayals of mothers, health-care facilities that fail to offer family care, congresspersons who will not vote to fund day care, universities that deny part-time study. We also have to act from our awareness of the many threats to our children's lives. We have many examples of mothers taking courageous public stands for their children's welfare: the mothers in Chile who help other families search for missing members, the mothers who demonstrate at the Pentagon against military buildup and nuclear arms, the mothers of Viet Nam veterans who counsel parents with draft-age sons, women of color who put long hours into fighting for decent education for all children.

NOTES

1. Reva Rubin. "Puerperal Change," in Nancy A. Lytle, ed. *Maternal Health Nursing*, Dubuque, IA: William C. Brown, 1967.

2. La Leche League International. "Breastfeeding, the Best Beginning," Publication No. 150, 1981. La Leche League International. "The Womanly Art of Breastfeeding," Publication No. 315, 5th ed., 1991.

3. La Leche League International. "The Womanly Art of Breastfeeding," Publication No. 315, 5th ed., 1991.

4. "OCs Said to Be Safe for Breastfeeding Mothers," *OB/GYN NEWS* (October 15, 1981).

5. Gail Brewer. "The Pregnancy After Thirty Workbook," Emmaus, PA: Rodale Press, 1978.

6. "Herbal Remedies in Pregnancy, and during and after Birth." Pamphlets available from *Birthday*, Cambridge, MA: M. Crowe, 1980.

7. William H. Masters and Virginia E. Johnson. *Human Sexual Response*, Boston: Little Brown and Co., 1966, p. 163.

8. Sheila Kitzinger. *Women As Mothers*. New York: Random House, 1978.

9. For an excellent discussion of challenges to older theories of postpartum depression, read Ann Oakley, *Women Confined*, New York: Schocken Books, 1980.

10. For a discussion of these physical-stress or hormonal theories, see D. A. Hamburg, R. H. Moos and I. D. Yalon, "Studies of Distress in the Menstrual Cycle and the Postpartum Period," in R. P. Michael, ed., *Endocrinology and Human Behavior*, London: Oxford University Press, 1968. See also J. A. Hamilton, *Postpartum Psychiatric Illness*, St. Louis: C. V. Mosby Co., 1962, quoted in H. F. Butts, "Psychodynamic and Endocrine Factors in Postpartum Psychosis," *Journal of the National Medical Association*, Vol. 60, No. 3 (May 1968), pp. 224–27. See the chapter on postpartum depression in Maggie Scarf's *Unfinished Business: Pressure Points in the Lives of Women*, New York: Ballantine Books, 1980.

11. R. E. Gordon, E. E. Kapostins and K. K. Gordon, "Factors in Postpartum Emotional Adjustment," *Obstetrics and Gynecology*, Vol. 25, No. 2 (February 1965), pp. 158–66. V. Larsen et al., "Attitudes and Stresses Affecting Perinatal Adjustment," final report, National Institutes of Mental Health, Grant No. MH-01381–01–02.

12. R. E. Gordon et al., "Factors in Postpartum Emotional Adjustment," pp. 158–66.

13. Rhona Rapoport, Robert N. Rapoport and Z. Strelitz. *Mothers, Fathers and Society*. New York: Random House, 1980.

14. M. Howell. *Helping Ourselves: Families and the Human Network*. Boston, MA: Beacon Press, 1975.

15. This research includes Harlow's work with monkeys (H. Harlow, *Learning to Love*, New York: Ballantime Books, Inc., 1971); the work of Spitz on hospitalized children (R. Spitz and K. M. Wolff, "Anaclitic Depression," *Psychoanalytic Study of the Child*, Vol. 2 [1946], pp. 313–42); and John Bowlby's work on separation and attachment (J. Bowlby, *Attachment and Loss*, New York: Basic Books, 1969).

16. Perhaps the most striking example of this brief, all-out approach to day care for working women is the story of the Kaiser aluminum plants during World War II. See M. S. Steinfels's account in *Who's Minding the Children: The History and Politics of Day Care in America*, New York: Simon & Schuster, 1973.

17. U.S. Bureau of Census data, 1989.

18. See also Lois Hoffman and F. E. Nye, *Working Mothers*, San Francisco: Jossey-Bass, 1974; and the *New York Times* (December 13, 1981).

19. For a discussion of the work options women can invent, see Chapter 8 in Boston Women's Health Book Collective, *Ourselves and Our Children*, New York: Random House, 1978.

20. Boston Women's Health Book Collective, *Ourselves and Our Children*, Chapter 8.

RESOURCES

Motherhood

Armstrong, P., and S. Feldman. *A Wise Birth*. New York: William Morrow, 1990.

Boston Women's Health Book Collective. *Ourselves and Our Children*. New York: Random House, 1978.

Chester, L., ed. *Cradle and All*. Boston: Faber & Faber, 1989.

Freidland, R., and L. Kort, eds. *The Mothers' Book: Shared Experiences*. Boston: Houghton Mifflin, 1981.

Grossman, F. K., L. Eichler and S. Winickoff. *Pregnancy, Birth, and Parenthood*. San Francisco: Jossey-Bass, 1980.

Howell, M. *Helping Ourselves: Families and the Human Network*. Boston: Beacon Press, 1975.

Kitzinger, Sheila. *Women as Mothers*. New York: Random House, 1978.

Lazarre, J. *The Mother Knot*. Boston: Beacon Press, 1976.

Lim, R. *After the Baby's Birth . . . A Woman's Way to Wellness*. Berkeley, CA: Celestial Arts, 1991.

Olds, S. W. *The Working Parents' Survival Guide*. New York: Bantam Books, 1983.

Richards, L. B., et al. *The Vaginal Birth after Cesarean Experience*. Westport, CT: Bergin & Garvey, 1987.

Exercise

Noble, E. *Essential Exercises for the Childbearing Years*. Boston: Houghton Mifflin, 1988.

Postpartum Disorders

Dix, C. *The New Mother Syndrome*. New York: Pocket Books, 1985.

Hamilton, J. A., and P. N. Harberger, eds. *Postpartum Psychiatric Illness*. Philadelphia: University of Pennsylvania Press, 1992.

Oakley, Ann. *Women Confined*. New York: Schocken Books, 1980.

Panuthos, C., and C. Romeo. *Ended Beginnings*. New York: Bergin & Garvey, 1984. Read the sections on postpartum issues.

Romito, P. "Unhappiness after Childbirth," in I. Chalmers, M. Enkin and M. J. N. C. Keirse, eds. *Effective Care in Pregnancy and Childbirth*. New York: Oxford University Press, 1989.

Breastfeeding

Guyer, R. L., and M. W. Freivogel. *Why Breast Feed?* Alliance for Perinatal Research and Services, Inc. Send $2.00 to Alliance for Perinatal Research and Services, P.O. Box 6358, Alexandria, VA 22306.
Kitzinger, S. *The Experience of Breastfeeding.* New York: Penguin, 1987.
La Leche League International. *The Womanly Art of Breastfeeding,* 5th ed. Franklin Park, IL: La Leche League International, 1991.
Prior, K. *Nursing Your Baby.* New York: Pocket Books, 1991.
Raphael, D. *The Tender Gift: Breastfeeding.* New York: Schocken Books, 1976.

Baby Care

Brazelton, T. B. *Infants and Mothers.* New York: Dell Publishing Co., Inc., 1983.
Howell, M. *Healing at Home: A Guide to Health Care for Children.* Boston: Beacon Press, 1978. A classic.
Leach, P. *Your Baby and Child.* New York: Alfred A. Knopf, 1989.
Pruett, K. *The Nurturing Father.* New York: Warner Books, 1987.
Spock, B., and M. Rothenberg. *Dr. Spock's Baby and Child Care: Fortieth Anniversary Edition.* New York: E. P. Dutton, 1985.
Stern, D. *Diary of a Baby.* New York: Basic Books, 1990.
Thevenin, T. *The Family Bed.* Wayne, NJ: Avery, 1987.

Child Care

Brazelton, T. B. *Working and Caring.* New York: Addison-Wesley, 1985.
Field, T. *Infancy.* Cambridge, MA: Harvard University Press, 1990.
Steinfels, Margaret O'Brien. *Who's Minding the Children: The History and Politics of Day Care in America.* New York: Simon & Schuster, 1973. Excellent.

Organizations

COPE (Coping with the Overall Pregnancy Experience)
53 Tremont Street
Boston, MA 02116
A Boston-based organization that provides a variety of support services for new parents.

Depression After Delivery
P.O. Box 1282
Morrisville, PA 19067
(215) 295-3994

The Family Resource Coalition
230 North Michigan Avenue, Suite 1625
Chicago, IL 60601
(312) 726-3750

International Cesarean Awareness Network (formerly called the Cesarean Prevention Movement)
P.O. Box 152
Syracuse, NY 13210
(315) 424-1942

La Leche League International
9616 Minneapolis Avenue
Franklin Park, IL 60131
(708) 455-7730
An international organization of nursing mothers that runs monthly support groups in many communities.

The Marcé Society
Queen Margaret College
Clerwood Terrace
Edinburgh EH 23-8TS
United Kingdom
(031) 339-8111

National Childbirth Trust
Alexander House
Oldham Terrace
Acton, London W36NH
United Kingdom
(01) 992-8637

Pacific Postpartum Support Society
1416 Commercial Drive
Vancouver, British Columbia V5L 3X9
Canada
(604) 255-7999

Post and Ante-Natal Depression Association (PANDA)
18 Elysee Court
Strathmore, Victoria
Australia 3041

Postpartum Support International
927 Kellogg Avenue
Santa Barbara, CA 93111
(805) 967-7636

Santa Barbara Birth Resource Center
1525 Santa Barbara Street
Santa Barbara, CA 93101
(805) 966-4545

22

Infertility and Pregnancy Loss

By Diane Clapp, with
Norma Swenson

With special thanks to Resolve, Inc.

This chapter in previous editions was called "Some Exceptions to the Normal Childbearing Experience" and was written by Jane Pincus and Barbara Eck Menning.

1992 Update by Diane Clapp, with Catherine Romeo and Norma Swenson.

Many of us have childbearing problems that cause us difficulty and emotional pain. After years of using birth control and being voluntarily childless, we are confronted with the reality that when we consciously decide to have children, we are unable to conceive or unable to carry a pregnancy. The following is a description of a totally unexpected miscarriage in the thirteenth week:

My husband held me and we cried together. It is not hard to remember what we were feeling. The deepest and most obvious was the sense of loss. Almost as strong was the fear. We did not understand what was happening and why—why it was happening to us. Did this mean something was wrong with one of us? Did this mean we could never have children? Had I done something wrong during the early months to cause the miscarriage? We were also frightened by the amount and look of what was pouring out of me. . . . It was terribly bloody. It wasn't bad enough that we were losing our baby, but in the midst of all that pain we had to stay strong enough to deal with all that blood. Why hadn't anyone given us any preparation? Since no one had ever told us about miscarriage, we had no tools to deal with it while it was happening.

We can learn to deal with potential problems and actual crises in two ways. First, we will want to have a general awareness that things may go wrong. We can tuck away such information to be used if necessary. The knowledge itself can't hurt us, but if it upsets us, we can hold dialogues with ourselves, our partners or our friends. Second, if we do suspect we can't conceive, if we miscarry or have another problem, we will want more specific information to answer our questions: What is happening? What shall I do? Where shall I get help? How shall I cope? What is my next step? What other questions shall I ask?

I was told by a doctor that he does not discuss miscarriage so that he will not frighten women who (he thinks) are not going to have them.

This kind of attitude insults our intelligence and undermines our emotional strength. We and our doctors are practicing sound preventive medicine when we ask our questions as strongly as we can and they answer them respectfully and to the best of their knowledge.

We can also seek out the physiological causes of our problems by reading all the available literature, learning about diagnostic procedures and available treatments, asking for test results and insisting on further tests if we are not satisfied.

We can develop emotional strengths to cope with what we are living through. Crises may produce feelings of isolation, fear, anger, grief, guilt and helplessness, as well as obsessions and fantasies. During such times we need sympathetic support from our partners, our friends and others who have had similar experiences. We need to be able to reach out to others.

This chapter is meant to be a first tool to help us acquire some of the information we need.

INFERTILITY

Infertility is defined by most doctors as the inability to conceive after a year or more of sexual relations without contraception. The definition includes women who become pregnant but can't maintain a pregnancy long enough for the fetus to become viable (able to live outside the mother). *Primary infertility* is when you have never had a full-term delivery. *Secondary infertility* is infertility subsequent to giving birth to a baby. Infertility may be a temporary or permanent state, depending on your problem and on the available treatments. Many people are surprised to learn that infertility is fairly common. About 4.9 million people in the United States are infertile, including about 8.5 percent of couples in their childbearing years. In 40 percent of these cases, male factors are responsible; in 40 percent, female factors are responsible; in 10 percent, combined factors are responsible, and 10 percent is unexplained.

Some major factors that cause infertility are: sexually transmitted diseases (STDs), which can lead to permanent damage to the reproductive system; the IUD, which sometimes contributes to infertility by causing pelvic inflammatory disease (PID) after insertion; women's decision to delay childbearing into their late thirties, when fertility decreases slightly; and the increase in environmental and industrial toxic products, which can affect both men's and women's reproductive systems. A badly done abortion or one which has not been properly followed up can cause infections that, if not treated, in turn affect fertility.

Though up until now one myth has held that infertility is the woman's problem, it has become clear that the man and woman must be diagnosed and treated together. If the man has the problem, then treatment of the woman alone has no value and usually involves many needless, painful and expensive tests. A man, because of his anatomy, is easier to diagnose: Semen analysis is one of the logical tests to perform first.

Another myth is that infertility is not treatable.

In fact, 50 percent of infertile people treated are able to achieve a pregnancy!

When you seek help for infertility, it is crucial to have a good relationship with your doctor. Find someone who specializes in infertility. The best infertility specialists are reproductive endocrinologists, who are obstetrician-gynecologists with two additional years of training in the field of infertility. If you don't have confidence in your doctor's methods, go elsewhere. Get a second opinion; that is your right.

It's important that your doctor be respectful of your body, mind and feelings; aware of your pain and strong emotions and available to you when you need him or her. It's the responsibility of your nurse and doctor to explain words and procedures so that you can fully understand—it may take you a while, because you are learning a new language and may be under stress. It is often helpful to make a written list of questions to take with you to each appointment and bring your partner or a friend with you.

You may need help from your partner, close friends or an infertility support group to obtain the necessary tests and diagnostic procedures you have learned about. Become as familiar with your own body's functions as you can.

Emotional Responses to Infertility

Infertility is a life crisis. It is usually unexpected; often we don't know how to cope with the feelings raised by the experience of discovering we are infertile. There is an initial reaction of shock and denial.

I, like every other woman in this society, always believed that I would have children without any problems—as many as I wished and when I decided it was the right time. Unfortunately, after four years of trial and error, tests, operations, et cetera, my husband and I are realizing that life does not always happen the way we plan it. I have found it quite hard dealing not only with our infertility problem but also with the reactions of people around me.

I'm sick of people telling me to "relax," "stop thinking it out," "adopt and you'll get pregnant," and all the other wonderful clichés that, although said to be comforting, ring of insensitivity. Friends and family can never possibly know the pain that I feel inside, the anger and resentment I feel every time I see a woman walking down the street with a big belly. How could they understand? How can anyone capable of having children understand?

Often it seems as if your life is on hold, as you postpone changing jobs, going back to school, and so on, because "six months from now you will be pregnant."

I quit teaching five years ago to become pregnant. When that did not happen, everyone wanted to know what I could possibly be doing at home all day if I didn't have kids. Neither a mother nor a career woman, I stayed in limbo because I kept thinking, Maybe it will happen this month! I was drifting, and it is hard to believe so much time has gone by with just this single purpose in mind.

When women you know have children, it may be hard for you to relate to them. Feelings of envy, jealousy and "why them and not me" are common. Because holidays are so child centered, they can become stressful, lonely and depressing times for you. You may feel isolated from friends and your mate. You may each react differently to the infertility crisis.

My husband is disappointed with our failure to conceive, but he could easily accept a child-free life. He says he understands my feelings and sympathizes but doesn't care to hear any more about the subject. His view is "play the cards dealt you"—you go on about your business no matter what. His disappointment is mitigated by involvement in a job he likes and other alternatives. I have not found a satisfactory alternative.

Anger is a common feeling, but it is hard to know where and toward whom to direct it. We tend to look for a reason for our infertility. We may feel that something we did in the past caused our present inability to conceive. Some people irrationally think that past abortions (even though properly performed), masturbation, unusual sex practices, and so on have caused this form of "punishment." They do not cause infertility, but our minds can trick us into believing it and make us feel terribly guilty.

Depression, sadness and despair are common.

What infertility seemed to do to me was to force a kind of confrontation with lifelessness or death. The fact that there would be no children meant that I was the last line of offense against death. Nobody to carry on who was living. The solution: Disconnect. So I numbed out. I invested back into work, which in the culture has been man's traditional way to combat mortality. If your work lives on, you haven't been wasting your time; there's a purpose to your life.

I grew up surrounded by the idea that if you were willing to work or study hard and always did your best, nothing was beyond your grasp. Generally I have found this to be true. The theory fell apart when I began to deal with my infertility problems. Not only did I become very depressed, but without the help of a friend of mine who shares the same problem, I

seriously doubt whether my marriage would have remained intact.

It is only through a great deal of pain and anguish that I have begun to accept the idea that I may never have children. After the initial shock wore off, my husband and I became closer than ever.

I wish that more doctors dealing with infertility would address themselves to the feelings of their patients instead of leaving them floundering, looking for their own resources.

Many women find the medical terminology used by doctors to be hurtful and even blaming in its tone. "Hostile cervical mucus," "habitual abortion," "incompetent cervix" and "blighted ovum" do not reflect any understanding of how difficult infertility or child loss can be.

Causes of Infertility

Fertility is based on several physiological events and their timing. Your partner must produce sperm of sufficient quantity, quality and motility (ability to swim). You must produce a healthy ovum. Sperm must be deposited in your vagina and move upward through cervical mucus to meet the ovum while it is still in the tube. (Timing of sexual relations is important, since an ovum may live as little as twelve or twenty-four hours, a sperm as little as one or two days.) Once the sperm and ovum have united, the resulting group of cells must implant properly in the uterine lining and proceed to grow. The usual order of tests done in an infertility checkup is based on an organized attempt to check all the links in this chain of events.

A man may be infertile because of the following:

1. Problems of production and maturation of the sperm may exist. These can be caused by previous infection, especially after puberty, such as mumps; undescended testicles; chemical and environmental factors; drugs; occupational hazards. Taking hot saunas and baths can cause overly high temperatures in the scrotal sac, an effect that lasts a few months. In addition, a varicocele (a varicose vein in the scrotum) can affect sperm production.

2. Problems with the movement (motility) of the sperm may exist. These may be due to chronic prostitis and abnormally thick or inadequate semen. In addition, certain drugs used to treat emotional disorders, stomach ulcers and hypertension can affect sperm motility.

3. Problems of conduction can result from scar tissue in the delicate passageways through which the sperm travel; this may be caused by infections or untreated STD. (Intentional blockage is accomplished by vasectomy.)

4. Inability to deposit the sperm into the cervix

can be caused by sexual dysfunction, such as impotence or premature ejaculation, as well as by structural problems in the penis, for example, when the opening is on either the top or the underside of the penis instead of at the tip. Spinal cord injuries and various neurological diseases can also contribute to this problem.

5. Other factors affecting male fertility are poor nutrition and poor general health. Researchers recommend that men eat well and increase their intake of zinc, vitamin C and vitamin E.

A woman may be infertile because of the following:

1. Mechanical barriers can prevent the union of the sperm and ovum, caused by scarring on the tubes or ovaries from previous PID or from certain IUDs. There is a 9 percent higher risk of developing PID if a woman is using an IUD. Untreated STD, such as gonorrhea and chlamydia, can also cause scarring and tubal blockage.

2. Endometriosis (see p. 586) can cause scarring, tubal blockage and possible immune responses.

3. Endocrine problems may exist. Failure to ovulate regularly or irregular menstrual periods may be due to a malfunction of the ovaries, pituitary, hypothalamus, thyroid or adrenal glands. Normally, several specific hormones are secreted at specific times in the menstrual cycle. If any one of these is not produced or produced in insufficient quantity, the whole cycle can be thrown off. In addition, when ovulation is unpredictable the chances of conception are decreased, as women cannot count on a consistent cycle with a known fertile time. Women often develop amenorrhea (absence of menstrual periods) following the use of birth control pills, which can result in infertility. Women who have irregular periods or who are older when they start their first menstrual periods seem to be more prone to this so-called post-Pill syndrome.

4. Structural problems in the uterus or cervix due to congenital problems or DES exposure *in utero* can cause infertility by preventing conception or affecting the normal growth and expansion of the uterus during pregnancy. If the cervix is affected, miscarriage may result.

5. Cervical mucus of an incorrect consistency or pH (an expression of acidity and alkalinity) can act as a barrier to the normal movement of the sperm up into the vagina.

6. Other factors, such as genetic abnormalities, extreme weight loss or weight gain, excessive exercise, poor nutrition and environmental and industrial toxins, may affect a woman's fertility. Infections, such as those caused by T-mycoplasma, can cause infertility by changing the quality of cervical mucus and possibly causing early miscarriage.

Infertility also takes the form of repeated miscarriage or stillbirths. In these instances conception is not the problem; there is an inability to carry a pregnancy to live birth.

A couple may have a combination of problems that results in infertility. Two shared causes are:

1. *Immunological response.* You or your partner may have sperm antibodies that tend to destroy the sperm's action by immobilizing them or causing them to clump.

2. *Simple lack of knowledge.* Neither of you may know when you are fertile, how often to have intercourse during this time or what to do during intercourse to make pregnancy more possible.

Finally, for 10 percent of infertile couples, physicians cannot specifically diagnose any cause for their infertility (unexplained infertility). These couples are told everything is "normal" and they can do nothing but wait. This finding can be one of the hardest to cope with—the idea that there is nothing that can be done. You may be told that your problems are all in your head. This kind of attitude is not helpful at all. Often you may be victims of a condition whose cause or cure has yet to be discovered. We must all press for more research.

Masters and Johnson stated that one out of five couples who attended their infertility clinic over a twenty-four-year period conceived within three months with no treatment other than use of this basic information: If your menstrual cycle is regular, whether it be long or short, you will probably ovulate fourteen days (give or take twenty-four hours either way) before the beginning of your next period. Using fertility awareness techniques (see p. 276), you can determine your most fertile times and have intercourse then. Spacing your lovemaking during this period is important. A man's sperm production decreases if he makes love too often, so you should have intercourse no more than once every thirty or thirty-six hours to keep active sperm in your genital tract during that period of time. It is wise to have intercourse two days before this three-day period to stimulate your partner's sperm production.

If your uterus is not tilted back, the most effective position for intercourse will be with your partner above and facing you and a folded pillow under your hips to raise them. (If your uterus is tilted back, use three or four pillows.) Use no artificial lubricant, such as jellies or creams, and never douche afterward. If lubrication is necessary, saliva is the safest choice. He should penetrate as deeply as possible, and when he reaches orgasm he should stop thrusting and hold quite still, deep in your vagina. Approximately 60 to 70 percent of the sperm are contained in the first part of the ejaculate. Since it usually takes only a few minutes for sperm to move through the cervical mucus up to the uterus and fallopian tubes, it is a good idea to stay on your back for about ten minutes.*

Many couples know that infertility and planned sex really affect their sexual life. Spontaneity in lovemaking decreases. You have to plan your sex life around your menstrual cycle; it becomes less an act of loving and pleasure and more a medically necessary response. Recording the time of your sexual relations on a temperature chart may make you feel like nothing is private or sacred in your life anymore!

I started with the temperature charts. This was quite taxing for me and mentally depressing. I felt very regulated and calculating, both with my own body and in my relationship with my husband. I need not say what it did to our natural sexual impulses. But a child at all cost—this was how we felt.

My husband woke me every morning at six A.M. so that I could take my temperature. Afterward, he charted it. I needed his involvement.

From your temperature chart or results from a urine test kit you can determine if you are ovulating or not and can time your sex to coincide. If you are ovulating normally, from the time of your last period until ovulation you'll have a fluctuating, low temperature (around 98 degrees Fahrenheit or less). About the time of ovulation there's usually a dip followed by a rise of half a degree or more. Some cycles show just a rise with no preceding dip. The higher plateau (usually around 98.4 degrees Fahrenheit) is maintained until the day before your next period, when it drops again. Your doctor will give you a chart, or you can get one from your nearest Planned Parenthood Association.

Urine test kits are available to monitor the amount of luteinizing hormone (LH) in your urine. When the level of LH rises, ovulation usually occurs in the next twenty-four to thirty-six hours. The kits that give specific guidelines concerning when to expect ovulation may make it even easier to predict your fertile time.

You must wait at least two cycles to begin to interpret your temperature chart or urine test results with any degree of accuracy.

Diagnosis

A complete infertility workup with all the diagnostic tests can take four or five menstrual cycles.

Many of the tests have to be scheduled at specific times in your cycle and can't be combined. An infertility workup is expensive, and unfortunately medical insurance coverage in most cases is poor, although some states now have laws mandating insurance coverage for infertility. The tests for women are invasive, painful, often undignified and emotionally exhausting.

Though the sequence of diagnostic studies will vary with both doctors and individuals, it will include some or all of the following:

1. *A general and medical history of both man and woman.*

2. *A pelvic examination of the woman.* Your reproductive tract, breasts and general development will be checked. You will want to tell your doctor about your menstrual history, including the onset and pattern of your menstrual periods; about any previous pregnancies, episodes of STD or abortions; about your use of birth control; about your sexual relations (frequency, position and related feelings); about where you live and what your job is, for environmental toxins may have affected you.

3. *Monitoring ovulation.* You will take your temperature daily with a special thermometer or use a urine test kit to record ovulation patterns.

4. *Semen analysis.* Your partner will ejaculate a sample of semen into a clean container. It must be kept at body temperature and examined as soon as possible under a microscope to determine the sperm count and motility. A count over 20 million sperm per cubic centimeter is considered in the normal range; below 10 million per cubic centimeter is considered poor. Yet men with low sperm counts *can* impregnate. The sperm must be able to swim in a forward motion and at least 60 percent should be normal in size and shape.

Special tests to check for movement and shape of the sperm are now available. If either motility or shape of the sperm is abnormal, additional tests such as a penetration test can be done to see if the sperm has the capacity to fertilize a specially prepared hamster's egg.

Repeat the semen analysis at least every six months, because a man's sperm can fluctuate in count and motility for many reasons. If the semen analysis is abnormal, your partner should pursue his own diagnosis before you have further tests done.

Any diagnosis of infertility can make things difficult for both man and woman.

My husband's sperm count was very low; we were both crushed. I don't think my husband believed it was actually happening. In fact, he often talked in the third person, not truly accepting the results. I love him and therefore hurt for him. I didn't know what to say. I couldn't say the typical, "Oh, it's all right," because we both knew it really wasn't all

---

*Some women douche with baking soda thirty minutes before intercourse to change the acidity of cervical mucus and make it less viscous. You can use litmus paper to test the acidity of your midcycle mucus. Do not douche if it is alkaline.

right. For some reason, I found I could handle a problem with myself but found it very difficult to handle my reaction to his problem. I was even more concerned that he couldn't handle his problem. Then we started seeing doctors for him.

If all male factors are normal, study of the woman will continue. You may need to have the following tests or procedures:

5. *A postcoital test (Sims-Hühner test).* Just before you expect to ovulate you will make love with your partner and within several hours will arrive at your doctor's office without washing or douching. The doctor will take a small amount of mucus from your vagina and cervix to be studied for the number of live, active sperm. A normal test result shows that sperm have the ability to penetrate cervical mucus and live in this environment.

6. *A uterotubogram, or hysterosalpingogram.* This allows for visualization of the tubes and provides a permanent record that can be used for comparison if future X-rays are needed. Doctors perform this procedure in the first part of the cycle, before ovulation, to prevent possible X-ray exposure of a fertilized egg if conception has occurred.* It involves injecting a harmless dye into the vagina and uterus. The dye should pass up through the uterus to the tubes and out into the abdominal cavity. A series of X-rays are taken during this process. The dye then passes out into the pelvic cavity and your body reabsorbs it. This test can be painful. Practitioners may give you local cervical anesthesia or an oral medication to help you relax before this test. Taking Motrin thirty minutes before the test can help reduce the cramping. Many clinics give women antibiotics for two to three days after the test to make sure no infection develops.

7. *Blood levels of hormones.* The blood levels of estrogen, follicle-stimulating hormone (FSH), LH, progesterone and prolactin will be done to determine if your hormone levels are normal and whether ovulation has occurred.

8. *An endometrial biopsy.* This is another test to determine whether you are ovulating. It can be done any time from a week after ovulation is suspected to the first day of your period.† The doctor inserts a small instrument into your uterus after partially dilating your cervix (this will cause some unpleasant cramping), scrapes a tiny piece of tissue from the lining of the uterus (endometrium)

*Remember that whenever you have X-rays, you are irradiating all future eggs.
†Many think that taking such a minute piece of tissue presents no danger to a new conceptus. Others avoid possible hazard to a pregnancy by having the woman come in on the day her temperature drops or even at the time her period starts. Some doctors advise using a condom during relations in this cycle so there will be no worry over a possible pregnancy.

and sends it to be examined microscopically. Tissue formed while progesterone is being produced (after ovulation) is different from tissue formed under the influence of estrogen (before ovulation) or in the absence of hormonal influence.

9. *Laparoscopy.* If s/he finds no problem, your doctor may want to do a *laparoscopy,* a hospital procedure that allows direct visualization of the tubes, ovaries, exterior of the uterus and the surrounding cavities. In laparoscopy, an incision is made near your navel. It is done under general or spinal anesthesia and can yield a great deal of information.*

A *hysteroscopy* may also be done at the time of the laparoscopy. A small telescope is inserted through the vagina and cervix into the uterus to allow the doctor to see the inside of the uterine cavity. If there is scar tissue or polyps present, they can be removed using the hysteroscope.

When you are going through these tests, once again your sex life comes under scientific scrutiny.

We were supposed to make love at seven o'clock in the morning and then I had to run to my doctor's for the postcoital test. Who feels like making love at seven in the morning during a busy week anyway?

Trying to work and find time to get these tests scheduled is difficult. Many women don't want their bosses to know about their infertility, so that adds another pressure—secrecy.

Relatives may ask you, "Well, has it happened yet?" Or, worse, they don't say anything, but they look at you and sigh a lot. People you hardly know may comment on your problem. Hopefully, during these times you can support each other and keep both your sense of humor and your sense of the awesomeness and privacy of sexuality.

Treatment

In 90 percent of the cases a reason is found for the infertility. Your doctor should talk with you both and outline a plan for treatment.

In general, male problems are more difficult to treat. However, various hormones, also used to treat female infertility (clomiphene citrate, human chorionic gonadotropin [HCG], human menopausal gonadotropin [HMG]), are now being tried with good success in the male. If there is a blockage in the tubes that bring the sperm from the testicle, sperm can be extracted with a needle, joined with your egg in a petri dish and replaced in your tube or uterus (see Chapter 18, "New Reproductive Technologies"). A varicocele can be corrected surgically, or in a nonsurgical procedure

*Some doctors prefer to do these procedures first; others do them as a last resort.

using a tiny balloon to block off the vein, with a rise in sperm count and motility usually seen three months after surgery. The stress of waiting to hear the results can take its toll on couples. If your mate's sperm count is low, insemination to the cervix or into the uterus (IUI) with your partner's sperm is sometimes done. This may be combined with ovulation-enhancing drugs such as clomiphene or HMG (Pergonal). If infection is causing a decrease in sperm motility, it is corrected by treatment with antibiotics.

For women, treatment for endocrine disorders currently offers the highest degree of success. Doctors use a variety of drugs to correct hormonal imbalances, help induce ovulation and correct problems in the luteal phase (after ovulation).

The main drugs used to induce ovulation are clomiphene citrate; HCG, a hormone extracted from the human placenta; and HMG, extracted from the urine of menopausal women. Pure FSH (Metrodin) and gonadotropin-releasing hormone (GnRH) agonists (such as Lupron or Synarel) may be used to improve the effects of Pergonal. The GnRH agonists can be taken via nasal spray form or by injection. This drug makes all your hormone levels temporarily drop and enhances the body's response to ovulation-triggering drugs like Pergonal or Metrodin. Some women experience hot flashes and vaginal dryness while on the medication, which can induce a temporary menopause-like state. Usually GnRH agonists are used from five to fourteen days.

Clomiphene citrate was introduced in the 1960s and is a commonly used infertility drug. It is taken orally on the fifth to the tenth day of the cycle. It appears to act directly upon the hypothalamus in the brain and causes it to produce more of the hormones FSH and LH, which then stimulate the ovary to ripen and release an egg. About 80 percent of women will ovulate with the help of this drug, and about 50 percent will become pregnant, with a 5 to 10 percent incidence of multiple births. Some women experience mood swings, breast tenderness, hot flashes, headaches, blurred vision and throbbing feelings in the ovaries at the time of ovulation while on clomiphene citrate. Clomiphene sometimes causes the midcycle cervical mucus to dry up, so make sure you get a postcoital test done if you are on clomiphene three or more cycles. A potential complication is hyperstimulation of the ovary, which, if undetected, may result in ovarian damage. Ideally, women on this medication should have a checkup at the end of each cycle to be sure this complication isn't developing.

HCG is often combined with clomiphene citrate and given intramuscularly near the time of expected ovulation. It acts like LH on the ovary and helps the developing egg ripen and release.

HMG is a very potent hormone used to induce ovulation, and should only be prescribed by an infertility specialist. Treatment with HMG involves frequent injections of the drug and often daily visits to a laboratory where blood and urine are examined for estrogen levels. Some doctors also use vaginal ultrasound to monitor the development of the ovarian follicle(s).* By monitoring these levels carefully, the danger of multiple eggs being released from the ovary and consequent multiple births is reduced. Ovarian hyperstimulation is also a possible complication of use of this drug.

Bromocriptine is another drug used to treat female infertility due to high levels of the hormone prolactin in the blood. In breastfeeding mothers, prolactin levels are normally elevated. Occasionally this hormone is elevated in the infertile woman as well. It appears that high prolactin levels can disturb normal ovulatory patterns. In such cases, bromocriptine is taken orally until prolactin levels fall and normal ovulation results.

Problems in the luteal phase of the cycle may be treated with any or all of the following: clomiphene citrate, HCG and natural progesterone. Natural progesterone is available in vaginal suppositories or given via intramuscular injections. You usually insert the suppositories twice daily, starting after ovulation. Synthetic forms of progesterone are not advised, as they can be harmful to fetal development in an unsuspected pregnancy.

Surgical techniques can often correct cervical weakness and various structural problems of the uterus. Microsurgery is a special type of surgery used to repair tubes and to remove adhesions. Laser surgery using the carbon dioxide or argon laser is also being used, often in combination with microsurgery, to remove scar tissue or endometrial adhesions. If there is significant tubal damage, *in vitro* fertilization (IVF) may offer more chance of a successful pregnancy than with surgical repair of the tubes, but even IVF has extremely low success rates (see p. 509 and Chapter 18). Endometriosis can be treated surgically and/ or with oral medications.

If there is a cervical mucus problem, you can douche to correct acidity, use estrogen to improve mucus quality and take cough syrup orally to treat very thick cervical mucus. Sperm antibody problems are usually treated by doing IUI or with low-dose steroids. However, steroids can mask infections in the body and can cause weakening of the bones in the hip joint. IVF and GIFT (see p. 390) have been used with some success for couples with sperm antibody problems.

Women often have a combination of problems, and their treatment may involve a combination of

---

*The effect of ultrasound on the ovary is unknown.

several medications, many of which are expensive. It is important to understand how these drugs work, how they affect you and how long you should use them. (See p. 59 for more information on the informed use of drugs.)

Shared infertility problems are usually treated by separate doctors. The man goes to a urologist and the woman to a gynecologist or infertility specialist. *Your doctors must communicate with each other.* For any couple with a shared problem, the potential to achieve pregnancy is improved dramatically if even one member of the couple can be treated and helped. If both of you can be helped, then your chances are excellent.

In all cases, there is a 5 percent spontaneous cure rate (a cure without any treatment whatever). Often, after many years of trying, pregnancy will finally occur. We do not understand these spontaneous cures well, but the fact that they do happen is a source of hope when all else fails.

In unexplained infertility there are usually no clear-cut medical reasons. It can be difficult for you and your doctor to know when to stop the tests or to stop various treatments. Your feelings of hopefulness may give way to depression, often a painful process.

In the case of *conclusive* or *absolute* infertility, such as premature ovarian failure, you have the facts. You must now adjust to that reality and re-examine your life. For some women, there is no clear ending. You may feel as if "the death of all your babies" has occurred. You may feel grief for the loss of a part of womanhood or manhood, for the parts of you that don't work or have been cut out of you. If you deny or repress this feeling of grief, you prolong the process of its resolution. Somewhere inside you are dealing with the experience. You have the choice of living it as consciously and directly as you can or suppressing these very natural but painful emotions. Sometimes the pain of infertility is never completely resolved but is accepted as a familiar ache that may recur, unpredictably, throughout life. Grieving often takes a long time.* To do your "grief work," the support of friends, family and other people who have experienced infertility can be helpful.

In July of last year I underwent hysterectomy at the age of twenty-nine. Needless to say, I was crushed with grief. I never had the chance to have a baby and then all hope was snatched away. In my case it had to be done—fibroid tumors had practically destroyed my uterus (there were twenty-one to be exact). I was very bitter for a while, but now I am healing.

That is not to say I don't hurt sometimes; I think a pain this deep will always come back from time to time.

After learning of my infertility five years ago, I experienced the usual shock and denial. Unfortunately, I pushed down all other stages and feelings by submerging myself in work. Eventually we adopted a son and all seemed right with the world. I thought I had everything together, as I rarely thought of my infertility and was very active.

Last fall, for no obviously apparent reason, my infertility again became a prominent concern, and all the feelings I had submerged five years ago resurfaced. After four unstable months I ended up in severe, crippling depression.

Only with the help of counseling have I been able to begin to work through the feelings and to come out of my depressed state.

It was relieving to meet and talk openly with other couples experiencing infertility. Each of us had our own specific difficulties, but our feelings and reactions were quite similar. After the initial nervousness that accompanied our first two meetings, I began to feel much more accepting and able to deal with the previous two and a half years that had given us two pregnancies and two miscarriages. My almost constant obsession with pregnancy was lifted. I began to feel in touch with myself and somewhat alive again.

MISCARRIAGE

Another form of infertility results from problems in carrying a pregnancy the full nine months. One in six pregnancies ends in miscarriage, 75 percent of these before twelve weeks. Miscarriage, then, is a fairly common event. We want to be at least minimally prepared to know how it feels and what to expect. Miscarriage is both a physical event for a woman and a serious emotional crisis that may be shared by both of you or experienced by each of you in very different ways. Miscarriages are usually unexpected the first time. They most often come at the joyful time of early pregnancy and thus are all the more of a shock.

When I found out I was pregnant, I danced around the house. My pregnancy was an easy one. . . . My body was slowly and pleasantly changing. Because it was a conscious and well-thought-out decision to have a child, I felt free to revel in my pregnancy and motherhood. It was a special time. I mention all of this because having a miscarriage has to do with the loss of something so deeply ingrained for so long that it is partially by understanding the depth of the joy that one can understand the depth of the loss.

---

*Some people immediately block this feeling of grief by planning to adopt. The adoption is more likely to be happy and successful if you can "work out" the grief.

The term for miscarriage before twenty-six weeks is *spontaneous abortion*. If it is a *threatened abortion*, the cervix is still closed but the woman is experiencing cramps and bleeding or staining. Often bed rest is advised, and your doctor may order specific blood tests to check your hormone levels. Ultrasound can be done as early as six weeks from your last period to evaluate fetal growth and to detect fetal heart movement. In *inevitable abortion*, bleeding becomes heavy, cramps increase and the cervix begins to dilate. The fetus, amniotic sac and placenta, along with a lot of blood, may be expelled completely intact. You'll probably know when this is happening. It's very important to say here that if you are not in a hospital, you must do the difficult task of collecting fetus and afterbirth, putting them in a clean container and taking them to a laboratory for examination. This will yield important information as to why you miscarried. Ask that specialized as well as routine tests be done, such as cultures for infection and genetic overview of tissues. If tests show you have lost a *blighted pregnancy* (where egg and sperm together have failed to divide correctly), then you can know that this has been a random event and that the chances of it happening again are small. If a study of the fetal tissue shows genetic abnormalities or suggests that you had an illness or infection, you'll work with your doctor on how to proceed. If the fetal tissue is normal, you may learn that your hormone levels were insufficient or that a weak cervix was at fault. Both of these conditions can be treated.

An *incomplete abortion* means that only part of the "products of conception" has been passed. Part remains within, and bleeding will continue. Usually a doctor will do a dilation and curettage (D and C) to clean out your uterus so that it will heal. A *complete abortion* means that everything in your uterus has been expelled. You will continue to bleed, but less and less. If you think you are bleeding too long, consult your doctor. (A D and C may be necessary.)

You may also experience a *missed abortion*. In this case, a fetus dies in the uterus but is not expelled. It can remain within for several months. Signs are lack of menstrual periods coupled with cessation of signs of pregnancy; sometimes there is spotting. Treatment is either a D and C or induction of labor.

Some possible causes for miscarriage are structural problems of the uterus, infection, weak cervical muscles, hormonal imbalances, environmental and industrial toxins, blood incompatibility between mother who is Rh negative and fetus who is Rh positive (there is now a drug, Rhogam, that can be given to women to prevent this reaction), and genetic error. Some research shows that 50 to 60 percent of all first-trimester miscarriages are caused by genetic abnormalities in the fetus. These miscarriages can be nature's way of screening out problems.

If you have had two or more miscarriages, blood tests can make sure that there is no immunologic cause for your pregnancy losses. These tests check for certain responses that affect blood clotting and for problems in the immune system.

Try to learn why you had a miscarriage. Some of the diagnostic procedures outlined earlier for infertility will be useful here. Ask to see the pathology report, and ask that all terminology be explained fully. If you are not satisfied with the explanation, ask if there are other tests that can be done. It is your right to learn as much as possible about your miscarriage.

One miscarriage does not mean you are infertile. There is a 70 percent chance that you will have a successful pregnancy even after two miscarriages. However, if you have two or more in a row, you may want to begin investigating. Plan with your doctor to check out each detail of your next pregnancy as it progresses. You will need encouragement in this project from your partner, friends and/or a support group.

The time following a miscarriage is difficult. Physically, your body may still feel pregnant for a while, your breasts full and tender, your stomach enlarged. You may continue spotting for several weeks. If you have increased flow or odd- or foul-smelling discharge or a fever, contact your doctor. It is usually safe to have sexual intercourse after four to six weeks when your cervix is closed and there is less risk of infection.

You may not believe what is happening. During the miscarriage, feelings of helplessness may develop as cramping and bleeding increase. Many women fear that they may bleed to death. Having to go to the hospital may intensify your anxiety and fear.

We went home from the hospital dazed and tired. I was weak and enormously sad. I don't know that I've ever experienced such deep emotional pain. The loss was so great and so complete in a way that only death is. For the first few days I couldn't talk to anyone, but at the same time it was painful to be alone. I would just cry and cry without stopping. One of the clearest reminders that I was no longer pregnant was all the speedy changes my body went through. Within two days my breasts, which had grown quite swollen, were back to their normal size. My stomach, which had grown hard, was now soft again. My body was no longer preparing for the birth of a child. It was simple and blatant. Tiredness was replaced with weakness. And then there was the bleeding. My body would not let me forget. I knew things would improve once we could make love again and would be even better when we were full of hope. But it seemed so far away.

You will almost always feel grief and anger. You will need family and friends.

Most people didn't know how to give me support, and perhaps I didn't really know how to ask for it. People were more comfortable talking about the physical and not the emotional side of miscarriage. I needed to talk about both. It was also difficult for my husband, because people could at least ask how my body was doing. Unfortunately, he would sometimes be completely bypassed when someone called to talk with us, despite the fact that he, too, was in deep emotional pain.

Feelings of grief are often complicated by guilt, which can cause tension between you and your partner. You may wonder if either of you did something "wrong" (too much activity, too much sex, not enough good food, etc.). You will be blaming each other unnecessarily, because such factors rarely cause miscarriage. Dispelling the tension will take a while, longer for some than for others. It is best if you acknowledge and talk out your feelings. The effects of the miscarriage can last for months. On the date when the baby would have been born, there is usually a resurgence of grief.

If you experience more than three miscarriages, it is important to see a doctor who specializes in this problem. Treatment for multiple miscarriages may involve hormonal treatment or taking a baby aspirin daily during your pregnancy if there is an immune problem that is affecting blood circulation in the placenta. If cultures show infection is present, a wide-spectrum antibiotic will be given to you and your partner. You will need a doctor who is skilled and also compassionate and understanding of the losses you have experienced.

Trying to conceive after several miscarriages can feel frightening. If possible, talk with women who have had the same experience.

ECTOPIC PREGNANCY

Ectopic pregnancy is another form of pregnancy loss, where the fertilized egg starts developing in the tube instead of in the uterus. Between 5 and 10 percent of women who have had previous tubal surgery may experience ectopic pregnancy, but it can happen to any woman. Ectopic pregnancies are on the rise because of the increased incidence of PID and use of IUDs, which can result in scar formation in the tubes (and greater likelihood of a fertilized egg getting stuck in the tubes) or inflammation of the uterine lining, which then "resists" implantation of the fertilized egg. If you're

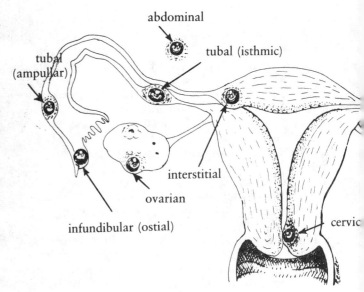

An ectopic pregnancy.   Nina Reimer

old enough to bear a child, have had intercourse and feel abdominal pains you don't understand, it's possible you have an ectopic pregnancy.

Because all the hormonal changes are similar to those of a normal early pregnancy, you can have all the early signs of pregnancy, such as fatigue, nausea, missed period and breast tenderness. As the pregnancy progresses, causing pressure in the tube, symptoms such as stabbing pain, cramps or a dull ache may become severe. Neck and shoulder pains also are common. In addition, you may or may not have menstrual-type bleeding.

To detect an ectopic pregnancy, hormonal levels are checked every day. If the levels do not double, an ultrasound should be done as early as possible to look for an embryonic sac in the uterus or tube. A blood pregnancy test should always be done after a suspected spontaneous abortion to make sure no fetal tissue is present in the tube. Ectopic pregnancy is sometimes misdiagnosed as an early spontaneous abortion. It is essential that any tissue passed from the uterus be checked for developing fetal tissue.

Ectopic pregnancy requires immediate treatment. There is danger of severe blood loss and shock if the tube ruptures.

If the doctor detects an ectopic pregnancy early enough, s/he may be able to remove the pregnancy and save the tube. This is often done through laparoscopy instead of doing major abdominal surgery. The anticancer drug methotrexate is also being used by some doctors. In these cases the drug is injected into the tube or given intravenously to dissolve the embryonic tissues. In some cases it is necessary to remove the whole tube and/or the adjacent ovary. Careful surgical technique is important; the less bleeding and consequent adhesions and scar tissue, the better the chance for a normal pregnancy later. In any case, if you have had a tubal pregnancy there is a higher risk of having another.

You may have all the feelings that result from a miscarriage. In addition, you may have had internal bleeding, and you will have had the trauma of an emergency surgical operation. The outlook for future pregnancies is somewhat changed by this experience: You may feel depressed and frightened by the possibility that this could happen again.

STILLBIRTH

Stillbirth is fortunately a rare occurrence. But if it happens to you, statistics mean nothing. Usually it is the result of the baby's oxygen supply failing before it can be safely born or failure of its lungs or heart to oxygenate its system after the cord is cut.

Your body knows nothing about stillbirth. It is elaborately prepared for the close contact and physical nurturing of a baby. Your breasts are filled with milk, never to be used. (In some cultures, women who lose babies at birth frequently hire out as wet nurses to nurture other babies in place of the ones they have lost. The wet nurse is an esteemed person in these cultures.) You and members of your family are also prepared for the event of a new baby.

Some considerations are in order if you suffer a stillbirth, beginning with the moment the death is expected or confirmed. If the baby's death takes place before labor and delivery, delivery in the quickest and least hazardous way possible is desirable. You should have the chance to decide if you want to go into labor spontaneously. Your partner should be present as long as either of you wish. Once the baby is delivered, birth attendants should handle her/him in a reverent manner and must be especially careful when autopsy is indicated to find the cause of death. You will need to decide if you want to see the baby, either immediately afterward or later on. It can help you accept the tragic reality of what has happened. Above all, if possible, you and your family must be allowed your grief in privacy if you need and want it. You may want a room away from the nursery; hospital personnel should be told that you have lost your baby. You may need to withdraw at first and not confront a reality that may be too much to bear. There may be a period of numbness. If you ask for help in grieving, we hope those around you will offer it intelligently and humanely. Platitudes such as "You'll have another baby before you know it" or "Think of your wonderful children at home" have no place in this situation. You are experiencing the death of this particular child—no other actual or potential children have any relevance. Perhaps the best help others can offer is sympathetic listening and close physical comforting.

It is important for you to understand exactly what happened to the baby. Most likely, whatever happened was totally beyond your control or the doctor's. (If you do suspect malpractice by your doctor, seek legal counsel quickly and have the facts analyzed.)

There is a tremendous sense of void and of loneliness following any pregnancy loss. Society has few ways of dealing with this particular type of loss and as a result you may feel alone in your grief.

ALTERNATIVES FOR INFERTILE COUPLES

Once it has been determined that you are infertile, you will wish to examine the possibilities and alternatives for the future. You may once again find yourself asking, Do I really want to be a parent? Take this time to redefine your goals and get on with living your life.

Donor Insemination

If male infertility or a transmittable genetic disease is the problem, donor sperm insemination is a possibility. (For more information, see Resources and the section on donor insemination in Chapter 18, "New Reproductive Technologies.")

In Vitro Fertilization

IVF is another alternative for some infertile women. More and more medical centers are offering this technique. At best, success rates for a successful ovulation, induction, fertilization, implantation and then a viable pregnancy are about 14 to 16 percent. The cost is $6,000 to $10,000 per ovulatory cycle and you may need to undergo the treatment for several cycles. Insurance coverage is very poor. Obviously, IVF is not a likely solution for the lower- or middle-income couple struggling with infertility. (For more information, see the section on IVF in Chapter 18, "New Reproductive Technologies.")

Adoption

Adoption (an institution that has been undergoing significant change) may be an alternative for many couples. But as the number of available children decreases, adoption becomes more difficult. It is most difficult to adopt Caucasian babies; many states have a five- to seven-year waiting list. Many couples consider adoption of children of color, infants or children from other countries, special-needs children and older children, as the waiting periods are much shorter.

The adoption process raises many negative feelings, often surprisingly similar to the ones experienced during the first stages of coping with infertility. Feelings of powerlessness, anger and frustration are common, especially during the time of the so-called home study, when the social worker is working actively with you. You may feel that s/he is evaluating and "testing" you on your potential as a parent. The home study can be lengthy and expensive (anywhere from $1,000 to $2,000) and often puts a strain once again on your relationship with your partner. Families and friends may not be as supportive as you would like, and you may go through periods of anxiety.

My husband and I found out we might become prospective parents in April. That gave us about seven to eight weeks to think about this. I had many things going through my mind. So many things could happen in the interim. The birth mother could still change her mind. I wondered what the child would be like. The baby's looks, personality, health—everything is unknown. . . .

I thought a lot about bonding. I wondered what I'd feel like when someone put an infant in my arms saying, "Congratulations! You are a mother. This is your child." Who is this stranger? How am I supposed to love someone I do not even know? How am I supposed to feel? I believe these are healthy feelings, but still it is frightening to think about. . . .

I believe couples facing adoption go through the same feelings that biological parents go through—the fears, insecurities, the great change of life-style. The only problem is that you do not have nine months to work your feelings through. It is like being told you are eight months pregnant.

While most adoptions occur through licensed social agencies and there are still *family* adoptions (where people adopt a relative's child), *private* or *identified* adoptions (arranged through lawyers or physicians) are now sharply on the rise. Foreign adoption policies vary and change, depending on the country, some imposing strict age or religious requirements. In many states a licensed home study is required for either an identified or foreign adoption. Adoption, either domestic or foreign, agency or identified, can range in price from $6,000 to $25,000.

It is helpful to talk with other adoptive parents and to join an adoption group (see Resources). Adoption should not feel second best; it should be a positive decision which you are comfortable with and excited about. When you decide to adopt, you will feel "pregnant," as excitement, anxiety,

vulnerability and joy infuse your daily life until the child is placed in your home. Like all new mothers, you will make the transition from being childless to having a child with a variety of responses. And, like any new family, you will all need the support of friends and family.

Adoption poses a number of problems that prospective adoptive parents need to think about in advance. At first, like many parents, you may be totally focused on the baby as a baby, getting to know her/him and learning how to cope. The future seems far away, and the child as an adult seems remote. But as adopted children start to grow up and reach their teens, they may have very powerful feelings about being adopted that they do not always express.

In recent years, more and more adoptees have begun speaking out about their experiences, demanding access to information about their origins and searching for—and sometimes finding—their birth parents. Many now believe it is a human right, if not a constitutional right, to be able to know one's biological origins. National organizations have been formed that support and assist searching adoptees. They also fight for changes in the laws and in the practices of social agencies that keep this knowledge secret. In many cases adoptive parents have become involved in helping their adoptive children with the search, as they have come to understand how important this knowledge and these experiences are to their children.

At the same time, the original parents, "birth parents" as they call themselves today, especially birth mothers, have also begun to speak out about their experiences, describing in many cases the abuse that the adoption experience was for them, including coercion by misleading information and by circumstances they could not control. As one said, "If the adoptees hadn't come out of the closet, we birth mothers probably never would have." Birth parents, too, have formed national organizations for support, for help in searching for their adult children and with their efforts to change the adoption laws. Birth mothers tell us they never forget (contrary to what many social workers insist), that they passionately desire to know about their children's welfare and to see them if possible. They tell us that they did not surrender their children because they *didn't* care about them or love them (as adoptive parents and social workers sometimes suggest to adoptees) but because they *did*. They surrendered them because they believed, as they had been told, that their children would have a better life with other parents. Many birth mothers can never begin to heal from their "surrender" experience until they have been reunited with their children.

Loyalty to their adoptive parents often prevents

many adoptees from expressing a desire to know their birth parents. Many adoptive parents fear that they will somehow "lose" their children and so become childless once again. Birth mothers or fathers fear rejection, not being "good enough" to measure up to their children's expectations, just as they once felt "not good enough" to become the parents of their offspring. Nothing can really alleviate these fears the way going through the experience of a reunion can, but no one is ready in exactly the same way or at exactly the same time as anyone else. Searching is not for everyone. Some never search and never express the desire. Many remain in this position for years until something happens to release in them the desire to know.

Reunions may be brief or temporary or may grow into more long-lasting relationships. Sometimes there are painful rejections on one side or another. But most who have been through it agree that any knowledge at all is better than no knowledge, even if the mother is found in a mental hospital, or the father dead, as some have found. "When I saw how much it meant to her, I wished we had done something about it sooner," one adoptive mother said. And if we are to believe the adoptees, the relationship with the adoptive parents usually improves.

Some adoptive parents and some of the larger social agencies in conservative areas have banded together and tried to stop this searching. They presume to speak for all adoptees and birth parents who, they claim, prefer the anonymity of the present situation. These groups are powerful and well organized and have spent hundreds of thousands of dollars to lobby legislatures all across the country to require records to be sealed tighter than ever. They have no good answers to the powerful feelings the adoptees and birth mothers express, but appeal instead to conservative adoptive parents and members of the social work profession to preserve the status quo.

Very few studies have been done to verify the assumptions and the dogma on which the practice of much adoption social work is carried out. These underlying assumptions usually are based on either traditional religious moral beliefs or Freudian psychoanalytic beliefs. The few studies that have been done demonstrate that these beliefs deny or neglect the true feelings and experiences of all those involved in the adoption process. We need to challenge the traditional assumptions and practices of social workers that have labeled certain feelings and desires "abnormal" and have distorted the experiences and needs of adoptees, birth mothers and adoptive parents alike.

The leadership in the social work profession today has begun to change; the emerging feeling seems to be that it is no longer possible for agencies to guarantee adoptive parents that they will never meet or hear from birth parents, or that adoptees will never be able to know their biological parents. As one social worker said, "We have forgotten who our real client is in all this controversy. It is the adoptee, and the needs of the adoptee, that should be uppermost in our thinking and planning."

Those involved in the movement to open records also help promote the trend to *open adoption* (currently less than 10 percent). Records are not sealed, and adoptive parents, birth parents and adoptees agree to visit and communicate, even though legal custody and the contact option remain, of course, with the adoptive parents.

Although many "open" adoptions are successful and avoid the traumas of secrecy, silence and searching, use of the term is still vague and may lead to misunderstandings. Not all work; in some cases the birth mother fails to resolve her relinquishment (she usually has more time to decide), or adoptive parents (who can cut down on waiting time dramatically) may decide to end contact against birth parent wishes.

As a potential adoptive parent, you owe it to yourself and your future adopted child to investigate these controversies and hear the issues from all sides, but particularly from the adoptees'. One important proposal to investigate is the idea of a separate legal contract, to be signed at the time of the adoption, in which you would agree to provide information to the agency from time to time about the child's progress, and in which the agency would agree to act as a go-between between you and the birth parents. In this way the agony of searching (often without success) would not be necessary, and adoptees could meet their birth parents easily as soon as they were ready. Birth mothers would be spared the torment of silence and lack of knowledge. "Just knowing that she is all right, doing well, would have been such a relief," one birth mother said. Most important of all, for the first time this would establish a mechanism to help protect against undetected abuses.

RESOURCES*

Infertility

Baran, A., et al. *Lethal Secrets: The Shocking Consequences and Unsolved Problems of Artificial Insemination*. New York: Warner Books, 1989. Explores effects on children and parents.

Carter, Jean, and Mike Carter. *Sweet Grapes: How to Stop Being Infertile and Start Living Again*. Indianapolis: Perspectives Press, 1989. About child-free living.

DeCherney, Alan, and Mary Lake Polan. *Decision Making in Infertility*. Philadelphia: B.C. Decker, 1988.

Franklin, Robert R., and Dorothy Kay Brockman. *In Pursuit of Fertility: A Consultation with a Specialist*. New York: Henry Holt & Co., 1990.

Glazer, Ellen, and Susan Cooper. *Without Child: Experiencing and Resolving Infertility*. Lexington, MA: Lexington Books/D.C. Health, 1988.

Hopkins, Ellen. "Tales from the Baby Factory," *New York Times Magazine*, March 15, 1991. Excellent discussion of the many problems and low success rates encountered by women seeking IVF.

Lasker, Judith N., and Susan Borg. *In Search of Parenthood: Coping with Infertility and High Tech Conception*. Boston: Beacon Press, 1987.

Menning, Barbara Eck. *Infertility: A Guide for the Childless Couple*, 2nd ed. New York: Prentice-Hall, 1988.

Noble, E. *Having Your Baby by Artificial Insemination: A Complete Resource Guide*. Boston: Houghton Mifflin, 1988.

Office of Technology Assessment. *Infertility: Medical and Social Choices* (GPD No. 052-003-010971-7). Washington, DC: U.S. Government Printing Office, 1988. Available from Superintendent of Documents, Government Printing Office, Washington, DC 20402-9325.

Salzer, Linda. *Surviving Infertility*. New York: Harper Perennial, 1991.

Pregnancy Loss

Borg, Susan, and Judith Lasker. *When Pregnancy Fails: Families Coping with Miscarriage, Stillbirth, and Infant Death*. Boston: Beacon Press, 1981.

Friedman, Rochelle, and Bonnie Gradstein. *Surviving Pregnancy Loss*. Boston: Little, Brown, 1982.

Panuthos, Claudia, and Catherine Romeo. *Ended Beginnings: Healing Childbearing Losses*. New York, NY: Bergin & Garvey/Greenwood Press, 1984.

Scher, Jonathan, and Carol Dix. *Preventing Miscarriage: The Good News*. New York: Harper & Row, 1990.

Shapiro, Constance. *Infertility and Pregnancy Loss*. San Francisco: Jossey-Bass, 1988.

Schweibert, Pat, and P. Kirk. *Still to Be Born*. Portland, OR: University of Oregon Health Sciences Center, 1986.

*Please see the Resources for Chapter 16, "If You Think You Are Pregnant: Finding Out and Deciding What to Do," for more information about adoption. See also Resources for Chapter 18, "New Reproductive Technologies."

Adoption

Elgart, Arty, and C. Berman. *Golden Cradle: How the Adoption Establishment Works*. New York: Citadel Press Books, 1991.

Gilman, Lois. *The Adoption Resource Book*. New York: Harper & Row, 1988.

Melina, Lois. *Making Sense of Adoption*. New York: Harper & Row, 1989.

Paul, Ellen. *Adoption Choices*. Detroit: Visible Ink Press, 1991.

Organizations

Compassionate Friends
P.O. Box 1347
Oak Brook, IL 60521
Chapters around the country, offers support after pregnancy loss or death of a child.

Concerned United Birthparents (CUB)
2000 Walker Street
Des Moines, IA 50317

Endometriosis Association
8585 76th Place
Milwaukee, WI 53223

National Adoption Information Clearinghouse
1400 Eye Street N.W., Suite 600
Washington, DC 20005

North American Council on Adoptable Children
810 18th Street N.W.
Washington, DC 20006

Pregnancy and Infant Loss Center
1415 East Wayzata Boulevard
Wayzata, NM 55391

Resolve, Inc.
1310 Broadway
Somerville, MA 02144
(617) 623-0744
National organization with over fifty chapters in the United States. Offers medical referrals, newsletters, fact sheets, and a telephone hot line. Has accepted funds from Serono Labs, which markets Pergonal.

Women Growing Older

23

Women Growing Older

By Paula Brown Doress, with Norma Meras Swenson, Robin Cohen, Mickey Friedman, Lois Harris and Kathleen MacPherson

With special thanks to Edith Fletcher, Ruth Hubbard, Barbara Krentzman, Lucile Longview Schuck, Anna Shenke, Anne Smith (all members of the Older Women's Group) and to Marian Saunders and Diana Laskin Siegal.

Menopause by Louise Corbett.

With special thanks to Tish Anisimov, Davi Birnbaum, Lorraine Doherty, Ruth Hubbard, Kathleen MacPherson, Audrey Michaud, Josephine Polk-Matthews and Diana Laskin Siegal (members of the Menopause Collective in 1983).

The "Menopause" chapter in previous editions was written by Meg Hickey, Irene Davidson, Pamela Berger and Judy Norsigian.

1992 Update by Diana Laskin Siegal.

My birthday started with my standing wet on the hilltop watching lightning zag straight down to the earth—moving from north to west—then work in the studio—then a friend with gifts, then two loved sculptor apprentices with flowers and a salad fresh with surprises and green and fruits like flowers....
And when well-wishers hoping to please me referred to this birthday as my 29th, I asserted my conviction that 78 was far more wonderful than 29![1]

Several groups of women participated in discussions about this chapter, which covers the decades in a woman's life from the forties through the eighties and beyond. The Menopause Collective wrote the section on menopause. An older women's group, ages fifty-two to seventy-eight, meeting over the course of a year, talked about their lives, provided important resources, pinpointed issues and contributed to the writing and editing. A midlife group, ages thirty-nine to fifty-six, met with us in a series of sessions and became a support group for each other; they also met with the older women's group a number of times to gain perspectives on their own lives and those of their parents.*

---

*The revisions of this chapter for this edition were done by one woman in consultation with others.

their skills and wisdom is particularly prevalent in times of rapid social and technological change, when we may forget that we can still learn a lot about living from those who have a greater reservoir of life experience.

Finally, a major source of ageism in our profit-oriented system is the devaluing of all those who don't "produce"—the old, the young, and their caregivers. For instance, some elders are pushed aside before we are ready to retire on the assumption that, once past a certain age, we can make no significant contribution.

Aging tends to exaggerate or deepen class differences. Wealthy elders are often able to maintain their economic position, while low-income persons inevitably grow poorer if they become ill and can't get paid work anymore. (This is especially true for women.)

Even as we ourselves age, we discriminate against older people. A woman in her seventies states:

I had always said, "Oh, I want to be with people of all ages, or with young people," but in fact I was avoiding being with people my own age—which would mean admitting I'm an old person—and missing out on a lot because of it!

I signed up for a weekend of hiking through the Elderhostel,* and that changed my mind. Everyone was so alert. We were all in sports clothes and we didn't have our hair waved just right. We're not Amazons by any means, just people interested in vigorous outdoor activity.

Midlife and elder women have taken action against stereotyped media images that foster ageism. The Gray Panthers and the Older Women's League conduct "media watches," and many individuals are keeping alert.

Every time I see a positive image of an older woman on TV, I write a complimentary letter to the sponsor of the program. And when I see something offensive, I let them know that, too.

There have been successes. For example, the images of midlife and older women depicted in medical journal ads have improved noticeably in the past decade.

Ageism, not age itself, is what limits elders. The fact that I can do things at seventy that when I was sixty

Bonnie Burt

Women experience so many changes—physical, social, economic and emotional—during these decades that we can't do justice to them in a short chapter. Yet, because older women's concerns are so often overlooked, even in feminist books, it is important to begin.*

THE CONTEXT IN WHICH WE GROW OLDER

Age and Ageism

Someday each of us will be old if we live long enough. Most of us want to live a long life, yet our ageist culture values neither aging nor being old and separates people by age and generation.

Ageism is systematic discrimination against persons because of their chronological age. It permeates our thinking in subtle and unconscious ways so that the discrimination against elders, which goes on in every one of our social institutions, appears to be "just the way things are"— until we name and confront it.

Ageism has several sources. First, our society denies the reality of infirmity and death, especially because many of us secretly cherish a belief in our own immortality. Infirmity threatens our national ideology of rugged independence. We isolate the aging and infirm to avoid acknowledging our ultimate interdependence and our own fears of infirmity and death. This massive denial discourages us from planning for our later years.

Second, isolation of elders and dismissal of

---

*Work on this chapter inspired a new book project by and for midlife and older women. *Ourselves, Growing Older: Women Aging with Knowledge and Power* by Paula Brown Doress and Diana Laskin Siegal et al., in cooperation with the Boston Women's Health Book Collective, was published in 1987 by Simon & Schuster.

---

*Elderhostel (see Resources for the address) is an adult education program for older people. Courses are given on a weekly basis, usually with living arrangements in dormitories. Many elders are also taking courses for credit and enrolled in degree programs. Further education is one of the greatest unmet needs of elders.

would have been frowned upon as inappropriate for an older woman shows how absurd ageism is, and how much difference changing social attitudes can make. Every time we speak out, we change attitudes. Affirming ourselves is something that's in the air now. That makes a lot more things possible.

The Feminization of Aging

The single most significant fact about our aging as women is that the population of older persons is overwhelmingly female. Women live, on the average, nearly seven years longer than men. And more people are living longer than ever before.*

The problems that arise with aging—chronic illness, insufficient economic resources, care-giving or needing care, surviving one's relatives and closest friends—are predominantly women's problems. Yet the researchers and policymakers have mainly been men who overlook older women's special concerns. Because we are statistically "invisible," the resulting programs don't address our needs.

RATIO OF WOMEN TO MEN IN THREE AGE GROUPS

Up to age 45 ♀ ♀ ♀ ♂ ♂ ♂

Numbers are equal—women 50 percent, men 50 percent. At age forty-five, the gap first begins to widen.

Over 65 ♀ ♀ ♀ ♂ ♂

By age sixty-five, women comprise 60 percent and men 40 percent. Women over sixty-five are no longer the fastest-growing segment of the U.S. population. Now the "baby-boomers," ages thirty-five to forty-four, are the largest bulge in the population. The women in this age group need to be concerned about the issues they will face as they age.

Over 75 ♀ ♀ ♂

Women's longevity rates continue to outstrip those of men. Women's life expectancy at birth is 78.3 years; men's is 71.5. Of those who survive to age sixty-five, women can expect to live to 83.6; men, to 79.9. Women are 65 percent of the population seventy-five years and over.[2]

A positive side of our growing numbers is our potentially greater clout as a political constituency. Women over forty now make up 20.5 percent of the U.S. population. The government and the press are paying more attention to us. We need to take advantage of this attention to create, demand and fight for programs that will be responsive to midlife and older women's needs.*

Married or single, we must take friendships with women more seriously, for it is women who will most likely sustain us when we are older. Large numbers of women outlive their husbands, often by a decade of two, and a significant number even outlive their eldest sons. A woman in her fifties states:

I was brought up to believe that the people in my biological family were the most important people in my world. I'm still very attached to immediate family members but I have consciously extended my family to include my "sisters" in the women's community.

According to a woman in her forties,

My loneliest times were during my marriage. I came out as a lesbian and my life with women has been a revelation. But so many women I meet don't understand my problems as a single parent and are younger than me. Coming to an older woman's meeting has made me realize that I want to meet more women my own age.

A woman in her sixties states:

I had never particularly liked women. When I was younger I remember thinking that men were where it was at; they were smart and they did things. I've rethought that a few times, especially after my experiences with death, divorce, major problems with children. We all have to deal with loss because we women are the ones who care for men when they are ill, and they are the ones who go first. It's given me a tremendous compassion for other women.

Ageism and Sexism
The Double-Edged Sword

The ageism we face is compounded by sexism and a double standard that considers women old at an earlier age than men.[3]

A sixty-two-year-old woman tells of her friendship with a sixty-year-old man:

It was hard for me to tell the man I have been going out with how old I am. When I told him, I felt ter-

---

*People sixty-five and over now make up 12.5 percent of the population of the United States and are expected to be 18 percent of the population by 2020.

*The Older Women's League is an important national organization to advocate for older women's concerns (see Resources).

Peter Menzel/Stock Boston

rible, as if I were telling him I had some socially disgraceful disease. You can't imagine!

In fact, women have greater vitality. In terms of life expectancy, it can be argued that women are "younger" than men of the same age.

This double standard for aging leads us to accept the view that while older men are craggy, women are wrinkled; gray hair, distinguished on a man, shows that a woman is "over the hill"; maturity makes a man sexually attractive, a woman grandmotherly.

I'm never going to be a "gray-haired old lady," never! People don't listen to what you say anyway because you are a woman, but if you are an old woman, forget it. I'm going to dye my hair until I die.

Our culture sees the sexuality of midlife women and elders as a source of humor—grotesque, threatening or inappropriate. Such a prejudice arises in part from falsely equating sexuality with reproductive capacity.

Poverty

After a lifetime of being either unpaid or underpaid, it is no accident that older women are considerably poorer than older men.* The poverty rate for women over sixty-five is more than *double* that for men over sixty-five. The median income in 1990 for an older white woman living alone was $9,946; for an older black woman living alone it was $5,920.[5] Although many older women lack

*Studies of poverty in the 1970s and 1980s found that the new poor are single women with children. In 1990 there are more women in this group. One out of four full-time working women do not earn enough to keep them out of poverty.[4]

basic necessities, many more are faced with being poorer than when we were younger, struggling to get by on limited funds.

- There is neither compensation, recognition nor pension eligibility for women whose work is homemaking. When we return to the workforce later in life, we often must take jobs that pay extremely low wages.* Many midlife and older women find themselves unemployable for lack of "recent" experience.†
- Due to sex discrimination, women earn less and receive less income from retirement plans.‡
- Women often work in the kinds of marginal jobs and industries that are not unionized and do not provide benefits such as pensions.
- Many women are not in the paid labor force for enough years or for the particular years required for pension eligibility. Many women workers are employed from age seventeen to twenty-five, leave to raise a family and return to work sometime between thirty-five and forty-four. Yet employees are not eligible to join pension plans in most companies until age twenty-five, while in other companies new employees over forty-five are excluded.[8] Even women who postpone having children and remain in the workforce until taking time off in their thirties and forties will have reduced pensions.
- Widowed or divorced women may find themselves ineligible for their husband's pensions. Many companies offer employees a choice of higher benefits in their lifetime or a reduced rate if spread over both spouses lifetimes. Now both spouses must sign the decision, giving women more power to protect themselves. Prior to this recent change, only 5 percent of widows collected on deceased spouse's benefits. Widows were 65% of the elderly poor in 1987.[9]

Economic Planning

Many of the women in the elder women's group talked about how important it is to take ourselves

*The majority of women over forty-five work in retail sales, unskilled or semiskilled factory work, private household work, other service jobs and clerical work. While men's earnings peak in the middle years, women may have difficulty establishing or maintaining employability.[6]
†The requirement of "recent" experience, as Tish Sommers (of the Older Women's League) pointed out, is not overtly sexist or ageist, but its effect is to exclude older women. If we are unable to find work during our middle years, we are also ineligible for most income supports and services which are designed for mothers with children under eighteen or elders over sixty-five. In response to this abysmal situation, the Displaced Homemakers programs, started by two such women, offer counseling, job training and placement (see Resources).[7]
‡In 1986, women with pensions collected an average monthly amount of $417; men collected $744.

seriously and do economic planning that lays the groundwork for having choices in our later years. Often we have to learn about money for the first time. The middle years—approximately forty-five to sixty-four—are critical for women economically. If we have not worked for pay before, in these key years we can work for pay, establish a retirement fund and plan for our older years as well.

According to a woman in her fifties with grown children,

I want to earn as much money as possible now before the potentials and the opportunities are completely gone. So I'm working harder, not necessarily because I want to but because I feel the time is getting shorter.

A woman in her forties who is divorced and the sole support of her children states:

I'm envious of people who can plan for the future— I know it's wise. But I'm blocking out thinking about getting older because I can't deal with any more than the present. If I tried to put away money for the future, I would have to do without the tiny creature comforts and little delights of life which I want now.

Because we all are growing older, we all have a stake in supporting older women's demands and concerns. We have to work on upgrading women's jobs and salaries as well as learning to plan for ourselves. Many social changes that would help older women to participate more fully in the workplace are similar to those needed by younger women with children: caregiving services for children and sick family members, better access to health care, flexibility in jobs.

I developed a new material for sculpting after my husband died. No one knew about it until a few years ago when I was invited to come to the university as a visiting artist. So I started my teaching career at seventy-two. I had two classes for fifty students and taught one day a week for three years. Oh, how I loved it! It was wonderful! Then they restructured the school and got rid of all the part-time teachers, and I couldn't possibly undertake to do a full-time teaching load, so I had to stop teaching.

Working a nine-to-five job is not the only way of being "productive." We know that we contribute to society whether we are working for pay, raising children or grandchildren, caring for a sick family member or working in our communities as volunteers. Whatever our differences, we must stand together as we fight for the changes that will recognize and reward our contributions to our families and communities.

THE MIDDLE YEARS

Exploration, Growth and Expansion

Midlife, the years approximately between forty-five and sixty-five, is more a life stage than a particular chronological period. Midlife often announces itself with a surge of new energy, perhaps simply restlessness, or with a growing recognition that we are coming to the end of familiar roles and ways of living. We take stock of our lives and desire to use our time and our abilities in new and different ways.

One day after twenty-odd years of marriage and three children I asked myself, "Who am I? What am I doing? Where am I going?" The only answer I could come up with was "I am a wife and mother." That was only part of me—not all of me. When I was younger I used to have fairly clear edges, but over the years being the mother and wife with unmatched fervor made those edges fuzzy.

I loved my work as a nurse. I'd never married or had children. I always denied that I experienced sexism until, when I was thirty-eight, a new male nurse was

from "Sylvia" by Nicole Hollander

promoted to head of my service. That left me fuming. I used my life savings and then some to go back to college and then medical school. I've never been sorry.

A woman in her forties:

I just want more! More time free of kids to focus on my work; more time to myself; more passion in my marriage, or from somewhere else!

This surge of energy may come with release from two decades of child rearing. Even while we miss our children, we can use freed-up time for refocusing—to acquire new skills, refine old ones, spend more time with people, get a job, work harder at our present job, enjoy time for reflection. It feels, as one woman puts it, like "getting ourselves back."

I am writing to assure women of middle age or beyond that it is not too late to attend school and begin a career or to switch careers.

All my life I had wanted to be a nurse but instead was a secretary. Finally, at age fifty-seven, when the youngest of our children graduated from college, I took a year from the workaday world to attend school and become a licensed practical nurse.

I made the highest grade in our class on the state board exam. I am not telling this to be boastful but to encourage others who might think they are too old to learn.

Seven years later, at age sixty-five, I am happily employed as an LPN—my lifelong dream.

I returned to college for several reasons—as a response to a suddenly very empty house (three sons going away to school at once) and a major change (we had just moved to the country from a large city), to increase my knowledge of rural social work and to finish a degree begun thirty years earlier. I wanted to prepare for what I dimly perceived might be the beginning of a new chapter—and what turned out to be a whole new edition!

The unexpected results were that I rediscovered my own intelligence and found skills I had been unaware of. I connected with much younger women and forged relationships that have continued long after graduation. I encouraged several contemporaries to jump in and try it! In my fieldwork in human services, I came in contact with various local and state decision makers and immediately found the door wide open for getting involved with community issues. This in turn enabled me to start an independent practice, working with and for elders and their families. I will never have to retire, and as my professional focus and confidence deepen and grow, I learn valuable lessons from those elders who are not only my clients but my teachers.

We may experience a change in our perspective—a heightened awareness of the passage of time and of the value of the time we have left. For today's women over forty, time at home or time devoted to full-time child rearing without some kind of paid work outside the home is increasingly rare. Poor women, who have always worked, and affluent women struggling to have it all may both find that only at retirement will they have the freedom to explore other interests or develop new skills, or just be at home.

A fifty-year-old woman states:

Now is the time to do the things I've always wanted to do. I'm no longer thinking in terms of "someday," but "soon."

It was a shock when a friend of ours, a middle-aged man, died suddenly. It got me thinking that I don't know how many years Dan and I have left together. I've been working hard and had some successes. Work is still very important to me, but I no longer want it to absorb my whole life. Now that we're in our forties, I want to spend time together and have fun.

When I was fifty I was the oldest person in my community and quite conscious of being older. I thought (this seems ridiculous now that I am seventy-six) that I certainly had to plan ahead because I wouldn't have much time left. In the next five or ten years I wanted to go to Africa and travel a lot before I died.

An eighty-five-year-old woman reflecting on her past choices:

Enjoy now as much as you can because there is almost never a tomorrow the exact way you would like to have it.

Losses During the Middle Years

In addition to growth and expansion, the middle years can bring a number of painful losses that, coming in quick succession, feel like "a crescendo of losses." Statistically, many of the important losses that women face cluster in the forty-five to fifty-five-year period. We mourn these losses and often don't know how to express our feelings or to whom.

Some losses undermine our image of ourselves as young, healthy, even immortal, as when diseases attack the very wholeness of our bodies. Breast cancer strikes one out of nine women, bringing the threat of surgery or even death. Thirty-seven percent of women are estimated to have had a hysterectomy by age sixty.* The rest of us lose our fertility at menopause at the average

---

*Cancer accounts for only 10.7 percent of all hysterectomies. Fibroids, the most common diagnosis, account for 27 percent.[10] Fibroids are stimulated by estrogen and so will generally shrink after menopause provided no estrogen is taken.

age of fifty. Our children are going through their adolescent years or leave home at about the same time that our fertility ends. Other important relationships may end or change: Our husbands may die, or, through divorce, they "pass on—to a younger woman." We may suffer one of the saddest losses—the loss of a child. Our parents may become ill or die. If we have to care for them or for our husbands, we may have to give up or postpone long-awaited changes or adventures. All these situations may leave us with less money and/or no health insurance and cause considerable stress and bereavement.

Changes in Body Image

Not as serious as threats to our health, but sometimes causing painful feelings of loss, are the surface signs of aging that eventually require us to develop a new body image. As we notice the changes or observe that others respond to us differently, we may keenly feel the loss of our youthful looks, in which we have been taught that much of our value resides.

When I walk down the street with my daughter now, I notice that when male heads turn in our direction they are looking at her. My pride in her blossoming young womanhood is bittersweet, because I miss getting that attention myself.

Employers may unfairly dismiss us as incompetent and useless if we don't present a contemporary (read "youthful") image and deny us opportunities if we "look our age" or have "let ourselves go" by refusing to diet or dye our hair. In our social groups and relationships youthful appearance may be overly valued.

A few months ago I let my white hair reemerge after some years of dyeing it. I thought it was more authentic. The man I am seeing now is about my age [sixty-two]. He said that because he doesn't have white hair, he would like me to continue coloring my hair. After thinking it over, I decided that I prefer it colored, too.

A fifty-two-year-old woman:

Most lesbians' culture is youth-oriented, and I feel better with my hair brown rather than gray. People don't look at me as though I'm old.

Some of us feel more confident when we can delay the outward signs of aging by using makeup and hair dyes.* Yet a growing number of us believe that our years and experience entitle us to wear

our graying hair, wrinkles or extra pounds— badges of mature womanliness—with pride. Being older provides a time to experiment with different colors, unconventional styles and new ways of presenting ourselves.

I look in the mirror and am always a little surprised that, with my graying hair and some new wrinkles, I don't feel what I'm "supposed" to be feeling.

If I were not constantly bombarded from reading, media and society in general with reminders that now that I'm fifty-three I'm supposed to be in crisis, withdrawing, feeling depressed, isolated, incapable or ashamed, these ideas wouldn't occur to me. I am simply building on what was before, seeking out new opportunities. I am, as always, energetic and involved.

I like being heavier. I take up more space. People listen to me more.

GRANDMOTHER ROCKING

Last night I dreamed of an old lover
I had not seen him in forty years.
When I awoke,
I saw him on the street,
his hair was white,
his back stooped.
How could I say hello?
He would have puzzled all day
about who the young girl was
who smiled at him.
So I let him go on his way.

—EVE MERRIAM

When Our Children Grow Up and Leave

At this time most of us feel the satisfaction of a job well done, or at least over.† Many women look forward to this time as a release from constant responsibility.‡ Yet we feel sadness, for we no longer have a daily relationship with our child(ren), some of whom had become close friends and confidants.

Divorced or single mothers of dependent children receiving child-support payments or welfare

---

*See Chapter 7, "Environment and Occupational Health," for a discussion of carcinogens in cosmetics, especially most commercial hair dyes.[11] Ingredients must now be listed on cosmetics. Those developed without testing on animals and with ingredients thought to be safe may be expensive.

†Child rearing is such a major part of so many women's lives that we cannot possibly do it justice here. For a whole chapter on parents' feelings when their children leave home, see *Ourselves and Our Children: A Book by and for Women* by the Boston Women's Health Collective, New York: Random House, 1978.

‡In Lillian Rubin's study of middle-aged women, at least one-quarter of the women expressed relief when the last child left home.[12]

may face economic dislocation when children leave home.*

When child-raising has been our main work and we haven't planned what to do next, we may be at loose ends. Identity crises have less to do with the "emptied nest" and more to do with the question, "What am I going to do with myself now?"

As we develop our own skills and interests, we can acknowledge missing our children, yet be glad of the extra time for our other pursuits.

The "Dependency Squeeze" of the Middle Years

Just when we are gearing up to focus on what *we* want, perhaps for the first time, new family demands may actually increase, with pressures for attention from both older and younger generations.

Caregiving has its own set of stresses. It is important for those of us who are caregivers to learn about supportive services available to our aging parents. This is particularly helpful for those of us caring for our parents long distance. It is helpful to join support groups not only to learn about services but to get support and nurturing for ourselves.†

As a single parent with young children and aging parents having health problems, I am pulled between two sets of needs. The pressures are most intense on Sundays when I "should" visit my parents. (They get home-care services on weekdays but none on weekends.) At the same time, since I work every day and go to school two nights a week, I want to do something wholesome and "outdoorsy" with my children. When Monday morning dawns I haven't had a day to sleep late, peruse the Sunday papers, bake bread or go for a walk with a friend—and when I try to take one I end up feeling guilty all the next week.

A further complication is that our mates or lovers may resent attention to aging parents just when children have left.

Because of financial pressures, some adult children are coming back home to live.‡ Some mothers wearily resume old parental roles and feel used and abused.

"I can't tell you how many times they have borrowed our car and wrecked it. Does that ring a bell?"

Sarah Putnam

"Are you kidding? Why do you think my car has all those different-color fenders?"

Other mothers, feeling newly independent, are better able to create new kinds of relationships.

After my children were grown and wanted to return home, I made it clear they were welcome only as equal adults bearing their share of the responsibilities of the home, not in a mother–child role.

You may have a respite between child rearing and the caregiving demands of the middle and later years.

One of the main reasons that I'm taking an extended trip is that I feel I have this golden moment when Deborah doesn't have a baby she needs help with and my parents are still well.

Often we don't have many choices. Yet even as we attempt to meet many demands on our time and energy, we are entitled to make some time for ourselves.

Loss of People We Love

As we watch our parents and relatives age, we begin to prepare ourselves for their deaths.

Two of my favorite uncles died a few years ago. Now my favorite aunt at seventy has cancer of the pancreas, and a third uncle has just had his second heart attack. I wept and wept about these real and threatened deaths of people who are like stalwart, familiar trees in the landscape of my childhood. I shouted, "No, I can't stand this; not my favorite aunt!" I know that it's inevitable. I dread my mother's phone calls now because every time she announces another

---

*Twenty-three million women who are divorced, separated, or widowed plus those who will lose AFDC benefits when their children leave home are in particularly difficult situations and often have trouble finding work. Government services have been created seemingly without these women in mind (see Displaced Homemakers in Resources).
†See Caregiving in Resources.
‡The stress of this return is sending some parents to therapists. (Roberta J. Apfel, MD, lecture on depression, Beth Israel Hospital, Boston, Spring 1982.)

illness, another death. Such present and imminent loss makes me value everyone I love and life itself.

My aunt said that every winter when she goes down to Florida a few more of her friends there have died. I said I can't imagine what that would be like; she said, "Well, that's just the way it is."

My mother now suffers both from a chronic and a progressive disease in an advanced state and from some of the debilitating effects of being in poor health and approaching eighty. She seems to be gradually fading away, her hair becoming whiter, her skin paler.

In my own life at the same time I have been going through a difficult transition—the end of a fifteen-year marriage—and experiencing some physical changes of midlife. For a while I equated them with my potential decay and imminent death, as a parallel to my mother's decline. My periods had become prolonged and heavy. I was anemic, looking pale (like my mother), and my hair was graying. I chipped a tooth twice in one month and began to worry about whether this meant my bones were becoming fragile. The bleeding got worse; I wore a pad for weeks each month because tampons were insufficient; it felt like a diaper, which is what my mother has to wear. My gynecologist recommended a hysterectomy. I felt totally sexless, listless and lifeless. Now I see that some of these changes were transitory health problems, which I got help for, and others simply the normal changes of middle age, with depression and stress exaggerating my feelings and fears.

Some of my relatives had criticized the decision to place my mother in a nursing home. Part of my identification with her decline came from guilt that I could go on and live and even enjoy my life when my mother was in such poor health.

One night during that time I dreamed of my own death. Instead of fear, I felt peace and completion. My work on earth had been accomplished. My only sadness was regret at not being able to attend my daughter's wedding. I transformed myself into a beautiful rainbow—nature's chuppah [Jewish wedding canopy]—and protected the festivities from bad weather. I could feel that my daughter recognized the rainbow as my gift to her.

When I awoke I was at peace with saying goodbye to my mother when the time came. I knew she would no more want to take me with her, scary as it is to die alone, than I would want my daughter's life to end with my death.

Widowhood

Three out of four women will be widows. Of 13.7 million widowed persons in the United States, 11.4 million are women,[13] and many more millions of women have lost "unofficial" partners, male and female, whom they had been loving or living with. A widowed woman lives, on the average, eighteen years after the death of a spouse. Chances of remarriage are low and decrease with age, because three out of four elderly men are married,* but only one out of three elderly women is.

The stress of widowhood is enormous, one of the most difficult life situations women live through. *Widows are particularly vulnerable to disease and often lose or cannot afford health insurance coverage just when it is most needed.* Grief is compounded when we

- Have found our main identity in being a wife.
- Are isolated and lonely after the initial mourning period.
- Find that most of our friends are in couples.
- Have to seek new friends as a formerly married person.
- Have to seek paid employment for the first time in decades.
- Need a crash course in financial planning.

We must negotiate all this while we are still numb with the shock of loss.†

We need people to call us up, visit, bring food, invite us to do things, shovel the car out and leave us alone when that's what we want. Yet some may pull back, especially after the initial formalized mourning period, embarrassed or frightened by our grieving or our neediness. Many women have found special support and understanding from other widows.‡ Ultimately we can build new lives.

When I was widowed at forty-nine, with five children ages twelve to twenty-two, my whole life was in turmoil. I had to cope not only with my own grief and insecurities but also those of his distraught parents and our children. I couldn't sleep nights for fear of the future. Would the children's lives be ruined, their educations shot; would I ever get over the emptiness on the other side of the bed? I developed giant hives, a swollen toe the doctor couldn't account for, lost fifteen pounds—even the dog developed allergies. Sleepless at night, I felt inadequate and aimless by day. Something had to be done, and I finally realized I was the only one who could do it.

I resolved to think objectively about each thing I felt unable to cope with. I started by reading the insurance policies in the long reaches of the night

---

*The majority who have lost their wives remarry. Those who remain single have higher death and illness rates. It is thought that women adjust better to widowhood despite the stresses because of our greater ability to make and keep friends.[14]

†The full impact of our loss may come months or even a year later. For some women it takes up to two years to feel pleasure and enjoy life again. Be wary of doctors who try to medicate away our normal grieving or label it pathological if it takes "too long."

‡See Widowhood in Resources for widow-to-widow groups.

when I couldn't sleep—I slept exhausted trying to make sense of the legalese. I read library books on the stock market and investments. I read Consumer Reports *on cars. I encouraged my children to get jobs and fill up their free time with income-producing activities. My twelve-year-old began baby-sitting and keeping track of her income and expenditures. The day she reached $1000 was a triumph for her. They all gained some sense of security from knowing they could produce their own clothes and spending money, even save some toward college tuition. They were too busy to get into teenage trouble. I rented our summer cottage instead of selling it—a stroke of genius, as it provided us in June and September a place to renew ourselves physically and emotionally. I made a list of the things I could have fun at without a man and did them. I took a part-time job, I set my life in order again—a very different order, but my own. I developed a new self-confidence and* joie de vivre. *It took about three years.*

When my husband died five years after our divorce, I experienced, with the utter finality of his death, the absolute end of our relationship. Suddenly the years of separation were obliterated and I mourned deeply the loss of my husband, the father of my children, and the ending of the whole life we had shared.

My husband died after a seven-year period when his health had been deteriorating and I had been his primary caretaker. My mother died within six weeks of his death. So, in addition to losing a husband and a mother, I lost a part of myself, my role as a helping, caring person.

I went out to my mother's farm and sat out there for six weeks. I did a lot of different things, but I spent a lot of time writing about what I had left now that I no longer had that identity: Who am I?

And what I had left was that I was a woman and I was growing older, and that was the beginning of both my feminism and my understanding of the concept of aging. That became a new identity for me.

A lot of us women are not reared to believe that we can make something of what we are. I had been my parents' child and my husband's wife and my children's mother. Now I had the opportunity to be a person in my own right.

Coping with a Series of Losses

This process is one of our most difficult midlife tasks.

A psychiatrist gave me Valium when I was in my forties. I took it or Equanil regularly or fairly regularly for about five to ten years. Now I think that tranquilizers suppressed or sent underground the pains of that period (divorce, death of mother, betrayal by a lover). These pains still surface with ag-

onizing strength. Maybe if I had fully faced them and "digested" them at the time they happened, this would not be the case.

When devastating losses occur in a cluster, we feel stunned and very much alone. Don't expect too much of yourself at this time. One of the best things you can do for yourself is accept your feelings as normal and not try to carry the load without help. Watch out for doctors who want to medicate away legitimate feelings of sadness and rage. It is a sign of strength to be able to acknowledge feelings of despair, anger, guilt, emptiness, fear, relief, anxiety, confusion. There is no right time or right way to grieve.* Each of us has her own unique rhythm. Talking with women who have "been there" often helps, as does reminiscing, writing or keeping a journal.

It takes enormous energy to rebuild your life. Don't exhaust yourself trying to take care of the emotional needs of others. Take special care of yourself. You will probably need more rest than usual. Go slowly—give yourself time to heal and to regain your trust in the world and in your own capacities.

MENOPAUSE

Prevailing Social Views

Stereotypical thinking about menopausal women includes many myths (many created and perpetuated by doctors and psychiatrists).

The first thing that comes to my mind about menopause is FALLACIES: Menopause is blamed for every mood change and unexplained feeling, the way menstruation is with younger women; also discrimination and derision—"she must be going through the change."

Helene Deutsch, a disciple of Freud, referred to menopause as women's "partial death." Mastering psychological reaction to menopause was, she said, "one of the most difficult tasks of a woman's life."[15] It would be more accurate to say that our most difficult task is mastering reaction to the cultural stereotype of menopausal women, a process that is complicated and made even more difficult by the fact that we cannot help internalizing that image to some degree.

The "raging hormones" myth describes menopausal women as so incapacitated by hormone fluctuations that they are incapable of rational thought and behavior and should certainly not

---

*In the professional literature you often find unhelpful prescriptive statements, like the assertion that if grieving lasts more than six months or a year it is pathological.

hold any kind of responsible position.* A more recent myth, part of the superwoman mystique, suggests that the usefully busy woman will hardly notice menopause at all. Neither extreme is accurate or helpful to women.

Particularly damaging is the myth linking menopause and depression. In the first half of this century, doctors and families hospitalized thousands of women for a "disorder" called *involutional melancholia,* a "mental disease" that supposedly occurred during or just after menopause. Some of us remember aunts, great-aunts or grandmothers who went into mental hospitals at menopause, some never to emerge again. Though contemporary studies fail to demonstrate that depression among midlife women is associated with menopause, the fear of going crazy at menopause is still part of our culture.[17] Yet involutional melancholia is not a disease but a myth.†

Even when a menopausal woman feels comfortable with herself, her family and others around her may resent her independence, mood swings or irritability, perhaps even fear these as signs of her growing older. They may urge drugs, surgery or psychotherapy on her rather than being willing to live with her through the changes.

Misogyny taints much of the medical literature. A well-known gynecologist/writer has referred to menopause as "a living decay,"[19] and another ob/gyn has said (in a federally sponsored symposium) that menopausal women are a "caricature of their younger selves at their emotional worst."[20] According to the same doctor (and author of a best-selling book), the menopausal woman is "not really a man but no longer a functional woman," and after menopause will "just be marking time until she follows her glands into oblivion."[21]‡ After helping to create the above stereotypes, doctors reinforce them by treating menopause as a deficiency disease to be managed with estrogen replacement "therapies," tranquilizers or surgery. In our efforts to counter such myths, we may unwittingly suggest that we can sail through menopause without even noticing its physical discomforts and emotional changes, not to mention the social realities facing midlife women. If we overlook the changes of menopause, we run the risk of trivializing our experience. Menopause is an important physical and emotional life transition, and we are different after we have gone through it. We can be strengthened and empowered by acknowledging the reality of our experiences and giving one another support during this transition.

Medical Definitions and Our Definition of Menopause

Definitions of menopause vary in medical literature, with little consensus on when it begins and ends and disagreement about its definitive signs. Texts refer to the "climacteric" as a fifteen-year period (from forty to fifty-five or forty-five to sixty) in the transition between reproductive ability and its ending: "The [female] climacteric is the gradual process of ovarian failure which normally precedes and extends beyond the last menses and within which menopause is only an event."[22] Menopause refers specifically only to the cessation of menses (menstrual periods). The current most widely used definition of menopause is a retrospective analysis—two years after the last menstrual period.[23]

Such textbook definitions fail to take into account the social and cultural context in which we live through menopause, our understanding of it and our varied emotional reactions. Going through menopause is experiencing the whole period that begins when we first have menstrual irregularities until menstruation finally stops completely and our bodies adjust to changes in estrogen production.

No one definition will satisfy every woman or cover all the varying aspects of menopause as we individually experience them.

I think of menopause as the psychological and emotional shifting of gears we experience when our hormone production changes, preparing us for a new stage of life.

Menopause is a slow turning in life. Your insides are changing but you remain the same person. Some people battle with this period as if trying to stop it. Some accept it and go through it more easily.

It's the end of periods and birth control. What a relief!

In the past twenty years, biomedical research into menopause has at last increased, partly because of the increased visibility of midlife women.

---

*Nineteenth-century doctors taught (and practiced on) the belief that the uterus was a source of disease and hysteria, especially once reproduction was over. Male doctors used myths about menopause to keep women out of medicine by casting doubt on their emotional stability.[16]

†Involutional melancholia has been dropped from the current edition of the *Diagnostic and Statistical Manual of Mental Disorders.* However, even up to the present time, women are subjected to treatments to cure depression presumably associated with menopause. "Over 70% of the population in mental hospitals is female. . . . Over 70% of those undergoing electroshock therapy are women, and more than 70% of those persons whose behavior is modified and controlled by therapy are women."[18]

‡Nothing has changed when *Physicians Weekly* associates menopause with "its wake of deadly and debilitating ills" (Alix Kerr, "A New NIH," Vol. 9, No. 2, [January 20, 1992] p. 1).

Women-initiated research on menopause chooses more relevant issues based on our own experiences.* Unfortunately most of the research has been conducted by drug companies based on women with problems who seek medical care[24] or studies of women in the general population looking back on the effects of drugs and/or surgery. Generalizations have often been drawn from the results without the further research needed on carefully matched groups.[25] Nineteen ninety-one brought increased funding by Congress for women's health issues, but advocates warn that the proposed research still requires careful scrutiny.

Physical Changes

Although medical and popular literature often discuss numerous menopause "symptoms," only three signs can be directly attributed to changes in estrogen production: (1) changes in menstrual cycle, (2) hot flashes and sweats (*vasomotor instability*) and (3) vaginal changes (decrease of moisture and elasticity in the vagina, sometimes called *atrophy*).[26]

Menstrual Changes

For most women the first signs of approaching menopause are changes in the menstrual cycle. Some of us menstruate more frequently than before, others skip periods or find that they are more widely spaced. We may have shorter periods with lighter bleeding or longer and/or heavier bleeding, sometimes with clots and "flooding."

The last time I flew in an airplane I perceived that I was flooding (though bolstered by a tampon and two pads) and rushed down the aisle to the bathroom. Blood flowed down my stockings and into my shoes. More dripped onto the carpet. Both bathrooms were occupied, of course. I waited, breathing deeply and resisting the very strong urge to kick in both doors.

Because very heavy or extended bleeding is such a frightening, disruptive and debilitating symptom, we can easily be pressured into taking drastic action, such as unnecessary surgery. (See the section on hysterectomy in Chapter 24, "Some Common and Uncommon Health and Medical Problems.") MDs think of heavy and irregular bleeding as a possible sign of cancer,[27] but this is true only in a small minority of cases.† It is a

possibility, so do check it out by asking for an endometrial biopsy, an office procedure. (See the section on uterine cancer in Chapter 24.) Because the training of MDs focuses so heavily on pathology and so little on the normal processes of women's bodies, many MDs have not learned that heavy, irregular or extended bleeding may simply reflect hormonal instability in women approaching menopause. Many women choose hysterectomy simply because of the disruption that the flooding causes in work and social life. However, many women are learning to cope by talking with other women who have this problem and by discovering new ways to decrease the flow, such as nonmedical approaches and alternative healing methods. If you want to consider these techniques, you should know that the most serious health risk you face, once cancer has been ruled out, is that of becoming anemic. Have your hemoglobin checked regularly and take iron only if yours is low.‡

Premenstrual symptoms may intensify or change, too, or begin to be noticeable for the first time.

The worst discomfort for me has been a great increase in premenstrual tension, extreme nervousness, breast soreness, headaches and insomnia for a week to ten days before my period.

One woman in five has no changes in her menstrual cycle at all until menstruation suddenly stops.[30]

It is hard to tell exactly when menstruation stops for good; periods may stop for several months, then start up again, and such fluctuations can last for a year or longer. Midlife women with irregular periods are at risk of pregnancy until they have been period-free for twenty-four months.

Hot Flashes

Another sign commonly associated with menopause is hot flashes (or flushes). Eighty percent of women report having hot flashes, but only 10 percent of these describe them as uncomfortable. Some women describe it as a sensation of heat in the face or moving through or across the upper half of the body. Sweating may follow, and sometimes you may experience a feeling like suffocation. Chills frequently precede or follow. Or the skin may feel "crawly." Hot flashes vary in intensity, duration and frequency. They can be aggra-

---

*See the work of Sonja McKinlay et al. (New England Research Institute, 4 Galen Street, Watertown, MA 02172), who have followed 2,500 randomly selected women before, through and after menopause.

†Only 6 percent of women develop uterine or ovarian cancer during the menopausal years, forty-five to fifty-four. The risk of cancer increases as we pass menopause, climbing to 14 per-

cent for ages sixty to sixty-four, the years of highest risk.[28] The risk is substantially increased if we have taken ERT, however.[29] (See the section on cancer in Chapter 24.)

‡You should not take iron unless a test shows you are anemic; you may take too much. (See p. 608 for guidance on iron supplements.)

vated by stress and diet. Some women get hot flashes when their bodies become overheated—during a heat wave, for example—when the thermostat is set too high, when they eat highly spiced food or drink coffee or alcohol.

During hot flashes, blood vessels dilate and constrict irregularly and unpredictably. No one knows exactly why this occurs. When ovarian estrogen production declines, the pituitary gland (located in the head) sends signals for the production of more estrogen. One theory is that hot flashes may be the body's attempt to respond.

Hot flashes may begin when menstruation is still regular or just beginning to fluctuate and continue after your periods end. Some women never experience them, whereas others have them off and on as late as their eighties. Many women are not bothered by their hot flashes. Some flashes are so mild that at first the woman experiencing them may think the room is too hot, there are too many blankets on the bed or the weather has changed. Some of us, however, are incapacitated by them. The sweating that follows can be so profuse that we need a complete change of clothes or bedclothes. Some women wake up five or six times a night or more, so that sleep may be seriously disturbed.

Some of us are embarrassed by hot flashes and particularly by their unpredictability, an embarrassment due in large part to the negative status of the aging woman as well as to the taboos, still prevalent, about "noticing" menstruation and menopause. Though you may feel hot or sweaty, most onlookers fail to notice what is usually a very slight change in coloring. Check your face in the mirror the next time you have a flash and you'll probably be reassured. Many of us find hot flashes less burdensome after we discuss them (and menopause in general) with other women. Some women carry folding fans to cool themselves, making themselves more comfortable and at the same time showing others that menopause is a perfectly normal occurrence.

Vaginal Changes

Changed estrogen levels may produce changes in the vagina (see p. 534).

Ovarian Function

When our ovaries no longer produce enough hormones to trigger the release of eggs or to build up menstrual blood and tissues on the inside wall of the uterus, both ovulation and menstruation eventually stop.* *Contrary to popular and medical*

---

*At press time, the discovery of a uterine hormone thought to control the time of menopause was announced. Called *inhibin*, its identification highlights how much we have yet to learn and how risky medical recommendations are often based on incomplete knowledge.

myth, these changes in ovarian function do not mean that our bodies or our ovaries stop producing estrogen. Long before the ovaries slow down, alternative sources of estrogen production are functioning in the fatty tissue of the body and in the adrenal glands, and the ovaries themselves usually continue to secrete small amounts of estrogen for ten years or longer after periods cease.

Adrenal Glands

Throughout life our adrenal glands help us cope with stress and maintain our resistance to disease. As estrogen from our ovaries begins to decline (beginning about age twenty-five), our adrenal glands gradually take over until they become our major source of estrogen after menopause. This is accomplished by converting a secretion called *androstenadione* into *estrone* (a nonovarian type of estrogen) in our blood and body fat. Exercising speeds this conversion process, and having a little fat on our bones makes it easier. While all living is stressful, we can make the adrenals' job easier by eating a healthy diet (including enough vitamins B and C) and getting adequate exercise and rest. Also, you may want to try relaxation practices and other ways of minimizing the effects of stress (see Chapter 5, "Health and Healing: Holistic Practices and Systems"). At this time in our lives comfortable habits, such as drinking coffee and alcohol and eating sweets, may actually become additional stresses on the adrenals, especially since the protection once provided by ovarian estrogen to heart, digestive organs, lungs, bones and skin must now come from the adrenals.

Other Changes

Some women cry more easily, feel irritable at times, are less patient or feel disorganized. Some of these emotional changes may be related to hormonal fluctuations. They may, however, also be a response to a culture that devalues older women or to the traumatic events that so often occur in midlife.

I definitely feel emotionally different. I am more assertive, my tolerance of people is lower. I get hurt and at times am confused about my feelings.

In what used to be a two-handkerchief movie, I may have to use four.

Minor physical changes also occur during these years, more or less at the same time as menopause. Our hair may thin, may turn gray, we may grow more facial hair, need reading glasses, gain weight. It is difficult to distinguish between signs of menopause and signs of aging; menopause itself is a sign of the aging of the female reproductive system. It is a common myth that all changes in midlife women are caused by menopause, with the implication that a woman's reproductive cycle is the major factor in her life and that once it stops, she is a changed person. In fact, men as well as women go through many of the changes, proof that they are not caused primarily by "estrogen deficiency."

Medical Approaches to Menopause

There is no growth without change. Menopause is a crucial stage in our psychic maturation.

A fifty-one-year-old woman:

I welcomed the end of my menstrual periods because for years I had experienced premenstrual tension and heavy bleeding. The hot flashes were not a bad trade-off if I could be free of periods at last. I have not had a period for four years; I feel healthier than ever, have an active and joyful sex life with no "dry vagina" problems, and do a lot of physical activities. This is definitely the best period of my life.

Though some practitioners are beginning to consider menopause a normal part of a woman's life and are learning about wholistic approaches, many doctors still think of menopause as a disease and offer medical solutions far more often than necessary.

The medical approach "protects" us from the natural discomforts and changes of outlook that accompany menopause and other transitions of the aging process. It leads us to believe that these changes are so painful or dangerous that we cannot get through them without drugs and/or surgery, that nonmedical alternatives are ineffective or that we are incapable of applying them systematically enough to benefit us. Many doctors do to menopausal women what they do to women in childbirth: They intervene in advance to prevent us from really *living* the experience of change.

Seeking Medical Treatment

Though many women are bothered by menopausal signs, most of us do not require treatment. It is only when these symptoms seriously interfere with our daily lives, when we have tried some nonmedical alternatives and they haven't worked, that we may consider getting medical help from a practitioner who will respectfully discuss the options.

Estrogen Replacement Therapy (ERT)

Since the 1940s, doctors, influenced by aggressive drug industry promotions and prestigious fellow physicians, have given what is known as *estrogen replacement therapy* (ERT), for menopausal "symptoms." Massive advertising campaigns conducted in the seventies made Premarin into the fifth most popular drug in the United States; by 1975, 6 million women were taking it.[31] By 1991, 10 million women were using estrogens and the most frequently prescribed brand, Premarin, moved into fourth place in sales of prescription drugs.[32] Articles and books celebrated ERT in the most extravagant terms, claiming that it prevented hot flashes, vaginal dryness, cancer, heart trouble and depression and reversed aging, unwrinkled the skin, heightened sexual desire and stopped osteoporosis.* Without adequate study, physicians prescribed it freely.

I had been using estrogen for about six months when I found it was making me depressed, so I stopped taking it. This was a rather brave thing for me to do at the time, because the doctor had been telling me it would "keep me young" for the rest of my life.

When it was first developed, ERT seemed to offer a miraculous cure for the "disease" of menopause.

In the mid-seventies studies showed that ERT is associated with a five-to-fifteenfold increased risk of endometrial cancer (cancer of the lining of the uterus), especially among women who have taken estrogen for more than a year,[33] an eightfold increase in gallbladder disease and twice as much gallbladder surgery,[34] and conflicting studies on its effects on breast cancer. An expert advisory group to the National Institutes of Health reported also that most of the claims made for ERT were inflated or incorrect.[35] In 1979, the FDA issued regulations requiring all estrogen products to contain an insert describing the risks of ERT.† It listed only two possible benefits: relief of hot flashes and of vaginal dryness, both of which are linked to loss of ovarian estrogen. The package insert (in such small print that many midlife women can't read it), warned that women with a history of cancer, breast cysts, blood clots or arteriosclerosis should not take estrogen; neither should women with kidney or liver disease. At that time the insert also warned that women with heart disease should not take estrogen. Use of estrogen is also contraindicated for women who have seizures. Some women also report new or increased migraine headaches. Thus millions of women have been the unwitting subjects of a mass experiment that the passage of time revealed to be life-threatening for some.[36] Prescriptions for menopausal estrogens fell drastically, leveled off and increased

---

*Osteoporosis is a disease in which the bones become thin and brittle and break easily, sometimes spontaneously. (See p. 544 for more on osteoporosis.)
†Only after consumer lawsuits successfully opposed the objections of the drug industry and the American College of Obstetricians and Gynecologists (ACOG).

again as drug companies, public-relations firms and physicians scrambled to minimize the findings, uncover new ways of proving estrogen "safe" from cancer risks and find still other uses for it.[37]

The campaign focused next on osteoporosis in women even though the fracture rate among women and men in their eighties is the same. (See pp. 544–46 for more about osteoporosis.) Sales are now being promoted anew with the publicity about the results of a study suggesting that women who took estrogen had less heart disease than women who did not.

With all the articles promoting estrogen use and the conflicting announcements about its benefits or its risks, it is difficult for women to get a total and balanced view in order to make their own decisions. We have space for only a brief review and suggest further sources including *Ourselves, Growing Older* and newsletters (see Resources).

Estrogen and Breast Cancer

One set of calculations made in 1982 had estimated that the long-term use of menopausal estrogens (seven to ten years) would increase the risk of breast cancer *two times* over what it is for women who do not take them. At that time, the general breast cancer risk was one in eleven and the resulting estimate was that approximately one in six women who take estrogens at menopause might develop breast cancer.[38] Although estrogen is not the only cause or facilitator* of breast cancer, the fact remains that ten years later, the lifetime risk of breast cancer in U.S. women is now *one in nine* and still increasing. Current estimates of the increased risk of breast cancer resulting from taking estrogen range from 30 to 50 percent.†

For more about breast cancer, see pp. 618–28. For current summaries of articles about breast cancer and hormones, read *The Network News* of the National Women's Health Network and *A Friend Indeed*, Vol. 8, No. 8 (January 1992) (see Resources).

Estrogen and Heart Disease

Death rates from heart disease for women rise after menopause, leading to speculation that estrogen may be a protective factor for women. Early trials giving estrogen to men were discontinued when nonfatal heart disease and overall mortality increased in the group given estrogen

---

*Economic incentives that promote the sale of drugs and hormones have dominated medical research. Public dollars have not been adequate for research to investigate suspected causes of breast cancer. These causes may include the drugs and hormones, fat and hormones in food, nuclear and X-ray radiation, pesticides and other toxic exposure and occupational hazards, as well as the effects of these factors at various ages of life especially at puberty when breast tissue is first developing. Hormone use later in life may also be a cofacilitator of cancer along with other causes suffered earlier in life.[39]
†Personal communication, Dr. Graham Colditz.

THE MEDICAL SCENARIO

To illustrate the "medicalization" of menopause, here is a sequence of medical events that can overtake a woman in midlife. This scenario describes extreme medical intervention, but variations of this scenario are unfortunately all too common.

At the beginning of menopause, the midlife woman may have irregular or heavy bleeding that she reports to her doctor. The doctor does a dilation and curettage (D and C) for diagnostic purposes, which may also reduce the bleeding temporarily. She is relieved to find out that her uterus is healthy. However, as the year passes, she may have more irregular or heavy bleeding. Her doctor advises another D and C; she follows his advice. Again, she finds nothing untoward, and there may be temporary relief.

More time elapses. Heavy or irregular bleeding returns and the woman may become anemic. The doctor now recommends a hysterectomy. At this point, the woman is frightened by her symptoms, confused about the exact state of her uterus and in all likelihood intimidated by what she feels is the doctor's superior knowledge of her body. So she has the hysterectomy, convinced by the physician to have her ovaries out, too, "in case" of future cancer. Because hormone levels commonly fluctuate after the operation, she may become depressed. For this, too, the doctor offers medical remedies: tranquilizers and estrogen, which can be "safely" administered because there is no longer a risk of uterine cancer. She may be referred to a psychiatrist. If the woman is anxious about the risk of breast cancer, either because she already is in a high-risk group or because she is taking estrogen, she may easily succumb to the suggestion of a prophylactic mastectomy. And here this scenario ends: Little more can be done to this unfortunate woman's body, gynecologically speaking. Paradoxically, she may feel grateful, not realizing that she has had dangerous and unnecessary medical "care."

over the control group. Still the myth of the value of estrogen persists despite women having lower rates than men at all ages, despite increases in heart disease resulting from the use of oral contraceptives and despite drops in heart disease among men resulting from changes to a healthier life-style.

The latest support for the continued use of estrogen comes from a study of a large number of women showing that women who took estrogen had lower rates of heart disease than women who did not take estrogen.[40] Because this is a study "after the fact" rather than a study of matched groups, it has been criticized on the grounds that the women who were given estrogen were healthier to begin with. The women who were not given estrogen may have been women who were already at high risk of heart disease (i.e., smokers and diabetics).[41] Recent extended analysis of these data show about a 50 percent reduction in heart disease, but not without the other increased risks already identified.*

What Every Woman Should Know About ERT and HRT

Women considering taking estrogen, progesterone, or combination treatments should consider the following:

1. The epidemic of breast cancer is affecting women past the age of fifty. In the last twenty-five years, breast cancer went up 74 percent in women over sixty years of age. Most of the increase involves cancers responsive to estrogen.[42]

2. Taking ERT interferes with, covers up, distorts and delays the body's natural adjustment to decreased estrogen levels, a transition which most women can pass through without major difficulty.

3. ERT is only effective against osteoporosis or the other "problems" of menopause for a few years (see below).

4. Taking estrogens can exacerbate any tendency toward uterine fibroids (already more common near menopause) and accelerate their growth, which can lead to other complications and thus increase the risk of hysterectomy.

5. Taking hormones can create vitamin deficiencies.[43]

6. Because of the risk of endometrial or breast cancer with estrogen use, many surgeons are more eager than ever to recommend prophylactic hysterectomies, oophorectomies and mastectomies in order to be able to offer estrogen "risk free."

7. Finally, being on hormones means that you rely on chemical substances whose effects need to be carefully monitored and may not be fully

---

*Colditz, G. et al., "Hormone Replacement Therapy and Risk of Breast Cancer," forthcoming in *American Journal of Obstetrics and Gynecology.*

CUMULATIVE EFFECTS OF ESTROGEN

Some women born between 1920 and 1930 have been exposed to one form of hormone after another since their youth. These women were given diethylstilbestrol (DES) at a time when doctors prescribed it more or less routinely to prevent miscarriage and to dry up milk after birth, often without telling women what they were taking. Some in the 1960s and 1970s took DES as a "morning-after pill" intended to prevent pregnancy after unprotected intercourse.

When the birth control pill first went on the market (at far greater dosages than were later found necessary or safe), members of this age group took it for long intervals, before studies resulted in warnings about its risks. As they grew older, many of these same women were given estrogen for "symptoms" associated with menopause.

The cumulative effect of so much estrogen over so many years on women now in their sixties and seventies is starting to be revealed. Women who were given DES during pregnancy have a significantly higher rate of breast cancer twenty years later. They, perhaps more than any other group of women, have reason to examine the literature about the effects of estrogen. If this has been your experience, you may want to be in touch with one or more the DES and menopause self-help groups. Many of them have information which your doctor may not have. Do everything you can to get your medical records. (See "Our Rights as Patients," p. 682.) Women who used birth control pills have a lower rate of ovarian cancer, but some studies show higher rates of breast cancer.

---

known for years, so that you need to be under the care of expert physicians, which may involve frequent and expensive office visits.[44]

When and How to Use ERT

If you are seriously troubled by hot flashes, and the nonmedical approaches (see below) don't work for you, you may want to consider ERT in as small a dose and for as short a time as possible. Choose a doctor who is expert in this and not responsible to a drug company (see Our Rights as Patients, p. 682). Keep a careful record of your medications and any unusual bleeding, discharge or breast swelling. Be sure to get a checkup from your doctor at least every three to six months while you are on ERT. Some women who have taken estrogen for short periods of time (two or three months) and then discontinued it feel relief from hot flashes; others report that the flashes have returned in full force or even stronger.*

I was placed on Premarin after surgical menopause. The medication was stopped after six months and severe night sweats began within a month. After three months of trying to wait them out, I went back on Premarin; then it was stopped again. The hot flashes then came at infrequent intervals and were easy to tolerate.

You may prefer to put up with the flashes, knowing that they are temporary and cause no permanent damage to your health.

The hot flashes go on and on, but I endure, can even say, "Hello, hot flash, my old friend...."

ERT also alleviates vaginal dryness. It has been suggested that estrogen creams or suppositories applied to the vagina or patches are not as risky as orally ingested estrogen.[45] Unfortunately, the body absorbs the estrogen through the vaginal walls and skin and though it bypasses the liver and gall bladder, the other risks are probably similar. (See p. 534 for self-help approaches to vaginal dryness.)

Progesterone Treatments

Doctors sometimes prescribe the hormone progestin, a synthetic progesterone (see below for risks), or Depo-Provera, an injectable progesterone (see Chapter 13, "Birth Control," for risks) to control excessively heavy or prolonged menstrual bleeding. Some women decide to take these in an attempt to avoid hysterectomy, but they don't always work.

Estrogen and Progestin Combined (HRT)

While we question estrogen use altogether and emphasize nonmedical alternatives, researchers and clinicians today continue to search for "safe" estrogen supplements. Studies show that administering artificial progesterone (generically called *progestin* or *progestogen*) in combination with estrogen reduces somewhat the risk of endometrial cancer. So, if you have a uterus, the recommendation to use estrogen should probably include the recommendation to use progestin as well (the combination is called hormone replacement therapy, or HRT). However, clinicians disagree over

dosages, sequences of administration and types of hormones. If given in higher dosages, monthly bleeding will occur. Lower dosages combined with

---

QUESTIONS TO ASK ABOUT HORMONE THERAPY

No one has to make a quick decision about taking hormones; you have time to read more and consider your decision. Remember that the literature of hormones and these various conditions appear in different journals. Busy physicians often read only within their own specialty and receive much of their information about a drug from the drug company sales representative. We recommend that any woman whose health-care provider suggests the use of estrogen, alone or with progestin, return with the following list of questions prepared by the National Women's Health Network (NWHN):*

1. If estrogen is being recommended to ease uncomfortable menopausal changes, how long does estrogen need to be taken? What are the alternatives? When might the changes subside on their own?

2. If estrogen is being recommended for prevention, what are my specific risks? What can I do to reduce those risks, other than taking estrogen? Are there any diagnostic tests that could give me more information about my risk of osteoporosis or heart disease? How long do you recommend estrogen be taken for prevention? What tests will you recommend for follow-up screening?

3. Are you recommending estrogen alone or in combination with progestin? Why? If you are recommending the combination treatment, how much is known about the effects of progestins on the condition for which I am taking estrogen?

4. To what percentage of your patients do you recommend estrogen?

If women are again to be subjects of experiments with hormones, we must at least be fully aware of the risks we run. If you choose this route, make sure your physician is closely monitored by researchers who are responsible not to a drug company but to a public board.

*See also the National Women's Health Network's *Taking Hormones and Women's Health: Choices, Risks, Benefits.*

---

*Some researchers think that if the estrogen is tapered off gradually, this problem can be minimized.

high calcium supplementation may also reduce bone loss with a reduced amount and frequency of bleeding.[46] It is not known yet if dosages low enough not to cause bleeding contain sufficient estrogen to slow bone loss or sufficient progestin to slough off the cells of the uterine lining stimulated by the estrogen.

While the body continues to produce estrogen even when the ovaries are removed, the production of progesterone ceases after menopause. The long-term effects of taking progestin are unknown. Progestin can cause changes similar to those of diabetes, can unfavorably alter blood cholesterol (raising low-density lipoproteins) and so may increase the risk of heart disease and strokes and may stimulate the growth of breast cancer cells. While studies are underway to determine effects of combined hormones, results will not be available for several years.

You will have to evaluate your own family and medical history and life-style habits with the conflicting evidence about bone mass, breast cancer and heart disease if you are considering hormone therapy.

Nonmedical Approaches

Nonmedical methods of dealing with menopause include exercise, diet, vitamin supplements, herbal therapy and various other techniques. These are much more under our control than medical approaches, and we may experience many kinds of benefits.

Eating well is essential. In addition to a good diet, many midlife women find vitamins and minerals helpful. Vitamin C, vitamin D and calcium are essential for bone formation. Vitamin A deficiency has been associated with heavy menstrual bleeding; supplements in moderate doses may help.* Magnesium can help relaxation. Some women find that vitamin E reduces leg cramps, and others note that it modifies or reduces hot flashes. Some women find that vitamin B complex reduces edema, and others that it helps joint pains and eases stress (see also Eating Well, p. 537).

Some women use herbal teas to reduce or control heavy menstrual bleeding and to reduce the discomfort of hot flashes and headaches. Since instructions vary or lack specificity about which herbs to use, how strong these teas should be and how much you should drink, consult an herbalist or holistic practitioner who knows about herbs. If you want to try these yourself, consult several books. Pay particular attention to any cautions, because some herbs can be harmful in large amounts.

Relaxation techniques, such as meditation, giving and getting massages and yoga, can reduce

stress and depression. Sex, including masturbation, can be relaxing and also helps prevent insomnia and vaginal dryness. Many women find these approaches, as well as acupuncture, helpful for head and neck aches, tension and lower back pain and especially for menstrual problems like heavy bleeding.

Finally, and most importantly, daily moderate exercise is essential for good health throughout menopause. (See Chapter 4, "Women in Motion," for strategies on how to start exercising even if you've been mostly sedentary for years.) *In fact, exercise, especially aerobic exercise, can produce in midlife many (if not all) of the things that the estrogen literature of the early seventies claimed would follow estrogen intake, including (for some women) reduction of hot flashes!*

During my vacation I hiked eight to ten miles a day in good, fresh country air. I cannot recall a single hot flash during that time, although I had them both before and after the trip. Perhaps I was tired enough to sleep without being aware of the flashes, but I don't think that was the case—I never felt healthier.

A few years ago when I was going through change of life I started having joint aches and swelling of hands in the morning. I increased the amount of exercise and took some mineral supplements and vitamin E, and the condition disappeared within a few weeks.

While these are all useful hints, they are not magic, and in most cases they are not enough by themselves. An equally important part of any nonmedical approach is to avoid or cut down your consumption of certain substances that tend to aggravate menopausal signs: alcohol, caffeine, sugar, chocolate, white-flour products, nutritional yeast, and so on, as well as many prescription drugs: tranquilizers, sleeping pills, antidepressants, and so on.

Support Groups for Menopausal Women

Women have always relied on one another for information and understanding. The networks of support groups that have proliferated in recent years are an especially important source of strength for midlife women. In these groups we get emotional support, increased understanding of our particular experience of menopause, and "body" information. Best of all, we reduce the sense of isolation so many of us have known as we recognize the social, economic and political context of our common condition.

I had never been in any kind of support group before. I thought it would be a discussion group and everyone would be an expert except me, and I'd be em-

---

*Vitamin A in high doses can be toxic. Try increasing foods containing carotene, with low-dose vitamin A (no more than 10,000 IU daily) first.

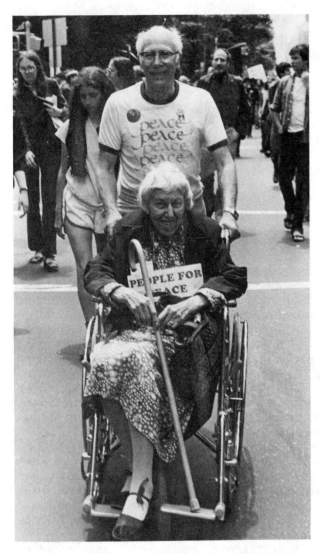

Julie Harper

barrassed because I wasn't an expert on anything. But that's not the way this group worked. There's a lot of mutual help; people really listen to each other and laugh a lot. Now I don't worry about menopause or growing older the way I used to.

Validated by the new knowledge that I had the same powerful physical and emotional experiences as all women, I was proud to have gone through menopause and some difficult life changes at the same time. For instance, creating a new life for myself after my divorce. I love my friends and know they have gone through similar changes.

MATURE WOMEN AND SEXUALITY

Sexuality continues throughout a woman's life. Some women first become fully aware of their sexuality in their middle years and have unexpectedly powerful sexual feelings. A fifty-year-old woman states:

I was shocked by being so horny after I was divorced, because it's not only sexual. It's aggressive. Certainly not what my mother taught me. It took me a long time to understand that I could lust.

A woman in her fifties:

I'm no longer worried about pregnancy; the children are gone; my energy is released. I have a new surge of interest in sex. But at the same time the culture is saying, "You are not attractive as a woman; act your age; be dignified," which means to me, be dead sexually. It's a terrible bind for a middle-aged woman. I say, acknowledge, applaud, enjoy sexuality! Get rid of stereotypes! Change the image of women to include middle-aged beauty and sexuality!

If you are sexually involved with men, keep using some form of birth control until you haven't had a period for two years. Birth control pills and the IUD are not recommended for midlife women.* Some midlife women consider the chances of pregnancy to be so low that they are willing to rely on abortion as a backup. But if you are certain you do not want to have a child and would not consider abortion, continue to use birth control. Practice safe sex to protect yourself from AIDS.

Many older women who would like to be sexually active with men lack the opportunity, especially since with each year of age there are fewer men in their age range.† A divorced woman in her sixties:

I have a great interest in sex, still, and a great desire for it. But what makes it most poignant that I don't have the right partner is that I am capable of giving now to a degree that I never achieved when I was young.

Even married, we may not be as sexually active as we might like if our partners lose interest in sex.

Our society admires older men who have relationships with women much younger than themselves but makes older women with younger partners the butt of jokes and derision. Yet some of us have younger men as partners.

It's hard to read the younger-man/older-woman thing. We have to send out signals if a sexual rela-

---

*For discussion of the Pill, see pp. 279–288. IUDs should be avoided by midlife women because they may trigger or exacerbate the heavy bleeding and flooding that sometimes precede menopause.

†A Duke University study showed that of older men interested in sex 87 percent were sexually active, while among interested older women only 60 percent were sexually active.[47] The implication in this study is that women can only be "sexually active" with men.

tionship is what we want. I've had a problem if the man is the same age as my son, though after thinking about it I've decided it's okay for me. What really bothers me is my vanity—exposing a middle-aged body to a beautiful younger man.

The joy of making love with a young man who is so full of energy and straightforward is wonderful.

Some midlife or older women are for the first time considering or having sexual relationships with women. A sixty-year-old woman:

Women and men have been socialized so utterly differently, and we have grown so different in the last decades, too, that if we restrict ourselves to heterosexual relationships, it's going to get harder and harder as we get older. I'm married and though my husband is considerably older than I, he's still very active. But if this relationship comes to an end—which would mean his death, because we're never going to separate—my sexual satisfactions would surely have to come either from myself or from other women. I can't imagine forming another relationship with a man.

Others of us have been lesbian for many years (see Older Lesbians, p. 191).
Many of us would rather not have sex at all or prefer to limit our sexual expression to masturbation and fantasy rather than changing our sexual orientation or a lifetime pattern of being involved in one special relationship. According to a seventy-three-year-old woman,

I frankly don't need it, and I don't miss it at all. I had a very, very full sex life—and I was mad about my husband, which is a nice way to be. When he died it was a real shock, but that's twenty-five years ago now. I've run around with a few men since, but nobody that I really wanted to connect with. You have to have a certain desire toward a person, and I haven't discovered another person that I had that desire for in twenty-five years now. I'm used to my life the way it is now, and I don't think that my life is incomplete.

Many single older women miss not just sex but touching, gentleness, closeness and the excitement of romance. A woman in her sixties states:

Some of you say you have husbands at home that won't go anyplace. I have buried three husbands, and I wish I had one to sit home with me now.

A woman in her seventies:

It's the intimacy that I miss more than the actual sex act. Shared jokes—you know. I'm finding this

with a number of women as well as with men, but the whole romantic aspect of my life seems to have gone by. I miss that.

Sex and Aging—Physiological Changes

We are physically able to enjoy sex more. With sexual experience we develop a large, complex venous system in the pelvic area that enhances our capacity for sexual tension and improves orgasmic intensity, frequency and pleasure.*
Elder women who seek any form of sexual expression, whether pleasuring ourselves or making love with others, face changes, too.

Vaginal Changes

Changed estrogen levels may produce changes in the vagina. Thinning of the vaginal walls, loss of elasticity, flattening out of ridges, foreshortening or narrowing of the vagina and especially dryness or itching may make intercourse less comfortable or even painful. These conditions may lead to irritation and increased susceptibility to infection. It is not clear whether these vaginal changes are caused by the changed estrogen levels of menopause or simply by aging. Some women never have this problem. Doctors, with their gift for nomenclature, call it *vaginal atrophy* and describe it in medical texts as occurring five or more years after menstruation ceases. Yet many women experience vaginal changes earlier in menopause, and others at age sixty or later. In addition, little is known about how long such a condition lasts, how troublesome it may become or how easily it can be corrected.[49]
Many "experts" recommend "regular intercourse" to maintain easy vaginal lubrication.

I asked a woman gynecologist with an excellent reputation, "Does it have to be intercourse? What about widows, or divorced women, or lesbians, or women whose husbands aren't too interested in sex or are ill?" I couldn't get a straight answer from her.

The fact is that we can maintain and improve our ability to lubricate through any type of arousing sexual activity.[50] There is nothing unhealthy about losing interest in genital sexual activity; we are not sex machines obligated to keep our bodies perpetually in condition for potential partners. There is also no evidence that vaginal dryness is irreversible. A woman in her sixties states:

I had a problem with dryness when I started having sexual intercourse again after a few years. In a month or two, my vagina began to get wet faster.

---

*Sexual activity with a partner or ourselves and pregnancy also contribute to the complexity of the pelvic venous system.[48]

You may take longer to become amply lubricated, or not lubricate at all. Saliva, vegetable oil and K-Y Jelly have long been used to reduce dryness. New lubricants (such as Astroglide) are available as gels, applicators or vaginal suppositories. The manufacturer of one nonhormonal moisturizer (Replens) suggests use three times a week with an applicator and claims the product has long-lasting effects in the vagina. Itching can be relieved by applying bancha tea or vitamin E oil topically to the pubic and vaginal area.

Sexual activity, masturbation and Kegel exercises (p. 406) also help maintain vaginal muscle tone.

Slower Arousal Time

The slower arousal time of older women and men has compensations. A woman in her forties states

When Jay used to lose his erection I would think that I had failed as a woman because I couldn't keep him aroused. But now I see that it can mean more time to play around and a chance to start over again so that lovemaking lasts longer.

Drugs and Disease

Drugs and disease can affect sexual behavior. Some drugs may affect sexual function or interest. Medication for high blood pressure can prevent erections, as can too much alcohol. (The depressive effect of alcohol becomes more pronounced as people get older.) Diabetes can make erections difficult for a man; its effect on the sexuality of women is not well understood.[51] L-dopa, prescribed for Parkinson's disease, may increase sexual interest. Ask your practitioner about the effects on sexual interest, arousal or functioning of any medications that are prescribed for you or your partner.

Changing Attitudes and Communication

Women now in their older years must shed years of training to act on the knowledge that there are alternatives to intercourse and that they can initiate sex. The physiological changes of aging invite both men and women to break through old patterns, assumptions, misunderstandings and miscommunications. Men may misinterpret their slowness to arousal as a sign that their sexual capacities are eroding and in panic seek out other (younger) women. Women may fear that their sagging bodies' diminished "attractiveness" has slowed their partner's arousal or interpret their own lack of lubrication as loss of attraction to their partner. It is important for both partners in a relationship, whether heterosexual or lesbian, to realize that changes are normal and to talk together

to find out what is pleasurable. Such communication may be difficult at first and requires practice. You may want to get some help.

If one or both of you have some physical difficulty, see p. 223. Do what pleases you and your partner, even if it seems unusual or strange. Chances are, if you like it, other couples do, too. A greater capacity for empathy and loving, developed through the years of living, can make sex better. A seventy-year-old woman, recalling a love affair at fifty, says:

My immense pleasure and response were for him an incredible high and that made me feel so marvelous. It was not just the physical part but our delight in each other that was so enormously exciting. It was a circular or spiral effect, because I had not realized that another person could enjoy my passion. Before this, I had experienced my passion and my partner would experience his passion. But this was different. And of course it's very much that way in a lesbian love affair, that delight in the other woman's total experience, the total emotional response. Danny took great pride in that just as a woman does with another woman. He thought it was marvelous that I was multiple-orgasmic. After he died, I was in a state of shock for over a year. The mutuality we shared was rare with a man. My subsequent love affairs have all been with women.

Some people continue to be sexually active in their seventies, eighties and even nineties.

I am seventy-four years old and have been married for fifty-two years. We are fortunate to have good mental as well as physical health. This is not entirely a matter of luck. We have worked at it. Our good times have been more numerous than our bad times. The medical profession has only recently discovered the healing power of laughter. In our fifty-two years together we have had a lot of laughs. A sense of humor is as important as food, especially within the confines of marriage. For us the sharing that comes with having a warm and loving sex life over so many years deepens our joy in one another.

AGING AND PREVENTIVE HEALTH— SPECIAL ISSUES

Although many people equate getting old with getting sick, the truth is more complex. Aging brings physical changes, most of which have little to do with sickness.

At sixty I am more vigorous and healthy than I was twenty years ago. My eighty-five-year-old mother shows me that by the eighties certain things in your body do start to give way, but even though she gets around less easily, she's certainly what I'd call healthy.

In our fifties and beyond, a lifetime of exposure to occupational health hazards may have caused a debilitating disease.* Yet while disease and chronic ill health are among the realities of the older years for many of us, they are not the only reality. And social factors can disable us more than is necessary: isolation from family and friends; caregiving for relatives and family without outside help; poor medical care, due to high cost, lack of insurance coverage, inadequate medical understanding of aging and maldistribution of doctors. Poverty is a special health issue for older women. Money worries due to being on a small, limited income and the fears of cutbacks to Social Security, Medicare and other government programs add greatly to the unhealthy stresses of daily living. Inadequate income also makes it harder to take care of our bodies in simple but crucial daily ways. It is difficult, for instance, to get enough exercise if we don't feel safe on the streets or have little access to indoor exercise facilities. A worsening economic situation and drastic cuts in social programs make it more difficult each month for thousands of older women to get adequate calories, let alone vitamins and special diets. Some already subsist partly on pet food. Many are starving.[53] Some are homeless or without adequate heat. Having insufficient money also severely restricts our access to medical care, especially in a time of reduced government aid. Four million American women between forty-five and sixty-five have no health insurance.[54] Without a major turnaround in social priorities and policies, the health of great numbers of older women will worsen drastically over the next few years, with more emergency hospitalization for anemia, dehydration and hypothermia† and collapse and deaths from all causes.

Here we will address special issues‡ for all older women as we seek to keep as healthy as possible.

Throughout our life we can take active steps to maintain good health and lessen the impact of illnesses or chronic conditions when we are older. We can rethink the ways in which we take care of ourselves and acquire new habits which will serve us well for the rest of our lives. We can stop smoking, exercise more, eat as well as possible, reduce our dependence on caffeine, sugar, alcohol, tranquilizers. Currently there is growing evidence that many of the changes of aging, even those once thought biologically inevitable, are preventable and even reversible with changes like these.[55]

The point is not simply to live longer but to have the highest possible quality of life as long as we live.

By reading many books and articles on women, mental health, nutrition and exercise I began to see that my life could and should change. The changes did not come easily. My husband resisted. After all, I was rocking the boat in which we had become quite comfortable. I took up Tae Kwon Do [Eastern self-defense]. To my amazement, after a few months of kicking and hitting an imaginary opponent, my chronic insomnia and stiff neck disappeared. Gone also were the painful attacks of gastritis. I began feeling more energetic. Encouraged, I decided to put into practice some of the nutritional advice that I'd been reading. I stopped eating white sugar in any form. No more of my favorite cream-filled doughnuts. No more processed food, including white bread, noodles, and spaghetti: in came more fresh vegetables and grains. Out went sleeping pills, aspirin and other medications: in came vitamins. It was not an overnight sensation. After all, I was trying to undo the damage done over forty-some years.

That was more than five years ago. Today, all the ailments I mentioned earlier are completely gone. No more of that headachy feeling from constipation— I count my blessings every day for being freed from this debilitating condition from which I suffered for so long. No more pains in my legs from varicose veins (some of my friends had surgery for this). No more stiff neck from internalized stress and tension. If you never suffered from chronic insomnia, you don't know the joy of being able to sleep all night, every night. All these things that I thought I would have to live with the rest of my life are gone.

Exercise

Exercise becomes increasingly important. Women begin to lose bone mass at around age thirty-five, yet this may be largely due to inactivity. Weight-bearing exercise increases bone density. Runners, for example, tend to have high thigh-bone densities.[56] Heavier women are less vulnerable to osteoporosis (see p. 545), possibly because their bones carry more weight.

Many of the benefits of exercise for older women are already evident. Exercise can lower blood pressure and reduce atherosclerosis, risks of heart attack and stroke, arthritis, emphysema and osteoporosis. It is central in finding and keeping a comfortable weight. It helps us sleep, improves

---

*One study of 1,100 persons over fifty in Ohio found that a main factor influencing health was occupation, past or present. "Those persons who have, or had, low-income occupations (and the disadvantages that go along with a lifetime of low income) were in poor health much more frequently than those with middle-income or high-income jobs."[52]

†Hypothermia is a condition in which the body temperature drops drastically. Older people are more vulnerable to cold.

‡Many of the more serious health problems that affect midlife and older women appear elsewhere in this book because they affect younger women, too: hypertension, cancer, arthritis, heart disease, diabetes, arteriosclerosis. The troubling but not life-threatening problems—visual impairment, hearing loss, difficulties in walking—along with osteoporosis, which primarily affects women over sixty, are discussed on pp. 541–46.

Deborah Wald

bowel functioning, maintains strength and good posture, often relieves depression and generally makes most people feel better.

My grandmother in her early nineties noticed that when she moved around more, her memory improved.

There seems now to be clinical evidence that after exercise blood rushes to the skin, bringing with it extra nutrients, and the skin's temperature rises as well. The collagen content then increases and skin actually thickens and becomes more elastic and less wrinkled. Delightfully, it is never too late to start exercising, and there are forms of exercise that fit almost any kind of physical limitation. A few tips: start slowly; watch less TV or exercise while you watch; better yet, exercise with a friend for company and support; try walking, yoga or swimming; take an exercise class to help you overcome sedentary habits. Review Chapter 4, "Women in Motion," for other ideas.

Eating Well

Although the same basic principles of healthy eating apply throughout life, nutritional requirements change somewhat with age. You need fewer calories (unless you are working or exercising hard), but the same nutrients and more of certain ones. See Chapter 2, "Food," for all but the following few items of special interest to older women and for sources of nutrients listed below.

Note: Some of the hints here and in Chapter 2 become less easy to follow in our older years, especially when we can't easily get out to shop or are on a small fixed income and cannot afford to buy fresh foods. If we have dentures or problems with teeth and gums, small changes in diet may be all we can manage—but even cutting down on junk foods can help a lot. If you put off cooking because you are just preparing meals for yourself, try designating one day per week as cooking day. Fix several dishes, including a main dish and a soup you like, and then eat them on alternate days, or freeze some in individual portions for later.

Because we absorb nutrients less well as we age and require fewer calories altogether, we may need supplements. (See the discussion of menopause on pp. 524–33.)

However, try to get as much of the nutrients you need from your food. See p. 37 in Chapter 2 for the advantages and risks of supplements. Though the particular balance needed by women over thirty-five sounds complicated, resources like the *Department of Agriculture Handbook (Composition of Foods* AH-8 and recent supplements), and the many new low-fat cookbooks can help you figure out whether you are eating well or what to change.

Protein

Because we don't absorb as much protein as we age, try to make protein foods a higher proportion of what you eat. However, be sure to balance with a sufficient amount of complex carbohydrates (whole grains, etc.; see p. 32).

Calcium, Magnesium and Phosphorus—A Balance of Nutrients

For postmenopausal women, calcium is an essential nutrient, as it prevents the bone loss that can lead to osteoporosis.* Unfortunately, women over thirty-five absorb calcium less easily,[57] so we must make a special effort to get more exercise (this is indispensable to helping our bodies absorb calcium), eat a calcium-rich diet, learn about the other nutrients that aid or inhibit calcium absorption and get the right balance of such nutrients.

- Phosphorus intake should equal but not exceed calcium. If phosphorus is too high, the parathyroid glands are stimulated to draw calcium from the bones. Most American women who eat meat and drink cola drinks probably have overly high phosphorus levels that inhibit calcium absorption. If you avoid milk because of its fat, replace it not with soda but with skim or part skim milk

---

*Calcium supplements can help us be sure we are getting the recommended 1,500 to 2,000 milligrams, but we need to balance this with about 750 to 1,000 milligrams of magnesium. Dolomite has often been recommended as containing the proper amounts of calcium and magnesium, but there have been reports of harmful trace minerals, such as arsenic and lead, found in some samples. Some women, therefore, prefer to buy calcium and magnesium supplements separately in a two-to-one ratio.

· or milk products. If your body can't tolerate dairy products (lactose intolerance), refer to Chapter 2, "Food," for nondairy sources of calcium. Lactose intolerance may increase with age.

- Magnesium intake should be half of calcium intake. If your magnesium level drops lower, calcium will be lost. There is some evidence that the older we are, the more magnesium we need (around 450 to 500 milligrams daily), especially when we are under stress.[58] Magnesium can help muscles and nerves relax—and is safer than tranquilizers. Fruits and vegetables contain magnesium.

- You need vitamin D, 400 to 800 IU a day, for calcium and phosphorus absorption.

Fiber

The fiber in vegetables, fruit, whole grains and bran helps with constipation (exercise helps, too). Fiber and oats may also lower cholesterol levels.

WEIGHT AND WEIGHT GAIN AT MIDLIFE AND LATER

As older women we are probably more preoccupied with food, eating and dieting than any other group in society, with the possible exception of teenage girls. One out of two of us puts on weight at midlife because our metabolism is slowing down and we no longer need as many calories to sustain us. Often, too, we are more sedentary than before, with fewer people in the household, fewer chores, less physical mobility, less exercise. If we continue the same food intake and get no more exercise (or even less) than before, we will tend to gain weight. In fact, women on the average gain almost ten pounds between thirty-five and forty-five and two more between forty-five and fifty-five. *There is good evidence that this weight has an important function:* the conversion of androgens into estrogen in our body fat is one of the three sources of estrogen after menopause. Some fat, therefore, is crucial: Women who are very thin have a higher rate of osteoporosis. It is also true that above a certain level, too many pounds can contribute to ill health—diabetes and high blood pressure in particular. There is controversy today, however, over what constitutes "too many pounds" (see Chapter 2, "Food"). Actuarial tables were changed when research showed that the ideal weights for older women and men were set too low.

Consider the several factors below in assessing your weight. If all these factors and their total combination are within the normal range and you feel well, your weight is probably fine.

1. Are you getting a reasonable amount of regular exercise?
2. Are you eating well?
3. Is your weight stable or changing slowly? Sudden weight gain or loss is dangerous at any age and more so as we grow older. If you plan to lose weight, do it slowly, as a result of long-term, permanent changes in eating and exercise patterns.
4. Is your blood pressure within normal range? After menopause, blood pressure tends to rise with increases in weight.
5. Is your blood sugar well within the normal range? As your weight increases, the likelihood of getting adult diabetes increases, and the disease often signals itself by slight rises in blood sugar.
6. How is your lung power and control? The lungs have been overlooked until recently as an indicator of general health. The simple, risk-free pulmonary function test is a good indicator and predictor of long-term health and longevity (for women better than for men). Usually done in a doctor's office as part of a general checkup, it measures lung power and control as you exhale. Yoga is a good way to build lung capacity.
7. Are your cholesterol readings normal? High cholesterol, by itself, is only an indicator of possible problems if it is a particular type of cholesterol. A special test measures lipid density, high-density lipoproteins (HDL) in high concentrations being a prognosticator of good circulatory health, and low-density lipoproteins (LDL) in high concentrations being an indicator of possible problems.* The test is expensive but worth asking for if questions have been raised about your health in relation to your weight.
8. Do you have signs of arthritis or osteoporosis? Either one can indicate that you need to change your diet and exercise patterns. Women who are overweight are more prone to osteoarthritis, whereas women who are underweight are at higher risk for osteoporosis.

*See Hypertension, Heart Diseases and Circulatory Diseases, p. 629, for more.

Fats

Aging makes us less able to resist the damaging effects of all fats. See Chapter 2, "Food," for which fats to eat and how to cut back.

Potassium

Plentiful in fresh fruits and vegetables, potassium becomes especially useful to women at midlife because it helps (1) heart action, which may be less effective during the estrogen transition;[59] (2) the elimination of fluid buildup, which continues cyclically for many postmenopausal women because of other sources of estrogen; (3) to balance sodium, which we may now have in greater quantities than we need; and (4) to lower blood pressure (along with a low-sodium diet). Coffee, tea, alcohol and too much sodium deplete potassium.

GETTING MEDICAL CARE

Despite the larger role that each of us can play in our own health care, at times we have to turn to the medical system. As midlife and older women, we face some special obstacles to good care.

Older women cannot count on the medical profession. Few doctors are interested in them. Their physical and emotional discomforts are often characterized as post-menopausal syndrome, until they have lived too long for this to be an even faintly reasonable diagnosis. After that they are assigned the category of senility.[60]

Inadequate Research

Medical research until very recently paid little attention to aging women's health concerns. Even today, medical literature focuses on menopause as the primary midlife health issue as though reproductive organs were the center of a woman's life. Failing to acknowledge women as workers outside the home, researchers have not studied occupational health issues for older women. Because the practitioner or clinic you visit may not have adequate information about the diseases and their prevention or the physical changes that affect older women in particular, you may have to educate the practitioners who treat you.

Physicians' Attitudes

The medical profession and other health personnel share the culture's negative attitudes toward the old. In a medical context this can take the form of active avoidance and dislike or a less obvious pattern of paternalism. . . . Physicians, like the lay public, are personally ambivalent and frightened by aging and death.[61]

The basic ageism that shapes many physicians' attitudes toward older patients is compounded by

sexism. The medical world seems to hold the underlying prejudice that once we can no longer have children, we have outlived our usefulness. Physicians and medical personnel discuss older women's complaints and health problems as neurotic or imaginary far more than men's, and at earlier ages. They have been heard to call aging women "old bags" and other insulting names. When such attitudes affect the quality of our medical care, they endanger our health.*

Inappropriate Sources of Care

At present, there are few practicing geriatricians.† Most ob/gyns are not particularly interested in women past menopause, especially when we have had a hysterectomy or refuse estrogen replacement therapy. Internists, family practitioners, physician assistants and well-informed GPs are often more appropriate physicians for older women—*when they have a positive attitude and enough information about aging.* Today interest in aging is growing and there are a number of geriatric centers and clinics, though these are mostly located near large medical centers.‡

Limits of the Medical Approach to Chronic Conditions

Many of the conditions we suffer from in the older years are not subject to outright "cure." Chronic diseases do not respond to the daring surgery or high-technology interventions that physicians are trained to prefer. The ordinariness of diet, braces, physical therapy and aspirin is boring, and doctors often give us less attention when these are what we need. Medical treatments that do help in some chronic conditions are often expensive,§ time-consuming and painful; sometimes they are dangerous and ineffective. This is another reason to look into nonmedical approaches to healing. (See Chapter 5 for alternatives.)

Misdiagnosis and Failure to Treat Reversible Conditions

Especially when we are past sixty, doctors tend to blame all our physical and emotional problems on aging and don't look for treatable disorders.

---

*These attitudes and practices are less blatant toward women who have ample financial resources and private physicians.
†Of 2,000 doctors surveyed 76.5 percent said training in geriatric medicine would help doctors give better care to elderly patients. Over half reported that at least one-fourth of their patients are sixty-five or older.[62]
‡There is a lively controversy today in medical schools and among health providers about whether geriatrics should be a medical specialty in its own right or whether geriatric training should be integrated with other medical specialties.
§Medicare and many private health insurance plans do not adequately cover care for chronic conditions unless they require institutionalization.

They'll interpret emotional or mental confusion as senility when these may be signs of poor nutrition, treatable physical malfunctions, grief or responses to inappropriate medication. Time after time physicians offer older women tranquilizers, sedatives, antidepressants and hormones instead of looking for what's really wrong. As one nurse puts it: "When a man complains of dizziness he gets a workup; an older woman gets Valium." We ourselves may play into this pessimism about whether we can actually get better.

I was afraid when I broke my wrist that it would take ages if ever to heal, and so I hesitated to do a more "aggressive" type of therapy for it. Now it's much better, and I'm going to begin that therapy. My fear and a stereotype of being old held me back.

Overprescription of Drugs

Many older people take several medications daily for various chronic conditions, often prescribed by different physicians. Most physicians don't realize that people over sixty are more sensitive to many drugs and should take lower doses of them if they take them at all.*

I can't tolerate any of the drugs I've been given for pain. When I take medication there's something in my system that feels dislocated, as if all my internal furniture has been piled up in the middle of the room or something. So I just live with the pain in my hands and get help with certain jobs.

Some drugs can cause depression (for which we may be offered more drugs) or mental confusion, though symptoms often stop when the medication is stopped.†

Practitioners frequently neglect the crucial step of finding out what medications a woman is taking before prescribing others. Elders have had so many bad reactions to taking too many medications that this "condition" has been given a name, *polypharmacy*.[64] Bring to your medical appointments a list of all the medications you are taking. A woman we know asked her doctor to review all her medications. As the doctor reviewed the list he began to cut down the dosage of most of them and cut a few out completely.

In nursing homes, many elders are literally "tranquilized" into quiet and compliance. If you believe that you or a relative or friend are being inappropriately or excessively medicated, do all you can to change the situation. Some states have a nursing home residents' advocate called an *ombudsman*.

I went to a visit a ninety-four-year-old friend who lives in a nursing home. She was recently diagnosed as having various ailments that require anywhere from three to ten pills a day. She was never told what the pills were or what they were for. When the nurse came to her room to give her the pills, my friend looked her squarely in the eye and said, "The doctor only knows my body and how it works for a short time. I know it for ninety-four years, and nothing is going in it until I know what it is!"

Making changes means, for many of us, turning around decades of a certain kind of dependency on doctors. It may involve changing their stereotype of us, asking more questions, going in with a friend for support and advocacy, learning all we can about our health problems and making informed decisions,* seeking second opinions more aggressively, checking the negative effects of all medications, looking for nonmedical alternatives, refusing unnecessary surgery. Physicians who are taken aback when younger women use these tactics may be even more surprised, and even hostile, when their long-time patients ("their girls") begin to change. It takes courage to break old patterns, especially when you are feeling sick or frightened. Probably the most helpful thing you can do is to join or create a self-help or self-health group of women your age—even two or three people—to talk openly about your body changes and go to doctor's appointments together to help each other get the best care you can. You can provide transportation and emotional support for each other when undergoing treatments that may be painful or scary.

The system itself must change, too, especially in research and medical training. Insurance, Medicare and Medicaid should pay for preventive measures, and for the devices—eyeglasses, hearing aids, canes, and so on—that help us deal with the daily limitations of chronic diseases and aging. Proud of the years we have lived and the contributions we have made to society, we must insist

---

*In older people, the ratio of fat to muscle is higher. The higher the fat, the longer drugs stay in the body. Because of this, the next day's dosage may be added to that still retained in the body from previous days, and the older person will become overmedicated.
†Drugs that are especially problematic for elders are reserpine, methyldopa, digitalis, procainamide, beta-blocking agents, all barbiturates, alcohol and tranquilizers.[63]

---

*Because we do not want to settle for mediocre or uninformed health care (especially when we have limited time and/or money or live in a rural area where choices in medical care are few), our best bet is learning as much as we can from women's health organizations, books and courses. If we are informed, we can tell health practitioners when we think their care or knowledge is inadequate. When we do so, we should be prepared to offer constructive and specific resources—books, articles, audiovisual materials—or know where they can be found.

on health and medical care that enable us to live our lives as fully as possible.

THE OLDER YEARS

Pleasures and Potentials

In our older years we may feel entitled to do what pleases and satisfies us, to slow down, to let go the strain of former obligations, to express our thoughts and feelings more strongly than ever before.

According to a seventy-eight-year-old woman,

Old age, because of its time perspective, can be a period of emotional and sensory awareness and enjoyment. I savor life more often. When I draw an iris, I see that iris more vividly than I did when my physical sight was better. When I read a book now, I read it more slowly. Several books I have reread, one I have just finished reading the third time.

Elemental things of life have assumed greater importance. I spend more time looking at sunsets. I am more aware of the importance to myself and others of touching (both physical and emotional), of communication, of tenderness.

Space and time for quiet reflection is more available for me now. In a strange way, impossible to put into words, I am experiencing a unity beyond space and time.

Sometimes I feel guilty to be happy when there are so many things wrong in the world and I'm not doing something about making joy possible for others. Yet the universe is going to have to get along without me sometime and so I don't have to change everything. Many of my companions are interested in a better, more compassionate world; I don't have to rush to do it all.

A seventy-three-year-old woman:

I know myself better and have more time to pursue my own interests. I enjoy less tempestuous relationships with children and grandchildren. I enjoy a personal growth not possible in my busier years.

Physical Impairments and Chronic Conditions

Some of us, however, miss these possible pleasures due to illness (often linked to low income) or to the loss of certain capacities.* The majority of women over sixty-five have some chronic health problem or condition that may limit activity over a period of time.[65] We should never automatically

---

*Recent research has shown that mental capacity stays the same or may increase; only the speed of reaction time decreases.

assume that *any* of these are the inevitable result of aging; instead we must investigate what we can do. Be suspicious of any practitioner who dismisses most complaints with "What do you expect at your age?" Many problems are as treatable now as they are at any age.

When we do have to give up a degree of independence or a cherished activity because we can't see, hear or move around as well as before, we may need time to get used to our limits and find alternative ways to manage.

Not to be able to drive (during day or night) may affect our independence, forcing us to give up cherished activities and even social relationships.

I loved my job and would have been happy to work for several years more, but it was getting more and more difficult commuting back and forth because my vision was so impaired. Driving back home in the dusk was scary. I felt as though I had my nose right up against the windshield.

Organized around the nuclear family and the individual automobile, this society magnifies the isolation of older women, so many of whom live alone. (In protest, one Gray Panther member came to a hearing with great difficulty to demonstrate that the lowest step of the elders' bus was not wheelchair accessible.) To live in more interdependent ways—sharing a house, organizing carpools—might be better for us. We must work for more and improved public transportation, and communities in which it is safe to walk around.

Eyes

Our eyes have less elasticity by midlife. If you are farsighted, you probably will need stronger glasses or perhaps glasses for the first time. Some nearsighted people can give up glasses, except for driving or other distance viewing; others may require bifocals. We may have trouble adjusting to them or feel embarrassed about wearing them.

If you experience sudden flashing light and black spots, get medical attention at once. These could be symptoms of a detached retina—an emergency. In our seventies and eighties or even earlier, cataracts (cloudy lenses) may develop. Although there isn't much evidence yet that these specific conditions can be prevented and not much is known about cause, eye repair is one of the few areas where medicine's heroics really pay off, restoring sight or improving it. Until cataracts are "ready" for surgery, however, the impaired vision can be limiting and discouraging. A second opinion is a particularly good idea for eye surgery, because some doctors will urge operations when they aren't necessary, or sooner (or later) than is appropriate. If you are having cataract surgery, also investigate postsurgery options in advance. Recent improvements include laser surgery and the possibility of *implants* placed at the time of surgery, rather than contact lenses or new glasses afterward. Be sure your *ophthalmologist* (a medical doctor who specializes in eye diseases) is experienced in this procedure.

Glaucoma is a chronic eye disease, usually appearing at midlife or later, in which the pressure of fluid inside the eye becomes too great. This excess pressure can damage the optic nerve and cause blindness if untreated. Because it affects women more than men and rarely causes early pain or symptoms, be sure your medical exams regularly include a test for glaucoma after age forty-five.

Tests, done with a *tonometer*, are quick and painless, but some are more accurate than others. *Optometrists*, who measure eye function, can perform some tonometry only in certain states. Ophthalmologists have the most accurate diagnostic equipment and skills.

If detected early, some mild glaucoma can be treated effectively with drops taken regularly. More severe glaucoma requires surgical treatment with regular follow-up, since there are no permanent cures.

Feet

If you've always been active, you probably take your feet for granted. If you begin to notice aches and pain, not just when walking but when you rest as well, this may be part of skeletal or bone changes. (See Osteoporosis, p. 544, and the section on arthritis in Chapter 24, "Some Common and Uncommon Health and Medical Problems.") But it is more likely to mean that you simply need more regular exercise to avoid stiffness. Some people swear they notice the effects of sugar and caffeine in their bones, especially their hands and feet.

Foot problems you already have may get worse as you age, especially if you have put on weight. Well-designed shoes with a firm, supportive arch may prevent fatigue as well as bunions* and other foot problems.

Most of us notice an increase in corns, calluses and other dry, scaly, hard skin on toes, heels and soles and a loss of flesh. Toenails often become much thicker, harder and sometimes yellower. This may be a sign of a fungus, so check with your practitioner. Soaking your feet regularly, an old-fashioned custom, is vastly preferable to harsh

chemicals or carving off dead skin with a razor blade. After a long soak, try a pumice stone to work off the excess skin. You can bleach yellow toenails, if they bother you, with ordinary household bleach, diluted, or cover them with opaque nail polish.

Caring for our feet, especially cutting our own toenails, may gradually become a near-impossible chore, especially if we cannot bend as well as we used to and must ask others to help us. It can be frustrating to need others for such simple acts. Insurance plans do not cover routine care by podiatrists, yet they will pay for care of problems and infections caused by neglect of routine foot care.*

You can do foot exercises with a friend or by yourself: rise on your toes, walk on them; flex heels and ankles, pick up a pencil with your toes, and so on.

Before going to sleep at night, give each foot a slight massage. It will warm your feet and help you to get to sleep more quickly, and the stretch may help you to maintain enough flexibility to care for your own feet. Find a "foot partner," massage each other's feet and help each other with grooming tasks.

Hearing

Hearing is a function we take for granted until we suddenly notice that we are missing what is being said or must ask people to repeat more often than feels comfortable.

Every once in a while I miss out on parts of a conversation or don't understand what I am hearing. When this happens, I discover to my later discomfort that, occasionally, I act as if I did hear—bright smile, nod of agreement. When this happens I feel so separate from people that I'm with.

Being hard of hearing is an invisible handicap. No one knows unless you tell them. You have a right to ask people to speak in a manner that enables you to understand.

One of the most important things a hard-of-hearing person can do for herself, I have discovered, is to be very assertive. Tell each person you talk with to speak louder or more clearly, and force yourself to keep reminding that person if she forgets.

Common as it is, hearing loss is not an inevitable accompaniment of aging, though it does seem to run in some families. The enormous increase in the volume and range of noise accom-

---

*Bunions are extremely painful, sudden misalignments of the cartilage under the tendon of the big toe. They can be caused by inadequate exercise and poor shoes or sometimes from the stress of sudden exercise, like running, without adequate preparation. Surgical treatment is not always successful.

---

*Medicare covers mainly acute conditions. Women have successfully lobbied for inclusion of mammograms and cervical Pap tests.

panying industrialization has contributed significantly to hearing loss in the present generation of over-sixty-fives, especially among factory workers and urban dwellers. Baby-boomers face additional risk from years of exposure to loud music.

It is crucial to obtain an accurate diagnosis of the cause of hearing loss, because treatment varies depending on whether one has nerve or conduction deafness. Conduction deafness, unlike nerve deafness, can often be corrected with surgery.

Urinary Incontinence and Urinary Tract Infections

Starting around the time of menopause, some women begin to notice a slight loss of urine as they cough, sneeze, laugh or exert themselves during strenuous activity.* The tissues around the urethra begin to thin out just as the vagina does, in response to reduced estrogen, sometimes making bladder control more difficult. Women who already have a history of this problem may find it getting worse. Kegel exercises (p. 406) and sit-ups or leg lifts to strengthen the abdominal muscles may help control this problem.

---

*This is called *stress incontinence*. This and other kinds of incontinence can be successfully managed or treated. See *Ourselves, Growing Older*, and Rebecca Chalker and Kristene E. Whitemore's *Overcoming Bladder Disorders*, New York: Harper & Row, 1990.

LIP READING

"Why a lip reading class?" my friends ask. The reason is a gradually increasing hearing loss I have had for several years. Unless I'm in a room with good acoustics and with people who speak clearly, I have trouble following the conversation.

In the meantime, here I am in the lip reading class of our community education program, learning a lot about how to face up to hearing difficulties. The mutual support of the group is reassuring.

While there's no magic cure, hearing aids, signing and lip reading can help. Lip reading is hard work. Many sounds can't be seen, so we are learning to be aware of other body clues and are improving our visual skills in general.

We are also planning strategies for better community understanding: distributing a leaflet titled "Tips for Talking to the Hard of Hearing" and doing a skit demonstrating some of the problems and issues.

As we age, the environment in the vagina and urethra becomes less acid; therefore more of us are vulnerable to urinary tract or bladder infections. Cutting back on white flour, sugar and caffeine products; drinking more clear fluids and fresh-fruit unsweetened citrus juices (especially plain cranberry) and adding vitamin C and magnesium sources may help (see the discussion of cystitis, p. 592).

Memory Loss and Confusion

It is frightening to become aware that simple everyday tasks have become a problem, or to notice a decline in your capacity for sound judgment. If you observe either an increasing confusion or loss of memory in yourself, a friend or family member, don't assume "That's it! It's all downhill from here."

What does it mean to have memory lapses? We may simply be slowing down, our memory declining just as vision or hearing do, so that we will have to work a little harder at remembering and

---

TIPS FOR TALKING WITH A PERSON WITH A HEARING DIFFICULTY

1. Don't talk from another room or from behind her.

2. Reduce background noise. Turn off radio or TV if possible.

3. See that the light falls on your face, so she can use visual clues.

4. Get her attention before speaking.

5. Face her directly and on the same level if possible.

6. Keep your hands away from your face. Avoid speaking while you are smoking or eating.

7. Don't shout. Speak naturally but slowly and distinctly—and continue that way without dropping your voice.

8. She may not hear or understand something you say. If so, try saying it in a different way rather than repeating.

9. Recognize that she will hear less well if tired or ill.

10. Be patient. Even hints of irritation or impatience hurt.

11. Be an attentive listener. It's probably easier for her to talk than to listen.

Hearing aids of many different types exist, but unfortunately there are hucksters who make their money from misleading older people with hearing loss. If you are considering a hearing aid, do some reading first (see Resources).

give ourselves more time. As we get older we have more memories, so retrieving a particular memory may be more difficult.[66] When we are depressed and haven't had a chance to express grief or other emotions, preoccupation with these feelings can interfere with memory.

As one who copes with considerable memory loss at age sixty-eight, my major aid is list-making. Knowing that I may well forget an idea or "to-do," I write it down immediately. As a result, I am far better organized than at any earlier time of my life and accomplish more.

Though we experience memory lapses throughout our lives, we worry about them more when we are older. It isn't helpful when younger persons say that they also forget things because it trivializes the fear older women experience.

We can exercise memory or prevent ordinary memory loss through "mindfulness," paying attention to everyday tasks, making small (and large) decisions for ourselves.

Severe memory loss and confusion are often diagnosed as *senility* (sometimes called *dementia*). There can be several reversible causes (whose physical signs or symptoms may not be obvious): drug toxicity (from overmedication or drug interaction), dehydration, hormonal disorders, vitamin deficiency, general malnutrition, chemical or mineral imbalance, hypothermia,* anemia or other blood disorders, fever or an acute infection, depression or grief, endocrine or metabolic disorders. A small stroke, a traumatic event or accident, a series of losses or an abrupt relocation can also trigger acute confusion and disorientation.

More precise means of diagnosis have recently identified Alzheimer's disease (*not* reversible), as a major cause of severe and permanent memory loss, confusion and depression. It is now believed that Alzheimer's disease accounts for 55 percent of all diagnosed senility.† Be sure to get a prompt and thorough assessment from your practitioner (a second opinion is often necessary) to avoid inappropriate labeling of senility.

For the small percentage of elders who are correctly diagnosed with some kind of organic brain disease, drug and other therapies are available. Although memory-enhancing drugs may have proved helpful to some, the search for effective treatment of Alzheimer's continues.

Depression

Please do not listen to doctors or others who imply that being depressed is typical of aging, because it need not be. If you lose your appetite, don't feel sexual, sleep too much or can't sleep and can't enjoy anything, if such symptoms continue for over a month and if talking to friends doesn't help much, you may need professional help. Fees are prohibitive for most older persons. Unfortunately, Medicare does not cover psychotherapy without a diagnosis of severe psychopathology, which you may not want to have on your record since this can be used to disqualify your judgment in legal matters or prevent you from getting needed insurance coverage.

It is deplorable, yet still true, that many mental-health professionals do not care to work with elders.* (They think it's depressing!) *You* may have to persist to find one who trusts your ability to grow.

Medication can sometimes help, but it should be taken with *extreme caution* because elders experience more and greater effects from psychoactive drugs, and some drugs may even cause or deepen depressions. *Medication should never be given as a substitute for psychotherapy and should always be carefully monitored.*

Osteoporosis

While bone loss in women and men is normal as we age, the exaggerated loss that characterizes osteoporosis (which is preventable) is not. Estrogen does have an effect in retarding some of the bone loss that women experience at menopause (we no longer need calcium reserves when we don't get pregnant). However, because agreed scientific standards for osteoporosis diagnosis don't yet exist so that any amount of bone loss is often labeled as osteoporosis, many doctors and women have confused the two conditions.

Similarly, the discussions about osteoporosis and preventing fractures are confused because the medical approach ignores what could be accomplished by preventing accidents and falls. The campaigns by drug companies have given the impression that all women will inevitably suffer fractures unless we take estrogen. In fact, most fractures are preventable and are not caused by severe osteoporosis. Now that the search is underway for drugs that can be given to men as well as to women, the reality that the fracture rate for men catches up to that of women later in life has become news.

Normally a woman's bone mass peaks at age thirty-five, after which she tends to lose about 1 percent of bone mass every year (10 percent per decade). At sixty-five the loss declines to 3 or 4

---

*See footnote on p. 536.
†To keep abreast of changes in the field, contact the Alzheimer's Association (see Resources).

*See Robert Butler's chapter, "Emotional Problems and Mental Illness in Old Age" in *Why Survive?* for a critique of psychiatry's failure to treat elders.[67] Also consult the numerous books on psychiatry's abuses of women.

percent every ten years.[68] We do not minimize the seriousness of fractures and the need to reduce their rate. Safety measures such as reducing over-medication (the main cause of falls in the elderly), eliminating hazards such as scatter rugs, making bathrooms and staircases safer and shoveling snow and sanding ice all reduce fractures.

The question of risk usually arises when a woman comes to menopause with already inadequate bone mass due to one or more of the contributing factors below.

Contributing Factors

Lack of important nutrients is a significant factor in two-thirds of cases. Osteoporosis may occur after both artificially induced menopause (surgical removal of ovaries or chemo- or radiation therapy that makes the ovaries nonfunctional) or natural menopause; this suggests that changing estrogen levels are at least *in part* responsible. Some long-term steroid medications, such as cortisone for arthritis, also contribute to osteoporosis.* The profile of a woman most at risk for osteoporosis includes the following characteristics: white, aged sixty and over, small-boned, slender and sedentary and her uterus and/or ovaries were removed. Usually she has exercised very little, taken in insufficient calcium during her growing years and breastfed several children in her teens and early twenties. Often she also smokes and drinks alcohol excessively.

Symptoms

During its early stages, osteoporosis produces no symptoms or only mild ones such as backaches or back-muscle spasms. An older woman may be unaware she has osteoporosis until she fractures her spine, hip or wrist in a simple fall. A possible sign in postmenopausal women is pain in the upper or lower spine lasting for several days and then stopping, which may be caused by disintegrated vertebrae that collapse spontaneously. In a more advanced form, these *compression fractures* in the upper spine cause a condition commonly called *dowager's hump*; the resulting shortened chest area may make digesting food more difficult.

Diagnosis

Although routine X-rays cannot clearly show signs of osteoporosis until 30 to 40 percent of bone is lost, they may show reduced bone mass caused by other conditions.† They do not make a defini-

tive diagnosis of osteoporosis possible. If either you or your health practitioner suspect early osteoporosis, it's best if you can go to a metabolic bone disease service, usually only found in a large urban medical-research center. Techniques to measure bone mass that are becoming more widely available are single-photon absorptiometry (SPA which measures forearm, wrist or heel), dual-photon absorptiometry (DPA which measures the hip and spine), dual-energy x-ray absorptiometry (DXA which measures hip, spine, and full body faster than DPA), and computerized tomography (CAT scan which measures only the spine and exposes the patient to higher doses of radiation than the other techniques).[69] Bone testing is not appropriate or cost-effective as a screening technique.

Treatment

Predictably, physicians emphasize treatment of existing osteoporosis, usually once a dramatic fracture occurs, and neglect early prevention.* They usually prescribe, after the fact, the very activities that might have prevented the condition from developing in the first place—replacement calcium, vitamin C and D supplements, exercises such as walking and swimming, special back-exercise regimens and physical therapy. Exercising in water offers beneficial resistance to movement while placing less stress on joints.[70]

The main sources of vitamin D are sunshine, fatty fish, fortified milk, and fortified cereals. Northerners who drink less than four glasses of milk a day may want to take a vitamin D supplement between October and March to bring their intake up to the Recommended Daily Allowance of 200 IU per day. Be sure to have 800 mg of calcium daily. Yogurt and cheese, while good sources of calcium, contain no vitamin D. If you have a history of kidney stones, check with your physician.[71]

Do not assume everything is known. For example, new research suggests that vitamin K may also have a positive influence on the absorption of calcium in bone.[72]

Controversial Medical Treatments

Medical research and practice seek prevention and treatment of osteoporosis through medical intervention with estrogen, sodium fluoride or other new experimental drugs. Research reports that rapid bone loss following premature menopause can be prevented for up to eight years by taking

---

*See footnote describing *iatrogenesis*, p. 652.
†*Osteomalasia* (rickets), when the bones are soft; an endocrine disorder such as hypothyroidism, diabetes mellitus, hypoglycemia and Cushing's syndrome; any of the four bone marrow tumors: plasma cell myeloma, Ewing's tumor, reticulum cell sarcoma and Hodgkin's disease of the bone.

---

*The American Society for Bone and Mineral Research has formally addressed osteoporosis prevention, announcing guidelines that stress adequate calcium intake, regular weight-bearing exercise and avoidance of smoking.

estrogen;* yet after eight years the positive effect ceases and bone loss actually increases.[74] For women going through a natural menopause at the usual age, the effectiveness seems to last for about four years.

These treatments are still controversial, so be sure to consider the risks of estrogen as discussed on pp. 528–32. The use of sodium fluoride, which builds bone mass of questionable quality and often causes other undesirable effects,[75] seems to be warranted only in severe cases and under careful monitoring. The safety and efficacy of other new drugs have not yet been established and must be demanded before they are marketed. A sixty-year-old woman:

When I read that women menstruate for an average of thirty-seven years, I realized that number came from fifty (average age of menopause) minus thirteen (average age of the start of menstruation). Since I started my periods at eleven and stopped at fifty-three, I have already had five more years of estrogen than average. That was one factor in my decision not to take ERT.

We believe that the major defenses against fractures are accident prevention safety measures to reduce falls; healthful food and exercise throughout life to build and maintain adequate bone mass; and avoidance of smoking, hysterectomies and oophorectomies, and other causes of bone loss. These measures are without risk. Then estrogen and other drugs for women and drugs for men can be considered by the very small number of women and men who have severe bone loss or are at special risk of severe bone loss.[76]

Coping with and Overcoming Impairments and Chronic Conditions—Some Examples

Four years ago, at age eighty-one, I got diabetes. It has impaired my living condition, but it doesn't get me down. In fact, I have always had the feeling that the more we have to fight and overcome, the stronger we are. Obstacles are here to be overcome. That's part of life, and it gives us a good feeling that we are not just little ants, we are fighters.

It's not only the physical impairment that has to worry you and the doctor. It is also your state of mind. The healthy mind creates the healthy body, and the healthy body creates the healthy mind. Sometimes a frail body can draw its strength from a courageous mind.

A seventy-eight-year-old woman states:

I coped with some of my feelings of loss about my diminished hearing by developing a new interest in foreign movies. I was missing a lot at the theater* and in American movies, but when I go to a foreign movie, I can read the subtitles so I don't miss a thing—and I'm expanding my horizons!

A woman in her seventies:

For a number of years I have been living with Paget's disease in my right hip.† The doctor gave me the feeling that there were a limited number of steps "programmed" for that hip and that I should give up many of the activities I enjoyed.

Fortunately others, professionals and lay friends, suggested I continue more or less as I was, testing limits and letting discomfort be the determining factor in what I did. When camping, I found I could take some of the easier hikes and avoid the strenuous ones. I had difficulty climbing stairs at a railroad station, so I found I could navigate them by putting both feet on a step before I went to another. If I had pain when I got up after sitting engrossed with a book, I consoled myself with the awareness that this, too, would pass as I limbered up. I accepted these limits to my flexibility and found I could live within them. Then, several weeks ago, I found that I didn't have to accept them as completely. It all began with borrowing a bicycle and relearning how to ride one. It took some getting used to, but I found out how to take advantage of my strong left hip and soon was braving traffic and riding, once more, with confidence. I experienced a new freedom, a new sense of my body's resources.

Then I learned from a hiking book that all my life I had been walking incorrectly. Soon I began changing, using a more productive method. I began to feel more grounded and, at the same time, freer.

CAREGIVING AND ALTERNATIVE LIVING ARRANGEMENTS

Caregiving—A Gap in Our Delivery of Health and Medical Services

Approximately 1.5 million chronically disabled people over fifty-five are confined to their homes in the United States. RNs provide only 18 percent of nursing care, such as bandaging and giving in-

---

*Signing is a way to make cultural events accessible to persons with hearing loss. If you are planning a cultural event, be sure to find someone who will sign.

†Paget's disease is a disease characterized by a softening and bowing of bones, which thickens and enlarges the deformed bones but leaves them structurally weak. Several million Americans may have it, but most do not require specific treatment. Some of those who have it require little attention, but in others the disease produces deformities and a wide range of complications.

---

*In a research study at the University of Washington in Seattle, nearly 1,000 women who had taken estrogen for six or more years reduced the risk of fractures by 50 to 60 percent.[73]

jections. Household members provide 80 percent of the home care their ailing relatives receive (bathing, dressing, feeding).

It is the plight of thousands of women (and some men), upon whom the health system depends, to care for the aged, the chronically ill, and the disabled. They are the invisible laborers without whom neither the health system nor the patient could survive.[77]

Women are nine or ten times more likely than men to care for an aging spouse or parent or spouse's parent. We often marry men who are older than we are; we maintain our health and live longer than they do. When caregiving is work we want to do, respected by our family and community, it can be rewarding. Too often, however, others simply expect it of us.

We planned for my husband—I was going to be the person who sustained him until his death. We never worked out who would care for me. It's an unseen social service that women do; if the wife dies first, he finds another woman.

Traditionally, women have cared for family members in their own homes. In modern times some of this care has shifted to nursing homes, where it is also carried out by women, paid at the lowest wage levels. However, a variety of services have been developed to help people remain in their homes, due to a growing awareness that it is best to avoid institutionalizing persons in need of care whenever possible. Unfortunately, though such services are not only desirable but cost-effective, they are not uniformly available and are often threatened by cuts in already meager government support. Thus family-provided care most often still means woman-provided care, in isolation, without pay or needed respite or support services, without the security of job-retraining, a pension or even health insurance when the person we care for dies.

For three years, I was confined caring for a sick husband twenty-four hours a day. Then my doctor said I had to send him to a nursing home because my blood pressure was rising.

We rushed my husband to the hospital with a stroke, and it was a medical miracle. Now I'm not so sure it was a blessing. He is not always rational and cannot be left alone. Naturally, I had to give up my job. Financially, we are in terrible shape, but disaster will strike when he dies. I am fifty-seven and won't be eligible for anything. I can't see any way out.[78]

For a growing number of us, caregiving demands conflict with our jobs. (Nearly half of the women now age sixty, 65 percent of those age fifty, and 75 percent of those age forty are in the labor force.) Clearly, we need services that would make continued employment possible, such as day centers or home-care workers. Short-term nursing-home placement—even for a weekend—would help relieve the pressure on a woman carrying a full-time job along with the second job of caregiving.* Some social service organizations have support groups for caregivers and some women have set up caring pools like babysitting pools.

When We Need Care

What if we had a different cultural perspective on dependency? What if instead of a Declaration of Independence we had a Declaration of Interdependence?

Women learn to accept and even expect that others will be dependent on us. Yet we fear becoming dependent ourselves. A fifty-five-year-old divorced woman with grown children:

After my recent eye surgery it took me ages to work up a head of steam to get back the energy level that I normally work at. I'm afraid that if I really got sick and couldn't work, there would be no one to help.

A woman in her seventies:

I have a great abhorrence for the ghettos of nursing homes. I would rather struggle with overcoming physical difficulties in my own house than be put in the hands of people that I'm paying and then having to please them so they'll be nice to me.

Chronic illness or a disability which occurs late in life may be a blow to our pride and our habits of self-sufficiency. It raises the question of who will be there to care for us and whether we feel we can accept care. On the other hand, we may feel perfectly entitled to receiving from others what we have given for many decades.

Learning to accept being cared for without resentment or loss of pride is one of the tasks of our later years. It helps when those caring for us can do so without taking over our lives or taking away all our choices. A sixty-five-year-old widow who helps with the care of her grandchildren on occasion states

The interdependence between my children and me is healthy. If I needed to be taken care of at some point,

---

*Some of us may want to care for a sick family member ourselves. When we do we should receive a salary and credit toward a pension. We may need a variety of services when the person we care for dies.

Michael Weisbrot/Stock Boston

unless they change radically, I might be able to tolerate that.

Making Plans

It is a good idea to plan beforehand with family members or friends the kind of care and living situation we want when we are no longer able to manage alone—ideally neither regimented nor paternalistic, offering a wide range of challenges, providing community, privacy and as much freedom as possible, where being old is only a *part* of who we are.

Nursing Homes

We ourselves, or our relatives, may have to go into nursing homes when we come to need fairly constant nursing care. (On a given day, only 5 percent of elders live in nursing homes, but 75 percent of those who do are women. Forty percent of those in nursing homes are eighty-five years of age and over. One-quarter of all women eighty-five years and over live in nursing homes. Forty-eight percent of all persons eighty-five years and older have Alzheimer's disease.)[79]

Nursing-home care is often poor, putting profits ahead of quality care, paying workers little, skimping on patient needs. Often, in the interest of "efficiency," the routines are set up to serve only the sickest residents, depriving healthier residents of a chance to use their full capacities. Having other people or pets to care for may sustain attentiveness and memory. Lacking any meaningful decisions to make, residents become confused and disoriented.[80] Physical and mental abilities deteriorate when we have neither mental stimulation nor chances to exercise and carry out simple tasks on our own.

We are critical of many aspects of nursing-home care—the skyrocketing costs, impersonal care, medicalization of everyday life and lack of privacy and choices for residents. Patients are often discharged as quickly as possible from hospitals while home-care services have been reduced. The result is waiting lists for nursing home admission for people who would rather stay at home and could if appropriate services existed. Some nursing home residents could return home if they still had homes or home-care services. Because nursing-home care is essential for some, we must work to improve quality of life and care and innovate ways that give residents more control.

Some recent innovations include regular visits from preschool children, waist-high garden plots for persons in wheelchairs, and private rooms for sexual activity, a right won after residents at a rest home instituted a lawsuit to obtain it.*

Support Services and Strategies for Living Independently or in Alternative Housing and Care Arrangements

As we grow older, it becomes more difficult to separate health, housing and socioeconomic needs into neat compartments. Those of us who live with chronic conditions know that we need concerned persons nearby to help us with everyday tasks that have become difficult. This can contribute more to our well-being and ability to live in the community than doctor visits or medical interventions.

Despite vast differences in our well-being, living conditions and income levels, most of us want to be self-sufficient as long as possible.

A variety of services can help us, as individuals or couples, to stay in our own homes even when we need occasional nursing services or help with everyday tasks. Meals on Wheels is a program that delivers hot lunches to elders, usually five days a week. Visiting nurses, physical therapists and home-care health aides may be available to perform needed services in the home. Home care in the form of health aides or homemakers is a highly beneficial and cost-effective program, yet it is not consistently available and is continually threatened with cuts. Emergency response systems permit older persons with potentially life-threatening conditions to live alone and some phone companies have special services. Some changes to work for to make continued living in one's home a reality are (1) converting part of a home to an accessory apartment for additional income and closer neighbors; (2) convincing banks to support home equity conversion. (This means that people who fully own a home that has appreciated in value, but do not have the cash to pay living expenses or upkeep, can turn to banks for a "reverse mortgage." Banks then own an increasingly greater

---

*See Resources for pamphlets on how to choose a nursing home and how to help your family member with a move to a nursing home.

share of the home and provide cash needed for living.) At some point for many of us, living alone is no longer feasible. We may experience physical changes, reduced energy or fewer resources; we may have problems that require having others nearby; we may be lonely. Yet we probably will not need twenty-four-hour care or medical services on a daily basis. Until recently, government reimbursement and financing policies encouraged institutionalization. However, there is a growing movement for alternatives, particularly in housing, often at its most innovative in rural areas where limiting red tape is at a minimum.

Living with others is not only cost-effective but care-effective, because housemates can participate in looking out for one another rather than paying others to do so. Cooperatives, intergenerational living with relatives or friends, congregate housing, turning part of a house into an accessory apartment, small group homes—these are all new patterns of living together. Total privacy is surely impossible, but we gain dignity, companionship and security. Many elders have the strength, will and independence of spirit to make the changes required for new living arrangements.

Congregate Housing

For the past year and a half, I have shared an apartment with four other persons, a man and three women, all of us older. I had some questions before I came in: Would I still have privacy? Would I be able to get along with persons I had not even met before? The answer to both is "Yes."

The technical name for this particular kind of living is congregate housing, but I am beginning to think of us as a "family of choice." We care for one another, celebrate special days and meals together. We have our differences, too, which we settle ourselves, growing in our decision skills. I think it would be impossible to make it work if those of us with few health problems had to take care of those who had more. One woman in our apartment, legally blind, needs a homemaker to help with shopping, cleaning, bathing, et cetera. Without home-care assistance, the responsibility would be too much for the others. But we can and do help each other in important little ways.

Life-Care or Continuing-Care Communities

These communities offer apartment living for people who are in relatively good health, with medical and social services nearby. Most include a nursing home on the premises. For a sizable entrance fee and monthly charges, residents are guaranteed a permanent place to live and a specified package of medical and nursing benefits to suit the resident's changing needs.

Obtain a written agreement specifying the care available, your rights to terminate the contract and receive a refund, the alternative provisions available and the conditions under which you might be discharged. Find out whether your assets remaining after your death belong to the owner or whether some equity passes to your heirs.

Some communities have closed, causing their residents hardships. Whether nonprofit or for profit, such communities need regulation. Be a prudent consumer: Obtain information in writing, and have the community's financial statement reviewed by your accountant, estate planner or lawyer.

Privately Run Retirement Homes

These may be appropriate alternatives for elders who do not need nursing care or case management but prefer not to be alone. In the words of a geriatric social worker describing her community:

Two women from Maine triumphed over midlife crises by going into a whole new field of endeavor. After being turned down by eight banks, they finally obtained funds for renovating an enormous old house in a small rural village. They provide room, board and laundry for a group of fourteen elders, most of whom have lived in the area for many years. Using the fruits of a large organic garden and orchard, bartering surplus seedlings for fish and other commodities, they acquired such a good reputation for their food that they were asked to cater weddings and parties. These activities in turn have enabled them to keep their costs—and their rents—fairly low and give the residents the option of participating in the food preparation or festivities.

We are impressed by the variety and innovativeness of support services for elders and their caregivers in other countries.

- The Scandinavian countries provide service buses to bring cleaning and laundry, hairdressing supplies, books and hot food to elders who wish to remain in their homes. Homemakers and personal care attendants are provided to those who need them. An alternative is the service house, where all such services are available on the premises to those who live there. The state pays family caregivers.
- In New Zealand, low-interest loans, services and subsidies are available to families who wish to care for elderly relatives at home.
- In England, clusters of about twenty apartments for elders are staffed by a state-employed "helper" who gets people to doctor appointments and so on. Respite care, short-term placement in nursing homes, is available to give

caregivers a breather. Caregivers are organized in an advocacy organization.

Many of these services or equally creative ones are available or potentially available to elders in this country. However, our programs exist as a patchwork of innovations in a crazy quilt of cutbacks and threatened cutbacks. For instance, chronically scarce funding, often awarded to innovative pilot programs, is not renewed after they succeed and are no longer "new." As a nation, we have not deliberately decided (as have the Scandinavian countries) to make the older years a good time of life, free from financial worry and deprivation. As an ever greater percent of the electorate enters the older years, we develop a growing base of support for such a national commitment.

DEATH

At all ages we struggle with the reality of death. We lose our parents; as parents we may lose infants and children. People we love die. If we become terminally ill at any age, we have to cope with our imminent deaths. But the impetus to accept this reality for ourselves comes for most of us as we grow older. A fifty-two-year-old woman:

We have the fear that if a person faces death that means she does not participate in life. Actually, it works the other way. The more we acknowledge and recognize death, the more we can live in the present.

A seventy-eight-year-old woman states:

I am more aware of a mystery and beauty in life since I have accepted death as a personal eventuality for me. Before then, I had thought of death out there; now I know that I am going to die. That has released me for more vivid living. I reach out more. Almost everything reminds me of its connections with other things; my present is many-textured. I do not look to the future with dread. It has to be shorter than my past but it does not have to be less rich.

Some of us continue to feel ambivalent and scared about acknowledging death or have difficulty coming to grips with the reality of it for ourselves. According to a seventy-four-year-old woman,

Intellectually I'm very glib about it, but in my gut I can't accept that one day I won't be here.

In our culture, discussion of death has been taboo until the last few years. Modern medical science often distorts our ideas of death. Many doctors view it as an adversary, an evil, a visible defeat. They often use every medical means possible to prolong life for its own sake without considering its quality or whether there is any hope of recovery, and without taking into account the ill person's wishes.

In response to the excessive medicalization of death, terminally ill people, their friends and relatives and concerned professionals have created *hospices*, a humane alternative to general hospital or nursing-home care. More than a place, a hospice is an idea and a service. The thing we fear most when we are seriously ill is prolonged and unmanageable pain. Hospice workers assist people to manage pain, to die at home or in special places neither home nor hospital. The patient and family together are the focus of attention. Hospices offer support, understanding and respite to everyone involved. Bereavement counseling may continue for a substantial period beyond the family member's death.

Taking Control of Our Own Death

We know we cannot control whether we die, so we often jump to the conclusion that there is *nothing* we can do about it—no control, no choice.

Yet we do have elements of control. Many of us can choose our place of death—at home or in a hospital or hospice. As long as we are able, we can fight for medical care that allows us to keep our dignity, instead of accepting care that is inappropriate for extreme pain and terminal illness. Only we can authorize a precise disposal of our property, donate vitally needed organs like kidneys and corneas for transplant if we wish and perform the little details that ensure an easier burden for relatives and friends.

Though legal, medical and theological controversies abound, many of us would like to participate fully in the decision about when and how we will die. The right to control our deaths is part of our basic right to have control over our bodies and our lives. A woman in her seventies:

I have been searching for a doctor who would let me participate not just in my health care but in my own death, too.

We want to be able to define for ourselves what we consider a tolerable quality of life, a worthwhile existence.

I've had a lot of things done to my body and I'm seventy-three. I've made up my mind that enough has been done to me. If something bad happens, something major, I'm not sure I want to be repaired again. No more tampering with my body! I don't want to live to be one hundred if I'm all botched up.

We may actively decide we want to avoid a long, drawn-out period of illness and dependency, to avoid a medicalized death in which life is prolonged by artificial means and/or to choose the occasion and means of our death. We can make a *living will** when we are well, stating what we want and do not want; however, there's no guarantee that these written wishes will be honored.

Laws vary from state to state. In many states it is not legal to decide how or when we want to die. All states, however, permit us, when we are well, to name a person who can make medical decisions for us if we become unable to make them for ourselves. We can name this person as part of a living will or in a separate document called a *durable power of attorney for medical affairs,* a *health-care proxy* or *an advance directive.*

To protect loved ones from possible prosecution as accessories, some dying persons have chosen to go off by themselves when taking a fatal substance. We may even have to forego some of the talking and planning we might want to do in order to protect our loved ones from legal harassment. A woman in her sixties:

I have for years kept a precious bottle somewhere. I talked with my daughter about it and she asked me, "Please, if you are ever ready to do this, tell me first." But I said I couldn't do that because I would be laying too heavy a burden on her; she would certainly feel that it was her job to dissuade me.

An important way to gain the power to choose our own deaths is by working to change the laws and social attitudes related to death and dying and by challenging legal, medical and religious control. Some organizations exist to help us raise these issues publicly and deal with them personally.

Claiming the right to control the ending of our lives in no way minimizes the seriousness or the finality of the decision, nor the pain and grief of those we leave behind. Yet the issues are complex. It is certainly more appropriate for the dying person rather than any outside authority to weigh all the factors involved.

SURVIVAL SKILLS

Many women are still going strong at seventy or seventy-five and beyond. We want to end this chapter with their voices as they tell of the "sur-

Photography class at Freedom House, Roxbury, MA.

vival skills" that keep them active, creative, involved and feeling good about themselves and their lives.*

In our mothers' time, the only acceptable role for a woman over sixty was a homebody, puttering around in the kitchen, not going out anywhere. We still have that image we can follow. If you don't question it, you may find that you are following a stereotype instead of your own true path. You have to go out and look for what really meets your needs. For myself, I look for activities that I can shape as well as contribute to and that get me out of the house. I enjoy my work visiting elders who can't go out; it makes me feel that I am contributing to others. My women's support group meets my needs as an older woman and is something that I can help define.

It is important to challenge the stereotypes of elders as rigid, unable to form new relationships or to experience change and growth.†

---

*Most of the older women we spoke with in preparing this chapter enjoy reasonably good health and adequate economic situations. Though this is not the case for large numbers of women, these experiences highlight the *potential* for the older years; a potential (the birthright of every person) denied to so many of us because of inadequate food, housing, care, transportation, health and medical care and the constant worry about how to pay for all of these.

†Professionals, researchers and practitioners have contributed to the stereotyping of elders by perpetuating the *disengagement theory*—the idea that elders gradually withdraw from life by divesting themselves of important roles and commitments as an appropriate adjustment to aging and approaching death. It would be more appropriate to say that disengagement is an inappropriate giving-in to ageism and the impoverishment of many elders. We have learned from the many lively, vital, elder women we spoke with that it is possible to live fully for as long as we live.

---

*Sample copies and other information available from Choice in Dying (see Resources). All hospitals and nursing homes now have advance directives available. See Patients' Rights in Chapter 25.

There's a discrepancy between my image of an older person in her seventies and the way I feel. In fact, there's no connection. My concept of a grandmother was of someone who didn't do much. But I became a grandmother at forty-seven. I started a vigorous exercise program at forty-three and am still running every day at seventy-six and love it.

A seventy-seven-year-old woman states:

The seventies have been the best decade of my life. From what I have seen with my friends, it is either the best or the worst. My creative work as an artist is what keeps me alive; my friends keep me happy and contented. If I had to give up people I would never have another happy day, but I would stay alive if I could work.

An eighty-five-year-old woman:

It is not so different to be over eighty, except that accidents and illness can make a change. If I had not broken my hip I would probably still be very active today, but I wouldn't have the insight I have. Being confined gives me more time for reflection.

I known I have grown in the last ten years, even at my age. I have become more optimistic. A lot of young people seem to be drawn to me. I don't know

Peter Simon

if I give more now than I used to or have more composure and insight. That sounds funny, but it is a fact.

I had to concentrate on getting well, and this makes you rather self-centered. Sometimes I catch myself thinking, I am too busy with my body. What about exercising my mind? That's why I think that intermingling with different kinds of people, young and old, is very important. The segregation of the aged is absolutely ridiculous, cruel, unproductive and costly.

Staying in Touch with Our Inner Selves— Nourishing the Spirit

Staying in touch with ourselves helps us reach out to others, cope with the hard things in our lives and keep on growing. There are many ways that we can stay in touch with ourselves—writing in a journal, reading a book, exercising, meditating, walking in the woods, a long hot shower or bath, camping. For some of us, being connected with a spiritual community helps, too.

Last week, at age seventy-three, I sat in a group of older women discussing religion and spirituality and was reminded of our midweek prayer meetings sixty years ago, except that no woman there was witnessing to the teachings of her childhood church indoctrination but was describing instead her "spirituality." The world's religions have all been founded by men and promote their beliefs, not to mention their reverence of dominance. I don't choose to have men control my moral and spiritual values. In looking within myself for what I value most, I discover I put honesty first, nurturing next, then striving for peace and justice in human relationships and cherishing our earth and universe. I nourish my spirit through music, nature study and meditation but mostly through relatedness to people I love.

A thought has come to me in the last few years. I doubt that when I die my life will be over—my life with all its loving and caring and striving. Can it be that all my loved ones—mother, sister, other relatives—can all this love be gone? Nothing in nature disappears. Out of our bones, our skeletons, new life comes in some other way.

Support Groups for Older Women

Friendship is valuable not only for happiness and mental well-being but for physical health and survival as well. Because aging in this country too often means increasing isolation, the middle and older years are a good time to create a support and friendship network if you don't already have one. A study at Yale found that, regardless of age, persons with strong social bonds (marriage, friends, group or organizational affiliations) had a mortality rate 2.5 percent lower than those who were relatively isolated. The other important finding was that friendship and support from *any* of these sources contributed to survival.[81]

I am open to the new adventure of meeting people. Once I was congratulated for having been one of the founders of the Boston Gray Panthers. I had to answer that I didn't deserve any thanks. The Gray Panthers deserve thanks from me. Those relationships and that connection mean so much that I am just plain grateful.

It is never too late to form a support group.

NOTES

1. Jean Tock (sculptor). Personal communication, 1982.

2. U.S. Department of Commerce, Bureau of the Census. *Statistical Abstracts of the United States 1991, The National Data Book.* Washington, DC: U.S. Government Printing Office, p. 73.
   U.S. Department of Commerce, Bureau of the Census. 1990 Census of the Population. "Projections of the Population of the U.S. by Age, Sex, and Race: 1988 to 2080," in *Current Population Reports,* No. 1018. Washington, D.C.: U.S. Government Printing Office, 1989, p. 25.

3. Susan Sontag. "The Double Standard of Aging," *Saturday Review of the Society,* Vol. 95, No. 39 (September 23, 1972), pp. 29–38.

4. Barbara Ehrenreich and Karin Stallard. "The Nouveau Poor," *Ms.* (August 1982), pp. 217–24. Paula Rayman. "Why Women Are Poor," testimony for House Select Committee on Aging, Brookline, MA, May 15, 1992.

5. U.S. Department of Commerce, Bureau of the Census. "1991 Current Population Survey," unpublished tables. Information from Arnold A. Goldstein.

6. Marilyn R. Block et al. *Uncharted Territory: Issues and Concerns of Women Over Forty.* College Park, MD: University of Maryland, Center on Aging, 1978, p. 144.

7. Tish Sommers. "Employment Problems of Older Women," pp. 3–4. Oakland, CA: Older Women's League.

8. Marilyn R. Block et al., *Uncharted Territory,* pp. 157–58.

9. Report of the National Commission on Social Security Reform, 1981. *Note:* This is a report that was prepared in the last days of the Carter administration and came out in early 1981. It was not widely circulated and was superseded by a subsequent report by the Reagan administration. The 1981 report contains important information for women. It is not easy to get, but it is possible to obtain a copy if you persist.

10. "Hysterectomies in the U.S. 1965–84." *Vital & Health Statistics,* DHHS Publication No. (PHS) 88-1753, December 1987.

11. *HHS News,* U.S. Department of Health and Human Services, October 31, 1980; *HEW News,* October 15, 1979.

12. Lillian Rubin. *Women of a Certain Age.* New York: Harper & Row, 1979.

13. Bureau of the Census. Statistical Abstracts of the United States 1991, p. 42.

14. Knud J. Helsing, Moyses Szklo and George W. Comstock. "Factors Associated with Mortality After Widowhood," *American Journal of Public Health,* Vol. 71 (1981), pp. 802–09.

15. Helene Deutsch. *The Psychology of Women: A Psychoanalytic Interpretation,* Vol. II. New York: Grune & Stratton, 1944.

16. Mary Roth Walsh. *Doctors Wanted: No Women Need Apply! Sexual Barriers in the Medical Profession.* New Haven, CT: Yale University Press, 1977.

17. Myrna Weissman. "The Myth of Involutional Melancholia," *Journal of the American Medical Association,* Vol. 242, No. 8 (August 1979), pp. 24–31. John B. McKinlay et al. "The Relative Contributions of Endocrine Changes and Social Circumstances to Depression in Mid-Aged Women," *Journal of Health and Social Behavior,* Vol. 28 (December 1987), pp. 345–63.

18. Janice G. Raymond. "Medicine as Patriarchal Religion," *Journal of Medicine and Philosophy,* Vol. 7 (1982), pp. 197–216.

19. Robert Wilson. *Feminine Forever.* New York: M. Evans and Co., 1966.

20. David Reuben. *Everything You Always Wanted to Know About Sex.* New York: David McKay Co., 1969.

21. David Reuben. *Everything You Always Wanted to Know About Sex.*

22. Patricia Kaufert. "The Perimenopausal Woman and Her Use of Health Services," *Maturitas,* Vol. 2, No. 3 (October 1980), pp. 191–205.

23. Sandra Ritz. "Growing Older Through Menopause," *Medical Self-Care,* Vol. 15 (Winter 1981), pp. 14–19.

24. Rosetta Reitz. *Menopause: A Positive Approach.* New York: Penguin Books, 1982. Barbara Seaman and Gideon Seaman. *Women and the Crisis in Sex Hormones.* New York: Bantam Books, 1977. *Consumer Reports* (November 1976), p. 642.

25. Comments by Diane P. Petitti, MD, School of Medicine, University of California at San Francisco, October 1991.

26. Vidal S. Clay. "Menopause," in Patricia Cooper, ed., *Women's Health and Medical Guide.* Des Moines, IA: Meredith Corp., 1981.

27. Vidal S. Clay. "Menopause." See also Patricia Kaufert, "The Perimenopausal Woman" in *Women's Health and Medical Guide.*

28. U.S. Department of Health and Human Services, Public Health Service. Surveillance, Epidemiology and End Results, Incidence and Mortality Data, 1973–1977, National Institutes of Health, Publication No. 81-2330.

29. Donald Smith et al. "Association of Exogenous Estrogen and Endometrial Cancer," *New England Journal of Medicine,* Vol. 293 (December 4, 1975), pp. 1164–67.

30. Vidal S. Clay. "Menopause."

31. Barbara Seaman and Gideon Seaman. *Women and the Crisis in Sex Hormones.* Survey by Pharmaceutical Data Services and *American Drug* magazine quoted in *Parade Magazine* (April 21, 1991), p. 12.

32. Survey by Pharmaceutical Data Services and

American Druggist reported in *Parade Magazine* (April 21, 1991), p. 12.

33. Kenneth J. Ryan. "Cancer Risks and Estrogen Use in the Menopause," an editorial in *New England Journal of Medicine*, Vol. 293 (1975), p. 1200.

34. Boston Collaborative Drug Surveillance Program. "Surgically Confirmed Gallbladder Disease, Venous Thromboembolism, and Breast Tumors in Relation to Postmenopausal Estrogen Therapy," *The New England Journal of Medicine*, Vol. 290 (1974), pp. 15–19. Diane B. Petitti, et al. "Increased Risk of Cholecystectomy in Users of Supplemental Estrogen," *Gastroenterology*, Vol. 94, No. 1 (1988), pp. 91–95.

35. Barbara Seaman and Gideon Seaman. *Women and the Crisis in Sex Hormones.*

36. S. M. Wolfe. Testimony of Public Citizens' Health Research Group, Washington, DC, August 1, 1979.

37. Sharon Lieberman. "New Discovery: Public Relations Cures Cancer," *Majority Report*, February 1977. See also S. Lieberman, "But You'll Make Such a Lovely Corpse," *Majority Report* (February 19–March 5, 1977).

38. Brian MacMahon. Personal communication, 1982. See also K. K. Steinberg et al. "A Meta-analysis of the Effect of Estrogen Replacement Therapy on the Risk of Breast Cancer," *Journal of the American Medical Association*, Vol. 265 (April 1991), pp. 1985–90.

39. Nancy Reider. Personal communication, 1991.

40. Meir Stampfer, et al. "Post-Menopausal Estrogen Therapy and Cardiovascular Diseases: Ten Year Follow Up from the Nurses' Health Study," *The New England Journal of Medicine*, Vol. 325 (1991), pp. 756–62.

41. Davi Birnbaum and Cynthia Pearson. Testimony to the Food and Drug Administration, June 14–15, 1990. Cynthia Pearson. Testimony before the Select Committee on Aging, May 30, 1991. Diane B. Petitti. Comments, October 1991.

42. Study published in the *Journal of the National Cancer Institute*. Reported by Richard A. Knox in *The Boston Globe* (April 19, 1991).

43. Barbara Seaman and Gideon Seaman. *Women and the Crisis in Sex Hormones.*

44. Lila Wallis. "Can Hormone Therapy of the Menopausal Syndrome Be Made Safe?" *Proceedings of the Women in Medicine Conference, Cornell Medical School*, 1981, pp. 89–92.

45. Barbara Seaman and Gideon Seaman. *Women and the Crisis in Sex Hormones.*

46. Ettinger, Bruce, et al. "Low-dosage Micronized 17B-estradiol prevents bone loss in postmenstrual women." *American Journal of Obstetrics and Gynecology*, Vol. 166, No. 2 (February 1992), pp. 479–88.

47. Quoted in Marilyn R. Block et al., *Uncharted Territory*, p. 43.

48. Mary Jane Sherfey. *The Nature and Evolution of Female Sexuality*. New York: Vintage Books, 1972, p. 102.

49. Jane Brody. "Personal Health: Sex in the Elderly," *The New York Times* (July 5, 1978).

50. Alice Lake. *Our Own Years: What Women Over 35 Should Know About Themselves*. New York: Random House, 1979, p. 98.

51. "How Your Health Affects Your Sex Life," *Family Circle* (June 8, 1982).

52. Robert C. Atchley. "Later Adulthood in Oxford Township." Summary of one-year data, Scripps Foundation Gerontology Foundation, Miami University, Oxford, OH, 1975.

53. Loretta Schwartz-Nobel. *Starvation in the Shadow of Plenty*. New York: G.P. Putnam's Sons, 1980.

54. *Growing Numbers, Growing Force: A Report from The White House Mini-Conference on Older Women*, 1980. Oakland, CA: OWL, 1980. Still available from the Older Women's League (see Resources) for $5.50 plus postage.

55. S.V. Saxon and M.H. Etlen. *Physical Change and Aging: A Guide for the Helping Professions*. New York: The Tiresiav Press, 1978. See also *Journal of the American Medical Association*, Vol. 247, No. 8 (February 26, 1982), pp. 1106–12.

56. J.F. Aloia et al. "Old Runners Overtake the Aging Process," *Medical World News* (April 30, 1979).

57. G. Donald Whedon. "Osteoporosis" (editorial), *New England Journal of Medicine*, Vol. 305, No. 7 (August 13, 1981), pp. 397–99.

58. Warren E.C. Wacker. *Magnesium and Man*. Cambridge, MA: Harvard University Press, 1980.

59. World Health Organization recommendations as quoted by Maggie Lettvin, personal communication, May 9, 1983.

60. Robert Butler. *Why Survive?: Being Old in America*. New York: Harper-Colophon, 1975.

61. Robert Butler. *Why Survive?* p. 178.

62. *Medical World News* (September 13, 1982), p. 70.

63. Alex Comfort. *A Good Age*. New York: Crown Publishers, Inc., 1976, p. 62. For a more complete list see *Health Facts*, Vol. VII, No. 34 (March 1982), p. 7.

64. *Beware*, a film about the dangers of overmedication for elders. Adelphi University Center on Aging, Garden City, NY 11530.

65. Robert Butler. *Why Survive?* p. 179.

66. Alice Lake. *Our Own Years*, pp. 215–16.

67. Robert Butler. *Why Survive?* pp. 231–35.

68. Donald G. Whedon. "Osteoporosis," pp. 397–99.

69. National Osteoporosis Foundation and Administration on Aging. "Testing Your Bone Health," *Bonewise*, 1991. See Resources.

70. Joseph Lane. "Postmenopausal Osteoporosis: The Orthopedic Approach," *The Female Patient*, Vol. 6 (November 1981), pp. 43–51.

71. Bess Dawson-Hughes. "Effect of Vitamin D Supplementation on Wintertime and Overall Bone Loss in Healthy Post-menopausal Women," *Annals on Internal Medicine*, Vol. 115 (1991), 99, pp. 505–512.

72. Natalie Angier. "Vitamins Win Support as Potent Agents of Health," *The New York Times*, March 10, 1992, pp. C1, C8.

73. Noel S. Weiss et al. "Decreased Risk of Fractures of the Hip and Lower Forearm with Postmenopausal Use of Estrogen," *New England Journal of Medicine*, Vol. 303, No. 21 (November 20, 1980), pp. 1195–98.

74. R. Lindsay et al. "Bone Response to Termination of Estrogen Treatment," *Lancet*, Vol. 1 (1978), pp. 1325–27.

75. B. Lawrence Riggs, et al. "Effect of the Fluoride/Calcium Regimen on Vertebral Fracture Occurrence in Postmenopausal Osteoporosis," *New England Journal of Medicine*, Vol. 306, No. 8 (February 25, 1982), pp. 446–50.

76. Richard L. Prince, et al. "Prevention of Post-

menopausal Osteoporosis: A Comparative Study of Exercise, Calcium Supplements, and Hormone Replacement Therapy." *The New England Journal of Medicine*, Vol. 325, No. 17 (October 24, 1991), pp. 1189–1195.

77. Elinor Polansky. "Take Him Home, Mrs. Smith," *Healthright*, Vol. II, No. 2 (Winter 1975–1976).

78. Tish Sommers. "A Feminist View of Death." Presented at Drake University Law School, Des Moines, IA, March 27, 1976.

79. AARP Women's Initiative. *Facts About Older Women. Housing and Living Arrangements*, 1989, p. 2. National Center for Health Statistics. *1985 National Nursing Home Survey, Use of Nursing Homes by the Elderly*, Bethesda, MD: Author, 1987. Alzheimer's statistic from Paul Raia, acting director, Alzheimer's Association of Eastern Massachusetts.

80. Ellen J. Langer and Judith Rodin. "The Effects of Choice and Enhanced Personal Responsibility for the Aged: A Field Experiment in an Institutional Setting," *Journal of Personality and Social Psychology*, Vol. 34, No. 2 (1976), pp. 191–98.

81. Syme, Leonard S. and Lisa Berkman. "Social Class Susceptibility and Sickness," in Peter Conrad and Rochelle Kern (eds.), *The Sociology of Health and Illness: Critical Perspective*. New York: St. Martin's Press, 1990. Earlier edition cited by Judy Foreman. "Friends: As Vital as Family," *Boston Globe*, February 3, 1982.

RESOURCES

Books

Alexander, Jo, et al. *Women and Aging: An Anthology by Women*. Corvallis, OR: Calyx Books, 1986.

Anderson, Beverly, and Adeline McConnel. *Single After 50: How to Have the Time of Your Life*. New York: McGraw-Hill, 1981. Not a feminist book, but full of useful tips for heterosexual women and men. Lively and empowering.

Block, Marilyn R., Janice L. Davidson and Jean D. Grambs. *Women Over Forty: Visions and Realities*. New York: Springer Publishing Co., 1981.

Bluh, Bonnie. *The "Old" Speak Out*. New York: Horizon Press, 1979. Interviews with women and men in their sixties, seventies, eighties, nineties and even past a hundred tell of the joys and pleasures as well as the struggles of the older years.

Boston Women's Health Book Collective. *Ourselves and Our Children: A Book by and for Women*. New York: Random House, 1978. See especially chapters "The Teenage Years" and "Being Parents of Grownups."

Butler, Robert N. *Why Survive? Being Old in America*. New York: Harper-Colophon, 1975. Essential reading, though the directory is outdated.

Butler, Robert N., and Myrna I. Lewis. *Sex After Forty: A Guide for Men and Women in Their Mid and Later Years*. New York: Harper & Row, 1986.

Chalker, Rebecca, and Kristene E. Whitmore. *Overcoming Bladder Disorders*. New York: Harper & Row, 1990. Excellent self-help and medical material for women and men on many subjects including incontinence and interstitial cystitis.

Clay, Vidal. *Women: Menopause and Middle Age*. Pittsburgh: Know, Inc., 1977.

Cohen, Leah. *Small Expectations: Society's Betrayal of Older Women*. Toronto: McClellan and Stewart, 1984.

Copper, Baba. *Over the Hill: Reflections on Ageism Between Women*. Freedom, CA: The Crossing Press, 1988.

Cunningham, Imogen. *After Ninety*. Seattle: University of Washington Press, 1977. Photographs of people over ninety along with interviews with those who knew and worked with Cunningham.

Geba, Bruno. *Vitality Training for Older Adults*. New York: Random House, 1974. A therapist working with elderly in nursing homes advocates masssage because many residents of nursing homes are starved for touch.

Harlow, Jan. *Good Age Cookbook: Recipes from the Institute for Creative Aging*. Boston: Houghton Mifflin Co., 1979.

Jacobs, Ruth Harriet. *Be an Outrageous Older Woman— A R*A*S*P* Remarkable Aging Smart Person*. KIT, 1131-0 Tolland Turnpike, Suite 175, Manchester, CT 06040, 1991. Full of humor, empowering suggestions and success stories.

Kübler-Ross, Elisabeth. *On Death and Dying*. New York: Macmillan Publishing Co., 1969.

Lake, Alice. *Our Own Years: What Women Over 35 Should Know about Themselves*. New York: Random House, 1979. Highly recommended.

Macdonald, Barbara, with Cynthia Rich. *Look Me in the Eye: Old Women, Aging, and Ageism*. San Francisco: Spinsters Ink, 1983.

Mace, Nancy L., and Peter V. Rabins. *The 36-Hour Day*. Baltimore: Johns Hopkins University Press, 1984. A family guide to caring for persons with Alzheimer's and related dementing illnesses and memory loss in later life.

Markson, Elizabeth, ed. *Older Women: Issues and Prospects*. Lexington, MA: Lexington Press, 1983. Academic in tone, but filled with useful information. The article on sexuality is especially useful.

Nickerson, Betty. *Old and Smart: Women and Aging*. All About Us Books, 3012 Yellow Point Road, RR #3, Ladysmith, BC, Canada V0R 2E0. 1991. $19.95 plus $2.50 postage and GST. U.S. ordering address: c/o Laurie Trieger, 443 Adams Street, Eugene, OR 97402. $16.95 plus $2 postage. Affirming book in large print.

Notelovitz, Morris, and Marsha Ware. *Stand Tall! The Informed Woman's Guide to Osteoporosis*, 1982. Triad Publishing Co., Box 13096, Gainesville, FL 32604.

Olson, Laura Katz. *The Political Economy of Aging*. New York: Columbia University Press, 1982.

Payer, Lynn. *How to Avoid a Hysterectomy*. New York: Pantheon Books, 1987.

Porcino, Jane. *Growing Older, Getting Better: A Handbook for Women in the Second Half of Life*. Reading, MA: Addison-Wesley, 1983. Highly recommended.

———. *Living Longer, Living Better: Adventures in Community Housing for Those in the Second Half of Life*. New York: Crossroad/Continuum, 1991.

Raphael, Beverly. *The Anatomy of Bereavement*. New York: Basic Books, 1984.

Robey, Harriet. *There's Dance in the Old Dame Yet*. Boston: Atlantic/Little, Brown, 1982.

Rubin, Lillian. *Women of a Certain Age: The Midlife Search for Self*. New York: Harper & Row, 1979.

Sanders, Katherine. *Grief: The Mourning After. Dealing with Adult Bereavement*. New York: John Wiley & Sons, 1989.

Sarton, May. *As We Are Now*. New York: W.W. Norton and Co., 1982. A novel about a woman placed without her consent in a badly run boarding home for elders.

———. *Kinds of Love*. New York: W.W. Norton and Co., 1980. A novel about the friendship between two older women and their bonds with each other, with family and others in their community. Celebrates caring and connection.

———. *A Reckoning*. New York: W.W. Norton and Co., 1981. A novel about a woman with terminal cancer who takes control of her death and ultimately finds it "a ripening"—one of the most interesting parts of her life.

Scott-Maxwell, Florida. *The Measure of My Days*. New York: Alfred A. Knopf, 1968.

Shapiro, Barbara. *The Big Squeeze: Balancing the Needs of Aging Parents, Dependent Children, and You*. Bedford, MA: Mills & Sanderson, 1991.

Shields, Laurie. *Displaced Homemakers: Organizing for a New Life*. New York: McGraw-Hill, 1981.

Silverman, Phyllis. *Helping Women Cope with Grief*. Beverly Hills, CA: Sage, 1981.

———. *Mutual Help Groups: Organization and Development*. Beverly Hills, CA: Sage, 1980.

———. *Widow-to-Widow*. New York: Springer Publishing Co., 1985. Reports on self-help groups for widows.

Skeist, Robert J. *To Your Good Health!* Chicago: Chicago Review Press, 1980. A practical guide for older people. Large print.

Slagle, Kate Walsh. *Live with Loss*. Englewood Cliffs, NJ: Prentice-Hall, 1982. Practical, compassionate techniques for coping with many kinds of loss and moving through grief to growth.

Thomas, Sherry. *We Didn't Have Much, But We Sure Had Plenty: Stories of Rural Women*. Garden City, NY: Doubleday/Anchor Books, 1981.

Wilson, Emily Herring. *Older Black Women of the South*. Philadelphia: Temple University Press, 1983.

Wolf, Deborah Coleman. *Growing Older: Lesbians and Gay Men*. Berkeley, CA: University of California Press, 1982.

Worden, J. W., and William Proctor. *Personal Death Awareness*. Englewood Cliffs, NJ: Prentice-Hall, 1976.

Periodicals

Broomstick
Options for Women Over Forty
 3543 18th Street, Suite 3
 San Francisco, CA 94110
A quarterly newsletter by, for and about women over forty.

A Friend Indeed—a newsletter for women in the prime of life. Janine O'Leary Cobb, editor
A Friend Indeed Publications, Inc.
 Box 515
 Place du Parc Station
 Montreal, Canada H2W 2P1

Published monthly except July and August. $30 per year. An international newsletter for women in menopause and midlife.

Hot Flash
Jane Porcino
c/o NAFOW
 Box 816
 Stony Brook, NY 11790-0609
A quarterly newsletter of the National Action Forum for Midlife and Older Women.

Membership Organizations and Sources of Printed Information and Referrals

Alzheimer's Association, Inc.
National Headquarters
 919 North Michigan Avenue, Suite 1000
 Chicago, IL 60611
 (800) 272-3900

American Association of Retired Persons (AARP)
 Program Department
 601 E Street NW
 Washington, DC 20049
 (202) 434-2277
Members receive their magazine, *Modern Maturity*, and newsletter, *Bulletin*. AARP has many subdivisions, including a women's division and a health division. The Institute for Lifetime Learning helps older persons pursue educational and/or career changes.

American Health Care Association
 1201 L Street NW
 Washington, DC 20005
 (202) 842-4444
"Thinking About a Nursing Home: A Consumer's Guide for Choosing a Long-Term Care Facility" includes a checklist of questions to ask.

American Self-Help Clearinghouse
St. Clares-Riverside Medical Center
 Denville, NJ 07834
 (201) 625-7101
Publishes *The Self-Help Source Book: Finding and Forming Mutual Aid Self-Help Groups*. $8. Send for complete publication list.

Elderhostel
 75 Federal Street
 Boston, MA 02110
 (617) 426-7788
Short-term, intensive campus-based educational experiences for older adults all over the world. Publishes three seasonal catalogs.

Gray Panthers
 1424 Sixteenth Street, NW, Suite 602
 Washington, DC 20036
 (202) 387-3111
An intergenerational membership organization. Advocates for concerns of elders and other social change issues. Their quarterly newsletter, *Network*, is available for $15 annually, $30 for organizations, libraries and foreign subscriptions.

National Osteoporosis Foundation
 2100 M Street, NW, Suite 602

Washington, DC 20037
(202) 223-2226
Send for *Bonewise,* a free information kit for older persons, published with the Administration on Aging. The kit includes *Boning Up on Osteoporosis,* which contains postural tips and exercises.

National Women's Health Network
1324 G Street, NW
Washington, DC 20005-2052
(202) 347-1140
Their educational and advocacy work on older women's issues has resulted in the publication of *Taking Hormones and Women's Health: Choices, Risks, Benefits,* available for $5 plus $1.50 costs. Membership includes the newsletter, *The Network News.*

Older Women's League
666 Eleventh Street, NW, Suite 700
Washington, DC 20001-4512
(202) 783-6686
A local and national membership organization that advocates for older women's concerns. Members receive the newspaper, *The OWL Observer.* For twenty-four-hour legislative update, call (202) 783-6689.

Special Resources on Selected Issues

Caregiving

Brody, Elaine M. *Women in the Middle: Their Parent-care Years.* New York: Springer Publishing Co., 1990.

Roberts, D. Jean. *Taking Care of Caregivers.* Palo Alto, CA: Bull Publishing Co., 1991.

Silverstone, Barbara and Helene Hyman. *You and Your Aging Parents: The Modern Family's Guide to Emotional, Physical, and Financial Problems.* New York: Pantheon, 1981.

Sommers, Tish and Laurie Shields. *Women Take Care.* Gainesville, FL: Triad Publishing Co., 1987. An important book on women as caregivers.

Children of Aging Parents (CAPS)
Woodbourne Office Campus, Suite 302A
1609 Woodbourne Road
Levittown, PA 19057
(215) 249-0509
A starter packet of materials is available for $25 including a national directory of caregiver support groups and professional geriatric care managers.

Eldercare Locator
A resource operated by the National Association of Area Agencies on Aging to help you find community services for the elderly in any community. The national toll-free number is 1-800-677-1116.

National Council on the Aging
1112 16th Street, NW
Suite 100
Washington, DC 20036
(202) 479-1200
Five brochures on caregiving are available for $1. They also have a *Directory of Support and Self-help Groups.*

Death and Dying

Choice in Dying
250 West 57th Street
New York, NY 10019
(212) 246-6962 or 6973
An educational and legal organization that publishes a newsletter and will send you a living-will form.

National Hospice Organization
1901 North Moore Street, Suite 901
Arlington, VA 22209
(703) 243-5900
Publishes a national directory.

Displaced Homemakers

National Displaced Homemakers Network
1625 K Street, NW, Suite 300
Washington, DC 20006
(202) 467-6346
This national office can help you locate the state and local programs. Send SASE for publication list.

Hearing and Hearing Aids

Marshall, Patricia. "Making Sure Hearing Aids Help," *FDA Consumer* (June 1976). Order from U.S. Government Printing Office, Washington, DC 20402, HEW Publication No. (FDA) 76-4003. Makes connections between aging and hearing loss.

Rudick, Joan, and Richard Bimont. "Tuning in on Hearing Aids," *FDA Consumer* (May 1980). Order from U.S. Government Printing Office, HHS Publication No. (FDA) 80-4024.

SHHH (Self-Help for Hard-of-Hearing People, Inc.)
7800 Wisconsin Avenue
Bethesda, MD 20814
(301) 657-2248

Lesbian and Gay Issues

Senior Action in a Gay Environment (SAGE)
208 West 13th Street
New York, NY 10011
(212) 741-2247
The oldest organization providing services to older lesbians and gay men. Services are available in N.Y.C. only, but the organization maintains a list of groups around the country and provides information for starting groups dealing with lesbian and gay aging. Newsletter available.

Menopause

Borton, Joan C. *Drawing from the Women's Well: Reflections from the Life Passage of Menopause.* San Diego, CA: LuraMedia, 1992. A personal and spiritual account.

Cobb, Janine O'Leary. *Understanding Menopause.* Toronto: Key Porter Books, 1988.

Coney, Sandra. *The Menopause Industry: A Guide to Medicine's "Discovery" of the Mid-Life Woman.* New York: Penguin Books, 1991. A New Zealand writer with a world view.

Greenwood, Sadja. *Menopause, Naturally.* San Francisco: Volcano Press, revised fourth edition forthcoming, 1995.

Menopause: A Self-Care Manual, 1989, and *La Menopausia* (Spanish edition), 1989. Order from Santa Fe

Health Education Project, Box 577, Santa Fe, NM 87501-0577. $6.50 each includes postage. Bulk rates available.

Reitz, Rosetta. *Menopause: A Positive Approach.* New York: Penguin Books, 1979. Still an excellent self-help resource.

Taylor, Dena and Amber Cloverdale Sumral. *Women of the Fourteenth Moon: Writings on Menopause.* Freedom, CA: The Crossing Press, 1991. An anthology showing the range of women's experiences.

Nursing Homes

Goldsmith, Seth B. *Choosing a Nursing Home.* New York: Prentice Hall Press, 1990.

Matthews, Joseph. *Elder Care: Choosing and Financing Long-Term Care.* Berkeley, CA: Nolo Press, 1991. Readable and helpful guide that is updated every two years. Also includes information about home care.

National Citizens' Coalition for Nursing Home Reform
1224 M Street NW, Suite 301
Washington, DC 20005
(202) 393-2018

A coalition of member groups and individuals, including nursing home residents and their families, committed to improving the quality of life and care for long-term-care residents.

Vladek, Bruce. *Unloving Care: The Nursing Home Tragedy.* Basic Books, 1980.

Widowhood

Widowed Persons' Service, AARP
601 E Street, NW
Washington, DC 20049

Recently bereaved persons can write for information describing services, help in locating a group in their area, referral, etc., as well as a free copy (in English or Spanish) of the pamphlet "On Being Alone." Bulk orders available.

PART VI

Some Common and Uncommon Health and Medical Problems

24

Some Common and Uncommon Health and Medical Problems

All sections below are by Mary Crowe, except where otherwise indicated. Most sections are based on work by Sarah Berndt, Edith Butler-Hallstein, Alice Downey, Susan Keady, Sandra Malasky and Betty Mitchell (all of the New Hampshire Feminist Health Center).

With special thanks to Norma Swenson, Judy Norsigian, Nora Coffee, Carol Englander, Craig Henderson, Jeanne Hubbuch, William Kaden, Rose Kushner, Charlotte Mayerson, Maryann Napoli, Gina Prenowitz and Leslie Walleigh.

This chapter in previous editions was called "Common Medical Problems and Practices" and was written by Terry Thorsos, Judy Norsigian, Meg Hickey and Norma Swenson.

Abnormal Uterine Bleeding; 1992 Update: Mitchell Levine

Anemia

Arthritis; 1992 Update: Carol Englender

Autoimmune Diseases and Disorders
  Chronic Fatigue Syndrome by Wendy Sanford
  Fibromyalgia by Beverly Richstone
  Scleroderma by Barbara Needleman, MD
  Sjogren's Syndrome by Barbara Henry
  Systemic Lupus Erythematosus by Barbara Horgan and Kathleen Quinlan

Breast Cancer and *Breast Problems* by the Breast Cancer Study Group: Laurie Ansorge, Cheri DesMarais, Jane Jewell, Elana Klugman, Annette Rosen, Jane Hyman Wegscheider and Nancy Zimmet
  With special thanks to Craig Henderson, Rose Kushner and Norma Swenson; 1992 Update: Mary Costanza, Sue Troyan, Linda Andrist, and Judy Norsigian

Introduction to Cancer by Jane Jewell

Cervix, with Adele Clark; 1992 Update: Adele Clark, Mitchell Levine

DES (Diethylstilbestrol) by Kris Brown, DES Action; 1992 Update: Margaret Lee Braun and Pat Cody, DES Action

Diabetes; 1992 Update: Ruth Thomasian, with David Nathan

Endometriosis by Jane Pincus, based on a work by the Endometriosis Association; 1992 Update: Mary Lou Ballweg, Endometriosis Association

Environmental Illness by Wendy Sanford

Gynecological Cancers; 1992 Update: Selma Mirsky, Lisa Whiteside

Gynecological Exams, Tests and Procedures

Heart Disease and Stroke by Sheryl Ruzek, with Norma Swenson; 1992 Update: Sheryl Ruzek

561

Hypertension; 1992 Update: Sheryl Ruzek

Hysterectomy and Oophorectomy by Mary Crowe, Edith Bjornson Sunley and Julia Doyle Sukenik; based on work by Edith Butler-Hallstein

Interstitial Cystitis; 1992 Update: Vicki Ratner

Pelvic Relaxation and Uterine Prolapse

PID (Pelvic Inflammatory Disease) by Debi Milligan With special thanks to Attila Toth, Connie Brooks and Ruth Tuomala; 1992 Update: Judith Wasserheit and Debi Milligan

Surgery

Toxic Shock Syndrome

Trichotillomania by Anonymous

Urinary Tract Infections

Uterus and Ovaries; 1992 Update: Carol Englender, Mitchell Levine

Vagina and Vulva; 1992 Update: Mimi Secor, Carol Englender

This chapter could have been a book in itself. We've had to choose only those health problems which affect large numbers of women or for which it is difficult to get reliable information elsewhere. Please be aware that information is constantly changing, and make use of the resources listed at the end of the chapter.

The entries in this chapter suggest nonmedical alternatives when possible—self-help techniques especially, and nonmedical practitioners. (See p. 82 for guidelines on choosing alternative practitioners.) Often, however, you will go to a doctor, nurse, clinic or hospital for treatment of the health problems discussed here. Please see Chapter 25, "The Politics of Women and Medical Care," for a discussion of the U.S. medical system and suggestions for choosing and using medical care.

GYNECOLOGICAL EXAMS, TESTS AND PROCEDURES

Medical practitioners consider a number of exams, tests and procedures to be part of good routine medical care. However, these procedures can sometimes be invasive, upsetting and even unnecessary.* The following suggestions may help you decide whether and when you need these tests.

Before giving your consent for any of the procedures and/or tests described below, ask your physician the following questions:

1. Why does s/he think you need the procedure?

---

*Some doctors order tests just to try to protect themselves against possible lawsuit.

2. What are the benefits of the procedure over others?

3. How is it done?

4. What are you likely to feel during and after the procedure?

5. What are the risks involved?

6. What are the negative effects, including effects on future fertility?

7. What may happen if you have no procedure done?

8. How experienced and skilled is the practitioner in doing this procedure? For instance, how many does s/he perform in a year?

Although no health practitioner can guarantee the outcome of any exams, tests or procedures, s/he has a responsibility to give you all the available information. If you have doubts or feel you need more information, seek another opinion.

The Physical Examination and Basic Tests

During any physical exam, a practitioner should take the time to explain exactly what s/he is doing and why. This enables us to learn more about our bodies and ask questions if we are unsure about anything. If your practitioner seems rushed or impatient, consider finding someone else. Bring a friend along to act as your advocate if that is what you want. With a practitioner who is respectful, gentle and informative, you will be able to relax more easily during the exam.

As part of a general examination, we should expect

- Questions about full family and personal medical history.
- An examination of the head (including eyes, nose and throat), skin and nails.
- A breast examination, with instructions in breast self-exam.
- Listening to the heart and lungs with the stethoscope placed in several positions and a breath exhalation test.
- A blood pressure and pulse check.
- A hematocrit for hemoglobin count and a CBC (complete blood count).
- A blood-sugar check if you have a family history of diabetes.
- A gonorrhea test and a blood test for syphilis.
- A urinalysis (this also can be used to check kidney function).
- A weight check (see Chapter 2, "Food").
- A Pap test.
- An abdominal exam.
- A pelvic exam, including a rectal exam (especially if you are over thirty-five).

Examination of Organs

The practitioner should examine your abdomen by touch (palpate) for any signs of liver or spleen

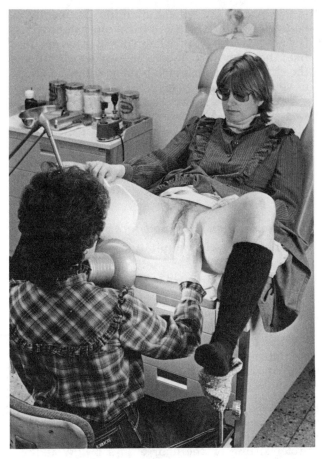

Virginia Coudron

Then the practitioner will insert a speculum into the vagina to hold the walls apart. (The speculum should be warmed metal or plastic and gently inserted.) S/he will examine your vaginal walls for lesions, inflammation or unusual discharge and will check your cervix (now visible) for unusual discharge, signs of infection, lesions, discoloration, damage or growths. S/he will take a Pap smear for abnormal cervical cell growth (a possible precursor of cancer), a culture for gonorrhea and sometimes a smear of discharge to examine under a microscope.

Some women experience pressure in the bladder or rectum with a speculum in place. Relaxing your muscles as much as possible may help. If not, ask the practitioner to readjust the speculum or try a different size.

Some practitioners keep a hand mirror available. If you wish to see your cervix, ask for help in positioning the mirror and light source. This is an opportunity to learn how and what to look for when examining your cervix in a self-exam.

After removing the speculum the practitioner will put on a clean plastic glove and insert two fingers of one hand into your vagina while placing the other hand on your lower abdomen. By pressing down on the abdomen and manipulating with the fingers in your vagina, s/he can locate and determine the size, shape and consistency of the uterus, ovaries and tubes. S/he can also locate any unusual growths, tenderness or pain.

Palpation of the uterus is usually painless, but

enlargement and check your back for any pain or tenderness in the area of the kidneys.

Pelvic Examination

This should include an examination of your external genitals (vulva), an internal exam using a speculum, a bimanual internal exam and a rectovaginal examination. If you have been doing regular self-exams (see p. 564), you will be more familiar with pelvic exams and can tell the practitioner of any changes you have noticed or simply help her/him understand what is normal for you. If it's your first exam, *say so*. Ask the practitioner to go slowly and explain what s/he is doing. Be sure to empty your bladder before the exam.

When examining the vulva, the practitioner will first check visually for irritations, discoloration, swelling, bumps, skin lesions, size and adhesions of the clitoris, hair distribution, lice and unusual vaginal discharge. S/he will then check internally with a finger for any Bartholin's gland cysts or pus coming from the Skene's glands. S/he will ask if you ever lose urine when you laugh or cough (urinary incontinence is a sign of uterine prolapse, rectocele or cystocele).

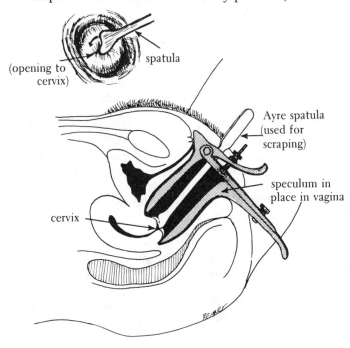

Placement of speculum for a pelvic exam. Spatula scrapes cervix for Pap smear (this is painless).

Nina Reimer

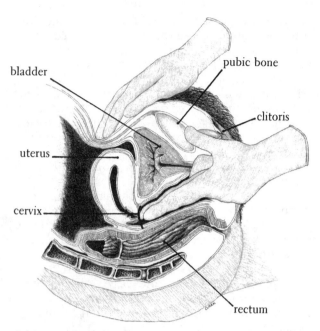

A bimanual pelvic exam.   Peggy Clark

palpation of the ovaries sometimes causes discomfort. The ovaries are difficult to find and often the twinge of pain you feel is the only way the practitioner is aware that s/he is touching your ovaries.

The bimanual examination will be more comfortable for you and easier for the practitioner if you are able to relax your neck, abdomen and back muscles and breathe slowly and deeply, exhaling completely.

To do the rectovaginal exam the practitioner will insert one finger into the rectum and one into the vagina in order to obtain more information on the tone and alignment of the pelvic organs as well as the ovaries, tubes and ligaments of the uterus. This exam can also help detect rectal lesions and test the tone of the rectal sphincter muscles. If you are over thirty-five, the practitioner should also check for masses or blood in the rectum (sometimes an early sign of colon cancer). Some women find the rectovaginal exam unpleasant; others don't mind it. You may feel as if you are having a bowel movement as the practitioner withdraws his/her finger from your rectum. Don't worry—you won't.

Some practitioners are much more sensitive and skilled in internal exams than others; some women find it easier to relax than others. You can do Kegel exercises (see p. 406) and practice inserting a tampon or speculum before an internal to help you practice relaxation.

Self-Examination

Over the past few years an increasing number of women have discovered the benefits of doing va-

ginal and cervical self-examination. By examining yourself regularly you can learn more about what is "normal" for you; what your discharges look like; the color, size and shape of your cervix and the changes in your mucus during different stages of your menstrual cycles.

Doing self-exam, we see parts of our bodies that we have learned to ignore or fear. By using a speculum ourselves we use a small part of medical technology to gain back some control over our bodies. Many women have taken self-examination a step further by talking about their experiences and sharing their knowledge with other women in self-help groups.

Self-Examination Tools and Techniques

For cervical self-examination you will need only a few basic items:

- A light source that can be directed, such as a strong flashlight.
- A speculum (plastic speculums are inexpensive and easier to get than metal; you can get one at a pharmacy that carries medical supplies).
- A lubricant, such as K-Y Jelly or Lubifax, or warm water.
- A mirror with a long handle.
- Antiseptic soap or alcohol.

Find a comfortable setting and get into a relaxed position on the floor or couch. Some women prefer sitting on the floor with a pillow at their back for support.

Familiarize yourself with the speculum and then lie back with your knees bent and your feet placed wide apart. You may want to lubricate the

Jean Raisler

speculum (see above). Hold the speculum in a closed position with the handle pointing upward. Some women prefer to place the speculum into the vagina sideways and then turn it. Experiment until you discover the most comfortable variation for you.

Once you have fully inserted the speculum, grasp the handle and firmly pull its shorter section toward you. This opens the blades of the speculum inside your vagina. Now hold the speculum steady and push down on the outside section until you hear a click; this means that the speculum is locked into place.

For some women placing the speculum and finding the cervix may take some effort. Breathe deeply and manipulate the speculum gently while looking into the mirror. Focus the light source on the mirror to help you see better. (A friend can help with this.) With the speculum in the correct position you will be able to see both the folds in the vaginal walls and your cervix, which looks pink, bulbish and wet. (If you are pregnant, your cervix will have a bluish tint; if you are menopausal or nursing, it may be quite pale.) Depending on where you are in your menstrual cycle, your secretions may be white and creamy or clear and stretchy. By learning what is "normal" for you, you will more easily be able to identify any changes that may indicate ovulation, an infection or pregnancy.

Some women prefer to remove the speculum while it is still in its open position, and others close the blades first. Clean it afterward with antiseptic soap or alcohol and store it for later use.

Pap Smear

The Pap smear is a method for distinguishing normal from abnormal cells of the vagina, uterus and cervix. It is most accurate in detecting cervical abnormalities. Since the recommended treatments for various kinds of abnormal cells detected by Pap smears remain controversial among practitioners, it will help to understand some basic facts about Pap tests and our treatment options (see p. 614).

To take a Pap smear a practitioner will, during the speculum exam, use a Pap stick or cotton swab to take one or more samples of cervical tissue from the outside of the cervix and just inside the cervical canal. You may feel a slight scraping sensation. S/he places the gathered cells on a glass slide and "fixes" them to prevent them from deteriorating. A good cell sample is essential for an accurate test. The slide goes to a cytology laboratory for analysis.

Dilation and Curettage (D and C)

A D and C is often used to find the cause of uterine bleeding or to treat it, especially in emergencies.

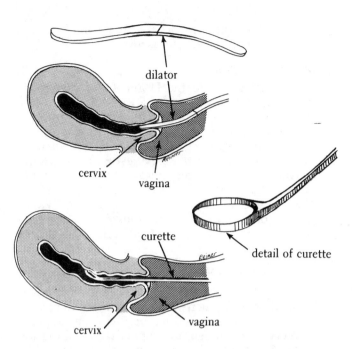

The dilator and curette, instruments for a D and C.

Nina Reimer

It is also used to diagnose uterine fibroids, endometrial polyps and uterine cancer. In addition, it may be part of a diagnostic workup for cervical cancer. It is often performed to prevent infection following an incomplete abortion or after delivery, if part of the placenta is left in the uterus. The diagnostic D and C is rapidly being replaced by vacuum (Vabra) aspiration or endometrial biopsy (see p. 566).

Many physicians still prefer to do a D and C in a hospital using general anesthesia, which creates total relaxation of the pelvic muscles and allows a more accurate pelvic exam. When such accuracy isn't necessary it can be performed on an outpatient basis using local anesthesia, thereby minimizing the risks and expense, which are both greater with general anesthesia.

D and C sometimes involves enlarging (dilating) the opening of the cervix by inserting a series of tapered rods that become progressively wider in diameter. Increasingly, laminaria (long stems of kelp) are inserted twenty-four hours before the D and C to dilate the cervix gradually and painlessly. The practitioner then inserts a long, thin metal instrument with a spoon-shaped end (curette) through the cervix into the uterus to scrape out some of the uterine lining. (The doctor sometimes takes a tissue sample from the cervical canal.) The procedure should take five to fifteen minutes.

Most women have some bleeding following a D and C and may also pass small clots and/or have cramps for a couple of days. The risks include infection, hemorrhage, perforation of the uterus or surrounding internal organs and complications related to the anesthesia used.

Vabra Aspiration

An alternative to the D and C for diagnostic purposes is Vabra or endometrial aspiration, which involves inserting a small cannula into the cervix and removing the uterine lining by means of low-pressure suction. This procedure can be done in an office with local anesthesia, thus eliminating the risks of general anesthesia. It usually causes the same mild to moderate cramping as the D and C. Some physicians recommend Vabra aspiration as part of a gynecological exam for all women at risk for endometrial cancer.

Cervical and Endometrial Biopsy

In a biopsy, a sample of tissue is removed to be examined under a microscope as an aid in diagnosis.

A *cervical biopsy* is done on abnormal areas of the cervix that appear through visual examination with or without Schiller's solutions or through the use of a colposcope (see Colposcopy, at right). An instrument that looks like a paper punch removes

cervix

A cervical biopsy.   Christine Bondante

endometrium

An endometrial biopsy.   Christine Bondante

the tissue sample from one or more sites on the cervix.

The biopsy may be done on an outpatient basis and generally without the use of anesthesia. Most women experience some cramping during the biopsy and spotting afterward.

In an *endometrial biopsy* (which can also be done on an outpatient basis with local anesthesia if necessary), usually a scraping instrument (curette) is inserted through the cervix to obtain a sample of the uterine lining. The procedure may be part of an infertility workup. It has a fairly high accuracy rate when used to diagnose cancer of the uterine lining (endometrium), but the Vabra technique is generally thought to be more accurate for this purpose.

Colposcopy

This procedure involves the use of a colposcope, a lighted magnifying instrument resembling a small mounted pair of binoculars, to examine the vaginal walls and cervix for abnormal cells. It is more accurate than a Pap smear since it can identify the specific areas where the abnormal cells are located. A biopsy can then be taken from those areas for accurate diagnosis. Colposcopy is useful in the diagnosis of abnormal bleeding. Regular colposcopy is recommended for all DES (diethylstilbestrol) daughters (see p. 583).

A colposcopy, easily done in a physician's office, usually involves little or no discomfort. However, it is often combined with a cervical biopsy, which may be painful. Also, it is a prolonged speculum exam, which for some women is physically or psychologically uncomfortable.

Conization or Cone Biopsy

Conization, used for both diagnosis and treatment, removes a cone-shaped section of the cervix. It is often recommended when a woman has severe dysplasia or cancerous cells confined to the cervix. A diagnostic conization may turn out to be therapeutic if it removes all the abnormal tissue.

A major surgical procedure, conization is done in a hospital under general anesthesia. Though the edges of the cervical area from which the cone is taken are sutured or cauterized, bleeding and infection are fairly common short-term complications. The removal of too many mucus-secreting glands may affect fertility by causing a decrease in cervical mucus. Sometimes pregnant women suffer a miscarriage after conization because of removal of muscle tissue, though *cerclage* treatment (which keeps the cervix from opening prematurely) may be possible.

A therapy that replaces cervical cone biopsy consists of *laser* treatments of the abnormal area of the cervix. Laser techniques cause few compli-

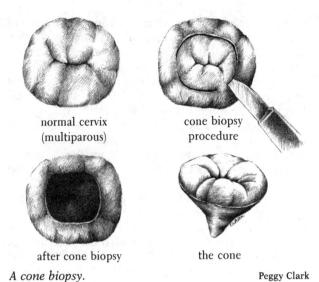

normal cervix
(multiparous)

cone biopsy
procedure

after cone biopsy

the cone

A cone biopsy.   Peggy Clark

cations and promote faster healing. Laser, however, destroys tissue, making it unavailable for laboratory analysis.

Schiller's Test

In this procedure an iodine solution is used to determine areas of the vagina or cervix that should be biopsied. Normal tissue painted with the solution will turn a dark brown color. Abnormal tissue will not absorb the stain. The Schiller's test is commonly used to help detect vaginal and cervical changes in women whose mothers took DES while pregnant.

Cauterization and Cryotherapy

Cautery involves destroying abnormal tissue through the use of chemicals such as silver nitrate or an electrically heated instrument. It is used by some doctors to treat abnormal cell development (dysplasia), cancer *in situ* or cervical erosion (a reddened area that develops around the cervical opening). Sometimes cautery is used to treat chronic cervicitis, vaginal or vulvar warts and endometriosis involving the cervix or vagina. Cautery can be done in a doctor's office, preferably right after your menstrual period. The practitioner inserts a speculum and applies the cautery tip to the affected area.* After treatment a scab forms, allowing healthy new tissue to grow. The scab falls off in a week or so, and complete healing takes seven or eight weeks. Side effects include swelling of the cervix, profuse discharge for two or three weeks and, rarely, infection or infertility if the cervical glands are damaged.

---

*No anesthesia is needed, since normally there are no nerve endings in the cervix.

Cryotherapy, often called *cryosurgery* and sometimes *cold cautery*, involves the use of liquid nitrogen to destroy abnormal tissue by freezing. It can be done in an office and takes only a few minutes. Cryotherapy causes much less damage to the cervical opening than cauterization. It may, however, cause a profuse watery discharge and temporary changes in the cervical mucus. It does not seem to cause infertility. Unfortunately, many doctors do not have cryotherapy equipment in their offices.

After either cauterization or cryotherapy, you should not douche, use tampons or have sexual intercourse for ten to fourteen days while your cervix heals. Until healing is complete, Pap smears will be inaccurate and difficult to interpret. *Note:* Cautery occasionally causes scarring, which makes all future Pap smears difficult to interpret.

Carbon Dioxide Laser

Laser is a technique sometimes used as an alternative treatment to cone biopsy, cauterization or cryotherapy. Done on an outpatient basis in the hospital, it involves using a laser beam to destroy cells in a small area and results in little or no damage to the surrounding cells. Laser treatment causes little or no bleeding and the treated area heals quickly. This technique is so new and expensive that it is currently available only at certain large hospitals or medical centers. As more doctors are trained in its use and the equipment becomes more widely available, laser treatment may replace the older methods.

After a laser treatment, a Pap smear may show atypical cells for four to six weeks. You should, however, have two follow-up smears at three-month intervals and two more at six-month intervals before returning to your regular Pap smear schedule.

Laparoscopy

The laparoscope is a lighted tubelike instrument that, when inserted through a small incision made below the navel, allows the physician to see the uterus, tubes and ovaries.

Laparoscopy is useful in the diagnosis of ovarian cysts, ectopic pregnancy, infertility caused by blocked tubes, unexplained pelvic pain or masses, and endometriosis, and in the recovery of an IUD that has perforated the uterus. It is also used in some female sterilization techniques. Laparoscopy is usually done in a hospital under either general or local anesthesia. Before inserting the laparoscope, the practitioner will inflate your abdomen with carbon dioxide to move the intestines out of the way and expose the pelvic organs to better view. With local anesthesia, you may experience an uncomfortable pressure or fullness. You may feel some pain under your ribs for the first few days after a laparoscopy as your body gradually absorbs the excess gas.

Anesthesia

It is as important to understand the type of anesthesia that you will receive as the type of surgery you will undergo. Before surgery you should ask the person who will be administering the anesthesia the following questions:

1. What type of anesthesia will be administered?
2. Why has s/he chosen this type or combination?
3. How will the anesthesia be given?
4. How may you feel after the surgery?
5. What are the possible risks and benefits of this type of anesthesia as compared to others?*

Be sure to tell the person who will be administering your anesthesia about any allergies to medication, prior anesthesia reactions, current medications you may be taking and information about your past and current health.

Anesthesia works by blocking pain. There are three types of anesthesia: *general*, in which you are unconscious; *regional* or *conduction* (including spinal and epidural), in which you are awake but numb in a specific region, usually the lower half (or a zone) of your body; and *local*, in which you are awake and only the area being operated on is numbed. General anesthesia makes you unaware of pain by working on the part of the brain that recognizes pain. Conduction and local anesthesia block the signals sent to the spinal cord and brain from the site which is anesthetized.

General anesthesia is administered by needle into a vein (intravenous), by inhalation or by a combination of both. When you get intravenous anesthesia, you will probably first be medicated with sodium pentothal (to induce deep sleep).† If you receive inhalation anesthesia, you will inhale it in gaseous form directly into the lungs via a tube inserted down your throat. Most types of anesthesia are administered after you are given medication to help you relax, which makes the procedure easier for the anesthesiologist and for you. If you are given gaseous anesthesia (such as halothane or nitrous oxide), adequate oxygen must be mixed with the gas, as general anesthesia lowers blood pressure and respiration rate. You may experience nausea, confusion or dizziness for

several hours or days after having either type of general anesthesia. Rarely (about once in 10,000 to 20,000 cases) there is a death or paralysis as a direct result of the anesthesia.

Spinal anesthesia (usually preceded by a local anesthetic) is injected into the spinal canal through the membrane that covers the spinal cord. You will feel numb in the legs, pelvis and possibly higher, depending on what anesthesia is needed for your surgery. Spinal anesthesia is most often used for operations within the abdominal cavity.

Anesthetic effects from spinals may last longer than those from general anesthesia. About one woman in twenty will get a postoperative headache that may last for several days, because of small losses of spinal fluid from the injection site. Lying flat on your back for eight to sixteen hours after surgery without lifting your head may help relieve your symptoms. You can also ask for a patch to be put over the hole (a "patch procedure") so that it doesn't leak.*

Epidural or caudal anesthesia is injected continuously into the space near the base of the spinal column but not into the canal itself. It works by bathing the nerve endings leading to large areas of the body such as the perineum and legs with anesthetic solution and is frequently used in childbirth. For more on epidural and caudal anesthesia (similar to epidural, sometimes used for rectal and genital surgery), see Chapter 20, "Childbirth." Always ask whether regional rather than general anesthesia is possible in your case, especially if you have a history of respiratory problems.

In *local anesthesia* a solution or jelly that numbs the nerve endings is applied to the mucous membranes, followed by an injection that blocks specific nerves (e.g., an injection of lidocaine given by the dentist).

Surgery

There are many different types of surgeons, calling themselves (and each other) by different names. General surgeons are a good choice *only* when they have special training for the procedures they perform.

Because there is a great deal of unnecessary surgery performed on women, we need to exercise great caution when deciding on an operation. Many public health researchers are convinced that excess surgery results from excess surgeons, since the United States has both the most surgeons and the highest rates of surgery in the world. An important part of surgical training is learning to persuade patients to agree to an operation. Because

---

*Anesthesia capability varies from hospital to hospital as well as from one anesthesiologist or anesthetist to another. Not all facilities offer a choice.
†However, you are not truly asleep, and you may hear or even remember conversations of those around you.

*This complication has become less common since the introduction of finer-gauge needles.

virtually all surgical procedures are reimbursed by insurance and graded according to their complexity, surgeons have strong financial incentives to perform a lot of surgery, especially the more difficult operations. Hospitals similarly benefit from concentrations of elective (i.e., nonemergency) complex surgeries. And, precisely because surgery has become so common, many people have internalized the surgical mentality ("When in doubt, cut it out") and are easily convinced that an operation is necessary.

Before giving your consent to surgery, you may want to take the following steps:

1. Get a second or even third opinion, preferably from a physician in a different specialty or who is *not* one of your doctor's close colleagues. (Many insurance policies and Blue Cross/Blue Shield programs will pay for this second opinion.) Try to find a doctor who is interested in helping you avoid surgery where possible. For example, internists may suggest nonsurgical alternatives not offered by ob/gyns and general surgeons. Such doctors are sometimes called "conservative," meaning that they don't resort to invasive measures unless they believe that it is absolutely necessary to do so. Procedures most frequently found unnecessary after a second opinion are hysterectomy, knee surgery, vein stripping, prostate removal, D and C, cataract extraction, breast surgery and gallbladder removal.* (See also Our Rights as Patients, p. 682.)

2. Ask your surgeon about studies that show improved *outcome* for the procedure in your case. For example, careful studies have shown that much coronary bypass surgery is useless and sometimes even shortens life, yet the popularity of this procedure is constantly increasing. (See the section on heart diseases, pp. 631–34.)

3. Ask also about the surgery's potential risks and negative effects.

4. Investigate in a self-help group or on your own what alternatives, medical and nonmedical, can be tried before or instead of surgery. Medical researchers themselves now suggest that at least seven common operations may no longer be necessary or may soon be replaced by other, less invasive, treatments: hysterectomy, tonsillectomy, cholecystectomy (gall bladder removal), appendectomy, cardiac revascularization, gastrectomy and radical mastectomy.

5. Ask whether the surgery has been widely performed, where and on how many people; check with your insurer to see if it is known and reimbursable. Because there is *no* regulatory or legal authority anywhere controlling surgery, new ex-

perimental procedures are constantly being launched without adequate testing and evaluation.

6. Ask specifically about mortality and morbidity rates in the institution where the surgery will be performed. (Call your state Department of Public Health or Health Systems Agency.) Some hospitals have more careful criteria and much better outcomes than others for certain procedures.

7. Carefully investigate the training and affiliations of the surgeon you are considering. Ask how often s/he performs the proposed procedure.

8. Ask if you can avoid general anesthesia (one of the major risks of most surgery) and hospitalization (a major source of postoperative infections) by having the surgery done as an outpatient or office procedure.

9. Talk all this over with your family and trusted friends.

10. Take the time you need to make a careful decision.

Before and After Surgery

Because surgery badly depletes the body of nutrients, you will need to eat a diet high in protein, vitamins and minerals to replenish these losses. You may also want to take supplements of Vitamins A, B, C and D, as well as zinc and iron. (See also the section on hospitalization, p. 681).

INFESTATIONS

Crabs, or Pubic Lice

Phthirus pubis is a roundish, crablike body louse that lives in pubic hair and occasionally in the hair of the chest, armpits, eyelashes and eyebrows. You can "catch" crabs by intimate physical contact with someone who has them or from bedding, towels or clothes that person has used. They are bloodsuckers and can carry such diseases as typhus. The main symptom of crabs is an intolerable itching in the genital or other affected area; they are easily diagnosed because they are visible without a microscope.

Though it may be difficult, try not to scratch. Scratching can transfer lice to uninfected parts of the body. Excessive scratching around the urinary opening can even lead to urinary tract infections.

Practitioners usually prescribe a lotion called Kwell,* available by prescription only. This drug should be used with caution: Follow the directions

*This conclusion is the result of second-opinion monitoring programs set up by insurance companies, Medicaid/Medicare and Blue Cross/Blue Shield.

*This drug should be used very carefully. Its active ingredient, lindane, is a potent pesticide that penetrates the skin and can cause allergic reactions. In addition, lindane has been found to cause tumors in laboratory animals. Pregnant women, infants and children should not use this drug.

carefully. Vonce, R.I.D., and A-200 Pyrinate are safe nonprescription drugs that are almost as effective as Kwell for crabs. Do not use any of these drugs in or around your eyes. If you have crabs in your eyebrows use an ophthalmic petroleum jelly.

Alternatively, you can try a very hot sauna, a treatment routinely used in Scandinavia. Either way, it's important that all intimate contacts, including lovers, family members and friends, be treated as well.

After treatment you should use clean clothing, towels and bed linen. Crabs will die within twenty-four hours after separation from the human body, but the eggs will live about six days. Previously used bedclothes, towels, and so on are safe after a week without use. Anything drycleaned or washed in boiling water can be used immediately.

As with scabies, the itch may persist for some time after treatment, especially if your skin is very irritated from scratching. Soothing skin preparations, such as aloe vera, can ease the symptoms and help your skin to heal faster.

The first time I got crabs I felt embarrassed and humiliated. I'd gone to visit my boyfriend at college and when I came home I began to itch. I couldn't believe that he would give me something like that—especially since I'd mistakenly associated crabs with people who didn't wash enough. I didn't know what to do so I just ignored them as long as possible. When the itching became really intolerable I went to a clinic. Once I learned how crabs are transmitted and that they are both very common and easy to cure, I felt a lot better. The next time I went to visit my boyfriend I took a bottle of A-200 with me. Turns out he hadn't known what to do either!

Scabies

Scabies are tiny parasitic mites that burrow under the superficial layers of the skin, depositing eggs and feces and causing intense irritation. Symptoms usually include intense itching (often worse at night) and red, raised bumps or ridges on the skin, which may be found on the hands (especially between the fingers), on or under the breasts or around the waist or wrists, genitals or buttocks. Scratching the area can break the skin, causing secondary bacterial infections.

Scabies is highly contagious. You can get it through sexual contact as well as from infested bed linen, towels, clothing and occasionally even furniture. If you've never had scabies, it may take a month or more for the skin reaction to develop. During this time you can pass it to someone else without knowing you have it. Once you've had scabies, however, your skin will react much more quickly, often within a day after reinfestation.

Diagnosing scabies can be tricky because it is easily confused with poison ivy, eczema, allergies and other skin conditions. Sometimes physicians will prescribe medication for scabies before they know what you really have. Because these medications can cause allergic reactions, do not apply them until you have a definite diagnosis (specially made by examining a small scraping of the irritated area under a microscope).

The most common and effective treatment is Kwell. Apply after a hot bath or shower (avoiding face, eyes and mucous membranes), leave on for twelve hours and carefully rinse off. If you need a second treatment, wait two weeks before reapplying.

An alternative to Kwell, often prescribed for pregnant women, is Eurax, whose active ingredient is crotamiton. It should be rubbed into the skin and reapplied after twenty-four hours.

An old-fashioned treatment using sulfur is making a comeback in popularity among dermatologists. It is especially recommended for treating infants, young children and pregnant women for scabies. It is considered less irritating than other chemicals that kill scabies, it seems to be less toxic and it seems to work.

The one disadvantage to the sulfur treatment is cosmetic. It smells like rotten eggs and can stain clothing.

For the adventurous, the recommended mixture is 6 percent sulfur, 3 percent balsam of Peru and the rest petroleum jelly. The mixture is put on the infected areas and left on for twenty-four hours, with a new application each night for three consecutive nights. Some pharmacists will mix the ingredients for you.

Treatment is important for any friends, lovers or family members with whom you've had intimate contact. You should also wash any clothing, towels, bedclothes, furniture covers, and so on, in very hot water and dry at the hottest possible temperature.

Even after treatment, you may continue to itch for several days or weeks. This doesn't mean you still have scabies; more likely your skin is still hypersensitive and needs some time for the irritation to die down. A soothing lotion (containing calamine or aloe vera) will ease the symptoms. If the itching is really intolerable, an antihistamine may help.

THE CERVIX

Cervicitis

Cervicitis is a term used loosely to describe an inflammation or infection of the cervix. The majority of Pap tests come back with *cervicitis* noted, but this does not necessarily represent a true disease or disorder. Cervicitis is often a sign that common vaginal infections, sexually transmitted diseases (STDs) or pelvic inflammatory disease (PID) is present. It can also result from a break in the tissue of the cervix caused by an IUD insertion, abortion or childbirth. Untreated, chronic cervicitis can cause fertility problems by blocking the passage of sperm or altering the cervical mucus.

Depending upon the severity and length of infection, you may notice an increased vaginal discharge, pain with intercourse, an aching sensation in the lower abdomen and/or the need to urinate more frequently. Severe infections may also bring fever.

Diagnosis

When you touch your cervix, it may feel warmer and larger than usual. Movement of your cervix with your finger may also be uncomfortable. If you examine yourself with a speculum, your cervix will look red and slightly swollen and you may observe a discharge. If only the cervical canal is affected, your cervix will look normal, but you may see a yellowish discharge coming from within the cervical opening.

If you go to a practitioner for an internal exam, be sure to tell him/her whether or not your discharge is normal. (Sometimes physicians mistake scar tissue and normal discharge for cervicitis.) A culture and wet mount will determine if the cause of the infection is bacteria or an STD. In some cases, a Pap smear will also be taken to rule out the possibility of cervical cancer.

Medical Treatments

If tests show that an STD such as gonorrhea, syphilis or chlamydia is responsible for the infection, you will get oral or injected antibiotics. For mild cervicitis involving no STDs, medical treatment may be pointless, as the condition is not serious and is likely to return after treatment. For more severe cases, some physicians recommend cryosurgery or electrocautery. Although these treatments work well when all other methods have failed, use them only as a last resort, as they can be painful, can lead to fertility problems and may take about six weeks for healing.

Self-Help Treatments

When symptoms are mild and not related to PID or serious STDs, the following remedies may help: goldenseal douche (a quarter of a teaspoon to one quart of water two times a day for two to three weeks), vitamin C douche (500 milligrams in one quart of water daily for three to four weeks) or vinegar douche. For more information on herbal remedies, see Resources.

To speed healing and strengthen the immune system and for future prevention, you may want to try oral doses of vitamin C (500 to 1,000 milligrams a day), zinc (twenty-five milligrams a day) and vitamin E (400 milligrams a day). You can also apply vitamin E directly to your cervix with your finger. You can use slippery elm as a douche or paste applied directly to the cervix in a diaphragm or on the end of a tampon.

No matter what treatment you use, try to combine it with extra rest and good nutrition. Avoid tampon use during menstruation.

Cervical Eversion

Cervical eversion is a common condition in which the tissue that lines the cervical canal grows on the outer vaginal portion of the cervix, making it red with a bumpy-looking texture smooth to the touch. It has almost a bandlike appearance. Eversion requires no treatment unless accompanied by infection. Those of us whose mothers took DES during pregnancy are more likely to have large eversion.

Most women do not have any symptoms; in those who do, the most frequent sign is a slightly increased nonirritating vaginal discharge. For common eversion no biopsy is necessary, unless there is an abnormal Pap smear. If the discharge is bothersome, use the self-help treatments listed under cervicitis.

Cervical Erosion

Cervical erosion looks like a large or small sore (benign lesion) on the cervix beside the cervical opening. It is usually pinkish red and sometimes rough-looking.

Cervical erosion has few symptoms, causes little discomfort and is quite rare. Most cases referred to as erosion in the past were really eversion.

Diagnosis

The first step in diagnosis is a Pap smear. If abnormal cells are present, some of the cervical tissue is removed and examined under a microscope (a biopsy). A biopsy will distinguish cervical erosion from cervical cancer.

Medical Treatments

Ordinarily, no treatment is needed unless an infection is present. Some physicians may suggest cauterization or cryotherapy, but this is not necessary if your Pap smear is normal. In addition, it is very difficult to interpret abnormal Pap smears accurately after these procedures.

Cervical Polyps

Cervical polyps appear as bright red tubelike protrusions out of the cervical opening, either alone or in clusters. They consist of excess cervical tissue that "heaps up" within the cervical canal. Polyps, which are very common, are often formed as the body attempts to heal itself after a cervical infection by growing new tissue or during pregnancy when hormonal changes stimulate excess cervical tissue to grow. Contact bleeding following intercourse, douching or self-exam is often the only symptom. Polyps sometimes bleed during pregnancy. Most contain many blood vessels with a fragile outer wall.

Medical Treatments

Polyps do not necessarily require treatment. When they are small and there is little or no contact bleeding you can usually just keep track of them with regular self-exams. You may want to have them removed if your symptoms change or the polyp begins to grow. Cervical polyps are rarely cancerous. Occasionally, however, they look like cervical cancer and produce similar symptoms. In that case you can have a Pap smear and biopsy to tell for sure.

A polyp can be removed in a doctor's office. The practitioner usually twists the polyp off and cauterizes the base. If your polyp is very large or if you have multiple polyps, you may have to go to the hospital for removal. Sometimes polyps recur after removal.

Cervical Leukoplakia

Leukoplakia, a white patch of tissue that forms on mucous membranes (inside the cheek, vagina, cervix, etc.), is our body's attempt to seal off an area that contains abnormal cells. If you see leukoplakia on the cervix, have the patch rubbed firmly during a Pap test. If your Pap test is normal but the area of whiteness is still present, most practitioners suggest removing it or biopsying it, as leukoplakia is thought by some doctors to be a precancerous growth. Increasingly, this term is no longer in use because of its lack of specificity.

Cervical Intraepithelial Neoplasia (Cervical Dysplasia)

Dysplasia means abnormal cell growth; *cervical dysplasia*, *cervical intraepithelial neoplasia* (CIN) and *squamous intraepithelial lesion (SIL)* are terms used to describe abnormal cells on or near the cervix. In most cases there are no symptoms, and the condition is detected by a routine Pap smear.

CIN is *not* cancer and does not develop into cancer in most cases. CIN occurs along a continuum: At one end the cells are all normal, while at the far-distant other end lies invasive cancer. The several stages or classes of CIN along the continuum can be difficult to distinguish; one stage or class blurs into the next, and different laboratories or physicians may "place" a given cell sample differently. Diagnosis is therefore often difficult, and treatment decisions can be controversial and hard to make. *Some* women with CIN will develop more severe changes (and at varying speeds), whereas most women's cells will return to normal. There is no way to determine in advance which will happen. Therefore, all cases of diagnosed CIN should be treated and/or watched closely with repeated Pap smears and other diagnostic tests.

Because we can't see CIN and we don't know what is going on, we often feel anxious when we are diagnosed as having it. There is no need to panic when a Pap smear comes back abnormal. Most cell changes like CIN are very slow. Some physicians may want to rush you into treatment. Because the diagnostic tests are not always accurate, and because practitioners vary in their diagnoses and preferred treatments, it is good to get the opinion of a second practitioner and a different laboratory about your condition. Most diagnosed cases of CIN are mild, and the cells return to normal spontaneously. We can monitor any changes by more frequent Pap smears or other diagnostic tests.

The results of Pap smears and other diagnostic tests are classified according to how much of the surface tissue (epithelium) of the cervix is affected and the kind and degree of cell changes that exist. There are four different classification systems currently in use. Below is a chart that compares all four systems, showing where they are the same or different. The four systems are named the *class system*, *dysplasia*, *CIN*, and *Bethesda/SIL*. The chart shows the continuum from normal healthy cells at the far left (negative smears) to invasive cancer at the far right. Many experts now believe that most CIN is caused by the human papillomavirus (HPV) (see p. 323).

Prevention

1. It is important to monitor your condition with repeated Pap smears or other tests in addition to employing preventive efforts. Studies show that using a barrier method of contraception (such as the condom or diaphragm) rather than oral contraceptives (the Pill) or an IUD may help to prevent CIN or cancer. One study showed that for some women already diagnosed as having CIN, use of condoms has been associated with a return to normal cervical cells.

2. Some sexually transmitted infections and diseases can contribute to abnormal cervical

Comparison of Cervical Cancer Classification Systems

	Class I	Class II		Class III		Class IV	Class V
The class system	Class I	Class II		Class III		Class IV	Class V
Dysplasia	Benign	Atypia	Mild	DYSPLASIA Moderate	Severe	CIS	Invasive cancer
Cervical intraepithe-lial neoplasia (CIN)	Benign	Atypia	CIN I	CIN II		CIN III	Invasive cancer
Bethesda/ squamous intraepi-thelial lesion (SIL)	Benign	Atypia	Low-grade SIL	High-grade SIL			Squamous cell carcinoma

changes. (See Chapter 14, "Sexually Transmitted Diseases," for methods of prevention.)

3. Eating foods high in vitamin C and/or taking supplements may help prevent CIN or cervical cancer. After a diagnosis of cervical abnormality, taking folic acid (ten milligrams per day) and vitamin C (a hundred milligrams per day) may help reverse the condition.*

4. We must insist on more research into the connection between occupationally and/or environmentally induced abnormalities and CIN and cancer, as well as the role of male partners in CIN and cancer.

Who Is at Risk of CIN (Dysplasia) or Cervical Cancer?

We don't yet know the causes of the cellular abnormalities that we call CIN and cervical cancer. However, certain factors may put you at higher risk for these conditions.

1. If you have an HPV infection (see p. 323), you are at a higher risk for CIN. The HPV, which causes condyloma warts, can also cause invisible flat lesions on the cervix. These lesions, which can show up as abnormal Pap smears or can be seen with a colposcope, are probably more common among women than the visible condyloma warts. Increasingly, evidence suggests that both forms of HPV infection are trigger factors to the onset of cervical cancer.

2. Recent studies suggest that a protein substance in sperm may cause cellular changes in some women. Women whose partners develop cancer of the penis are also at greater risk.

3. Being exposed to synthetic hormones (such as DES or the Pill) may increase your chances of developing CIN or cancer, because it increases the area of the cervix vulnerable to HPV.

4. Recent studies have linked cervical cancer with smoking.

5. If you began intercourse at an early age, your risks may be greater. Physical changes in the types of cells which line the vagina occur especially during our teens: As we age, more vulnerable softer cells are gradually replaced by tougher (squamocolumnar) cells. If we began intercourse before those changes were mostly complete, our cells are more vulnerable to whatever may cause cellular changes.

6. If either you or your partner or both of you had multiple sexual partners, your risks of developing abnormal cervical cells may be somewhat greater. Barrier contraceptives (especially condoms) may reduce such risks. This pattern has sometimes been used to "blame" women for sexual activity that "caused" their cellular changes. First, we do not know what causes such changes. Second—and often ignored—the number of sexual partners of a woman's *mate* (not the woman herself) may affect the degree to which she is at risk of cervical abnormalities. Third, some women who have only had one partner have developed cellular changes. Last, *neither* early age at first intercourse nor many partners *causes* cellular abnormalities. Blaming the victim with such abnormalities certainly won't cure them.

7. If you or your partner works at a job that involves contact with carcinogenic substances (such as those in the mining, textile, metal or chemical industries), you may be at higher risk for cervical abnormalities.

8. Finally, poorer women who do not have access to healthful living and working conditions have a much higher incidence of CIN and cancers, and are more likely to develop such problems at an earlier age than middle-class women. This may also be related to the greater occupational hazards

---

*A hundred milligrams per day should prevent any major deficiency of vitamin C, but many women will want to take more if they are often exposed to conditions that destroy vitamin C in their bodies, such as smoke.

faced by poorer women and/or their partners as well as their lack of access to good nutrition.

Diagnosis

The first step is the Pap smear. If you have an abnormal result, indicating CIN (not just inflammation), then your physician or nurse-practitioner should perform a colposcopy. In many cases, the colposcopy will show no abnormalities, because some labs have a high false-positive rate. Where an abnormality does appear, your physician or nurse practitioner may perform a tissue (punch) biopsy. Both Pap smears and colposcopies may be repeated for diagnostic monitoring. With mild dysplasia there may be a 30 to 50 percent spontaneous regression rate.

Medical Treatments

Treatments for dysplasia and/or CIN vary from very mild to more serious. What you want is to get appropriate treatment for the condition you have and to avoid unnecessary or inappropriate treatment or surgeries. Different physicians or practitioners may have varying "preferred" treatments for each diagnosis. This is why second and even third opinions may be important in deciding on your treatment.

It is important that procedures such as colposcopies, punch biopsies and cones be done by practitioners who have special training, skills and experience. The mildest treatment is the "wait and see" approach with repeat Pap smears and/or colposcopies (see p. 566) and punch biopsies. Regular condom use may also help. The next step up the treatment ladder is destruction of abnormal cells either by cryotherapy or laser. Cryotherapy is an office procedure in which suspicious cells are frozen and then slough off, allowing new healthy cells to replace them (see p. 567). Many physicians prefer carbon dioxide laser (see p. 567) over cryotherapy.

Another type of treatment is the loop electrosurgical excision procedure (LEEP). In this method, a low-voltage, high-frequency radio wave is run through a thin wire loop, which is used to remove the abnormal tissue from the cervix. The loop works by scooping out the dysplastic tissue in a matter of seconds. The excised tissue is then examined pathologically for indications of cancer. A major advantage of LEEP is that it combines diagnosis and treatment in the same visit to your practitioner. The procedure is done with local anesthetic and may involve minor discomfort. Cervical healing takes about a month for routine cases.

When repeated Pap smears or colposcopies confirm severe dysplasia or cancer *in situ* (CIS, or localized cancer) and if the abnormal area extends into the cervical canal (and therefore cannot be reached for colposcopy or cryotherapy), a cone bi-

---

DES DAUGHTERS AND CIN

The type of cancer, squamous cell, that CIN *may* develop into should not be confused with clear cell cancer, which is linked to DES exposure. It is not known at this point whether DES daughters are or will be at a higher risk for CIN or squamous cell cancer. Still more research is needed.

DES daughters who have been diagnosed to have dysplasia should be aware of two issues:

1. One study of a small number of DES daughters who had cryosurgery showed results of cervical stenosis (narrowing of the cervical canal, which can affect menstruation and childbirth) in varying degrees of severity. Non-DES-exposed women in the same study did not experience these side effects from cryosurgery.

2. Metaplasia, a normal process whereby tissue changes from one form to another, may be present in a larger area in DES-exposed than in non-DES-exposed women. Why is this important? Some people feel that the changed tissue may be more vulnerable to precancerous or cancerous change and pathologists may mistakenly interpret the change as abnormal (dysplasia or CIN). Such misdiagnosis can lead to unnecessary treatment and the possible harmful effects of cervical stenosis.

Kris Brown

---

opsy (conization or conical) is often recommended. The cone-shaped piece of tissue removed by this surgery in the hospital is examined to ensure that all borders of the abnormal area were removed. If the abnormal area extends beyond the edge of the removed cone, the physician may recommend a second conization (to remove a larger area). Hysterectomy is generally recommended as the appropriate treatment for invasive cancer (see p. 626). It involves major surgery and some risks.

Some of these treatments can be uncomfortable and occasionally somewhat painful. After a cone or punch biopsy, cryotherapy, laser treatment or LEEP, do not use tampons, douche or have intercourse for at least three weeks. (This minimizes pain and the risk of infection.) Some women experience cramping, tenderness, bleeding and/or discharges.

A cone biopsy involves some risk of future infertility because it may weaken the cervix. A hysterectomy permanently ends a woman's reproductive capacity. Both surgeries can be appropriate and save women's lives. However, if such a treatment is recommended, it is important to seek a second or even third opinion on whether it is appropriate and what other treatment options may be available, especially for severe CIN or cancer *in situ*.

BENIGN BREAST CONDITIONS

In adolescence, when our breasts first begin to develop, we usually feel both pleased and awkward. We worry about whether they will be too big or too small, attractive or unattractive. At this age, we sometimes walk hunched over, clutching schoolbooks to our chests in the hopes that no one will notice our newly maturing breasts. Other times we may stuff tissues into training bras and wear tight sweaters. Our self-images quickly become tied up with our own and others' reactions to our breasts. These reactions can be as confusing and contradictory for grown women as they are for teenagers. Many of us discover that our breasts can be intensely pleasurable to us as well as to those who look at us or with whom we make love. A few women can even experience orgasm from breast stimulation alone. At other times, however,

we may be embarrassed or inconvenienced by our breasts. In addition, many of us develop fears concerning our breasts—from the simple fear of sagging to the often overwhelming fear of disease and loss of a breast.

These feelings, both positive and negative, are reinforced by our society's obsessive fixation on breasts. Provocative images of bared breasts are on billboards and magazines everywhere. They are used to sell everything from cars to whiskey. They can also be a factor in getting or keeping jobs. Many men feel free to whistle or stare at our breasts or even to touch them uninvited. Some women may resent or pity us because of our "size." What should be a short-lived adolescent confusion over growing up is prolonged into a lifelong concern with breast size and shape. This sexual context often makes it difficult for us to think about our breasts as functioning parts of our bodies that need health care. It also makes breast problems particularly disturbing.

Wide Range of Normal Breasts

Women have breasts of all sizes and shapes—large, small, firm, saggy, lumpy. One woman's breast may be different in size or shape from her other breast. Nipples may be prominent or inverted. The areola (the area surrounding the nipple) may be large or small, darker or lighter, and usually has little bumps just under the skin. Sometimes there are long hairs near the edge of the areola.

These individual differences, along with the changes caused by age and menstrual cycles, often produce needless anxiety. Unfortunately, we do not usually have sufficient information about what is normal, either in appearance or function, to be able to tell when something is abnormal and requires further attention. This lack of information often results in a fear that every change or pain is a symptom of cancer, when in fact *most conditions causing change, lumps or pain are not cancer.* The following are some of the common *benign* (noncancerous) conditions.

Fibrocystic Condition

(This is also called, or includes, *cystic mastitis, mastodynia, mastasia, sclerosing adenosis* and *ductal dysplasia*.) At least half of us experience some swelling, discomfort or lumpiness in our breasts that comes and goes with our periods. During ovulation and just before menstruation, hormone levels change, often causing the breast cells to retain fluid. Cysts (small sacs filled with fluid or semifluid materials) often develop. If you examine your breasts during these times, you may find a series of rather sore lumps in one or both breasts, es-

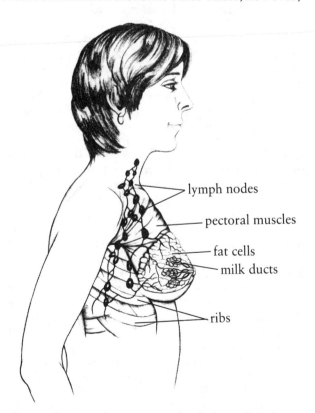

A breast, showing the structure of milk ducts, lymph nodes and fat cells.   Christine Bondante

- lymph nodes
- pectoral muscles
- fat cells
- milk ducts
- ribs

pecially in the areas nearest the arms. Most lumps will usually decrease or disappear within a day or two of the start of your period.

Some women have this fibrocystic (also called *cystic*) condition from their very first period. Others develop it in their twenties or thirties. The condition may continue—some months slightly better, others worse—until it disappears around menopause. For a few women, the condition is progressive, increasing slowly over the years from a monthly mild soreness to a constant state of sharp pain and lumpiness. Many of us, especially as we get older, find that while the pain and fullness still come and go with our periods, some of the lumps have become permanent. These lumps may or may not shrink after menopause.

"Condition" or "Disease" Controversy

Until recently, most doctors referred to this hormonally induced, cyclical pain and lumpiness as a "disease," partly because they thought it was abnormal and partly because insurance will often pay for the treatment of "diseases" but not "conditions." Now an increasing number of physicians and laywomen argue that this inaccurate terminology causes needless anxiety in millions of women about a normal aspect of the menstrual cycle that is no more a disease than menstruation, menopause or pregnancy. (Nursing a baby can be uncomfortable and complications can occur, but we do not call it "lactative disease.") Referring to it as a disease can also lead to overtreatment.

Though traditional medical opinion has been that a fibrocystic condition increases your chances of getting breast cancer, now some newer studies, plus reinterpretation of old data, cast serious doubt on that conclusion. Most women who have benign lumps do *not* develop cancer.

Fibroadenomas

If you are in your teens or twenties and find a lump that does not fluctuate with your period, it is most likely a fibroadenoma. Fibroadenomas rarely develop in women past their thirties. Those that appear early may last throughout life. Women may develop one or more fibroadenomas in one or both breasts. The cause of these growths is unknown, though some research suggests that they may be related to fat consumption. Occasionally a fibroadenoma will grow large enough to interfere with circulation or to distort the breast's shape. Such fibroadenomas are usually removed surgically. Sometimes the fibroadenoma will grow back, though not necessarily as large as previously. These growths sometimes shrink at menopause, an indication that they may be a normal occurrence. (Cancer rarely, if ever, shrinks.) The

main problem with fibroadenomas is that they often feel like cancer. The younger you are, the more likely your doctor will assume that any lump you may have is a fibroadenoma and not a cancer, but there is no way to be certain except by microscopic examination involving a needle or surgical biopsy. At present, nothing specifically links fibroadenomas with an increased risk of breast cancer.

Breast Self-Exam

Breast self-exam is a technique by which you examine your own breasts for suspicious lumps. It is recommended by most physicians as a method for the early detection of cancer.

For a while, after someone I knew got breast cancer, I checked my breasts regularly. But it was so confusing. Sometimes there were lumps and sometimes there weren't. At first, every time I'd find one, I'd run to the doctor and he'd say, "Oh, it's nothing. Don't worry. You're too young to have breast cancer." So I quit examining my breasts. I'll probably start again when I'm older.

I just feel so uncomfortable touching myself there.

I'm afraid of what I'll find. . . . I can't stand the thought of having my breast removed.

I seem to go by spurts and spells. For several months, I'll be very conscientious and examine my breasts carefully after each period. Then something comes up and I'll skip a month. Then I guess I just forget and several months or even a year will go by before I get around to doing it again. But I never seem to be able to make it a habit. I feel guilty and then get angry with myself. Why can't I find time for something so important? Why do I have so little self-discipline? Then I think about what will happen if I get breast cancer. I probably won't find it in time and it will be my fault if I die of it.

American women (60 percent or more) do not practice breast self-exam regularly, although many have tried to and almost all of us believe that we should. Study after study has shown that women who begin the routine usually discontinue it after a few months. Those who learn the technique from a health care practitioner are more likely to continue than those who learn it from another source.

The authors of this chapter found that no one in our group of seven regularly examined her breasts (although two of us have had mastectomies and are at high risk for breast cancer). Extending our informal survey, we found that almost no one we knew examined her breasts regularly.

Most had tried to develop the habit and many were actively involved in women's health issues.

Why does this issue raise so many emotions? Why is it hard to do something that we believe in and that is supposed to help save our lives? In most women's minds, a lump means cancer and cancer means losing a breast, a frightening prospect to many women.

In recent years more women have been doing breast self-exam. Now 85 percent of lumps are found by women themselves. Although breast self-exam has not been proven to decrease mortality, it has helped to detect cancers at an earlier stage.

What to Do If You Find a Lump

There are no adequate words to describe the panicky anxiety that follows the discovery of a distinct lump that wasn't there before. Cancer is the first thought that flashes into our minds, along with a lot of wild, confused thoughts about "why this should be happening to me." Some women rush immediately to the nearest doctor. Others remain quiet about their lumps, afraid to go to the doctor for fear it is cancer. They can't face the thought either of having the disease or of having to undergo a mastectomy, often mistakenly assuming that it is the only treatment course.

It is important to remember that 80 to 85 percent of all lumps are not cancer. This is especially true for younger women. One possible first step in finding out is self-screening.

Self-Screening

There are some self-screening techniques that can help you distinguish between lumps more likely to be benign and those that probably require medical evaluation. The following steps may be especially helpful to women with lumpy breasts for whom it would be both impractical and very costly to see a doctor whenever lumps appear.

First, if you are still having periods and have no previous history of either lumps or cancer, observe whether the lump disappears or fluctuates in size during your monthly cycle—a sure sign that it is not malignant. It is common medical practice, especially for younger women, for a doctor to recommend first watching the lump for a month or two. *There is no evidence that this will make any difference in length of life, even if the lump does prove cancerous.* Do not feel the lump every day or you may not be able to tell if there is any change. The best times to check are during the

---

*Many oncologists and other expert researchers have agreed with this statement, especially since we have so little evidence of treatment benefit. Certainly, if this active watching makes you anxious, seek a biopsy as soon as possible.

PREVENTION OF BREAST CANCER

At this point there is no known way to be sure that you will never get breast cancer, but there are ways in which you can protect yourself against environmental factors that may cause or encourage the disease. You can also strengthen your immune system to fight it. It is logical that the younger you are when you make any changes aimed at prevention, the more likely they are to be effective. (Remember that breast cancer may develop for as long as twenty years before it shows up.)

Cutting down on the fat in your diet is probably the single most important thing you can do. High incidence rates of breast cancer are apparently related to diets high in fat, and in the standard American diet fats (from meats and dairy products) make up 40 percent of the total calories. The American Cancer Society, the National Cancer Institute and the National Academy of Sciences have all issued guidelines and recommendations concerning the high-fat diet and cancer. Try to substitute foods high in fiber (fruit, vegetables and whole-grain cereals) for fatty foods.

The breast is highly vulnerable to cell damage through X-rays at younger ages. If possible, avoid unnecessary X-rays, especially during puberty or pregnancy. You can protect your breasts with breast shields during X-rays of the lower back. For dental X-rays, a lead apron and collar should be provided to protect the body. X-rays of the arms and legs are less dangerous (see also p. 611).

---

three or four days before and, for comparison, three or four days after the first day of your period.

You can also try changing your diet. Many women have found that they can reduce or totally eliminate certain noncancerous lumps this way. Some medical studies have supported links between diet and benign breast conditions, but more definitive studies are needed.

Here are some suggestions on diet and vitamin supplements that may help reduce breast lumps:

1. Avoid fatty and fried foods.

2. Reduce salt in your diet.

3. Eliminate foods and beverages containing caffeine—coffee, tea, most colas, chocolate and many brands of aspirin and cold remedies.

4. Don't smoke.*

5. You may want to try daily supplements:

- Vitamin E: 400 to 800 IU (already widely prescribed by many physicians for fibrocystic conditions).
- Vitamin B₆: 100 to 200 milligrams.
- Evening primrose oil: two to four grams.

While dietary changes bring lump reduction in some women within just one cycle, others must continue the diet for up to six months to get improvement. If after two months the lump has not definitely decreased, you should proceed to medical screening.

Medical Evaluation of a Lump

When seeking professional screening, the proper selection of a physician or medical facility is essential. Although your lump will probably turn out to be benign, on the outside chance that it *is* cancer, it is best to go to a breast specialist who has considerable experience with both cancer and benign conditions, not necessarily a gynecologist. Even though you may have a good relationship with your own doctor, chances are high that s/he does not keep up with current research on diagnosis and treatment options. You may find that your loyalty to your doctor is locking you into diagnoses and treatments that may be inappropriate for you. A local women's health center or the Cancer Information Service listed in Resources may help you find a sympathetic and more experienced physician. If you live in a small town, you may want to consider going to the nearest large city with a research or university hospital. The National Cancer Institute (see Resources) sponsors an increasing number of hospitals with breast-evaluation centers where you can have your lump evaluated by a team of specialists. The advantage of going to such a team is that they can be more flexible about diagnosis and treatment, as they are much more likely than local doctors to keep up with current research. Of course, a disadvantage is that you may have to travel far from your home (see Introduction to Cancer, p. 609).

Avoid scheduling your appointment just before or during the first few days of your period or around ovulation. Your breasts may be more lumpy during these times, and the doctor may miss a more suspicious lump hidden by the general swelling.

The doctor should examine your breasts carefully as you raise your arms over your head and then lower them to your sides while you are sitting up and again while you are lying down. This procedure is very important, as a lump can sometimes be felt in only one of these positions. The examination may be uncomfortable but is generally not painful. The physician will make a professional, though inevitably somewhat subjective, judgment on whether the lump feels like cancer. Cancers are usually more irregular, harder and less freely moving than benign growths, but *only a biopsy* (a procedure to remove part or all of a lump and examine some cells under a microscope for evidence of cancer) *can tell for sure, even if a mammogram is also done.* (See the section on mammography, p. 581).

Needle Aspiration—The First Step

Needle aspirations, when possible, are the best first procedure for suspicious lumps. Most lumps turn out to be benign fluid-filled cysts, and it is simple for the doctor to test for these with an aspiration, an office procedure. The aspiration avoids the problems of minor surgery associated with a surgical biopsy, and it is quicker and less painful as well. The physician inserts a fine needle into the lump. Many physicians give a novocaine shot first; others don't. Some women feel that the novocaine shot is as painful as the procedure itself. If the lump is a cyst, fluid is drawn off and it collapses.

If the lump does not yield fluid when it is aspirated, it may still be a cyst or other benign growth. An ultrasound can determine if it is a simple cyst, in which case a biopsy would not be necessary. A biopsy would be indicated if any of the following occurs: The cyst fluid is not normal in appearance (for example, if it is bloody or thick), the lump does not disappear with aspiration, an ultrasound reveals possible echoes within the cyst (fluid should have no echoes), or the cyst continues to recur following repeated aspiration.

The use of aspiration as the first step in evaluating a lump is increasing but is not yet routine everywhere. Because most lumps (well over 95 percent) turn out to be cysts, aspiration as a first step saves much time, expense and anxiety. If your doctor does not suggest an aspiration at first, you may want to request one. A few lumps, however, are buried so deeply within a generally lumpy or large breast or may "feel" so much like cancer that some doctors will recommend a surgical biopsy first rather than an aspiration. Others may want to try a needle biopsy first (see below).

Biopsy

This procedure involves removing all or part of a lump and examining it for cancer. Biopsies can be needle biopsies (removing cells), incisional biopsies (surgical removal of only part of the lump) or excisional biopsies (removing all of the

---

*One study found that all the women who got no relief from eliminating salt and caffeine were also smokers. The women who then quit smoking subsequently found their lumps noticeably reduced.

lump through surgery). Core needle biopsies are called *Tro-car* or *Tru-cut* biopsies. These can be done as simple in-office procedures. After applying a small amount of anesthesia to the breast (similar to the novocaine that dentists use), the doctor inserts a needle that carves out a small part of the lump. The withdrawn sample of breast tissue is sent to a laboratory for cancer testing. Besides leaving less of a scar, this needle biopsy technique is less expensive and time-consuming than a surgical biopsy.

However, the results of any incisional biopsy (needle or surgical) can only be completely trusted if they are positive, that is, if cancer is found. There is always the possibility that an incisional biopsy may miss the malignant part.

Still, a needle biopsy may be a good second step for a woman under thirty with no significant risk factors. Cancer is extremely rare in these younger women and their lumps, even those that do not fluctuate with their periods or yield fluid when aspirated, almost always turn out to be benign. Such a young woman may decide that she is satisfied with the incisional needle biopsy, especially if the results show that the lump is a fibroadenoma.

Attitudes toward the biopsies vary enormously among physicians. Some physicians biopsy everything just to be sure. Others avoid the procedure. In general, your physician should use aspiration and/or ultrasound to determine whether or not a lump is a cyst. If a lump is solid, then a biopsy is necessary. Some physicians recommend mammography at this point in order to see if there is other suspicious tissue that should be biopsied at the same time. (Note that a normal mammogram reading does not change the original recommendation to biopsy the solid lump.)

If you have a biopsy, you need to decide on the type of biopsy and whether to have it with general or local anesthesia.

If a woman tends to develop a lot of lumps, it is much easier to check them with a needle biopsy than to cut each one out completely. Frequent surgical excisional biopsies can leave the breast scarred and distorted and can build up confusing scar tissue within the breast. However, the age when women develop the most lumps is in their thirties and forties. Although most of these lumps are benign, the incidence of breast cancer rises steeply after age forty. Consequently there is increasing risk that a needle biopsy will miss a cancer after age forty, even though such instances are rare.

Anesthesia

Needle biopsies are almost always done with local anesthesia. Surgical biopsies, which may be excisional or incisional, can be done with either local or general anesthesia. Some women consider it too stressful to be awake during the biopsy and thus prefer general anesthesia. Others choose a local because they prefer being awake and/or because they are concerned about the serious health hazards of general anesthesia (see p. 568).

You may meet resistance if you want local anesthesia. Some surgeons recommend the general out of habit, because they think people are too frightened by the idea of a local, because insurance is more likely to pay or simply because they themselves are uncomfortable with a person who is conscious.

About 10 percent of the time, the size or depth of the lump or a very large or lumpy breast makes the surgery more complicated, and general anesthesia may be required.

Before the Biopsy

We do not advise the one-step biopsy, in which you sign a release allowing a mastectomy before you even know whether or not your lump is cancerous. In this procedure, the doctor removes the lump and examines it by the frozen section method while you are still under general anesthesia. For this test, the lump is frozen immediately upon removal. Technicians cut a thin slice of the lump and examine it under the microscope for signs of cancer. The results of a frozen section (always tentative) are usually available within twenty minutes. If cancer is found, your doctor proceeds with a mastectomy. The major problem with the one-step is that occasionally the quick-frozen section test is inaccurate, and women's breasts have been removed when they did not have cancer. Even if you do have cancer, the one-step gives you no time to consider your options. For example, mastectomy might be an inappropriate treatment for your type of cancer. You can prevent any misdiagnoses or unwanted treatments more easily when the biopsy is separated from any other treatment and the permanent section is used as the determining test for cancer. The permanent section takes several days but is more accurate and gives additional information about the type of cancer which may be helpful in deciding what further treatments, if any, to take. The National Cancer Institute specifically advises against the one-step biopsy (followed immediately by a mastectomy), although many doctors still practice it.

Before the biopsy, you may want to ask the surgeon to cut so as to leave the smallest possible scar. Sometimes doctors are not careful about this, because they assume the breast will be removed later during a mastectomy. (However, you may not choose mastectomy even if you do have cancer.) Depending on the size and location of the lump, the incision can sometimes be made along natural wrinkle lines or along the edge of the areola, or under the arm. Any scar, discoloration or distortion left by the biopsy usually becomes less noticeable over time, though this varies significantly from one woman to another.

Be sure that estrogen and progesterone receptor (ER and PR) assays are planned. These tests, which indicate how much a tumor is influenced by the hormones estrogen and progesterone, must be done *immediately* after the lump is removed. The information can make a big difference in treatment decisions (see below). By now ER and PR assays should be routine everywhere. You may also want to ask about other important tests for special tumor characteristics, such as flow cytometry or oncogene expression. Flow cytometry is a way of measuring the rate of cell division in a tumor. Oncogenes are special genes that appear to increase the rate of cell growth in a tumor.

Results of Biopsies

Waiting for the results of a biopsy can be an excruciating experience. Ask when the results will be ready and whether the doctor's office will call or you should call them. If you haven't heard by the appointed day, call. If the results are *negative*, that means you do not have cancer. *Positive* results mean that cancer was found (see Breast Cancer, p. 616).

If the Results Are Negative

Most likely (in 80 to 90 percent of all biopsies) the tests will be negative. If you are premeno-

---

WHEN A BIOPSY IS NEEDED

1. When needle aspiration or ultrasound does not clearly demonstrate that a lump is a cyst.
2. When mammography shows a suspicious mass or suspicious calcifications.
3. When other symptoms that may indicate cancer are present. These include hard, swollen lymph glands in the armpit area, a skin rash on the breast, nipple discharge or dimpling or puckering of the skin around the nipple.
4. If a lump persists after one or two menstrual cycles.

Many women have good instincts about which changes, especially lumps or thickening, are harmless and which are dangerous. One cancer specialist said he always listens to his patients' intuitions, as they are often correct.

---

pausal, the doctor is likely to say that the lump is just *fibrocystic*, a term that has unfortunately become a catch-all term for noncancerous lumps in younger women. You may be so relieved that you don't have cancer that you don't want to bother with any more medical terms. However, you should ask the doctor exactly what *fibrocystic* means in terms of *your* lump. You need to know the precise name, whether this type tends to recur and whether it is ever related to cancer. Your doctor may not know or be willing to share this information, so you may have to be very persistent.

You have a right to obtain and examine a copy of all your medical records, and it is a good idea to get a copy of the biopsy test results. The information may be helpful in years to come as new data become available as to which, if any, types of lumps are associated with cancer. Having your own copy helps when getting second opinions or changing doctors. It also provides protection against the common problem of loss of medical records.

Prophylactic Mastectomies

Prophylactic (preventive) mastectomies are being performed in increasing numbers on women who do not have breast cancer but are considered to be at high risk for the disease (see p. 581). Unfortunately, the type of surgery used in most prophylactic operations (the subcutaneous mastectomy) does not guarantee that the woman will avoid breast cancer. In the subcutaneous mastectomy, approximately 80 to 95 percent of the breast tissue is removed, leaving the skin, nipple and some underlying fat intact. A saline implant may be inserted at the same time to replace the breast tissue and give a more normal appearance, but complications frequently occur. Some women will develop cancer in the small amount of remaining breast tissue. Keeping this in mind, any woman who is considering a prophylactic mastectomy should probably consider having a simple mastectomy rather than the more cosmetic subcutaneous mastectomy. However, even this will not provide complete assurance. It is always possible that an undetected cancer had already developed in the breast and was present in other parts of the body before the mastectomy.

A few women request prophylactic mastectomies but more frequently doctors suggest it. Yet even women labeled at high risk, the usual candidates for prophylactic mastectomies, are more likely not to develop breast cancer than they are to develop it. Prophylactic mastectomy is a radical step that should not be taken without a second opinion from a breast cancer specialist.

Only when medical science can predict with total accuracy who will get breast cancer might

THE "HIGH-RISK" CONTROVERSY

It is extremely important to inquire carefully about the basis for any high-risk label assigned you by your doctor. Few doctors have adequate training in epidemiology or genetics, and most are too busy to keep up with today's sophisticated risk studies. Inappropriate labeling may lead to unnecessary, dangerous and expensive tests and procedures, as well as the emotional stress of believing you are in greater danger of developing breast cancer than the average woman. Remember, of every one hundred women who develop breast cancer, less than 25 percent will have some identifiable risk factor.

The American Cancer Society has reevaluated its list of factors believed to be associated with an increased or high risk of developing breast cancer. In reality only a few factors are truly known to increase one's risk, and even these cannot *predict* breast cancer. For example, only if a mother or sister had a confirmed diagnosis of breast cancer *before age fifty* does a woman's risk increase significantly, more so if the cancer was in both breasts. Exposure to radiation and DES have increased risk in a relatively small number of women.

Menopausal estrogens have been shown in numerous studies to increase breast cancer risk, but the subject is still controversial. A previous personal history of breast cancer increases the likelihood of discovering new cancer (not a metastasis) in the other breast (by about 1 percent per year, or 15 to 20 percent over a lifetime).

Women is this country face a one in nine lifetime risk of developing breast cancer, but the risk of developing breast cancer *within the next decade* will vary greatly and depend upon a woman's age as well as other factors. After the age of fifty, a woman's age is the most important risk factor. An excellent resource for helping to determine your own breast cancer risk is *Understanding Breast Cancer* by Patricia Kelly (Philadelphia: Temple University Press, 1991).

As the incidence of breast cancer continues to rise, a more constructive way for us to think about our risks is to disregard the outmoded and misleading studies of the past and think about our future by taking prevention seriously. (See p. 577, Prevention of Breast Cancer, and p. 611, A Program to Reduce the Risk of Cancer. See also Chapter 7, "Environmental and Occupational Health.")

prophylactic mastectomy become more generally appropriate.

Mammograms

Mammography (taking X-rays of the breast) is a means of *detecting*, not a means of *preventing*, breast cancer. Worldwide evidence now shows that routine mammography screening with or without a clinical exam reduces mortality among women over fifty years by 30 to 50 percent. Recommendations vary as to how often (every year versus every two years) and at what ages (somewhere between forty and fifty years) a woman should begin to get regular mammograms.

Before the biopsy of a lump, your doctor may want you to have a mammogram to help determine whether other areas should be biopsied as well.

Advantages and Disadvantages of Mammography

Mammograms do offer important advantages, such as detecting some cancers which aren't yet palpable (easily felt), serving as a map or guide to surgeons and providing a baseline against which later mammograms can be compared to see if any unusual changes have taken place in recent years. When mammograms detect cancers that are not yet invasive, the cancers are more likely to be successfully treated. There are also serious drawbacks to the procedure, including misdiagnoses, both through missing cancers that are there and mistakenly identifying benign lumps as cancerous. The cost of the procedure and the time taken off from work or other activities may be disadvantages as well. With modern mammography equipment one case of breast cancer is induced per million women examined per year.

There have been cases where false positives (mistaken diagnoses of cancer) from mammograms combined with false positives from quick-frozen section biopsy tests (see previous section) resulted in the removal of breasts from women who didn't have cancer. Remember that mammograms only indicate *possible* cancerous areas. A *permanent section test* (surgical biopsy) on a sample of that area is required to confirm the diagnosis of cancer (see Biopsy, p. 578).

The quality of mammography services has a

critical influence over both advantages and disadvantages. Poorly calibrated equipment may expose a woman to unnecessary radiation or increase the rate of false negatives. Inadequately trained technicians may produce inaccurate results. It is important to get your mammogram in a facility accredited by the American College of Radiology. As of late 1991, however, only 36 percent of mammography services had obtained such accreditation (see box on legislation).

Who Should Have Mammograms?

If you are over fifty years old or if you have already had one or more breast cancers detected, the advantages of mammography have clearly been established. Current studies are investigating whether the same benefits hold for younger women.

The breast tissue of premenopausal women is denser and does not show up as well in a mammogram. Overall, mammography has a false-positive rate (indicating cancer where there is none) of about 7 percent. Estimates of false negatives (missing a cancer that is present) vary from 4 to 30 percent. These false positives and false negatives are more common among premenopausal women.

There is also evidence that the breasts of younger women may be more susceptible to radiation damage than those of older women. In addition, any woman who starts annual or frequent mammograms at twenty-five or thirty-five is clearly increasing the amount of radiation exposure over her lifetime, thus increasing her chances of breast cancer. If a radiation-induced cancer takes twenty years to develop, a fifty-five-year-old woman might develop breast cancer at seventy-five, but a twenty-five- or thirty-five-year-old woman may develop it at forty-five or fifty-five.

The decision to have or not to have a mammogram is more complex if you are under fifty and have no suspicious lumps but are considered to be at high risk for breast cancer. (See the section on risk controversy, p. 581). Many doctors argue that high-risk women have the most to gain from mammography—they are more likely to have cancers that mammography can detect. But it may also be that they have the most to lose from it. Perhaps being at high risk means greater vulner-

ENSURING THE QUALITY OF MAMMOGRAPHY SERVICES

As of early 1992 there were no regulations to govern the quality of mammography services. Under voluntary accreditation programs about one-third of mammography facilities failed to pass on their first attempt, and only slightly more than one-third of mammography services were accredited by late 1991.

The Breast Cancer Screening Act of 1991, proposed by U.S. Representative Patricia Schroeder and others, called for all mammography facilities to be certified by a national accreditation body. This body would inspect mammography equipment annually and require that only certified persons operate the machines and that only qualified radiologists interpret test results. Similar legislation has been proposed at the state level. Such regulation is essential in order to reduce unnecessary exposure to radiation, poorly interpreted test results and other problems.

MAMMOGRAPHY: BREAST X-RAYS

1. Recommended for follow-up of women of any age who already have breast cancer.
2. Shown effective in reducing breast cancer death rates only for women over fifty.
3. Effectiveness for women under fifty is unproven. Research continues.
4. Problems with mammography:

- When older, poorer-quality equipment is used, the radiation used may cause cancer.
- There are occasional false negatives which are falsely reassuring.
- There is an increasing ability to detect preinvasive cancers—a type that has not yet spread or become life-threatening. Although this may result in unnecessary treatments that further distort the cure and survival rates, it also makes possible a real cure in some cases.

5. Advantages of mammography:

- It detects many cancers before they can be felt and thus expands options for breast conservation.
- It serves as a map or guide to the surgeon.
- Baseline mammograms may be compared with later mammograms for suspicious changes.

ability, less resistance than other people to carcinogens such as radiation. Should this be the case, then high-risk women would be advised to avoid mammography more than average women. At this time, neither interpretation of high risk is proven.

Most European countries now recommend mammography every two years. In the United States, most professional groups recommend yearly mammograms for women over forty. The U.S. Preventive Health Services Task Force recommends every one to two years. Because breast cancer incidence appears to be rising among women in their thirties and forties, more women are obtaining regular mammograms before the age of fifty. They and their physicians hope that earlier detection and earlier treatment of breast cancer will make a positive difference. Current research soon will offer more definitive answers to questions about the benefits of mammography for younger women.

Even if mammography does turn out to be effective for younger as well as older women, this usefulness may still be bought at the price of inducing a small number of cancers in some women exposed to inadequate mammography equipment. This is no boon to any woman who may die from radiation-induced breast cancer. For this reason, we believe that researchers should emphasize developing truly safe screening methods.

Remember that a mammogram should never substitute for direct examination of a lump, as described earlier in this section.

DES

A DES daughter with clear-cell cancer:

October will be three years since I was diagnosed with clear-cell adenocarcinoma. At that time I underwent a seven-hour operation to remove my uterus, vagina, fallopian tubes, an ovary and many lymph nodes. A split-thickness skin graft was used to reconstruct my vagina. As of this date I'm still trying to understand what clear-cell cancer is, what happened to my body and how it could have happened to a healthy twenty-five-year-old in the first place. I especially got mad when I found out that there was a reason why this cancer happened and that it never would have happened if DES had been properly tested. It is amazing to me that the people involved in the marketing of DES are so callously indifferent to the fact that it causes cancer.

Overview

DES (diethylstilbestrol) is a powerful synthetic estrogen prescribed to 3 to 6 million American women over a thirty-year period, between 1941 and 1971. DES was prescribed in the mistaken belief that it would prevent miscarriage. In fact the drug was untested for pregnancy use and aggressively marketed until 1971—when the link to a rare form of vaginal cancer in DES daughters was established. DES was manufactured under more than 200 brand names and used throughout the United States, Canada and Europe in pills, injections and suppositories.*

DES crosses the placenta and damages the reproductive system of the developing fetus. A range of reproductive tract injuries are linked to DES exposure. DES may also affect other body systems (endocrine, immune and cardiovascular), but there is little research under way. Although the majority of DES-exposed are still in their thirties, DES research has dwindled to practically nothing.

Who Is Exposed and How to Find Out

Several million people (mothers, daughters and sons) have been exposed to DES, most without knowing it. If you were born after 1940, ask your mother if she had problems with any of her pregnancies or if she remembers taking anything when she was pregnant with you. (It is generally believed that DES was most widely used between 1947 and 1965 when wonder drugs were so popular.)

I didn't remember taking anything besides vitamins during my pregnancy, but when my daughter asked me, we checked, and there it was on the medical record.

If a woman doesn't know whether she took DES, she can check with the doctor she saw at that time. However, many doctors no longer have their medical records, and some refuse to give the information. You may find something in the medical records at the hospital where the birth took place.

Any woman who is not sure whether her mother took DES can get a special exam (see below) from a medical-care provider knowledgeable about DES exposure.

Medical Problems and Medical Care

DES Daughters

Clear-cell adenocarcinoma is a rare type of vaginal or cervical cancer linked to *in utero* exposure to DES. Before 1970 clear-cell cancer had only

---

*Use of DES in European countries continued throughout the 1970s (until 1975 in England and the Netherlands, until 1977 in France) and in some countries into the 1980s (until 1981 in Spain and Italy, until 1983 in Hungary). DES was prescribed in every country where U.S. drug companies had markets.

rarely occurred in medical history, and never in women so young. It is estimated that 1 out of every 1,000 DES daughters will develop clear-cell cancer of the vagina or cervix. The cancer has occurred in girls and women between the ages of seven and forty, with the peak at ages fifteen to twenty-two. Although clear-cell cancer cases have declined in the last ten years (mirroring the decreased use of DES in the 1970s), clear-cell cancer is still being diagnosed in 1991, and the upper age limit for developing the cancer is unknown.[1]

Regular DES exams can find clear-cell cancer early so that it can be treated. Clear-cell cancer is fast-growing and, in the early stages, sometimes symptomless. The typical treatment for the cancer includes a radical hysterectomy, surgical removal of all or part of the vagina (vaginectomy) and reconstruction of the vagina. Radiation treatment is often used in conjunction with surgery. Eighty percent of the patients survive, but the adjustment to the extreme treatment is a difficult one.

Structural changes, such as cervical "collars" or "hoods," are also common among DES daughters. They do not need treatment and may disappear after age thirty. DES daughters are also more likely than others to have a T-shaped uterus. Some structural changes may contribute to pregnancy problems (see below).

a normal uterus

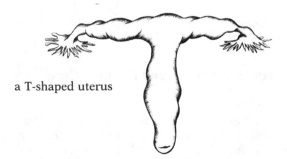

a T-shaped uterus

A T-shaped uterus is one of the abnormal changes often found in DES daughters. The uterus may also be smaller than normal. The unusual size and shape may contribute to pregnancy problems for DES daughters, most notably preterm labor.   Christine Bondante

Metaplasia is a normal process whereby tissue changes from one form to another. Although all women have areas of cells undergoing metaplasia around their cervix, this area of changing tissue may be larger in DES daughters with adenosis. This metaplasia raises two concerns: First, some suspect that this area may be more vulnerable to precancerous or cancerous changes. Second, pathologists may mistakenly interpret the change as abnormal (dysplasia). Such misdiagnosis can lead to unnecessary treatment with possibly harmful effects.

Most researchers do not find dysplasia (see p. 572) to be more common among DES daughters. However, DES daughters who do have dysplasia may want to approach treatment recommendations with caution.*

Squamous cell carcinoma, usually of the cervix, is a slow-growing cancer that is sometimes preceded by dysplasia. Research is needed to ascertain whether DES daughters will be at a higher risk for this cancer in later years.

Pregnancy problems are more common in DES daughters, partially due to abnormalities in the uterus and/or cervix. They may have trouble conceiving or carrying a first pregnancy to term due to miscarriage, premature delivery or tubal pregnancy (pregnancy in the fallopian tube instead of in the uterus). Early in pregnancy, watching for signs of a tubal pregnancy may help prevent serious problems. Later on, a pregnant DES daughter should receive high-risk obstetrical care.

When I got pregnant, I found out that the doctor who was doing my DES exams didn't know anything about pregnancy problems for DES daughters. So I brought him seven articles that DES Action gave me. We both read them and, as a result, he checked my cervix at every prenatal visit. It took fifteen seconds and took away tons of anxiety.

Other problems, such as endometriosis, menstrual irregularities and PID, have been reported by many DES daughters. There is as yet no research on whether these problems are more significant among DES-exposed women.

Contraception for DES daughters poses some special considerations. Birth control pills may be inadvisable due to the possible effects of further estrogen exposure on someone who is already at increased risk of a hormone-related cancer.[3] IUDs for DES daughters are questionable because of the

---

*One study of a small number of DES daughters found that cryosurgery (a common treatment of freezing the affected tissue) resulted in sometimes serious aftereffects in these women that did not occur in nonexposed women.[2]

possible cervical and uterine abnormalities. Barrier methods are often the overall safest choice.

The DES Exam

DES-caused changes do not usually show up in regular pelvic examinations or Pap smears. Starting with your first period or any signs of trouble (discharge or bleeding), see a medical-care provider experienced in DES screening. Ask whether the person who examines you is following other DES daughters and if s/he is familiar with the techniques described below.

A DES exam consists of

- A careful visual inspection of the vagina and cervix for physical abnormalities.
- A gentle palpation of the walls of the vagina.
- A four-sided (quadrant) Pap test of the cervix *and* vagina.
- Iodine staining of the vagina and cervix (normal tissue stains brown, adenosis tissue does not stain) (see Schiller's Test, p. 567).

The clinician may also do further tests or refer you to a special doctor or special clinic for more tests. These may include biopsy (p. 578) and colposcopy (p. 566).

DES Mothers

Some of the few studies available suggest that DES mothers have an increased incidence of breast cancer and cancer of the uterus, cervix or ovaries and of noncancerous tumors of the uterus. Most studies agree that there is a time lag of ten to twenty years between taking DES and developing a related disease.

If you are a DES mother, get a professional breast exam every year in addition to performing monthly breast self-examination.

DES Sons

Ongoing studies report several areas of concern for DES sons: underdeveloped testes, benign (noncancerous) cysts on the epididymis (the part of the testicle that stores mature sperm), undescended testicles (which may increase the risk of testicular cancer) and sperm and semen abnormalities (which may cause fertility problems). Concerned sons can be examined by a urologist and DES sons can practice regular self-examination of the testes.

Emotional Issues

For the DES-exposed, all of these physical effects often generate emotional effects as well. Living with the necessity of frequent medical examinations, a fear of cancer, knowledge of deformities and worry about the ability to have a healthy child adds to the revictimization of DES-exposed people.

Not surprisingly, some DES mothers feel guilty

DES Action

when they find out that something they took may have harmed their children. Some find it difficult to tell them, though it is essential to do so. Many mothers describe relief after telling their children and talking about the health care they need.

I read about the report on DES and its link to cancer back in 1971. I cut the article out of the paper and stuck it in my bureau drawer. Five years later my daughter was fourteen and I knew I had to do something soon. So I found a doctor who knew about DES and how to do the exam, and I finally told my daughter. What a relief!

It really helped me to talk with other DES daughters. We compared notes and I went back to my next medical appointment with a list of questions and a friend for moral support. We had a long discussion with the doctor, who was surprised at how much we knew.

DES, which has caused me so much pain, has at least allowed me new and needed understandings. I know to keep myself informed. I would like to work with my doctors. I know that they haven't always read the medical journals. I know that they cannot care about the outcome of my case nearly as much as I do.

Although we know much more about DES than we did ten years ago, daughters, sons and mothers face unanswered questions about their future health. More research is needed in all areas. Furthermore, some doctors still do not know about the DES exam, special pregnancy problems and other recent medical findings; their ignorance can result in serious overtreatment or undertreatment. Finally, we need to tell the DES story so that people who have been exposed can receive the medical care they need and so that we can help prevent similar medical mistakes from happening in the future.

DES Action USA and the DES Cancer Network

DES Action USA (1615 Broadway, Suite 510, Oakland, CA, 94612, 510-465-4011) is a national consumer organization which provides information and medical referrals to DES-exposed persons. The DES Cancer Network (P.O. Box 10185, Rochester, NY, 14610, 716-473-6119) is a national resource for information on clear-cell cancer, providing research advocacy, patient-to-patient support, and information about DES cancer issues.

ENDOMETRIOSIS

Endometriosis, which can be an extremely painful disease, occurs when some of the tissue that usually lines the uterus (endometrium) grows in other parts of the body. This "normal tissue in an abnormal location," sometimes referred to as *growths*, *nodules*, *tumors* or *lesions*, most commonly develops in the pelvic area—on the ovaries, the lining of the pelvic cavity (peritoneum), ligaments or fallopian tubes. Growths may also occur on the bladder, intestines or even distant parts of the body—in the arm, lung or head.

Like the lining of the uterus, endometrial growths usually respond to the hormones of the menstrual cycle. They build up tissue each month, break down, and cause bleeding. Internal bleeding, inflammation and formation of cysts and scar tissue results. The immune system appears to be involved in some as yet unknown way.

Endometriosis may cause severe pelvic pain around menstruation, ovulation and/or sexual activity; excessive menstrual flow; fatigue; painful bowel movements with periods; lower back pain with periods; diarrhea and/or constipation and other intestinal upset with periods; and infertility. It can also cause other severe health problems, including ruptured ovarian cysts; adhesions; increased risk of ectopic pregnancy and general debilitation. And yet some women experience no symptoms except perhaps infertility.

A thirty-three-year-old woman describes her experience:

I experienced the first symptoms of endometriosis (in my case, very severe pain when having a bowel move- *ment) when I was nineteen years old. About five years later I began to have the same kind of pain at midcycle and during my periods. I mentioned this to several doctors, and they seemed unconcerned. A year or two later I began to have premenstrual spotting, which increased in duration as time progressed. I went to at least four different doctors. No one even mentioned endometriosis. . . . At the age of thirty I had new symptoms: chronic, low-level pelvic pain and pain on intercourse, in addition to pain on pelvic examination. At this time the word "endometriosis" was first mentioned, and a diagnosis by laparoscopy followed a few months later.*

A particularly difficult aspect of the disease for many women is that it is chronic. In one survey, 60 percent of 200 women said that they were unable to carry on normal work and activities, usually for one to three days at a time and sometimes for weeks or even months, not including the time lost for surgery. One woman calculated that three days lost to pain each month for twenty years added up to a staggering two years of her life. While most people would not make light of two years lost to illness, the recurring nature of this condition—the fact that it comes and goes with the menstrual period and gets better and worse—means that women often don't get recognition and sympathy for the difficulties it causes. A twenty-four-year-old woman states:

The biggest problem is looking very healthy. People don't seem to understand pain and sickness unless they can see physical evidence. This makes you feel absolutely desperate.

Causes and Risk Factors

The cause of endometriosis is not known. A number of theories have been advanced, but no one of them seems to account for all cases. One theory is the retrograde menstruation theory—that during menstruation some of the menstrual tissue backs up through the fallopian tubes, implants in the abdomen and grows. Research has shown that many women experience some menstrual tissue backup and that an immune system problem and/ or hormonal problem allows this tissue to take root and grow in women who develop endometriosis. In addition, many women have implants but no sign of disease, according to another research study. It is possible the definition of endometriosis will be changing in coming years, as studies such as these imply that the immune system factors in those women who develop endometriosis are more important than simply the presence of endometrial tissue outside the uterus. Since the Endometriosis Association's research has found many other signs of immune problems in women with severe endometriosis and their families, the understanding of endometriosis as primarily an immune disease may help us understand many of the puzzles surrounding endometriosis.

There are numerous other theories about the cause of endometriosis but none proven at this time. Of importance to women with endometriosis is a genetic theory that suggests that certain families may have predisposing factors to endometriosis. The association is following families with the disease and related health problems. These include a range of problems related to *Candida albicans* (both vaginal yeast infections and other signs and symptoms throughout the body), allergies, asthma, eczema, hay fever, food sensitivities, a history of mononucleosis and a higher than normal incidence of immune system diseases, including lupus and thyroid-related problems. Some of these findings are very new and will take much more research to determine exactly what is happening. Also, women who have cycle lengths of twenty-seven days or less and periods lasting one week or more and those who started their periods early are at greater risk of developing endometriosis. In addition, orgasm during the menstrual period has been found to be a risk factor: It is thought that the contractions of the uterus may cause more endometrial tissue to back through the fallopian tubes. This is directly contrary to the old advice that women should engage in sex or masturbate to orgasm to relieve menstrual cramps and associated problems of primary dysmenorrhea. Finally, cone biopsy has recently been linked to endometriosis of the cervix.

In addition, women with endometriosis generally have a history of primary dysmenorrhea; indeed, it is impossible to tell where primary dysmenorrhea ends and endometriosis begins. Given the chronic pain and other difficulties that both primary dysmenorrhea and endometriosis cause, it would be wise to attempt to control primary dysmenorrhea with the antiprostaglandin preparations available (ibuprofen is used most commonly). If you or your family have other risk factors, you may also want to control them to improve your health and perhaps decrease your risk for endometriosis. Again, much more research is needed before we will have solid answers on the cause, prevention and cure for endometriosis.

Myths impede both diagnosis and treatment of endometriosis. The classical "psychological profile" of the endometriosis sufferer still crops up in both medical literature and popular media, labeling this "the career woman's disease" and blaming the victim as an upwardly striving, white, educated, egocentric woman in her late twenties or early thirties who has postponed pregnancy in favor of her career. The anachronistic view probably exists because these were the women who tended to have the financial resources, education, sense of entitlement and private doctors necessary to obtain a correct diagnosis. However, women of color do develop the disease, though the medical system has historically overlooked that fact. Also, it is *not* true that the disease typically begins in the late twenties and early thirties. In a very large study from the association's data registry, 60 percent of the women experienced their first symptoms of the disease before age twenty-five. Also, contrary to medical myth, early pregnancy—even teenage pregnancy—does not confer immunity to the disease.

Another myth is that menstrual pain is primarily psychological. Many doctors still don't take it seriously, which makes them slow to diagnose endometriosis. Any teen or woman with severe menstrual cramps or other menstrual problems should seek a very sensitive and knowledgeable physician. The Endometriosis Association offers a special information kit to help you with diagnosis.

Diagnosis

Though physicians can sometimes feel endometrial implants during a pelvic exam, a laparoscopy is needed for a definitive diagnosis. Endometriosis is sometimes confused with other disorders and diseases (for example, PID, ectopic pregnancy, cysts, cancer, appendicitis or diverticulitis) that have similar symptoms. Thus, proper treatment cannot occur without proper diagnosis.

Treatments

Choosing a treatment is rarely simple. A number of factors may enter into your decision, among them your age, location of the endometriosis and its severity, your desire for pregnancy, past experiences with hormones and family history.

The aim in treating endometriosis with hormonal treatments is to stop the ovary from working and producing estrogen and also to stop menstruation. Although doctors often recommend pregnancy as a treatment, it is certainly a dubious one. It is, of course, best to have a child because you want to, not to cure a disease. Pregnancy is not a cure anyway, though it may offer temporary relief. And it is not always possible to become pregnant, as women with endometriosis have higher than average infertility. If you have the disease and know you want a child, be aware that delay may make pregnancy less likely if the disease advances.

Hormonal treatments include gonadotropin-releasing hormone (GnRH) analogs, various synthetic progesteronelike drugs (Provera) and oral contraceptives. The drugs most commonly used by specialists—danazol and the GnRH analogs—are very expensive. All of the hormonal treatments cause problematic side effects for some women.

THE ENDOMETRIOSIS ASSOCIATION

The Endometriosis Association, founded in January 1980, is an international self-help organization with three major goals: supporting and helping women with endometriosis, educating the medical community and public about the disease and conducting research.

The association offers lectures and support group meetings, crisis telephone services, networking for special problems (especially for finding sensitive and knowledgeable physicians) and a wide variety of informative, accurate and highly acclaimed literature on endometriosis and related health problems. The association's literature includes its popular book entitled *Overcoming Endometriosis: New Help from the Endometriosis Association*, videotapes, audiocassette tapes of speeches by experts on the disease, a "How Can I Tell If I Have Endometriosis?" kit to help those not yet diagnosed who suspect they have the disease and other literature.

The association headquarters is located in Milwaukee, Wisconsin; members, chapters and groups are scattered worldwide. Ending the feeling of being alone, sharing with others who understand what you are going through, counteracting the lack of information and misinformation about endometriosis and learning from each other are ways those affected by the disease help each other.

Since 1980 the association has been gathering information from thousands of women who have endometriosis and maintains the world's largest data registry on the disease. Information from this registry is used in preparing association literature, in the association's research, and also by other researchers.

For additional information, call the association at (800) 992-3636 in the United States and (800) 426-2363 in Canada, or write to the Endometriosis Association, 8585 North 76th Place, Milwaukee, WI 53223.

Also, all tend to work while the woman is on the drug, but recurrence of the disease within a relatively short time after discontinuing the drug is the rule.

Surgery to treat endometriosis includes a wide range of treatments, from conservative (scraping, cutting, cauterizing or lasering the growths) to radical (hysterectomy, with or without removal of the ovaries). Radical surgery has been said to be the definitive cure for endometriosis, but the Endometriosis Association's research has found a high rate of continuation/recurrence of the disease even with removal of the uterus and ovaries. Surgery through the laparoscope, called *operative laparoscopy*, is rapidly replacing major abdominal surgery in the United States and will probably also do so in other countries.

According to a twenty-eight-year-old woman:

The hardest part in deciding treatment is picking the lesser of two evils.

In the words of a thirty-three-year-old woman describing eleven years of intensifying symptoms:

Doctors seemed unsympathetic about the fact that by this point I was in almost constant pain. They suggested that I try to get pregnant; I mentioned that intercourse was now quite painful. They shrugged and suggested a few drinks or a few aspirins a day.

Some women, searching for cure and relief from pain (sometimes they have to use prescription painkillers for extended periods of time) have turned to alternative forms of healing—visualization, meditation, acupuncture, chiropractic, homeopathy, herbs and nutritional therapies among them. The Endometriosis Association is evaluating these methods and requests that women with endometriosis write them about their experiences.

The Endometriosis Association keeps careful records of these reports as well as reports on medical treatments. In gathering and sharing information, we work to build mutual support so that women will not feel isolated. Together we hope to encourage researchers to build on what we have learned, to find better solutions and cures and to recognize endometriosis as the serious health problem that it is.

PELVIC INFLAMMATORY DISEASE

I obtained a copy of my medical records and discovered that I had been complaining of the same problem—pain in my lower right abdomen—for a couple of years.

I tried several different doctors, none of whom took it seriously or were very sympathetic. If any-

thing, they made me feel unclean, almost to the point of being ashamed. I had severe menstrual irregularities, fevers, bleeding between periods, bleeding after intercourse, pains and general malaise. Several times I was treated with antibiotics, which brought only some temporary relief. Never was the issue resolved as to what was causing this. Never were my sexual partners or practices mentioned.

Pelvic inflammatory disease (PID) is a general term for an infection that affects the lining of the uterus (endometritis), the fallopian tubes (salpingitis) and/or ovaries (oophoritis). It is primarily caused by sexually transmitted diseases that spread up from the opening of the uterus to these organs (see Chapter 14). Annually, nearly 1 million women in the United States are reported to develop PID. In addition, 300,000 women are hospitalized. The cost for treating PID and PID-related problems was more than $4.2 billion in 1990. These statistics probably greatly underestimate the amount and consequences of PID now occurring. This is primarily because so much PID is undiagnosed.

Symptoms

PID symptoms vary. They may be so mild that you hardly notice them, but the primary symptom is pain. For instance, you may be aware of tightness or pressure in the reproductive organs or an occasional dull ache in the lower abdomen. On the other hand, the pain may be so strong that you may not even be able to stand. You may feel pain in the middle of your lower abdomen or on one or both sides of the lower abdomen.

You may have some, most or none of these other symptoms:

- Abnormal or foul discharge from the vagina or urethra.
- Pain or bleeding during or after intercourse.
- Irregular bleeding or spotting.
- Increased menstrual cramps.
- Increased pain during ovulation.
- Frequent urinating, burning or inability to empty bladder when urinating.
- Swollen abdomen.
- Sudden high fever or low-grade fever that can come and go.
- Chills.
- Swollen lymph nodes.
- Lack of appetite.
- Nausea or vomiting.
- Pain around the kidneys or liver.
- Lower back or leg pain.
- Feelings of weakness, tiredness, depression.
- Diminished desire to have sex.

The intensity and extent of the symptoms depend upon which microorganisms are causing the

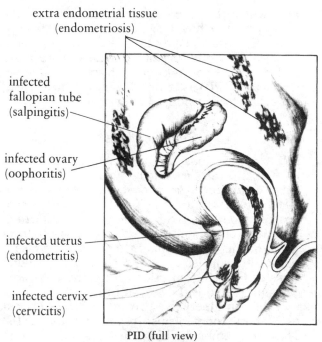

extra endometrial tissue (endometriosis)

infected fallopian tube (salpingitis)

infected ovary (oophoritis)

infected uterus (endometritis)

infected cervix (cervicitis)

PID (full view)

infected fallopian tube and ovary

normal fallopian tube and ovary

Christine Bondante

PID can cause a sharp pain at the most infected site and/or can cause pain throughout all or part of the abdomen. Christine Bondante

PID, where they are (uterus, tubes, lining of the abdomen, etc.), how long you have had it, what if any antibiotics you have taken for it and your general health, that is, how much stress you are under and how well you take care of yourself. Doctors characterize PID as acute, chronic or silent (when a woman doesn't notice her symptoms).

Complications

PID complications can be very serious. If untreated, PID can turn into *peritonitis*, a life-threatening condition, or a tuboovarian abscess. It can affect the bowels and the liver (perihepatitis syndrome). Months or years after an acute infection, infertility or ectopic pregnancy can result from tubes having been damaged or clogged by scar tissue. PID can also cause chronic pain from adhesions or lingering infection. In the most extreme cases untreated PID can result in death.

Ninety to ninety-five percent of PID is caused by the microorganisms responsible for STDs. These may enter the body during sexual contact with an infected man or woman* and also during an IUD insertion, abortion, miscarriage, childbirth, procedures involving the uterus such as endometrial biopsy, hysterosalpingogram (X-ray of the reproductive tract) or donor insemination when there has not been careful screening for all STDs. It is not uncommon for male sexual partners of women with PID to have no or few symptoms but to be carrying the organisms that can cause it, so they must be tested and treated as well and should use a condom.

My husband had no symptoms at all, although I had been suffering from chronic PID for years. Neither of us could figure out how I got sick. It took us a long time to find a doctor who cultured both of us for organisms. I finally got over it when we both started getting tested and treated according to what organisms were found: chlamydia, mycoplasma, staph, strep.

Doctors may lead women with chronic PID to believe that they are at fault for not responding to antibiotic treatment when in fact it is their sexual partners who need treatment also.

You are at higher risk for developing PID if you are exposed to infected secretions—especially infected semen—during menstruation and ovulation, when your cervix is more open and your mucus is more penetrable. Some researchers hypothesize that certain bacteria can attach themselves to moving sperm and get into the uterus and fallopian tubes. (Birth control pills seem to create dense cervical mucus that prevents sperm

from entering the uterus and so reduces the risk of developing PID.) Women using IUDs are also at higher risk during the first four months after insertion. In parts of the country gonorrhea still causes most PID. However, in other areas chlamydia, mycoplasma and a number of aerobic and anerobic microorganisms (those that need oxygen and those that don't) are being found more and more frequently in cervical, endometrial and tubal cultures taken from women with PID. These organisms may reside in the genital tract for years.

Diagnosis

It would be ideal if, when you got PID, you could know right away exactly which organisms were causing it so you could get the appropriate antibiotics. But such exactness is rarely possible because pinpointing the organisms often takes some tests that may not be readily available and may be expensive (though it may cost less to get a culture done in the first place than to go to doctor after doctor). Even when you can find a doctor and lab that culture for organisms such as chlamydia and mycoplasma, you often cannot trust a negative culture result; these organisms are difficult to culture. Sometimes the organisms infecting the uterus and fallopian tubes will not show up in a cervical culture. Although some doctors rely on blood tests, especially sedimentation rates and white blood cell count, to indicate whether or not you have an infection at all, these are not reliable for diagnosing PID. Sometimes an endometrial biopsy can be useful if hard-to-culture organisms are suspected and not found in a cervical or vaginal culture. However, such a biopsy, if not performed carefully, can further spread organisms from the cervix and vagina to the uterus. In some cases ultrasound, including vaginal ultrasound, may also be useful. A definitive diagnosis often requires laparoscopy (see p. 567).

If you have PID and a male sexual partner, he must get a test done, too. Frequently, men are diagnosed as having NGU (nongonococcal urethritis). Some of the organisms causing these infections in men (chlamydia and ureaplasma, for example) can cause PID in women. In men, the specimen can be obtained by a urethral swab or by masturbating into a sterile jar, and it must immediately be put into culture mediums (different for different organisms). The latter method may be important, because men's urethral specimens (like cervical specimens from women) may not contain the organisms living in other parts of the male reproductive or urinary systems.

At the present time, most experts seem to agree that since your health and fertility are at stake, you should not delay getting treatments while waiting for test results.

---

*The incidence of PID is very low among lesbians.

There is now growing awareness among gynecologists and urologists about the importance of prompt testing and treatment for PID. Additional research is needed to develop improved, less invasive diagnostic approaches. Some STD clinics and fertility specialists are giving accurate and up-to-date tests and treatments for PID. Call the National STD Hotline, (800) 227-8922, to find out about tests and clinics.

Treatments

PID must be treated just as STDs are; that is, both you and your partner must be treated. If you are treated alone and your partner continues to carry the microorganism(s), you will be reinfected.

When you do start on antibiotics, you cannot be accurately cultured again until you have been off them for at least a couple of weeks. Taking the wrong drugs can make organisms more difficult to get rid of. However, it is impractical to suggest that all women with PID wait until cultures are available to them to take antibiotics. The practical course is to take thorough cultures, begin treatment and then adjust the treatment according to what is found. Treatment recommendations recently have changed dramatically and include antibiotics such as cefoxitin, doxycycline and ceftriaxone. The minimum duration of therapy is ten to fourteen days because PID is a serious infection. You should receive two different kinds of antibiotics, since more than one organism is often involved. Remember to take all your antibiotic, even if your symptoms are gone. You or your doctor can contact the Centers for Disease Control in Atlanta for the most up-to-date information about effective antibiotics.

Antibiotics can cause yeast overgrowth in the vagina. Treatment may be needed to keep the yeast in check while trying to cure the much more serious PID. Try yogurt or acidophilus for yeast.

I felt like crying today as I filled my prescriptions for antibiotics for PID and suppositories for subsequent yeast. The money is one thing, the visits to the doctor another, but the frustration is the worst. I feel like I'd never have sex again if I knew I'd be cured.

According to the Centers for Disease Control, hospitalization should be strongly considered when (1) the diagnosis is uncertain, (2) surgical emergencies such as appendicitis and ectopic pregnancy must be excluded, (3) a pelvic abscess is suspected, (4) severe illness precludes outpatient management, (5) the woman is pregnant, (6) the woman is unable to follow or tolerate an outpatient regimen, (7) the woman has not responded to outpatient therapy, (8) clinic follow-up after forty-eight to seventy-two hours following the start of antibiotic treatment cannot be arranged or (9) the woman is an adolescent. Many experts recommend that *all* women with PID be hospitalized for treatment.[4] Unfortunately, many physicians do not follow these recommendations.

Most women are hospitalized for PID or possible PID when they have acute attacks. In the hospital you can get intravenous (IV) antibiotics that provide a sufficient concentration of medication in your body to fight the infection. When antibiotic treatment is not successful even then, it is probably because the antibiotics were not the correct ones for the infection and/or you were reinfected because your sexual partner was not treated successfully. IV antibiotics may also fail because of problems such as pelvic abscess, septic pelvic thrombophlebitis (an infection of the pelvic veins) or an incorrect diagnosis. Instead of cystitis accompanying or preceding PID, you may be told that you have chronic cystitis caused by trauma to the urethra during intercourse and to try intercourse in another position; instead of having a sexually transmitted infection, you may be told that you have infected yourself with organisms from your colon by wiping yourself from back to front; you may be told that you have a spastic colon or that you have an emotional, not a physical, problem.

You and your doctor may decide you should have surgery to try to restore fertility by opening closed, scarred tubes (tuboplasty). You may have *adhesions*, fibrous bands of scar tissue caused by infections. These can bind your internal organs together, causing pain and infertility. In this case, you may decide to have a laparotomy to cut them out. Remember that surgery itself can cause adhesions. Remember, also, that physicians sometimes attribute pain solely to adhesions and fail to recognize the presence of infection.

You may be urged to have a hysterectomy if the doctor thinks PID has ruined your pelvic organs beyond repair. Also, emergency hysterectomies are done in some cases of acute PID. If the infection is in your urinary tract, which it often is, then hysterectomy does not eliminate it. Some women elect to have hysterectomies in order to get over persistent, debilitating PID, but hysterectomies are rarely necessary for PID.

Personal Issues

Many of us have felt guilt and anger about our own or our partner's sexual experiences that have led to the constant physical problems and pain of PID. We are also angry at a medical system that is not prepared to deal adequately with the growing numbers of women getting STDs, more and more of whom are coming down with PID. Asymptomatic sexual partners may not want to have tests and treatments or not understand that we need to avoid intercourse with them. They may look for other people to have sex with, which may feel like punishment to us and puts us in further danger of exposure. Unfortunately, instead of expressing our anger outwardly we may just become depressed. It is also enormously frustrating to deal with a doctor who is not willing to pursue thorough diagnosis. Some doctors do not recognize that we are sexually active, and they disapprove of us for contracting what is so often a sex-related disease or doubt the severity and significance of our pelvic symptoms. Finding ourselves untrusted and judged by the medical world can add to the physical and emotional pain we suffer from PID.

It feels like a dirty trick was played on me, doctor after doctor telling me my pain was not in my pelvis but in my head. How many times did I conscientiously and politely ask about getting further tests? I am still mad and sad and bitter. It took months and a lot of pain before I found a doctor who would do what was necessary.

There are many things you can do to help heal yourself while you wait for test results to come back and antibiotics to take hold and work. Very hot baths and heat applied directly to the lower abdomen help relieve pain and bring disease-fighting blood and drugs to your pelvis. A heating pad can be your best friend at this time. Close your eyes and visualize your reproductive organs as healthy, pink, oxygenated and relaxed. Do not use tampons or douche; to do so may force microorganisms up into your uterus. Do not reuse a douche bag that may be harboring infectious organisms. Have intercourse *only* when you feel completely well through an entire monthly cycle and your partners have had negative tests for *all* STDs. Sometimes it takes months to feel better after PID. Some women have short bouts of PID months after the initial infection is cleared up, particularly if they abandon their daily health routines or are under too much stress. Acupuncture may help control pain and rebalance energy. You can soak cotton cloth in castor oil, place it on the abdomen, cover it with plastic to prevent greasiness and then cover it with a heating pad or hot water bottle to bring a maximum amount of heat to the pelvic area. Ginger root compresses and taro root poultices may relieve pain, help eliminate accumulated toxins, keep the area loose and freer from adhesions and dissolve already formed adhesions. (These are strong medicines and best used with the guidance of a holistic health practitioner.) A number of herbs and teas are useful against infection of the reproductive and urinary tracts. Raspberry leaf tea strengthens the reproductive system. Eliminate sugar and cut down on dairy products (to lessen mucus production); take plenty of vitamins C, A, D and B complex and zinc and other minerals. Eat wholesome, fresh foods; avoid stress as much as possible. Eliminate alcohol, tobacco and other drugs that lower your resistance to disease, and reduce coffee consumption. You may be unusually tired and rundown. Get plenty of sleep. Complete bed rest is recommended, but difficult to achieve. Remember, the most critical element in your healing will be the antibiotic treatment.

To prevent PID, follow these guidelines:

Prevention of PID is like prevention of STDs, because so much PID is caused by sexually transmitted organisms. Birth control foams, creams and jellies kill some bacteria that can enter the vagina during intercourse. If possible, avoid having intercourse without using a barrier method (condom, diaphragm) of birth control, especially if you have already had an STD or PID. Have your male partners use condoms and avoid using an IUD, particularly if either of you have more than one sexual partner.

Be aware that PID is an extremely serious problem that needs prompt and skilled attention.

URINARY TRACT INFECTIONS

Urinary tract infections (UTIs) are so common that most of us get at least one at some point in our lives. They are usually caused by bacteria, such as *Escherichia coli*, which travel from the colon to the urethra and bladder (and occasionally to the kidneys). Trichomoniasis and chlamydia can also cause UTIs; low resistance, poor diet, stress and damage to the urethra from childbirth, surgery, catheterization, and so on can predispose you to getting them. Often a sudden increase in sexual activity triggers symptoms ("honeymoon cystitis"). Pregnant women are especially susceptible (pressure of the growing fetus keeps some urine in the bladder and ureters, allowing bacteria to grow), as are postmenopausal women (because of hormonal changes). Very occasionally, UTI is caused by an anatomical abnormality or a prolapsed (fallen) urethra or bladder, most common in older women or women who have had many children.

Cystitis (inflammation or infection of the bladder) is by far the most common UTI in women. While the symptoms can be frightening, cystitis in itself is not usually serious. If you suddenly have to urinate every few minutes and it burns like crazy even though almost nothing comes out, you probably have cystitis. There may also be blood in the urine (hematuria) and pus in the urine (pyuria). You may have pain just above your pubic bone, and sometimes there is a peculiar, heavy urine odor when you first urinate in the morning.

It is also possible to get mild temporary symptoms (such as urinary frequency) without actually having an infection, simply because of drinking too much coffee or tea (which are diuretics), premenstrual syndrome, food allergies, anxiety or irritation to the area from bubble baths, soaps or douches. As long as you are in good health and not pregnant, you can usually treat mild symptoms yourself for twenty-four hours before consulting a practitioner.* Cystitis often disappears without treatment. If it persists more than forty-eight hours, recurs frequently or is ever accompanied by chills, fever, vomiting or pain in the kidneys, consult a practitioner. These symptoms suggest that infection has spread to the kidneys (pyelonephritis), a serious problem that requires medical treatment. Some researchers estimate that 30 to 50 percent of women with cystitis symptoms also have silent kidney infections. Consult your practitioner if cystitis symptoms are accompanied by any of the following: blood or pus in the urine, pain on urination during pregnancy, diabetes or chronic illness, a history of kidney infection or diseases or abnormalities of the urinary tract. Untreated chronic infections can lead to serious complications, such as high blood pressure or premature births (if they occur during pregnancy).

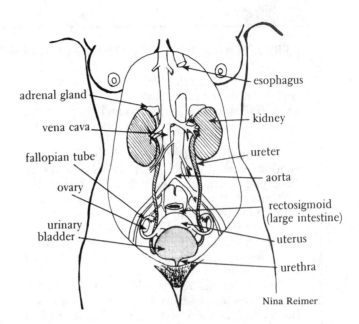

Nina Reimer

Diagnosis

When cystitis does not respond to self-help treatments within twenty-four hours or recurs frequently, get a urine test. An ordinary urinalysis is not sufficient to test for cystitis—make sure your practitioner takes a clean voided specimen† and does a pelvic exam to rule out other infections. Your urine will be examined for evidence of blood and pus and a culture will be taken. Sometimes, even when you have symptoms, the culture may come back negative (i.e., not show a cause for the infection). False-negative cultures may be due to mishandling or overly dilute urine; you may also get a false negative if your cystitis is caused by something other than bacterial infection (such as anxiety or stress). On the other hand, a negative culture accompanied by white cells in the urine (called *acute urethral syndrome*) may indicate a chlamydial infection. (See Chapter 14, "Sexually Transmitted Diseases.") Sometimes women have bacteria in their urine (bacteriuria) without symptoms. If bacteriuria shows up during a routine urine test, you should be treated to prevent kidney infection and other complications.

A sensitivity test, which shows what kind of antibiotics to use, is not always necessary unless you have had many infections or severe symptoms indicating pyelonephritis. Women who have had pyelonephritis repeatedly may be tested for abnormalities of the urinary tract. The usual test is an IVP (intravenous pyelogram) in which a dye injected into the bloodstream collects in the kidneys, showing any blockages or obstructions on an X-ray.

Treatments

For symptoms that are severe or indicate a kidney infection, medications are usually started immediately. For milder infections, many practitioners prefer to wait for culture results before prescribing a drug.

Most UTIs respond rapidly to a variety of antibiotics. Drugs commonly used include antibiotics such as ampicillin, nitrofurantoin, tetracycline or sulfonamides (Gantrisin). (Women who may be glucose-6-phosphate alhydrogenase deficient should not take sulfonamides; see Hereditary and Other Types of Anemia, p. 608.) The medication may be given in a single large dose or may be spread out over three to ten days. If symptoms persist for more than two days after you start taking drugs, see your practitioner again.

Antibiotics often cause diarrhea and vaginal yeast infections. Eating plain yogurt or taking acidophilus in capsules, liquid or granule form helps to prevent this diarrhea by replacing the normal bacteria in your intestines killed by the drugs. See pp. 604–7 for information on preventing and relieving vaginal infections.

*See the box on UTIs and *Cystitis: The Complete Self-Help Guide* by Angela Kilmartin (New York: Warner Books, 1980).
†Wash the area carefully, urinate a little, then collect the rest of your urine in a sterile jar.

PREVENTING UTIS, TREATING MILD INFECTIONS AND AVOIDING REINFECTIONS

1. Drink lots of fluid every day. Try to drink a glass of water every two or three hours. (For an active infection, drink enough to pour out a good stream of urine every hour. It really helps!)

2. Urinate frequently and try to empty your bladder completely each time. Never try to hold your urine once your bladder feels full.

3. Keep the bacteria in your bowels and anus away from your urethra by wiping yourself from front to back after urinating or having a bowel movement. Wash your genitals from front to back with plain water or very mild soap at least once a day.

4. Any sexual activity that irritates the urethra, puts pressure on the bladder or spreads bacteria from the anus to the vagina or urethra can contribute to cystitis. Make sure that you and your lover have clean hands and genitals before sex and wash after contact with the anal area before touching the vagina or urethra. To prevent irritation to the urethra, try to avoid prolonged direct clitoral stimulation and pressure on the urethral area during oral–genital sex or masturbation. Make sure your vagina is well lubricated before intercourse. Rear-entry positions and prolonged vigorous intercourse tend to put additional stress on the urethra and bladder. Emptying your bladder before and immediately after sex is a good idea. If you tend to get cystitis after sex despite these precautions, you may want to ask your practitioner for preventive tablets (i.e., sulfa, ampicillin, nitrofurantoin); a single dose of a tablet after sex has been shown effective in preventing infections and is usually not associated with the same negative effects as prolonged courses of antibiotics.

5. Some birth control methods can contribute to or aggravate a UTI. Women taking oral contraceptives have a higher rate of cystitis than those not on the Pill. Some diaphragm users find that the rim pressing against the urethra can contribute to infection. (A different-size diaphragm or one with a different type of rim may solve this problem.) Contraceptive foams or vaginal suppositories may irritate the urethra. Dry condoms may put pressure on the urethra, or the dyes or lubricants may cause irritation.

6. If you use sanitary napkins during your period, the blood on the pad provides a convenient bridge for bacteria from your anus to travel to your urethra. Change pads frequently and wash your genitals twice a day when you are menstruating. Some women also find that tampons or sponges put pressure on the urethra.

7. Tight jeans, bicycling or hoseback riding may cause trauma to the urethra. When you engage in sports that can provoke cystitis in you, wear loose clothing and try to drink extra water.

8. Caffeine and alcohol irritate the bladder. If you don't want to stop using them, try to drink less of them and drink enough water to dilute them.

9. Some women find that routine use of unsweetened cranberry juice, cranberry concentrate supplements or vitamin C to make their urine more acid helps to prevent urinary tract problems. (If you have an infection, try combining 500 milligrams of vitamin C and cranberry juice four times a day; you can substitute a half cup of fresh cranberries in plain yogurt for the juice.) Whole grains, meats, nuts and many fruits also help to acidify the urine. Avoid strong spices (curry, cayenne, chili, black pepper).

10. Diets high in refined sugars and starches (white flour, white rice, pasta, etc.) may predispose some women to urinary tract infections.

11. Women use a wide variety of herbal remedies to prevent or treat UTIs. Drinking teas made of uva ursi, horsetail or shavegrass, barberry, echinacia, cornsilk, cleavers, lemon balm or goldenseal may be beneficial to the bladder. You may want to consult a herbalist.

12. Keep up your resistance by eating and resting well and finding ways to reduce stress in your life as much as possible.

13. Vitamin B_6 and magnesium-calcium supplements help to relieve spasm of the urethra that can predispose to cystitis. This is especially helpful for women who need to have their urethras dilated repeatedly.

14. If you have an infection, soak in a hot tub two or three times a day; try a hot water bottle or heating pad on your abdomen and back.

For pain with UTIs, there is a prescription drug called Pyridium, a local anesthetic that relieves pain but does not treat the infection itself. It dyes the urine a bright orange, which will permanently stain clothing. Pyridium can cause nausea, dizziness and possibly allergic reactions. Self-help remedies are probably better.

Have a follow-up urine exam when you finish taking the drugs (a culture if you have repeated UTIs) to be certain the organism is gone.

Sometimes chronic cystitis will involve the Skene's glands (at the opening of the urethra). In such cases you may think you are cured, then the glands are squeezed (as in intercourse, for example) and release some pus, which starts the cystitis symptoms all over again. Sometimes the Skene's glands are removed (meatotomy) to solve this problem, though specialists disagree about the need for this operation. (Recovery takes about a month.)

Your practitioner may recommend other surgical procedures, such as stretching the urethral opening and/or making a slit in the urethra to help drainage (internal urethrotomy). Ask for documentation of their effectiveness. Surgery is often recommended to correct a prolapsed bladder or urethra, which can be connected with chronic UTIs. Kegel exercises (see p. 406) can avoid the need for this surgery and help prevent future infections.

Even with drugs and/or surgery, many women continue to have recurrent urinary tract infections. Sometimes it helps to treat chronic infections with long-term, low-dose medications. Better diet and reduced stress may also help avoid infections.

INTERSTITIAL CYSTITIS

Interstitial cystitis (IC) is a painful and debilitating bladder disease that affects approximately 450,000 people in the United States, 90 percent of whom are women. Formerly thought to be a postmenopausal condition, studies now indicate that IC occurs in women of all ages. The average age of onset is approximately forty years old, and 25 percent of women are under the age of thirty.

IC is an inflammatory condition of the bladder wall whose symptoms are similar to the common UTI known as cystitis. However, routine urine cultures are negative and there is usually no response to antibiotics. The symptoms of IC include pelvic pain and pressure, and the urgent need to urinate, sometimes as often as sixty to eighty times a day. There may also be associated vaginal and rectal pain. Pain during sexual intercourse is common. Symptoms may vary from mild to severe.

Because of confusion in defining and understanding IC, many patients have difficulty obtaining the correct diagnosis. IC may be incorrectly diagnosed as urethral syndrome or trigonitis, or patients may be told that there is nothing wrong and that they have a "sensitive bladder." The diagnosis of IC is usually made by a urologist. A complete battery of urologic tests is typically negative. Conditions that have symptoms resembling IC include bladder infections, kidney problems, vaginal infections, endometriosis and STDs. If no infection is present (i.e., urine cultures are negative), and no other disorder is identified, a cystoscopy should be performed, during which a cystoscope, which allows the urologist to look directly inside the bladder, is inserted into the urethra. This must be done under regional or general anesthesia so that the bladder may be distended enough to see the pinpoint hemorrhages characteristic of IC. A biopsy is taken at this time to rule out bladder cancer.

There is no consistently effective treatment or cure for IC. However, treatments are available that may temporarily alleviate symptoms. The most commonly used treatments include the following:

1. Bladder distention, in which the bladder is stretched by filling it with water while the patient is under regional or general anesthesia.

2. Oral nonsteroidal anti-inflammatory medication, antispasmodics and antihistamines.

3. Antidepressants, such as amitriptyline (Elavil), appear to have antipain properties.

4. Elimination of caffeinated beverages, alcohol, artificial sweeteners, spicy foods, citrus fruits and tomatoes may alleviate symptoms.

5. Dimethyl sulfoxide (DMSO, Rimso 50), a medication instilled directly into the bladder that acts as an anti-inflammatory agent.

6. Sodium pentosanpolysulfate (Elmiron), an oral medication believed to coat the bladder wall and protect it from irritants in the urine (FDA approval is anticipated in 1992).

7. Nalmefene, an oral medication currently undergoing FDA-supervised clinical trials.

8. Oxychlorosene sodium (Clorpactin), when placed directly into the bladder appears to decrease symptoms. Administration of regional or general anesthesia may be necessary for its instillation.

9. Transcutaneous electrical nerve stimulation (tens unit), a small portable unit worn on the body that is thought to block pain through low electrical nerve stimulation.

10. Surgery (partial or complete removal of the bladder). These surgical procedures pose a substantial risk of complications and should be performed only as a last resort when all other conservative treatments fail.

The Interstitial Cystitis Association (ICA) (see

Resources), a patient advocacy group, provides information, education and support to IC patients and their families. The organization is dedicated to raising funds for research and educating the public as well as the medical community about the disease.

UTERUS AND OVARIES

Abnormal Uterine Bleeding

Abnormal uterine bleeding is a term used to describe a variety of unusual bleeding patterns. You may have unusually light or very heavy periods, bleeding or spotting between periods, cycles that vary widely in length. Abnormal bleeding is frequently due to hormonal changes and is most common in teenagers just beginning to menstruate or women just entering menopause. Many women in their thirties experience light spotting at the time of ovulation, due to the sudden drop in estrogen. Doctors use a particular term, *dysfunctional uterine bleeding*, to describe abnormal bleeding due to a menstrual cycle in which ovulation did not occur—an anovulatory cycle. Women who don't ovulate regularly may have late periods and very heavy bleeding due to a buildup of estrogen. Other possible causes of prolonged, heavy or irregular bleeding include the IUD, birth control pills, PID, ectopic pregnancy, polyps, fibroids, endometriosis and cervical or uterine cancer. (See the sections on each of these conditions for information on their treatments.)

In postmenopausal women, abnormal bleeding may be caused by estrogen replacement therapy, vaginitis or overgrowth of the endometrial tissues (endometrial hyperplasia), or cancer.

Sometimes, even after extensive testing, no clear-cut reason for bleeding is found.

Self-Help Treatments

If you are premenopausal, you may be able to stabilize your menstrual flow by reducing stress and changing your diet. Cutting down on animal fat and adding fiber helps to restore normal hormonal balance by lowering cholesterol (which is converted to estrogen in your body). In addition, supplements of vitamins A, E and C with bioflavinoids, as well as zinc, copper and iodine, can help regulate heavy bleeding. Consult a holistic nutritionist, if available, to advise you on dosage. Acupuncture can also help to restore hormonal balance. If you are bleeding heavily, increase your iron intake to prevent anemia (see p. 608).

Medical Treatments

If you are premenopausal and having light, irregular bleeding, your practitioner may suggest waiting a month or two to see if your system rights itself. (Sometimes stress can contribute to hormonal imbalances.) If abnormal bleeding persists, particularly in women over forty, an endometrial biopsy or D and C should be done to check for endometrial hyperplasia or endometrial cancer. (Finding cancer is very unusual except in women over fifty.) If there is no precancerous or cancerous condition, a woman may choose not to have further therapy. If the bleeding is bothersome, hormonal therapy (with progesterone and/or estrogen) may correct the problem. If you want to avoid taking hormones and the bleeding isn't too heavy, you may want to continue self-help measures while observing the amount of bleeding carefully. If you are anovulatory and wish to become pregnant, you may consider taking a fertility drug that stimulates ovulation. Be sure you are informed of the risks associated with such fertility drugs.

Pelvic Relaxation and Uterine Prolapse

Pelvic relaxation is a condition in which the muscles of the pelvic floor become slack and no longer adequately support the pelvic organs. In severe cases, the ligaments and tissues that hold the uterus in place may also weaken enough to allow the uterus to "fall" or "prolapse" into the vagina. Women sometimes experience pelvic relaxation and/or uterine prolapse after one or more very difficult births, but the tendency can also be inherited. Uterine prolapse is often accompanied by a falling of the bladder (cystocele) and rectum (rectocele) as well.

Often the first sign of pelvic relaxation is a tendency to leak urine when you cough or sneeze or laugh suddenly. If your uterus has fallen into your vagina you may have a dull, heavy sensation in your vagina or feel like something is "falling out."

Prolapsed uterus.   Christine Bondante

These symptoms are usually worse after standing for long periods.

Prevention and Self-Help Treatments

The best way to prevent pelvic relaxation and uterine prolapse is to do regular Kegel exercises and leg lifts, which strengthen the muscles of the pelvic floor and lower abdomen (see Chapter 20, "Childbirth"). One way of determining whether your pelvic muscles are in good shape is to try starting and stopping the flow of urine when you go to the bathroom. If you can't stop the flow, you need to do more Kegels. Some practitioners recommend doing up to a hundred a day, especially during pregnancy when the pelvic muscles are under particular stress. You may also strengthen a slightly prolapsed uterus by relaxing in the knee–chest position (kneeling with your chest on the floor and your bottom in the air) several times a day. Some women find that certain yoga positions, such as the shoulder and head stands, relieve discomfort from a prolapsed uterus.

Medical Treatments

Medical intervention is usually not necessary for pelvic relaxation or even mild uterine prolapse. If the prolapse is severe enough to cause discomfort, you can have a pessary (a rubber device that fits around the cervix and helps to prop up the uterus) inserted. The disadvantages include difficulty in obtaining a proper fit, possible irritation or infection and the need to remove and clean the pessary frequently. A surgical procedure called a *suspension operation* can lift and reattach a descended uterus and often a fallen bladder or rectum as well. Many physicians recommend hysterectomy for prolapsed uterus, but it is frequently unnecessary and should be done only as a last resort.

Uterine Fibroids (Lieomyomas, Myomas)

Fibroids are solid benign tumors* that appear on the outside, inside or within the wall of the uterus, often changing the size and shape of it. About 30 percent of all women will develop fibroids by the time they are thirty-five, and they are more likely to affect black women. Although they are of unknown cause, these growths seem to be related to estrogen production: If you are pregnant or taking oral contraceptives or menopausal estrogens (all of which raise estrogen levels in the body), fibroids are apt to grow more quickly.

---

*The word *tumor* is very scary to most of us. It is part of an older language of illness that was used by many of our grandparents, both patients and doctors, to disguise the mention of cancer. Actually, tumors are growths of cells that serve no purpose. Over 90 percent of all tumors are benign and harmless.

Fibroids (benign growths).　　　Karen Norberg

uterine wall

Fibroids may be discovered during a routine pelvic exam. Because fibroids keep growing, ask your practitioner how many you have and how big they are. If they have grown no further when you have a second exam six months later, a yearly checkup will be sufficient.

Small fibroids are usually symptom-free. However, very large or numerous fibroids may cause pain, bleeding between periods or excessive menstrual flow. (Because they usually do not cause abnormal bleeding, if you do have fibroids and abnormal bleeding, be sure to be carefully checked for other causes.) Depending on their size and location, fibroids can also cause abdominal or back pain and urinary problems. Large fibroids rarely make it difficult to conceive or to sustain a full-term pregnancy.

Self-Help Treatments

You may be able to reduce large fibroids by eliminating your intake of synthetic estrogen (found in birth control pills) and stopping estrogen therapy (ERT). Yoga exercises may ease feelings of heaviness and pressure. If your fibroids cause heavy bleeding, see the nutritional therapy section in Abnormal Uterine Bleeding (see p. 596). Visualization techniques may be helpful in dealing with fibroids. Some women try to prevent fibroids by avoiding the hormones usually found in commercial meat, dairy and egg products.

Medical Treatments

In many cases no treatment is necessary, but if you have excessive bleeding, pain, urinary difficulties or problems with pregnancy, you may want to have the fibroids removed. *Very* occasionally this can be done during a D and C, but usually a *myomectomy*, which removes fibroids and leaves the uterus intact, is necessary.* In approximately 10 percent of cases, the fibroids will return.

Many physicians recommend hysterectomy as a treatment for fibroids in women who are past

---

*A new technique, called *hysteroscopic resection*, in which the fibroid is shaved off may also be done for smaller fibroids inside the uterine cavity.

childbearing age or who do not want more children. This surgery may be unnecessary, particularly for women nearing menopause, when the natural decline in estrogen levels usually shrinks fibroids. Moreover, hysterectomy can have serious consequences for women, including sexual dysfunction and ovarian failure (even when the ovaries are preserved). Myomectomy—done by a surgeon skilled in this procedure—poses no greater risks than hysterectomy and avoids some of the problems associated with hysterectomy. Even large fibroids can be removed with a myomectomy.

For women near menopause, sometimes the drug Lupron is recommended to help shrink fibroids. (Lupron induces an artificial menopause, suppressing the production of estrogen, which promotes fibroid growth.) However, Lupron is generally not used for longer than six months. Fibroids will grow back after Lupron is discontinued unless the natural onset of menopause continues this lowered estrogen state.

Ovarian Cysts

Ovarian cysts are relatively common and often don't cause any symptoms or discomfort. Most ovarian cysts are functional (physiological) and will resolve on their own. A cyst usually develops when a follicle has grown large—as one or more do every month during ovulation—but has failed to rupture and release an egg. Most of these cysts are filled with fluid. Cysts may be accompanied by symptoms such as a disturbance in the normal menstrual cycle, an unfamiliar pain or discomfort in your lower abdomen at any point during the cycle, pain during intercourse and unexplained abdominal swelling. Found by a routine bimanual pelvic exam, cysts usually disappear by themselves, though some types may have to be removed.

To determine whether a cyst requires treatment, wait a cycle or two for it to disappear. If it persists, a practitioner may use ultrasound to see if it is likely to be a pathological cyst, such as a dermoid cyst, a cyst of endometriosis or cancer. Such pathological cysts should be removed. Practitioners disagree about the necessity of removing benign cysts, but small functional cysts do not usually cause problems and may be left alone.

If your physician advises removal of the ovary along with the benign cyst, get a second opinion. This conventional practice is, in many cases, unnecessary. Ovaries perform many functions, even after menopause.

Recurrent cysts may indicate a hormonal imbalance or life stresses. Changing your diet, learning how to reduce stress and acupuncture may also help to get your system back in balance.

HYSTERECTOMY AND OOPHORECTOMY

Each year about 650,000 women in this country have a hysterectomy (removal of the uterus). Sometimes it is done along with an oophorectomy (removal of the ovaries), when in fact it is often not necessary.* Today, the vast majority of hysterectomies and oophorectomies are elective— that is, performed by choice and not as an emergency or lifesaving procedure.† Several careful studies have shown that at least 30 to 50 percent of these operations are clearly unnecessary and another 10 percent or more can probably be avoided by using alternative therapy (see p. 599, When Is Hysterectomy Necessary? and p. 603 on indications for oophorectomy.[5] The incidence of this surgery rose by 25 percent between 1971 and 1975, dropping off at the 1971 level by 1980. But the rise was fastest for younger women: Between 1970 and 1978, 3.5 million women under forty-five had hysterectomies. In 1990 the hysterectomy rate had fallen about 20 percent since the mid-1970s, but one in three women can still expect to have a hysterectomy by the age of sixty. Every woman faces the possibility that hysterectomy and/or oophorectomy will be recommended.

Both procedures are considered major surgery; we are only beginning to understand their long-term effects on our health, sexuality and life expectancy. Certainly, they have saved lives and restored health for many women. But they also involve significant risks—both immediate and long-term—that we need to be aware of. Because of the controversy over hysterectomy and oophorectomy rates, many insurance plans now require a second opinion from another physician before agreeing to pay for the procedures.

Why are so many women having so many hysterectomies and oophorectomies? More are being done for conditions that would not have "required" surgery ten years ago. Too often surgeons recommend them (and women agree to them) as an easy solution to routine gynecological problems,

---

*Some women do not know whether they have had their ovaries removed. Others agreed to the removal without realizing that it is an *elective* procedure or without realizing the disadvantages. If you are uncertain about the extent of your surgery, obtain a copy of your medical record from the hospital. Also *write* to your surgeon (keeping a copy of your letter) and ask for a reply in writing.
†The elective nature of many hysterectomies is highlighted by the fact that different groups of women have different rates of hysterectomy. The U.S. has twice the rate of England and Sweden. Doctors' wives, for example, have more hysterectomies proportionally than any other group. Traditionally, women of color have had twice as many hysterectomies as white women (often a form of sterilization abuse, also a problem for poor white women [see p. 301]); recently the rate for young white women has risen sharply. The highest rate of hysterectomies is found in the South and West, where gynecologist-surgeons tend to cluster in large numbers.

simply a way of preventing cancer and a permanent method of birth control. Some gynecologists still recommend the procedure for sterilization ("hysterilization").

Physicians frequently attribute the sudden spurt of pelvic surgery to the apparent increase in endometriosis, uterine bleeding, pelvic infections and endometrial cancer. (Ironically, the increased use of estrogen replacement therapy [ERT] may have partially caused the increased rate of endometrial cancer—and also unmanageable fibroids that indicate hysterectomy.) The surgery increase may also be connected with the increased availability of health care via more health insurance and more federal monies going into the medical system. In some cases, poorer women are now more able to get needed (or needless) surgery.

Ob/gyns and surgeons have powerful economic incentives to perform hysterectomies and oophorectomies. They are more profitable than less complicated, often less dangerous procedures and provide a source of income to compensate for the declining birth rate and resulting loss of obstet-rical fees. Surgeons' fees and hospital fees for the procedures are expensive—the average cost of a hysterectomy varies from $3,000 to $6,000 (approximately five times the cost of a tubal ligation). Health care analysts believe it is no accident that hysterectomies occur far less frequently under prepaid insurance plans (such as HMOs) than under indemnity plans such as Blue Shield. Most hysterectomies and oophorectomies are performed as part of a private practice, where the surgeon and woman alone make decisions, often consulting no other physician.* Why are women willing to risk their lives in surgery? What factors should they consider?

Risks and Complications of Hysterectomy and Oophorectomy

Surgeons recommending hysterectomy seldom tell us that the rate of death from hysterectomy is

*See Diana Scully's study of ob/gyn training, *Men Who Control Women's Health: The Mis-Education of Obstetrician-Gynecologists*, (Boston: Houghton-Mifflin, 1980) for an important analysis of how these decisions are made.

WHEN IS HYSTERECTOMY NECESSARY?

A number of life-threatening conditions require hysterectomy, including

1. Invasive cancer of the uterus, cervix, vagina, fallopian tubes and/or ovaries (8 to 12 percent of hysterectomies are performed to treat cancer).

2. Severe, uncontrollable infection (PID).

3. Severe, uncontrollable bleeding.

4. Life-threatening blockage of the bladder or intestines by the uterus or growth in the uterus.

5. Conditions associated with rare but serious complications during childbirth, including rupture of the uterus.

If you have any of these conditions, hysterectomy may not only save your life but free you from significant pain and discomfort.

Some conditions that are not life-threatening but may justify hysterectomy include

1. Precancerous changes of the endometrium (hyperplasia).

2. Severe, recurring pelvic infections (see the sections on STDs and IUDs in Chapter 13, "Birth Control").

3. Extensive endometriosis, causing debilitating pain and/or involving other organs.

4. Fibroid tumors that are extensive, large, involve other organs or cause debilitating bleeding.

5. Pelvic relaxation (uterine prolapse).

Depending on their severity, many of these conditions can be treated without resorting to major surgery.* Fortunately, new diagnostic techniques, such as sonography, Pap smears and laparoscopy, make it possible to avoid or delay many hysterectomies that might have been done in the past. Unfortunately, most surgeons do not make frequent enough use of such techniques, believing that there is no advantage to saving a uterus, especially if a woman is past her childbearing years.

Hysterectomies are frequently performed unnecessarily for the following reasons:

1. Small fibroids that are not causing problems.

2. Abortion (during the first and second trimesters).

3. Sterilization.

4. Cervicitis.

5. Mild dysfunctional uterine bleeding.

6. Pelvic congestion (menstrual irregularities and low back pain).

These problems can usually be treated with cheaper and safer alternative therapies. If your doctor insists on hysterectomy for one of these, consider changing physicians.

*See individual sections for alternative treatment, also N. Lauersen and Eileen Stulcane's *Listen to Your Body: A Gynecologist Answers Women's Most Intimate Questions* (New York: Berkley, 1983).

fairly high, between 1 and 2 women in 1,000;* that as a sterilization method, hysterectomy has ten to twenty times the complication rate of tubal ligation with its contraceptive failure rate of 1 to 2.2 percent. Women unknowingly play an enormous gambling game, assuming that we will not suffer from complications of anesthesia or surgery or from serious aftereffects.

Forty to fifty percent of all women who have hysterectomies have surgical complications, including

1. *Infection.* Most can be treated successfully with antibiotics, but some infections can be severe or even uncontrollable and may result in death. Many surgeons now order antibiotics routinely before surgery.

2. *Urinary tract complications.* Almost half of the women who have hysterectomies will have a kidney or bladder infection following surgery. In most cases the problem is not serious, but sometimes additional surgery is necessary. In radical hysterectomy, sensory nerves may be cut (sometimes unnecessarily) and women can lose both the sensation of having to urinate and control over bladder functions.†

3. *Hemorrhage.* More than one in ten women require transfusions, some due to undetected preexisting anemia.

Less common surgical complications include

1. *Bowel problems.* These can occur if there is damage to the intestines during surgery. Two percent of all women who have a hysterectomy need further surgery to remove scar tissue from the bowel.

2. *Blood clots.* Clots are rare but always dangerous because of the possibility of the clot traveling to the lungs or brain, which can be fatal.

3. *Death or paralysis from anesthesia.*

4. *Postsurgical complications.* These can include abnormal bleeding, postsurgical infection, improper healing that can cause narrowing of the vagina, and heavy discharge.

Long-Term Risks

Current evidence suggests that for women who are premenopausal, removal of the uterus *with or without* removal of the ovaries approximately doubles the risk of heart attack.[6] However, use of replacement estrogen appears to reduce this risk.

Even if your ovaries are *not* removed, there is a slight chance of sudden or premature menopause.‡ Most physicians assure us that we can

---

*This works out to between 600 and 1,200 women annually, some of whose hysterectomies were unnecessary.

†Injury to the ureters or urinary tract occurs in 2 to 5 percent of every 1,000 cases.

‡This is usually due to the decreased supply of blood to the ovaries, which causes them to lose their ability to produce hormones—either immediately or over a period of time.

I hope you can justify this hysterectomy to my women's health group.

avoid these risks and symptoms by taking ERT, which has its own risks. (See the sections on ERT, p. 528, and menopause, p. 524.)

Hormonal responses vary from one woman to the next, for reasons not yet established. Some women suffer severe hot flashes and lack of lubrication. Others are more fortunate.

After my hysterectomy-oophorectomy, I went home with my prescription for estrogen to await the worst. I started to read a lot about ERT being harmful to women. The reasons for not taking ERT seemed to be a lot stronger than my fears of menopause, so I quit the program cold turkey. Lubrication was a problem at first after discontinuing the estrogen. We kept the tube of K-Y Jelly on the night table. My own glands took over and lubrication is rarely a problem now.

Some women continue on ERT while still others may wish to follow the more gradual reduction suggested by Susanne Morgan (see Resources; see also Vaginal Changes, p. 534).

Hysterectomy, Oophorectomy and Sexuality

Many women are concerned about the effect that hysterectomy with or without oophorectomy will have on sexual response. Physicians and popular literature tend to be blandly reassuring and state that any sexual difficulties we may experience are "all in our heads." Only recently has the physiological basis of women's sexuality begun to be understood. In fact, from 33 to 46 percent of women have difficulty becoming aroused and reaching orgasm after this surgery.[7] Moreover, we now know why these changes occur.

First, many women experience orgasm primarily when the penis or a lover's fingers push against the cervix and uterus, causing uterine contractions and increased stimulation of the abdominal lining (peritoneum). Without the uterus or cervix, there may be much less of this kind of sensation.

Second, if the ovaries are removed, ovarian *androgens*, which affect sexuality, may be greatly reduced, thus lowering sexual response. *These hormones cannot be replaced by ERT* (for replacement options, see below). Even when the ovaries are not removed, this hormonal change may occur because the surgery may interfere with the blood supply.

I had a hysterectomy two years ago at the age of forty-five. I went from being fully aroused and fully orgasmic to having a complete loss of libido, sexual enjoyment and orgasms immediately after the surgery. I went to doctors, all of whom denied ever having seen a woman with this problem before and told me it was psychological. Before surgery my husband and I were having intercourse approximately three to five times a week, simply because we have an open and loving relationship. Now I find that I have to work at becoming at all interested in intercourse. And I no longer have the orgasm that comes from pressure on the cervix, although I still have a feeble orgasm from clitoral stimulation.

Third, vaginal lubrication tends to lessen after oophorectomy.

Fourth, local effects of surgery may occasionally cause problems. If your vagina has been shortened (see the section on vaginal hysterectomy, p. 602), intercourse may be uncomfortable. Scar tissue in the pelvis or at the top of the vagina from either the vaginal or abdominal procedure can also cause painful intercourse.

Some of us will find sex unchanged or more enjoyable after hysterectomy. In the words of a woman who had a hysterectomy because of huge fibroids:

I had terrible cramps all my life and genuine feelings of utter depression during my periods. My ovaries were not removed and my libido was not affected. My sexual response, if anything, improved. I also had for the first time no fear of unwanted pregnancy and more general good health.

Sex may be better when the operation helps to relieve a painful condition such as infection, endometriosis or heavy bleeding.

Many women do experience genuine loss of sexual desire or response or both, so you must weigh the benefits of surgery against the sexual risk that is *not* "all in the head" and cannot necessarily be predicted in advance.

One self-help group (at the Elizabeth Blackwell Women's Health Center in Philadelphia) exchanged information about what increased their desire and ability to orgasm during intercourse with a male partner. Their suggestions included:

- More strong and deliberate "turning on" by themselves or their partner, through humanely erotic (not pornographic) reading, pictures, films; verbal lovemaking; massage; sexy clothing; candlelight; change of location, partners or techniques; dancing; (play) wrestling and activities that physically move the pelvic area.
- More effort in intercourse to push the penis hard against the far end of the vagina in order to stimulate the peritoneum. Deep penetration is helped by the female-astride position or the man-on-top position with the woman's legs on the man's shoulders and pillows under her hips.
- Use of coconut oil or K-Y Jelly to lubricate the clitoris and vagina.
- More experimentation with oral sex or delicate manipulation of the clitoris.
- Learning to use penetration with fingers first (gentle internal stimulation to prepare for intercourse with a penis); this helps lubrication occur more rapidly.
- Relearning a new pace for lovemaking, moving more slowly, respecting the fact that arousal may take longer.
- Trying the testosterone pellet (see below) to restore the ability to become aroused.

Androgen replacement therapy is at least partially effective in restoring sexual response. When testosterone (one of the androgens) is administered orally or through injection in a dosage sufficient to restore libido, masculinizing effects may occur, such as lowered voice, acne and facial hair. However, another way of administering testosterone, with greatly lowered side effects, is through a small slow-release pellet inserted under the skin in the hip region by a simple office procedure every six months.[8] This procedure is quite readily available to British women, but American women have difficulty finding a physician familiar with it. One woman who has received this kind of therapy says:

In the last week we've made love oftener than in the past two months. It's a great feeling! We've giggled and rolled on the floor like a couple of kids. Previously, I'd shied away from any physical contact that would end up in bed. My body is much more sensitive, though I don't have the same deep internal orgasms as before. Sometimes I think if I'd had the help of hormones a few years ago, I'd never have appreciated the feelings I have now. I know there will still be times when I am depressed and longing for the deep orgasms I once had, but I'll be able to remember the three years when I had no feelings at all and it won't seem bad.

We have our doubts regarding *any* hormone therapy. Keep looking for new information about them.

Even if you were prepared for hysterectomy and

HYSTERECTOMY PROCEDURES

These are the common procedures for hysterectomy. Rather than simply accepting the *name* of the procedure your surgeon proposes, ask for a complete description with a diagram.

· *Total hysterectomy,* sometimes called *complete hysterectomy.* The surgeon removes the uterus and cervix, leaving the fallopian tubes and ovaries. You will continue to ovulate but will no longer have menstrual periods; instead the egg is absorbed by the body into the pelvic cavity.

· *Total hysterectomy with bilateral salpingo-oophorectomy.* The surgeon removes the uterus, cervix, fallopian tubes (*salpingo*) and both ovaries (*oophor*).* *Bilateral* means both sides, though sometimes one ovary may be left if it is not diseased. In rare cases (usually to treat widespread cancer), the surgeon will remove the upper part of the vagina and perhaps lymph nodes in the pelvic area. This is sometimes called *radical hysterectomy.*

Abdominal Versus Vaginal Hysterectomy

Removal of your uterus can be done either through an abdominal incision or through the vagina. The surgeon will have to recommend an abdominal incision if your ovaries are to be removed, if there is a large tumor in your uterus or if you have chronic pelvic disease. (Surgeons usually prefer an abdominal approach because it enables them to see the pelvic cavity more completely. However, in an abdominal hysterectomy they are more likely to remove healthy ovaries because they are more accessible.) The incision is made either horizontally across the top pubic hairline (called a "bikini" incision) or vertically between the navel and pubic hairline. Vertical incisions (across the grain of the muscle) tend to heal more slowly. Discuss with your doctor whether you can avoid one.

Vaginal hysterectomy, useful in cases of prolapsed uterus (when the uterus bulges into the vagina; see p. 596) and for a number of other conditions, has the advantage of a shorter recovery period and faster healing. In addition, because the incision is made inside the vagina, you will have no visible scar. However, since vaginal hysterectomies are performed less frequently and require greater skill, it is important to find a surgeon who does this procedure regularly. Mistakes during surgery can result in permanent urinary tract difficulties. Other disadvantages include a possible shortening of the vagina, which can result in painful intercourse afterward, and possible temporary severe back pain as a result of being placed in a lithotomy position (head down, bottom up) during surgery.

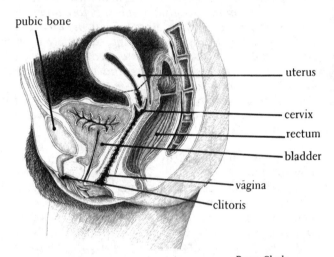

Peggy Clark

A partial hysterectomy. The uterus is tipped to show line of surgical incision; the ovary is hidden. After surgery the cervix and the stump of the uterus remain, requiring regular Pap tests.

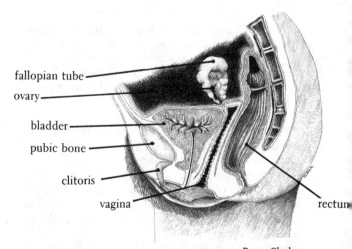

Peggy Clark

A complete hysterectomy. The uterus is removed, including the cervix (ovaries and tubes are attached to top of vagina).

---

*Very occasionally a physician will leave the cervix, but because this procedure carries the risk of infection or cancer in the cervix, it is considered largely outmoded.

A large, well-researched study by the Centers for Disease Control suggests that the 50 percent complication rate of abdominal hysterectomy may be anywhere from two to four times higher than that of vaginal hysterectomy. The exception: Women who have had previous cesareans have a nearly 65 percent complication rate after vaginal hysterectomy.

Oophorectomy: Reasons and Risks

Oophorectomy means removal of the ovary—either one (unilateral) or both (bilateral); the fallopian tube(s) may be removed as well. When both ovaries are removed, a hysterectomy is usually performed at the same time. Common reasons for oophorectomy include ectopic pregnancy, endometriosis, benign or malignant tumors or cysts on the ovary and PID.* An enlarged postmenopausal ovary may be cancerous and urgently requires a checkup.

If only one ovary is removed and not your uterus, you will continue to be fertile and have menstrual periods. If both ovaries are removed, however, you will experience surgical menopause. Even if one or both ovaries are retained, you may experience symptoms of hormonal loss because of loss of blood supply to the ovaries.

Many surgeons routinely remove the ovaries of women during hysterectomy, whether or not the ovaries are diseased,† if the woman is past forty-five or so. For decades, this practice had been one of the most controversial in gynecology. Those in favor argue that oophorectomy prevents the possibility of future ovarian cancer, which strikes 1 in 100 women over forty and has a cure rate of only 10 to 20 percent. On the other side, studies show that the actual risk of developing ovarian cancer following hysterectomy is very small (about 1 in 1,000). Other physicians think the cancer risk is insignificant compared to the risks involved in losing ovarian function: circulatory disease, premature osteoporosis and sudden menopause, all of which raise the difficult question of ERT (see the sections on ERT, p. 528, and menopause, p. 524).

Oophorectomy affects the hormonal balance of both postmenopausal and premenopausal women, since the ovaries usually continue to produce significant amounts of hormones after menopause (see p. 599, Risks and Complications of Hysterectomy and Oophorectomy).

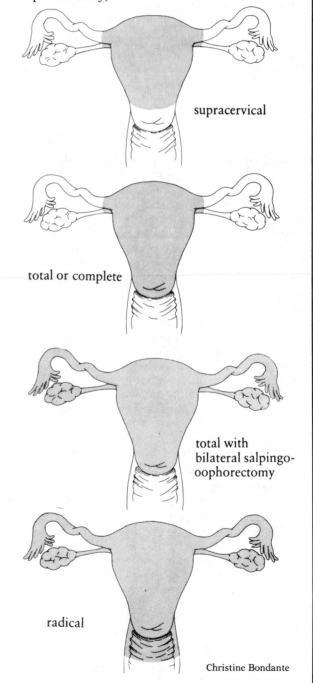

supracervical

total or complete

total with
bilateral salpingo-oophorectomy

radical

Christine Bondante

---

*Rarely, ovaries were removed in cases of cancer of the uterus, breast, cervix or abdominal cavity because ovarian secretions are known to increase the chances of developing recurrent cancer in these areas. This strategy is now outmoded and has been replaced by chemotherapy (see the section on cancer, p. 613).

†The terms *diseased* and *healthy* are frequently used carelessly by surgeons when referring to ovaries. Given the rarity of ovarian cancer, ask carefully in advance whether an ovary with a cyst or mild fibrous involvement would be removed as "diseased."

did not expect to feel depressed, you may cry frequently and unexpectedly in the first few days or weeks after surgery. This may be due to sudden hormonal changes. Many women are upset. Losing any part of ourselves, especially a part that is so uniquely feminine, is bound to have an impact. You may feel robbed. If you are premenopausal, you may bitterly resent the fact that you cannot have children. Acknowledging feelings of anger and grief after losing a part of yourself or losing some of your sexual responsiveness is an important part of the recovery process.

Thousands of women like me must confront the depression that comes with the loss of their sex lives and the anger they feel when they finally find out that this loss was a side effect of surgery that may have been unnecessary to begin with.

We or our caregivers may or may not recognize posthysterectomy depression promptly. Many gynecologists recommend psychiatric help and prescribe tranquilizers (or other habit-forming drugs) but almost never encourage treatment of underlying physical or sexual conditions caused by the surgery.* Tranquilizers taken together with estrogen therapy may produce negative effects, yet many physicians routinely prescribe both.

If you are depressed, try to find a women's support group where you can talk about your feelings in a supportive atmosphere. If you can't find a group through a local women's health center, consider starting a postsurgery group of your own. (For information on support groups you can contact, see Resources.)

Some women feel only relief following hysterectomy or hysterectomy/oophorectomy, especially when the operation eliminates a serious health problem or chronic, disabling pain.†

Self-Help—Recovering from a Hysterectomy or Oophorectomy

After a hysterectomy you may be in the hospital for five to seven days, depending on the kind of procedure and the amount of anesthesia you had. For the first day or two you will probably have an IV and a catheter inserted. You will usually be given medication for pain and nausea. Within a day you will be on your feet and encouraged to do exercises to get your circulation and breathing

back to normal. You may also be told to cough frequently (to clear your lungs). (Holding a pillow over an abdominal incision or crossing your legs if you had a vaginal incision will help to reduce pain.) When your bowels become active again (usually on the second day), you may also have gas pains to contend with. Walking, holding on to a pillow and rolling from side to side in bed and slow deep-breathing exercises will help. By the third or fourth day you can begin to have light solid foods as well as fluids.

After you go home, you will have light vaginal bleeding or oozing that gradually tapers off. You may also have hot flashes caused by estrogen loss. (Even if your ovaries were not removed, estrogen may be lost due to the disruption of blood flow to the ovaries during surgery.) You will probably continue to have some pain as well that pain-killers may not relieve entirely. Consult your practitioner if you have excessive pain accompanied by fever or discharge, as this may signal an infection.

Try to arrange for someone to take care of you for the first few days. For at least the first few weeks, ask family and friends for help with household chores and children.

Your practitioner may tell you to avoid tub baths, douches, driving, climbing or lifting heavy things for several weeks. If you have to drive or have small children at home who need to be carried, ask for suggestions as to how to do these tasks safely. Most practitioners also recommend waiting six to eight weeks before resuming intercourse and/or active sports. Some women return to these activities much earlier. Start with light exercise (such as walking) and gradually build up to your old routines. Visualizing yourself as healthy and active can speed the recovery process. Full recovery generally takes four to six weeks, but some women feel tired for as long as six months or even a year after surgery.

VAGINA AND VULVA

Vaginal Infections (Vaginitis)

All women secrete moisture and mucus from membranes that line the vagina. This discharge is clear or slightly milky and may be somewhat slippery or clumpy. When dry, it may be yellowish. When a woman is sexually aroused, under stress or at midcycle this secretion increases. It normally causes no irritation or inflammation of the vagina or vulva. If you want to examine your own discharge, collect a sample from inside your vagina—with a washed finger, of course—and smear it on glass.

Many bacteria grow in the vagina of a normal, healthy woman. Some of them help to keep the

*Despite publication of the 1981 study of Zussman et al. (see note 7), many surgeons continue to believe that all posthysterectomy problems are psychological/emotional in origin. Medical school texts and courses remain similarly unaffected.
†For information on recovering after these operations, see Susanne Morgan's book *Coping with Hysterectomy* (particularly the chapter entitled "After Surgery").

vagina somewhat acid, which keeps yeast, fungi and other harmful organisms from multiplying out of proportion. These harmful organisms may secrete wastes that, in large amounts, irritate the vaginal walls and cause infections. At such times there may be an abnormal discharge, mild or severe itching and burning of the vulva, chafing of the thighs and, occasionally, frequent urination.

Some of the reasons for vaginal infections are a general lowered resistance (from stress, lack of sleep, bad diet, other infections in our bodies); too much douching; pregnancy; taking birth control pills, other hormones or antibiotics; diabetes or a prediabetic condition; cuts, abrasions and other irritations in the vagina (from childbirth, intercourse without enough lubrication, tampons or using an instrument in the vagina medically or for masturbation). Postmenopausal women are particularly susceptible. We can also get many of these infections during sex with a partner who has them (see Chapter 14, ''Sexually Transmitted Diseases'').

Prevention

1. Gently wash your vulva and anus regularly. Pure, unscented mineral oil is a good cleanser and does not dry out the tissues as soap tends to. Pat your vulva dry after bathing and try to keep it dry. Also, don't use other people's towels or washcloths. Avoid irritating sprays* and soaps (use special nonsoap cleansers for skin very sensitive to plain soap). Avoid talcum powder.†

2. Wear clean, white, all-cotton underpants. Avoid nylon underwear and pantyhose since they retain moisture and heat, which help harmful bacteria to grow faster. Launder all underwear in hot, soapy water. Be sure to rinse thoroughly.

3. Avoid pants that are tight in the crotch and thighs.

4. Always wipe your genital and anal area from front to back (so that bacteria from the anus won't get into the vagina or urethra).

5. Make sure your sexual partners are clean. It is a good practice for a man to wash his penis daily and especially before making love. Using a condom can provide added protection. If you or your male partner is being treated for a genital infection, make sure he wears a condom during intercourse. Better yet, avoid intercourse until the infection is cleared up.

6. Use a sterile, water-soluble jelly if lubrication is needed during intercourse (something like K-Y Jelly, for example, *not* Vaseline). Also, recent studies show that birth control jellies slow down the growth of trichomonads and possibly monilia. Using these jellies for lubrication and/or general prevention is a good idea, especially with a new partner you may not know very well. Most lubricants contain propylene glycol, which may cause irritation to a woman or her partner.

7. Avoid sexual intercourse that is painful or abrasive to your vagina.

8. Cut down on coffee, alcohol, sugar and refined carbohydrates (diets high in sugars can radically change the normal pH of the vagina).

9. Although some women have used unpasteurized, plain yogurt to alleviate mild symptoms of vaginal infections, this practice can prevent proper diagnosis and may even contribute to chronic vaginal complaints.

10. Avoid douching of any kind unless specifically recommended by your practitioner.

11. Take care of yourself. Not eating well nor resting enough makes you more susceptible to infection. Continue most of these practices even after you get an infection.

12. Avoid tampon use, especially if you have a history of frequent vaginal infections.

Medical Versus Alternative Treatments

The usual treatment for vaginitis is some form of antibiotic or sulfa drug, which kills infection-causing bacteria. In the process, however, these drugs disturb the delicate balance of bacteria in the vagina and may actually encourage some infections (such as those caused by yeast) by altering the vagina's normal acid/alkaline balance. Some of these drugs also have unpleasant or even dangerous side effects.

As an alternative to antibiotics for vaginitis, many women are turning to natural and herbal remedies that help to restore the normal vaginal flora and promote healing. For example, you can use herbs to make soothing douches, poultices or sitz baths. (You should not rely on these remedies, however, if you have a serious STD [see Chapter 14] or an infection that involves your uterus, tubes or ovaries.)*

Yeast Infections (Also Called Candida, Monilia or Fungus)

Candida albicans, a yeast fungus, grows in the rectum and vagina. In a healthy vagina, the presence of some yeast may not be a problem. When your system is out of balance, yeastlike organisms may grow profusely and cause a thick, white dis-

---

*Feminine hygiene sprays may irritate or cause an allergic reaction in the skin of the vulva. They are at best unnecessary and often harmful. The FDA has suggested and may soon require that all feminine hygiene sprays carry a warning on the label.
†Studies indicate that it may cause ovarian cancer.[9]

---

*For more information on alternative remedies for vaginitis, send for ''Home Remedies for Vaginitis,'' Santa Cruz Women's Health Center, 250 Locust Street, Santa Cruz, CA 95060. Send a stamped, self-addressed envelope and 50¢.

charge that may look like cottage cheese and smell like baking bread. If a woman has a yeast infection when she gives birth, the baby will get yeast in its throat or digestive tract. This is called *thrush* and is treated orally with nystatin drops.

Candida grows best in a mildly acidic environment. The pH in the vagina is normally more than mildly acidic (4.0 to 5.0), except when we take birth control pills or some antibiotics, are pregnant, have diabetes and when we menstruate (when the pH rises to between 5.8 and 6.8, because blood is alkaline). Obviously, we often find ourselves with a vaginal pH favorable to candida, so preventive measures are especially important.

Microscopic analysis of vaginal secretions (known as a *wet mount*) is the only way to be sure that the infection is candida and not something else. Several other conditions (such as cytolytic vaginosis) may respond temporarily to candida treatments and then recur a short time later, so accurate diagnosis is important.

Once candida sets in, treatment usually consists of some form of vaginal suppository or cream. Use of antifungal external creams such as chlortrimazole may reduce or even eliminate symptoms, sometimes without actually curing the infection. (A yeast culture and vaginal wet mount can determine if the infection is really gone.) For severe, chronic cases some of the newer oral antifungal medications may be necessary. Suppositories and creams have fewer side effects than oral medications, and they can be used during pregnancy, but they may not be strong enough to cure severe yeast infections.

Another treatment for candida involves painting the vagina, cervix and vulva with gentian violet. This is bright purple and it stains, so a sanitary pad must be worn. This procedure really helps, except in occasional cases when there is a severe reaction to gentian violet.

Self-Help Treatments

Some of us have had success with the following remedies: yogurt in the vagina; garlic suppositories (peel but don't nick a clove of garlic, then wrap in gauze before inserting in the vagina); and acidifying your system by drinking eight ounces of unsweetened cranberry juice every day or taking cranberry concentrate supplements. An effective and inexpensive treatment for candida is potassium sorbate, commonly used as a preservative in the home brewing of beer. A cotton tampon is dipped into a 3 percent solution (fifteen grams of dry potassium sorbate in one pint of water) and then inserted into the vagina at night and removed in the morning.

For a long time I felt as though I were on a merry-go-round. I would get a yeast infection, take Mycostatin for three weeks, clear up the infection and then find two weeks later that the itching and the thick, white discharge were back. Finally, I discovered that reducing my sugar intake and drinking unsweetened cranberry juice would help prevent repeat infections.

Trichomoniasis

Trichomonas vaginalis, or trich, is a one-celled parasite that can be found in both men and women. Many women have trich organisms in their vaginas, though often they are without symptoms. Usually women with trich have a thin, foamy vaginal discharge that is yellowish green or gray in color and has a foul odor. If another infection is present along with trichomoniasis, the discharge may be thicker and whiter. Trich is usually diagnosed by examining vaginal discharge under a microscope. It can also cause a urinary infection. It is most often contracted through intercourse (thus trichomoniasis can be considered an STD) but can also be passed on by moist objects such as towels, bathing suits, underwear, washcloths and toilet seats. Sometimes emotional stress can cause symptoms to flare up or recur.

The usual treatment for trich is oral doses of metronidazole (Flagyl). We think that women should use this drug with great caution, as metronidazole has caused gene mutations, birth defects and cancer in animal studies. Women with blood diseases, central nervous system disorders or peptic ulcers should *not* take this drug. Pregnant and nursing mothers should also avoid metronidazole, as it can pass through the placenta and breast milk to the baby. Many women who take this drug experience unpleasant effects such as nausea, headache, diarrhea, joint pain and numbness of arms or legs. In addition, anyone taking metronidazole should avoid alcohol, as the combination can make the effects of both worse.

In some cases, you can treat trich successfully with sulfa creams (low efficacy), Betadine or self-help remedies (see below). Chlortrimazole may be used (60 percent cure rate), but its use during pregnancy has not been proven safe. Unless you detect the infection early, however (and often even when you do), these treatments are not always as effective as Flagyl. If you have a stubborn case that has not responded to other treatments and decide to use Flagyl, ask for a single oral dose instead of the usual three- to seven-day course of pills. Studies show that one dose has a 98 percent cure rate and far fewer negative effects. Because men can also carry and transmit the infection, many practitioners believe male partners should be treated at the same time.

Self-Help Treatments

1. Although some women have used douches made from vinegar, goldenseal-myrrh, chickweed and other substances, douching can push organisms further up into your reproductive system, causing even more serious problems. Douche only with the recommendation and guidance of your practitioner.

2. Garlic suppositories inserted every twelve hours (see above).

One trichomoniasis specialist advises that taking tub baths, wearing loose clothing (since exposure to air destroys parasites causing infection) and avoiding tampons, douches and vaginal sprays will help prevent recurrences.

Bacterial Vaginosis (Formerly Called Gardnerella or Hemophilus)

The *Hemophilus* bacterium is one of the most common causes of vaginitis. Like candida, it thrives when the normal pH of the vagina is disturbed. You can get it through sexual intercourse, and possibly via washcloths, etc. The symptoms are similar to those of trich, though the discharge tends to be creamy white or grayish and especially foul smelling (often "fishy") after intercourse. Although the bacterium is fairly easy to recognize on a wet mount, it is sometimes diagnosed incorrectly.

The Centers for Disease Control recommend metronidazole as the treatment of choice. Another possible treatment is clindamycin vaginal suppositories (1 or 2 percent) at bedtime for one week. Hemophilus can be transmitted sexually, so your partner should use a condom until your infection is cured. Your partner may also need to be treated.

Untreated bacterial vaginosis is associated with pregnancy problems and other reproductive problems such as abnormal vaginal bleeding, abnormal Pap smears and UTIs.

Self-Help Treatments

Self-help treatments include (1) acidifying your system by drinking eight ounces of unsweetened cranberry juice every day or taking cranberry concentrate supplements; (2) garlic suppositories changed once a day; (3) taking extra vitamins B and C; (4) minimizing the use of tampons (to help prevent recurrences); (5) using condoms (this may prevent recurrences by protecting you from the alkaline effect of semen).

Vulvitis

Vulvitis, an inflammation of the vulva, may be caused by external irritants; oral sex; a bacterial or fungal infection; injury or allergy to common commercial products such as soaps, powders, deodorants, sanitary napkins, synthetic underwear, pantyhose and medications. Vulvitis often accompanies other infections such as vaginitis or herpes. Stress, inadequate diet and poor hygiene can make you more susceptible to vulvitis. Women with diabetes may develop vulvitis because the sugar content of the cells is higher and the pH is higher in the vagina; these factors cause susceptibility to infection. Postmenopausal women often develop vulvitis because, as the hormonal levels drop, the vulvar tissues become thinner, drier and less elastic, making them susceptible to irritation and infection.

Vulvitis symptoms include itching, redness and swelling. Sometimes fluid-filled blisters form that break open, ooze and crust over (these may resemble herpes). Scratching can cause further irritation, pus formation and scaling, as well as secondary infections. Sometimes, as a result of scratching, the skin whitens and thickens. In diabetic vulvitis the skin may look beefy red; in postmenopausal vulvitis, sores and red, irritated areas often appear.

Women with this problem tend to overclean the vulva, contributing to further irritation. Using mineral oil or shortening (such as Crisco) as a substitute for soap may reduce irritation.

Prevention

See the section on preventing vaginitis, p. 605.

Medical Treatments

If you have a vaginal infection or herpes, treating these problems will usually clear up the vulvitis as well.

Depending on the cause of vulvitis, your practitioner may prescribe antifungal creams. If itching is severe, s/he may prescribe cortisone cream or other soothing lotions. (Low-dose cortisone creams are good for a short period of time. Fluorinated ones cause thinning and atrophy of the skin if used for a long time.) Postmenopausal women may be given topical estrogen cream or ERT but should not use this for prolonged periods without also adding progesterone (to reduce the risk of uterine cancer).

If the vulvitis persists or worsens, you may need a vulvar biopsy to rule out the possibility of cancer. This can be done in an office under local anesthetic.

Self-Help Treatments

Discontinue using any medications, soaps, powders, deodorants, tampons, toilet paper, and so on, to which you may be sensitive. Keep your vulva clean, cool and dry. Hot boric acid compresses and hot sitz baths with comfrey tea are soothing. Use unscented white toilet paper and soft cotton or linen towels and underclothes to prevent chafing. Cold compresses made of plain natural yogurt or cottage cheese also help relieve itching and soothe irritation. Calamine lotion also helps relieve itching. Aveeno colloidal oatmeal bath can be very soothing. Use a sterile, nonirritating lubricating cream such as K-Y Jelly during intercourse and other genital sex. Finally, try to eat well, get more rest and find ways of coping with stress.

ANEMIA

Anemia results from a shortage of red blood cells and/or a low hemoglobin content of these cells, and occurs four times as often among women as among men. (The hemoglobin molecule carries oxygen to every part of the body. When we are anemic, our tissues get less oxygen.) Often vague, symptoms may include chronic fatigue, irritability, dizziness, memory problems, shortness of breath, headaches and bone pain. Dark-skinned women may look gray, light-skinned women very pale. Mild anemia may have no noticeable symptoms.

Iron-Deficiency Anemia

Iron-deficiency anemia is by far the most common form in women, often caused by heavy menstrual periods as well as bleeding associated with miscarriage, abortion, childbirth or surgery for fibroids. Pregnant women are especially prone to anemia because the fetus absorbs much of the iron the mother takes in.

Prevention and Treatments

The best preventive is an iron-rich diet (see the chart on pp. 38–39). Cooking foods in iron pots increases their iron content. If despite eating an iron-rich diet you are still anemic, you may want to take supplements. (Some practitioners recommend that pregnant women routinely take iron supplements.) Ferrous gluconate and chelated iron are the most easily absorbed forms of iron. They work best on an empty stomach, but if they cause nausea or cramps take them with food. Taking vitamin C at the same time will increase absorption. Even so, some women find through subsequent hematocrits that they cannot absorb iron pills. Eating blackstrap molasses has helped some women. Iron pills can cause tarry stools or constipation, which can be remedied by eating more whole grains, bran and fruit and drinking lots of water. Iron interferes with the absorption of vitamin E. If you are taking vitamin E supplements, be sure to take them at least six hours before the iron. Iron can be given by injection for severe deficiency.

Vitamin-Deficiency Anemias

Pregnant women, women who have had many children, women on oral contraceptives and malnourished women can become anemic due to a lack of folic acid (an essential B vitamin). You can prevent or treat this deficiency by eating whole grains and dark green vegetables and/or taking folic acid supplements. Vegetarians who eat no animal or dairy products sometimes suffer from pernicious anemia caused by lack of vitamin B_{12} (present in all animal products). Symptoms may include burning or weakness in the legs. Adding brewers' yeast (which often contains B_{12}), a fortified cereal like Grape-Nuts, spirulina (a microalga) or fermented foods like miso, tempeh or fermented sprouts to the diet will help. Women who lack a protein called the *intrinsic factor*, necessary for oral absorption of vitamin B_{12}, will need monthly injections of this vitamin.

Hereditary and Other Types of Anemia

Some forms of anemia can be inherited. Sickle cell anemia is found in some people of African ancestry and thalassemia affects people of Mediterranean descent. Also, some African and Mediterranean (especially Italian) women inherit a deficiency in an enzyme called glucose-6-phosphate-dehydrogenase, which causes them to develop hemolytic anemia (which may be fatal) if they take sulfa, aspirin or antimalarial drugs.

Finally, anemia can result from chronic illness such as kidney disease, thyroid disease, arthritis or cancer. Exposure to certain drugs, chemicals, metals or radiation can occasionally cause anemia.

Testing for Anemia

The hematocrit is a basic screening test for anemia. In this cheap and simple test, blood is taken from a prick on your finger and the percentage of red blood cells is measured. The normal hematocrit for a woman who is not pregnant is 37 to 47 percent. An annual test is a good idea; it will enable you to get an idea of changes from year to year. If your hematocrit is low, ask for a complete blood count, a lab test done on blood removed from a vein in your arm. In some cases other specialized expensive tests may be needed.

ARTHRITIS

Although arthritis encompasses over a hundred different joint diseases, women, who get arthritis twice as often as men, most often develop either osteoarthritis or rheumatoid arthritis. The former is a degenerative disease in which the cartilage, usually in the knees, hips, ankles or spine, gradually wears away. Common symptoms are swelling, redness and stiffness around the joints. Osteoarthritis, which is most common among older women (affecting about 25 percent), is not usually a crippling disease.

In rheumatoid arthritis, which affects about 3 percent of adult women, the body manufactures antibodies that attack the membranes covering the joints. In severe cases, the heart, lungs and kidneys can be affected. Symptoms include pain, swelling and redness in the fingers, knees, hips and back; fatigue; anemia; fever and weight loss. They may be mild or severe, spreading to many joints and getting worse over time. In severe cases, the joint supports (cartilage, ligaments and tendons) become inflamed and the joints themselves may begin to degenerate. A blood test can distinguish rheumatoid arthritis from other forms of the disease.

Prevention and Self-Help Treatments

(See *The Arthritis Helpbook* in Resources.) Exercise, relaxation and nutrition can both prevent and treat arthritis, sometimes reducing or eliminating the need for medical treatment. Regular exercise, such as yoga, walking or swimming, stretches, strengthens and preserves the joints. Daily rest is especially important when arthritis is severe. Some studies suggest that a diet low in fats can dramatically reduce pain, swelling and stiffness.[10] Since many foods (such as beef, pork, milk, sugar, chocolate, monosodium glutamate, pepper, alcohol and artificial preservatives) actually trigger attacks, determining what these are and then eliminating them from your diet can be the key to preventing arthritic attacks. Some women find that regular consumption of alfalfa alone (in tea, sprout or pill form) prevents flare-ups of osteoarthritis, but alfalfa may cause rheumatoid arthritis to worsen. Acupuncture and vitamin C supplements may also be helpful.

Arthritis pain can also be related to stress and depression, making us less motivated to take care of ourselves and thus causing more pain, setting up a cycle that is difficult to break. Meditation, yoga, relaxation exercises and biofeedback may help us break the stress-depression-pain cycle. Symptoms sometimes abate temporarily during pregnancy.

Medical Treatments

The most common treatment for mild arthritis is aspirin, which relieves both inflammation and pain. Too much aspirin, however, can cause stomach irritation and bleeding. (Taking aspirin with food reduces this irritation.) Ibuprofen, an anti-inflammation drug now more commonly used for arthritis, has less risk of bleeding and is also available over the counter.

For severe or crippling rheumatoid arthritis, your physician may recommend surgery to repair or replace damaged joints. Other treatments sometimes used for severe rheumatoid arthritis include gold-salt injections, antimalarial drugs, immunosuppressant drugs (such as methotrexate) used in cancer therapy, steroids and other powerful antiinflammatory agents. These drugs, which can have dangerous side effects, should be recommended only when all other methods have failed.

INTRODUCTION TO CANCER

Most of us (about two-thirds) will never get cancer. Many who do are cancer-free years after their original diagnosis. Why does this illness hold so much terror for us? It is partly due to the constant media attention, treatments that seem almost as bad as the disease, and the uncertainty of cure (60 percent of those who do get cancer die within five years).[11] For women, there is the added factor that cancer often develops in our sexual or reproductive organs (breasts, ovaries, uterus). Because the conventional treatment, for example, in breast cancer, has been surgical removal, we may fear losing our attractiveness or womanliness in a society that so often locates a woman's identity in her physical attributes. We may also face the loss of certain sexual pleasures. (See the discussion of hysterectomy on p. 600, for example).

Then there is the shame, the "What have I done to deserve this?" feeling that so often sweeps over someone who has cancer. And no wonder! All around us, the word *cancer* is used to describe any particularly immoral or illegal situation. Drugs and juvenile delinquency are "cancers" in our society. Watergate was the "cancer of democracy," not the "heart attack."

This fear and shame means that many of us avoid thinking about cancer even when we ourselves have it. Because of this avoidance, we do not always make the best medical decisions or live as full a life as possible.

What Is Cancer?

Through a process not completely understood, normal cells sometimes become abnormal and begin to grow out of control. These abnormal cells may spread (metastasize) throughout the body, taking over organs and preventing them from functioning. Some cancers are fast-growing, others are slow. Each type of cancer has its own particular pattern of growth, spread and probability of cure or survival time.

Who Gets Cancer?

Although people of all ages can get cancer, it is most often found in older persons, as the disease can take as long as twenty years to reach a detectable state.

Over the past twenty-five years, the death rate from cancer has increased 50 percent among the black population and only 10 percent in the white population. The incidence (number of new cases) is also higher among blacks; in some cases (such as cervical cancer) the rate is twice as high for black women as for white women.[12] At least part of the reason for these differences must be the discrimination that causes many black people to be exposed more frequently to workplace and environmental carcinogens (cancer-causing substances) than whites, to have less access to high-quality medical care, nutritious food and decent living conditions.

Women develop less cancer and die less frequently from it than men do; the gap (except for lung cancer) is widening.* At least part of this difference exists because until recently men consumed much more tobacco and alcohol and were more often exposed to workplace carcinogens. It may also be that as women we are better able to handle stress and thus keep our immune (disease-fighting) systems stronger. Or there may be something inherent in our immune or metabolic systems which increases our ability to fight cancer.

Terminology

The following terms are frequently misunderstood or misused, even by medical personnel. Ask for careful explanations—it is your right to know exactly what is going on.

Mortality (death) rates tell how many people died from cancer per 100,000 population per year.

Survival rates, generally given for five-, ten- and twenty-year periods, report how long people with specific kinds of cancer usually live. Survival rates are always calculated from the date the cancer was first diagnosed. These rates are most helpful when they are subdivided according to such factors as how far advanced the cancer was at first diagnosis, the type of treatment received, and the age, sex, race, socioeconomic status and occupation of the people involved.

Cure rates purport to tell how many people are completely cured of their cancers. However, cure rates are generally based on survival rates, resulting in the misleading impression that many people are "cured" who have merely survived for a specified (usually five-year) period. For example, physicians usually consider a five-year survival a cure in breast cancer, even though many women die of the disease in the sixth or seventh year.

Remission is sometimes used loosely to refer to any improvement, other times in a more technical sense with very strict criteria regarding amount of change in tumor size and blood tests. Some cancer therapies will produce technical "remission" of certain symptoms but do not increase cure or survival rates. Remission rates are usually given as percentages of persons "going into remission" after receiving various types of treatments.*

We should keep in mind that while statistics provide useful information, they can't really predict what will happen to us as individuals.

Causes

Cancer rates increase with exposure to carcinogens (such as radiation, asbestos, some pesticides), smoking, alcohol or particular dietary habits (see below). Certain genes and viruses have caused cancer in laboratory animals and similar processes are suspected but not conclusively proven in some human cancers. Yet it is not clear how these substances cause cancer or why everyone

---

Long-term remission refers to a specific number of disease-free years and is preferred to *cure*, as people with cancer are often considered to have their disease under control rather than to be entirely cured.

FIVE-YEAR SURVIVAL RATE PERCENTAGES (ADJUSTED FOR NORMAL LIFE SPANS) NATIONAL CANCER INSTITUTE—1981–87

Type of Cancer	Rates for Women Only (%)		
	Localized	Regional	Distant metastasis
Lung	48	16	2
Colon	90	60	6
Rectum	84	50	4
Breast†	92	71	18
Uterus/cervix	88	52	14
Uterus/internal (corpus or endometrial)	93	70	27
Ovary	87	39	19

†While breast cancer is mistakenly thought to occur only in women, a small number of cases (less than 1 percent) occur in men.

---

*From 1950 to 1985, there was a 30 percent increase in men's cancer death rates and a 6 percent decrease in women's. However, as women's smoking has increased, our lung cancer rate is also increasing, and is now the leading cause of cancer death in women.[13]

who develops the same kind of cancer does not respond in the same way, either to the disease or to treatments. There are also unexplained cases of spontaneous remission: Approximately 7 to 8 percent of people with terminal cancer suddenly recover and live out their lives apparently free of the disease. These different responses show that our individual immune systems are very important factors.

It seems most likely that cancer is caused by a buildup of one or more factors to the point (different for each person) where the body's immune system can no longer handle the load. Thus smoking will not guarantee that you will get cancer, but it will increase your chances. (Smoking or smoking combined with heavy alcohol consumption accounts for 30 percent of all cancer deaths.[14]) Add smoking to heavy drinking, repeated X-rays, constant stress, exposure to pollution* or excessive overweight, and the risk of cancer goes up.

Both environmental and hereditary elements appear to cause cancer. *Heredity* refers to the traits and tendencies passed on to us by our parents in our genes, whereas *environment* includes all that we eat, breathe or come into contact with. Most researchers now believe that environment is responsible for the development of 85 to 95 percent of all cancers.

Prevention

Although we can do many things to reduce our risk of cancer (such as stopping smoking, limiting X-rays), many other factors, such as air pollution and the many environmental carcinogens that bombard us in our daily lives, are not so clearly under our personal control. Even diet changes can be expensive and resisted by family, friends and physicians.

Thus cancer prevention means restructuring both our personal lives and the society at large so that a clean environment, safe jobs, healthy food and less stressful living become top priorities.

A Program to Reduce the Risk of Cancer

In the list below, factors that seem to be related to breast cancer are marked with an asterisk.

*1. Don't smoke, and avoid smoke-filled environments.

2. Avoid frequent X-ray exposure, especially at earlier ages.

*3. Avoid estrogen replacement therapy at menopause and any other medication with estrogen such as the morning-after pill (DES). The relationship between oral contraceptives and breast

cancer is very controversial. Some studies have shown that women who begin taking birth control pills at a young age and continue for a long period have a higher risk of breast cancer. Other studies indicate that the Pill lowers women's chances of developing uterine and ovarian cancers. To be on the safe side, women concerned about their risk of breast cancer may want to avoid oral contraceptives.

4. Minimize consumption of smoked, salted or pickled foods, such as bacon. Avoid additives, preservatives and refined flour.

*5. Keep fat consumption low—about 15 to 20 percent of total calories; reduce both saturated and unsaturated fats while making sure that both are supplied in the diet.

6. Limit or eliminate alcohol.

*7. Research has shown that people who are overweight (more than 40 percent above the old "norms") get more cancer and die more frequently from it. In breast cancer, this may be related to ovarian estrogen levels. Many studies point to high levels of estrogen as a precipitating factor in breast cancer. There is evidence that fat tissue manufactures its own estrogen. Although this process may be helpful during and after menopause as a natural form of ERT, it may also be dangerous to a woman who is very large or who already has elevated estrogen levels.

8. Maintain frequent and regular bowel movements. Increasing exercise and dietary fiber may help.

*9. Avoid hair dyes made from petroleum bases.

10. Eat a diet high in organic whole grains, vegetables and fruits rich in bran and fiber.

11. Eat food high in beta-carotene (a vitamin A precursor found in carrots and other yellow and dark leafy vegetables as well as some yellow fruits). Or take supplements of beta-carotene. *Be wary of large doses (greater than 10,000 to 15,000 IU daily) of vitamin A, as it can be toxic and is not a substitute for beta-carotene.*

12. Eat foods high in selenium (brewers' yeast, eggs, garlic, onions, liver, asparagus, tuna, mushrooms, shrimp, kidney, whole grains and brown rice). Selenium can be toxic in high doses, so be careful of any megatherapy or supplementation.

Costs

The total costs to the U.S. economy of cancer research and treatments is many billions of dollars per year. Medical treatment for cancer can reach tens of thousands of dollars for an individual, not including hidden costs like transportation, babysitters and loss of income.

Unfortunately, the profit motive affects how this country tackles cancer. Major research has emphasized high-profit treatments rather than

*See Chapter 7, "Environmental and Occupational Health," for more on environmental and workplace carcinogens.

prevention. (Chemotherapy, for instance, can cost up to a thousand dollars per session.) These benefit hospitals, doctors and the pharmaceutical, insurance and medical-equipment companies, but have not yet brought significant progress in eliminating cancer. Government and industry do little to clean up the environment, the workplace or hazardous consumer products or to discourage the profitable dietary and smoking habits that contribute to cancer. In fact, the government subsidizes tobacco production. One cancer researcher remarked that a cure for cancer may never be found because too many people depend on it for a living.

What to Do If You Have Cancer

Inform yourself. The first thing to do is learn all you can. Unfortunately, there is no reliable cure for most cancers, and all the once-accepted theories and treatments in the field are now under question. It helps to be persistent and aggressive in seeking the most up-to-date information and to have someone you trust do it with or for you.

Resist the pressure to rush. Your doctor or your family may pressure you to begin treatment immediately. Yet most cancers have been developing for two to twenty years before being discovered. Several studies have shown that a short delay of three or four more weeks while you get adjusted to the idea, seek out information and get second or third opinions should not make any difference in the ultimate outcome of your disease. If you decide then to follow your doctor's original advice, you will feel much better about the decision. If you decide to take another course of action, you may have saved yourself unnecessary treatment or considerable regret at not having made your own choice.

Talk to others with cancer. Try joining (or starting) a group for people with cancer. Being with those who understand and have faced the same problems can provide the kind of practical information and emotional support that is simply not routinely available from those providing conventional medical cancer treatment.

Joining my cancer discussion group is one of the best things that has happened to me since my diagnosis.

In a group founded by those who have cancer rather than one started by professionals at a hospital or a service organization, you may feel freer to confront all aspects of your situation. These include critical evaluation of traditional and alternative therapies; the problems surrounding child care, insurance, jobs and marital relations and ways of coping with your own fears as well as those of family and friends. If you can't find or

create such a group, talk with individuals—people in waiting rooms, people suggested by your doctor, friends or clergy. Don't hesitate to call persons you haven't met. Many people with cancer are glad to talk about their experiences.

Factors to Consider When Deciding on Conventional Medical Treatment (Surgery, Radiation and Chemotherapy)

Unfortunately, there has been little progress over the years in effective cancer treatment. Many doctors and hospitals have one preferred treatment that they will urge you to accept. Some specialists tend to recommend their own approach; for example, surgeons promote surgery and radiologists radiation. Yet new research indicates that many factors—age, sex, previous health history, type and stage of cancer—can influence how well a treatment works. The data are changing rapidly and even those doctors who are familiar with the most recent research often can't agree on how to interpret the information. Ideally, you should have access to a team of specialists to be sure of getting the treatment most appropriate for your cancer and for you.

Because so many variations exist, we cannot give a comprehensive guide to cancer treatments. What we can do is discuss some of the issues and indicate what you need to know in order to make informed decisions. Where no one treatment has proved best, it often makes sense to choose the one that will disrupt your body and your life the least.

Although everyone wants the benefits of the most current therapies, it is tragic to give false hope, waste limited finances or subject already ill persons to painful treatments unless there is good reason to believe that the treatment will pay off with either increased survival time or improved quality of life remaining. We urge anyone considering surgery, chemotherapy, radiation or any of the alternatives to study carefully what can be reasonably expected from the treatment in her particular case (see also Chapter 25, "The Politics of Women and Medical Care.")

There are other factors to consider. Choosing anything but the most conventional and locally available treatment often involves traveling quite a distance. This may separate you from loved ones and a familiar environment, important factors in the healing process. Also, most forms of treatment are very expensive, and pursuing a less available treatment may mean even more expense—for second-opinion medical visits, travel, noninsured costs. Many women (perhaps having internalized the culture's view of women as secondary) feel guilty about using their own or their family's money on themselves. In making this difficult decision, every woman deserves both the clearest, most current information and the strongest possible support from family and friends.

Surgery

Surgery has been the mainstay of cancer therapy for over a century. It helps with local control of the disease and seems to be effective in a few types of cancer (such as nonmelanoma skin cancers and cervical cancer). But surgery is not always the best treatment, and it takes the body a long time to recover from it. See p. 568 for some things to consider before consenting to surgery.

Surgery and Early Detection

Until very recently, most doctors believed that surgery would work if they caught the cancer before it had a chance to spread. For this reason, when possible they would cut a sizable area around the cancer to "be sure to get it all." They based this approach on the theory that cancer begins in one place (e.g., the lung or breast) and spreads from there.

However, over the past twenty years or more, cancer has been detected earlier and earlier with, in most cases, no corresponding drop in the death rate (see Early Detection, p. 618). This has made many physicians question the entire notion of early detection. Now many doctors are beginning to view some cancers as systemic diseases that tend to show up first in certain areas but are already microscopically present throughout the body. There is evidence to support both theories, and the final answer may lie somewhere in between. However, the treatment you are offered will reflect the theory preferred by the doctor or hospital you go to.

Radiation and Chemotherapy

Radiation (via high-power X-rays or internal implants) and chemotherapy (chemicals taken by pill or injection) are supposed to kill cancer throughout the body in places that surgery can't reach. They themselves have carcinogenic (cancer-causing) potential, yet are theoretically more harmful to cancer cells than to normal cells. So far neither therapy has been very successful in curing or prolonging life in regard to the common cancers such as breast, colon and lung cancer, although they have reduced some cancer symptoms.

Negative effects common to both chemotherapy and radiation include nausea, fatigue and diarrhea. In addition, chemotherapy may result in amenorrhea (cessation of menstruation, usually permanently), alopecia (hair loss, usually not permanently), heart damage and suppressed immune systems (seriously lowering resistance to infections). Radiation may cause skin burns, extreme

sun sensitivity, weakened bones and sudden bone fractures, as well as ulcers (body sores that do not heal). Some drugs lessen these symptoms, but they may have their own negative effects. Marijuana often helps reduce the nausea and pain and is now legal in certain situations for people with cancer. Both forms of treatment involve repeated trips to a medical center or hospital.

Chemotherapy and radiation were formerly used only when cancer recurred in the same organ or metastasized elsewhere. Increasingly, doctors recommend radiation and/or chemotherapy immediately after surgery even when there is no evidence of spread (e.g., breast lumpectomy with radiation). A few physicians try chemotherapy and radiation without surgery (if the cancer is too advanced for surgery).

We feel some concern that physicians are overusing chemotherapy and radiation in instances where there's no proven benefit—almost as though they were miracle cures. This is understandable. Most doctors genuinely want to help their cancer patients and are frustrated by the lack of a reliable cure. Most people with cancer feel more reassured when they and the doctor are doing *something*. Overtreatment is psychologically appealing on both sides; both want to hope that "this time" treatment will make the difference.

Popular articles about cancer often give the impression that chemotherapy is working wonders with all types of cancer. This image makes people more likely to accept treatment under the false notion that it will increase their survival time also. It has shown significant results in a few of the less common types.* In addition, recent evidence shows that chemotherapy offers significant benefits for some women with breast cancer (see Breast Cancer, p. 616). *It is important to check that chemotherapy has been proven effective for your type of cancer.*

It is also important to find out exactly *how much* increased survival time can be gained. Sometimes the percentages doctors or researchers give are misleading: What is called 50 or 100 percent increased survival time may mean only two or three more months, or it may mean two or three years more. See the questions below.

Many people question whether the possibility of longer survival times is worth the negative effects of these therapies. Others feel that even one

---

*Chemotherapy has produced dramatic increases in five-year survival rates in childhood leukemia, young-adult Hodgkin's disease and other lymphomas. A child treated for leukemia may gain many precious years of life. However, s/he may get another form of cancer later on, caused by the chemotherapy chemicals themselves. It may be inappropriate to call the leukemia treatment a cure in all cases.[15]

more day of life is worth any price. Only you can make this difficult decision with the support of those who love you.

Questions You Need to Know the Answers to

An asterisk indicates those questions that doctors frequently do not or cannot give sufficient answers to. Press your doctor to find out and let you know, but also check books, medical journals and resource centers and speak to others who have had the same form of cancer as you.

*1. Exactly what form of cancer do I have? Is it slow- or fast-growing?

*2. What therapies are available?

*3. How effective is each therapy? What is the probability of cure? What definition of *cure* is used?

4. What benefits can I expect? Longer life? Reduced symptoms? Reduced pain, and so on?

*5. Can the therapy prolong life by months? By years?

*6. What percentage of people treated benefit from the therapy—25 percent? 50 percent? 75 percent? How is that benefit measured?

7. Will I be able to continue my regular activities during the therapy? What about sex? Working? Athletics?

8. Will the therapy require overnight stays in the hospital, or can it be done on an outpatient basis?

9. What are the potential negative effects? How serious are they? What percentage of people get them? Are they permanent? Are there any drugs that will help alleviate these effects? Do these drugs themselves cause any negative effects? How long does any symptom usually last? How soon after receiving treatment are symptoms likely to begin? (For example, does nausea generally start immediately, within twenty minutes or several hours later?)

10. How long will the therapy last? Each session? How many sessions?

*11. How many people get recurrences after this treatment, and how soon?

*12. Are there survival, cure, mortality and remission rates for this therapy for my type of cancer, broken down by such factors as type of cancer, age, sex, race, socioeconomic status, occupation, geographical location and so on?

13. What are the costs involved? Does insurance usually cover them?

*14. May I speak with some of your other patients? Do you know of any local groups for people with cancer? Any groups for family members and friends?

Alternative Therapies

The medical establishment as a whole regards most alternatives to surgery, radiation and chemotherapy with great caution or outright hostility. Yet women are increasingly seeking out unconventional approaches because the conventional therapies have not significantly improved survival rates and have many disadvantages. To date, alternative therapies are most often used along with conventional ones or as a last resort for advanced cancers after conventional treatments have failed. A few physicians are willing to work with combined approaches.

What alternatives are available and what can we expect from them? This is not an easy question to answer because we don't have reliable statistics on survival, recurrence and mortality for the alternative therapies.*

Alternative therapies are often reported in what is called *anecdotal style:* One particular person who was cured of cancer (or greatly helped) by a certain treatment tells her/his story. This style, which makes for inspirational reading, presents great problems. It is hard to confirm individual case histories. Even when it is determined that the person involved did use the treatment and recovered from cancer, there is still no proof that it was the treatment that caused the cure; some people have spontaneous remissions. The important issue is what percentage of people treated with a certain therapy recover or improve and how that compares with other therapies. Physicians, while they decry the use of the anecdotal style regarding alternative approaches, often resort to it to convince people under their care. Also, it is frequently through looking at the unusual cures that we find ideas for new or improved treatments. By all means ask the same questions about these alternative therapies that you ask about conventional methods.

The following list of alternative cancer therapies is more detailed than the above description of surgery, radiation and chemotherapy because this information is often hard to find. Keep in mind that the alternatives have not been tested in large-scale, long-term trials.

The Gerson Diet and Detoxification Therapy

Perhaps the most promising of the nontoxic alternatives is the Gerson diet and detoxification

---

*Supporters of nonconventional treatments contend that their therapies might show better results if 90 percent of their patients weren't already terminally ill, with immune systems suppressed by radiation and chemotherapy. Meanwhile, it is equally important to remember that the statistics we do have on conventional medical treatments do not themselves show significant improvements in overcoming cancer.

therapy. The diet consists of organically grown fresh fruits and vegetables. It forbids salted, processed or refined foods and fat. Meat is not allowed in the early stages of treatment. In most cases, the therapy includes tablets and injections of various nutrients, especially potassium and pancreatic enzymes. The Gerson therapy, developed in Austria in the 1920s and 1930s, is one of the few alternatives for which there are records and reports of long-term survival rates. For more information, contact the Gerson Institute of California, run by Dr. Gerson's daughter (see Resources).

The therapy itself is very rigorous and should be followed precisely for at least a year and a half. It is not sufficient to merely eat more healthily.

Physicians and various health practitioners have developed other diet therapies. Most of them are similar to the Gerson diet, though there are some discrepancies, especially between raw and cooked foods. Most also include procedures for detoxification (removing wastes from the body through skin, bowels, etc.) and spinal adjustments (see Chiropractic, p. 91). Many people who use these diets experience periods of nausea and headache and occasional pain and fever. The therapy's supporters attribute these to the removal of toxins that created the conditions for cancer.

Meganutrition Therapies

Two-time Nobel prizewinner Linus Pauling states that large daily doses of vitamin C, as high as fifty grams, can aid in both preventing and treating cancer. A study in Scotland supported his claim, but many doctors have vehemently attacked Pauling because similar studies in the United States have shown no improvement. Pauling and his associates believe that the American studies are faulty because they are based on people who had already had chemotherapy (which represses the immune system and may inhibit the vitamin's action).

Other researchers have found evidence that megadoses of other nutrients, especially vitamins A and B complex, the previtamin beta-carotene and trace minerals such as potassium and selenium, can help in the prevention and treatment of cancer. Carlton Fredericks' *Winning the Fight Against Breast Cancer, the Nutritional Approach* (New York: Grosset & Dunlap, 1977) contains a good summary of this research.

Care must be taken with any of the megatherapies. Some vitamins, such as A and D, can be toxic at high levels, and for this reason many doctors argue strongly against all megatherapies. Advocates, on the other hand, contend that what would be a toxic dose in a healthy person is needed by someone whose system is trying to deal with cancer.

Laetrile

The most controversial and probably best known of all the unconventional therapies is laetrile therapy. Produced from apricot pits, laetrile releases a cyanide into the system. Like chemotherapy and radiation, it is toxic to the body. Thousands of people have credited laetrile with their recovery from cancer. (See above for the limits of anecdotal reporting, however.)

Opponents point out cases where people who might have received good results from the traditional therapies chose laetrile instead and succumbed to their disease. Despite a blanket condemnation of laetrile by the prestigious Sloan-Kettering research center, some studies at that very institute showed that laetrile delayed metastases of breast cancer in mice.[16] The case for or against the drug is still not resolved. It is illegal in many states.

Hydrazine Sulfate

Hydrazine sulfate is an inexpensive substance that several researchers have found to help control the process of cachexia, or wasting away, which is the actual cause of death in over 50 percent of cancer cases. The doctors studying it think that if the other bodily systems can remain healthy and not be drained by the cancer, then any cancer therapy, traditional or alternative, will have a better chance of working. Overdoses can cause serious side effects, but at the proper dosage level there are few or no adverse effects.

Psychological/Spiritual Alternatives

Visualization, meditation and other psychological/spiritual approaches to cancer are gaining favor with both doctors and the general public. These emphasize people's self-healing capabilities and the ability of the mind to influence the body's recovery (see also Chapter 5, "Health and Healing: Alternatives to Medical Care").

The Simonton Technique

Probably the best known of these is the Simonton visualization technique in which the person with cancer learns to picture her/his body's defense system cleansing the body of cancerous cells and replacing them with healthy cells. Some hospitals offer counselors who teach this and other aspects of the Simonton approach. Although too new to have long-term survival statistics, this therapy appears to have been a major factor in the recovery of many people with cancer, including some for whom the conventional treatments had failed.[17]

Prayer

Many of us have found that prayer, meditation or other spiritual approaches can help to transform our experiences with serious illness from a terrifying, hopeless time into a period of personal growth and fuller enjoyment of life. Sometimes this spiritual healing includes "cure" and sometimes it does not.

Faith Healers and Psychics

If you are considering visiting a psychic or faith healer, try to find out as much as possible about the healer in advance. Making your own decision here is just as important as in any other type of treatment. Do not be rushed into a commitment by well-intentioned friends or deterred by ridicule from nonbelieving friends. We do caution anyone to avoid any faith or psychic healer who charges exorbitant fees or insists that you must "prove your faith" by refusing all other treatments.

Danger of Blaming the Victim

When using psychological/spiritual approaches such as the Simonton technique or faith healers, we need to be careful not to blame the victim for getting cancer—"she brought it on herself, all that repressed anger"—or condemning her if she doesn't get well—"she just isn't strong enough; she doesn't really want to get well; she doesn't have enough faith." Those of us who have cancer need the support and help, not the judgment, of our friends, families and health practitioners.

Problems in Getting Alternative Therapies

When a woman asks her doctor about nonconventional approaches, she often receives ridicule and warnings. Doctors often sincerely believe they are protecting their patients in this way, for medical journals expose them only to the negative side. Of course, there *are* people—in both conventional and alternative fields—who try to take advantage of the fear and desperation of some people with cancer. But doctors' warnings may also reflect the medical establishment's resistance to theories and treatments that do not follow the line of drugs, radiation and surgery.

In large part due to opposition from the medical world, alternative clinics are not well funded or widely available. A decision to go to one usually means added and noninsured expenses for treatment, travel, child care, housing and so on.

Friends and family who disapprove of therapies may withdraw emotional or financial support. Still, many women have found it worthwhile to push past these obstacles to find alternative sources of healing.

Some kinds of cancer are very painful near the end, while others aren't. Often women feel that it is a sign of weakness to take any medicine for the pain, or they are afraid of addiction. Occasionally doctors have these same inhibitions. If pain is pre-venting you from living as normally as possible and from enjoying the company of family and friends, you should feel no hesitation in asking for relief. Morphine and codeine are usually used, and there is an increasing acceptance of marijuana.

Remember that metastasis does not inevitably equal death. But if death does seem to be imminent, you can do much to ensure that you live your remaining time as fully as possible.

I don't want to die, but since I accepted the fact that I probably will, I am more at peace. It's as if my energy had been used up denying the reality of my own impending death and, when I stopped struggling against the idea, I suddenly felt free. I could begin to think about living again, about what to do with the time I do have. I have my down days, when I ask, "Why me? Why can't I die twenty years from now? Why can't I live to see my children grow up, my grandchildren born?" But these days are fewer and fewer. In a sense, I'm lucky to know about my death in advance. I won't be like those who die unexpectedly with things left unsaid and undone. I've planned what I want to do, who I want to see. I've started working on projects that I had always wanted to do but was too busy for. I can't afford to travel or do much special, but then anything I do now seems special.

I am not dying of cancer; I am living with cancer. I try to deal with the problems caused by my cancer in my daily life, but my emphasis is on the living, not the dying.

BREAST CANCER

If you turned to this section, we hope you will go to the beginning of Benign Breast Conditions (p. 575) and read from there. If you ever do have a breast cancer diagnosis following biopsy, you will be much better able to cope with it and to decide what to do next if you have done some reading and thinking beforehand.

Because breast lumps are so common and most of them are not dangerous, it is important for us to familiarize ourselves with ways of recognizing and dealing with them.

If the Biopsy Results Are Positive

No one who has not had the experience can understand the waves of shock, disbelief, fear and anger that overcome you after finding out you have cancer. This emotional trauma comes exactly when you need to focus all your energy on learning about your treatment options.

The usual first reaction is to do whatever your doctor suggests. This is appealing at a time when you may need to feel that you are being taken care of, but it has not always resulted in the best of care. Although most doctors are well intentioned, they tend to offer only the treatment they know best. Physicians as a whole have been slow to accept new therapies even when numerous studies have demonstrated that the new approaches have the same or better effectiveness with fewer negative effects. Many are unwilling or unable to discuss all the available therapies. Only several states, including Massachusetts, California and Minnesota, have laws that require that women be informed of all the medical options.

At this point, it is advisable to get a second opinion from a medical oncologist before committing yourself to a course of treatment. The National Cancer Institute (see Resources) sponsors many centers where your case can be evaluated by a team of specialists. Medical oncologists (cancer specialists), surgical oncologists and radiation oncologists work together to prescribe the best combination of treatments for your individual situation. They are more likely to be up-to-date on research. This team approach helps to avoid the tendency of most physicians to promote their own specialty: surgeons using surgery, radiation oncologists presenting radiation as the best solution and so on. Such centers may also offer more treatment choices, possibly including experimental therapies (see Our Rights as Patients, p. 682).

Remember, there is no rush. You can take several weeks to adjust and find out about your options. If you had an excisional biopsy, the main cancer is already out. In some cases, this could be the end of surgical treatment within the breast. You can always decide later to have further treatment such as mastectomy, radiation or chemotherapy. Some doctors will try to rush you into a decision by stating that the biopsy may have "stirred up" the cancer and it is therefore important to proceed immediately with mastectomy. This is an outmoded theory.

There is a tendency to rush women into treatments before they have a chance to get second opinions and learn about all the available options. No one knows for sure how long you can safely wait before beginning treatments, and doctors' opinions on this issue may vary widely. In order to decide upon optimal treatment, both locally and systemically, you need to know the total size of the tumor, the status of your lymph nodes, the hormone status of your tumor, and other tumor characteristics (see following pages). Evaluating these factors with a team of specialists helps you to explore your treatment options most effectively.

The entire field of breast cancer medicine is changing rapidly as old, established theories and treatments are coming under question while newer techniques have not been used long enough to be completely evaluated. While we cannot tell you which therapy will be best for you, we can

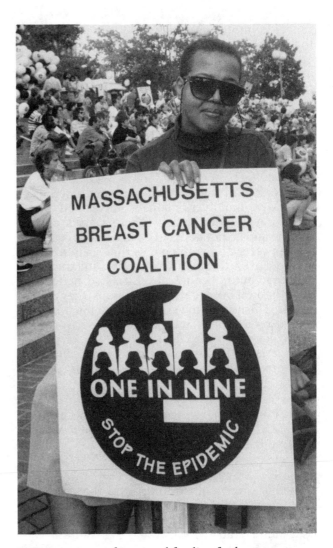

Rally in support of increased funding for breast cancer research.   Ellen Shub

point out some directions to pursue and pitfalls to avoid.

A good place to begin is the reading list in the Resources. *Dr. Susan Love's Breast Book* by Susan M. Love (Reading, MA: Addison-Wesley, 1990) is especially good (although not cautious enough on the subject of breast implants).

Stages of Breast Cancer

There are several systems for staging cancer, the most commonly accepted based on the three elements called TNM—*t*umor size, number of malignant *n*odes and whether or not you have distant *m*etastases (cancer in other parts of your body). When you are first diagnosed, you are staged *clinically* (by physical exam and tests). Following your local surgical treatment you are staged *pathologically* (by microscopic analysis). The stage of the cancer is important because doctors usually base their recommendations for treatment on how well other women with cancer at the same stage and a similar personal history have responded to the treatments.

Clinical Stages*

When physicians think that a particular lump "feels" like cancer, they estimate the size of the suspected cancer by the apparent size of the lump and the "feel" of nearby lymph nodes and other organs. In addition, they should order blood tests, chest X-ray and liver or bone scans to see if cancer exists beyond the breast. (These tests are often routine and do not necessarily mean that your cancer has spread.) Lymph nodes that seem to be involved are frequently merely inflamed or hardened but not cancerous. Likewise, nodes may be malignant but not palpable; that is, they cannot be felt. This estimated clinical stage must be confirmed by a biopsy and permanent section. *It is not wise or necessary to submit to a bone scan or other tests until there is a diagnosis of cancer obtained by tissue diagnosis.*

Stage 0

This refers to noninvasive breast cancer, either ductal carcinoma *in situ* or lobular carcinoma *in situ* (see below).

Stage I

In this stage a small lump (less than or equal to three-quarters of an inch or two centimeters) does not appear to have spread to either the lymph nodes under the arms or to more distant parts of the body. Eighty-five percent of women with Stage I cancer are still living five years after diagnosis.

Stage II

Nodes are palpable and/or tumor size is larger (between two and five centimeters or between three-quarters of an inch and two inches). There is no evidence of distant metastases. Sixty-six percent of women with Stage II cancer survive five years from diagnosis. Larger tumors are now included in this stage if the lymph nodes are not involved.

Stage III

The lump is large (greater than two inches or five centimeters), and the lymph nodes appear by palpation to be involved, although there is no evidence of more distant spread. Smaller tumors are included in this stage if they are attached to the chest wall or have invaded the skin. For women with Stage III cancer, the five-year survival rate is 41 percent.

Stage IV

This is the same as Stage III, except that there is evidence also that the cancer has metastasized and is growing in other parts of the body. At this stage, a cancer is not considered curable. Mastectomy is not useful unless the breast is infected or ulcerated. Ten percent of women with Stage IV cancer live five years after diagnosis.

Pathologic Stages

The pathologic stage is based on the TNM system but with microscopic evaluation of removed lymph nodes. A surgeon removes several lymph nodes positioned at lower levels in the axilla (underarm area) nearest the breast with the malignancy. This is usually done during the main breast surgery—lumpectomy or mastectomy. Occasionally, the lymph node dissection is done as a separate operation. General anesthesia is preferred for lymph node surgery because the operation can be painful and lengthy.

Removing the nodes is not an attempt to cure or halt the spread of cancer. Its only purpose is to see if the cancer has gone beyond the breast, but node status also predicts survival most accurately. Cancer in the nodes is an indication that undetected cancer *may* exist elsewhere in the body. Removing more than the lower level of nodes may increase the likelihood of developing arm swelling in the future. Level 1 and 2 lymph node dissection is the recommended procedure. The number of lymph nodes in the area varies markedly from women to woman with most being from eight to eighteen, but some women have fewer or more. Some cancer experts also believe that the nodes serve a protective function, delaying or slowing metastases.

Other factors relating to your type of cancer include the location of the tumor (central, lateral or medial); presence or absence of estrogen and progesterone receptors and the grade of malignancy, including differentiation (whether or not cells still retain the characteristics of the normal breast cell rather than the embryonic appearance of the advanced cancer cell), pleomorphism (variety of cells in the same area), mitotic rate (growth rate) and oncogene characteristics (*oncogenes* are a genes that cause and/or promote cancerous changes in normal cells). Research on these and other aspects of tumors is in progress.

Early Detection

Almost all (90 percent) of lumps are discovered by women or their partners, either through breast self-exam or incidentally while washing, dressing,

---

*For all stages (I to IV), see Jay Harris et al., *Breast Diseases* (Philadelphia: Lippincott, 1991).

making love and so on. Today those lumps that do turn out to be malignant tend to be smaller and much less likely to be associated with disease in lymph nodes or other organs than the breast cancers doctors used to see regularly years ago. However, this earlier detection through breast self-exam has not brought a corresponding improvement in survival or cure rates.

The situation is different for mammography screening, which has become more common since the late 1980s, although not universal. For women over fifty, there is unequivocal evidence that early detection through mammography screening *does* increase survival and that this longer survival time is not just the result of *lead-time bias*, that is, not simply a result of finding the cancer earlier and thus counting the years of survival from an earlier point.

Early detection through mammography screening has *not* been shown to improve overall survival for women under fifty. But for some women under fifty, with cancers that do respond to treatment, early detection can increase their survival. Until there are more effective ways to distinguish among the various cancers and to make a more accurate prognosis, there is no way for a woman to know whether or not, in her case, early detection will actually increase survival (see p. 581).

Most experts now view breast cancer as a systemic disease of varying types that requires a combined treatment approach, both local and systemic.

For some of us, the systemic view has a special personal meaning. Those of us who have cancer have often blamed ourselves (or felt blamed by others) for not "finding it early enough," for not practicing breast self-exam faithfully or for not choosing to have periodic mammograms or regular medical checkups. Paying attention to breast changes and lumps is important, but we don't need to take on the extra burden of guilt for something that is out of our control, namely, the type of cancer we have.

If cancer is found, be as assertive as you can in demanding that the type of treatment you receive is appropriate for the type of cancer you have and that it meets your needs.

Treatments

A Brief History of Breast Cancer Treatments

In the United States, for many years the standard practice upon doing a breast biopsy and finding malignant tissue was to proceed immediately ahead with a mastectomy. Several years of hard work, especially on the part of activist and journalist Rose Kushner (who has since died from breast cancer), resulted in a landmark National Cancer Institute (NCI) recommendation in 1979 that breast biopsies be done as part of a two-step procedure in most cases. That is, NCI advised that a diagnostic biopsy specimen first be studied with permanent histologic sections, and then a woman discuss her treatment options (including nonsurgical approaches) in order to make an informed decision. This NCI recommendation represented an important step forward in the treatment of breast cancer and also increased general awareness of the importance of nonsurgical treatments.

For the better part of this century, almost everyone agreed that the Halsted radical mastectomy was *the* way to treat breast cancer. In 1960, over 90 percent of women in the United States who had surgery for breast cancer underwent this operation, which removes the entire breast plus the underlying muscles and the nearby lymph nodes. The Halsted radical leaves a woman with a sunken chest wall and usually a swollen, less mobile arm. Believing that cancer begins locally and then spreads in a predictable, gradual manner, physicians assumed that the more tissue they removed, the more likely that they would "get it all" and thus prevent the spread of the disease. Yet as the years went by, statistics failed to support this theory. Survival and mortality rates did not improve significantly.

Some doctors and laywomen began to question both the use of the radical mastectomy and the idea it was based on. They pointed to growing evidence that cancer may not begin locally and then spread in a predictable manner but may be microscopically present throughout the body from the very beginning of the disease (the systemic theory: see Early Detection, p. 618). In a number of countries, including Canada, England and the Scandinavian countries, physicians were removing much less breast tissue than in the Halsted radical procedure and were getting almost identical survival rates. Slowly, American surgeons began to try these less extensive operations. In 1979, the NCI declared that the Halsted was no longer the preferred treatment except in a few rare cases, and today the Halsted radical accounts for 5 percent or less of breast cancer operations.[18]

Now most physicians have retreated far from the theory behind the Halsted radical. The most

Histological Stages National Surgical Adjuvant Breast Project		
	Percent Survival	
Number of Cancerous Nodes	5 Years	10 Years
None	78.1	64.9
1–3	62.2	37.5
4 or more	32.0	13.4

common treatment for breast cancer in the United States is still the modified radical mastectomy, which removes the entire breast and some lymph nodes. This is less disfiguring and leads to fewer subsequent health problems. However, most of the above arguments against the Halsted also apply to the modified radical. Numerous studies have shown that this modified operation, like the Halsted before it, does not provide better survival than some less extensive surgeries with radiation therapy.

In 1990 a National Institutes of Health Consensus Development Conference[19] concluded that certain treatments that offered greater breast conservation (see below) were preferable to total mastectomy. However, there are still hospitals in the United States that have never performed anything but a mastectomy.

Treatment Issues

Breast cancer treatment is one of the most controversial areas in medicine today. There are currently two main questions. First, how much surgery is necessary—must the surgeon remove just the lump, the lump plus some surrounding tissue or the entire breast? The second concerns the role of systemic therapies such as chemotherapy and radiation.

Because most invasive cancers are eventually associated with distant metastasis and shortened survival (see p. 618), systemic therapy aimed at eradicating presumed distant disease does make sense. Currently, there is very strong evidence that chemotherapy in premenopausal women (whether lymph nodes are positive or negative) will reduce mortality from breast cancer by 25 percent. Hormone therapy in postmenopausal women (whether the lymph nodes are positive or negative) will reduce mortality by 15 percent.

Systemic therapies, which should begin shortly after the diagnosis of breast cancer is made, are called *adjuvant therapies*. Current unanswered questions are how much chemotherapy to give, when exactly to begin therapy (presurgery or postsurgery), what is the best combination of drugs, are chemotherapy and hormone therapy more effective if combined and so on.

Be sure to discuss whether and what adjuvant therapy is most appropriate for your situation at the same time that you are deciding about definitive local therapy (mastectomy or lumpectomy and radiation therapy). Be sure you have a consultation with a medical oncologist shortly after the diagnosis of breast cancer is made. The decision to have systemic (adjuvant) therapy rests on how large your risk of getting recurrent (metastatic) disease is. For women who have tiny (less than one-half centimeter) tumors, with very good

prognostic factors, adjuvant therapy may have little additional benefit. But for women with poor prognostic factors, systemic treatment is indicated. Because most women will be at some risk for metastatic recurrence, all women should review their personal risks with a medical oncologist. Ask about ongoing clinical trials, which usually study the latest in treatments.

In making treatment decisions, women frequently feel caught between well-intentioned but competing factions with no way to determine what is best in their particular situation.

After I and the guy I live with had spent almost two hours with the surgeon, we came away convinced that simple mastectomy was the only sensible treatment. I so wanted to be sensible about it all. Then I went to Boston for a second opinion. I went up full of skepticism, feeling that they could never be as convincing as my New York surgeon, but that I must go through the motions to satisfy myself that I had heard the "other side" [in this case, for lumpectomy plus radiation]. It turned out that the "other side" was equally convincing, and I went back to New York feeling really torn. I felt like a statistic that was being wooed by both sides to show how successful their treatments were. "Good instincts," commented an oncologist friend. "That's precisely what it's all about." [This woman, after more research and much agonizing, went back to Boston for a lumpectomy plus radiation.]

The decision of what treatment to take is never easy. Sometimes one physician seems more reasonable. Sometimes your intuition will point strongly to a certain option. Sometimes one hospital is more conveniently located. Sometimes a friend's experience is influential. All these factors and more will enter into your final choice, which is often a compromise. In the end, each woman will make the decision in her own way, ideally with the most informed and friendly support possible.

Most women receive a combination of the four types of conventional medical treatments—surgery, radiation, chemotherapy and/or hormone therapy. The *primary therapy* is the first treatment to the primary site of the cancer (the breast). *Adjuvant therapies* are any additional systemic treatments following the primary treatment. Lumpectomy plus radiation therapy or mastectomy is usually considered a primary treatment and chemotherapy and/or hormone therapy an adjuvant.

Lumpectomy, mastectomy and radiation are *local therapies*, limited to the breast or other specific body area. In contrast, chemotherapy and hormone therapy are *systemic therapies* that circulate throughout the entire body, hopefully eliminating stray cancer cells that may already exist in other parts of the body.

The goals of your various treatments depend on the stage of the cancer, its type and other factors such as your age and general health. Some treatments are intended to cure, some to prolong life, some to produce remission of symptoms. Although these treatments may not result in increased survival time, quality of life may be improved. Other therapies primarily relieve pain or the side effects of the other treatments. *It is important that you ask your doctor to clearly explain the goal of each recommended treatment, its possible adverse effects and the most likely physical consequences of not taking the treatment.* Try to find out the statistical *five-, ten- and fifteen-year disease-free survival and mortality rates* for women with the same type and extent of disease (local, regional, metastatic), in the same menopausal status, who have selected the same treatment your doctor is recommending. You can then compare this information to results of other available treatments. (See questions in the general cancer section, p. 614). All this will help you decide which treatments, if any, are best for your individual case.

Treatment Options for Local Disease (Usually Clinical Stages 0, I and II)

The following *primary treatments* (surgery and radiation) are listed in order from the least disfiguring and debilitating to the most.

Procedures That Remove Less than the Entire Breast

1. *Lumpectomy* (also called *tylectomy, wide excision, segmental resection* or *partial mastectomy*) removes the lump and a varying amount of surrounding tissue. Adverse effects include scarring and some disfiguring of the breast (though this may be only slightly more than that caused by the original biopsy), depending on the size of the lump and the size of the breast.

2. *Radiation therapy* involves lumpectomy plus radiation. Therapy usually consists of radiation treatments to the breast five days a week for five to six and a half weeks after the lump is removed. Radiation may be boosted by an external electron beam. Adverse effects while undergoing treatment include fatigue; muscle pain; dry, red, itchy skin and extreme sun sensitivity. (Sun should be carefully avoided. A painful burn can occur even through a white blouse.) Occasionally (in 5 percent of women receiving the treatment) the radiation causes ribs to become more brittle and thus more prone to fracture. Another 10 percent develop a lung ailment similar to bronchitis that lasts about a month, generally does not recur and is painful but not life-threatening.[20]

Quadrantectomy removes the quarter of the breast with the tumor and is usually followed by radiation. This surgery is performed mostly in Europe. Problems occur that are similar to those resulting from lumpectomy, but there is more breast disfigurement.

Procedures That Remove the Entire Breast— Mastectomy

These are again listed from least to most disfiguring and debilitating.

1. *Simple mastectomy* (also called *total mastectomy*) removes the entire breast but leaves the chest muscles and lymph nodes. The adverse effects include the emotional trauma of losing a breast, numbness of the skin, scarring, and posture and balance problems related to the size and weight of the remaining breast.*

2. *Modified radical* (also called *total mastectomy with axillary node dissection*) is the simple mastectomy plus lower axillary lymph node dissection to stage the cancer. Adverse effects are the same as in simple mastectomy, with occasional arm problems such as fatigue and swelling and the inability to raise the arm completely or to lift and carry heavy items, plus less overall resistance to infection. Although this procedure formerly involved the removal of some muscle, this no longer should be done.*

3. *Radical mastectomy* (Halsted) involves removal of the breast and underlying muscle and extensive removal of lymph nodes. As of 1979, this operation is not recommended by the NCI (see p. 619). Adverse effects include all of the above. Arm problems tend to be severe and constant. The ribs and lungs, no longer protected by a layer of muscle, are more vulnerable to injury and illness.

There are variations within each surgical type and a multitude of different names for the same operation. Doctors also tend to use the terms differently. Thus one doctor's "modified radical" is

---

*These procedures usually offer the option of reconstruction, however.

A woman with a tatoo over her mastectomy scar.

Hella Hammid

another doctor's "total mastectomy plus lymph node dissection." This makes it difficult to compare advice from different physicians. Sometimes the distinctions between procedures are blurred for insurance purposes. A few surgeons may cut (or report that they cut) a little bit more than the whole breast in order to qualify for the higher fees granted the more extensive surgery. In order to be sure you understand how much your surgeon intends to remove, *ask to see diagrams and photographs and have her/him explain why this particular surgery is being recommended for your type of cancer.*

In Situ (Noninvasive) Cancer

Ductal carcinoma *in situ* (DCIS) and lobular carcinoma *in situ* (LCIS), classified as Stage 0 diease, represent noninvasive forms of breast cancer. How to treat DCIS—the noninvasive proliferation of malignant breast cells—is now one of the most controversial areas of breast cancer treatment. Theoretically, since the cancer is not yet invasive, local excision should be 100 percent effective. But it is not. Studies show that local excision alone is associated with a 10 percent chance of recurrence of DCIS and a 10 percent chance of developing invasive cancer in the same part of the same breast within ten years. (It is the latter, of course, that is of concern.) Adding radiation therapy to lumpectomy reduces the risk of recurrence of DCIS and the risk of the development of invasive cancer by about one-half.

For comparison, a fifty-year-old woman in this country who has not had DCIS and who does not have any family history of breast cancer has a 1½ percent risk of developing invasive breast cancer by the time she is sixty years old.

Although mastectomy is the most effective treatment for DCIS, it may be too much. Current studies are evaluating the impact of tamoxifen (an antiestrogen drug) on improving recurrence rates after lumpectomy plus radiation.

LCIS is uncommon and *not* considered to be invasive, but it is currently thought to be a warning that *either* breast is at higher than usual risk for developing invasive cancer. Careful observation of LCIS is wise.

If you have DCIS or LCIS, try to get second opinions from specialists who are following this rapidly changing area of treatment.

Must I Have a Mastectomy?

In most cases, no. For Stages I and II breast cancer (which account for 90 percent of all cases), there appears to be no difference in long-term (fifteen- and thirty-year) survival rates for radical mastectomy, modified radical mastectomy, simple mastectomy, lumpectomy, and lumpectomy plus radiation. Thus the least debilitating and dis-

figuring surgeries—lumpectomy with or without radiation or simple mastectomy—seem to be enough. A large-scale comparison of these therapies—modified radical, lumpectomy plus radiation and lumpectomy alone—found no difference in survival rates. Local recurrence is much higher, however, for lumpectomy alone than for the other two therapies. Most surgeons prefer some form of mastectomy because that is the operation they were originally taught and have experience with.

Doctors may try to dissuade women who want radiation therapy (lumpectomy plus radiation) by telling them that it hasn't yet been proven over the long term. In fact, it is only relatively recently that lumpectomy with radiation has been studied in the United States. In Canada and Europe, doctors have statistics showing that mastectomy and lumpectomy plus radiation have equivalent survival rates for twenty-five years from diagnosis.

If preserving your breast is not a central issue for you or reconstruction is an option (see p. 623 for information on breast implants) or if the lump is large and your breast small, mastectomy may be your best choice.

If lumpectomy plus radiation seems a reasonable choice for you, it's necessary to look for an experienced physician and a hospital with the needed equipment and staff experienced in the technique.

Reconstruction After a Mastectomy

After a mastectomy your options are leaving your chest as it is, using an external prosthesis or having one of two types of surgical reconstruction. Some women find that doing nothing is the most comfortable choice, while others want to hide the fact that they have had surgery, usually because the visible reminder of their mastectomy provokes anxious reactions in themselves and others.

Nothing can restore the sexual and nursing function of your breast but you can have the appearance of a breast. Because of the mastectomy surgery, some women find that their chest area is numb; others find that their skin sensation returns.

With an external breast prosthesis, you may look as if nothing has changed as long as you have on your bra, which holds the prosthesis. The prosthesis may shift under your clothes, or feel hot or heavy, especially in warm weather. Obviously, when you take off your bra, the surgery will be apparent. Some women find this a disturbing reminder that they have had cancer. The advantage of an external prosthesis is that it does not require more surgery and thus eliminates the possibility of further complications.

You can have surgical reconstruction done at the time of the mastectomy or at any time later.

Although most women use an external prosthesis, some women find surgical reconstruction is very important for their psychological recovery. Some want immediate reconstruction, but if you feel that you have too many decisions all at once—trying to sort out your cancer therapy as well as determining the best method of reconstruction for you—don't rush into it. Take the time to decide what is best for you. A number of years ago doctors often felt that women who wanted reconstruction were inordinately vain. Now the situation is often reversed, with the doctor advising the woman that she will feel better if she has immediate reconstruction. In neither case are individual differences among women taken into account.

Surgical reconstruction involves either using an implant (see below) under the chest muscle or moving your own tissue, which involves moving muscle, fat, blood vessels, and adjacent tissue from your back, abdomen, or buttocks to your chest area. Sometimes an implant is used to supplement the tissue transfer operation. The tissue transfer operations are long and difficult. If you decide on this method, check your plastic surgeon's credentials carefully and speak to several women who have had the same operation you want with this particular surgeon. If well done, this is the best operation cosmetically. But if it is poorly executed, you may be disabled. If you are active, ask the surgeon if you will be able to continue to do the particular activities you do. Since muscle is taken from one place and moved to where it is no longer functional, you will lose strength at the original site. Also ask your surgeon in what percentage of cases for him or her the transferred tissue dies (necroses). If you are a smoker or diabetic, this operation is probably not appropriate for you since the blood vessels are narrower or damaged and healing is more difficult.

An implant is a rubberlike silicone envelope filled with saltwater (saline) or silicone gel, which may contain as much as 90 percent silicone oil. Tiny amounts of this oil leak from all gel-filled implants. Silicone oil was banned by the Food and Drug Administration in the 1960s for injection into humans unless done under FDA-approved clinical trials. New types of implants made of other materials may come on the market. The reconstruction process involves putting an empty silicone envelope under the chest muscle first. The doctor adds salt water incrementally over a few months through a tube from the implant to the outside of your skin until the skin is stretched to the desired size. Some implants are designed to remain after being filled and others, called expanders, need to be replaced after the skin is stretched. The replacement implants can be filled with salt water, silicone gel or perhaps some other material that the FDA will approve.

Although silicone envelope implants with various fillings, especially silicone gel, have been used since the early 1960s, the rates of complications are not well documented. Thus, this device is essentially experimental. The FDA formally acknowledged this in April 1992 when it decided that silicone gel–filled implants may be used only in tightly controlled studies for a limited number of women who want them for breast enlargement. All who want them for reconstruction will be able to get them, but their plastic surgeons are supposed to see them for follow-up visits regularly thereafter. The FDA is supposed to call for studies showing the safety and effectiveness of saline-filled implants sometime toward the end of 1992, after which the manufacturers have almost three years to produce the data.

The most common problem with implants is a hardening of the scar tissue around them. For many women this is not bothersome but others report pain and baseball-like breasts. When you have implants, you are likely to need further surgery to correct this hardening, cosmetic problems of improper placement or removal of broken implants. The implants last a variable amount of time. Some research indicates that the breakage rate increases dramatically after seven years. If the implant is salt water–filled and it breaks, it will deflate and your body will harmlessly absorb the salt water. All silicone gel–filled implants leak small amounts of silicone oil, even when intact. This silicone can be transported by the lymph system and possibly the bloodstream to other parts of your body. No one really knows yet what the consequences of this are, but anecdotal reports are disquieting. If a gel-filled implant breaks it should be removed as soon as possible in order to keep large quantities of silicone from leaving the breast area. Gel-filled implants, however, can rupture silently; that is, you will not notice any obvious change right away. No reliable method of detecting rupture in gel-filled implants exists now although researchers continue to investigate mammography and ultrasound. The most worrisome long-term complication is a possible development of various autoimmune diseases, such as scleroderma (see p. 637) or lupus (see p. 638), as a reaction to the silicone. The connection between silicone and autoimmune diseases is as yet unproven, but some animal studies and reports from rheumatologists create concern. Most cases of the development of autoimmune disease after implant use involve silicone gel–filled implants. A few women with saline-filled implants also report autoimmune symptoms which may be linked to the silicone envelope. In addition, animal studies and a recent human study associate silicone with various cancers. Although currently undocumented, the authors are hearing of a possible increase in cardiovascular problems with gel-filled implants. Symptoms include heart palpitations, severe headaches and stroke. For the many other possible complications, ask your surgeon for the *doctor* package insert that comes with the implant. You should also be given an informed consent statement that lists many of the complications. Ask the doctor about any medical terms you don't understand. Make sure you keep a copy of the manufacturer, model and lot number of the implant that comes on a sticker for attaching to your medical records. Then if there are problems with a particular implant you will know if it is the type you have. As with any implant, you should make a point of having regular medical checkups and be sure to inform your practitioners that you have implants.

With all types of reconstruction, after the surgeon creates the breast shape, you can also have darker skin grafted or a tattoo to make a nipple and areola. Sometimes, with one breast removed, the plastic surgeon will recommend that the remaining breast be reduced or changed in shape to more closely match the reconstructed breast. You need to investigate the possible problems that can result, including loss of nipple sensation, before you agree to do this.

All methods of reconstruction have problems. We need to demand better methods with fewer complications.

Chemotherapy and Hormone Therapy

These adjuvant treatments, viewed more and more as the key to increased survival, are usually given in addition to one of the primary local therapies listed above for local disease.

Chemotherapy

Chemotherapy uses injections or tablets of anticancer drugs to reach malignant cells that are circulating or lodged throughout the body. Some of the chemotherapy agents have very serious side effects; others are mild. Chemotherapy can cause early menopause, an important consideration for younger women who want to bear children. (See the discussion in the general cancer section, p. 613.)

Currently, only women up to the age of sixty have shown much improved survival (about 25 percent) with chemotherapy. Women over sixty have fared as well without chemotherapy as with it. Many researchers think this is because the right combination of drugs has not yet been found for postmenopausal women. This may be the case, but postmenopausal women taking this therapy should know that the effectiveness of chemotherapy is unproven for their situation and that they cannot necessarily expect the treatment to prolong their lives.

Therapy using a combination of drugs, especially the combinations called CMF (cyclophosphamide, methotrexate and 5-fluorouracil) and CAF (cyclophosphamide, adriamycin and 5-fluorouracil), have given better results than the use of single agents (one drug used alone).[21]

Tamoxifen, an antiestrogen drug, should be avoided (unless as part of a controlled study) by premenopausal women with ER (estrogen receptor) negative readings, as one large trial showed that such premenopausal women receiving it actually had decreased survival times.[22]

How soon chemotherapy should begin and how long it should continue are still unknown. Some evidence indicates that any benefit that occurs happens early on. This evidence supports early chemotherapy after diagnosis and casts doubt on long courses of treatment.

Hormone Therapy

The purpose of hormone therapy is to repress or eliminate estrogen's effect on breast tumor growth. It is useful for most women with estrogen-dependent cancers (also called ER + or estrogen positive, estrogen-rich or high-estrogen) and for a few women (approximately 10 percent) with ER − cancers. Both surgery and drugs are used in hormone therapy.

- *Drugs.* The antiestrogen drugs used most frequently, tamoxifen and megestrol (a progesterone), often induce an early and sometimes permanent menopause. Some doctors include these drugs as part of chemotherapy, so you may not know that you are receiving them unless you ask.
- *Surgery. All the following are considered outmoded*, as drugs can generally produce the same effects without the major problems associated with surgery. Some doctors try surgery when drugs and other treatments have not been successful:

  An *oophorectomy* (surgical removal of the ovaries) is usually done only after chemical hormone therapy has been tried, but it is of almost no value in postmenopausal women or women under thirty-five. It sometimes helps in premenopausal women over age thirty-five.

  Adrenalectomy (removal of the adrenals) or *hypothalectomy* (removal of the hypothalamus) are other techniques to limit estrogen production.

Treatment Options for Metastatic Disease (Stage IV)

Once the cancer has metastasized, there is no known cure. All the above treatments are used in attempts to control the disease and prolong life. For example, radiation and chemotherapy may be used to relieve pain and shrink tumors. Mastectomy is probably unnecessary unless the primary tumor is very large. A few women live beyond five or ten years with metastatic cancer.

What Are Your Chances? (The Prognosis of Breast Cancer)

Overall, the prognosis for breast cancer is not very encouraging. The mortality (death) rates presented in the literature are confusing. One group of researchers reports that one-third of women who get breast cancer die from it. This figure is based on the data reported to health authorities that show that each year approximately 175,000 new cases of breast cancer are diagnosed while about 45,000 women die from the disease. Studies that follow the course of breast cancer from diagnosis to death (whether from cancer or other causes) of a large number of individual women find that almost 80 percent of women who develop breast cancer eventually die from it or with it. This rate has not changed significantly since the 1930s. However, some women live with the disease for as long as twenty or thirty years; although they do eventually die of breast cancer, their life spans have not been shortened. Many physicians no longer speak in terms of cure. Instead they refer to long-term remission or survival rates. According to this view, breast cancer, like diabetes or other chronic diseases, may be controlled but not yet cured.

Research has found that some groups of women do better than others. You are more likely to be among those with long-term survival if

1. You have no malignant lymph nodes. This is the most important single predictor found so far (see Histological Stages, p. 619).

2. Your cancer is estrogen dependent (has high levels of estrogen receptors). These ER-high (also called *positive*) cancers tend to have fewer or later recurrences no matter what type of treatment is used, although the difference is only 6 to 8 percent. ER-high cancer is more common in postmenopausal women.

3. You have one of the following types of cancer and no positive nodes. These cancer cell types tend to grow and metastasize very slowly. They account for about 20 percent of all breast cancers.

- Adenoid cystic carcinoma.
- Colloid carcinoma.
- Medullary carcinoma.
- Papillary carcinoma.
- Tubular carcinoma.

4. Your tumor cells are highly differentiated; that is, they retain the characteristics of normal breast cells rather than the embryonic appearance of advanced cancer cells.

Even with these indicators, it is difficult to make predictions for any specific woman. Some

ONGOING STUDIES

The NCI is conducting a number of high-priority clinical trials that you may be interested in joining. To find out more about which trials are ongoing, which trials are still open to new participants and how you might benefit, contact the NCI Cancer Information Service: (800) 4-CANCER.

Several trials ongoing in the early 1990s include

1. Tamoxifen with lumpectomy and radiation for noninvasive breast cancer. This study will "evaluate whether the drug tamoxifen can prevent the occurrence of invasive breast cancer in both the same and the opposite breast in women treated by lumpectomy and radiation therapy for [noninvasive] cancer that is contained within the duct of the glandular portion of the breast."[23]

2. Evaluation of high-dose consolidation chemotherapy with autologous bone marrow transplantation for Stage II or III breast cancer. "This study compares standard adjuvant chemotherapy (treatment using anticancer drugs following surgery) versus standard chemotherapy with high-dose chemotherapy and autologous bone marrow transplantation (ABMT) in patients with Stage II or Stage III breast cancer. ABMT involves taking bone marrow from the patient before high-dose chemotherapy and reinfusing it into the patient after treatment."[24] (This procedure is followed because the high-dose chemotherapy is potentially lethal to the blood-forming cells of the bone marrow.)

3. High-dose chemotherapy with autologous bone marrow transplantation for Stage II or III breast cancer. The purpose of this study is to "determine whether the high-dose chemotherapy treatment following standard chemotherapy treatment can delay or prevent recurrence and prolong survival of patients with primary breast cancer whose breast tumor and axillary lymph nodes have been removed."[25]

women (about 15 percent) with very good prognoses die quickly from the disease, whereas a few (about 7 to 8 percent) of those whose conditions have been called terminal recover and live normal life spans. There are still many unknown factors. It may well be that an individual's particular immune system and general health as well as her emotional attitude may be as important as or more important than the treatment chosen.

It is estimated that more than 1.5 million women will face a diagnosis of breast cancer during the 1990s. Although all cancers are frightening, breast cancer seems to hold the most terror for us as women. The available information is confusing and the experts often disagree. This makes it even more important that we become active participants in all stages of detection, treatment and decision making. The information in this section is necessarily brief. You owe it to yourself to take the time to research all the available options and get additional opinions. If you have not read it already, we recommend turning to the general section on cancer next. It has more information on treatments (including alternatives to the accepted trio of surgery, radiation and chemotherapy). In this section, we have tried to make definite recommendations wherever possible, but so many areas are still unsettled that we can only indicate the issues involved and urge you to find out what new data have become available since the publication of this book.

WITHOUT

Without breasts
a woman's heart
rounds and softens her body,
bears her milk.

Without hair
a woman can fully
receive sunlight,
is crowned with the smoothness
of her scalp.

Without legs
a woman moves
with song and thought.

Without ears
she hears
what words
obscure.

Without eyes
she is not limited
by the confusion
of objects, color.

Without uterus, ovaries,
she spawns wisdom
with the turn of the moon.

Without her life's breath
a woman becomes earth,
the bearer of herb and seed,
rock and ground root.

ELANA KLUGMAN

GYNECOLOGICAL CANCERS

Invasive Cancer of the Cervix

If severely abnormal cells have spread beyond the upper tissue layer (surface epithelium) of your cervix into the underlying connective tissues, you have invasive cervical cancer. A Pap smear followed by a biopsy can determine this. At first the spread is very shallow and may not involve the lymph or blood systems. In its early stages, cervical cancer is 100 percent curable.

Most physicians recommend a hysterectomy (removal of the uterus) with close follow-up. If the cancer has spread into the lymph or blood system, physicians usually suggest radiation or hysterectomy/oophorectomy. (Chemotherapy is not as effective as local radiation.) Sometimes a combination of the two is used.

Radiation treatment is given in two ways. If the tumor is large, you will be given external radiation daily over a period of several weeks. During treatment you will have to make daily trips to the medical center or hospital, which, depending on how far away you live, can be exhausting and cause you considerable inconvenience. This is a time to ask family and friends to help with your other commitments and as traveling company and support. Negative effects of the radiation treatment include diarrhea, skin changes, rectal bleeding and fatigue. Because each person reacts to radiation differently, the amount may have to be increased or decreased depending on your response. The negative effects of the radiation therapy are thought to be short-lived. When the radiation treatment has reduced the size of the growth, internal radioactive materials are placed inside your uterus or in the upper portion of your vagina. You will be hospitalized and given general anesthesia for this procedure. The implants are left inside your body from one to three days while you are in the hospital. This type of treatment directs a greater amount of radiation to a smaller area. Radiation treatment for early invasive cancer has a 60 to 90 percent survival rate, depending on the size of the tumor and the amount of spread. (See pp. 609–10 for a general discussion of cancer and survival rates.)

Surgical treatment for invasive cancer usually involves a radical hysterectomy.

You should be involved in your treatment and have the final say in all decisions concerning your cancer. If you have any doubts about treatments recommended by your physician, get a second and third opinion if you can.

Ovarian Cancer

Ovarian cancer affects 20,700 new women a year in the United States. The incidence increases with age, with a high percentage of cases found in postmenopausal women. The exact causes are still unknown, but researchers have suggested possible risk factors: a family history of ovarian cancer; few or no pregnancies; a history of breast, colorectal or endometrial cancer; exposure to industrial products, including asbestos, or to high levels of radiation; the use of talcum powder in the genital area; a diet high in fat and the use of estrogens other than the birth control pill. In fact, oral contraceptive use and multiple pregnancies may exert a protective effect.*

Diagnosis

Symptoms are not always present with ovarian cancer. However, there are warning signs that can be vague and are frequently dismissed as "stress" or "nerves." Persistent symptoms indicate the need for a thorough physical evaluation for ovarian cancer. Symptoms may include indigestion, gas, constipation or diarrhea, loss of appetite or weight, a feeling of fullness, lower abdominal discomfort or pain, frequent urination, fatigue, backache, nausea, vomiting, nonmenstrual vaginal bleeding, enlargement or bloating of the abdomen or an unusual growth or lump.

The process of diagnosing ovarian cancer begins with a review of symptoms; the medical and family history; a complete physical checkup, including a pelvic and rectal exam;† and blood tests, especially the tumor marker, CA-125. Other diagnostic tests include pelvic and transvaginal ultrasound, CT or CAT scan (computerized tomography), magnetic resonance imaging (MRI) and surgery, which is the only conclusive diagnostic tool. (For more information, see Resources.)

Medical Treatments

Treatment depends on the stage of the disease at the time of diagnosis, the type of cells that make up the tumor and how fast the cancer is growing. Current medical options for treating ovarian cancer include surgery, chemotherapy and/or radiation therapy. Biological therapies are also now available. These therapies are evolving as a result of research, which continues to offer hope for improving the outcome of treatment for women with

ovarian cancer. (See Introduction to Cancer, p. 609, and Resources for more on treatments.)

Cancer of the Uterus

Cancer of the lining of the uterus (endometrial cancer) is the most common pelvic cancer, affecting 14 out of every 10,000 women yearly. Most women who develop this cancer are past menopause and in their fifties; 10 percent are still menstruating. If you are very heavy; if you have diabetes, high blood pressure or a hormone imbalance that combines high estrogen levels with infrequent ovulation or if you take synthetic estrogen, your risk of developing uterine cancer is increased. During the early 1970s there was a sharp rise in the incidence of uterine cancer due to increased use of ERT to relieve symptoms of menopause (see pp. 528–32). Bleeding after menopause is the most common symptom of uterine cancer. For women who are still menstruating, increased menstrual flow and bleeding between periods may be the only symptoms. Unfortunately, the Pap smear is unreliable in detecting the abnormal cells of uterine cancer. If you are premenopausal, your practitioner may suggest a D and C as the first step because it not only screens for cancer but frequently relieves abnormal bleeding from a variety of less serious causes. If you are postmenopausal, you will probably have an aspiration or endometrial biopsy (an office procedure), and if the biopsy is not conclusive, your practitioner may suggest a D and C. Before agreeing to a D and C, however, make sure that you have both considered the risks and discussed alternatives for diagnosis and treatment of abnormal bleeding (see p. 596).

Prevention and Self-Help Treatments

Because endometrial cancer appears to be influenced by factors such as obesity, hypertension or diabetes, controlling these conditions with self-help methods may prevent this type of cancer from developing or spreading.

Medical Treatments

Medical treatment for uterine cancer includes surgery, radiation and chemotherapy. There is wide disagreement about which is best. Outside the United States radiation is used frequently with good results. In this country radical hysterectomy is the most common treatment, sometimes with follow-up radiation after surgery if the tumor was large, if spread to lymph nodes was suspected or if the cellular changes were more excessive than usual. If you should have a return of the cancer after one of the above treatments, progesterone treatments may help slow its spread.

---

*Removal of the ovaries has been proposed as an option to protect women against ovarian cancer. Although the benefit of prophylactic oophorectomy has not yet been established, some specialists do suggest this surgery for high-risk women, who have two or more close blood relatives with ovarian cancer. Due to the risks and long-term side effects, this procedure should be considered with caution (see Hysterectomy and Oophorectomy, p. 598).

†A Pap smear should be part of the pelvic exam. It may occasionally reveal malignant ovarian cells, but it is not a reliable test for ovarian cancer.

When uterine cancer is found early, the success rate of conventional treatments is very high.

DIABETES

Diabetes, a common chronic metabolic disorder more prevalent among women than men, changes the way our bodies break down and use starches and sugars (glucose). Normally insulin, a hormone produced in the pancreas, helps to store glucose in a form that can later be released for energy.

Eighty to ninety percent of diabetes is non-insulin-dependent diabetes mellitus (NIDDM), in which the pancreas produces insulin, but not enough to overcome the insulin resistance that characterizes this type of diabetes. Formerly called *maturity-onset diabetes*, NIDDM most often occurs in people over forty who are very heavy.

NIDDM symptoms usually develop slowly and may include weakness, headache, a vaguely sick feeling, extra hunger and thirst, more frequent urination, itching and minor skin or vaginal infections. Hypoglycemic pills, which increase insulin secretion from the pancreas, or insulin is used for people with NIDDM who cannot stay on a strict diet or for whom diet alone does not lower glucose to an acceptable level.

Less common is *insulin-dependent diabetes mellitus* (IDDM), where an absolute deficiency of insulin requires replacement by daily injections of insulin. Formerly called *juvenile-onset diabetes*, IDDM usually develops in childhood or early adulthood and accounts for less than 10 percent of diabetes. It is characterized by severe and rapidly developing symptoms, which include greatly increased hunger, excessive thirst and urination and a sudden, dramatic loss of weight. People with IDDM may face coma or death from either inadequate insulin replacement (hyperglycemia and/or ketoacidosis) or relatively too much insulin (hypoglycemia—low blood sugar), the major risk of insulin therapy.

A third form of diabetes that is specific to women is called *gestational diabetes mellitus* (GDM). It is similar to NIDDM, develops in 3 percent of previously nondiabetic women during the last trimester of pregnancy and disappears after delivery. Diagnosis is made with an oral glucose tolerance test (OGTT) between weeks 24 and 28 of pregnancy. The OGTT is recommended for all pregnant women. As many as one-half of the women with GDM will redevelop diabetes later in life.

You can control all types of diabetes through factors such as food intake, exercise, body weight, blood sugar monitoring and, where necessary, medication. All of these can affect your blood sugar level. More intensive therapy, especially with IDDM, generally results in closer to normal blood sugar levels.

The National Institutes of Health is conducting research to determine if intensive treatment, aimed at maintaining normal blood sugar levels, can prevent or lessen the long-term complications of IDDM. These complications include disease of the retina that can result in blindness (diabetic retinopathy), kidney disease that can result in kidney failure (diabetic nephropathy), disease of the nervous system (diabetic neuropathy) and peripheral and cardiovascular disease.

No one fully understands the underlying causes of IDDM and NIDDM, but both have hereditary components. In addition, NIDDM seems to be closely associated with being overweight and often disappears with weight loss. Other factors, including decreased exercise, are associated with an increased risk of developing NIDDM.

Diagnosis

Most cases of IDDM are readily evident with the appearance of dramatic symptoms accompanied by an elevated blood glucose. NIDDM may not have significant symptoms and is sometimes diagnosed on the basis of a routine blood test showing abnormally high levels of sugar. Although an abnormal fasting blood sugar level is often sufficient to diagnose NIDDM, a glucose tolerance test, which measures blood sugar levels before and after you drink a large quantity of glucose, may be necessary.

Treatment and Self-Management

Although there is no cure for diabetes, people with diabetes are able to live healthy and productive lives. The key is to eat the right amount and kinds of food, exercise regularly, maintain your weight in proportion to your height and body type and, when necessary, administer medication and monitor blood sugar. Blood glucose test strips purchased over the counter enable you to monitor your own blood sugar levels. The majority of people with NIDDM can control the disease through diet and exercise alone, whereas people with IDDM must also take an active role in administering insulin and monitoring their blood glucose levels.

Prevention and Self-Help

The currently recommended diabetic diet is a balance of carbohydrates, fat and protein that encourages high fiber and low fat. For the majority of people with NIDDM who are overweight, weight loss is the primary dietary goal. People with IDDM must aim for consistent and regular dietary intake. Food exchange lists can help you with substituting one type of carbohydrate, fat or protein for another.

Sugar, often identified as the one ingredient that diabetics must avoid, is actually a category of sweeteners that includes barley malt, brown sugar, corn syrup, dextrose, fructose, honey, maltose, molasses and even sorbitol. Avoid too much simple or refined sugar, because it will raise blood glucose levels. Keeping sugar intake low, however, is no guarantee that glucose levels will remain low. If insulin is not present to metabolize carbohydrates, glucose levels will rise and will "spill" into the urine.

The basic diabetic diet is one of the healthiest since it emphasizes low fat, low cholesterol and high fiber. It is important for people using insulin to eat consistent and regular meals in order to avoid large fluctuations in blood glucose. If the blood glucose level drops too low, people may develop hypoglycemia, which can result in sweating, tremulousness, lightheadedness, lack of concentration or, if severe, seizures or loss of consciousness.

People using insulin must carry a ready supply of carbohydrate, preferably orange or apple juice or glucose tablets in case food is not readily available. In this way, they are prepared for emergencies that could cause considerable anxiety or harm. Fad diets will, in general, cause problems.

Since eating is so much a part of our interactions with other people whether it be family, friends or colleagues, it is important to communicate your food needs to the people around you if you have diabetes. They need to understand why you are particular about what and when you eat.

Regular exercise, such as walking, jogging or yoga, further reduces the body's need for insulin and therefore helps to prevent NIDDM as well as control diabetes. Exercise can also help with weight loss, which in turn decreases the amount of insulin needed to metabolize carbohydrates. A consistent exercise routine is most beneficial.

Wear an ID bracelet, such as Medic Alert, that states you have diabetes and provides a telephone number for use in an emergency. In the event you are not able to speak for yourself, this will identify your medical condition.

If you have IDDM, teach family members and friends how to help you if you show signs of low blood sugar. Always carry juice, glucose tablets or hard candy with you for emergency situations when your blood sugar level drops below normal. It is also helpful to carry blood-testing strips with you to determine your blood sugar level. These are simple ways to avoid the potentially life-threatening situation of being immobilized by low blood sugar.

Diabetes can lead to complications over time, so it is important to schedule regular follow-up visits with practitioners, including ophthalmologists and dieticians. This enables you to get prompt attention for any complications that develop.

Before I found out I had diabetes at the age of twenty-four, I never had a serious illness or a major operation. So I was stunned to think that my "perfect" body was "falling apart" in my youth. But I quickly realized how lucky I was that diabetes could be diagnosed and controlled through medication, food intake and exercise.

Now twenty-two years later, I am in the best of health probably because health care and feeling well top my priorities. Diabetes, rather than dominating my life, is my reason for achieving good health.

HYPERTENSION, HEART DISEASES AND CIRCULATORY DISEASES

Hypertension, or high blood pressure, and *atherosclerosis* (sometimes called *hardening of the arteries*) are diseases that increase women's risk of heart disease and stroke, the leading causes of death in women over age fifty. Despite the importance of these diseases to women, little research included women until very recently. During the past few years, medical scientists have discovered many differences in the way women and men are treated for heart disease. For example, women are referred for coronary bypass surgery at a later stage of disease than men, and this may be what accounts for their higher death rate from this surgery. Women also receive less complete diagnostic workups and are less likely than men to receive coronary bypass surgery. Among women who have had heart attacks, researchers have found women had many more risk factors and suffered more chest pain before their heart attack than men but are only about half as likely to have had a cardiac catheterization to assess their heart disease. Dr. Bernadine Healy, appointed director of the National Institutes of Health in 1991, believes that the new research provides evidence of sex bias in the management of coronary heart disease. What is unclear is whether women are undertreated or men overtreated. Although less attention is focused on the lack of research on hypertension and atherosclerosis in women, these underlying disease conditions are equally ignored by medical researchers.

Hypertension

Hypertension (high blood pressure) is sometimes called "the silent killer" because it is often symptomless and, when untreated, can lead to heart disease and strokes, the leading killers of both men and women in the United States. Untreated, it can also affect the brain and eyes and cause serious problems during pregnancy.

About 20 percent of women of all ages in this country develop hypertension at some point in their lives. (Even children may do so.) No one yet knows how hypertension in women thirty-five and under affects life expectancy, an increasingly important question as larger numbers of women who are or have been taking oral contraceptives move into this age range. (About 25 percent of all women who use oral contraceptives develop hypertension.) In addition, blood pressure tends to rise naturally with age.

Women of color, especially blacks, have a higher incidence of hypertension than white women. This is due to a combination of environmental, behavioral, dietary, stress and possibly genetic factors.

Symptoms

Severe cases of hypertension may be accompanied by warning symptoms such as headache, dizziness, fainting spells, ringing in the ears and nosebleeds. However, most women have no symptoms of hypertension, so periodic blood pressure readings are important to ensure detection of hypertension in the early stages.

Cause

Approximately 5 percent of all cases of high blood pressure are caused by glandular or hormonal abnormalities. But in the other 95 percent, no single obvious cause is found. This is called *essential hypertension*. Causes other than oral contraceptives and smoking are still being investigated, including diet, properties of the water supply, person's size, stress, behavioral patterns and heredity. Many of these factors may interact to cause hypertension.

Diet, and excess salt intake in particular, is thought to play a key role in causing hypertension. The average American diet contains ten to fifteen grams of sodium a day (about five to ten times as much salt as our bodies need). Meat and dairy products contain a fair amount of salt naturally, and canned and processed foods, fast foods, snacks and soft drinks have large amounts of salt added during processing.

Cadmium, a trace element found in white-flour products and in many water supplies, has been strongly linked to hypertension. Hypertension is much more common in areas where water is soft.

Research shows that those of us who are very overweight are at increased risk for developing hypertension. The stress associated with being fat in a "thin" society may also be an important factor. Although some studies show that losing weight can be effective in controlling hyperten-

sion, others indicate that regular exercise is much more important than the amount of weight loss.

Stress is also linked to hypertension. When we are under pressure or tense, blood pressure, breathing rate and heartbeat all tend to increase. When our lives are continually stressful, we have a greater chance of developing high blood pressure.

Finally, those of us with a family history of hypertension are at somewhat greater risk.

Diagnosis

Blood pressure is described by two numbers (for example, 120/70). The top number is the systolic pressure (the force of the blood in the arteries when the heart is pumping blood out). The bottom number is the diastolic pressure (the force of the blood in the arteries when the heart is filling with blood). In general, a systolic pressure of above 140 or a diastolic pressure above 90 is considered a sign of hypertension.

Blood pressure varies with the time of day, activity and stress. Only a *consistent* elevation of the blood pressure is considered hypertension. At least three elevated blood pressure readings, taken days or weeks apart, should be obtained before hypertension is diagnosed and treated. Some researchers think that a diagnosis of mild or borderline hypertension should be delayed until consistent readings have been obtained over a period of years, since slightly elevated blood pressures fall by themselves within a few years in a majority of cases. Also, since women normally have higher blood pressure than men, the distinction between normal and borderline hypertension is difficult to interpret. For example, it is normal for blood pressure to rise during pregnancy (temporarily) and after menopause and to fluctuate more as part of the aging process.

Because the stress related to a medical exam or procedure may raise blood pressure, make an effort to check your blood pressure when you are not anxious—perhaps at home, at work or at a neighborhood health center. Large women should be sure to use a cuff big enough to fit around the arm; otherwise they may get a false inflated reading. Taking blood pressure is an easy skill to learn. (Kits with stethoscope and blood pressure cuffs are available in drugstores and many discount and department stores.) Increasingly, libraries, senior centers and shopping centers are also providing this screening service, but *don't* rely on coin-operated machines, which can give false readings.

Prevention and Self-Help Treatments

You can often prevent hypertension in a number of simple ways and also lower mildly raised blood pressure—enough, in many cases, to eliminate the need for potentially risky drug treatments.

1. Diet is probably the single most important factor in preventing and treating mild hypertension. Gradually restrict salt intake by avoiding processed foods and eliminating salt during cooking and at the table. Replace white flour with whole grains whenever possible and make sure to include enough protein, potassium and calcium in your diet (see Chapter 2, "Food"). Eating garlic can also help to prevent or reduce slightly elevated blood pressure. Keep alcohol consumption down to two ounces a day or less. Some people also recommend vitamin B and potassium supplements to help the body excrete excess fluids and sodium.

2. Avoid smoking. Studies show smoking contributes to heart disease.

3. Get together with people in your community to investigate the water supply. If you find that it contains cadmium, try to eat less of this trace mineral in foods (especially white-flour products).

4. Avoid combination oral contraceptives and other estrogens. If you do take the Pill, insist on finding out your blood pressure both before and a few months *after* starting. If it is initially high, don't take the Pill; if it rises, switch to another contraceptive.

5. Regular aerobic exercise (such as fast walking, jogging or bicycling) often brings elevated pressures down to normal.

6. Losing weight if you are very large can prevent or lower high blood pressure. It is most effective in conjunction with exercise. Crash dieting, however, is *not* recommended.

7. Try to reduce stress in your life. Biofeedback, meditation and relaxation therapies may help.

Medical Treatments

When the above methods do not work or hypertension becomes severe, you may need drugs. Diuretics (which eliminate water from the tissues) are the most commonly used. Diuretics can have side effects that lead to digestive disorders and exhaustion. They may also affect cholesterol and blood sugar levels. Newer drugs include beta-blockers, angiotensin inhibitors and calcium channel blockers. These drugs reduce the constriction of the arteries, the amount of blood pumped from the heart, or relax the blood vessels. Often a combination of drugs is used. (See p. 59 for guidelines in taking drugs.) Hypertension drugs treat only the symptoms of the disease; they do not cure it. You will probably have to take medication for life. Be cautious when physicians recommend drug therapy without attempting less risky methods first. If your hypertension is severe, you will have to evaluate the risk of taking medication against the benefits of preventing a crippling or life-threatening stroke.*

Heart Diseases and Circulatory Diseases

Most people typically think of men, not women, as having heart attacks. Most research on the subject, therefore, has been on men. Although men do suffer more heart attacks than women, heart disease is the most frequent cause of death in women over the age of fifty. In addition, a greater percentage of women who have heart attacks die from them. In the Framingham heart study, one of the few longitudinal studies of heart disease in women, 45 percent of the women with symptomatic heart attacks died within one year compared to only 10 percent of the men. Stroke remains the third most common cause of death in the United States. Women have twice as many strokes as men and black women have a 43 percent higher death rate from stroke than white women. Stroke is directly related to high blood pressure, which becomes much more common after menopause and is more chronic among women.

What Are These Diseases?

Many forms of heart and circulatory diseases are related to atherosclerosis, a slowly developing disease process in which the passageway through the arteries becomes narrowed and roughened by fatty deposits called *plaques*. In the most common type of heart disease, called *coronary artery disease* or *ischemic heart disease*, the development of plaque blocks one or more of the arteries that supply the heart muscle with blood. When sufficient blood can no longer reach the heart, part of the heart dies from lack of oxygen and other nutrients. This is a "heart attack," or what physicians call a *myocardial infarction* (MI), *coronary thrombosis* or *coronary occlusion*. When the artery blockage is partial it may cause chest pain, a condition referred to as *angina*.

Atherosclerosis can also lead to a narrowing of the blood vessels that supply blood to the brain. Called a *stroke*, or *cerebral hemorrhage*, this leads to the death of that part of the brain.

Less common types of circulatory disease are congenital heart disease, phlebitis, hypertrophic disease, valvular heart disease and cardiomyopathy. The causes are similar for all and may lead to congestive heart failure or arrhythmia (irregular heartbeats).

---

*Most doctors have little interest in nondrug approaches. However, studies comparing people treated by drugs with others treated by diet alone do show comparable effects and a longer life span among the diet-treated group.

Who Is at Risk?

The more of the following risk factors a person has, the more likely she/he is to develop atherosclerosis and subsequent heart disease, circulatory problems or stroke. The first four (in that order) are the best-established risk factors at present.

- Over age fifty (heart attack is uncommon in women under the age of fifty).
- High blood pressure (hypertension).
- Smoking.
- Elevated serum (blood) cholesterol.
- Diabetes.
- Taking oral contraceptives (particularly if the woman also smokes) (see Chapter 13, "Birth Control").
- A family history of coronary artery disease *and* a husband with a history of heart attack.
- Hysterectomy before age forty-five (see p. 600).
- Certain "personality" factors (habitual impatience, hostility, high competitive drive) and stress.

Prevention

Considering the seriousness of these diseases, we are disturbed that so few resources are directed toward prevention as compared to emergency care and treatment. We are also concerned that very little is known about how to prevent heart disease and stroke specifically for women. The "experts" have assumed until very recently that what is good for men must be good for women, too. Reducing the risk of heart disease and stroke is very similar to risk reduction for hypertension. Consider rethinking your current health practices in the following areas.

1. *Smoking.* The more you smoke, the more likely you are to have a heart attack. Women smokers who take oral contraceptives have a 40 percent increase in risk of developing cardiovascular disease. We urge you to give up smoking. For particulars on women and smoking, see Chapter 3, "Alcohol, Mood-Altering Drugs and Smoking."

2. *Diet.* Diet is an important factor in preventing heart disease, if it reduces "bad cholesterol," low-density lipoproteins (LDLs) and increases "good" high-density lipoproteins (HDLs). LDL is associated with coronary heart disease risk, whereas HDLs appear to protect against heart disease in men in whom it has been studied. The relationship between diet and LDLs and HDLs is not yet fully understood, but eating saturated fats tends to raise LDLs so cutting back on these fats (see p. 35 in Chapter 2, "Food") may help prevent heart disease. However, the food industry has been capitalizing on the low-cholesterol issue by promoting highly processed hydrogenated foodstuffs as beneficial because they are polyunsaturated. Many scientists now question the value of eating more polyunsaturates and are increasingly concerned about the negative health effects of highly processed foods.

Current medical advice to avoid foods high in cholesterol and saturated fats may pose problems for women. In an effort to reduce fat intake, some women may eliminate or cut back on dairy products, which may be their main source of calcium. (Inadequate calcium is a factor in the development of osteoporosis and hypertension.) No prevention study has included women, a serious flaw considering that hormonal factors are believed to affect the ways in which dietary cholesterol is converted into serum cholesterol, which increases the risk of heart disease.

3. *High blood pressure.* Preventing or treating high blood pressure (see p. 630) will reduce the risk of both heart attack and stroke.

4. *Exercise.* Regular exercise is believed to reduce the risk of heart attack, can definitely lower blood pressure and, in some cases, raises beneficial HDL cholesterol levels (see Chapter 4, "Women in Motion"). Women who are sedentary and get little physical activity have three times the risk of developing heart disease than those who exercise even moderately three days a week.

5. *Weight.* Excess weight itself does not directly affect the heart, but it may increase blood pressure, cholesterol and blood sugar levels, which increases the risk of heart disease and stroke. A combination of general weight reduction and exercise can be an important strategy for reducing the risk of cardiovascular and circulatory disease in some women.

6. *Oral contraceptives.* Women over forty who use oral contraceptives have five times the risk of heart attack and seven times the risk of stroke. If you have other risk factors, including a family history of cardiovascular disease, carefully consider your decision to use oral contraceptives.

7. *Estrogen replacement therapy.* Controversy continues over the benefits of ERT for preventing heart disease. There is speculation that women's rate of heart disease rises rapidly after menopause when women lose the protective effect of estrogen. Current thinking is that giving estrogens after menopause decreases the LDL level and increases the HDL level, increasing the body's ability to cleanse itself of cholesterol that could be deposited in arteries. Some cautious supporters of estrogen note that there has not been adequate surveillance of vascular disease in women to assess the real effects.

8. *Stress reduction.* The effects of work-related stress on heart disease in women have not been researched adequately, but it is theorized that multiple role demands on women may play a role in heart disease. All stress is implicated in cardiovascular disease. Changing one's life circum-

stances may not always be possible, but women can often moderate the effects by using stress reduction techniques.

9. *Regular medical examinations.* Dr. Marianne J. Legato, a cardiac researcher and specialist on women and heart disease, recommends that women have an annual physical examination in part to get to know their doctor well enough to feel comfortable calling and reporting possible symptoms of heart disease. In addition to checking blood pressure, she suggests that an annual electrocardiogram is critical to detect silent heart attack; over one-third of all heart attacks in women go unreported. Researchers have noted, however, that even when heart disease symptoms are detected by noninvasive diagnostic procedures, doctors are less likely to refer women than men for follow-up diagnostic procedures. Both women and health providers need to alter their perception of the seriousness of cardiovascular disease symptoms in women.

Heart Attack

Recognizing the Signs of Heart Attack

Unfortunately, the first sign of heart disease can be sudden death from heart attack, especially for women. One-fourth of all people who have heart attacks had no previous warning or knowledge of heart disease, and 60 percent of heart-attack deaths occur before the person reaches the hospital.

Some describe the pain as viselike or constricting, like a rope being pulled around their chest. Others describe the pain as feeling like a heavy weight crushing their chest. It is useful to know that chest pain can also come from conditions other than heart attack.* Heart pains that occur with exertion but go away with rest indicate angina, a condition that may not be immediately life-threatening but should be evaluated by a physician.

Getting Help

If you or anyone you are with experiences heart-attack symptoms, CALL A PHYSICAN OR AMBULANCE OR GO TO A HOSPITAL IMMEDIATELY. DO NOT WAIT TO SEE IF THE SYMPTOMS GO AWAY! As women, we may be afraid of being seen as "hysterical" or feel that we

---

*Chest pain can also come from muscles in the chest, the lungs, the diaphragm, spine or organs in the upper abdomen. Often it is difficult even for practitioners to determine the pain's precise origin. Shooting pains that last a few seconds are common in young people, and a "catching" sensation at the end of a deep breath does not need attention. Chest-wall pain, rarely present at the same time as a heart attack, can often be identified by pressing a finger on the spot, which increases the pain. Hyperventilation (too rapid breathing that changes the carbon dioxide balance in the blood) can cause both dizziness and chest pain.

SYMPTOMS OF HEART ATTACK

Do you have *one or more* of the following for more than two minutes:

1. Chest pain and shortness of breath?

2. Irregular pulse?

3. Sweating, dizziness or faintness?

4. Severe pain in your jaw, neck, shoulder or arm?

5. Severe feelings of indigestion that do not go away with an antacid or burping?

If so, seek medical attention immediately.

---

will be ridiculed for going to the hospital unless we have something "really serious." To ignore heart-attack symptoms is to risk our lives.

Most cities have ambulances staffed by paramedics who are trained to administer cardiopulmonary resuscitation (CPR)* and to monitor the heart rate and rhythm and administer intravenous drugs on the order of physicians with whom they are in contact by radio. It is important to keep calm. Medical personnel often give the person an analgesic drug such as morphine to induce relaxation and relieve chest pain. Oxygen may also be given.

Most urban hospitals have special coronary care units where sudden changes in the rhythm of the heart can be detected immediately and treated, reducing both damage to the heart and the likelihood of death. Every effort should be made to seek emergency medical care from a well-equipped and well-staffed hospital.

Treatments

For women who have had a heart attack or who have been diagnosed as having coronary artery disease or angina, there are two approaches to treatment: medical and surgical. Within the medical and scientific communities, there is considerable controversy over the relative effectiveness of these two approaches.

Coronary bypass surgery, popular in recent years, is done primarily to relieve chest pain. Coronary bypass surgery involves removing a vein from the leg or a mammary artery and attaching it to the coronary artery to "bypass" the obstructed area. Some people experience dramatic relief of pain and can lead physically active lives

---

*CPR is an emergency procedure combining mouth-to-mouth resuscitation and closed-chest heart massage. In some U.S. cities, CPR is credited with saving as many as 200 lives a year. To learn CPR, call your local chapter of the American Red Cross or American Heart Association.

after surgery. There is no evidence, however, that surgery increases life expectancy.* Nonetheless, over 100,000 procedures are done each year in the United States, at a cost of over $1.5 billion.

Several excellent studies have shown that more conservative treatment is equal or superior to bypass surgery for most people.† This medical approach to treatment focuses on *heart conditioning*—a program of progressively more strenuous exercise combined with a low-fat diet, relaxation techniques and drug therapy. Blood pressure is lowered and participants are urged to stop smoking. (For some participants, any exercise at all is dangerous.)

Before having bypass surgery, even for seemingly intractable pain, a woman may want to consult with a cardiologist who specializes in the *medical* treatment of heart disease. If your family doctor or a clinic refers you to a heart surgeon who advises surgery, try to get a second opinion from a medically oriented cardiologist who is not part of your surgeon's immediate colleague network. This will ensure that you get a truly different treatment perspective. A final note of caution: The death rates for heart surgery vary enormously from hospital to hospital. Generally, well-known university-affiliated medical centers with specialized coronary surgery teams have the best records. The more frequently the teams operate, the less often their patients die. *Never consider undergoing bypass surgery at a hospital where fewer than 200 bypass operations are performed each year* (see the section on surgery, pp. 568–69).

Stroke

Because high blood pressure is easily detectable, stroke is among the most preventable of the causes of sudden death. Yet true prevention, as described above, must begin *before* high blood pressure appears.

Strokes may be very mild, so mild that you or your practitioner may not recognize them. They may cause only minor or temporary impairment. These are called *transient ischemic attacks* (TIAs). When an artery bursts because of high blood pressure, either damaging part of the brain or impairing its function due to the pressure of pooled blood, the result is a *cerebral hemorrhage*. Depend-

---

*For an excellent discussion of the controversy with reference to the medical literature, see Marcia Millman's *The Unkindest Cut: Life in the Backrooms of Medicine* (New York: William Morrow, 1978), pp. 215–52. See also Office of Technology Assessment, U.S. Congress, "Assessing the Efficacy and Safety of Medical Technologies," GPO Stock No. 052-003-00593-O, September 1978.

†For only one group, those with obstruction of the left main coronary artery, does surgery improve chances of survival.

SYMPTOMS OF STROKE

1. Numbness, tingling, weakness or loss of strength in an arm, leg or side of the face or difficulty walking.
2. Blindness in one or both eyes.
3. Speech problems.
4. Intense, mounting headache lasting many hours.

---

ing on the type of stroke you have, if you survive, you may experience speech loss, paralysis or other loss of mental and physical function. Rehabilitation and therapy sometimes achieve remarkable results by helping undamaged parts of the brain to "take over," but there is no way of reversing the brain damage itself, and frequently there is no improvement.

Signs of Stroke or TIA

Any one or more of the symptoms listed in the box call for action, even though they may happen over several hours. Go immediately to a hospital emergency room or call your regular physican. While less can be done to save a life than in the case of heart attack, prompt treatment may reduce impairment, prevent another stroke (they tend to come in threes) and maximize future functioning.

AUTOIMMUNE DISEASES AND DISORDERS

Chronic Fatigue Syndrome/Chronic Fatigue Immune Dysfunction Syndrome*

In November 1988, I came down with a bad flu— or so I thought at the time. My whole body hurt . . . I was so deeply exhausted that a trip to the kitchen for more juice would leave me on my back for hours, without the energy to speak or even keep my eyes open. I called my office and told them I'd be out of work for the week . . . I never made it back. Three years later, my life is still about the business of getting well.

About 3 million women and a smaller number of men and children suffer from *chronic fatigue immune dysfunction syndrome* (CFIDS), also called

---

*Thanks to Gail Kansky of the Mass CFIDS Association, Lee Liberman, Laurel Berger, Wendy Sanford and others who wish to remain anonymous. Thanks also to Julianna Simon and Marya Grambs for their writings in "Chronic Fatigue: A Serious Epidemic," *Sojourner: The Women's Forum* (December 1991).

chronic fatigue syndrome. Often starting with a sudden, intense bout of flu, CFIDS is marked by two months to several years of a relentless and immobilizing exhaustion that can make even turning over in bed feel impossible. There is a wide and often puzzling array of other symptoms, including low-grade fever, headaches, sleep disorders (insomnia or a tendency to sleep a great deal), swollen glands, muscle pain and weakness, nerve pain, allergies, sore throats, thyroid inflammation, digestive difficulties, sensitivity to light and cold, mood swings, irritability, depression and (for women) yeast infections and menstrual problems, including severe PMS. There can also be significant cognitive symptoms: memory loss, confusion, an inability to think clearly or to concentrate and loss of IQ.

Symptoms

Many of the wide-ranging CFIDS symptoms suggest a chronically activated immune system (the system in the body that fights off infections). A major study released in January 1992 implicated a virus or viruses as the cause and stated that the triggering factors may be genetic or environmental (such as stress or exposure to toxins).[26] It is not clear whether CFIDS is passed from one person to another, but sometimes several family members or coworkers contract it at the same time, which suggests that genetic or environmental factors may well be operating.

Diagnosis

Diagnosing CFIDS has been a problem. For years most health-care providers did not believe CFIDS was an illness, because its symptoms could be ascribed to other illnesses and it did not show up on standard medical tests. Sexism led some providers to dismiss women's complaints: "I keep being told it's all in my head," one woman reported. Some practitioners speculated that the illness was psychiatric: Depression, in fact, is known to cause fatigue. Yet those in the growing CFIDS support network insist that the depression diagnosis doesn't fit, and recent studies cite a viral, not a psychiatric, origin. As one woman said, "Of course it's depressing not to be able to do the things I'm used to doing. But I didn't start out depressed." Initially the media made things worse by belittling CFIDS as the "yuppie flu." Yet people of all ages and of every imaginable kind of work and living situation have CFIDS.

Meanwhile many persons with CFIDS—often people in their most active and fruitful years—have had to stop working and for years at a stretch have been unable to carry on with life. Yet it has been difficult to qualify for health insurance or disability payments because they haven't had a medically diagnosable illness.

Finally the federal government and more of the medical profession have begun to take CFIDS seriously. A few studies have been initiated, at least one funded by the National Institutes of Health. Serious questions about causes, treatment and transmission are finally receiving public attention. More and more physicians know about CFIDS, and there is printed information for those who want to learn.

Treatments

If you have CFIDS, you may feel not only frequently exhausted and sick but also alone with it. If you have found health-care providers who understand CFIDS or are willing to learn, it helps. But family and friends may have pulled away from you in ignorance and confusion about your illness. In our society, women are expected to take care of everyone else, so family members may feel resentful of your need. Or you may have pulled away from them, because even the briefest visit or phone call may be exhausting to you. Also it can be upsetting to need help, when many of us have prided ourselves on being independent. Whatever the cause, the isolation and loneliness can be painful, but there is fortunately a strong, active CFIDS support network with hotlines, support groups, doctor referrals, a buyer's club for vitamins and other holistic treatments, as well as publications that can inform you, your health-care providers, family and friends.

There is no one treatment or approach for CFIDS. The following steps have worked for some women.

1. Rest is primary. Try to arrange to get a tremendous amount of rest. Don't rush back to work thinking that if you just try hard enough the energy will return. This may involve rearranging your life, but it has helped others to improve. One woman writes:

Regular periods of uninterrupted rest have been essential, particularly in acute phases of the illness. That means periods of time with no phone calls, no doorbells to answer, no unexpected decisions to make, people to deal with or problems to solve. . . . It was hard for me to arrange, but I do not believe I could have made progress without it.

2. Do what you can do to help your body heal: Eat a healthy diet, with plenty of vegetables and complex carbohydrates (avoiding yeast-encouraging carbohydrates like bread if you suffer from yeast infections). Avoid stress. Vitamins, acupuncture, meditation, bodywork and homeopathic remedies may help lessen the symptoms.

3. Although no one medical approach seems to work in all cases, many providers use gamma globulin to help increase antibodies to fight infection; low dosages of certain antidepressants seem to work on a variety of symptoms, including insomnia, muscle fatigue and pain, as well as depression. Antibiotics may be used for certain infections, but they aggravate yeast problems, and repeated use can slow down the improvement of other symptoms; some providers are experimenting with more powerful antibiotics that are less likely to required a repeat application.

4. Apply for insurance and/or disability benefits with the assistance of a doctor who understands the illness (see Resources).

5. Know that you are not crazy.

6. Get yourself some support by calling one of the phone numbers listed in the Resources for phone counseling or a support group referral. Contact with people who know what you are going through and are familiar with current research and treatments can make a big difference in your ability to cope.

7. If you have energy to spare, join a group that works to educate the public and to change public policy about CFIDS (see CACTUS in the Resources). Even if you merely sign up, knowing that you are part of such a group may be a boost.

Rest and treatment cost money. This is why changing public policy about medical insurance and disability benefits for persons with CFIDS is crucial. As one woman put it, "This epidemic manages to trigger all the inadequacies and prejudices of American's health-care system, particularly in relation to women." For those of us *without* CFIDS, it should be clear where some of our precious energy needs to go.

Fibromyalgia

Symptoms and Diagnosis

Fibromyalgia (originally called *fibrositis*) is a syndrome of diffuse pain, aching and stiffness of the muscles, often accompanied by fatigue and sleep disturbance. By a conservative estimate, at least 6 million people in the United States suffer from fibromyalgia, the majority of whom are women from twenty to fifty years old. Fibromyalgia can be distinguished from other chronic pain syndromes by the presence of a well-defined characteristic pattern of *tender points*, which are unusually painful spots in muscles and in areas where muscles join tendons. The diagnosis is established by applying pressure to each of these sites and observing the person's pain response. A finding of at least eleven out of eighteen painful tender points, with a history of widespread pain for at least three months, establishes the diagnosis. Lab tests, neurological and joint exams are generally found to be normal in the absence of other disease.

While the location of tender points is generally consistent from one person to another, the everyday pain experienced by each person varies considerably in location and intensity and may not always correspond to tender point sites. The quality of pain can also vary from intense aching to widespread burning. Pain often results from exercise intolerance, which causes muscles to remain tired and stiff after exertion, sometimes for several days. However, short periods of inactivity, such as standing or sitting in one position, can also cause pain and stiffness, which may be somewhat relieved or prevented by frequent changes in position. Most people also report morning stiffness upon arising, which may wear off in several hours or last throughout much of the day.

Other symptoms of fibromyalgia can include irritable bladder, headaches, sensations of numbness and tingling, mouth sores, a subjective sense of peripheral swelling without objective signs of swelling, difficulty concentrating and generalized hypersensitivity to environmental phenomena, such as changes in temperature, humidity, barometric pressure, as well as noise, odors and so on.

Cause

Despite the large numbers of persons—especially women—suffering from fibromyalgia, relatively little research has been conducted to determine its causes. Recent years have brought increasing demand for further investigation, due to the rising numbers of people reporting fibromyalgia symptoms. The earlier bias of physcans toward a psychological explanation, which was named *psychogenic rheumatism*, has been challenged by growing scientific evidence that fibromyalgia has a physical basis. Studies have repeatedly shown that the central features of fibromyalgia occur independently of psychological status, although the severity of pain may increase with stress, as in other illnesses. Research has uncovered some potentially fruitful areas of investigation, although there are no definitive answers at present. Some studies of neurotransmitters have detected elevated levels of substance p, a pain transmitter, and decreases in the levels of at least one chemical messenger, serotonin. Some researchers have hypothesized increased autonomic nervous system arousal. Studies have also investigated muscle metabolism, exploring insufficient oxygen levels and reduced energy reserves, as evidenced by decreased levels of adenosine triphosphate. Some muscle biopsies have shown alterations in the structure of affected muscle areas, suggesting that there may be an increased tendency toward muscle microtrauma (injury of the muscle cell membrane). Research measuring amino acids has demonstrated low levels of some of these protein building blocks.

Treatments

With no clear cause identified, treatment for fibromyalgia has been difficult to establish. The following approaches have been used with varying success: stretching or special muscle exercises, low-impact graded aerobic exercise (swimming, walking), gentle massage, heat, techniques to reduce stress and posture correction via physical therapy. Doctors may prescribe antidepressants in small doses for their sleep-enhancing and pain-relieving properties. It is important to note that these doses are often one-tenth of those used to treat depression, suggesting that the benefit is not based on the alleviation of masked depression. Anti-inflammatory medications, systemic corticosteroids and narcotic analgesics have not been found to be effective in the treatment of fibromyalgia. Injection at tender points with a local anesthetic or a corticosteroid is also generally not effective or recommended.

Given that fibromyalgia is a chronic, relapsing condition, a long-lasting response to one of these treatment approaches is rare. It is generally agreed that learning as much as you can and becoming actively involved in your own treatment decisions is the best way to achieve as much recovery as possible. Support groups, which have proliferated all over the country, can be extremely helpful in providing up-to-date information, doctor referrals and encouragement in coping with this chronic and often disabling condition (see Resources).

Note: Until research proves otherwise, it is best not to assume that fibromyalgia and CFIDS are identical disorders, although a person with fibromyalgia may also exhibit symptoms consistent with CFIDS and vice versa.

Another syndrome often confused with fibromyalgia is myofascial pain syndrome. Although it has similarities to fibromyalgia, it is distinguished by localized rather than difuse pain and tenderness. Rather than tender points, it has trigger points that, when palpated, are associated with referred pain at other locations. The referred pain can usually be eliminated by injection at the trigger point with a local anesthetic.

Scleroderma

Scleroderma is an autoimmune disease of unknown cause characterized by activation of the immune system, excessive deposition of connective tissue and damage to blood vessels. The deposition of excessive connective tissue and the damage of blood vessels cause thickening and scarring (fibrosis) of the skin and malfunction of internal organs, such as the lungs, gut, heart and kidneys.

Three out of every four people with scleroderma are women, who are typically in their thirties or forties when the disease begins. Patients with *limited scleroderma* have less skin fibrosis and, early in their disease, usually have problems with Raynaud's phenomenon (sensitivity of the hands and feet to cold), digital ulcers and heartburn. Patients with *diffuse scleroderma* have more widespread skin involvement, such as on the chest and abdomen, and early on tend to have more scarring of the lungs, heart damage and reduced kidney function.

Although some women do quite well despite their disease, scleroderma can devastate the lives of others. Changes in physical appearance and loss of hand function are common problems. Five-year survival is 60 to 70 percent, with lung, heart and kidney involvement the leading causes of death. There is no cure, so treatment is usually targeted against those organs that are severely involved. Much more research is needed to better understand this disease and to develop effective treatments.

For more information, contact the United Scleroderma Foundation or the American College of Rheumatology (see Resources).

Sjogren's syndrome

Sjogren's syndrome is an autoimmune disease in which the body's immune system reacts against itself. Lymphocytes and autoantibodies invade and destroy the exocrine glands as though they were foreign bodies. This results in decreased or absent production of tears and saliva, because the glands producing these secretions have been impaired or destroyed.

Nine times as many women as men have Sjogren's syndrome. It occurs most commonly among women thirty-five to sixty years old. The chance of a patient with Sjogren's having a first-degree relative with Sjogren's is about 12 percent. Fifty percent of people who have rheumatoid arthritis are also believed to have Sjogren's.

The confusing and often debilitating symptoms of Sjogren's include dry eyes, with a gritty sandy feeling, itching, burning, photophobia, blurry vision of varying degrees and in severe cases corneal abrasions; dry mouth with a burning tongue, cracked lips, swollen and painful parotid glands, rampant tooth decay and periodontal disease, teeth erosions, loss of teeth, difficulty chewing, swallowing and speaking, sores and lesions of the soft tissues of the mouth and tongue, susceptibility to infection and a dry cough; musculoskeletal problems, including fatigue and flulike pains throughout the body; and central nervous system problems, including carpal tunnel syndrome, sensory neuropathy and cognitive impairments.

Treatment of Sjogren's syndrome is dependent upon severity of symptoms. It also can mimic or coexist with many other autoimmune diseases. Early diagnosis and treatment are a must to prevent major debilitating problems from occurring.

For more information, write to the National Sjogren's Syndrome Association (see Resources).

Systemic Lupus Erythematosus

Systemic lupus erythematosus (SLE), a connective tissue disease characterized by inflammation, can affect different parts of the body, especially the skin, joints, blood and kidneys. Its cause is unknown, though certain predisposing traits may be inherited. (These may or may not result in the actual development of SLE.) Certain drugs (including birth control pills), stress, exposure to sun, infections and pregnancy can trigger SLE, though the mechanism is unknown. SLE is an autoimmune disorder, which means that the body's immune system becomes defective and produces antibodies against *normal* parts of the body, causing tissue injury. A hallmark of this disease is often unusual fatigue, a sign of generalized inflammation. As with arthritis, people with SLE have both flare-ups and remissions (symptom-free periods).

Close to a million women in the United States have SLE—*ten times more than the number of men affected.* Two out of every three of these women are African-American, Native American or Asian-American. These factors may explain why research into SLE has been so inadequate.

Because SLE is so often misdiagnosed and therefore mistreated, it is important for women to learn about the characteristics and symptoms of SLE. Any four of the following could indicate the presence of SLE: (1) facial rash ("butterfly" across the cheeks); (2) other disclike lesions or rash marks (discoid lupus); (3) whitening of fingers after exposure to cold (Reynaud's phenomenon); (4) hair loss; (5) mouth or nasal ulcers; (6) arthritis *without* deformity; (7) inflammation of the lining of the lungs or heart (pleuritis or pericarditis), often indicated by shortness of breath and/or chest pains; (8) light sensitivity; (9) convulsions; (10) anemia, low white blood or platelet count; (11) presence of cells without nuclei (LE cells); (12) chronic false-positive tests for syphilis; (13) excessive protein or cellular casts in the urine. You can detect the last few symptoms only through lab tests, which you should request if you think you have SLE. Other characteristics include fever, muscle weakness, joint pains and/or redness as well as fatigue. While many women with lupus have these symptoms, others simply don't feel well but can't put their finger on a specific problem.

Treatment for SLE will vary from woman to woman. Extra rest, a good diet and avoiding the sun will help somewhat. The following can provide effective relief from the SLE symptoms,

though they sometimes cause other problems: anti-inflammatory drugs such as aspirin, antimalarial drugs (which can cause irreversible retina damage, so regular eye exams are necessary to detect this problem early on) and steroids (which can cause high blood pressure, ulcers, swelling and other negative effects—use with caution!). Gynecologists tend to know little about SLE, so it is wiser to consult an internist or other physician with special knowledge of autoimmune diseases (rheumatologist).

SLE is *not* usually life-threatening, although it can be extremely disabling. The ten-year survival rate is higher than 90 percent. Kidney involvement is the most serious complication and can require kidney dialysis as part of the treatment. Pregnancy is potentially problematic since women with SLE have a higher-than-average rate of miscarriages and often experience flare-ups after the birth.

Because symptoms are often invisible, vary a lot in severity and usually come and go (as with many chronic diseases), women with lupus are often accused of being hypochondriacs. Physician ignorance, job discrimination, lack of support from family and friends and the need to restrict activities are just some of the problems experienced by women with SLE.

Support groups are a key resource for women coping with lupus. If you have lupus, ask your doctor about other women who have this problem or contact the Lupus Foundation (see Resources).

When I first found out I had SLE ten years ago, I was immediately faced with many changes: I had to drop out of school, was hospitalized three times that summer, gave up running five miles a day and lost twenty pounds by fall. In the years that followed I learned to cope with my limitations and regain my strength. When my ninety-year-old grandmother complains about not being able to do what she used to, I sympathize. For me that happened at twenty-five. Today, after returning to complete a second graduate degree, I work full-time. I control my illness by taking medication daily but I am still afraid to tell my employer and hate to miss days because of flare-ups. I maintain my health with regular exercise (I swim three-quarters of a mile a day), a good diet and rest. Acquaintances and even good friends don't always understand when I cancel plans, leave early or wear long sleeves in summer. But the other lupus patients in a support group I attend understand me; we speak the same language.

ENVIRONMENTAL ILLNESS

As the environments in which we live and work become more polluted, a large number of people, the majority of them women, have developed a debilitating illness that is commonly called *environmental illness* (EI). Persons with EI suffer from an acute sensitivity to commonly occurring environmental toxins. The chemicals in many different substances can make them sick: in food, air, tap water, medicines, clothes or building materials used in homes and offices (particle board and synthetic carpets, for example).

The symptoms of EI vary, sometimes according to the particular toxin and sometimes according to the individual; symptoms can include breathing difficulty and lung pain, digestive disturbances, food sensitivities, headache, joint pain, incapacitating exhaustion, drowsiness and a host of other problems. The condition has also been called *multiple-chemical sensitivity* and *total allergy syndrome*. Many persons with EI have been treated for one allergy or another; but there are indications that EI is more than a single allergy or even a string of them; it is a systemic sensitivity to toxins. It is not yet clear why more women than men suffer from EI.

Most of the medical world has not so far considered EI to be a discrete, identifiable illness, perhaps because, as one woman with EI remarked, "the medical model wants one cause, one set of symptoms and one cure." Many practitioners of holistic medicine, however, take EI seriously and have developed a variety of treatment approaches, including acupuncture. Whatever the treatment chosen, dealing effectively with EI involves a major shift in life-style to eliminate the toxins: One woman had all her kitchen cabinets ripped out because the formaldehyde used as a glue in particle board was damaging her lungs, many have switched to organic foods to avoid the chemicals in fertilizer and many say they feel better on a macrobiotic diet.

Because we have insufficient space to discuss EI further, we refer you to the Resources. See also Chapter 7, "Environmental and Occupational Health."

U.S. industry introduces hundreds of new chemicals each year, making EI a health hazard for workers. Observers have suggested that those who suffer from EI are like the canaries that miners used to send into the mines to test for deadly fumes. A dead canary signaled danger to humans. There is a sense among many persons with EI that in finally becoming acutely reactive to particular chemicals, their bodies are showing the cumulative effects of a lifetime of the same chemical assaults that we all experience. For those who have EI now, and perhaps for us all, the ultimate "treatment" is cleaning up the environment.

TOXIC SHOCK SYNDROME—A CONTINUING PROBLEM

Toxic shock syndrome (TSS) is a rare but serious disease that mainly strikes menstruating women under thirty who are using tampons. (Menstrual sponges, contraceptive sponges and diaphragms used during the menses have also been associated with TSS.) Although only a small number of menstruating women have gotten TSS (one to seventeen per 100,000 menstruating women), a few of them have died. An increasing number of non-tampon-related cases are showing up in postoperative (male and female) and postpartum patients in hospitals.

TSS is probably caused by a strain of the bacterium *Staphylococcus aureus,* which infects some part of the body, often the vagina, and produces toxins (poisons) that go into the bloodstream, causing a bodily reaction. No one yet knows why some women with *S. aureus* bacteria in their vaginas get TSS and others don't. We wonder if a woman's vaginal secretions and the type of birth control she uses, which significantly affect the vaginal pH, are factors. Higher-absorbency tampons are more likely to be associated with TSS.

This disease is a syndrome, or group of symptoms. At present, only those people who have *all* the symptoms are officially counted as having TSS. However, there are reports of people with a few of the symptoms who may have a milder form of the same disease. The symptoms are

- A high fever, usually over 102 degrees Fahrenheit.
- Vomiting.
- Diarrhea.
- A sudden drop in blood pressure that may lead to shock.
- A sunburnlike rash that peels after a while. The rashes are easiest to see on a person's trunk and neck, and the peeling is obvious on the palms of the hands or the soles of the feet.

Treatments

If you get any of the aforementioned symptoms during your period and you are using a tampon, remove it immediately. Do not use tampons or any other internal method for catching menstrual blood until you get a culture showing that you have no *S. aureus* in your vagina. TSS can progress extremely rapidly, within hours. It's a good idea to get in touch right away with a medical person, preferably at a medical facility, who can keep track of what is happening to you. For a mild case, the most important thing is to drink lots of fluids and rest if possible.

TSS involving severe dehydration or very low

blood pressure may require hospitalization. Although antibiotics do not seem to affect the symptoms once the disease has started, they can still significantly reduce the chance of recurrence. Because this type of *S. aureus* is penicillin and ampicillin resistant, beta-lactamase-resistant antistaphylococcal antibiotics must be used.

TRICHOTILLOMANIA

Trichotillomania, or compulsive hair pulling, is a disorder that primarily affects girls and women. Although once thought to be very rare, it may occur in up to 8 million Americans alone. Psychoanalytic theorists have seen it as a sign of unresolved conflicts, whereas behavioral psychologists have treated it as a habit disorder. The diagnostic manual of the American Psychiatric Association classifies it as an impulse disorder. Current research by the National Institute of Mental Health has found the medications clomipramine (Anafranil) and fluoxetine (Prozac) to be effective treatments for some hair pullers, which points toward a biochemical component of the disorder. At this time researchers agree that there is no one cause of trichotillomania and that it may result from a combination of genetic predisposition and precipitating stress factors.

Although some hair pullers begin the behavior as children, onset is usually during adolesence, often in conjunction with a traumatic event. Adolescent onset may be triggered by hormonal changes. Pulling sites may include the scalp, eyebrows, eyelashes and pubic hair. Hair pullers usually play with the hair or root in some way, and some eat the hair, resulting in an indigestible hairball in the stomach, which can, in rare cases, require surgery.

REMEMBER THE DIGNITY OF YOUR WOMANHOOD. DO NOT APPEAL, DO NOT BEG, DO NOT GROVEL. TAKE COURAGE, JOIN HANDS STAND BESIDE US FIGHT WITH US...."

CHRISTABEL PANKHURST
ENGLISH SUFFRAGIST, (1880-1958)

Karen Norberg

Hair pullers commonly have a deep sense of shame and isolation. Women will often go to great lengths to keep their hair pulling a secret, using wigs, scarves and heavy eye make up and limiting their activities to avoid the risk of exposure. Its effect on identity, body image, self-esteem and sexuality can be devastating and long-term. Hair pullers may also be ridiculed by others and may become the center of conflict in their families if members cannot understand why they are unable to stop the behavior. Many hair pullers appear to the outside world to be functioning very well, while coping with internal feelings such as low self-esteem, depression, shame, anxiety and avoidance of intimate relationships.

A combination of treatment approaches seems to be most helpful. For some people, medication and cognitive behavioral therapy used together are effective. Other treatments that hair pullers have used in addition with varying degrees of success (though they have not been researched) include hypnosis, insight-oriented psychotherapy, biofeedback, acupuncture and relaxation training.

Recently, hair pullers have begun to form support groups, including professionally run groups, leaderless self-help groups and twelve-step groups.

NOTES

1. A. L. Herbst. *University of Chicago DES Program Follow-Up of Mothers and Offspring. 1990 Newsletter.* Chicago: University of Chicago, 1990.
2. G. Schmidt et al. "Reproductive History of Women Exposed to Diethylstilbestrol *in Utero*," *Fertility and Sterility*, Vol. 33 (January 1980), p. 21. G. Schmidt. Dervical Stenosis Following Minor Gynecological Procedures in DES-Exposed Women," *Obstetrics and Gynecology*, Vol. 56, No. 33 (September 1980), p. 334.
3. See DES Task Force. "Summary Report," NIH Publication No. 82-1688, 1978. (Reprinted in October 1981.)
4. U.S. Department of Health and Human Services, Public Health Service, Centers for Disease Control, Division of Sexually Transmitted Diseases. "Sexually Transmitted Diseases Treatment Guidelines, September 1989." *Morbidity and Mortality Weekly Report Supplement*, Vol. 38, Nos. 5–8 (September 1, 1989).
5. S. Ruzek in Resources for Chapter 25, "The Politics of Women and Medical Care."
6. Julie Palmer, Lynn Rosenberg, and Samuel Shapiro, "Reproductive Factors and Risk of Myocardial Infarction," *American Journal of Epidemiology* (on press for later 1992).
7. L. Zussman, S. Zussman, R. Sunley and E. Bjornson. "Sexual Response after Hysterectomy-Oophorectomy: Recent Studies and Reconsideration of Psychogenesis," *American Journal of Obstetrics and Gynecology*, Vol. 40, No 7 (August 1, 1981), pp. 725–29.
8. Margaret H. Thom and J.W. Studd. "Hormone Implantation," *British Medical Journal*, March 22, 1980,

p. 848. Margaret H. Thom and J.W. Studd. "Ovarian Failure and Ageing," *Clinics in Endocrinology and Metabolism*, Vol. 10, No. 1 (March 1981), p. 105. The latter article has a long and useful bibliography.

9. See Brigham and Women's Hospital Study by D. W. Cramer, M.D. et al., reported in *Cancer*, "Ovarian Cancer and Talc," (July 15, 1982). See also D. L. Longo and R. C. Yound, "Cosmetic Talc and Ovarian Cancer," *Lancet*, Vol. 2 (August 1979), pp. 1349–51.

10. See also Dava Sobel and Arthur Klein, *Arthritis: What Works—Treatments That Really Work.* (New York: St. Martin's Press), 1989.

11. American Cancer Society. *Cancer Facts and Figures, 1990.*

12. American Cancer Society. *Cancer Facts and Figures, 1990.*

13. American Cancer Society. *Cancer Facts and Figures, 1990.*

14. American Cancer Society. *Cancer Facts and Figures, 1990.*

15. American Cancer Society. *Cancer Facts and Figures, 1990.*

16. Ralph W. Moss. *The Cancer Syndrome.* New York: Grove Press, 1980.

17. O. Carl Simonton et al. *Getting Well Again: A Step-by-Step Self-Help Guide for Overcoming Cancer for Patients and Their Families.* New York: Bantam Books, 1978.

18. National Cancer Institute. NIH Consensus Development Conference Summary, "The Treatment of Primary Breast Cancer: Management of Local Disease," Vol. 2, No. 5 (June 1979).

19. National Cancer Institute. NIH Consensus Development Conference, June 18–21, 1990. Free copies of the "NIH Consensus Statement on the Treatment of Early-Stage Breast Cancer" are available from NCI, Bethesda, MD 20892.

20. Craig Henderson, et al. "Cancer of the Breast—The Past Decade (Medical Progress)," Parts I and II, *The New England Journal of Medicine*, Vol. 302 (January 3, 1980), pp. 17–30; (January 10, 1980), pp. 78–90.

21. B. Fisher et al. "Disease-Free Survival at Intervals During and Following Completion of Adjuvant Chemotherapy: The NSABP Experience from Three Breast Cancer Protocols," *Cancer*, Vol. 48 (September 15, 1981).

22. B. Fisher et al. "Treatment of Primary Breast Cancer with Chemotherapy and Tamoxifen," *The New England Journal of Medicine*, Vol. 305 (1981), pp. 1–6.

23. National Cancer Institute, Office of Cancer Communication. "High Priority Clinical Trial" announcements, December 1991.

24. National Cancer Institute. "High Priority Clinical Trial" announcements.

25. National Cancer Institute. "High Priority Clinical Trial" announcements.

26. Dedra Buchwald et al. "A Chronic Illness Characterized by Fatigue, Neurologic and Immunologic Disorders, and Active Human Herpesvirus Type 6 Infection," *Annals of Internal Medicine*, Vol. 116, No. 2 (January 15, 1992).

RESOURCES

General

Federation of Feminist Women's Health Centers. *A New View of a Woman's Body*, illustrated by Suzann Gage. New York: Simon & Schuster, 1981. Available from Womancare, 2850 6th Avenue, Suite 311, San Diego, CA 92103.

———. *How to Stay Out of the Gynecologist's Office*, illustrated by Suzann Gage. Culver City, CA: Peace Press, 1981. Available from Womancare, 2850 6th Avenue, Suite 311, San Diego, CA 92103.

Gartley, Cheryle, ed. *Managing Incontinence.* Ottawa, IL: Jameson Books, 1985.

Hasselbring, Bobbie, et al. *The Medical Self-Care Book of Women's Health.* Garden City, NY: Doubleday & Co., 1987.

Hepburn, Cuca, and Bonnie Gutierrez. *Alive and Well: A Lesbian Health Guide.* Freedom, CA: Crossing Press, 1988.

Melpomene Institute for Women's Health Research. *The Bodywise Woman: Reliable Information About Physical Acitivity and Health.* New York: Prentice Hall Press, 1990.

National Center for Health Statistics. *Health United States, 1990.* Hyattsville, MD: Public Health Service, 1991.

National Women's Health Network. *Taking Hormones and Women's Health: Choices, Risks and Benefits.* 1989. $5. Available from National Women's Health Network, 1325 G Street NW, Washington DC 20005.

Nissim, Rina. *Natural Healing in Gynecology: A Manual for Women.* NY: Pandora Press, 1986. Available from HarperCollins Publishers, P.O. Box 588, Dunmore, PA 18512-0588.

Ratcliff, Kathryn Strother, ed. *Healing Technology: Feminist Perspectives.* Ann Arbor: University of Michigan Press, 1989.

Shangold, Mona, and Gabe Mirkin. *The Complete Sports Medicine Book for Women.* New York: Simon & Schuster, 1985.

Thornhill, Annette. *Ask Your Doctor Ask Yourself.* Gloucester, MA: ParaResearch, 1986.

White, Evelyn C., ed. *The Black Women's Health Book: Speaking for Ourselves.* Seattle, WA: Seal Press, 1990.

Worcester, Nancy, and Mariamne H. Whatley, eds. *Women's Health: Readings on Social, Economic, and Political Issues.* Dubuque, IA: Kendall/Hunt Publishing Co., 1988.

Organization

National Headache Foundation
5252 North Western Avenue
Chicago, IL 60625
(312) 878-7715
(800) 843-2256

Chronic Fatigue Syndrome

Readings

Bell, David S. *The Disease of a Thousand Names.* 1991. $22.50. Available from Pollard Publications, P.O. Box 181, Lyndonville, NY 14098.

Casanova, Kenneth. *How to Apply for Social Security Benefits If You Have CFIDS.* $4.00. Available from Mass CFIDS Association, 808 Main Street, Waltham, MA 02154.

Feiden, Karen. *Hope and Help for Chronic Fatigue Syndrome.* Englewood Cliffs, NJ: Prentice Hall Press, 1990.

Mass CFIDS Association. "CFS: A Primer for Physicians and Allied Health Professionals." 1992. Available from Mass CFIDS Association, 808 Main Street, Waltham, MA 02154.

Stoff, Jesse. *Chronic Fatigue Syndrome.* New York: Random House, 1988. Not recommended. This book has much inaccurate information and is outdated.

Organizations

CACTUS—CFIDS Action Campaign for the U.S.
P.O. Box 2578
Sebastopol, CA 95473
(707) 823-0725
Goals: to secure federal money for research, treatment and rehabilitation; reform of health provision, disability, Social Security and insurance systems. Bimonthly publication.

CFIDS Association
P.O. Box 220398
Charlotte, NC 28222
(704) 362-2343
Toll-free information line: (800) 442-3437
Toll information line: (900) 988-2343 ($2 first minute, $1 each additional minute)
Publishes a national journal of research and advocacy information. Offers information about support groups and physicians.

CFIDS Foundation
965 Mission Street, Suite 425
San Francisco, CA 94103
(415) 882-9986
Provides information and referral, printed information for health-care providers, telephone counseling, advocacy and public policy development.

Mass CFIDS Association
808 Main Street
Waltham, MA 02154
(617) 893-4415
Publications, support group information. Call-in hours several times a week.

United States Public Health Service Centers for Disease Control
Atlanta, GA 30333
Information hotline: (404) 332-4555
Free articles on CFIDS.

Disabilities

National Clearinghouse on Women and Girls with Disabilities. *Bridging the Gap: A National Directory of Services for Women and Girls with Disabilities.* New York: Educational Equity Concepts, 1990.

Pitzele, Sefra Kobrin. *We Are Not Alone: Learning to Live with Chronic Illness.* New York: Workman Publishing, 1986.

Saxton, Marsha, and Florence Howe, eds. *With Wings: An Anthology of Literature By and About Women with Disabilities.* NY: Feminist Press, 1987.

Webster, Barbara. *All of a Piece: A Life with Multiple Sclerosis.* Baltimore, MD: Johns Hopkins University Press, 1989.

DES

Books

Apfel, R., and S. Fisher. *To Do No Harm: DES and the Dilemmas of Modern Medicine.* New Haven, CT: Yale University Press, 1984.

Glendinning, C. *When Technology Wounds: The Human Consequences of Progress.* New York: William Morrow, 1990.

Meyers, R. *DES: The Bitter Pill.* New York: Seaview Putnam, 1983.

Articles

Anderson, B., et al. "Development of DES-Associated Clear Cell Carcinoma: The Importance of Regular Screening," *Obstetrics and Gynecology,* Vol. 33, No. 3 (March 1979), pp. 293–99.

Dieckmann, W., et al. "Does the Administration of Diethylstilbestrol During Pregnancy Have Therapeutic Value?" *American Journal of Obstetrics and Gynecology,* Vol. 66, No. 5 (November 1953), pp. 1062–81.

Greenberg, E.R., et al. "Breast Cancer in Mothers Given Diethylstilbestrol in Pregnancy," *New England Journal of Medicine,* Vol. 311, No. 22 (November 29, 1984), pp. 1393–98.

Herbst, A.L., et al. "Adenocarcinoma of the Vagina: Association of Maternal Stilbestrol Therapy with Tumor Appearance in Young Women," *New England Journal of Medicine,* Vol. 284 (April 22, 1971), pp. 878–81.

Kaufman, R.H., et al. "Upper Genital Tract Changes and Infertility in Diethylstilbestrol-Exposed Women," *American Journal of Obstetrics and Gynecology,* Vol. 154, No. 6 (June 1986), pp. 1312–1318.

Robboy, S.J., et al. "Cooperative Diethylstilbestrol Adenosis (DESAD) Project," *Obstetrics and Gynecology,* Vol. 53, No. 3 (March 1979), pp. 309–17.

Wingard, Deborah L., and Judith Turiel. "Long-Term Effects of Exposure to Diethylstilbestrol," *Western Journal of Medicine,* Vol. 149, No. 5 (November 1988), pp. 551–54.

Organization

The DES Cancer Network
DES Action USA
1615 Broadway
Oakland, CA 94612
(510) 465-4011

Endometriosis

Ballweg, Mary Lou, and The Endometriosis Association. *Overcoming Endometriosis: New Help from the Endometriosis Association.* New York: Congdon and Weed, 1987.

Kennedy, Stephen H., et al. "A Comparison of Nafarelin Acetate and Danazol in the Treatment of Endometriosis," *Fertility and Sterility,* Vol. 53, No. 6 (June 1990), pp. 998–1003.

Weinstein, Kate. *Living with Endometriosis: How to Cope with the Physical and Emotional Challenges.* Reading, MA: Addison-Wesley, 1987.

Organization

The Endometriosis Association
8585 North 76th Place
Milwaukee, WI 53223
(800) 992-3636 (in the United States)
(800) 426-2363 (in Canada)

Environmental Illness

De Schepper, Luc. *Peak Immunity: How to Fight Epstein-Barr Virus, Candida, Herpes Simplex and Other Immune-Suppressive Disorders and Win.* Santa Monica: LDS Publications, 1989.

Leviton, Richard. "Environmental Illness—A Special Report," *The Yoga Journal* (November/December 1990), pp. 42–53 and 95–99. This article cited, as a further resource, the American Academy of Environmental Medicine, P.O. Box 16106, Denver, CO 80216, (303) 622-9756.

Rogers, Sherry. *Environmental Illness.* 1986. Available from Prestige Publishing, Box 3068, Syracuse, NY 13220, (315) 455-7862.

———. *You Are What You Ate.* 1988. Available from Prestige Publishing, Box 3068, Syracuse, NY 13220, (315) 455-7862. Although poorly edited and indexed, these books provide useful material.

———. *Tired or Toxic.* 1989. Available from Prestige Publishing, Box 3068, Syracuse, NY 13220, (315) 455-7862.

———. *The Cure Is in the Kitchen.* 1991. Available from Prestige Publishing, Box 3068, Syracuse, NY 13220, (315) 455-7862.

Fibromyalgia

Readings

Ediger, Beth. *Coping with Fibromyalgia.* Available from Fibromyalgia Association of Texas, Inc., 5650 Forest Lane, Dallas, TX 75230, (214) 363-2473.

Journal of Musculoskeletal Pain. Haworth Press, Inc., 10 Alice Street, Binghamton, NY 13904. This new professional journal pertaining to musculoskeletal pain syndromes will be inaugurated at the end of 1992.

Organizations

The Fibromyalgia Association of Central Ohio
Riverside Hospital
3545 Olentangy River Road, Suite 8
Columbus, OH 43214
(614) 262-2000

Fibromyalgia Network
7001 School House Lane
Bakersfield, CA 93309-2768
Quarterly newsletter gives comprehensive listing of support groups throughout the United States and Canada, as well as summaries of the most recent research studies.

USA Fibrositis Association
P.O. Box 1483
Dublin, OH 43017-0549
(614) 846-8344

Interstitial Cystitis

Interstitial Cystitis Association
P.O. Box 1553
Madison Square Station
New York, NY 10159
(212) 979-6057

PID/STDs

"STD Treatment Guidelines, Sept. 1989: Pelvic Inflammatory Disease," *MMWR,* Vol. 38, Nos. 5–8 (September 1, 1989).

STD Bulletin, Vol. 10, No. 1 (July 1990). Entire issue on PID.

Vancouver Women's Health Research Collective. "PID: Pelvic Inflammatory Disease." 1983. Available from VWHRC, 1501 West Broadway, Vancouver, British Columbia, Canada V6J 1W6. A comprehensive, illustrated thirty-four-page booklet with extensive bibliography. Very useful.

Wasserheit, Judith N. "Pelvic Inflammatory Disease and Infertility," *Maryland Medical Journal,* Vol. 36, No. 1 (January 1987), pp. 58–63.

Scleroderma

The United Scleroderma Foundation
730 Thompson Road
Kangaroo Beach, Stevensville, MD 21666

The American College of Rheumatology
60 Executive Park South, Suite 150
Atlanta, GA 30329

Sjogren's Syndrome

The National Sjogren's Syndrome Association
Barbara Henry, president
3201 West Evans Drive
Phoenix, Arizona 85023
(800) 395-6772

Trichotillomania

National Institute of Mental Health
9000 Rockville Pike
Building 10, Room 3, D41
Bethesda, MD 20892
(301) 496-3421

Obsessive Compulsive Foundation
P.O. Box 9573
New Haven, CT 06535
(203) 722-0565

Trichotillomania Learning Center
1215 Mission Street, Suite 2
Santa Cruz, CA 95060
(408) 457-1004

UTIs

Chalker, Rebecca, and Kristene E. Whitmore. *Overcoming Bladder Disorders: Compassionate, Authoritative Medical and Self-help Solutions for Incontinence, Cystitis, Interstitial Cystitis, Prostate Problems, Bladder Cancer.* New York: HarperCollins, 1991.

Kilmartin, Angela. *Cystitis: The Complete Self-Help Guide.* New York: Warner Books, 1980.

Sant, Grannum R. "Interstitial Cystitis," *Monographs in Urology*, Vol. 12, No. 3 (1991), pp. 37–63.

———. "Interstitial Cystitis: Pathophysiology, Clinical Evaluation, and Treatment," *Urology Annual*, Vol. 3 (1989), pp. 171–96.

Sant, Grannum R., and Edwin M. Meares, Jr. "Interstitial Cystitis: Pathogenesis, Diagnosis, and Treatment," *Infections in Urology* (January/February 1990), pp. 24–30.

Hysterectomy and Oophorectomy

Readings

Costa, Barbara, and D. Dilanni, "Sudden Changes: Post-Hysterectomy Syndrome," 29-min. color video. Examines the reasons for the high number of hysterectomies performed on women every year, the alternatives available, the side effects and aftereffects. Includes interviews with doctors, other professionals and women who have undergone the operation. Available from The Cinema Guild, 1697 Broadway, New York, NY 10019.

Davies, Mary E. "A Consumer's Guide to Hysterectomy," *Medical Self-Care* (Summer 1983), pp. 33–37.

Morgan, Susanne. *Coping with Hysterectomy.* New York: Dial Press, 1982.

Payer, Lynn. *How to Avoid a Hysterectomy: An Indispensable Guide to Exploring All Your Options—Before You Consent to a Hysterectomy.* New York: Pantheon Books, 1987.

Organization

Hysterectomy Educational Resources and Services (HERS)
422 Bryn Mawr Avenue
Bala Cynwyd, PA 19004
(215) 667-7757

Vaginal Infections (Vaginitis)

Hasselbring, Bobbie. "Every Woman's Guide to Vaginal Infections," *Medical Self-Care* (Summer 1983), p. 45.

Santa Cruz Women's Health Center. "Home Remedies for Vaginitis." Available from The Santa Cruz Women's Health Center, 250 Locust St., Santa Cruz, CA 95060.

Arthritis

Books

Lorig, Kate. *The Arthritis Helpbook.* Reading, MA: Addison-Wesley, 1990.

Sobel, Dava, and Arthur Klein. *Arthritis: What Works—Treatments that Really Work.* New York: St. Martin's Press, 1989.

Organization

Arthritis Information Clearinghouse
P.O. Box 34427
Bethesda, MD 20034

Provides information on professional, patient and public education materials on rheumatic diseases and related topics. Publishes a bulletin.

Cancer

Books and Articles

American Cancer Society. *Cancer Facts and Figures—1991.*

American College of Obstetricians and Gynecologists. "Cancer of the Ovary," *Technical Bulletin*, No. 141 (May 1990), pp. 287–289.

Andolf, Ellika, Connie Jorgensen and Birger Astedt. "Ultrasound Examination for Detection of Ovarian Carcinoma in Risk Groups," *Obstetrics and Gynecology*, Vol. 75, No. 1 (January 1990), pp. 106–9.

Atack, D.B., et al. "CA 125 Surveillance and Second-Look Laparotomy in Ovarian Carcinoma," *American Journal of Obstetrics and Gynecology*, Vol. 154, No. 2 (February 1986), pp. 287–89.

Averette, Hervy E., and Daniel M. Donato. "Ovarian Carcinoma: Advances in Diagnosis, Staging and Treatment," *Cancer*, Vol. 65 (February 1, 1990), pp. 703–8.

Brady, Judith, ed. *1 in 3: Women with Cancer Confront an Epidemic.* Pittsburgh: Cleis Press, 1991.

"Breast Cancer: The Retreat from Radical Surgery," *Consumer Reports*, January 1981, pp. 24–30. An excellent discussion of factors leading to the lumpectomy plus radiation approach.

Butler, Sandra, and Barbara Rosenblum. *Cancer in Two Voices.* San Francisco: Spinsters Book Co., 1991.

Coney, Sandra. *The Unfortunate Experiment: The Full Story Behind the Inquiry into Cervical Cancer Treatment.* Auckland, New Zealand: Penguin Books, 1988.

Cramer, Daniel W. "Lactase Persistence and Milk Consumption as Determinants of Ovarian Cancer Risk," *American Journal of Epidemiology*, Vol. 130, No. 5 (1989), pp. 904–10.

Cramer, Daniel W., et al. "Ovarian Cancer and Talc: A Case Control Study," *Cancer*, Vol. 50 (1982), pp. 372–76.

Dollinger, Malin, Ernest H. Rosenbaum and Greg Cable. *Everyone's Guide to Cancer Therapy*. Toronto: Somerville House Books Ltd., 1991.

Epstein, Samuel. *The Politics of Cancer*. New York: Anchor Books, 1979. Describes the cancer industry, which makes millions of dollars in profits from research and treatments that have done little to help cancer patients.

Gorback, Sherwood L., and David R. Zimmerman. *The Doctors' Anti-Breast Cancer Diet*. New York: Simon & Schuster, 1984.

Greenspan, Ezra M. *What Every Woman and Her Doctor Could Discuss About Ovarian Cancer*. 1990. Available from The Chemotherapy Foundation, 183 Madison Avenue, New York, NY 10016.

Gwinn, Marta L., et al. "Pregnancy, Breast Feeding, and Oral Contraceptives and the Risk of Epithelial Ovarian Cancer," *Journal of Clinical Epidemiology*, Vol. 43, No. 6 (1990), pp. 559–68.

Henderson, Brian E., Ronald K. Ross and Malcolm C. Pike. "Toward the Primary Prevention of Cancer," *Science*, Vol. 254 (November 22, 1991), pp. 1131–254.

Howell, Stephen B., et al. "Intraperitoneal Cisplatin-Based Chemotherapy for Ovarian Carcinoma," *Seminars in Oncology*, Vol. 18, No. 1 (February 1991), pp. 5–10.

Jacobs, Ian, and David Oram. "Prevention of Ovarian Cancer: A Survey of the Practice of Prophylactic Oophorectomy by Fellows and Members of the Royal College of Obstetricians and Gynecologists," *British Journal of Obstetrics and Gynecology*, Vol. 96 (May 1989), pp. 510–15.

Kelly, Patricia T. *Understanding Breast Cancer Risk*. Philadelphia: Temple University Press, 1991.

La Vecchia, Carlo, et al. "Dietary Factors and the Risk of Epithelial Ovarian Cancer," *Journal of the National Cancer Institute*, Vol. 79, No. 4 (October 1987), pp. 663–69.

Love, Susan M. *Dr. Susan Love's Breast Book*. Reading, MA: Addison-Wesley, 1990.

Lorde, Audre. *The Cancer Journals*. San Francisco: Spinsters, 1980. Important testimony of a lesbian feminist poet's personal and political reckoning with breast cancer and mastectomy.

McGinn, Kerry. *Keeping Abreast: Breast Changes That Are Not Cancer*. Palo Alto, CA: Bull Publishing, 1991.

Napoli, Maryann. *Mammography Screening: A Decision-Making Guide*. 1990. Available from Center for Medical Consumers, 237 Thompson Street, New York, NY 10012.

National Cancer Institute. *Cancer of the Ovary, Research Report*, Bethesda, MD: NIH Publication No. 89–3014. March 1989.

———. *Ovarian Cancer, PDQ (Physicians Data Query) State-of-the-Art Cancer Treatment Information*. March 1, 1991. Available from Office of Cancer Communications, Building 31, Room 1024, 9000 Rockville Pike, Bethesda, MD 20892.

———. *What Are Clinical Trials All About?* NIH Publication No. 88--2706. April 1988. Available from Office of Cancer Communications, Building 31, Room 1024, 9000 Rockville Pike, Bethesda, MD 20892.

Newell, Guy, and Neal Ellison, eds. *Progress in Cancer Research and Therapy*, Vol. 17, *Nutrition and Cancer: Etiology and Treatment*. New York: Raven Press, 1981.

Ramstack, Janet L., and Ernest H. Rosenbaum. *Nutrition for the Chemotherapy Patient*. Palo Alto, CA: Bull Publishing, 1991.

Stocker, Midge, ed. *Cancer as a Women's Issue*. Chicago: Third Side Press, 1991.

van Negell, John R., et al. "Transvaginal Sonography as a Screening Method for Ovarian Cancer," *Cancer*, Vol. 65 (1990), pp. 573–77.

Villard-Mackintosh, Laurence, Marin P. Vessey and Leslie Jones. "The Effects of Oral Contraceptives and Parity on Ovarian Trends in Women Under 55 Years of Age," *British Journal of Obstetrics and Gynecology*, Vol. 96 (July 1989), pp. 783–88.

Williams, Wendy. *The Power Within. True Stories of Exceptional Patients Who Fought Back with Hope*. New York: Harper & Row, 1990.

Yoder, Linda H. "The Epidemiology of Ovarian Cancer: A Review," *Oncology Nursing Forum*, Vol. 17, No. 3 (1990), pp. 411–15.

Organizations

American Cancer Society
  19 West 56th Street
  New York, NY 10019
  (212) 586-8700
Provides information, booklets, Reach to Recovery (one-on-one counseling by women with histories of breast cancer).

Breast Cancer Action
  P.O. Box 460185
  San Francisco, CA 94146
  (415) 922-8279
Provides education, political advocacy, direct support.

Command Trust Network
  Cosmetic Surgery Division
  P.O. Box 17082
  Covington, KY 41017
Provides contact with women regarding breast implant concerns.

Encore
  Contact your local YWCA.

Foundation for Alternative Cancer Therapies
  P.O. Box 1242
  Old Chelsea Station
  New York, NY 10113
  (212) 741-2790

Gerson Institute of California
  P.O. Box 430
  Bonita, CA 91908
Advocates diet as alternative therapy.

Lesbian Community Cancer Project
  2524 North Lincoln Avenue, Suite 199
  Chicago, IL 60614
  (312) 549-4729

Livingston Foundation Medical Center
   3232 Duke Street
   San Diego, CA 92110
Offers alternative cancer therapies with strong focus on diet.

Mautner Project for Lesbians with Cancer
   P.O. Box 90437
   Washington, DC 20090
   (202) 332-5536

National Alliance of Breast Cancer Organizations (NABCO)
   1180 Avenue of the Americas, 2nd Floor
   New York, NY 10036
   (212) 221-3300
Provides written information, resources; lobbies for legislative concerns. Also the contact for the Breast Cancer Coalition.

National Cancer Institute
   Office of Cancer Communications
   Building 31, Room 10A24
   9000 Rockville Pike
   Bethesda, MD 20892
   Hotline: (800) 4-CANCER
Hotline answered at all times except 12:00 midnight to 8:00 A.M.; general cancer and PDQ information available.

National Coalition for Cancer Survivorship
   323 Eight Street SW
   Albuquerque, NM 87102
   (505) 764-9956
Provides education and advocacy.

Reach for Recovery
   Contact your local American Cancer Society.

Women's Cancer Resource Center
   P.O. Box 11235
   Oakland, CA 94611
   (415) 548-WCRC

Women's Community Cancer Project
   c/o Women's Center
   46 Pleasant Street
   Cambridge, MA 02139
   (617) 354-9888

Diabetes

Books

Clinical Center Communications. *Diabetes in Adults.* October 1990. Available from National Institutes of Health, Building 10, Room 1C255, 9000 Rockville Pike, Bethesda, MD 20892.
Milchovich, Sue K., and Barbara Dunn-Long. *Diabetes Mellitus: A Practical Handbook.* Palo Alto, CA: Bull Publishing Co., 1990.

Organization

American Diabetes Association
   National Service Center
   1660 Duke Street
   P.O. Box 25757
   Alexandria, VA 22313
   (703) 549-1500
A private voluntary organization fostering public awareness of diabetes and supporting/promoting diabetes research.

Hypertension, Heart Diseases and Circulatory Diseases

Books and Pamphlets

Douglas, Pamela S. *Heart Disease in Women.* Philadelphia: F.A. Davis Co., 1989.
Eaker, E.D., et al., eds. *Coronary Artery Disease in Women.* New York: Haymarket Doyman, 1987.
Legato, Marriane J., and Carol Colman. *The Female Heart: The Truth About Women and Coronary Artery Disease.* New York: Prentice Hall Press, 1991.
National Heart, Lung, and Blood Institute. *NHLBI Kit '90,* Manual A, *Information for Program Planners;* Manual B, *Information for Consumers.* Bethesda, MD: Public Health Service, 1990. Available from NHLBI Education Programs Information Center, 4733 Bethesda Avenue, Suite 530, Bethesda, MD 20814-4820.

Articles

Ayanian, John Z., and Arnold M. Epstein. "Differences in the Use of Procedures Between Women and Men Hospitalized for Coronary Heart Disease," *New England Journal of Medicine,* Vol. 321 (1989), pp. 221–25.
Eaker, E.D., et al. "Epidemiology and Risk Factors for Coronary Heart Disease in Women," *Cardiovascular Clinics* (1989), Vol. 19, No. 3, pp. 129–45.
Hardman, A.E., et al. "Brisk Walking and Plasma High Density Lipoprotein Cholesterol Concentration in Previously Sedentary Women," *British Medical Journal,* Vol. 299 (1989), pp. 1204–10.
Healy, Bernadine. "The Yentl Syndrome," *New England Journal of Medicine,* Vol. 321 (1989), pp. 274–75.
Khan, Steven S., et al. "Increased Mortality of Women in Coronary Artery Bypass Surgery: Evidence for Referral Bias," *Annals of Internal Medicine,* Vol. 112, No. 8 (1990), pp. 561–69.
Lerner, D.J., and W. Kannel. "Patterns of Coronary Heart Disease Morbidity and Mortality in the Sexes: A 26-Year Follow-up of the Framingham Population," *American Heart Journal,* February 1986.
Matthews, K.A., et al. "Menopause and Risk Factors for Coronary Heart Disease," *New England Journal of Medicine,* Vol. 321 (1989), pp. 641–46.
Steingart, Richard M., et al. "Sex Differences in the Management of Coronary Artery Disease," *New England Journal of Medicine,* Vol. 325 (1991), pp. 226–30.
Tofler, G.H., et al. "Effects of Gender and Race on Prognosis After Myocardial Infarction; Adverse Prognosis for Women, Particularly Black Women," *American College of Cardiology,* Vol. 9 (1987), pp. 473–82.
Wenger, Nanette K. "Gender, Coronary Artery Disease, and Coronary Bypass Surgery," *Annals of Internal Medicine,* Vol. 112 (1990), pp. 557–58.

Organization

American Heart Association
  7320 Greenville Avenue
  Dallas, TX 75231
Offers many free pamphlets, etc.

Systemic Lupus Erythematosis (SLE)

Readings

Chester, Laura. *Lupus Novice: Toward Self-Healing.* Barrytown, NY: Station Hill Press, 1987.
Lupus News. 111 Pleasant Street, Watertown, MA 02172. A publication of the Lupus Foundation of America.
NIAMS Task Force on Lupus in High Risk Populations.

What Black Women Should Know About Lupus. July 1991. Available from the National Institute of Arthritis and Musculoskeletal and Skin Diseases, Box AMS, 9000 Rockville Pike, Bethesda, MD 20892.

Organizations

American Lupus Society
  3914 Del Amo Boulevard, Suite 922
  Torrance, CA 90503
  (213) 542-8891
  (800) 331-1802

Lupus Foundation of America, Inc.
  4 Research Place, Suite 180
  Rockville, MD 20850-3226
  (301) 670-9292
  (800) 558-0121

PART VII

Women and the Medical System

25

The Politics of Women and Medical Care

By Hilary Salk, Wendy Sanford, Norma Swenson and Judith Dickson Luce
Our Rights as Patients by Sherry Leibowitz and Joan Rachlin

With special thanks to David Banta, Gene Bishop, Mary Fillmore, Mary Howell, Judy Norsigian, Sheryl Ruzek and Karen Wolf 1992 Update by Amy Alpern, Robin Blatt, David Clarke, Judy Norsigian, Kathy Simmonds, Norma Swenson and Nancy Worcester.

This chapter in previous editions was called "The American Health Care System" and "Choosing and Using Health and Medical Care" and was written by Barbara Perkins, Lucy Candib, Nancy Todd, Mary Stern and Norma Swenson.

THE AMERICAN MEDICAL CARE SYSTEM

I've repeatedly described my symptoms to physicians—disconcerting symptoms to say the least: sudden menses cessation, elevated temperature, weight loss, anxiety, extreme fatigue, nausea, joint pain, vertigo—but the doctors have made only the catch-all diagnosis of "menopause," unsupported by any testing. They advised me to go into counseling, expecting me to "live with it," despite the fact that I have told them that the symptoms seem extreme, are increasing and have impaired and even curtailed my work, my studies, my personal relationships.

From a letter to the Women's Health Collective in Providence, Rhode Island:

I think you would have been proud of the way I handled the situation with the surgeon. Despite a fair amount of crying on my part (to top it all off, my husband was away when all this happened), I was able to demand a second opinion for my diverticulosis treatment and the most conservative treatment possible. My surgeon was appalled when I balked at surgery Monday without what I felt was adequate time to discuss the situation or get another opinion. By Friday I was able to deal with him, but it took about all I had. I really think that if it wasn't for my experience with the Women's Health Collective and the support of my friends and family, I would have a temporary colostomy right now.

I, extremely well informed, well connected, verbally aggressive, have had to summon all my resources to get what I wanted in my treatment for breast cancer: medical care that was consistent with the findings of the latest literature and that took into account my needs as a woman.

As a young woman interested in one day having a family, I was never told that cimetidine "should not be used in pregnant patients or women of child-bearing potential unless, in the judgment of the physician, the anticipated benefits outweigh the potential risks." I should have been informed of this and given the opportunity to make the decision myself in consultation with the doctor. This is one more indication of my rights and indeed my body being violated. My family raised me to trust doctors, but I no longer can do that.

In the words of a visiting nurse:

I learned to listen to patients, to speak their language, to let them set their own priorities for care, to teach them when they were ready. I also learned to evaluate the health care system through their eyes. Each day I confronted an irrelevant, noncaring, inadequate health care system that refused to consider the personal, social, cultural and economic needs of the patient.

It is a sobering time for women using the medical system in this country. Although some women are satisfied with the medical care they get, many are not.* The women quoted above are only a few of the thousands speaking out about the physicians and other medical personnel in medical settings who have

- Not listened to them or believed what they said.
- Withheld knowledge.
- Lied to them.
- Treated them without their consent.
- Not warned of risks and negative effects of treatments.
- Overcharged them.
- Experimented on them or used them as "teaching material."
- Treated them poorly because of their race, sexual preference, age or disability.
- Offered them tranquilizers or moral advice instead of medical care or useful help from community resources (self-help groups, battered women's services, etc.).
- Administered treatments which were unnecessarily mutilating and too extreme for their prob-

lem, or treatments which resulted in permanent disability or even death (*iatrogenesis*).*
- Prescribed drugs which hooked them, sickened them, changed their entire lives.
- Performed operations they later found were unnecessary and removed organs that were in no way diseased.
- Abused them sexually.

Why Focus on Women and the Medical System?

Women are part of the medical care system, either for ourselves or our children, spouses or aging parents, more than twice as often as men are. We are 85 percent of all health care workers in hospitals and 75 percent in the system as a whole.† We carry out most doctors' orders—treatment regimens like special diets, medications and bed rest, and so on—either as unpaid workers at home or as paid workers. We teach about health both in the home and in the system—what is good and not good for you. At home we are usually the first to be told when someone doesn't feel well, and we help decide what to do next. Some health care analysts even call us "primary health care workers" or the "layperson on the team." Most "patient" communication for and about family members flows through women: We report signs and changes, symptoms, responses to treatments and medications. The system also depends on women: Our direct reporting forms the basis of much of what medicine calls "scientific results," and our bodies provide the raw material for experimentation and research (e.g., the birth control pill), often without our knowledge and consent.[2]

Yet despite our overwhelming numbers and the tremendous responsibility we carry for people's

---

*We are basing the analysis in this chapter both on thousands of personal accounts and on the work of a wide range of people and groups: feminist writers and other investigative journalists; feminist, radical and progressive physicians; public health researchers; health workers and practitioners of all kinds; medical historians and medical sociologists; public interest groups and government specialists; as well as social and feminist critics of many different persuasions.

Iatrogenesis is the process by which illness, impairment or death results from medical treatment. Some examples are cancers caused by DES, pelvic inflammatory disease (PID) or hysterectomy caused by an IUD, death or disability due to anesthesia accident (particularly when the surgery may not have been necessary), electrocution or burns from hospital equipment, infection from respirators, crippling or fatal strokes due to the birth control pill, addiction to tranquilizers and illness or death resulting from infant formula feeding in hospitals.
†While ailing men do report many of the same problems with the medical care system as women, men use the system less. They do not, like women, have to consult physicians for normal events in the reproductive cycle, such as pregnancy. Men tend to come into the system only during crises. Many different studies have shown that medical care providers treat male patients with more respect than women and offer fewer tranquilizers and less moral advice.[1] Also, since only 17 percent of doctors are women, most women see male physicians, a situation which severely exaggerates male-female power imbalances.

health, we still have limited power to influence the medical system. Policymakers, usually male, have designed the system primarily for the convenience and financial gain of physicians, hospitals, administrators and the medical industries. *We believe that women, as the majority of consumers and workers, paid and unpaid, should have the major voice in health and medical care policy-making in this country.*

A previous edition of *Our Bodies, Ourselves* expressed considerable optimism that women would be able to work together to change medical care. In fact, women of all ages have joined together in local communities and nationwide: The resulting women's health movement has significantly changed the way many women look at medical care and is successfully fighting in legislatures, hospital administrations and law courts for improvements (see Chapter 26, "Organizing for Change: U.S.A."). Yet change comes slowly. The medical care system is too often unresponsive to women, deeply entrenched as it is in American economic, political and social structures, and the influence of medicine* in people's lives continues to grow. For example, the insurance and drug industries continue to make unrestrained profits, and physicians are still among the highest paid and among the least accountable of all U.S. professionals.† Despite a few governmental programs—Health Systems Agencies (HSAs) and neighborhood health centers—the medical establishment‡ has the money and status to contain most citizen attempts to achieve community control.

Our critique of medicine has taken on a new dimension. We see basic errors in its fundamental assumptions about health and healing. Although conventional medical care may at times be just what we need, in many situations it may be bad for our health because it emphasizes drugs, sur-

gery, psychotherapy (especially for women) and crisis action rather than prevention.* It is not enough to provide or improve medical care, to have more women physicians, to stop the abuses or to increase access to existing health and medical care for the poor and elderly—even though we support absolutely equal access to care for all classes and groups (see p. 683). We want to reclaim the knowledge and skills that the medical establishment has inappropriately taken over. We also want preventive and nonmedical healing methods to be available to all who need them. We are committed to exposing how the medical establishment works to suppress these alternatives (home birth and nurse-midwifery, for example), contrary to the spirit of the antitrust laws of this country.

Pessimistic as we are about the present system, we believe in the healing powers within all of us—our ability to help one another by listening, talking, caring, touching—and in the power of small groups as sources of information sharing, support and healing. We still believe that we, as women, are the best experts on ourselves. The more we understand how vulnerable we become—both to disease and to dependency on experts—when isolated from one another, the more we see group experience and action as essential resources for health, from small consciousness-raising or self-help groups to large numbers of women organized for political action.

In this chapter we warn you of some of the dangers of this system and offer strategies to make it work for you as well as possible. We hope that you will feel entitled to demand more information about your health and medical needs, more able to distinguish when to turn to professionals, more empowered to take care of yourself and others when that is appropriate and more deeply convinced that good health is a fundamental right worth fighting for.

The Power of Medicine in Society

Why do most people have an almost religious belief in American medicine? Despite numerous bad or disappointing experiences, so many women say, "It must be my fault" or "I must just have had the wrong doctor," and fail to see that the system itself has serious faults. The institution and ideology of American medicine has penetrated so totally into the fabric of our lives over the past fifty years that most of us aren't even aware of its influence. Its

---

*We use "medicine" to mean both the *tangible* personnel and institutions of the medical system like physicians and hospitals, and the discipline, field or profession of medicine. We also mean the *intangible* institution of beliefs, ideology and assumptions that influence or control our daily habits in ways most of us are not aware of (as do "the family" and "religion").
†Accountability in the case of the medical profession would mean that they be more responsive to our perceived needs and wishes in recognition of the fact that, as taxpayers, we support medical education, research, hospital construction and much of the medical care given in hospitals, nursing homes and clinics.[3] See also the footnote on p. 660 which discusses accountability.
‡By *medical establishment* we mean the cluster of organized physician, hospital, drug and insurance groups like the AMA (American Medical Association), the ACOG (American College of Obstetricians and Gynecologists), the AHA (American Hospital Association) and the PMA (Pharmaceutical Manufacturers Association), which pay large sums to influence public opinion, legislation and policy on health and medical matters.

---

*Women consume far more prescription drugs, undergo much more unnecessary surgery and are referred for psychotherapy much more often than men, though crisis care is medicine's model for both sexes. (See relevant chapters for details.)

power rests mainly on several widely held myths, which have in good part been created by an aggressive and highly successful public relations campaign of the wealthy AMA and other such groups.* Brought up as most of us were to "believe" in medicine, it is hard at first to realize how influenced (even at times manipulated) we have been by medical propaganda.

Myths and Facts

Myth: *American medical care is the best in the world.*

Fact: The United States spends more money on medical care, uses more medical technology per capita than any country on earth and has one of the highest ratios of doctors and hospitals to people. Yet it lags behind other industrialized countries in life expectancy and ranks twenty-fifth in infant mortality rates, two crucial basic indicators of health in the general population.[4] Clearly, we are not getting our money's worth.†

Myth: *Medical care has been responsible for the major improvements in world health.*

Fact: Many dread infectious diseases‡ were "conquered" in the past century, but this was most likely because of improved nutrition and sanitation, not medical care. *Their incidence rates were already falling* when medical treatments and vaccines were introduced. With the exception of smallpox, vaccines helped speed the decline of these diseases only minimally. *The disappearance of these diseases is the major source of our greater life expectancy in this century, leaving the chronic diseases, for which medicine has provided no cures.* Difficult as it is to believe, mortality from most of the chronic diseases, which are our leading causes of death today, has remained virtually unchanged throughout the century.[6]

Careful studies reveal that medical care has *not* been the most important factor in improving infant mortality rates. Factors such as education, income and race continue to be the most accurate predictors of whether infants live or die. *General improvements, especially in nutrition and fertility control, have contributed most to improvements in neonatal mortality rates.*

Myth: *Medicine is a rigorous science.*

Fact: Medicine has prestige largely because it is associated with science in the public mind and claims objectivity and neutrality. Much of the theory on which modern medical practice is based actually derives from the untested assumptions and prejudices of earlier generations of medical leaders. Even though medical schools vaunt their "scientific method," they never actually teach it.[7] Furthermore, the scientific method is difficult to apply to human beings, since it is rarely possible or ethical to experiment on them as one would on inanimate objects or substances.* (However, animal researchers sometimes produce useful results.)

Myth: *Medical treatments in current use have been proven safe and effective.*

Fact: Most accepted treatments, therapies and medical technologies today have never been *scientifically* evaluated in terms of benefit.† Fetal monitors and radical mastectomies are only two examples of technology coming into widespread use before being fully evaluated. Scientific evaluation (in the form of randomized or controlled clinic trials [RCTs, CCTs])‡ is difficult, time- and labor-consuming and expensive and gets little funding from public sources. Most doctors have had no training in how to evaluate medical treatments and technology and often base their recommendations simply on what they think may work. As we were told by an assistant professor of medicine at Harvard Medical School:

---

*Misleading tactics have been applied by organized medicine and the drug industry in a variety of situations through their skilled manipulation of the media. Gullible reporters have announced breakthroughs and false reassurances for anything from reselling menopausal estrogens to claiming that the Pill is now totally safe.

†Some physician apologists have claimed that black and minority groups "drag down" our international standing in infant mortality (a clear case of racism and blaming the victim); however, even some of the most racially homogeneous U.S. communities lag considerably below Europe's best.[5] Furthermore, the resources we do spend have not improved certain disparities in health status. For example, in 1990 the National Commission to Prevent Infant Mortality reported that the death rate for black babies in the United States was twice that for white babies (17.9 deaths per 1,000 live births vs. 8.6). Also, from 1980 to 1987 the number of pregnant women not receiving prenatal care increased 50 percent.

‡The diseases were typhoid, smallpox, scarlet fever, measles, whooping cough, diphtheria, influenza, tuberculosis, pneumonia, diseases of the digestive system and poliomyelitis.

---

*There are always physicians willing to try if allowed to, which is one reason why ethical review boards have been set up in many institutions to set standards which all investigators must abide by (see Our Rights as Patients, p. 682).

†"No class of [medical] technologies is adequately evaluated for either cost effectiveness or social and ethical implications."[8]

‡Although there are other methods of evaluation, RCTs or CCTs are preferable. For these, very large numbers are required. Such trials also require that one group receiving treatment be compared with another (control) group receiving a different treatment or no treatment. This is the most difficult concept for the practicing physician, for whom the withholding of treatment is abhorrent. Without such evaluation, however, there is no way of *proving* that a certain type of medical treatment is effective, even if some people do seem to get better. "Only 10–20 percent of all procedures used in medical practice have been shown by Controlled Clinical Trials to be of benefit."[9]

Too frequently practicing physicians indulge in "cookbook medicine": They open the latest medical journal and inflict the latest recipe on patients, assuring their patients that on the one hand they are receiving "the latest thing" and on the other hand that they are "not guinea pigs."... In fact, the practicing physician is often extending some scientist's last experiment into the community setting—and without obtaining the patient's informed consent! At the same time, the scientist who performed the original experiment five years ago and who wrote the paper two or three years ago has long abandoned that approach in favor of something with more promise for a real cure.

Fact: Most nonreproductive medical research has been done only on men and the results have been applied to women. Such a process is also far from scientific. In 1990, the National Institutes of Health (NIH) issued new guidelines to ensure that women would be adequately represented in all NIH-funded research of potential relevance to women. Thus, this situation should improve.

Myth: *Medical care keeps us healthy.*
Fact: Although deep down many of us believe that medicine has created and sustained our health through the technological advances of the past fifty years, public health* studies show that our health is primarily the result of the food we eat, the water we drink, the air we breathe, the environment we live in, the work we do and the habits we form. These factors in turn result primarily from the education we have, the money we are able to earn and the other resources we are able to command. Still other factors contribute to good health and long life: control over one's personal life, influence over the larger forces that affect all our lives, loving friendships and a supportive community.

Drugs, surgery and medical technology (kidney dialysis machines or blood transfusions, for example) are invaluable tools, and many people would not be alive today without them. While few of us would want to live without these skills and emergency resources available to us and our families, it is fundamentally what *we* do or don't do, not what medicine does, that keeps us healthy.

By focusing on more profitable crisis care after people get sick rather than using its tremendous resources to help us prevent illness before it happens, the medical establishment shows itself unwilling to consider what really can and must be done to keep people healthy. This is a political

issue, not simply a medical one, although many medical spokespeople argue that medicine is apolitical, scientific or politically neutral. Because Americans spend increasing health dollars on treating symptoms, we have less to spend on preventing chronic diseases in the first place.* *To consider reallocating the money available would force all of us to confront our economic, political and social system as major contributors to our ill health.*

When we go to a physician, clinic or hospital, every one of these myths encourages us to *trust* professionals, to lean on their reassurances and to follow their orders. Especially when we are sick, it is difficult to be anything but trusting and compliant; being sick is frightening and we *need* to feel comforted. Because medical professionals offer false reassurances more often than we'd like to think, we *must* be as critical as we can, get all the information possible and ask friends and family to help us in doing this.

Poverty, Racism and Health

Poverty is the most basic cause of ill health and early death in our society. The poor, who are mostly women and children and disproportionately people of color, have more illnesses and die in greater numbers and earlier than people with more income and education.[10] Many of their health problems are diseases that result from malnutrition, workplace dangers, inadequate housing, environmental pollution or excessive stress.

The medical system blames poor people for suffering the effects of poverty; for instance, accusing poor women of not taking proper care of themselves or their children and seeing alcoholism and depression in working-class families as individual, preventable failures. Medicaid and Medicare programs, which offered the poor and elderly at least minimal access to medical care, have been cut drastically and will take decades to reinstate.† The very programs that reduce people's need for costly medical care—job training, food-assistance programs, health education to the community—have been cut as well. The almost inevitable result will be increasing illness and death among the poor.‡ The United States and South Africa are the only modern industrialized nations without a universal health service or a national health program.

Public health, which is the study of diseases or conditions in groups of people, is to be distinguished from *medicine*, the study and treatment of disease in the individual. *Epidemiology* is the basic science of public health.

*Prevention could reduce our illnesses by about half. (See Derek Bok, *Harvard Magazine*, May–June 1984, p. 430.)
†As it is, Medicaid covers only about 40 percent of the poor. Some states have expanded coverage for pregnant women beyond Medicaid through state-funded programs.
‡In Michigan, which has one of the highest unemployment rates in the country, the infant mortality rate in Detroit increased 5.4 percent from 12.8 per 1,000 in 1980 to 19.7 in 1990.

Poor women are increasingly turned away from health facilities.

Racism is a serious threat to health and in some instances creates more barriers to obtaining needed care and to survival than does social class.[11] For example, even allowing for social class, black babies still die at higher rates than white babies living in the same geographic area, due mainly to low birth weight among black babies, which is almost entirely preventable.[12] In many communities, medicine's response to the widening infant death gap between those who are getting adequate nutrition and prenatal services and those who are not is to propose even more costly neonatal centers.* What's needed is not more expensive machines but a serious attempt to counter the effects of racism or class discrimination on the health of expectant mothers. Leadership for such an effort will not come from the medical establishment, which is heavily invested in technological and pharmacological solutions to problems, not social change.

Although people of color need medical care more often than white people do, they frequently get less. For example, black people are less likely to get the most modern specialty treatment and follow-up care for cancer and do not survive as long after diagnosis. Similarly, even though hypertension is 82 percent higher among women of color, they do not receive any more treatment than white women.[13] Poor women and women of color often receive more abusive and damaging care than other women and are more likely to be used as "teaching material" in hospitals, so that physicians in training can practice the craft they will use later on wealthy private patients.[14] Sterilization abuse is far more frequent. When clients do not speak English fluently, they are often treated as though they are stupid. Stereotypes so govern practitioners' responses that a minority or poor patient who has the same symptoms as a white middle-class person will receive a different diagnosis and different treatment. In the words of a woman depicted in the film *Taking Our Bodies Back:*

It almost doesn't matter what I came in for, the place they send me is the "L" clinic ["L" is a code for sexually transmitted diseases]. They say, "She's black, she's got bladder trouble or a vaginal infection, she must be a prostitute—send her to the 'L' clinic."[15]

When poor women are badly treated, they don't have the money to sue. They may hesitate to complain assertively, fearing that then they will get no care at all, since "free" care may be cut off at any time. Paradoxically, when women decide not to return for care, their absence gives rise to the health administrators' accusation that "they just won't come," although services are available. Again, women are blamed. Poor women also have little access to the more costly nonmedical alternative practices.

Though we are more critical than ever of the present medical system, at the same time we are working for the right of every woman, regardless of race or income, to have access to that system. Above all, we want to promote those social programs that would reduce people's need for expensive medical interventions and work for the deeper societal changes that will help eliminate poverty and racism.

Medicalization and Social Control of Women's Lives

Everywhere you turn, medical professionals are claiming expertise in matters never before considered medical: in criminality, adolescence, overactivity in children, sex, diet, child abuse, exercise and aging. In this takeover, called *medicalization*, medical people become the "experts" on *normal* experiences or social problems.[16] Surely the most striking example of this process is the medicalization of women's lives.

Consider how often we are expected to go to physicians for normal life events. For our early sexual encounters we may expect to go to gynecologists for most birth control devices and perhaps even for advice about sex.* During pregnancy we are urged to see obstetricians to be sure all is proceeding normally, and few of us have any alternative but the hospital for giving birth (see Chapter 20, "Childbirth"). The medicalizing of childbirth has become so complete that it resembles treatment for a severe, life-threatening illness. When birth goes well, we are often grateful to the physician and give her or him the credit for

---

*For example, during the economically depressed period of the early 1980s, Rhode Island's Women and Infants Hospital proposed building a $50 million hospital to include a high-technology neonatal intensive care unit to save low-birth-weight infants in distress. Despite massive opposing testimony from citizens who argued that such deaths were preventable through community-based nutrition and midwifery-care programs, the building was approved. Such costly endeavors have become the national trend, displacing funds that could be used not only for nutrition and midwifery programs, but for drug treatment and AIDS prevention efforts as well, which pose increasing threats to women and their children.

---

*Men do not go to urologists for their basic medical care; children are not segregated by sex when visiting pediatricians. Yet for decades many of us are expected to go to an obstetrician-gynecologist to obtain our basic care. We learn to do this without realizing that by doing so we begin to define ourselves and all our bodily needs in terms of our sex organs and reproductive capacities.

our success; when it goes badly, we are even more grateful for the interventions we believe saved us and our babies. And once the baby is born, we shift our gratitude and dependence to the pediatrician, so that even the first moments of mothering are conducted with an immediate sense of what our pediatrician thinks is right and proper.

When we are depressed or having difficulties in our personal relationships, we are encouraged to seek the advice and help of a psychiatrist instead of talking with friends. Women see psychiatrists in far greater numbers than men (see Chapter 6, "Psychotherapy").

Medicine has stepped up its treatment of menopause and of aging as diseases. In a sense, the medical world defines women as inherently defective throughout life, in that we "require" a physician's care for all our normal female functions.

Medical "care" offered often extends to value judgments about our behavior, as we hear how a good girl, a good wife, a good mother should behave.

After advising me on when to put in my diaphragm ("Dinner, dishes, diaphragm," he said), my ob/gyn went on to speak about the fairly serious postpartum depression I was experiencing. "I like to tell my new mothers to get out to the library once in a while to keep their minds alive, but basically to find their happiness in the fact that they are taking care of their husbands and raising a new generation."

When I told my doctor (foolishly) that I'm a lesbian, the whole visit turned into a moral lecture and he never really paid attention to my problem. I walked out when he recommended a psychiatrist.

These moral judgments carry a weighty power, though they are no more "scientific" than the judgments of a priest or rabbi.[17]

We don't question the role that the physician has taken in our lives because, for one thing, our exposure and acceptance began early. When we were little, our mothers took us regularly to "the doctor," an extremely busy and important person, who may have ignored what our mothers said, and certainly what we said, and had their own answers. It may have seemed that our mothers allowed doctors to do all kinds of embarrassing or uncomfortable things to us and even that they did some of the same things themselves later on on the doctor's orders. Our mothers were very passive and compliant, in part because by the twentieth century male physicians had become the "authorities" on health. They had led a successful campaign during the late nineteenth and early twentieth centuries to eliminate midwives and sharply reduced the number of female physicians. For the first time in the history of the world,

women were forbidden by law to be responsible for other women's childbirths and were replaced almost exclusively by male physicians (see p. 692). When this happened, women lost both female role models and caregivers and also the support of a whole system of woman-to-woman guidance (see Women as Healers, p. 689).

During the mid-twentieth century, the gradual further moving of childbirth out of the home and into the hospital continued the process of isolating women from one another. Perhaps we have yet to measure how deeply our self-confidence as women may have been damaged by the loss of midwives as role models and respected sources of information and female authority.

All these factors together have brought us into an extreme and enforced dependency on professional experts—usually male physicians or those trained by them.[18]

Through these many medical encounters in the course of our normal life experiences, physicians gradually initiate women into the medical belief system, warning us against listening to other women, belittling the advice of our mothers, aunts, grandmothers and midwives—female lore—by calling it "old wives' tales." In this way, physicians prepare us to be their disciples. As we carry their message into our families and communities, we further contribute to the medicalization of society and a narrow, biological/technological perspective on the solution of human problems.*

It is difficult for most of us to recognize how "allopathic" medicine's proponents historically used women and women's central life experiences to initiate our entire society into a belief in and dependency on medicine. Despite much evidence to the contrary, most physicians believe sincerely that modern medicine has always helped women and that it deserves credit for society's overall health improvements since the turn of the century. Thus they tend to feel it is women's moral duty to teach children to place their faith in medicine.

Medicine as an Institution of Social Control

All societies establish institutions of social control, vested with the authority to define what is right or wrong, good or bad, sick or well. The schools, courts, and churches all play a role in defining our morality, but perhaps none more thoroughly than medicine does today. When we "deviate"—fail to conform to norms of woman-

---

*For a thorough analysis of medicalization and iatrogenesis, see Ivan Illich, *Medical Nemesis: The Expropriation of Health*, New York: Pantheon Books, 1976; Bantam Books, 1977.

hood—we discover how powerful medicine is.* Consider the ugly pronouncements medical authorities have made over the years, in the name of "science," about so-called inferior groups of people like women and blacks, and the way these pseudoscientific statements have been used to deprive these groups of social control and political power. For example, in the nineteenth century physicians claimed that to become a midwife or a doctor would "unsex" a woman: She would see things that would taint her moral character, cause her to "lose her standing as a 'lady' " and, because of the unusual physical and nervous excitement, "would damage her female organs irreparably and prevent her from fulfilling her social role as a wife and mother."[20] About blacks, a nineteenth-century physician wrote:

The grown-up Negro partakes, as regards his intellectual faculties, of the nature of the child, the female, and the senile White . . . [21]

This misuse of power and these pronouncements continue today: Physicians dismiss females as too much "at the mercy of their hormones" to be trusted with serious responsibility, and cite blacks' "low-degree expectations" as a hurdle to parity in medical schools.†

Partly through the sanctity of the private physician–patient relationship, medicine (primarily obstetrics/gynecology and psychiatry) also achieves social control by encouraging us to see personal problems as individual isolated experiences rather than as problems we have in common with other women.

The Doctor–Patient Relationship

The relationship between a woman and her doctor is usually one of profound inequality on every level, an exaggeration of the power imbalance inherent in almost all male–female relationships in our society. The scales are even more unbalanced if the doctor is an ob/gyn with special knowledge about and power over our most intimate bodily selves or a psychiatrist with the authority to label us crazy or sane, to decide whether we can keep our children or not. *Doctors also frequently doubt our word simply because we are women.*

As in any relationship in which we are less powerful, we tend to evaluate what happens in a medical encounter in terms of *our* behavior rather than the doctor's. For example, if we don't understand something, we feel inadequate. Often we believe that a doctor's superior education, training, experience, sex and (sometimes) age automatically produce infallible judgment. "Well, he must know," many women say.

Many of us want to believe that we are in the hands of superior physicians—even though this may well not be true.

I knew that my doctor had a reputation for being one of the best in the city, and it made me feel good when I said his name and other people would say, "Oh, right, I've heard of him." I expected that he was going to do the best job he could possibly do. When he criticized me, I shrank inside. Sometimes I'd be annoyed that I had to travel so far for him to look at my stomach. But the mysteries still held. He was going to give me the baby. Once he confused me with someone else, and I was very depressed.

There may always be something about the "laying on of hands" that calls up the child in us and makes us feel dependent, especially when pain and fear are present. Many physicians deliberately work to increase this natural phenomenon into a special kind of dependency (psychiatrists call it *transference*) in which the patient turns to the physician for guidance in all kinds of personal problems. Many medical schools and residency training programs teach techniques for eliciting this dependency as a useful way of "managing" patients, using the parent–child relationship as a model.* When a woman raises real, matter-of-fact questions, a doctor is apt to say, "What's the matter, don't you trust me?" For most doctors, the fact that the transference develops is justification for it—that is, a woman becomes overly dependent because she "needs" or wants to be.

---

*For example, many poor women are sterilized without their knowledge or consent because they are unmarried or a physician thinks they have "too many babies" (see Sterilization, p. 300). Physicians have forced some women to accept cesarean sections, declaring them "unfit mothers" in court when they refuse a recommended section (despite the risk to the mother's own life); some women have had their children taken from them by the courts because a physician judged them "potential child abusers" for refusing medical treatments during pregnancy.[19]

†The kinds of biological (rather than societal) explanations for behavior and social position popular in the nineteenth century are becoming influential once again. Reinforced by such notions as "sociobiology," these myths have dangerous consequences for women, people of color and the poor.[22]

*As Diana Scully describes in her 1980 landmark study of obstetrician/gynecologists,[23] the training process prepares the surgeon to gain the patient's trust and confidence primarily for the purpose of controlling or "managing" her and then to *manipulate* her into doing something *the physician wants her to do*—undergoing surgery, for example, or some other procedure. Often, this is done either to gain experience or to generate income and is frequently not in her interests. (See the section on hysterectomy, p. 598, and other relevant procedures.)

Dr. G. sighed when he saw me. After examining me he sat down and said, "Let me be direct with you, hon." (I flinched at the "hon.") "You have called me or been here no less than four times this fall. You are complaining about a pain that has no apparent organic basis. Quite frankly, my guess is that there are areas of your life you are having trouble facing, and the result is a funny pain in your chest and shoulder that flits around and is sometimes here and sometimes there and sometimes not anywhere at all."

"But I can feel exactly where it is," I broke in.

"Why don't you just leave the worrying to me?" he admonished. "I am the doctor. I have everything under control."[24]

The work of feminist sociologists such as Sue Fischer and Alexandra Todd shows the importance of changing this imbalance and improving communication. Our stories are crucial for correct diagnoses as well as for control over treatment options.

We can start needed change by pressing for real answers to our questions, using other sources of information besides our doctors (books, magazines, friends, nurses), seeking second opinions (not from a doctor who is our doctor's close colleague, on the same hospital staff or in the same specialty) and by bringing a friend to medical visits. Immersed in the propaganda about women's "need" for dependency, and comfortable with the fatherly, authoritarian role, many physicians react with surprise and even hostility at our "aggressiveness" when we insist on being partners in our health and medical care decisions. We must not let their reactions prevent us from persisting.

Occasionally, over time, you can build a satisfactory relationship with a doctor.

Friends now marvel at my close relationship with my current doctor and my ability to talk back, question and disagree with him and his colleagues. He respects me and trusts me to tell him what is going on, and I in turn trust him to listen, make suggestions and consult with me before any action is taken. When I don't want a procedure done or feel the psychological burden of making yet another trip to the lab or to his office is just too much for me on an occasion, I will tell him and he understands me most of the time. I have finally after many many years found someone willing to take into account my whole medical history and apply it to my current situation.

Sexual Abuse

Not only have women reported increasing numbers of cases of rape by their doctors, but between 5 and 10 percent of doctors have admitted in sur-

veys and interviews to having sexual relations with their patients, sometimes saying that they believed such relations were either harmless or actually beneficial or "therapeutic" to the women involved. Because of the unequal power relationships involved, this sexual abuse may produce severe damage, akin to father–daughter incest.[25] When the woman turns to or is referred to a psychiatrist, she may be blamed for having "caused" the abuse.* Worse still, a few psychiatrists seduce the woman once again.[26]

It takes enormous courage for women to come forward and speak out about sexual abuse by doctors. Frequently no one believes them, and in one case, even nurses reporting their eyewitness experiences of patient abuse for three years were ignored by hospital administrators until another physician caught his anesthesiologist colleague in the act.[27]

The few cases that do reach state boards of registration in medicine frequently drag on for months and are then resolved with inadequate controls on future abuse. In spite of the fact that the Hippocratic oath and the ethics codes of all medical societies specifically forbid sexual relations with patients, doctors have made no serious effort to discipline those who breach the code. In fact, the medical profession often appears more concerned with covering up for a colleague who commits what are tactfully called "indiscretions." In the words of a woman psychiatrist:

I reported a psychiatrist who had had sex with two of his patients to the medical society. I called back two months later to find out what had been done. They told me the doctor denied everything, and it was his word against the patients'; so they were dropping the matter. When I persisted, the chairman of the ethics committee told me, "You know, my dear, we are not a consumer organization."

Physicians themselves may arrange for a problem physician to go to another community, without telling the unsuspecting new community about his assaultive behavior. In one famous case, medical school faculty members wrote glowing letters of recommendation for a convicted rapist who had moved to a new community.[28]

It is common for women who are sexually abused by a doctor to be persuaded that he has fallen in love with them. This is not a sign of naiveté or psychopathology on our part. The physicians involved have abused a trust that every

---

*Another 20 percent believe this. In California alone, one survey reported 36 percent of psychiatrists and 46 percent of psychologists had admitted affairs with clients during therapy.

woman has learned to place in them (see also Chapter 8, "Violence Against Women").

We want to encourage women to notice any peculiar or irresponsible behavior and discuss these experiences with one another, to feel entitled to take action if necessary, protect ourselves and others and get our genuine needs for trust met appropriately. Keep a record of what happens; call a local women's group or rape crisis center; give serious consideration to mentioning your experience to a reliable lawyer.

The Profit Motive in Medical Care

Why doesn't the present U.S. medical system provide affordable services and emphasize prevention and primary care? The profit motive has to be the main reason. From the many individuals who still want to be paid "fee for service" and build up a lucrative practice to the profit-making drug and insurance companies, medical care is now an industry in itself—the second-largest in the country—and a virtual monopoly.

The Medical Monopoly

Our present type of medicine created a monopoly at the turn of the century through its control over state licensing laws which defined what the practice of medicine should be and who could be called a doctor. The laws provided state-sanctioned penalties for those who were not "properly" trained and licensed. At the same time the medical profession also gained absolute control over its education process, thus becoming a "legally enforced monopoly of practice."[29] Today medicine continues to set its own priorities and terms, with physicians controlling the majority of the medical decision-making and resource allocation processes. The profession decides what will be taught in medical schools, what medical services will be offered and how and where.* Surgeons generate most of their own income by self-referral ("I recommend this procedure and I will also perform it"), a practice judged unethical in other countries. Patients or third-party payors pay for services rendered. In many situations there is still no one but another doctor to decide whether or not these services are necessary, and no way of knowing whether or not they are effective. When review of costs occurs (as in the case of insurance), it is often only physicians who undertake that review.

Medicine's monopoly was further consolidated when the government made federal funds available for hospital construction (Hill-Burton law), and the "Blues" (Blue Cross/Blue Shield) were created to reimburse in-hospital care. (Many of the Blue Crosses were created originally by local medical societies and are still physician dominated). Backed up by the private insurance industry, hospitals became the base of medical care in this country. Substantial federal funding for Medicare, Medicaid and medical research increased the volume of federal money flowing into medicine. At the same time, profit-making hospital and nursing-home chains also began to proliferate. Today, expenditures for medical care grow faster than anything else. The whole system is completely out of control, despite growing cuts. Medicine has been allowed to expand continuously, and virtually without limits or accountability.*

In addition, there has been a phenomenal rise in the "corporatization" of medical care; that is, profit-making medical care chains that operate laboratories, "emergency rooms," mobile CAT scanners and so on, in addition to hospitals and nursing homes—a proliferation of separate services purely for profit.† Academic centers, medical schools and teaching hospitals have themselves created new and unprecedented arrangements amounting to millions of dollars with profit-making drug firms, all in the name of "scientific research"[30]—the medical-academic-industrial complex.

Those who profit from our illnesses are well organized politically and use their ample resources to keep the medical system free from gov-

---

*Because medical care should always involve so much more than the application of technical skills and because it always occurs in a social context, society should be able to influence both the quality and quantity of medical care available. For example, we have too many specialists crowded into affluent communities and entirely more doctors than we need, although many inner city and rural areas in greater need have severe shortages of physicians. Yet 95 percent of physicians now specialize, despite a continuing shortage of primary-care physicians. Medical schools take no leadership in rectifying the problem, which leaves millions with inadequate access to quality care.

*Because so much of our tax money is involved, we expect public utilities and our public education system, for example, to be somewhat accountable to the users. Through a public process we participate in decisions about cost, services and salaries, and sometimes even the budget itself. Though medical education, research and hospital operations are heavily subsidized by our taxes at all levels, we have virtually no say in how this money is spent. A few federally funded attempts were made in the past to make medicine more accountable, such as the formation of HSAs, but further attempts will now have to depend on local funding and initiative.

In addition, when there are errors or abuses in medical practice, physicians insist on "policing" themselves, leaving our range of options for redress short and unsatisfactory (see Medical Education and Training, p. 663, and Our Rights as Patients, p. 682).

†For example, recent surveys show that half of U.S. physicians are now on salary, many in profit-making corporations that are often physician owned. The fee-for-service system is changing, but not necessarily for the benefit of consumers, because only a few salaried doctors work in nonprofit settings such as health centers.

ernment intrusion. Although they do not always agree among themselves, an informal coalition—physicians' lobbying groups like the AMA and ACOG, the pharmaceutical industry, hospital associations, the big voluntary "health" associations (Heart Association, Cancer Society, etc.), among others—tend to support the profit motive, the fee-for-service reimbursement system and the present crisis-care medical model.*

Health care has become a commodity or economic good, with profit as a blatant and legitimate goal. However inadequate government involvement in medical care was, it did make it possible for us to partially evaluate the system. It increased access to the system in some regions for a percentage of those who most needed it, and helped us to monitor or check a few of the system's most flagrant abuses. Government agencies were forced to respond *somewhat* to citizen pressure in the name of public interest. But federal regulations have been evaporating, with the result that profit-making enterprises have increased in number and monitoring their practices will be more difficult.

Our best hope is to form groups of workers and friends in the community and to work at the state level, making sure that reasonable options for care remain open to as many as possible at reasonable prices.

Insurance

The insurance principle has become increasingly influential in shaping U.S. medical care. All third-party reimbursement systems, whether through private, profit-making insurance systems, nonprofit Blue Cross/Blue Shield (the "Blues") or public programs (Medicare, Medicaid), reward doctors and hospitals by reimbursing them for doing the most expensive and complicated procedures on a fee-for-service basis. Yet they pay nothing or even require us to pay out of pocket for basic well-woman or preventive care. The insurance system thus acts as a kind of "blank check": We pay the premiums, directly or through our taxes (both continually rising); the doctors and hospitals bill the third parties (sometimes doctors also bill us for the "difference" between what insurance covers and what their real charges are), and there is no one looking to see if something cheaper or better (or sooner) might have been done. Medical costs skyrocket as a result. The chief beneficiaries of the insurance system are actually

*The Center for Science in the Public Interest has played an important role in recently challenging how these extremely wealthy national organizations spend the money donated to them and in urging them to play a more effective role in health policy directed toward prevention. We can work locally by getting onto boards of chapters to help influence local projects (see Resources in Chapter 26, "Organizing for Change: U.S.A.").

the doctors and stockholders, whose incomes and profits are all guaranteed.[31]

The insurance industry discriminates blatantly against women both as health and medical care workers and as consumers. Programs often do not reimburse directly for the services of nonphysician workers like nurse-midwives, nurse-practitioners, physical therapists and nutritionists, the majority of whom are women (this is changing now). Instead they reimburse the physicians, health departments or hospitals who hire or supervise them and indeed profit from their labor.

The Drug Industry

Almost nowhere is the inherent conflict between profit-making and public safety more obvious than with the manufacture and sale of prescrip-

---

WHERE DOES THE MONEY GO?

- About 12 percent of the U.S. gross national product, or $666 billion, now goes for health and medical care.
- This 12 percent is at least 25 percent more than Sweden or Canada, two-thirds more than Japan and twice that spent in Great Britain. Yet our infant mortality rate is higher and life expectancy lower than in all these countries.
- Per capita spending on hospital and physician services for the insured are 25 to 50 percent greater than for the uninsured.
- Nursing home costs increase more than 10 percent annually, inching toward $50 billion.
- Unnecessary services, administrative and advertising costs amount to at least $200 billion annually. Administrative costs, due largely to the many health insurers (over 1500), different billing systems and variations in coverage plans, account for more than 20 percent of total health and medical care expenditures—more than in any other nation.
- Physician earnings and hospital costs continue to rise well ahead of inflation; for many, profits are increasing.
- Technological innovations, largely of unproven value, account for 70 percent of health and medical care costs.
- Our tax dollars now support more than half the medical enterprise in all its forms, including medical education.

---

tion drugs. Yet it is difficult to control the drug industry, which lies at the heart of both the medical system and the capitalist system. According to Dr. James L. Goddard, former commissioner of the Food and Drug Administration (FDA):

An American buying prescription drugs buys on faith what his doctor has prescribed. He is like a child who goes to the store with his mother's shopping list, which he cannot even read. He is totally unsophisticated as to the workings of the $5,000,000,000 [1972 figures] industry to which he is contributing and which his tax money is already helping to support. The consumer of drugs pays up and takes his medicine, and the Drug Establishment, about which he knows nothing, scores again.[32]

Prescription drug sales in 1987 were estimated at about $23 billion, averaging twenty prescriptions per family in the United States. Pharmaceutical companies regularly show a return on investment of over 26 percent, outperforming any other part of the industrial sector. The drug industry is more than three times as price inflationary as all other U.S. industries. Americans have to pay more than twice or three times what Canadians and Europeans spend for drugs.

Although some drugs do save lives and enhance the quality of life for many sick people, research reveals increasing numbers of both new and older drugs to be dangerous or useless.* The GAO (the government's General Accounting Office) reports that Medicare/Medicaid pays $40 million a year for drugs shown to have no effectiveness. Each year, at least 1.5 million people go into the hospital because they have adverse reactions to drugs. Women receive about two-thirds of all prescription drugs, and the most profitable drugs made by the industry are oral contraceptives, injectable contraceptives (like Depo-Provera) and tranquilizers, all risky in some ways and all targeted mainly for women.

The drug industry spends 25 percent of its resources ($10 billion) on marketing—*more than on research*—and most of it for prescription drug promotion targeted to physicians.[34] Despite recent legislative efforts to curb gifts to medical students, the industry continues to woo successfully both practicing physicians, medical residents and medical schools by offering "research" opportunities and luxurious travel symposia, as well as sponsoring educational programs in hospitals and schools. Because medical school training in phar-

macology is largely inadequate, doctors become permanently dependent on drug companies for information (or misinformation). As a result, physicians often cannot or do not protect us from ineffective or dangerous drugs. Often they don't know the possibly serious negative effects, or they continue to prescribe the drugs anyway,* based on personal observation or the belief that any negative findings (always challenged by the drug companies) have been inaccurate. Doctors also tend to prescribe the advertised brand-name drugs, which are more profitable to the drug companies, rather than using generic drugs, cheaper for the consumer, and often encourage patients' notions that a visit to the doctor is not complete without a prescription to "solve" the problem.

Regulation
The FDA was ostensibly designed to protect the public from the dangers of adulterated food and harmful or useless drugs. (See Chapter 2, "Food," for more on the FDA.) Over many years, the efforts of some conscientious FDA staff, prompted and encouraged by the pressure of consumer groups, activists, investigative reporters and members of Congress, have sometimes led to effective, though limited, protection, as well as increased consumer participation in the regulatory process.

▪ Barbara Seaman, a founder of the National Women's Health Network and an early researcher on the Pill and menopausal estrogens, helped alert the public to the risk of these drugs in her testimony before Congress.
▪ Doris Haire, founder of the American Foundation for Maternal and Child Health, has repeatedly challenged the FDA, Congress and physician experts to demonstrate the safety to the infant and mother of drugs administered routinely during pregnancy, labor and delivery.
▪ Ralph Nader's Health Research Group has publicized the dangers and ineffectiveness of many drugs, successfully pressured the FDA to get them off the market, testified in Congress and worked extensively with the FDA staff on behalf of consumers.

However, these achievements are being increasingly threatened by the antiregulatory climate of a conservative government and also by the fact that the FDA's small budget has never been able to compete against the huge financial resources

---

*An industry-sponsored study of all drugs approved between 1938 and 1962 showed only 12 percent to be effective for their prescribed use and at least 15 percent to have no effectiveness whatsoever. *Yet most of these drugs are still on the market.*[33]

*For instance, physicians continued to prescribe progestin for pregnancy tests despite the discovery of a link to birth defects. The FDA warned against the use of the drug in the early stages of pregnancy, yet 75,000 prescriptions for progestin tests were given in 1978, years after the first FDA warning (testimony of Sidney Wolfe before Senator Edward Kennedy's Senate Health subcommittee August 1, 1979).

the drug industry musters for lobbying, court cases and the production of new products. The FDA is no match for many of the "best" drug companies, which often have substantial criminal records involving bribing of officials in foreign governments, falsifying of test data and failing to comply with FDA requirements to report adverse reactions to drugs.[35] Because drug companies are themselves required to test new drugs for safety and effectiveness, they also hire most of the researchers; if the research lab or doctor can make data look favorable to the company, it is more likely to continue to obtain funding.

At the very least, the drug industry should be required to submit to certain basic reforms, such as the severing of financial connections to those researching the safety and efficacy of the drugs they want to market, and the payment of much more severe penalties for misconduct. Consumer and public-interest groups have to be better watchdogs than ever before and also must serve as pressure groups to establish better regulatory systems at the state and local levels.

Medical Education and Training

Physicians have unusually broad powers. They decide which patients will be treated and where, who goes to the hospital, what treatment is given and for how long and which drugs are administered and in what quantities. They also have enormous influence in our most personal decisions. Why do many physicians misuse their power, consciously or unconsciously? Many of the behaviors we complain about in physicians—their authoritarian manner, their insensitivity and condescension—can be traced back to their education and training as doctors.

Who Gets into Medical School?

Traditionally, upper- and upper-middle class white men have been the ones to survive the fierce competition for medical school entrance. In the words of one prestigious medical educator, "The years of premedical education, once considered so rewarding, have become a battleground of ruthless competition."[36] Some students tear out textbook pages so others cannot read them, and distort their fellow-students' experiments. Some also cheat, and it is known that those who do so will continue their deceptive behavior as doctors. Experienced educators have believed for some time that medicine is no longer attracting the best and brightest students, one reason being that they are repelled by the typical premed who would become their colleague. Although 1960s and 1970s activism resulted in a surge of women, poor and minority students, this number peaked around

1977 for poor and minority students, in part due to cutbacks in federal funding and in part to the fact that most medical schools were accepting these other candidates only under pressure.* Therefore, most physicians train alongside people more or less exactly like themselves, with teachers formed from the same mold. The result is a kind of cloning: The medical profession reproduces itself.

The Training

Medical schools ask students to absorb an enormous quantity of highly technical information in compressed form, largely through one-way lectures. They place little emphasis on thinking and reasoning and none at all on questioning, criticizing or arguing. Few could learn to think critically in this environment if they did not know how before medical school. Students "are being driven to absorb an enormous amount of science at the sacrifice of just about everything else." Recall is poor after even a short period, however, and many in academic medicine admit that much of this material, irrelevant to competent medical practice, has crowded out crucial skills and subject matter. In the words of a woman physician:

The training program is disease-oriented, with life-threatening or rare conditions receiving the most attention, and the acquisition of skill in doing procedures (biopsies, punctures) and using diagnostic machines (EKG, X-ray, lab tests) being prized. The day-to-day ills of the public are ignored as "minor problems." The promotion of health and the prevention of disease are neglected almost entirely.[37]

The training usually does not challenge students to become more aware of the social and political realities affecting people's health or to work through their own sexism, homophobia, class bias, ageism and racism. A woman doctor who does have a political awareness, wrote:

When I show a student her own cervix with a mirror, she is fascinated. When she is with me as a student and I offer my white middle-class patient the opportunity, the student thinks it is great. But when I offer a sixty-year-old woman the chance or a twenty-five-year-old working-class black woman, the student is amazed that "that kind" of patient would want to see her cervix. When I say, "This could be done in the clinic and would make women feel more in control," students say to me, "Oh, no, there's no time" (one extra minute?) or, worse, " 'Those people' wouldn't be interested."

---

*Enrollments for women are still increasing, however.

Glaringly absent from medical training are most of the values, concerns and skills often thought of as "feminine": nurturance, empathy, caring, sensitive listening, encouraging others to take care of themselves, collaboration rather than competition. The medical hierarchy relegates these values and skills to the domain of nurses, other aides and (female) family members of the patients—physicians have "more important" things to attend to. Patients deprived of these elements of caring may not be as quick to recover, may miss absorbing important information about aftercare or preventive care and may end up feeling depressed about their experience because no one has paid attention to the emotional impact of their health problems. Women often complain bitterly of cold, abstract, impersonal or authoritarian doctors. A major study by the Institute of Medicine found that a majority of families were dissatisfied with their doctors and up to half had changed them as a result.[38] These qualities may have less to do with the physician's original personality than with the one-sidedness of her or his training. Similarly vital knowledge needed for optimum patient care—how to evaluate studies and risks accurately, what tests and treatments really cost, how to recognize a patient's rights and identify the ethical issues involved in medical decisions, what patients could do for themselves to prevent illness—is either absent altogether or relegated to

the status of an elective. Students get the message: This material is not important.[39]

Many medical educators are now alarmed over the erosion of clinical skills caused by the overemphasis on technology in today's training, that is, by the increasing inability of younger physicians to make judgments based on experience, examination and careful listening to the patient rather than on readings from tests and machines.

The focus narrows further at the residency stage, where students aim to specialize because specialization promises more money, prestige and control over one's work.

Specialization and the rapid rate of advancement of knowledge and technology may tend to pre-empt the attention of both teachers and students from the central purpose of medicine, which is to heal the sick and relieve suffering.[40]

Residency programs are grueling, low-paid, often demanding as much as thirty-six hours at a stretch and a hundred hours a week in consistently understaffed conditions, undesirable for both residents and patients alike. Teaching becomes haphazard, and not surprisingly, all types of residents have shown declining scores and performances in recent years, particularly in basic skills.

In short, specialty training is a dehumanizing process. Few working conditions in the industrial age have survived with so little change. Composed of one part sleep deprivation, one part shutting off of all feelings and one part automatic response to orders in what is probably the most militaristic of all civilian disciplines, this training resembles a kind of brainwashing.* The stress contributes to physicians' high rates of mental breakdown, drug addiction, alcoholism, suicide and family disruption.[41] Rates of incompetence among physicians in practice have also grown alarmingly. In addition to errors, they both perform many useless procedures and fail to perform needed ones.[42]

Studies have shown that while medical students may begin medical training with idealism and a sincere desire to help people, after years of training in the closed worlds of medical school and residency they become almost invariably more cynical, detached and mechanistic than at entry.[43] Their ability to communicate has actually deteriorated during the process.[44] Because of the enormous personal sacrifice medical training requires, and because most of the teachers and the doctors they admire are highly paid specialists,

A Lady as a physician.   The Feminist Press

---

*The term *brainwashing* has been used repeatedly by medical educators, students and physicians in conversations with the authors. See also Allan Chamberlain, "Night Life: Sleep Deprivation in Medical Education," *The New Physician* (May 1981), p. 30, for use of this term.

young physicians feel entitled to earn very large sums of money and to command interpersonal authoritarian power once the training is completed. Here is how another distinguished medical educator puts it: "What emerges are physicians without inquiring minds, physicians who bring to the bedside *not* curiosity and a desire to understand but a set of reflexes that allows them to earn a handsome living."[45]

These criticisms are not new; indeed, many

TOP PRIORITY FOR THE 1990S—A NATIONAL HEALTH PLAN

Except for South Africa, the United States is the only industrialized country in the world without a national health plan. During the 1990s this country will debate different legislative proposals designed to secure universal access to health and medical care. The National Women's Health Network and the Boston Women's Health Book Collective, along with other progressive organizations, believe that any successful system of universal access must include the following features:

- Comprehensive services, including preventive, routine, long-term care and independent living services;* noninstitutional alternatives, and access to caregivers such as midwives, chiropractors and homeopaths. For women, this means inclusion of such services such as Pap smears, birth control, mammography, and access to homebirth and freestanding birth centers (for low-risk childbearing women) and home-care services.
- Funding from a single source, publicly controlled, with most funds raised through progressive taxation.
- More systematic technology assessment, so that new (and increasingly more expensive) technologies will come under closer scrutiny before becoming accepted medical practice. (The internal fetal heart monitor is an excellent example of inappropriate and wasteful routine use of technology as a result of inadequate assessment.)
- No barriers to obtaining care, such as copayments, deductibles and exemptions for previously existing conditions.
- Some significant degree of community input and control over the nature and type of services offered. This will require better education of the public about the most important determinants of health, so that increased community involvement will translate into improved decision making;
- Complete elimination of the fee-for-service model (which has encouraged unnecessary and often harmful treatment, especially for women). Already, close to half of U.S. physicians are on salary, so this may be a far less radical proposal today than twenty years ago.
- More equitable distribution of services and facilities to underserved populations and regions.
- A greater decision-making role for women and minorities, at least proportional to their presence in the community.
- High-quality, free and inexpensive resources for health- and medical-care information geared to laypersons.

The tremendous influence of the insurance industry, the current antitax climate and organized medicine may limit the political viability of some of these measures. The over 1500 insurance companies in the United States are especially opposed to the single-payor model, because it would essentially eliminate their current role in the provision of health and medical care. They, of course, prefer minor reform of the current insurance system. Interestingly, many members of Congress have expressed support for a "pay or play" approach (whereby employers either provide coverage to their employees or pay into a general fund that will cover their employees), usually because they state it is the most politically viable. Pay-or-play plans, as currently proposed, discriminate against part-time employees and thus hurt women more than men.

Surveys of the public show an overwhelming preference for the single-payor model (similar to that in Canada), suggesting that political viability is determined more by large lobbying interests than what the citizenry want. We hope that expanded public debate and activism on the question of a national health program will bring needed change before the turn of the decade—despite the opposition of powerful lobbies such as the insurance industry.

*Long-term care and independent living services for people with chronic illness and physical and mental disabilities are especially important for women given our longer life span. These services must include durable equipment, personal assistance services under the control of the individual, and backup hospice care.

were voiced as soon as the medical monopoly was created nearly a century ago. When *Our Bodies, Ourselves* came out in 1973, the then president of the American Association of Medical Colleges said every medical student should read it.

A number of proposals to reform medical training have emphasized the importance of good communication skills and medical care that is culturally, linguistically and racially appropriate. For example, in response to pressure from the women's health movement, which had protested teaching medical students how to do pelvic exams on anesthetized women (often without their consent) and prostitutes, some medical schools now involve specially trained gynecological teaching associates (GTAs) in the teaching of the pelvic exam. These women can offer important, immediate feedback about how well a student is doing an exam, when s/he is doing something that may be hurting and so on.*

Even if educational reforms were to be realized, without substantial input from consumers and their communities, the experience of health and medical care will continue to be frustrating for women. Meanwhile, we can look to the many alternative and neighborhood facilities created by women and men over the past twenty years or so for examples of successful efforts to integrate competence, caring and community partnership (see Chapter 26, "Organizing for Change: U.S.A.").

Women Physicians

Today about 17 percent of all MDs in the United States are women, and this percentage may rise to 25 percent by the year 2000. Women express over and over again the hope and belief that female physicians will be different from their male colleagues, that they will listen and understand and be sensitive and caring. How realistic is this hope?

Within five years of the beginning of the second wave of feminism, women began applying to medical schools in record numbers. Since the 1960s, female enrollments have been increasing, sometimes passing 40 percent. The leadership of medicine, almost entirely male, was at first clearly appalled at this influx and tried every kind of psychological intimidation to discourage women from applying.† Camouflaging a basic fear of women as economic competitors, arguments

against women being doctors focused (as in the nineteenth century) on women's supposed biological inappropriateness for the role of physician: The menstrual cycle causes emotional instabilities, women in the classroom distract males, women marry and have children and prove their training a waste. In the 1970s, it took a class-action lawsuit charging discrimination against every medical school in the country, plus many individual lawsuits and affirmative action legislation, to get medical schools and residency programs to accept women in anything but token numbers.[47]

Once in school, women students "have to work twice as hard as men to be accepted . . . to be considered equal."[48] Very few women are on the faculty.

Women students must also endure hostility from their male colleagues. In one Ivy League school in 1982 women found obscene and angry graffiti left on their bulletin boards: "Scrotum breaths" and "You are pigs, but we like that in a woman." Plates of excrement appeared outside their doors.[49]

Perhaps worse, women students continuously encounter the demeaning and objectifying way women patients are presented in classrooms, textbooks and actual clinical settings.

I have been told by a surgeon that a twenty-five-year-old female with abdominal pain was by definition an "unreliable historian."

A professor who had included a nudie slide in his lecture [said] . . . "Men need to look down on women, and that's why I show the slide."

Often women are portrayed as hysterical or as nagging mothers or as having trivial complaints. Men are almost never pointed to as having a psychological component to their illnesses.[50]

Such indignities present women students with a painful dilemma. As one said, "Every day we must choose between speaking up in a sexist situation or suffering in silence." The only other alternative is to block off any personal identification with other women students or with women patients.

Many women students keep silent, deciding to concentrate first on performing well:

I felt as a medical student you played by the rules of the game, otherwise you weren't going to keep moving.

Later, when fully credentialed, they plan to use their authority to challenge and perhaps change the distressing practices they saw as students. Un-

---

*For more information on GTAs, contact the Program in Introduction to Clinical Medicine, Tulane University Medical Center, 1430 Tulane Avenue, New Orleans, LA 70112.

†Margaret Campbell completely catalogues the many forms of discrimination women experienced during the 1970s. In a major study of attitudes toward female applicants, some of the replies from medical schools were "too outrageous to be published."[46]

IMAGES OF WOMEN IN MEDICAL TEXTBOOKS

Medical students and physicians in residency training are often referred to ob/gyn and psychoanalysis textbooks as sources of authority on how to determine the character of and how to "manage" women patients. Most practicing physicians today absorbed as students considerable sexist, judgmental and paternalistic dogma from these books.[51] Although there have been some improvements in recent years, the following excerpts are from recent texts currently used in leading medical schools today. The tone of these comments clearly encourages doctors to think of themselves as skilled and powerful counselors who have the right and even the obligation to act as our judges and moral guardians. It is ironic that doctors are looked upon by society as experts on women's psyche and sexuality, yet are typically so ignorant and poorly trained. These passages help perpetuate both the attitudes and errors passed down from one generation of doctors to the next.

1983 *The evaluation of the patient's personality need not be a lengthy matter. It begins as she enters the consultation room and sits down. Character traits are expressed in her walk, her dress, her makeup, her responses to questions, and in almost every action, both verbal and non-verbal in nature. The observant physician can quickly make a judgment as to whether she is overcompliant, overdemanding, aggressive, passive, erotic or infantile....*

Many physicians hesitate to delve into a patient's emotional state because they fear a negative reaction from the patient or even that their questions might make the patient feel worse. If they question patients gently and watch for signs of resistance, no harm can be done. Certainly the patient who responds with anger or disgust should be allowed to keep her own confidences, but this response in itself indicates that an emotional problem may exist . . . [52]

1981 *With the dawn of female suffrage and equality, the professional prostitute has begun to disappear, but the nonprofessional prostitute has appeared....*

*In Western culture, education in sexuality had as its proper aim the development of a mature, responsible adult who was, therefore, prepared to enter into a happy, monogamous marriage and become a responsible parent. [Repeated sim-*ilarly in four places.] ... In the Jensen *Handbook, it is advised to discuss certain abnormalities of the sex drive, such as homosexuality, exhibitionism and child molesters. [Emphasis ours.] ... The topic of masturbation, however, is one which might be casually introduced as a normal adolescent habit pattern which disappears as the individual reaches adulthood. . . . One should know that intercourse is habit-forming. The nervous system of an adolescent is still plastic, therefore habits are easily established. This is one reason why it is especially unwise for individuals still under the age of 21 to use habit-forming addictive drugs, such as alcohol, pot, glue, etc., likewise with the habit of intercourse. . . . The frequency of intercourse should depend primarily upon the male sex drive, for the male physiology involved requires active physical stress.*

The female should be advised to allow her male partner's sex drive to set their pace and she should attempt to gear hers satisfactorily to his. Lack of consideration for the male partner's inherent physical drive is a common cause of impotence and reflects an immature attitude of the female who is using her partner for self-gratification.

The patient should be encouraged to discuss her attitude towards intercourse in order that the physician may evaluate her maturity and knowledge. . . . Sexual frigidity, by which is meant the inability to respond sexually, is not frequent in the female, although there seems to be little doubt that libido, which is well developed among normal males, appears to be somewhat less highly developed among females . . . [53]

1978 *Many women complain bitterly of severe, persistent lower abdominal pelvic pain, which is completely out of proportion to the physical findings. The pain is real to the patient, but she is totally unable to convey to the gynecologist any clear-cut description of its nature, its point of origin or its path of radiation....*

It is a difficult matter to pinpoint the trigger mechanism for the production of pelvic pain due to functional *cause. In general, there seems to be agreement that this kind of pain is related to some form of emotional disorder. The actual cause of the pain is similar to that noted in patients who suffer from hysteria. [Emphasis ours.] ...*

continued

continued

To get a maximum response in the patient with dysmenorrhea it may be necessary to alter her attitude toward femininity and encourage the patient to accept her maturing womanly status with pride. If you can accomplish this the patient may come to feel that the monthly cramps are not so intolerable as she formerly believed. Simple analgesic drugs may then be effective. It is alleged that black women are more likely to take pride in their womanhood and as a consequence have much less dysmenorrhea. . . .

It has been stated and confirmed by compe- *tent authority that more successful pregnancies stem from an informative discussion of the problem coupled with a complete physical examination than from any other form of therapy for sterility. . . . The woman who consults her physician because of failure to conceive has an emotional problem, however well adjusted she may appear at first. The measure of success in helping the infertile woman to become pregnant is in direct proportion to the physician's ability to bring about a release from her emotional tension through sympathetic understanding.[54]*

fortunately, medical training cuts so deeply into one's prior values that many women may well lose their desire to work for change. Others have no such desire.

A number of women—feminists, minority women and women slightly older than average—have tried to challenge the offensive behavior directed toward women or minority patients or against themselves. For doing so, some have been dismissed, threatened with dismissal or forced to resign their posts. A few have taken their cases to court. If only one or two women speak out, it is easy for a school or hospital to label them as misfits or troublemakers. Yet overworked women medical students find it difficult to carry out sustained organizing. And the highly individualistic nature of the training also leads them further and further away from the habit of working in groups, which is so central to successful organizing. An equally challenging dilemma for many women is the effort to conform to male styles of emotional detachment. As Jean Baker Miller reports, most women carry with them the socialization to be highly sensitive to others.[55] However, the very qualities medical reformers claim they are seeking in students—sensitivity, empathy, honesty, humility—are instantly suspect if displayed by women, as signs of their possible clinical or intellectual incompetence. This tremendous resource women are bringing into medical schools is being smothered by the training. Similarly, more general criticisms of the training process are much less likely to be raised openly by women.

Analysts of the situation insist that once there is a "critical mass" of women, their sheer numbers will put them in a position to make real changes in the system. Although it is doubtless true that few changes can be initiated until women no longer feel isolated, unless they resist their training no new consciousness will result. Simply

taking over leadership positions as presently constituted, even if that were possible, is not what critics usually mean by change, either. Wisely, few women are choosing the most grueling specialties; their preference is to live like human beings. Unfortunately, most of the influential leadership of medicine is not drawn from specialties women favor. It is only a critical mass in *leadership* positions that may give women power, but only if they all want the same things.

Women in medical training need a tremendous amount of support from friends outside the medical world just to be able to survive the training whole, much less resist the injustices. Even experienced women physicians who are already prominent in their field face discrimination and sexual harassment that white males rarely encounter.

Women residents find their work even more arduous. The exhausting routine, originally set up for men who have women at home to take care of them, allows no flexibility for other commitments like family or sick relatives. Many women are unprepared for the deep isolation of the final years of training. They postpone having children or forgo motherhood entirely. Those who are mothers find it enormously stressful to combine childbearing and/or marriage with medical training. Part-time residencies are few.

The emotional cost of medical training for most women is tremendous, more so than for most (white) men, because of discrimination, lack of support and intensity of outside demands. With these stresses added to the already dehumanizing training, many women emerge from the process expecting prestige and position just as male MDs do. What's more, many are eager to prove that they can be as good as any male physician according to the male-centered criteria of the profession: clinical competence, emotional detachment and financial success. Because they have not chosen to question the underlying medical ideology, they are virtually indistinguishable from their male counterparts. These women physicians can be a great disappointment if the patients' expectations are high.

At the medical plan I belong to, I chose one of the two women doctors because I believed a woman would be less likely to push drugs and surgery, would look with me first for the less invasive nonmedical alternatives. In the first visit, she suggested not only thyroid medication but also a "routine" X-ray; she talked crisply, rapidly, coolly, with many complicated medical terms. I felt like I was sitting across from a medical school curriculum.

It is a mistake, therefore, to assume that women physicians are the answer to the inadequacies of the medical system. The very existence of women physicians may deceive people into believing that medicine has indeed reformed. Unfortunately, the public and even the medical community have quickly elevated women doctors to the status of "experts" on the feelings, experiences and health needs of all women. In health books, talk shows, conferences and magazines, female physicians are replacing the voices of women speaking their own truths. Women MDs sometimes study and write about us, the "patients," in exactly the objective way we once criticized male doctors for doing.

Yet there are also women doctors who have survived the training, kept alive their warmth and compassion and remember what it's like to be a woman patient. They can make a great difference.

For the first time I left a doctor's office feeling absolutely wonderful. I felt that she was genuinely concerned for my well-being as a person. I knew that if I had any further complications, I could call and discuss them with her without feeling like I was "eccentric."

Rate a woman physician as you would any doctor—for skill, honesty, quality of communication, flexibility, intellectual curiosity, ability to really listen and respect for you as a person.

Women as Workers in the Medical Care System

The medical system in this country is a pyramid, with mostly highly paid male doctors and administrators at the top and women—underpaid and undervalued—forming the vast base. While about 83 percent of doctors are men, *more than 80 percent of all medical-care workers are women:* nurses, physical therapists, medical technicians, secretaries and other clerical workers, service and

maintenance staff and more. When we go for care, particularly to a hospital, we encounter mainly women—women whose freedom to offer care and healing is often limited by lack of power.

Women health workers are part of a medical system we strongly criticize; like most physicians, some are overly medicalized, focused on technology, too busy or seemingly uncaring. Yet at the same time women health workers, like most other women workers, work within a structure over which they have little or no control, which means tremendous frustration and overwork. We want to support these women as they fight within the system to be able to deliver more humane, person-oriented care, for better working conditions and for more control over their work.

Nursing

Since the male-physician takeover of health and medical care at the turn of the century, nursing has been one of the few options open to women who want constructive and useful health-related work. Today, of 1.4 million nurses—registered nurses (RNs) and licensed practical nurses (LPNs)—97 percent are women. Nursing has historically been a low-status occupation like other women's jobs. In 1992, only $60 million of federal funds were appropriated for nurse training, although $119 million had been authorized—the largest gap ever. Nurses have been seen as doctors' servants or handmaidens, and doctor–nurse relationships have embodied all the worst in male–

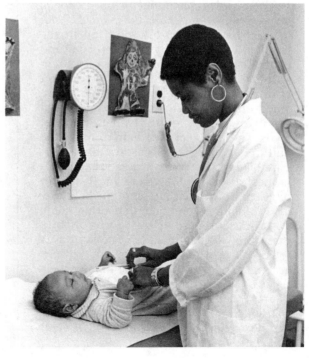

Ellis Herwig/Stock Boston

female inequalities: The female must be obedient and dependent, whereas the male is (or pretends to be) knowledgeable and has the prestige and power. Class differences exaggerate this imbalance: Most nurses come from the middle and lower classes, most physicians from the upper middle or upper classes.

Hospitals, which employ 68 percent of nurses, now offer nurses better salaries, although not necessarily better working conditions. Nurses still have inadequate control over nursing rules and regulations, which are often set in the interests of convenience, profit and prestige for doctors and for the hospital itself. Working conditions for nurses are often poor, with severe and growing understaffing, occupational hazards and insufficient job mobility. Within hospitals, nurses are the chief coordinators, administrators and monitors of the patients' experience. Despite this huge responsibility, they lack overall administrative power, as do workers in most other hospital departments.

Nurses themselves see nursing as distinct from medicine. In the "caring versus curing" dichotomy that fragments medical care today, nurses traditionally do the caring—the day-to-day, hands-on work with patients and their families, the listening, soothing, teaching, with a special emphasis on prevention. Partly because hospitals undervalue this work, nurses who want job pro-

motions and higher pay have to move into supervisory or administrative roles. Nurses active in working for change stress that they *want* to be able to care directly for patients and to be valued and paid well for this work. They believe *medical* care will improve dramatically with this shift, because caring plays much more of a role in actual "curing" than medicine has so far been willing to admit.*

Nurses have also increasingly been delegated *medical* functions—doing physical examinations, conducting tests, drawing blood, starting IVs, doing EKGs and so on. Yet they do this medical work without much acknowledgment or control. For instance, many nurses have become skilled in using diagnostic and treatment machines; many see this as a form of expertise that will help them professionally. But physicians retain full control over who uses the technology, when it is used and what diagnoses are made. It is still dangerous to go beyond "doctor's orders."

My friend Jeanie works in a nursing home. One of her patients had a terrible case of bedsores. Both of us have used aloe vera† to cure ourselves of similar kinds of skin irritations. I suggested she use the remedy. "No way," she said. "I could get fired for using something not prescribed by the doctor."

Nurses, who see patients far more than physicians do, have been "making diagnostic decisions for years but protect themselves with elaborate games, which cast physicians in a decision-making role even when the decision has been made by the nurses."[56] To make things worse, a nurse can be sued if she does something that harms a patient, even if she is only obeying doctor's orders.‡

Many nurses are now looking for work, and some nursing schools are closing down. The nursing shortage is over, creating an employers' market and more difficult working conditions. Economic hard times have reduced hospital staff and kept down turnover.

Nurses' frustration with the nursing role is on the rise, partly because the women's movement has affirmed women's capabilities and worth and inspired women to express their entitlement to

---

Physical and occupational therapists, social workers, nutritionists and other allied health workers have such a low position in the medical-care hierarchy in terms of pay and control that the public usually sees them as less skilled or valuable than doctors. Yet each is a profession separate from medicine, setting its own standards and training its own workers in distinct and vital skills. These workers can help us make the daily changes often necessary for a real cure or for preventing illness. Their techniques speed healing, help us live with physical limitations and ease the helplessness, loneliness and fear that often come with sickness. Yet they can rarely fully use their knowledge and skills. The system is set up so that patients do not have easy access to them and often don't know their services exist unless their doctor tells them. *You will have to learn more about what they do. Remember to ask to see one of these workers if you think they might be at all helpful to you.*

---

*As Mary Howell, Michelle Harrison and other feminist physicians have pointed out, medicine undervalues caring because of sexism (women's work is less valuable), because of medicine's continual fascination with ever more complex technology and because hospitals are increasingly becoming big businesses. Caring work doesn't use medical supplies, drugs or expensive machines or generate profits.
†A simple house plant whose juice has healing properties.
‡Nurses often have to obtain patient cooperation to carry out many painful procedures ordered by doctors, whereas doctors more often carry out their far more invasive procedures behind the shield of anesthesia.[57]

better conditions. Their frustration has led to a number of developments.

1. Within nursing there has been a move toward professionalism. The American Nurses Association, the most influential of nursing's professional associations, has made a recommendation that all nurses obtain a baccalaureate degree (BS), which would put an end to training nurses at the diploma level.* Certified nurse-midwives, nurse-anesthetists and nurse-practitioners have been developing extra skills and a strong professional identity.

Hospitals themselves have tried to attract nurses by promoting various degrees of professionalization; most recently they have developed the idea of the "primary-care nurse," who has full responsibility for providing twenty-four-hour nursing care to a certain number of patients, a situation that may be more satisfying but also more stressful.

Many aspects of professionalization are controversial among nurses themselves, because professionalism emphasizes more education and credentials as well as a doctorlike relationship to patients. Nurses also express the concern that extra responsibilities and functions do not always bring additional recognition or compensation.

Professionalism teaches us to see ourselves as unique and better than other health care workers. The more we talked about professionalism, the more we saw that it was used by administrators to make us work in certain ways which are not beneficial to us or our patients. In other words, professionalism can be used to exploit nurses.[58]

Still other critics believe that dividing up nurses as health care workers into increasingly specialized or professionalized subgroups continues to rob nurses of their collective unity and power to work for significant change.

Professionalism doesn't guarantee control over working conditions, job security or access to clients. When specially trained nurses threaten to compete with physicians—when nurse-midwives or nurse-practitioners, for instance, start to attract the same affluent clients who used to fill doctors' private offices (instead of sticking to poor communities where most doctors don't want to practice)—their existence becomes precarious. Their freedom to work is still in the hands of physicians, administrators and legislators. Nurse-practitioners (about 1 percent of nurses) became popular a

Sarah Putnam

decade ago because they saved private physicians' and health maintenance organizations' (HMOs') time, often bringing in more money than they were paid. Fortunately, the current national health care reform debate has created greater public awareness and support for nurse practitioners and other non-physician primary care providers such as physician assistants and midwives.

2. In some regions nurses are joining temporary nursing agencies. Modeled after Kelly Girl secretarial agencies, they offer a chance to travel if desired, more money in most cases and freedom from the daily hassles and responsibilities of a staff position in hospitals. The effect of these agencies on the aspirations for nursing as a whole, however, can be disastrous as, for instance, when agency personnel are "imported" to break nursing strikes.

3. Collective action: Nurses are seeking change and taking more risks, speaking out against injustices to themselves and to patients. Nurses and other hospital workers are beginning to organize and go out on strike more frequently, asserting their demands for better conditions, higher pay and improvements in patient care. Some are joining unions.*

4. Legislative action: A number of nursing organizations are lobbying increasingly actively at state and national levels, and groups like Nurses-NOW (a part of the National Organization for Women) seek effective political and legislative strategies. One goal is third-party reimbursement by insurance companies and by Medicaid for nurs-

---

*The National League for Nursing, whose larger membership includes more "diploma nurses," strongly disagrees with this trend.

---

*Unionization poses another set of problems because traditional unions tend to be controlled by men, have a blue-collar image and are not very responsive to women's problems in the workplace. The public, which often has mixed feelings about unions, may become less sympathetic.

ing care, which would make a big difference in the autonomy and job satisfaction of many nurses with specialized training, even though this perpetuates the fee-for-service system. Nurses have far fewer financial resources for lobbying and for political action than does the medical establishment; legislative change will, at best, be slow, and needs the combined efforts of both consumers and other supportive professionals.

The growing mix of frustration and assertiveness among nurses comes through vividly in the words of one nurse:

The nursing shortage means more than overwork. It means ignoring loneliness, suffering and pain in the people the nurse works with, their friends and families. The dollars and cents demand that you maintain a semblance of giving the necessary physical, technical and miracle care while ignoring the human beings. Nurses watch people live and die alone because they don't have the time to really be with the people they work for.

We have put up with so much. Our contributions are barely mentioned, the labor of our backs is never recognized. We have come to the point where we actively discourage others from becoming nurses. We are beginning to question whether we want to continue to be the mainstay of the "health industry" and all its concomitant pollutants.

We nurses must begin to believe in ourselves. We must look at our numbers and consider the sum total of our shared experiences. We must rejoice that our hands can soothe, that our arms can lift those that cannot move, that our eyes can show what is in our hearts. . . . They have made us handmaidens—we will not be machines! The dictatorship of the dollar must end. It is time that we nurses start to define the structure of our work. We can be creative. We know we are strong. And we know we are right.[59]

SURVIVING THE SYSTEM: CHOOSING AND USING MEDICAL CARE

Where to Find (and Not to Find) the Information We Need

To have some control over our lives and to be informed participants in our health and medical care, we need information about our bodies and about the caregiving system. Knowledge gives us the ability to make choices, and some of the control we desire.

Often when we visit doctors, what we really come for is solid, factual information, not medical attention. When we have appropriate factual information and even a little skill or a few tools or can get access to them quickly, we are in a much better position to cope with minor emergencies and to decide whether or not we really need to spend the time and money on a medical visit. Illnesses like toxic shock syndrome, pelvic inflammatory disease, strep throat and some ear infections can have serious complications, so we should be aware of the symptoms and get them treated early. Many simple infections and even more complex ones like sexually transmitted diseases are to some extent preventable.

Today there is much more health and medical information available than there was fifteen years ago, some of it trustworthy, some of it not; this section offers guidance in selecting the most reliable sources. It is crucial for our health that we get information from sources that are both *accurate* and *independent*, that is, sources able to evaluate the material from technical, user *and* feminist perspectives.

Ourselves

We know a lot about our bodies; we must listen to and trust what our bodies are telling us. Our awareness of change in ourselves or our children is the first and most important indicator of sickness. Most of what doctors learn about us we tell them. We learn much from the women in our lives: our mothers, sisters, aunts, grandmothers and friends.

Reading

Reading is important, but we must make sure that our sources are as accurate as possible. Magazines and newspapers, a common resource, have their problems (see below). Consumers can also buy the *Physicians' Desk Reference* (PDR) or ask for it in local libraries to find out what the drug industry says about the drugs it manufactures. *Be sure to see consumer guides to drugs as well* (see Resources in Chapter 26, "Organizing for Change: U.S.A."). Beware of booklets and brochures in your doctor's office.*

Self-Help Groups

These are one of the most important sources of both courage and information. Different from medically run self-care groups, these small informal groups of women are meeting throughout this country to help each other learn about birth control, fertility awareness, menopause, breast cancer, DES, cervical self-exam and many other topics as well.

---

*Usually prepared by drug companies, medical foundations or guilds and the large national health charities, these items tend to downgrade nonmedical or nonpharmacological approaches and are slow to present innovative alternatives or prevention orientations.

Such groups are organized in ways that reflect values important to us. They are nonhierarchical; every member plays an equal part. Information is free. Implicit in these groups is the belief that we *can* understand medical information, that it "belongs" rightfully to us. Group members' experiences are an important source of information about health, illness and treatment. By comparing notes and trading stories with other women, we learn best how to use the information we get from both medical and nonmedical sources. Independent of medical-care institutions and professionals, these groups are not hampered in exploring nonmedical therapies and practitioners or in questioning, challenging and evaluating accepted ones.

When groups focus on one specific issue, they are often better able than many physicians to keep abreast of the most current research. Some groups already exist (see Resources in Chapter 26). We have to initiate others as the need arises. When you find one or two other women who want to get together, that is a good beginning.

The Media

These days the media carry more women's health and medical information than ever before. A few women's magazine articles and TV shows are excellent, well researched and responsible in their outlook. Most often, however, a "medical expert" (usually a physician) presents only the medical point of view, with no consumer representation. Reporters, awed by medical "expertise," may spread inaccuracies by quoting as fact what are actually the doctor's opinions or assuming the doctor is always up-to-date in her/his information. Sometimes public relations firms hired by drug companies or medical specialty groups pay for such TV shows and articles. And the media cater to the human fascination with drama, highlighting the spectacular "cures" and treatments, the most daring surgery, the most expensive and highly technical procedures. Media coverage usually perpetuates the mistaken assumption that medicine and spectacular medical technology create good health. Look for presentations that focus on what *you* can do. Remember that experts often disagree.

Health Information Centers

There are a few good (and fairly stable) independent health information centers women can turn to. Examples are our Women's Health Information Center in Somerville, Massachusetts, devoted to all aspects of women and health; the Center for Medical Consumers and Health Care Information in New York City; and Plane Tree Health Resource Center in San Francisco. In these centers, a cross between a library and a hotline, anyone can come to read, learn and sometimes talk about health and medical care—what the controversies are, what home remedies women have tried, the risks and possibilities of various medical and nonmedical treatments. They may also try to help you select a practitioner and put you in touch with women who have gone through experiences similar to yours. Many women's health centers and community groups offer similar services on a more limited basis.

Health Information Centers of the Future— Our Vision

As community funds dry up and hospitals take on a larger corporate existence, more and more health information centers will not be community run but hospital run, with all the limits outlined below. We strongly believe that health information centers should be part of each neighborhood and/or region, located in public libraries or other community settings. They should be community controlled, with a definite consumer perspective and plentiful information on where to go for additional resources. We will have to fight for them and convince others they are worthwhile and worth paying for.

Sources Within the Medical Establishment

Doctors

Although most of us learned while growing up to turn mainly to doctors for health and medical information, our experience reveals that they have limits to what they can or will tell us. Some doctors are happy to give over-the-phone common-sense information that can be extremely helpful. Others send complete reports in writing after a checkup. But the information we get from doctors can be limited by

- The sexism, racism and homophobia of their training.
- How little time they budget to teach patients.
- Their mistrust of our ability to understand or make good use of complex information.
- Their tendency not to keep up with the latest research or their inability to evaluate it.*
- Pressures from drug company representatives to push certain medications.
- The desire to control information as "belonging" rightfully to MDs.
- The desire to appear "sure" and "dependable," which creates an unwillingness to admit to uncertainty or controversy.
- Their unfamiliarity with and distrust of nonmedical alternatives.

---

*Doctors often are not taught skills to enable them to analyze new information.

- Overspecialization: training to focus on an organ or system and not to take into account the whole person.

It can be frustrating, even humiliating, to try to get information over the phone or in person from doctors who don't want to give it, who think of most women as dumb and women who ask a lot of questions as "pushy." We may try to get test results and find that the doctors will not give them to us. We may leave an office or clinic with many questions.

We must remember in these situations not to blame ourselves. We have a right to be treated with respect and to get the information we need.* See What Can One Woman Do? (p. 678) for suggestions.

Nurses

Nurses, especially nurse-practitioners, learn in their training to consider teaching patients as one of their roles. If your doctor's office has hired a nurse-practitioner or if one has set up an independent practice in your community, s/he may be more informative and sensitive than a physician. S/he may, however, be unfamiliar with nonmedical alternatives and too busy to keep up-to-date on innovative or controversial treatments.

Health Educators

These medical workers, usually hired by hospitals or large medical centers, can help those of us with chronic conditions when we need to change daily habits and adjust to physical limitations. Often, however, the health educator simply makes sure that patients understand and accept medical routines and treatments. As employees, they are frequently restricted in what they are able to say about controversial matters. Also, they are often available only after a person is sick and not always for preventive care.

Classes or Groups Sponsored by Hospitals, Physicians or HMOs (Often Called Self-Care Groups)

Some of the more practical physicians and medical centers have recognized, mainly because of pressure from women's and consumer health activists, that patients want and can use more information than they are getting. One popular solution is groups or classes in everything from childbirth to smoking cessation to weight management or posthysterectomy adjustments. These groups help up to a point, mainly because they give you a chance to talk with other people in your situation, trade ideas, feel less alone and perhaps learn a few skills. Such groups often emphasize "self-care," that is, those activities *doctors* and *nurses* have decided you can carry out for yourself. Be aware that these classes and groups have a major limitation: Their main goal is a smoothly functioning medical system with compliant patients who are, in one self-care expert's words, "members of the health care team."[60] They rarely offer nonmedical alternatives or a chance to criticize accepted practices.

Living with Uncertainty

In giving up our unquestioning trust of the information we get from doctors and other medical personnel, we also give up the (often false) comfort that comes from their frequent reassurances that we are getting "the best treatment possible." Often we and our health practitioners have to make decisions without complete information, because no one, not even the "experts," knows enough yet about certain problems to suggest that one approach is necessarily better than another. Yet physicians often believe that they have to act *sure* even when they are not. Especially when we are scared, it can be deeply reassuring to believe them. Learning about the controversies and alternatives rather than blindly trusting what our doctors tell us, therefore, may mean living without the particular kind of certainty or hope that they offer.* Often what we need most is courage in the face of uncertainty.

Choice

When we need medical care, we want as much choice as possible. As in most aspects of our lives, economic status, sex and race limit our choices. There is a severe maldistribution of doctors. Prepaid medical programs, although sometimes convenient, limit our choices. Profit-making incentives limit choice even more for people who need medical care most. For example, more and more hospitals are turning away women in labor if they cannot prove they can pay. In many settings, the elderly are forced to pay for many of their drugs and increasing amounts of their care. Women who are poor, women of color, working-class women, lesbians, older women and disabled women seeking medical care have often faced particular language or culture barriers, physical-ac-

*Lab or X-ray results may be available as part of your hospital record, depending on your state's laws.

*A very few doctors are learning to admit their uncertainties and share the decision-making with patients. For a sample of how this kind of thinking works in practice, see H. Bursztajn et al., *Medical Choices, Medical Chances*, New York: Routledge, 1990.

cess barriers, prejudice and abuse. As our choices evaporate, it becomes more necessary to improve our skill at evaluating care and to create fair and equitable complaint and grievance systems wherever medical care is given.

Practitioners

Primary-Care Practitioners*

Primary care refers to a basic, general form of caregiving that emphasizes prevention. Ideally we would seek care first from primary-care practitioners who would then refer us to specialists as necessary. A good primary-care practitioner is trained to give well-person care and checkups. S/he monitors mild, uncomplicated conditions and recommends appropriate treatments, recognizes more serious complications that require more expert evaluation and treatment, coordinates specialists' care and institutional treatments, helps act as an advocate in decisions about medical treatment, provides continuity and helps to evaluate our experience afterward.

Nurse-Practitioners or Certified Nurse-Midwives

You may want to rethink the whole question of seeking a physician as your first choice of practitioner for normal childbirth or well-woman gynecological care. A skilled nurse-practitioner (NP) or nurse-midwife (CNM) may well be more satisfying and appropriate and less expensive. Both handle routine exams and problems. Although both NPs and CNMs always work in consultation with MDs, some have agreements that permit relatively autonomous practices, referring to their backup doctors only rarely; others work within doctors' offices, hospitals or clinics and are in daily consultation with them. Depending on the situation, a specially trained nurse may be able to make referrals and give out health and medical-care information relatively independent of doctors. Some have better performance records than doctors.

Many physicians fear that these specially trained nurses threaten both their accustomed roles in medical care and their incomes. However, some doctors accept them when they discover how skilled the nurses are at routine, time-consuming care and answering patients' questions and that a solo office practice can generate much more income when even one such worker is included. To improve your access to NPs and CNMs, get involved in state legislation and regulation.

Physician Assistants

You may also want to consider seeking primary care from a physician assistant (PA), who always works in a practice with one or more physicians. This consultative model frequently offers more time for counseling and questions. In many states PAs can make referrals and write prescriptions.

Family-Practice Physicians

These practitioners are specialists, different from old-time general practitioners in that they have gone through a residency in family medicine and perhaps taken a specialty board examination as well. Family practitioners treat both families and individuals of all ages, and some specialize in delivering babies, frequently with fewer interventions than their ob/gyn counterparts. Some family-practice physicians set up an office and have admissions privileges at a hospital. Others are prevented by specialists from getting hospital admitting privileges.

Primary-Care Internists

Another reasonable choice for primary care might be an internist, a specialist with residency training in internal medicine. However, most internists actually subspecialize (circulatory, heart, digestive problems, etc.), and only a few have had special training in primary care. Inquire about the kind of diseases and patients s/he is interested in. Traditionally some internists have had an unspoken "gentleman's agreement" to refer most women to ob/gyns for routine care, whereas they themselves prefer to care for male patients. However, women have serious nonreproductive medical problems that the internist, not the ob/gyn, is specifically trained to treat—work-related or environmental illnesses, for instance; difficulties with basic body functions, such as metabolism, elimination, breathing and so on, as well as problems created by contraceptive or tranquilizer use.

Physician Specialists

Today about 90 percent of practicing physicians are specialists (graduate training after the MD degree) in fields like surgery, radiology, psychiatry, cardiology, neurology.* Most doctors regard spe-

---

*Primary-care practitioners are often looked down upon by specialists.

*This results in serious, dangerous shortages of primary-care doctors.[61]

cialty medicine as more important and more dramatic than primary care; it is more lucrative and prestigious. Specialists are less likely to see you as a whole person or oversee your total care than a primary-care practitioner would. However, because there is a shortage of primary-care practitioners and an excess of specialists, most of us rely on non-primary-care specialists. Three have particular relevance for women: obstetrician/gynecologists, psychiatrists and surgeons (see Surgery, pp. 568–69, and Chapter 6, "Psychotherapy").

Obstetrician/Gynecologists

Today the majority of ob/gyns are seeing healthy women who turn to them for routine well-woman care, and they attend 95 percent of births. *Yet their training is neither necessary nor appropriate for this service.* Ob/gyns are surgical specialists, trained especially to diagnose and treat diseases of the reproductive organs, manage childbirth complications (about 5 to 15 percent of births) and perform gynecological surgery. With this kind of training and a tendency to suspect a psychological origin for the physical pain women report, ob/gyns may miss important nonreproductive illnesses. They may overprescribe tranquilizers and refer to psychiatrists inappropriately. They are also likely to offer treatment solutions more drastic, invasive and permanent than is always necessary—hyster-

ectomy, for example—and may offer few alternatives, medical or nonmedical. But we often need their surgical talents. Many know little about women past menopause and may not appreciate the nonhormonal aspects of the midlife transition or of aging; they are often insensitive to women's emotional needs while giving birth and to the health concerns of lesbians. Yet, though they have neither the training nor the competence for the role, they are socially sanctioned life advisers and sexual counselors for women. The fact that obstetrician/gynecologists see only women as patients—are "specialists in women"—has caused the public to confuse their surgical skills and knowledge of female reproductive disease with expertise on female sexuality, character and proper place in society (see The Doctor/Patient Relationship, p. 658).

Largely because we return to them so often for expensive, routine office visits, for delivering babies and for surgery, ob/gyns have among the highest incomes of any physicians in office-based practice. As a result, ACOG (American College of Obstetricians and Gynecologists) is one of the most effective medical specialty societies, with the financial resources to maintain lobbyists in an office in Washington, DC.

General Surgeons

See Chapter 24, "Some Common and Uncommon Health and Medical Problems."

Health and Medical-Care Treatment Settings Other than the Practitioner's Office

Clinics

These institutions are generally outpatient departments or ambulatory care centers attached to nonprofit hospitals. Wealthy industrialists and their wives used their philanthropy to found clinics around the turn of the century. They were spurred by doctors who needed teaching material and saw free care for the poor as an ideal solution.

Almost all specialist physicians (residents), interns and even medical students still get at least part of their training in these teaching-hospital settings.* Because university medical centers' interests are primarily research, teaching or profit, they find ways to attract or discourage patients who do or do not fit in with these priorities. Many centers provide two different types of clinic care: one for the public and poor patients and another for the more affluent.

REPORTING PROBLEMS

Tongue depressors, Band-Aids, tampons, diaphragms, IUDs and cervical caps, as well as the more obvious things like kidney dialysis machines, are classified by the FDA as medical devices. If you have any problems, even minor ones, with a medical device or prescription or over-the-counter drugs, report them to the FDA, which records complaints in publicly available databases.* (Your name will not appear in the public report.) These reports are the only way to make public the problems women are having and to assess their frequency. Manufacturers are supposed to pass on reports of problems to the FDA but often do not. The FDA acts only in response to complaints. It will not initiate investigations. Write to the FDA, 5600 Fishers Lane, Rockville, MD 20857. Keep a copy of your complaint for future reference.

---

*Reporting a problem to your physician alone does not guarantee that the FDA will learn about it.

---

*There are nonteaching-hospital clinics in many smaller cities that are staffed by fully trained doctors who spend part of their week providing care for poor people for less than their customary fee. Some of the most punitive and moralistic charity may be given at these institutions.

There are a few clinics (some in hospitals, some not) that offer very high-quality care for all who come. They often attract excellent workers, many of them women drawn to primary care. Workers in these clinics tend to be comfortable in a team-work situation where one's judgments are always on view and subject to checks and balances by others, health workers and physicians alike. Patients can benefit from this type of setup.

Profit-making enterprises are setting up a wide variety of freestanding walk-in clinics offering hypertension monitoring, primary care, emergency rooms and so on as specific limited services. These are often located in shopping malls. Ask other clients and friends in the community about their experiences (see Evaluating Health/Medical-Care Settings).

Women's Health Centers and Clinics

An excellent option in some cities* and often a good model for quality care, women-run health centers specializing in well-woman care, gyn exams, birth control and abortion services are worth hunting for. The atmosphere is usually different from that of conventional clinics, because clients may see a health worker first and may have a chance to talk with other women clients either informally or in an organized group. Physician care, when needed, is available on site or by referral. The quality of information in many centers is very high; staff will usually answer questions or make information available even if you do not choose to use their services.

At the same time, women-run health centers should be scrutinized with the same care as any other health facility. The informality of some settings and personnel may be uncomfortable for some women accustomed to conventional care, whereas others may find it reassuring. Because they are run on a not-for-profit basis without regular sources of funding, centers are often under-staffed by women who may be underpaid. Services may sometimes suffer as a result.

Some centers also run self-help groups, film showings and classes in addition to offering health and medical services. Most are also involved in political work to improve women's health through legislation, demonstrations and mailings.

Emergency Rooms

If they are part of hospitals, emergency rooms (ERs) are required by law to take all comers. Accidents and emergencies, alcoholism, drug abuse

---

*Though many have closed, new centers are opening each year. Be alert for both conventional medical facilities and anti-abortion centers that masquerade as women-controlled centers by using similar names but do not subscribe to self-determination in either reproductive health or medical care.

EVALUATING HEALTH/MEDICAL-CARE SETTINGS

1. Who is in charge? (Owners, administrators, board?) Do users have a strong voice in planning and evaluating the services? Is management provided by an outside corporation hired by the board or by people within the medical facility itself? Who makes decisions about care, services, staffing and so on, and to whom are the decision makers accountable? How does one become a board member? Does the facility put out public reports and make its records public?

2. Is there a mechanism that brings users/consumers together to discuss common concerns and raise issues to bring to the management or staff? Do clients and management meet together?

3. Is there a grievance procedure and, if so, how does it work? Are nonphysicians involved in reviewing physicians' judgments? What is the ultimate recourse of a dissatisfied client?

4. How are staff members selected and evaluated, and what input, if any, do they have? What are staff working conditions?

5. Is there a directory that describes training and background of providers and staff?

6. If this is a freestanding facility, what are its hospital backup arrangements?

7. Do costs and quality of care change over time?

These are only some of the questions you might ask.

---

and mental illness bring many people into ERs, sometimes on a regular basis. For this reason many people who cannot afford doctors and have no insurance turn to ERs for routine care, which can be surprisingly expensive.

The ER staff makes judgments about the legitimacy of both your complaint and your claim on the facilities. Their judgments directly affect the speed with which you are seen and whether or not you receive adequate care. To improve ER care, try to bring someone with you who can explain your emergency and advocate for your care. Try to establish your ability to pay as soon as possible. If you have any contact with regular staff inside the hospital (doctor, nurse or social worker), get in touch with that person as soon as possible; s/he may also advocate for you with the ER staff. Ask for bilingual assistance whenever you need it.

WHAT CAN ONE WOMAN DO?*
THREE STEPS TO BEGIN TO GET BETTER MEDICAL CARE

STEP 1: BEFORE YOUR VISIT

Talk to many other women about individual doctors and clinics. Contact women's groups or consumer groups to get more information about costs, attitudes and medical competence of a number of practitioners or clinics (see Practitioners, p. 675, and Evaluating Health/Medical-Care Settings, p. 677).

STEP 2: AT YOUR VISIT

Know your own and your family's medical history. If possible, bring a written record of your own. If you have a problem, write down when it began, symptoms, and so on. When you are in the waiting room, or before that, write down any questions that you want to ask about it.

Bring a friend or relative with you.

Firmly ask the practitioner to explain your problem, treatments, tests and drugs in a clear and understandable fashion.

Take notes, or ask your friend to do so. (A tape recorder, if you have or can borrow one, will help in the case of long, complicated explanations.) Such record-keeping can be invaluable, so try to be assertive even if your doctor reacts defensively.

Ask the doctor to prescribe drugs by their generic names rather than brand names (e.g., aspirin, *not* Bayer's). This will save you money.

Talk to nurses and assistants. They are often sources of valuable information and support and may explain things better than the doctor.

Ask for a written summary of the results of your visit and any lab tests.†

*Adapted from HealthRight, Inc.
†Because laboratory quality varies considerably, be sure to ask for at least one more test from a different lab to verify results, especially before agreeing to undergo any invasive procedure.

Remember, you have a *right* to a second opinion. If a series of expensive tests or surgery is recommended, you can tell the doctor to wait until you consult another doctor. This may prevent unnecessary treatment.

Don't forget—it's your life and your body. You have a right to make decisions about drugs, treatments, methods of birth control, and so on.

STEP 3: AFTERWARD

After the visit, write down an accurate account of what happened. Be sure you know the name of the doctor and/or the other people involved, the date, the place and so on. Discuss your options with someone close to you.

"Shop" drugstores, too. Studies have shown that many drugstores in poorer neighborhoods charge more than those in richer neighborhoods.

Ask to see the pharmacist's package inserts listing medical indications and contraindications. Request detailed information about interactions with certain foods, beverages, alcohol, aspirin, and other drugs and get warnings taped onto the medication container.

Have clear instructions written on the label, because of the risk to others who may take it in error and also because when traveling abroad you may be challenged for possession of pills.

If you get poor treatment, if you are given the wrong drugs, if you are not listened to, it is important for your own care and that of other women that you *protest* (see Our Rights as Patients, p. 682). Then write a letter describing the incident to one or several of the following:

Neighborhood Health Centers

These facilities are part of a program begun in the sixties; some still exist in parts of the United States, though many are closing due to shrinking federal monies. This model of care has demonstrated several important principles: (1) that comprehensive, primary care at the community level is feasible and improves outcomes as well as reducing hospitalization; (2) that people in an eco-nomically or racially mixed neighborhood can receive a single standard of care; (3) that health and medical care services can be managed and made accountable to the community (through a representative board) in a way that is mutually satisfying to both consumers and providers. Many medical care analysts and consumers feel that NHC care is superior to that given in either hospital clinics or doctors' offices. Consumers can use

- The doctor involved.
- The doctor who referred you.
- The administrator or director of the clinic or hospital.
- The director of community relations of the clinic or hospital.
- The local medical society.
- The organization that will pay for your visit or treatment (e.g., your union, your insurance plan or Medicare).
- Organizations that may be paying this doctor for treating other patients (such as Medicaid or Medicare).
- The local health department.
- The neighborhood health council or community boards.
- Community agencies.
- Local women's groups, women's centers, magazines, newspapers (see also The Doctor–Patient Relationship, p. 658).

And about a hospital:

- Joint Commission on Accreditation of Healthcare Organizations, One Renaissance Boulevard, Oakbrook Terrace, IL 60181.
- American Hospital Association, 840 North Lake Shore Drive, Chicago, IL 60611.

However, it is hard for one woman to keep working alone. The medical profession and health institutions are very strong and powerful and will always defend themselves against complaints from the outside. Patients must work together to get the treatment and services they need.

So, to get changes made:
WORK WITH A GROUP . . .
FIND ONE OR START ONE.

the principles and standards established by such centers as a yardstick for judging other types of services.

Group Practices

You might want to choose a group practice rather than a solo doctor in office practice. Yet in some places group practice may be almost as rushed and crowded as a clinic, and you may never see the same doctor twice. Some group practices charge so much more than clinics that you may not find them as desirable. On the other hand, when doctors in a group practice exchange opinions and judgments with each other, they will probably give you better diagnoses and treatment options than a physician in solo practice.

There are two kinds of group practice, with important differences. In one, a group of the same type of specialist has banded together to share the load and better manage their time and profits by seeking more patients. (Most ob/gyns in metropolitan areas are in this type of practice.) In the other, a collection of different specialists sets out to offer families and individuals more comprehensive care. Yet even this type of group practice is not primary care, but specialty medicine dominated by physicians for those who can afford the office fees or prepayment fees supporting it.

Health Maintenance Organizations

One of the most important options for comprehensive health and medical care is the HMO. Subscribers enroll as members for an annual premium paid in advance and, except for nominal sums for visits or special services, receive all office or outpatient visits and hospitalizations for this same fee. In principle, the advantages are obvious: "one-stop shopping" for all office visits, which are "free" or obtainable at a nominal fee; one price that you can budget in advance; if you do need specialized services, your HMO will arrange and coordinate them for you, as any primary-care practitioner will do. You are protected from unnecessary hospitalization by an incentive program in which physicians lose money when they hospitalize patients too often.

HMOs: How They Work

HMOs do work in many respects: Rates of hospitalization are 51 percent lower, regardless of the procedure involved and independent of whether clients are more or less sick to begin with. They are cheaper than conventional hospital insurance plus out-of-pocket payments, and research suggests that medical outcomes are as good as those associated with conventional, fee-for-service care. It is frequently alleged that HMOs cost less because they engage in "skimming," that is, they provide coverage only to the young and healthy. There is evidence, however, that the lower costs have to do with the less hospital-intensive style of medicine practiced in HMOs than that in the fee-for-service system. HMOs control their costs mainly through these mechanisms:

- Outpatient surgery.
- Prescreening hospital admissions (to make certain they are necessary).

- Performing most tests prior to admission.
- Putting physicians on salary.
- Bonus payments to physicians as incentives to keep costs down.
- Extensive use of home health-care and nursing-home programs.
- Watching the length of hospital stay carefully.
- Utilization review and quality assurance programs.

HMOs are also able to moderate their costs by limiting the choice of health-care provider. In contracting with selected providers rather than with all providers in an area, the HMO is able to negotiate lower reimbursement rates because it is able to guarantee a predictable amount of patient volume to the selected providers. These savings are passed on to the consumer in the form of lower health insurance premiums. More important, however, is that in contracting only with selected providers to provide care to their members, HMOs are able to ensure that those providers meet certain quality standards. Traditional insurers are unable to do this, and the fee-for-service system must rely on peer review and voluntary credentialing beyond licensure status.

We have talked with people in HMOs in different parts of the country. Most of them agree that it is a far better system with respect to preventive care and care during mild illnesses than what is available through more expensive conventional health insurance. However, many describe unpleasant or frightening incidents when they tried to get treatment during a crisis, couldn't get through an overloaded switchboard or were discouraged by receptionists or doctors by telephone and later found that serious medical conditions had been ignored. Others who had to get emergency care at other than the designated facilities were later denied coverage by the plan, even when the emergencies did turn out to be justified. Others deplore their loss of choice, either when they'd prefer to use a different facility but would have to pay or when they tried to get some flexibility in procedure during hospitalization for maternity or pediatric care. Some HMO practitioners leave out important tests because they are too expensive. From too much doctoring for profit, we may be moving toward too little (also for profit).

Another serious flaw in all group and HMO systems is that a group of physicians or practitioners may decide together that a patient is "deviant" or simply an untrustworthy informant—"a crock," in their language. When they reinforce one another's convictions in this way, there is little a woman can do to reinstate her credibility or to win an advocate from among them.[62]

Because we want HMOs to be sensitive and responsive to women's needs for primary care and

better information, we will have to strive within our workplaces and communities, as well as in the state legislatures, for (1) one-third consumer representation on HMO boards or on the boards of the corporations that control them at a distance; (2) *open enrollment*, which allows individuals to join a plan (enrollees in some states must come in as part of employee groups, which excludes the small-shop or part-time employee, the poor, elderly, chronically ill or disabled); and (3) requirements that HMOs be developed in underserved areas.

Hospitals (Tertiary Care, Acute-Care Institutions)

The so-called nonprofit, private voluntary hospital run by a board of trustees with a separate medical staff is still the most common. However, profit-making or investor-owned (proprietary) institutions are growing fast. Most nonprofit hospitals were constructed at least in part by federal Hill-Burton funds, which obliged them to provide free care to those who cannot pay. Most serve a wide range of patients through a variety of reimbursement mechanisms and use the payments of the affluent to help offset the costs of servicing the sicker and poorer clients. In order to maximize income and enable expansion to take place, most private, nonprofit hospitals concentrate on providing well-reimbursed and elective (nonemergency) services. *Investor-owned hospitals* take *only* the paying customers and offer an even narrower range of the most profitable services. Neither type of hospital has any internal mechanisms for accountability for its policies and practices to either the public or its users; however, both have been accused of compromising patient-care quality through cost cutting, primarily through reducing nursing staff. (Profit-making hospitals may also be more unhealthy.)

Public hospitals, meanwhile, are caring for the overwhelming majority of the poor and "medically indigent" and most are also teaching hospitals. Funded by tax money, they have been hovering on the edge of collapse for almost two decades, as city, county and now federal governments suffer increasing cutbacks. Under further Medicaid cuts, some may actually go under, to be taken over by profit-making corporations. Some have already made alliances with state governments to contract for exclusive care of the poor (as teaching material in what may well become a twentieth-century version of the charity wards and clinics of the last century). There are many such schemes afoot, and we as taxpayers must get involved in shaping and monitoring them. Our tax dollars and the well-being of large segments of the population are at stake.

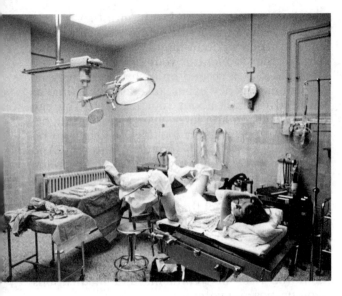

James Holland/Stock Boston

The Hospitalization Experience—Problems and Survival

The major problems of hospitalization for us as women and consumers have to do with costs, risks, isolation and the lack of provider accountability in almost all settings. Because most of us will continue to use hospitals, we have to be aware of how to use them as well as possible.

First of all, make sure you need to be hospitalized. If the procedure is elective (postponable, nonemergency), get a second or even third opinion. Some insurance and some Medicaid programs will pay for this. Investigate outpatient surgical possibilities, which may be less invasive, use local anesthesia and may be cheaper. Consider medical *and* nonmedical alternatives.

Once hospitalization seems necessary, find out from your doctor, friends and neighbors what hospitals you can use and what their policies are. For example, one mother was upset to discover that the hospital would not allow her to stay with her seriously ill child; another woman learned that her partner could not be with her during her cesarean section; still another woman discovered that her lesbian lover was excluded from the intensive-care unit because she was neither "family" nor spouse and therefore had no "legitimate" claim.

If possible, bring someone with you when you are being hospitalized who can act as your advocate and help you make decisions (see Our Rights as Patients, p. 682). Once you are hospitalized, the following information may be helpful:

- *Whenever you are in a hospital, you have a right to know the name of one doctor in charge of your case.*

- Whenever tests or X-rays are proposed, be sure to ask why. The rapid expansion of technology in hospitals vastly increases overall hospital cost and further depersonalizes care; such technology is often applied inappropriately, creating iatrogenic illnesses and problems.

- Try to forge an alliance with the nursing staff. Nurses are the true coordinators of your total care and keep their own records that are separate from the doctors'. Nurses' judgments can influence the whole course of your care. Remember that they work under constraints that may severely limit their ability to advocate for you. Also, just because a nurse is a woman does not necessarily mean that she will be able to empathize with you.

- There are nearly continuous outbreaks of infection in most hospitals that are increasingly resistant to antibiotic treatments.* Such infections complicate surgeries, delay recoveries and may cause secondary illnesses that necessitate further treatments; sometimes they are fatal (as in the case of some newborns). If you are hospitalized, try to go home as soon as is reasonable.

- In a wide range of operations, local anesthesia can be used instead of general anesthesia. Local anesthesia enables you to recover more quickly, and doesn't carry the same risk of death (see Surgery, pp. 568–69).

- Because rates of error in administering medications remain high, find out as soon as you can what medicines have been prescribed for you, by whom, for what purpose and how often you must take them. Ask nurses which medications they are giving you, try to keep a record of these and cross-check with your doctor(s). Resist *routine* tranquilizers and sleeping pills if at all possible. Try milk at bedtime instead of juice, because it contains L-tryptophan, a natural relaxant.

- Because hospital food is frequently not nutritious, ask friends to bring you good food daily. Hospital water at the bedside has repeatedly been shown to be contaminated by bacteria, such as salmonella, so bottled spring water is also a good idea. Also consider taking vitamins, especially vitamin C, unless your doctor(s) has objections on the grounds that they would interfere with medications or other treatment.

- Wearing your own sleepwear, robes, and so on, may make you feel more like yourself.

- As you leave the hospital, ask for a copy of your

---

*Called *nosocomial* infections, they are not brought in from outside the hospital, as many hospital personnel imply, but are produced within the hospital environment and carried, largely by doctors and nurses, some of whose antiseptic techniques are careless.

records; they may be useful in the future, and some hospitals destroy records after a short period of time. (They will send them to your home.)

Nursing Homes

Although the majority are profit making and many are funded through Medicaid and Medicare, there is a substantial though dwindling number of community-based homes. The quality of nursing homes varies enormously. The past decade has been witness to continuing scandals involving abuse and substandard care in many different parts of the country. Presently, slightly less than 10 percent of the elderly are in nursing homes, but the majority are women. If you are considering nursing-home care for a member of your family, or home care, be sure to investigate carefully. In addition to a tour of the facility, inquire among different caregivers and social-service agencies in the community about what home-care options are really available and possible before you decide on a nursing home. If there is an HSA (Health Systems Agency) in your region or state, find out what kinds of standards have been established for licensed nursing homes, home care or hospice care in your state. Or call the public health department, because many federal regulations are being dropped. Several books and brochures have been prepared to help you evaluate different settings* (see Chapter 23, "Women Growing Older").

Our Rights as Patients

Each of us has specific and inviolate legal rights that protect us in our daily lives, including a number of particular rights as consumers of medical-care services.

In a medical setting, your most important right is the right to control what happens to your body. This includes the right of informed consent, which means that before you permit anyone in a medical or mental-health setting to do anything to you, they must first inform you fully as to (1) what is being planned, (2) the risks and potential benefits of that treatment plan and (3) the alternative forms of treatment, including the option and outcome of no treatment at all. For consent to be truly informed, you must also understand all that is being explained. It is not enough for a provider to simply catalogue the risks and benefits in a quick or complicated manner, to do it when you are under the effects of medication or in English if it's not your first language. You should ask as many

questions as you have and wait until they are answered to your satisfaction before proceeding. You might ask for a written statement of the treatment plan in order to monitor your care or in case you choose to seek a second opinion later. Where no medical emergency exists, take as much time as you need to think about your decision. You can make a decision and later change your mind, because informed consent includes the right to refuse *during* as well as before any treatment. And you must agree *voluntarily*, without any coercion or pressure applied by physician, family members or others.

Yet despite the fact that it is the *physician's legal duty* to ensure informed consent, many doctors and hospitals do not do so. Insist on an unpressured discussion with your provider. It is not uncommon for patients to be told little or nothing about the risks of treatments and medications being proposed for them.

Once you decide to seek medical care or are admitted to any facility, you run the risk of trading away some of your rights. Sometimes hospitals will tell you that unless you sign a *blanket* consent form that authorizes the hospital or physician to do whatever they consider "necessary," you will not be admitted. Physicians and hospitals frequently take advantage of the few legal exceptions to the informed consent requirements.*

It is essential to read any consent form very carefully and to inquire about any vague or technical terms before signing, because your signature suggests—often incorrectly—that you *were* informed. Some hospitals ask patients to write out their understanding of the proposed procedure in their own words. You may cross out, reword or otherwise amend a prepared form before signing. Insist on getting a second opinion if you have any unanswered questions about proposed treatment or surgery. Remember that signing a general or blanket consent form does not prevent you from refusing a treatment at any time or from bringing a

---

*The National Women's Health Network has prepared a "Nursing Home Resident's Bill of Rights" (see Resources in Chapter 26, "Organizing for Change: U.S.A.").

*(1) In the event of a "medical emergency" (trauma/shock, for example), the physician is supposed to seek the consent of a relative, but if none is available, s/he can proceed without consent. Staff in mental institutions sometimes abuse the informed consent principle by claiming that a medical emergency exists so as to give psychiatric medications or other treatments without patient consent. (2) The so-called therapeutic privilege permits a physician—in very limited circumstances—to withhold information when s/he feels that disclosure would have an adverse effect, usually when dealing with critically ill or acutely depressed persons. Many physicians abuse the therapeutic privilege, assuming that it is in patients' best interest not to know the truth. (3) Each state, and very often each hospital, has its own laws or policies governing at what age and to what procedures minors can consent. (Abortion consent laws now in effect in at least thirteen states are examples.)

suit afterward.* Be sure to ask for a copy of any form you sign.

Why do abuses occur? Medical schools teach little about informed consent or respect for patients' rights. Some physicians believe that these rights challenge their superior knowledge, whereas others resent the loss of total control. Some fear that with full and accurate information the patient will decline treatment or take her/his business elsewhere. Others prefer to discuss treatment choices with the patient's family as well. Many say, "I'm simply too busy to sit down with each person and go into a detailed explanation. . . ."

Some state legislatures or courts have specified what a physician's obligation is with respect to patient consent,† but it is usually up to *us*, the patients, to insist on adequate and accurate information. We are the best, and in most situations the only, advocates available (see A Model Patients' Bill of Rights, pp. 686–87).

Experimentation

Under certain conditions medical personnel are obligated, legally and ethically, to give us much more detailed and complete information before we give our consent to treatment, as when

- The provider uses an unproven (experimental) medical, surgical or psychiatric treatment, and the outcome in this case is therefore unknown (see the discussion of technology evaluation, p. 654).
- A study is being carried out that may involve giving certain people *no* treatment or a treatment that may be inferior, in order to compare results with a newer treatment.
- A drug may be used in a research project for a purpose not approved by the FDA. (Check the *PDR* or package insert for the approved purposes.) *This situation is extremely common among women, because most routinely used obstetric drugs, many hormonal preparations and some psychiatric drugs are given for purposes not specifically approved by the FDA.*

Because so much research goes on in teaching hospitals, it is important to determine whether or not you are being treated with standard or experimental therapies. Also, the line between treatment and experimentation is often unclear, and because researchers are so poorly prepared or unwilling to protect us, we must continually ask questions about recommended treatments in order to make certain we are not unknowingly participating in research. Experimental situations require that researchers keep a record of our statements that we understand and agree to the experiment and realize that the *probability* of a good outcome is uncertain. If the research is taking place in an institution that derives part of its support from public funds, federal regulations require a special committee called an *institutional review board*, which includes both medical personnel and nonmedical community representatives, to be created. This board must first grant approval to the project, and then make certain that we are adequately informed and clearly consenting. In this instance the researcher is obligated to give you a copy of any informed consent form you sign.[63]

What Other Rights Do We Have?

The law does not yet recognize all the rights we feel we should have, although women's and consumer health activists are working to expand these rights through lawsuits and legislation. We believe that physicians and institutions should recognize *all* of our rights and not just the ones legally defined.

Certain rights are guaranteed by laws, including the Constitution, federal and state laws and case law, which is developed through lawsuits, and federal or state agency regulations (such as those of the U.S. Department of Health and Human Services and the FDA, Medicare, Medicaid and so forth). A number of decisions made by hospitals or other private groups may also affect our rights as consumers.*

Reproductive Rights

The U.S. Constitution implicitly guarantees each one of us a right to privacy, and the U.S. Supreme Court has ruled that this right protects a woman's ability to make personal decisions concerning abortion, sterilization, contraception and other reproductive matters. Although the Court has delegated to each of the fifty states the right to limit women's reproductive rights where a "compelling state interest" exists, it has confirmed a woman's right to privacy in seeking an abortion. The Supreme Court has, however, determined that this right to privacy is not absolute, and that the fifty states have a certain amount of power to limit the exercise of this right. Presently, both federal and state governments are attempt-

---

*This is true even though signed forms are sometimes used as evidence of informed consent.
†Check with your local branch of the American Civil Liberties Union.

*Many national hospital organizations and local hospitals have issued their own patients' "bill of rights" as public-relations gestures, but these statements can neither give nor take away our constitutional rights, though they may help inform both patients and staff.

ing to limit women's access to abortions. Should they succeed, women's already limited choices as consumers of reproductive-related services will be further restricted (see Chapter 17, "Abortion").

The Right to Refuse Treatment*

Each of us has a legal right to refuse medical treatment at any time, even if we have consented to it previously. In life-or-death matters, however, physicians and hospitals often resist a person's choice to refuse treatment. Many states have passed laws that, through the use of a *living will* or other means, allow terminally ill patients to authorize the withholding or withdrawal of medical treatment, even though such an order may lead to their death. These statutes enable both patients and their families to seek death with dignity and also protect hospitals from any lawsuits that might result.

Courts have generally found that a competent individual has the right to refuse even life-saving treatment, and procedures have been developed to determine whether a person is competent to make such a decision. A person is competent if s/he understands the nature of the illness, the risks and benefits of the proposed treatment and the outcome of nontreatment. Simply disagreeing with your physician's recommendation does *not* mean that you are incompetent. The whole area of medical decision making and competence becomes even more difficult when we are required to make treatment choices for persons who clearly are incompetent, such as children, or elderly parents who may be senile or comatose. Many courts have refused to permit parents to withhold treatment that would save the life of their child.† This dilemma is most acute in the case of severely handicapped newborns.

Merely seeking medical care in a teaching hospital places you in a subtly coercive environment that sometimes makes it increasingly difficult to refuse the proposed treatment. As a result, it is often difficult to assert your right to refuse, and you must be prepared to explain your position. Remember, too, that accepting one part of the treatment plan does not mean that you must accept it all, and you always have the right to leave the hospital if your wishes are not respected. Enlisting the support of a family member or other advocate may be particularly helpful in such situations.

The Right to Receive Care

The laws in our country do not recognize an affirmative right *to* treatment, except in the case of medical emergencies seen in a hospital emergency room. *If either transfer or discharge will threaten or adversely affect a patient's condition, then treatment must be rendered, regardless of ability to pay.**

The lack of a legal right to treatment, when combined with the high costs of medical care, means that many people receive either inadequate care or no care at all. There are a few programs for pregnant women and low-income, elderly or physically challenged persons, although many of these are being cut back—for example, Medicare or Medicaid payments (which are constantly being cut and the eligibility requirements made more stringent) and monthly Social Security payments for those who are temporarily disabled, regardless of age. All hospitals which have received public monies for construction† must allocate a certain amount of money each year to the provision of free care. Contact your local legal services office for a full list of the various programs and their eligibility requirements.

We hope that some day everyone's right to receive quality care will be guaranteed, but we realize that such a prospect is not immediately likely. Women's health activists and organizations will continue to advocate for these rights; meanwhile, they may make available lists of nongovernmental resources for those affected by cutbacks.

Rights Regarding Medical Records

In most states, patients have a legal right to see, obtain or have access to their hospital records. But in reality, many patients are never informed of this right and find it difficult and costly to obtain their records. In addition, many facilities keep medical records only for the limited period of time specified by state law. There are also variations from state to state as to medical versus psychiatric records, hospitals' versus doctors' or nurses' records and minors' versus adults' records. It is advisable to have copies of all medical encounters for future reference.

Theoretically, your records are private and only personnel directly involved in your care may see them. However, with the rise of computerization and the large numbers of staff persons with access to records, violations of rights to confidentiality are becoming more common.

Physicians' records, on the other hand, are the

---

*See also the Patient Self-Determination Act, p. 685.
†The Chad Green case is the best-chronicled of this type.[64]

*Hospitals refusing such treatment to poor women in labor often assume they will not have the knowledge or resources to bring suit.
†Called Hill-Burton funds.

NEW LAW IN UNITED STATES NOW ENCOURAGES DISCUSSION ABOUT "ADVANCE DIRECTIVES"

Beginning December 1, 1991, the 1990 federal Patient Self-Determination Act required almost all health and medical care providers to give patients or residents written information on our rights under state law to make decisions concerning medical care. These include the right to accept or refuse medical or surgical treatment and the right to complete an *advance directive* (see below). They must also give us copies of the institution's written policies concerning implementing these rights.

All hospitals, HMOs, hospices, nursing homes and home-care agencies funded by the federal Medicare or Medicaid programs should now be asking their patients on admission: Have you completed an advance directive? *Advance directive* is the collective name for a variety of legal forms that allow competent adults to express their health and medical care preferences *before* a possible time of incapacity. Because advance directives are all dictated by individual state law (there is *no* one form accepted in all states), they differ widely in name, requirements and application. Generally speaking, however, there are two kinds:

1. A *living will*–type directive is a statement of one's health-care preferences in the event of a terminal illness—often taken to mean "within six months of dying." Individual state living wills vary widely, although most include a statement that in the event of a terminal illness, the person completing the form wishes to avoid or forgo extraordinary life-sustaining treatment. North Carolina, for example, has as Statement of a Desire for a Natural Death; California has a Natural Death Act; and Florida has a Life-Prolonging Procedures Act. As of January 1992, forty-four states had some form of a living will law.

2. Most states also have some kind of proxy law that allows competent adults to choose another person to make health-care decisions for them in case they become unable to make or communicate their own health-care preferences. Whether called a Health Care Proxy, Health Care Power of Attorney or Durable Power of Attorney for Health Care, these proxy forms share common features. They become effective *only* if and as long as the principal (the person completing the form) becomes in-capacitated and unable to make or communicate health- and medical-care decisions. They allow the health care agent (or attorney-in-fact)—the person chosen as decision maker—to act not just in cases of terminal illness, but at any time the principal cannot act on her own behalf. The health care agent must follow the principal's wishes. The principal can also give the agent explicit instructions about treatment preferences based on the principal's personal values or beliefs.

If you have completed an advance directive, it must be noted in your medical record. Health and medical facilities are also required to provide education about advance directives not only to their own staff members, but also to the wider community. Providers cannot condition the provision of care or discriminate against a person based on whether or not a person has completed an advance directive. Advance directives work best when we discuss them with our physicians, family and named agent *before* the directive must be put into effect.

Most advance directives are consumer-friendly forms that do not need the services of a lawyer, although some people will want legal advice. Forms should be available from your local health-care facility (the social services, patient care and/or admissions department), your HMO member services office or from various nonprofit organizations such as the local medical society, a senior citizen organization or a voluntary health agency.

David B. Clarke, JD, MPH
Director, Massachusetts Health Decisions
P.O. Box 417,
Sharon, MA 02067-0417

doctors' property, though states vary in requiring physicians to make them available to patients. Some physicians will give you copies of your records and test results if you ask, and a few may send you reports voluntarily. Otherwise, your only recourse is to hire a lawyer who will demand the records through either a letter or, in rare circumstances, a lawsuit. When selecting a physician, you might ask how s/he feels about making records available.*

How Can We Enforce Our Rights?†

Our rights as patients mean little if we are unable to enforce them effectively. The method of enforcement will depend on state laws and the right involved. Listed below are some of the most common ways to exercise and enforce our rights.

Patient Advocacy

One way to safeguard your rights is to bring someone as an advocate to all medical encounters. Your advocate may be a friend, relative or women's health worker—anyone you trust enough to share confidential health information with and who will help you assert your rights. Before your medical visit, discuss with your advocate what you expect—and what you *want*—to happen. Make sure you both understand what kinds of diagnostic tests, treatments or surgery are being proposed. Ask your advocate to keep a record of events that occur while you are unable to be aware of them. Try to anticipate those situations that, in the past, made you feel powerless or inadequately informed. Make a list of the questions you want to ask. If there is more than one physician involved in your case, your advocate can help coordinate your care. If the medical staff raises questions about your emotional or psychiatric stability (and thereafter dismisses your concerns and complaints), an advocate can speak up for you.

Although some private physicians do not mind the presence of a relative or friend during office visits or examinations, hospitals may be more restrictive. Be as firm as you can about wanting your advocate with you, and if your provider refuses unreasonably, you may want to make a change if you can. Some hospitals have specific policies about advocates.

Large hospitals may employ *patient advocates* or *patient representatives* who can be helpful in cutting through red tape. Yet because they rep-

Following is a *model* patients' bill of rights developed by George Annas for the American Civil Liberties Union. This bill applies to hospitals and clinics, not to doctors in private offices. Its language is precise: Where the phrase "legal right" is used, the right is one well recognized by case law or statute. The term *right* refers to one that probably would be recognized if the case were brought to court. "We recognize the right" refers to "what ought to be."

The model bill is set out as it would apply to a patient in his/her chronological relations with the hospital: sections 1–4 for a person not hospitalized but a *potential* patient; 5 for emergency admission; 6–15 for inpatients; 16–22 for discharge and after discharge; and 23 relating back to all twenty-two rights.

A MODEL PATIENTS' BILL OF RIGHTS

Preamble: *As you enter this health-care facility, it is our duty to remind you that your health care is a cooperative effort between you as a patient and the doctors and hospital staff. During your stay a patients' rights advocate will be available to you. The duty of the advocate is to assist you in all the decisions you must make and in all situations in which your health and welfare are at stake. The advocate's first responsibility is to help you understand the role of all who will be working with you and to help you understand what your rights as a patient are. Your advocate can be reached at any time of the day by dialing———. The following is a list of your rights as a patient. Your advocate's duty is to see to it that you are afforded these rights. You should call your advocate whenever you have any questions or concerns about any of these rights.*

1. The patient has a legal right to informed participation in all decisions involving his/her health care program.

2. We recognize the right of all potential patients to know what research and experimental protocols are being used in our facility and what alternatives are available in the community.

3. The patient has a legal right to privacy regarding the source of payment for treatment and care. This right includes access to

---

*All federally qualified HMOs must make records available.
†Further information and possible assistance can often be obtained by contacting local women's health groups, consumer groups or legal services organizations (see Resources in Chapter 26, "Organizing for Change: U.S.A.").

the highest degree of care without regard to the source of payment for that treatment and care.

4. We recognize the right of a potential patient to complete and accurate information concerning medical care and procedures.

5. The patient has a legal right to prompt attention, especially in an emergency situation.

6. The patient has a legal right to a clear, concise explanation in layperson's terms of all proposed procedures, including the possibilities of any risk of mortality or serious side effects, problems related to recuperation and probability of success, and will not be subjected to any procedure without his/her voluntary, competent and understanding consent. The specifics of such consent shall be set out in a written consent form, signed by the patient.

7. The patient has a legal right to a clear, complete and accurate evaluation of his/her condition and prognosis without treatment before being asked to consent to any test or procedure.

8. We recognize the right of the patient to know the identity and professional status of all those providing service. All personnel have been instructed to introduce themselves, state their status and explain their role in the health care of the patient. Part of this right is the right of the patient to know the identity of the physician responsible for his/her care.

9. We recognize the right of any patient who does not speak English to have access to an interpreter.

10. The patient has a right to all the information contained in his/her medical record while in the health-care facility and to examine the record on request.

11. We recognize the right of a patient to discuss his/her condition with a consultant specialist, at the patient's request and expense.

12. The patient has a legal right not to have any test or procedure, designed for educational purposes rather than his/her personal benefit, performed on him/her.

13. The patient has a legal right to refuse any particular drug, test, procedure or treatment.

14. The patient has a legal right to privacy of both person and information with respect to the hospital staff, other doctors, residents, interns and medical students, researchers, nurses, other hospital personnel and other patients.

15. We recognize the patient's right of access to people outside the health-care facility by means of visitors and the telephone. Parents may stay with their children and relatives with ter-

minally ill patients twenty-four hours a day.

16. The patient has a legal right to leave the health-care facility regardless of his/her physical condition or financial status, although the patient may be requested to sign a release stating that he/she is leaving against the medical judgment of his/her doctor or the hospital.

17. The patient has a right not to be transferred to another facility unless he/she has received a complete explanation of the desirability and need for the transfer, the other facility has accepted the patient for transfer and the patient has agreed to transfer. If the patient does not agree to transfer, the patient has the right to a consultant's opinion on the desirability of transfer.

18. A patient has a right to be notified of his/her impending discharge at least one day before it is accomplished, to insist on a consultation by an expert on the desirability of the discharge and to have a person of the patient's choice notified in advance.

19. The patient has a right, regardless of the source of payment, to examine and receive an itemized and detailed explanation of the total bill for services rendered in the facility.

20. The patient has a right to competent counseling from the hospital staff to help in obtaining financial assistance from public or private sources to meet the expense of services received in the institution.

21. The patient has a right to timely prior notice of the termination of his/her eligibility for reimbursement by any third-party payor for the expense of hospital care.

22. At the termination of his/her stay at the health-care facility we recognize the right of a patient to a complete copy of the information contained in his/her medical record.

23. We recognize the right of all patients to have twenty-four-hour-a-day access to a patient's rights advocate who may act on behalf of the patient to assert or protect the rights set out in this document.

As is apparent from the preamble of this document, it is my view that a statement of rights alone is insufficient. What is needed in addition is someone, whom I term an advocate, to assist patients in asserting their rights. As indicated previously, this advocate is necessary because a sick person's first concern is to regain health, and in pursuit of health patients are willing to give up rights that they otherwise would vigorously assert.

resent the hospital, these advocates are simply not free to represent your interests when they conflict with the interests of the hospital or doctor. Although they may help with small or administrative complaints, they are not generally able to provide the kinds of information and control that are essential to pursuing and enforcing your rights.

Complaint Mechanisms

If you are unhappy with the results of a medical encounter, do not be afraid to complain. Make a written record of the events as soon as they occur and draft a letter that clearly states what happened and when. If friends or family members have firsthand knowledge of the events, ask them to record their thoughts and observations right away. If your complaint is against a licensed health professional, send it to the appropriate licensing board, and send a copy to the relevant county and state professional societies. You can also contact a local women's health group for assistance and encouragement. When complaining about a facility (hospital, nursing home, clinic, etc.) that is licensed by the state, contact the appropriate licensing agency, as well as the consumer protection division of the attorney general's office. If you have reason to think you have received an experimental drug or experience a strong drug reaction, report this to your local FDA (see Resources in Chapter 26). The Joint Commission on Accreditation of Hospitals in Chicago should also be sent a copy of any correspondence dealing with the facilities they accredit (see Resources in Chapter 26).

It is sometimes useful to discuss your intentions with the provider before actually lodging any complaints, because this may provide the incentive necessary to improve the situation. Make certain, though, that all your medical records and supporting materials are in order prior to discussing the matter with your provider, because once they are put on notice as to your discontent, they may become more defensive and limit or manipulate the information included in your record.

Litigation and Malpractice

The number of malpractice suits is increasing rapidly, largely because patients have no other way of expressing their dissatisfaction with medical care. The dollar amounts in damages awarded are also rising, though not as much as insurance companies would like us to believe. These increases give the companies an excuse to raise malpractice insurance premiums, which results in many physicians being unable to afford the hikes. When we analyze the actual lawsuits, however, we find that:

- Obstetrician/gynecologists are sued more than any other type of doctor.
- Seventy-five percent of all malpractice claims originate from treatments given in hospitals.
- A *few* doctors are being sued several times, most doctors never.
- The majority of suits are unsuccessful, largely due to doctors' refusal to testify against one another, even when malpractice is obvious.*

Rather than police their colleagues, most doctors prefer to pass the cost of increased premiums on to their patients in the form of higher fees and work with the state legislatures to restrict patients' ability to sue.

Contrary to the protestations of the medical profession and the insurance companies, patients are not responsible for the skyrocketing cost of malpractice insurance, which in turn drives up the cost of medical care. Doctors who practice bad or careless medicine are responsible, and malpractice suits are one way we as patients can be compensated for the harm those doctors cause. Litigation, though, is an expensive, time-consuming and often frustrating means of recourse. Unless you have suffered serious injury, lost earnings (past *or* future), incurred large medical bills or experienced serious emotional harm, litigation will probably not be worth the effort.

In order to recover in a lawsuit against a provider or drug/device manufacturer, it is necessary to show (1) that the defendant provider had a responsibility to you, the patient (which generally exists as a matter of law); (2) that that responsibility was breached; (3) that you were harmed; and (4) that the harm was a direct result of the breach or negligent behavior.

If you feel you have been injured, you will probably want to seek a lawyer. Lawyers, like doctors, tend to specialize. Make sure that your lawyer has had extensive experience with malpractice cases. Both NOW and the American Civil Liberties Union usually maintain reliable attorney referral lists. Many attorneys will take malpractice cases on a *contingency fee* basis and will not charge clients for pursuing the matter unless they win (in which case they claim a percentage of the recovery), whereas others charge the clients for expenses regardless of outcome.

Legislation

Changing or enacting a law is a difficult and time-consuming process,† requiring both the skill

---

*The AMA Principles of Medical Ethics urge doctors to "strive to expose those physicians deficient in character or competence, or who engage in fraud or deception."
†For example, it took many years of hard work to pass the Americans with Disabilities Act of 1990 (see p. 695).

necessary to negotiate the legislative process and the political clout that comes from forming alliances among diverse groups. Only strong and sustained support can help you resist the attacks of the powerful and well-organized opponents many advocates for women's health have faced across the country. Whereas the legislative route is difficult, it does offer the promise of more permanent and broader solutions than most groups can achieve at the local level.

WOMEN AS HEALERS

The history of women as healers is our history. It tells us where we have come from and casts a revealing light on our present condition. It puts us in touch with a power that has rightfully belonged to women throughout the ages and which we now legitimately reclaim. Without a past, our image is incomplete, and part of our deepest selves is lost.

We are just beginning to discover the true history of women and healing, because history as men have written it ignores women. In particular, midwives and "wise women" (healers) have been primarily poor and working class and as such have

A midwife attending a childbearing woman seated on obstetrical stool, sixteenth century. The Feminist Press

not been recognized as significant matter for history. Women's research is uncovering the missing pieces of our story, and so we learn about ourselves from the way churchmen and medical men viewed women. Many of us have internalized these views.

What has happened in the evolution and suppression of women as healers is critical to our understanding of the relationship between medicine and women today. It helps us to see the vast difference between healing and medicine.

Below are a few selections from early writings by and about women healers and from recent historical works by women. In the space allotted in this book, all we can do is open a door. *This is our history. These are our historians.*

Foreword

Medicine, like war, is an extension of politics. The story of the old wife is not the story of an inferior practice losing ground with the advances of medical science and technology; rather, it is a story which concerns the politics of medicine—a story of control and access.
     —Mary Chamberlain, a modern historian[65]

The Healers

About 3000 B.C., Near East
The practitioners of healing in the preclassical cultures of the Near and Middle East were also the religious guardians.

In nearly all areas of the world, goddesses were extolled as healers, dispensers of curative herbs, roots, plants and other medical aids, casting the priestesses who attended the shrines into the role of physicians of those who worshipped there.
     —Merlin Stone

In Sumer, Assyria, Egypt and Greece until about the third millenium the practice of healing was almost exclusively in the hands of priestesses.
     —Mary Chamberlain[66]

About 1550 B.C., Egypt
The Ebers Papyrus, which contains guidance on midwifery, indicates that knowledge of gynaecology and obstetrics was quite advanced, including not only childbirth and abortion but a range of other problems from breast cancer to prolapse of the womb.
     —Mary Chamberlain[67]

About 129–201 A.D., Rome
The conversion of the Roman empire to Christianity crystallised attitudes towards women and women

healers. *The Roman gods were replaced by one all-powerful God whose duties included healing, and who delegated the role of healing to His chosen successors. Thus men were confirmed in their role as official healer and Galenic medicine . . . was confirmed as Christian medicine.*

—Mary Chamberlain[68]

11th–12th century, Europe
In fact, the wise woman, or witch, as the authorities labeled her, did possess a host of remedies which had been tested in years of use. Liber Simplicis Medicinae, *the compendium of natural healing methods written by St. Hildegarde of Bingen (A.D. 1098–1178), gives some idea of the scope of women healers' knowledge in the early middle ages. Her book lists the healing properties of 213 varieties of plants and 55 trees, in addition to dozens of minerals and animal derivatives.*

—Barbara Ehrenreich and Deirdre English,
modern historians[69]

14th–16th century, Europe
For all but the very rich healing had traditionally been the prerogative of women. The art of healing was linked to the tasks and spirit of motherhood; it combined wisdom and nurturance, tenderness and skill. All but the most privileged women were expected to be at least literate in the language of herbs and healing techniques; the most learned women traveled widely to share their skills. The women who distinguished themselves as healers were not only midwives caring for other women, but "general practitioners," herbalists, and counselors serving men and women alike.

—Barbara Ehrenreich and Deirdre English[70]

15th century, England
And although women have various maladies and more terrible sicknesses than any man knows, as I said, they are ashamed for fear of reproof in times to come and of exposure by discourteous men who love women only for physical pleasure and for evil gratification. And if women are sick, such men despise them and fail to realize how much sickness women have before they bring them into this world. And so, to assist women, I intend to write of how to help their secret maladies so that one woman may aid another in her illness and not divulge her secrets to such discourteous men.

—Unknown writer[71]

14th–16th century, England
They [Old Wives] were the custodians of communal and community medical knowledge. But this knowledge was free and freely given. With little or no money at stake there was no need to preserve a "closed"

Devil seducing a witch.
The Feminist Press

profession in terms of entry, training and dissemination of knowledge.

—Mary Chamberlain[72]

Suppression

The Witch Trials

14th century, Europe
An acquaintance of herbs soothing to pain, or healing in their qualities, was then looked upon [by the Church] as having been acquired through diabolical agency. In the fourteenth century the Church decreed that any woman who healed others without having studied, was duly a witch and should suffer death.

—A 19th-century feminist historian[73]

14th century, Europe
The exclusion of women from the universities, and therefore from access to learning, was justified on the grounds that their intellects were deficient, largely because they were governed by the senses rather than by reason.

—Mary Chamberlain[74]

All witchcraft comes from carnal lust which is in women insatiable. . . . Wherefore for the sake of fulfilling their lusts they consort even with devils. . . . It is sufficiently clear that it is no matter for wonder that there are more women than men found infected with the heresy of witchcraft. . . . And blessed be the Highest who has so far preserved the male sex from so great a crime.

—Dominican monks Frs. Sprenger and Kramer,
authors of the Inquisition's Malleus
Maleficarum[75]

1484–1700s, Europe and England
And if it is asked how it is possible to distinguish whether an illness is caused by witchcraft or by some

690

natural physical defect, we answer that there are various methods. And the first is by means of the judgment of doctors.
                              —*Frs. Sprenger and Kramer*[76]

Moreover... it was shown... that the greatest injuries to the Faith as regards the heresy of witches are done by midwives: and this is made clearer than daylight itself by the confessions of some who were afterwards burned.
                              —*Frs. Sprenger and Kramer*[77]

1608, England

For this must always be remembered, as a conclusion, that by Witches we understand not only those which kill and torment, but all diviners, charmers, jugglers, all Wizards, commonly called wise men and wise women ... and in the same number we reckon all good Witches, which do no hurt but good, which do not spoil and destroy, but save and deliver. ... It were a thousand times better for the land if Witches, but especially the blessing Witch, might suffer death.
                    —*William Perkins, the leading English Witch Hunter*[78]

15th–16th century, Europe

The extent of the witch craze is startling: in the late fifteenth and early sixteenth centuries there were thousands upon thousands of executions—usually live burnings at the stake—in Germany, Italy, and other countries. In the mid-sixteenth century the terror spread to France, and finally to England. One writer has estimated the number of executions at an average of six hundred a year for certain German cities—one or two a day, leaving out Sundays. In the Bishopric of Trier, in 1585, two villages were left with only one female inhabitant each. Many writers have estimated the total number killed to have been in the millions. Women made up 85 per cent of those executed—old women, young women, and children.

The targets of the witch hunts were, almost exclusively, peasant women, and among them female lay healers were singled out for prosecution.
                    —*Barbara Ehrenreich and Deirdre English*[79]

15th–16th century, Europe and England

Because the Medieval Church, with the support of kings, princes and secular authorities, controlled medical education and practice, the Inquisition constitutes, among other things, an early instance of the "professional" repudiating the skills and interfering with the rights of the "nonprofessional" to minister to the poor.
                    —*Thomas Szasz, a modern psychiatrist and historian*[80]

The witch trials established the male physician on a moral and intellectual plane vastly above the female healer. It placed him on the side of God and the Law, a professional on a par with lawyers and theologians, while it placed her on the side of darkness, evil, and magic. The witch hunts prefigured—with dramatic intensity—the clash between male doctors and female healers in nineteenth-century America.
                    —*Barbara Ehrenreich and Deirdre English*[81]

The Intellectual Arguments

17th century, Europe and England

Between the twelfth and seventeenth centuries the theological arguments which held that the spiritual deficiency of women laid them open to temptation by the Devil were translated into lay terms. By the seventeenth century spiritual deficiency had become intellectual deficiency: women were not merely open to the temptations of sensuality but were motivated by illogicality and irrationality. In both arguments, women's bodies were seen to be the cause of their fundamental weakness.
                              —*Mary Chamberlain*[82]

The Hippocratic (medical) tradition held that women were governed by the womb and were therefore "naturally" incapable of logic and reason. Moreover ... women took advantage of the sick!
                              —*Mary Chamberlain*[83]

1612, England

Such persons are the curse of God and the sinne of man [for they that] persuade the sicke that they have no needs of the Physition, call God a lyar, who expressly saith otherwise! And make themselves wiser than their creator, who hath ordained the Physition for the good of man.
                    —*John Cotta, an early 17th-century physician*[84]

18th century, England and Europe

The intellectual mood of the eighteenth century meant a move away from the "arts" of the Middle Ages and towards the cognitive sciences and ideas of progress and enlightenment. With this came the desire to protect those areas of knowledge from those unable to comprehend its complexities. Knowledge itself began to be institutionalized, and became expertise. Knowledge without expertise became skillful deceit. "Cunning" changed its meaning from "knowledge" to "craftiness," and the cunning woman, once an expert, was now a charlatan.
                              —*Mary Chamberlain*[85]

An early nineteenth-century ovariotomy.

The Feminist Press

A doctor delivering under a sheet, for modesty's sake.

The Feminist Press

North America

18th–19th century, U.S.A.
The North American female healer, unlike the European witch-healer, was not eliminated by violence. No Grand Inquisitors pursued her; flames did not destroy her stock of herbs or the knowledge of them. The female healer in North America was defeated in a struggle which was, at bottom, economic. Medicine in the nineteenth century was being drawn into the marketplace, becoming—as were needles, or ribbons, or salt already—a thing to be bought and sold. Healing was female when it was a neighborly service, based in stable communities, where skills could be passed on for generations and where the healer knew her patients and their families. When the attempt to heal is detached from personal relationships to become a commodity and a source of wealth in itself— then does the business of healing become a male enterprise.
—Barbara Ehrenreich and Deirdre English[86]

Late 19th century, U.S.A.
But the American medical profession would settle for nothing less than the final solution to the midwife question: they would have to be eliminated—outlawed. The medical journals urged their constituencies to join the campaign: "Surely we have enough influence and friends to procure the needed legislation. Make yourselves heard in the land; and the ignorant meddlesome midwife will soon be a thing of the past."
—Barbara Ehrenreich and Deirdre English[87]

Late 19th–early 20th century, U.S.A.
The obstetrician thought of her as ". . . The typical, old, gin-fingering, guzzling midwife with her pockets full of forcing drops, her mouth full of snuff, her fingers full of dirt and her brains full of arrogance and superstition" (Gerwin, 1906); "filthy and ignorant and not far removed from the jungles of Africa" (Underwood, 1926); "a relic of barbarism" (deLee, 1915); "pestiliferous" (Garrigues, 1898); "vicious" (Titus in Huntington, 1913); "often malicious" (Emmons and Huntington, 1911); "[with] the overconfidence of half-knowledge . . . unprincipled and callous of the feelings and welfare of her patients and anxious only for her fee" (Emmons and Huntington, 1912); "[earning] $5,888,888 . . . which should be paid to physicians and nurses for doing the work properly" (Ziegler, 1913); and lastly "un-American" (Mabbott, 1907).
—Neal Devitt, modern physician and historian[88]

A gynecological exam.   The Feminist Press

The medical system we have inherited today has certain intrinsic features which were accentuated in the struggle for dominance over what came to be termed "illegitimate" practitioners. These practitioners were largely women and the struggle for dominance was, I believe, fundamentally a gender struggle. To that extent, modern medicine is "masculine" medicine, and some of its most dominant features are reactions against healers' practice.

                    —Mary Chamberlain[91]

An Alternative

The year 2000 and beyond

This is the vision that is implicit in feminism—a society that is organized around human needs: a society in which healing is not a commodity distributed according to the dictates of profit but is integral to the network of community life . . . in which wisdom about daily life is not hoarded by "experts" or doled out as a commodity but is drawn from the experience of all people and freely shared among them.

          —Barbara Ehrenreich and Deirdre English[92]

The Consequences

20th century, U.S.A. and the Western world

With the elimination of midwifery, all women—not just those of the upper class—fell under the biological hegemony of the medical profession. In the same stroke, women lost their last autonomous role as healers. The only roles left for women in the medical system were as employees, customers, or "material.". . . The male takeover of healing had weakened the communal bonds among women—the networks of skill and information sharing—and had created a model for professional authority in all areas of domestic activity.

        —Barbara Ehrenreich and Deirdre English[89]

It is perhaps inevitable that childbirth and areas related to women's sexuality should have become those areas most susceptible to aggressive medical techniques. For not only are these areas ones in which the old wife remained a challenge but they are also areas in which women, as women, remain a challenge to men.

                    —Mary Chamberlain[90]

Men doctors teaching about a woman patient.

                    The Feminist Press

693

THE HUMAN GENOME PROJECT

The Human Genome Project (HGP) is a fifteen-year, three-billion-dollar international "mega-science" project coordinated by the U.S. Government. It is not a single study but an amalgam of many research investigations carried out in public and private laboratories, universities and governmental agencies. The major goal of the HGP is to determine the location of all the genes on chromosomes and to identify the chemical sequences of the DNA in the chromosomes. Another goal is to develop new technologies that will give the United States a competitive edge in the global marketplace.

The HGP is expected to shed new light on relatively rare conditions traditionally viewed as genetic, such as sickle cell anemia, cystic fibrosis and Huntington's disease. It may also provide insight into the mechanisms of more common conditions, such as heart disease, cancer, behavioral and neurological conditions, and into biological processes associated with aging to the extent that hereditary components are involved. Some expect the HGP to facilitate the development of pharmaceutical and gene therapy treatments for inherited conditions. But we must be careful not to allow such attention to genes overshadow the importance of political and economic measures needed to improve people's health and well-being. Politicians and other policymakers still must work toward universal access to good nutrition, housing, and routine medical care.

Even as the HGP was just getting under way in late 1990, people who were likely to develop inherited conditions have already begun to experience discrimination from employers, insurance companies, adoption agencies and other institutions. Such genetic discrimination has been irrespective of whether these people exhibit symptoms, or indeed will ever do so, or whether their symptoms would interfere with their daily lives.

As increasing numbers of people receive genetic predictions, the potential for genetic discrimination will increase. Furthermore, without strict regulations, which will be hard to monitor and enforce, the storage of genetic information in databanks threatens all of us with major invasions of privacy by insurers and by law enforcement or other public and private agencies.

Potential outcomes of the HGP may have more dire implications for women than for men, particularly in the area of prenatal genetic testing. While predictive genetic tests are often portrayed as increasing our reproductive options, they actually may end up limiting our choices. The identification of numerous genes and the development of technologies that will result from the HGP will make it possible to screen, diagnose and eventually perhaps treat an increasing number of conditions in fetuses and newborns. Although it is rarely possible to predict the degree of disability from a genetic condition, the availability of new prenatal technologies will increase the pressure on pregnant women to submit to tests and therapies, most of which involve invasive medical and surgical interventions. In addition, many of the new DNA-based tests often involve other family members.

To explore some of the ethical, legal and social implications, 3 percent of the HGP's budget has been set aside for research to deal with such concerns. For more information about the HGP and about grants to explore the implications for women and how the project might be adapted to meet women's needs, contact The National Center for Human Genome Research, Program on the Ethical, Legal and Social Implications of Human Gene Research, National Institutes of Health, Building 38A, Room 613, Bethesda, MD 20892, (301) 402-0911.

by Robin Blatt and Ruth Hubbard

Additional Resources:
GeneWATCH, bimonthly publication of the Council for Responsible Genetics, 19 Garden Street, Cambridge, MA 02138. (617) 868-0870.
The Genetic Resource, a publication of the Massachusetts Genetics Program, Massachusetts Department of Public Health, 150 Tremont Street, 4th Floor, Boston, MA 02111. (617) 727-5121.
Hubbard, Ruth, and Elijah Wald. *Exploding the Gene Myth*. Boston: Beacon Press, 1993.
Lippman, Abby. "Prenatal Genetic Testing and Screening: Constructing Needs and Reinforcing Inequities," *American Journal of Law and Medicine* Vol. 17, Nos. 1 and 2, 1991.
Reilly, Philip. "New Genetic Tests and Our Right to Privacy," *Journal of Medical Ethics* 4(1):7, 10 (1989).

AMERICANS WITH DISABILITIES ACT OF 1990

The Americans with Disabilities Act of 1990 (ADA) gives civil rights protections to individuals with disabilities that are like those provided to individuals on the basis of race, sex, national origin and religion. It guarantees equal opportunity for individuals with disabilities in employment, public accommodations, transportation, state and local government services and telecommunications. Public accommodations include women's health clinics, day-care centers, schools, community services, city and state government offices, haircut salons, stores and all kinds of places where women may want to be.

The ADA will have a profound effect on the lives of women with disabilities. Because of the overlap of discrimination against disabled people and sexism, disabled women are even more likely to be unemployed or underemployed than disabled men and therefore need legal protection to combat job discrimination. Women with disabilities often have lower incomes and therefore depend more on public transportation. Mothers who are disabled or who have children with disabilities need housing, transportation, communication systems, community facilities and services that can accommodate their own and their family's needs.

For more information regarding the ADA, contact the Civil Rights Division, U.S. Department of Justice, P.O. Box 66118, Washington, DC 20035-0301, (202) 514-0301/(202) 514-0381-3(TDD).

NOTES

1. Barbara Bernstein and Robert Kane. "Physicians' Attitudes Toward Female Patients," *Medical Care*, Vol. 19, No. 6 (June 1981), pp. 600–08. See Chapter 3 and Images of Women in Medical Textbooks and Women Physicians, on pp. 666 and 667.

2. Gena Corea. *The Hidden Malpractice: How American Medicine Mistreats Women*. New York: Harper & Row, 1985.

3. Arthur Owens. "Who Says Doctors Make Too Much Money?" *Medical Economics* (March 7, 1983), pp. 66–67. See also Peter Conrad and Rochelle Kern. *The Sociology of Health and Illness: Critical Perspectives*, 3rd ed. New York: St. Martin's Press, 1990. See figures quoted elsewhere in this chapter for taxpayer expenditures for medical care and training.

4. See United Nations Population and Vital Statistics Report in *U.N. Demographic Yearbook 1988*. In 1988 the U.S. infant mortality rate of 10 per 1000 live births was double that of Japan (5 per 1000 live births). The cities of Detroit, Washington and Baltimore all had rates above 19 deaths per 1000 live births. See also U.S. Department of Health and Human Services, *Report of the Secretary's Task Force on Black and Minority Health*, Vol. 6, *Infant Mortality and Low Birth Weight*, January 1986. Low-birth-weight babies are the major cause of high infant mortality rates. In poorer communities, there is what Professor Edward Sparer has called an "infant death gap" between haves and have-nots, which is getting wider.

5. Kathleen Newland. *Infant Mortality and the Health of Societies* (Worldwatch Paper #47). 1981, pp. 6–11. Available from Worldwatch Institute, 1776 Massachusetts Avenue NW, Washington, DC 20036. See also U.S. Department of Health, Education and Welfare, *Factors Associated with Low Birth Weight*, Hyattsville, MD: HEW, April 1980, p. 2.

6. John B. McKinlay and Sonja M. McKinlay. "Medical Measures and the Decline of Mortality," in Peter Conrad and Rochelle Kern, eds., *The Sociology of Health and Illness: Critical Perspectives*, New York: St. Martin's Press, 1981, pp. 12–30. Thomas McKeown. *The Role of Medicine: Dream, Mirage, or Nemesis*. London: Nuffield Provincial Hospitals Trust, 1976. René Dubos, *Mirage of Health: Utopias, Progress, and Biological Change*. New York: Harper Colophon, 1979, p. 23 ff.

7. Lack of teaching of scientific method in medical school is documented in David H. Banta, Clyde J. Behney and Jane Sisk Willems, *Toward Rational Technology in Medicine*, New York: Springer Publishing Co., 1981, p. 30. Additional discussion of the unscientific nature of modern medicine may be found in Rick Carlson, *The End of Medicine*, New York: Wiley-Interscience, 1976. A discussion of how medical decision making might be brought more into line with modern scientific thinking is presented in Harold Bursztajn, Richard I. Feinbloom, Robert M. Hamm and Archie Brodsky, *Medical Choices, Medical Chances*, New York: Routledge, 1990.

8. The Congressional Office of Technology Assessment. "Strategies for Medical Assessment," Publication 052-003-00887-4. Quoted in *The Nation's Health* (November 1982). Available from the U.S. Government Printing Office, Washington, DC 20052.

9. David H. Banta et al. *Toward Rational Technology in Medicine*, p. 122.

10. Leonard S. Syme and Lisa F. Berkman. "Social Class, Susceptibility, and Sickness," in *The Sociology of Health and Illness*.

11. National Academy of Sciences, Institute of Medicine, Division of Health Care Services. "Health Care in a Context of Civil Rights: A Report of a Study," No. 1804. Washington, DC: U.S. Government Printing Office, 1981.

12. Wornie L. Reed. Racism and Health: The Case

of Black Infant Mortality," *The Sociology of Health and Illness*, pp. 34–44.

13. S. Woolhandler et al. "Medical Care and Mortality: Racial Differences in Preventable Deaths," in Phil Brown, ed., *Perspectives in Medical Sociology*. Belmont, CA: Wadsworth, 1989, pp. 71–81.

14. Diana Scully. *Men Who Control Women's Health: The Miseducation of Obstetrician-Gynecologists*. Boston: Houghton-Mifflin, 1980. (See the footnote on p. 658, col. 2.)

15. *Taking Our Bodies Back: The Women's Health Movement*, a 33-minute 1973 color film. Available from Cambridge Documentary Films, Box 385, Cambridge, MA 02139.

16. Irving Zola. "Medicine as an Institution of Social Control," in *Socio-Medical Inquiries—Recollections, Reflections, and Reconsiderations*. Philadelphia: Temple University Press, 1983, p. 262 ff.

17. See Janice Raymond, "Medicine as Patriarchal Religion," *The Journal of Medicine and Philosophy*, Vol. 7 (1982), pp. 197–216.

18. See Barbara Ehrenreich and Deirdre English, *For Her Own Good: 150 Years of the Experts' Advice to Women*. New York: Doubleday/Anchor Books, 1978.

19. George J. Annas. "Forced Cesareans: The Most Unkindest Cut of All," *The Hastings Center Report* (June 1982), pp. 16–17. Also personal interviews with the authors of *Our Bodies, Ourselves*.

20. Dorothy Wertz and Richard W. Wertz. "The Decline of Midwives and the Rise of Medical Obstetricians," in *The Sociology of Health and Illness*, pp. 173–74.

21. Barbara Ehrenreich and Deirdre English. *For Her Own Good*, p. 117.

22. Estelle P. Ramey. "Men's Cycles (They Have Them Too, You Know)," in A. Kaplan and J. Bean, eds., *Beyond Sex-Role Stereotypes*. Boston: Little, Brown, 1976. See also Ruth Hubbard, Mary Sue Henifin and Barbara Fried, *Biological Woman—The Convenient Myth: A Collection of Feminist Essays and a Comprehensive Bibliography*, Cambridge, MA: Schenkman Publishing Co., 1982 (entire volume).

23. Diana Scully. *Men Who Control Women's Health*. See also Michelle Harrison, *A Woman in Residence*. New York: Random House, 1982.

24. From a woman who was later operated on for a rare form of cancer that had spread to her lungs. Stephani Cook, *Second Life*, New York: Simon & Schuster, 1981.

25. Anita Diamant. "Bedside Manners: Of Doctors, Patient Abuse, and Regulation. Again," *The Boston Phoenix* (November 10, 1981), Section 2, p. 14.

26. Personal communication, women's medical association members investigating physician sexual misconduct. See also "Therapist-Patient Sex Has Negative Effect for Most," *Ob/Gyn News*, Vol. 16, No. 24; D. Sobel, "Sex with Therapist Said to Harm Client"; John Kelly, "Sexually Abusive Doctors"; Ronald Kotulak, "Doctor-Patient Sex."

27. "New Case Alleges Sex Abuse by an M.D. at Rock's Sacramento," *Medical World News* (September 3, 1979), pp. 38–39. See also Anita Diamant. "Bedside Manners," p. 13.

28. "Harvard Medical School Dean's Statement on Letters of Recommendation," *Harvard Medical Area FOCUS* (October 8, 1981), p. 5. See also Fox Butterfield. "Doctors' Praise Assailed for Peer in Rape Case," *The New York Times* (September 24, 1981).

29. E. Freidson, quoted in Peter Conrad and Rochelle Kern, *The Sociology of Health and Illness*, p. 161.

30. Harvard University News Office for the Medical Area. "$6 Million Du Pont Gift for Genetics Research" (September 12, 1981), p. 8; "Johnson & Johnson Gives $500,000 for Basic Research" (September 12, 1981), p. 8; "Gift for Unrestricted Cancer Research from Bristol-Meyers" (April 8, 1982), p. 5. *Harvard Medical Area FOCUS*, 25 Shattuck Street, Boston, MA 02115. See also Barbara J. Culliton, "The Hoechst Department at Mass General (Hospital)" (News and Comment, second in a series on the Academic-Industrial Complex), *Science*, Vol. 216 (June 11, 1982), pp. 1200–03. For a critique, read Arnold S. Relman, "The New Medical-Industrial Complex" (Special Article), *New England Journal of Medicine*, Vol. 303, No. 17 (October 23, 1980), pp. 963–70.

31. William K. Stevens. "High Medical Costs Under Attack as Drain on the Nation's Economy," *The New York Times* (March 28, 1982), pp. 1, 50. Sandra Salmans. "Critics Say Lack of Incentives Hurt Insurers' Efforts to Curb Medical Costs," *The New York Times* (March 31, 1982).

32. *Science for the People*, Science and Society Series, No. 1 (November 1973).

33. Maryann Napoli. *Health Facts*, p. 15. See also "Ineffective Drugs," *The Public Citizen, 1981 Annual Report* (winter 1982), p. 22; Sidney M. Wolfe, Christopher M. Coley and the Health Research Group, *Pills That Don't Work: A Consumer's and Doctor's Guide to Six Hundred Prescription Drugs that Lack Evidence of Effectiveness*. New York: Warner Books, 1982.

34. Staff Report of the Special Select Committee on Aging, U.S. Senate, 102nd Congress, 1st Session, Committee Reprint. Washington, DC: U.S. Government Printing Office, 1991.

35. "Informed Consent," *Health Facts*, Vol. 4, No. 22 (July/August 1980), p. 3. See also Chapter 5, "Bribery and Other Strategies," in Milton Silverman, Philip R. Lee and Mia Lydecker, *Prescription for Death: The Drugging of the Third World*, Berkeley: University of California Press, 1982, pp. 119–30; Barbara Seaman and Gideon Seaman. *Women and the Crisis in Sex Hormones*, New York: Rawson Associates, 1977, pp. 73–74; Mark Dowie et al., "The Illusion of Safety," *Mother Jones* (June 1982), pp. 39, 43, 46–48; Ivan Illich, "The Pharmaceutical Invasion," in *Medical Nemesis*, New York: Pantheon Books, 1976, pp. 63–76; "Eli Lilly is Accused in FDA Documents of Not Reporting Adverse Drug Reactions," *The Wall Street Journal* (August 4, 1982), p. 6.

36. Dr. John Z. Bowers, as quoted in *Medical Area FOCUS* (Harvard Medical School), February 11, 1982.

37. Cynthia Carver. "The Deliverers," in Shelly Romalis, ed., *Childbirth: Alternatives to Medical Control*. Austin: University of Texas Press, 1981, p. 135.

38. Derek Bok, "Needed: A New Way to Train Doctors," president of Harvard University, in his annual report to the Board of Overseers, April 1984, *Harvard Magazine* (May–June 1984), p. 43.

39. Derek Bok, "Needed: A New Way to Train Doctors."

40. "Curriculum Review Panel for Medical School Education Initiated by the Association of American Medical Colleges," *The New York Times* (October 21, 1982).

41. Jack D. McCue. "The Effects of Stress on Physicians and Their Medical Practice," *New England Journal of Medicine*, Vol. 306, No. 8 (February 25, 1982), pp. 458–63.

42. President's Commission for the Study of Ethical Problems in Medicine and Biomedical Research. Washington, DC: U.S. Government Printing Office. *Securing Access to Health Care.* 1983. Also see Marcia Millman, *The Unkindest Cut: Life in the Backrooms of Medicine,* New York: William Morrow, 1977.

43. Howard S. Becker, E.C. Geer, Everett C. Hughes and Anselm L. Straus. *Boys in White.* Chicago: University of Chicago Press, 1961. Though over thirty years old, this classic study appears to apply to most of today's male students as well. No comparable work has yet been done on women. The work of psychiatrist Harold Lief, MD, at the University of Pennsylvania over a twenty-year period has provided similar corroboration, with special reference to sexuality. (The SKAT [Sex Knowledge and Attitude Tests] for physicians, was developed by Dr. Lief.) See also Bryce Nelson. "Can Doctors Learn Warmth?" *The New York Times* (September 13, 1983).

44. Derek Bok. *Harvard Magazine,* p. 70.

45. Dr. J. Michael Bishop, in a speech to the American Association of Medical Colleges, November 8, 1983.

46. Margaret Campbell. *Why Would a Girl Go into Medicine?* New York: The Feminist Press, 1974.

47. Gena Corea. *The Hidden Malpractice,* p. 40.

48. Comment made to a Boston Women's Health Book Collective member by four different women physicians between 1988 and 1991.

49. Personal communication to members of the Boston Women's Health Book Collective in a meeting with women medical students at their school.

50. Mary C. Howell. "What Medical Schools Teach About Women" (Sounding Board), *New England Journal of Medicine,* Vol. 291, No. 6 (August 8, 1974), pp. 304–07.

51. See Diana Scully, *Men Who Control Women's Health* for excerpts from texts of the past two decades.

52. Robert J. Willson and Elsie Reid Carrington. *Obstetrics and Gynecology,* 6th ed. St. Louis: C. V. Mosby, 1979, p. 51.

53. Edmund R. Novak. *Novak's Textbook of Gynecology.* Baltimore: The Williams and Wilkins Co., 1981, pp. 847, 849, 851.

54. Langdon Parsons and Sheldon C. Sommers. *Gynecology,* 2nd ed. Philadelphia: W. B. Saunders, 1978, pp. 331, 352 and 378.

55. Jean Baker Miller. *Toward a New Psychology of Women.* Boston: Beacon Press, 1976.

56. Bonnie Bullough. *American Journal of Public Health* (March 1976).

57. Mary Daly. "American Gynecology: Gynocide and the Holy Ghosts of Medicine and Therapy," Chapter 7 in *GYN-ECOLOGY: The Meta-Ethics of Radical Feminism,* Boston: Beacon Press, 1978. For decisions establishing liability of hospital personnel, see Darling vs.

Charleston Community Hospital, 33 Illinois, 2d 326, 211 N.E. 2d 253, 1965.

58. Boston Nurses Group. "The False Promise: Professionalism in Nursing" (reprint). Somerville, MA: The New England Free Press, Union Square. Reprinted from *Science for the People,* Vol. 10, No. 3 (May/June 1978), pp. 20–34.

59. Rachal Lynch. *New Women's Times* (November 1981).

60. Quoted in Lowell Levin et al., *Self-Care: Lay Initiatives in Health.* New York: Prodist, 1976. For a critical review, see Norma Swenson, "Self-Care" (review), *Social Science and Medicine,* Vol. 12 (May 1978), pp. 183–88.

61. D. Steinwachs et al. "Changing Patterns of Graduate Medical Education," *New England Journal of Medicine,* Vol. 306, No. 1 (January 7, 1982), pp. 10–14.

62. Personal communications to members of the Collective.

63. See The President's Commission for the Study of Ethical Problems in Medicine and Biomedical and Behavioral Research, *Protecting Human Subjects: The Adequacy and Uniformity of Federal Rules and Their Implementation.* GPO 040-000-00452-1, December 1981. Write to Superintendent of Documents, U.S. Government Printing Office, Washington, DC 20402.

64. Barry Chowka. "Update!" *New Age Journal* (May–June 1980), p. 16.

65. Mary Chamberlain. *Old Wives' Tales: Their History, Remedies, and Spells.* London: Virago Press, Ltd., 1981, p. 139.

66. Mary Chamberlain. *Old Wives' Tales,* p. 11. (Contains a quote from Merlin Stone, *The Paradise Papers,* London: Virago/Quartet, 1976, p. 19.)

67. Mary Chamberlain. *Old Wives' Tales,* p. 13.

68. Mary Chamberlain. *Old Wives' Tales,* p. 29.

69. Barbara Ehrenreich and Deirdre English. *For Her Own Good,* p. 36.

70. Barbara Ehrenreich and Deirdre English. *For Her Own Good,* p. 34.

71. Richard Smith. "A Fifteenth Century 'Our Bodies Ourselves,'" *British Medical Journal,* Vol. 283, No. 28 (November 1981), pp. 1452–53.

72. Mary Chamberlain. *Old Wives' Tales,* p. 3.

73. Matilda Joslyn Gage. *Woman, Church and State: The Original Exposé of Male Collaboration Against the Female Sex.* Watertown, MA: Persephone Press, 1980 (original ed. 1893), p. 104.

74. Mary Chamberlain. *Old Wives' Tales,* p. 44.

75. Jacob Sprenger and Heinrich Kramer. *Malleus Maleficarum (The Hammer of Witches).* Germany, 1484. Translated by Montague Summers. London: John Rodker, Publisher, 1928, p. 47.

76. Jacob Sprenger and Heinrich Kramer. *Malleus Maleficarum,* p. 87.

77. Jacob Sprenger and Heinrich Kramer. *Malleus Maleficarum,* p. 140.

78. William Perkins. *A Discourse of the Damned Art of Witchcraft.* England, 1608. As quoted in Christina Hole, *Witchcraft in England.* New York: Collier Books, 1966, p. 130.

79. Barbara Ehrenreich and Deirdre English. *For Her Own Good,* p. 35.

80. Thomas Szasz. *The Manufacture of Madness: A*

Comparative Study of the Inquisition and the Mental Health Movement. New York: Harper & Row, 1970; Harper Torchbooks, 1984 (paper), p. 91.

81. Barbara Ehrenreich and Deirdre English. *For Her Own Good*, pp. 31–32.

82. Mary Chamberlain. *Old Wives' Tales*, pp. 31–32.

83. Mary Chamberlain. *Old Wives' Tales*, p. 46.

84. John Cotta. *A Short Discoverie of the Unobserved Dangers of Severall Sorts of Ignorant and Unconsiderable Practisers of Physicken in England.* London, 1612, p. 29.

85. Mary Chamberlain. *Old Wives' Tales*, p. 79.

86. Barbara Ehrenreich and Deirdre English. *For Her Own Good*, p. 41.

87. Ann Sablosky. "The Power of the Forceps: A Study of the Development of Midwifery in the United States." Master's thesis, Graduate School of Social Work and Social Research, Bryn Mawr College, May 1975, p. 17. Quoted in Barbara Ehrenreich and Deirdre English, *For Her Own Good*, pp. 96–7.

88. Neal Devitt. "The Transition from Home to Hospital," in *The Elimination of Midwifery, 1900–1935*, p. 8. Unpublished manuscript, Information Center, Boston Women's Health Book Collective, Somerville, MA.

89. Barbara Ehrenreich and Deirdre English. *For Her Own Good*, pp. 98, 191.

90. Mary Chamberlain. *Old Wives' Tales*, pp. 153–54.

91. Mary Chamberlain. *Old Wives' Tales*, p. 139.

92. Barbara Ehrenreich and Deirdre English. *For Her Own Good*, p. 324.

26

Organizing for Change: U.S.A.

By Judy Norsigian, with
Jane Pincus

With special thanks to all the
groups who sent us descriptions of
their history, projects and ways of
working together

*This chapter in previous editions was
called "Coping, Organizing, and
Developing Alternatives" and was
written by Norma Swenson.*

*1992 Update by Judy Norsigian and
Rachel Lanzerotti.*

GETTING TOGETHER

There is no one recipe for finding others to work with. Sometimes we come together spontaneously, galvanized by a need to learn something about ourselves or to improve a situation that touches all our lives.

In the early seventies, after working in the antiwar movement, I began to talk with other women about the kind of care doctors gave us and also about our bodies, the quality of our sex lives. I'd thought I was the only one to have questions and problems about birth control and childbirth. But it turned out that many other women were concerned with the same things. Our personal discussions began in our living rooms and kitchens. They then blossomed into many kinds of health groups and projects. We all moved easily back and forth between expression of needs and ideas and political action. I felt absolutely elated that what was so important to me personally could also form the basis for political action in this immediate way. My work created tension in my family: I was away at meetings so often, kept making discoveries that shook up my family as well as myself. Yet my life was so much richer than before, one reason being that woven into every day were friendships that quickly became strong and deep because we touched so many dimensions of our lives through talking, working and playing together.

Why do I keep at it year after year, when progress seems so slow? I keep thinking of how much worse it might be for women in our community if our health information group weren't around. We may not always give out as much information as we would like to or succeed as we fight for changes in public policy to improve people's health and well-being, but we are always able to raise the issues we believe everyone should be thinking about.

Knowing what I know about the injustices pervading our society and seeing how racism and sexism ruin the lives of so many, especially women, how could I not contribute at least some of my time and energy to efforts that might change the status quo? It seems immoral not to do so. As long as I don't push myself too much or forget about my own and my family's day-to-day needs, the work I do enriches my whole life. I love the women in my group, respect the way our collective skills keep creating new solutions to new problems and value how we change and grow together over the years.

You can meet other women working on health issues through friends and neighbors, at your workplace, at a public meeting or by placing an

Ellen Shub

- How many women are affected?
- What research has been done already? By whom?
- Are the women most affected centrally involved in efforts to create solutions?
- Who and what is the opposition?
- What approaches to the problem are we considering? What is the possibility of success with these approaches?
- Are there already other organizations or individuals working on the problem?
- Will our work give women a sense of power? Will our work help inform the public and motivate it to work for more improvements in women's health? Will it tangibly improve the quality and accessibility of good health and medical care for women?

The Group

- Should we close it to new members or keep membership open? (The former increases stability and minimizes the need to keep orienting new people, whereas the latter allows for valuable new resources and energies.)
- How should we make decisions? By consensus? By majority vote?
- When, how often and where should we meet? (It is difficult for mothers of young children to attend dinnertime meetings; inaccessible locations may prevent women with certain physical disabilities from attending.)
- Do we want our group to have diversity in terms of race, class, age and physical ability? How can we go about achieving this?
- How much money do we need? How can we get it? What resources other than money do we need? How much can we achieve without money?
- How will we handle conflict among ourselves? Will we be able to stop discussing business to deal with strong, unresolved, maybe even unvoiced feelings or personality clashes?

Some Resources and Tactics

1. *Using the media effectively*—knowing when and how to get publicity when we need it—is essential to all our efforts to bring about change, since most people get almost all their information from TV, newspapers, radio and magazines. To get the best media coverage possible it is essential to develop your *speaking skills* for press conferences and interviews with media people both "on" and "off" stage, *writing skills* for press releases and newspaper articles and *graphic skills* for flyers, posters and brochures.

ad in a newspaper, a notice on a bulletin board. If you already belong to an organization, you may want to become part of a subgroup within it, like the Women's Caucus of the American Public Health Association or the reproductive rights committee of a local NOW chapter. You can work from within the system as health workers or from the outside as a "consumer" pressure group seeking institutional change (e.g., a local childbirth group).

Once your group starts to meet, your need for information and for taking effective action generates its own energy and fuels your enthusiasm. At first, women may drift in and out, but usually the group settles down to a steady number of people. After you choose a focus (or it chooses you!) and continue to work together, you'll want to ask and answer the many questions that come up about how to proceed. Here's a sampling:

The Issue(s)

- What will be the scope of our work? What is the background of the issue?

In our group very few women had experience speaking publicly to or before the media. So we set aside some meetings to role-play, to practice speaking before a group and to learn how to say the most important things in the least amount of time. We also practiced saying the things we wanted people to hear even if it was not related to the interviewer's question. Doing all this is a great way to break through shyness and stage fright.

Working with the media can have serious drawbacks. Inevitably, distortions occur, even when you are careful about what you say. You may be quoted out of context or misquoted so badly that you seem to be saying the opposite of what you intended. When this begins to happen frequently, you may need to pull back for a while. But try again. Over time it becomes clear which reporters are most reliable, sympathetic and trustworthy.*

2. *Allies inside government agencies and health institutions* can be useful sources of information (e.g., about upcoming meetings, proposals for new technologies, studies) and can help to develop strategies for achieving specific goals. Sometimes these contacts can offer invaluable advice about how best to approach a key official. By offering assistance from the "inside," these women and men who support the women's health movement can make significant contributions.

3. *Writing letters* to legislators and key officials about specific legislation, institutional policies and regulatory proposals is an effective way to

---

*An excellent media resource is *Promoting Issues and Ideas: A Guide to Public Relations for Non-Profit Organizations.* $24.95. Available from The Foundation Center, 79 Fifth Avenue, New York, NY 10003-3050.

influence policymakers. Write clearly and concisely, as a group or as private individuals, and point out why your position is in the best interests of women and possibly other constituents of the official addressed.

When I heard that the Massachusetts Medical Society was actively lobbying against the bill that would allow nurse-midwives to practice in freestanding birth centers [birth centers outside of hospitals], I picked up my pen and wrote to my state senator for the first time. I got several friends to send letters and make phone calls, too. I wasn't sure it would help much, but when I saw that the legislature overrode the governor's veto and passed the legislation, I knew that enough of us had spoken up to make a difference.

It is important to thank officials for their efforts on your behalf. There will always be a next time!

A National Women's Health Network activist testifying before Congress.   Robert Frazier

Working together with other women to keep *Manushi* alive has been a joyful experience in spite of many, many setbacks and difficulties, because the way *Manushi* is being received (both the love and hostility it provokes) fills me with the hope that, however far away, the future is ours—it belongs to women.

The most encouraging and rewarding aspect of our work is that wherever *Manushi* is reaching, it is acting as a catalyst in the emergence of new women's groups. When the news of struggles in some particular areas reaches areas where women have not yet started organizing, they seem to get the feeling, "If women in that place could do it, why can't we do it here?" And that is often the beginning of a new women's group.

Ever since *Manushi* started, I feel accountable for every minute of my life and feel every day filled with purpose. And through *Manushi*, getting to see and know the strength that is in us as women, and in myself, I feel my struggle has become more joyful.

—Madhu Kishwar of *Manushi*, an Indian women's magazine

For more on what women are doing internationally, see Chapter 27, "Developing an International Awareness."

THE WOMEN'S HEALTH MOVEMENT

There are now thousands of women in the women's health movement. Many of us began working on health issues with several other people. Some groups have remained small, whereas others have expanded into much larger organizations. You will find excellent models to pattern your own group after from the wide range of existing groups and organizations below.

Self-Help Groups

People have always banded together to help one another deal with everyday problems. Self-help means discussing feelings and experiences, supporting each other to learn together; finding out what we *do* know, what we do *not* know, what we *want* to know and exploring from there; demystifying health professionals' "expertise" and our own bodies; making choices based on our own valid experience and knowledge. Through sharing knowledge, we develop certain skills that enable us to meet medical professionals halfway and reverse the doctor-as-only-authority versus patient-who-knows-nothing roles. Self-help also stresses that the *ways* in which we learn—from one another in settings where we feel equal, comfortable and respected—are as important as *what* we learn. Finally, self-help is political in that it challenges the medical hierarchy's monopoly of information and care. It gives us more control over what we allow to be done to our bodies.

Self-help groups may be action-oriented; the possibilities are endless, depending only on our needs and creativity.

Carol Downer and Lorraine Rothman, founders of the Feminist Women's Health Center in Los Angeles, began one of the first gynecological self-help groups in 1971. Each woman examined her vagina and cervix with a mirror, speculum and flashlight, seeing for the first time those formerly unmentionable, mysterious parts of her own body. They learned to distinguish what was normal for each of them. On the East Coast, Washington Women's Self-Help held community workshops, participated in radio programs, provided cervical caps and generally aimed to give women tools for self-education. Another such group, the Menopause Collective, began in the late 1970s when several women affiliated with a feminist health center in the Boston area started a series of discussion groups about menopause. Members of these groups, in their thirties, forties and fifties, continued working together to offer more self-help groups for community women and to research and write about menopause and other health concerns of older women. In New York City, women in the Lesbian Illness Support Group met to give each other understanding and courage in the face of severe illness. This group had future plans others might like to consider.

. . . inviting health workers to speak to the group, a Speakout on Lesbians and Illness, a resource listing of readings and doctors' names we have found useful, the creation of group rituals, joining class action suits against the government and taping some of the meetings to share with other groups.[1]

Some more suggestions:

- Focus on a specific topic such as infertility, pelvic inflammatory disease (PID), endometriosis, being teenagers, herbal remedies.
- Organize a "Know Your Body" course.
- Start a hotline for birth control and abortion information, postpartum support, help for women who are raped or beaten.
- Publish listings of the better community resources where women can go for basic well-woman care, breast cancer treatment, abortion services, infertility help, midwifery care and so on. Start a childbirth education group to provide information about both hospital and out-of-hospital birthing options.
- Work to change a local health care facility.
- Get child care/day care into clinics and hospitals.
- Mobilize with other parents around issues concerning children's health—immunizations, cost of medications, street safety, violence on TV and in films, and so on.

You can also start a *health information center*. The Health Book Collective's present information center began in one room of a group member's house and overflowed into the rest of the house as more information and women kept coming in. Books, periodicals, medical journals, newsletters, and newspaper clippings piled up. People began phoning for specific health information or to get support in their dealings with the medical profession. It was only after five years that we rented an office in the basement of a church. We acquired more filing cabinets and hired more staff to help answer phone calls, send out information, file and manage the office.

Women's Health Centers

On a different scale, you can start a *women-controlled health center*. These centers offer a supportive atmosphere for such services as well-woman care and abortions. Some stress learning to do as much as you can for yourself and encourage women to learn about their bodies and health care together in groups. For example, the New Hampshire Feminist Health Center began in 1974 as the first freestanding clinic in New Hampshire to offer abortions. Now, as the Concord Feminist Health Center, it provides many services, including gynecological care, women's health courses, a community outreach and education program and an excellent nationally distributed publication called *WomenWise*. These centers can be incredibly exciting places to create and to work in. Still, there are many difficulties and frustrations, including conflicts between the desire to provide skilled, compassionate unhurried services to all women regardless of ability to pay and to earn adequate income to keep workers and centers going. Another conflict arises when workers want to reach out and care for lots of women and are also committed to taking time for group process. In the words of the women of the New Hampshire Feminist Health Center:

For over two years now, we have closed our doors on Thursdays and held day-long staff meetings. . . . Some have called it a waste of time; a more friendly critic calls it idealistic but cost-ineffective. Still, it is the way we . . . choose to do our work, make our decisions and run our affairs.

Some women's health centers, through their abortion rights work, media outreach, research and participation in the National Women's Health Network, have become resources for others around the country. Those that have been picketed, harassed and invaded by antiabortion groups may face constant pressure and challenges. For example, staff at the Vermont Women's Health Center in Burlington fought in the Vermont state legislature to preserve the apprentice physician's assistant system* and to fight the procession of restrictive antiabortion laws that have come up these past few years.

Alliances and Coalitions

Some groups, after working awhile on a single issue, take up other issues as well. As you learn more and meet with more women (and men), you may create or become part of *alliances*, larger networks of groups and individuals in which you exchange new information and ideas, compare different strategies for change and sometimes even organize into a larger organization or movement. In the Northeast, women working in feminist health centers and health information groups from Vermont, New Hampshire, Massachusetts, Connecticut, Maine, Rhode Island and Philadel-

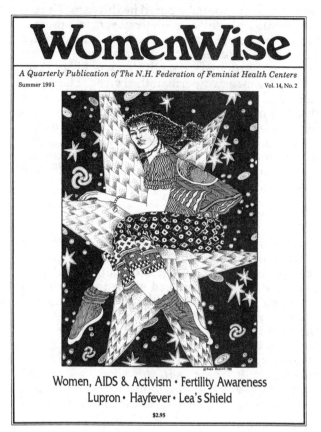

WomenWise

A Quarterly Publication of The N.H. Federation of Feminist Health Centers
Summer 1991   Vol. 14, No. 2

Women, AIDS & Activism • Fertility Awareness
Lupron • Hayfever • Lea's Shield

$2.95

phia occasionally meet to discuss problems and provide mutual support. From Atlanta, the National Black Women's Health Project helps to coordinate activities of self-help affiliates around the country.

In some cities, groups that hold widely different views come together to work on a particular local issue. These *coalitions* may form and dissolve as needed. The Coalition for Reproductive Freedom in Boston consisted at one point of more than thirty groups, among them lawyers', teachers', physicians' and community action groups.

In Oakland, California, a community organization called the Coalition to Fight Infant Mortality worked to lower the scandalously high infant mortality rates in poor and minority neighborhoods.* From 1978 to 1980, coalition members conducted a community-based investigation of the problem of infant mortality and, in particular, the quality of care at the county's only public hospital offering obstetrical services to the low-income community. They presented their results to the entire community and finally forced the trustees of the hospital to recognize the problem officially and make certain changes, such as the addition of obstetricians who had a strong com-

---

*Being licensed as a PA after apprenticing to a physician, rather than going through a special course of studies at school.

---

*There were 26.3 infant deaths per 1000 live births in 1976 as compared with 3.5 per 1000 in nearby, more affluent, Piedmont.

mitment to community-based health care. The coalition also sought a midwifery service and expanded bilingual services. The community clinics also began to offer early prenatal care and the state legislature passed a bill that would help create comprehensive perinatal services. The coalition and the community fought together to demand quality services accessible to all regardless of ability to pay. They were strongly aware that high infant mortality rates reflect racism and discrimination against women and the poor as well as the profit orientation of the health and medical system.

Two Model Organizations

The Coalition for the Medical Rights of Women (not a coalition in reality), a remarkably successful project based in San Francisco, California, began as a small group concerned about the absence of state and federal laws regulating the testing and marketing of IUDs. In the 1970s and early 1980s, the Coalition grew into a large membership organization of both consumers and providers. One of their publications, *The Rock Will Wear Away: Handbook for Women's Health Advocates*, offered invaluable advice to those forming new women's health groups. It described how the Coalition itself

Hope Zanes

was structured, how its main issues were selected and how several "issue committees" worked on specific problems. Despite its demise in the late 1980s, the Coalition remains a model for how to develop and build a structure that will allow work to be done as effectively as possible without losing a feminist workstyle. They had a small, part-time paid staff and many volunteers, did effective fundraising and held periodic membership meetings.

The National Women's Health Network, this country's only national membership organization devoted exclusively to women's health, influences health policy at the local and national level. Founded in 1975, its membership has grown to over 20,000, including several hundred organizations that represent a constituency of half a million people. Today the annual budget is $450,000,

THE PROJECT ON WOMEN AND DISABILITY

The Project on Women and Disability (PWD) grew from a project of the Boston Women's Health Book Collective in 1988 to become a nonprofit organization serving women whose lives are affected by disability. This includes women with disabilities, mothers, partners and friends of disabled people and women working in disability services.

The mission of PWD is to eliminate sex and disability bias in our society, promote women with disabilities as equal and active members of the workforce and the community and to enlist men and women as our allies. Among our primary goals are quality health care and reproductive rights for disabled women. PWD provides training, discussion and support groups, information and referral and a quarterly journal on women and disability issues, called WILDA (Women in Leadership/Disability Issues).

Where do you go for help if you're a divorced mother of two and you're disabled and can't find housing? I've called all the women's hotlines and centers and none of them could comprehend my disability. It seems that women's services don't understand disability, and disability agencies don't understand the needs of disabled women. *In this group, it was such a relief to talk to each other about what it really means to be a* female with a disability.

with five staff members at its national headquarters in Washington, DC, and dozens of interns and volunteers. The members of the network's board of directors come from different geographical areas, diverse racial and ethnic backgrounds and span forty years in age. Its many committees work on a wide range of women's health concerns, such as reproductive health; occupational and environmental health; alcohol, smoking and drugs; concerns of women of color; breast cancer; disabled women; health planning; health law and regulations; international issues; lesbian health; midlife and older women's health; women and nutrition; rural women's health; and holistic health care.

NOTES

1. Nancy Johnson. "NY Lesbian Illness Group: What Being a Lesbian Means in the Deepest Sense," *Off Our Backs* Vol. 11, No. 5 (May 1981), pp. 8–18.

RESOURCES

Books

Annas, George. *The Rights of Patients: The Basic ACLU Guide to Patient Rights*. Second ed.; Totowa, New Jersey: Humana Press, 1992.

Burgess, Ann W., and Carol R. Hartman, eds. *Sexual Medicine*, Vol. 4, *Sexual Exploitation of Patients by Health Professionals*. New York: Praeger, 1986.

Bursztajn, Harold J., Robert M. Hamm and Archie Brodsky. *Medical Choices, Medical Chances: How Patients, Families and Physicians Can Cope with Uncertainty*. New York: Routledge, 1990.

Coalition for the Medical Rights of Women. *The Rock Will Wear Away: Handbook for Women's Health Advocates*. Out of print, but photocopies of it are available from the Boston Women's Health Book Collective.

Conrad, Peter, and Rochelle Kern, eds. *The Sociology of Health and Illness: Critical Perspectives*, 3rd ed., New York: St. Martin's Press, 1990.

WOMEN OF COLOR ORGANIZING FOR CHANGE

The National Black Women's Health Project (NBWHP), a self-help and health advocacy organization, promotes the health and wellness of African-American women, girls and their families. The NBWHP involves women who live in public housing in self-help groups through the Center for Black Women's Wellness. The new presence of an arm of the NBWHP in Washington, DC, will continue and strengthen advocacy by speaking out on public policy issues and developing positions consistent with the NBWHP philosophy of self-empowerment through self-help.

Part of the broader coalition African-American Women for Reproductive Rights, the 1990 NBWHP conference on reproductive health attracted women from around the world. Internationally, SisteReach is a new program of the NBWHP with the goal of exchanging health information and resources with women of color in self-help projects worldwide.

Opened in 1988, the Native American Women's Health Education Resource Center (NAWHERC) offers community-based activities—support and self-help groups, youth tutoring services and advocacy/outreach—as well as health education information. In September 1991, the NAWHERC helped open the Women's Lodge/Shelter, a shelter for abused women and/or children.

Working through the resource center, the Native Women's Reproductive Rights Coalition, a coalition of women from over eleven Northern Plains nations, came together in 1990 to create an agenda and statement of reproductive rights for Native women.

The National Latina Health Organization was formed to raise Latina health consciousness. The NLHO promotes self-help methods and self-empowerment processes as a vehicle for Latinas taking greater control of health practices and life-styles.

The NLHO is committed to work toward the goal of bilingual access to quality health care and the self-empowerment of Latinas through educational programs, outreach and research. All programs are bilingual.

The NLHO, in coalition with other organizations and individuals through Latinas for Reproductive Choice, is taking an active role in ensuring Latinas' legal right to abortion and expanding the abortion issue. Reproductive choice encompasses access to quality health care, bilingual information and education on sexuality that is culturally relevant, affordable birth control, early prenatal care to ensure healthy babies and freedom from sterilization abuse.

santa cruz women's health center

250 locust street
santa cruz, ca 95060
(408) 427-3500

Corea, Gena. *The Hidden Malpractice: How American Medicine Mistreats Women*, rev. ed. New York: Harper & Row, 1985. Remains the most stunning investigative journalism extant on American medicine's shameful history toward women.

Dreifus, Claudia, ed. *Seizing Our Bodies*. New York: Vintage Books, 1978. A useful selection of classic articles on women's health issues from the early days of the women's health movement.

Dubos, René. *Mirage of Health: Utopias, Progress, and Biological Change*. New York: Harper & Row, 1979. A readable classic, basic for demystification of health, disease, science and medicine.

Ehrenreich, Barbara, and Deirdre English. *Complaints and Disorders: The Sexual Politics of Sickness*. Old Westbury, NY: The Feminist Press, 1974. A vivid portrait of nineteenth-century class struggle and the role of medicine and women in it.

———. *For Her Own Good: 150 Years of the Experts' Advice to Women*. New York: Doubleday/Anchor Books, 1978. No other book makes modern women's manipulation by succeeding generations of male experts appear so credible or so devastating. Exposes the unscientific basis of "scientific" expertise used to control women.

———. *Witches, Midwives, and Nurses: A History of Women Healers*. Old Westbury, NY: The Feminist Press, 1972. One of the classics of the second wave of feminism, this powerful booklet explains the medieval witch burnings of the Church as the suppression of female sexuality, female organizing and female healing, in a move to consolidate patriarchal power.

Fisher, Sue. *In the Patient's Best Interest: Women and the Politics of Medical Decisions*. New Brunswick, NJ: Rutgers University Press, 1986.

Gage, Matilda Joslyn. *Woman, Church and State*. Original printing 1893. Watertown, MA: Persephone Press, 1980. A remarkable account of systematic oppression of women by Christian church teachings (including Judaic influences) through the centuries. By one of the major feminists of the nineteenth century.

Gordon, Linda. *Woman's Body, Woman's Right—A Social History of Birth Control in America*, rev. ed. New York/Middlesex, England: Penguin Books, 1990. Traces the history and development of the birth control movement in the United States, covering political, social and economic aspects. An excellent feminist analysis.

Harrison, Michelle. *A Woman in Residence*. New York: Random House, 1982. A seasoned woman physician in ob/gyn specialty training at a major teaching hospital describes how the quality of patient care is undermined by training priorities.

Hornstein, Francie, and Judith Waxman, eds. *Birthrights: An Advocate's Guide to Ending Infant Mortality*. Los Angeles: National Health Law Program, 1983.

Hubbard, Ruth. *Politics of Women's Biology*. New Brunswick, NJ: Rutgers University Press, 1990.

Hubbard, Ruth, Mary Sue Henefin and Barbara Fried, eds. *Women Looking at Biology Looking at Women*. Cambridge, MA: Schenkman Publishing Co., 1979. Valuable reflections on the contributions of biology and social sciences to the denigration of women, and refutations of the "scientific" basis for it.

Illich, Ivan. *Medical Nemesis: The Expropriation of Health*. New York: Pantheon Books, 1976; Bantam Books (paper), 1977. A rich and provocative analysis of iatrogenesis (medically induced illness) on many levels.

Inlander, Charles B., and Ed Weiner. *Take This Book to the Hospital with You: A Consumer's Guide to Surviving Your Hospital Stay*. Emmaus, PA: Rodale Press, 1985.

Institute of Medicine. (U.S.) *Medical Professional Liability and the Delivery of Obstetrical Care*, Vols. I and II. Washington, DC: National Academy Press, 1989.

Lewin, Ellen, and Virginia Oleson. *Women, Health and Healing: Toward a New Perspective*. New York: Tavistock Publications, 1985.

Lorber, Judith. *Women Physicians: Career, Status and Power*. New York: Tavistock Publications, 1984.

Millman, Marcia. *The Unkindest Cut: Life in the Backrooms of Medicine*. New York: William Morrow, 1977. An eyewitness study of doctors' handling of errors, and each other, when peer review is instituted.

Physicians' Desk Reference. Oradell, NJ: Medical Economics. The industry-sponsored guide to drugs, on which most doctors depend for information. Published annually.

Ratcliff, Kathryn J., ed. *Healing Technology: Feminist Perspectives*. Ann Arbor: University of Michigan Press, 1989.

Roberts, Helen. *The Patient Patients: Women and Their Doctors*. London: Pandora Press, 1985.

Ruzek, Sheryl. *The Women's Health Movement: Feminist Alternatives to Medical Control*. New York: Praeger Publishers, 1978. A fine feminist study of self-help and its role in changing fundamental attitudes toward medical care.

Scully, Diana. *Men Who Control Women's Health: The*

Miseducation of Obstetrician-Gynecologists. Boston: Houghton-Mifflin, 1980. This three-year study of ob/gyn training at two leading U.S. hospitals is outstanding; it shows how all aspects of training ultimately prepare surgeons to manipulate women to accept surgery and control by doctors during childbirth.

Seaman, Barbara. *The Doctor's Case Against the Pill*, rev. ed. New York: Doubleday, 1980. Classic background to the Pill cover-up.

Seaman, Barbara, and Gideon Seaman. *Women and the Crisis in Sex Hormones.* New York: Rawson Associates Publishers, 1977; Bantam Books (paper), 1978. A detailed account of the development of major birth control methods.

Todd, Alexandra D. *Intimate Adversaries: Cultural Conflict Between Doctors and Women Patients.* Philadelphia: University of Pennsylvania Press, 1989.

Walsh, Mary Roth. *Doctors Wanted—No Women Need Apply: Sexual Barriers in the Medical Profession 1835–1975.* New Haven, CT: Yale University Press, 1977. An excellent history of U.S. women doctors and why feminism is essential to their survival, now as then.

Wertz, Dorothy C. *Ethics and Human Genetics: A Cross-Cultural Perspective.* Heidelberg, Germany: Springer-Verlag, 1989.

Wertz, Dorothy, and Richard Wertz. *Lying-In: A History of Childbirth in America*, rev. ed. New York: Free Press, 1989. The most comprehensive history of the takeover of childbirth by male-dominated technology and medicine from women and midwives.

White, Evelyn J., ed. *The Black Women's Health Book: Speaking for Ourselves.* Seattle, WA: Seal Press, 1990.

Articles

Atkinson, Carla, and John Geiger. "Just Say No? When Drug Companies Make Offers Doctors Can't Refuse," *Public Citizen* (March/April 1991), pp. 12–14.

THE SANTA CRUZ WOMEN'S HEALTH CENTER

The beginning of 1982 marked a turning point in the Santa Cruz Women's Health Center (SCWHC) as the Bilingual Outreach Program was launched. Our mobile health unit, a van equipped with medical and educational supplies, provides health information, counseling and referrals directly to three Latino neighborhoods in North Santa Cruz County. The mobile health unit also serves as a link between Latina women and the bilingual health services offered at the SCWHC.

We consist of a multiracial group of women who designed and developed this project for the SCWHC. This project has, from its beginning, been a project for Latina women, designed by Latina women and initiated by a multicultural group of women.

The dream was to create a bilingual outreach program that would serve the desires and needs of Latina women in our community. The goal of the program is to bring basic information about women's health care to the Latino and low-income community, to give women the information they need to have/take more control over their lives and the lives of their children and families.

Our process has been based on the exchange of information, knowledge and experience; we have learned an enormous amount from the women whom we are serving. We started our project by going to the four designated areas in North Santa Cruz County as a team, literally knocking on every door and talking to women about our dream to bring a mobile health unit to the community. We met with women once a week and our question was always, Is this service something you feel you can use? The answer was always overwhelmingly yes; the women always encouraged us.

The mobile health unit contained a minilab and a library and served as a resource center with health information and community referrals. The mobile unit provided health education classes and counseling in nutrition, high blood pressure, anemia, pregnancy counseling, prenatal care, birth control and abortion counseling.

—Rosemaria Zayas and Martha Ways
(excerpts from a letter to the MS Foundation)

1992 Update: The mobile health unit ultimately provided a catalyst for the historic and present-day ethnic and cultural diversification of the staff, clients and board of the SCWHC. In general, the mobile van created and strengthened the outreach services of the SCWHC, which continue to be integral to their programs. The work of the mobile van also culminated in the formation of Familia Center, a community center run by and for Latinos in the barrio of Santa Cruz; once a project of the SCWHC, the Familia Center is now a successful, community-organized, independent project.

For current publications of the SCWHC, see Resources.

SELECTED EARLY ACCOMPLISHMENTS OF THE NATIONAL WOMEN'S HEALTH NETWORK

▪ Testified at numerous U.S. Senate and House hearings on unsafe birth control pills and devices, drug reform laws, contraceptive research priorities, nurse-midwifery practice, treatment for DES daughters and unsafe hospital childbirth practices.

▪ Won, with other groups, a precedent-setting lawsuit requiring drug companies to publish patient information on the risks of menopausal estrogen drugs.

▪ Initiated a national campaign to locate women's health activists to become consumer representatives at FDA hearings.

▪ Testified at U.S. Department of Health, Education and Welfare hearings on sterilization abuse and recommended safeguards to ensure informed consent and bilingual patient information.

▪ Testifed before the U.S. Senate against proposed bills that would outlaw abortion services.

▪ Organized the first major rural women's health conference in Appalachia in June 1981.

▪ Successfully pressured the federal government to spend $1.5 million to study the effectiveness of the cervical cap and make it available to women nationwide.

▪ Brought a lawsuit in federal court challenging the Catholic Church's antiabortion political and lobbying activities.

▪ Filed a worldwide class-action lawsuit against the A. H. Robins company on behalf of all women damaged or potentially damaged by the Dalkon Shield IUD.

▪ Testified at FDA hearings against approval of Depo-Provera for contraceptive use in the United States and also filed a class-action suit against Upjohn Company on behalf of women injured by this drug.

Joining the network is an important way women and men can support the goals of the women's health movement. For more information about current activities write to the National Women's Health Network, 1325 G Street NW, Washington, DC 20005.

Bell, Susan. "Political Gynecology: Gynecological Imperialism and the Politics of Self-Help," *Science for the People* (September/October 1979), pp. 8–14. The article focuses on the experiences of a group of feminists involved in a program to teach pelvic examinations to medical students.

Conrad, Peter. "Medicalization and Social Control," *Annual Review of Sociology*, Vol. 18 (1992), pp. 209–32.

Gladwell, Malcolm. "Public Health Experts Turn to Economic Ills," *Washington Post* (November 26, 1990), p. A3.

Lipnack, Jessica. "The Women's Health Movement," *New Age Journal* (March 1980). An excellent and thorough review of major aspects of the U.S. women's health movement in the 1990s, including historical background.

The National Black Women's Health Project. *Self-Help Developers' Manual*, rev. ed. 1990. Available from the Project at 175 Trinity Ave SW, 2nd Floor, Atlanta, GA 30303.

Rodin, Judith, and Jeanette R. Ickovies. "Women's Health: Review and Research Agenda as We Approach the 21st Century," *American Psychologist*, Vol. 45, No. 9 (September 1990).

Schwartz, Richard. "The Physician and the Social Contract," *Obstetrics and Gynecology*, Vol. 79, No. 1 (January 1992).

Smith, Beverly. "Black Women's Health: Notes for a Course," in G. T. Hull, P. B. Scott and B. Smith, eds., *All the Women Are White, All the Blacks Are Men, but Some of Us Are Brave: Black Women's Studies*. New York: The Feminist Press, 1982.

Weaver, Jerry, and Sharon D. Garrett. "Sexism and Racism in the American Health Care Industry: A Comparative Analysis," in Elizabeth Fee, ed., *Women and Health: The Politics of Sex in Medicine*. Farmingdale, NY: Baywood Publishing Co., 1983, pp. 79–104.

Periodicals

Health Facts
Center for Medical Consumers
237 Thompson Street
New York, NY 10012
Regular, clear, in-depth, referenced discussion of key issues for consumers.

Healthsharing
Women Healthsharing
14 Skey Lane
Toronto, Ontario, M6J 3S4 Canada
Excellent quarterly newsletter covering many women's health concerns.

International Journal of Technology Assessment in Health Care
Cambridge University Press
110 Midland Avenue
Port Chester, NY 10573
Each issue has a thematic section. For example, Vol. 7, No. 4 (Fall 1991), includes a special section on Obstetric Technology: A Future Perspective.

The Medical Letter on Drugs and Therapeutics
The Medical Letter, Inc.
  1000 Main Street
  New Rochelle, NY 10801
The single best independent source of professional drug
  evaluation.

Medical Self-Care
  349 Healdsburg Avenue
  Healdsburg, CA 95448
  (707) 431-1100
Each issue on a special theme, with many articles and
  resources.

Off Our Backs
  2423 18th Street NW, 2nd Floor
  Washington, DC 20009
A feminist newspaper with excellent regular coverage
  of women's health issues.

Women and Health
The Haworth Press, Inc.
  10 Alice Street
  Binghamton, NY 13904-1580

Women in Medicine Newsletter
Women in Medicine Task Force
American Medical Student Association
  1890 Preston White Drive
  Reston, VA 22091

WomenWise
Concord Feminist Health Center
  38 South Main Street
  Concord, NH 03301
An excellent quarterly.

Special Publications

*Bridging the Gap: A National Directory of Services for
  Women and Girls with Disabilities.* National Clear-
  inghouse on Women and Girls with Disabilities. New
  York: Educational Equity Concepts, 1990.
Children in Hospitals 1992 Consumer Directory. Available
  from Children in Hospitals, Inc., c/o Federation for
  Children with Special Needs, 95 Berkeley Street,
  Boston, MA 02116. Updated every two years.
Haire, Doris. *How Safe Is Safe?* Available from National
  Women's Health Network, 1325 G Street NW, Wash-
  ington, DC 20005. (202) 347-1140. A special report on
  how the FDA determines drug safety and what con-
  sumers need to know to protect themselves.

Audiovisual Materials

Healthcaring from Our End of the Speculum, a 35-minute
  film. A good introductory film covering many different women's health concerns. Available from Women
  Make Movies, 225 Lafayette Street, New York, NY
  10012.
Nursing: The Politics of Caring, a 22-minute 16-mm 1978
  film. A documentary about the struggles of nurses to
  increase their voices in the system. Available from
  Fanlight Productions, 47 Halifax Street, Jamaica
  Plain, MA 02130.
La Operación, a 40-minute 16-mm film. A powerful documentary about sterilization abuse, particularly

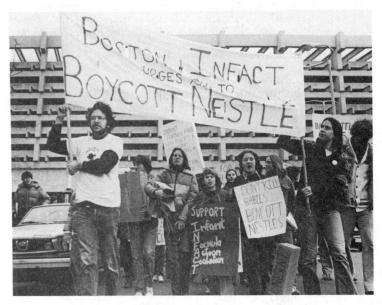

Ellen Shub

among Puerto Rican women. Available from The Cinema Guild, 1697 Broadway, Suite 802, New York, NY
  10019.
Taking Our Bodies Back: The Women's Health Movement,
  a 33-minute 1973 film. A classic general film on wom-
  en's health. To be updated in the early 1990s. Available from Cambridge Documentary Films, Box 385,
  Cambridge, MA 02139.

Organizations

American Medical Women's Association (AMWA)
  801 North Fairfax, Suite 400
  Alexandria, VA 22314
  (703) 838-0500
The AMWA is a national organization of 12,000 women
  physicians and medical students dedicated to promoting the personal and professional well-being of
  women physicians. The organization has as a primary mission the promotion of improved health care
  for women and is active on such issues as reproductive rights, domestic violence, breast cancer and osteoporosis.

Asian Health Project
T.H.E. Clinic for Women, Inc.
  3860 West Martin Luther King Boulevard
  Los Angeles, CA 90008
  (213) 295-6571
Provides multilingual health information and a wide
  range of health services to Asian and Pacific communities in Los Angeles County. Multilingual publications on sexual and reproductive health and hygiene for both women and men.

Boston Reproductive Rights Network (R2N2)
  P.O. Box 686
  Jamaica Plain, MA 02130
A grassroots feminist reproductive rights organization.
  Organizes demonstrations, picket lines, coalitions,

leafletting, clinic defense, conferences and media campaigns. Publishes *Reproductive Rights Newsletter*.

Bread & Roses Women's Health Center
5825 West Capitol Drive
Milwaukee, WI 53216
A health center providing gynecological health services with a commitment to change the conditions of women's lives by providing quality professional health care and by upholding the recognition of patient's rights.

Center for Science in the Public Interest
1501 16th Street NW
Washington, DC 20036
(202) 332-9110
Excellent resources, including posters on food and nutrition. Publishes *Nutrition Action*.

Choice in Dying
250 West 57th Street
New York, NY 10107
(212) 246-6962
Works through educational, judicial and legislative action for recognition of the right to die with dignity. Provides information and advice for consumers and professionals concerned with dying and the development of a living will.

Concord Feminist Health Center
38 South Main Street
Concord, NH 03301
(603) 225-2739
Publishes an excellent quarterly, *WomenWise*, which covers a wide variety of topics on women and health.

Ethical Treatment in Health Care (ETHC)
P.O. Box 112
Weston, MA 02193
(617) 646-3322.
Nonprofit organization promoting ethical health and mental health care for the public. Supports victims of medical and therapeutic sexual/emotional malpractice.

The Federation of Feminist Women's Health Centers (FFWHC)
633 E. 11th Avenue
Eugene, OR 97401
(503) 344-0966
The FFWHC is an association of women's health projects, working to secure reproductive rights for women and men, to educate women about the healthy functioning of our bodies, and to improve the quality of women's health care. Members of the FFWHC include Atlanta Feminist Women's Health Center, Atlanta, GA; Chico Feminist Women's Health Center, Chico, CA; Sacramento Feminist Women's Health Center, Sacramento, CA; Redding Feminist Women's Health Center, Redding, CA; Santa Rosa Feminist Women's Health Center, Santa Rosa, CA; Womancare: A Feminist Women's Health Center, San Diego, CA; Womancare South: A Feminist Women's Health Center, San Diego, CA; Portland Feminist Women's Health Center, Portland, OR; Yakima Feminist Women's Health Center, Yakima, WA; Cedar River Clinic: A Feminist Women's Health Center,

Renton, WA. These health centers offer abortion and gynecological services. Some are involved in research on contraceptive methods.

The Foundation Center
79 Fifth Avenue
New York, NY 10003-3050
(212) 620-4230.
Publishes *Promoting Issues and Ideas*.

Gray Panthers
1424 16th Street NW, Suite 602
Washington, DC 20036
(202) 387-3111
Nonprofit advocacy organization working on national health and medical care reform.

Health/PAC (Health Policy Advisory Center)
47 West 14th Street, Suite 300
New York, NY 10011
(212) 627-1847
Analyzes health issues from a radical perspective. Produces a variety of publications, including the periodical *Health/PAC Bulletin*.

Health Research Group
2000 P Street NW
Washington, DC 20036
(202) 833-3000
Ralph Nader–affiliated research and advocacy group. Publishes consumer-oriented books and manuals on drugs, medical devices, occupational and environmental health, health insurance and benefits programs and related topics.

International Childbirth Education Associates (ICEA)
Box 20048
Minneapolis, MN 55420
(612) 854-8660
Offers extensive annotated lists of publications and audiovisual resources; their monthly newsletter covers a wide range of childbirth issues.

Lyon-Martin Women's Health Center
1748 Market Street, Suite 201
San Francisco, CA 94102
(415) 565-7667
Offers primary care at a community clinic staffed and run by women. Committed to serving all women, focusing on lesbians, with special outreach to women of color, low-income women, older women and differently abled women. Works with the goal of providing quality, affordable, accessible, nonjudgmental, comprehensive health care in a way that demystifies health care and empowers women.

Montreal Health Press
Box 1000
Station G
Montreal, Quebec H2W 2N1 Canada
(514) 272-5441
Publishes *A Book About Birth Control, A Book About Menopause, A Book About Sexually Transmitted Diseases, A Book About Sexual Assault*, and poster kits on female and male reproduction, birth control methods and abortion. English and French.

National Association for Public Health Policy (NAPHP)
c/o The Marin Institute
24 Belvedere Street
San Rafael, CA 94901
(415) 456-5692
Develops health policy and legislation, with the goal of establishing a progressive national health program. Publishes the *Journal of Public Health Policy*, an excellent quarterly that covers women's health.

THE NORTHWEST COALITION FOR ALTERNATIVES TO PESTICIDES

Since 1977, the Northwest Coalition for Alternatives to Pesticides (NCAP) has been coordinating the activities of seventy-five groups throughout the Northwest working to decrease pesticide exposure. Their work involves educating the public about pesticide effects, promoting the use of pesticide alternatives and sustainable resource management and intervening in the public processes determining pesticide use. They provide the information and strategic advice necessary for citizens to effectively challenge exposure to these toxic chemicals.

NCAP's first efforts, following investigations of miscarriages that occurred after nearby herbicide spraying, helped instigate a national emergency suspension by the Environmental Protection Agency of dioxin-containing 2, 4, 5-T and Silvex on forest lands.

*Women and children are most clearly affected by herbicide exposure and it is therefore women who have provided the impetus and strength for our organization. Women in NCAP are generally either rural residents or forest workers who have united through their communities' NCAP member groups in activities opposing herbicide spraying on the forest lands they live adjacent to or work in. This is a survival issue for us.**

The staff and membership of NCAP primarily are women. Women in NCAP have done most of the local community organizing and intervention in government pesticide-use processes.

---

*The complete statement is available from NCAP, P.O. Box 1393, Eugene, OR 97440.

National Black Women's Health Project (NBWHP)
1237 Ralph Abernathy Blvd., SW
175 Trinity Avenue SW, 2nd Floor
Atlanta, GA 30310
(404) 758-9590
See p. 705.

National Clearinghouse on Women and Girls with Disabilities
Educational Equity Concepts, Inc.
114 East 32nd Street
New York, NY 10016
(212) 725-1803
Actively promotes equal opportunities through educational programs and materials that address the intersections of race, disability and low income. Special concerns: teenage pregnancy and parenting and sex role stereotyping; the special educational needs of women and girls with disabilities.

National Health Law Program
2639 South La Cienega Boulevard
Los Angeles, CA 90034
(213) 204-6010
Publishes the *Health Advocate* newsletter and other materials. Covers many issues of concern to women.

National Latina Health Organization (NLHO)/Organización Nacional de la Salud de la Mujer Latina
P.O. Box 7567
Oakland, CA 94601
(415) 534-1362
See p. 705.

National Women's Health Network
1325 G Street NW
Washington, DC 20005
(202) 347-1140
A national consumer/provider membership organization; monitors and works to influence government and industry policies. Publishes *Network News*.
See p. 708.

National Women's Studies Association
University of Maryland
College Park, MD 20742-1325
Large membership organization promoting feminist and women's studies in all educational institutions as well as the larger community.

Native American Women's Health Education Resource Center (NAWHERC)
P.O. Box 572
Lake Andes, SD 57356
(605) 487-7072
See p. 705.

New Day Films
121 West 27th Street
New York, NY 10001
(212) 645-8210
A cooperative distribution organization of independent media producers who distribute their own films and videotapes about social, political and cultural issues. Films and video tapes about women's experience and health.

Northwest Coalition for Alternatives to Pesticides (NCAP)
P.O. Box 1393
Eugene, OR 97440
(503) 344-5044
See p. 711.

Nurses for National Health Care
P.O. Box 441021
Somerville, MA 02144
(617) 739-2923
Nurses working together with consumers and other health-care workers to support the creation of a national health-care program in the United States that promotes the health of every person.

The Project on Women and Disability
One Ashburton Place, Room 1305
Boston, MA 02108
(617) 727-7440
See p. 704.

Santa Cruz Women's Health Center
250 Locust Street
Santa Cruz, CA 95060
(608) 427-3500
See p. 707.

Taller Salud
Apdo. 2172
Hato Rey, PR 00919
A self-help and activist collective in Puerto Rico.

Vancouver Women's Health Collective/Le Collectif de la Sante des Femmes de Vancouver
1720 Grant Street, Suite 302
Vancouver, British Columbia V5L 2Y7 Canada
(604) 255-8285
A resource center promoting a self-help approach to health care. The Information Center offers files, books and journals on all aspects of women's health. The collective also offers a practitioner referral directory and phone line for questions or referrals. Workshops on health topics.

Women's Health Action Mobilization (WHAM)
P.O. Box 733
New York, NY 10009
(212) 713-5966
WHAM is a direct-action group demanding, securing and defending reproductive freedom and quality health care for all women. Their actions range from escorting women into clinics to dropping banners off the Statue of Liberty. Contact the New York group for affiliates in other cities.

Women's Legal Defense Fund (WLDF)
1875 Connecticut Avenue NW, Suite 710
Washington, DC 20009
(202) 986-2600
Through legislative channels, policy-making and advocacy, works to shape a society that offers equal opportunity to every person, that responds to women's basic economic and health needs and that embraces policies that enable women and men to live with dignity and participate fully in every aspect of family and community life.

American Academy of Physician Assistants
950 N. Washington Street
Alexandria, VA 22314

Association of Physician Assistants in Obstetrics and Gynecology
P.O. Box 1109
Madison, WI 53701

27

Developing an International Awareness

By Vilunya Diskin

With special thanks to Norma Swenson, Judy Norsigian, Anita Anand, Asoka Bandarage, Elizabeth Coit, Jane Cottingham, Marilee Karl, Una MacLean and Annie Street.

1992 Update by Judy Norsigian and Norma Swenson, with Betsy Hartmann and H. Patricia Hynes.

A s feminists, we feel a strong bond with all women. We value the solidarity that comes when women in different countries meet, listen and exchange experiences with one another. We believe that feminism as a political perspective must look across national boundaries to address all the issues that affect women's lives.

All of us have been systematically denied access to crucial information about our bodies, bodies that are similar whether we inhabit them in the United States, Africa, Asia, Australia, Latin America or Europe. We all have fundamental needs for water, food and shelter.

Denial of reproductive rights, domestic violence, rape, sexual harassment in the workplace or on the street, racism, sexism, repression of lesbians, occupational hazards, economic exploitation and the horrors of war—none of these respects national boundaries. From a rural women's health and education group in South India:

When we read about women like us, rural, poor, from other parts of the world, we begin to feel women are similarly placed all over the world. The cultural contexts may differ, but the exploitation of women is the same everywhere.[1]

Women in the United States lack information from and about women throughout the world; women in industrialized countries know little about Third World women. There are few communication channels for useful and honest dialogue. An Asian woman observed: "American and European feminists, by being uninformed about their sisters in other countries, contribute unwittingly to their exploitation."[2] Living and voting in the most affluent and industrialized country, we have to take responsibility for the ways this country's policies affect the lives of women elsewhere. For example, if we succeed in removing dangerous contraceptives or other consumer products here, manufacturers may dump them on unsuspecting Third World women, as was the case with the Dalkon Shield and the high-dose estrogen pills. Our activism must include organizing with women of other countries to prevent such abuses.

Opening our eyes to common issues and being aware and respectful of our different realities, women around the world can better understand and help one another.

SEXISM

Sexism, or discrimination on the basis of sex, is a universal problem. There are differences in the varying forms and degrees, but all patriarchal societies (those dominated by men and organized around their activities and goals) circumscribe girls' and women's basic rights and opportunities. They thereby lose the benefit of our skills, talents and energies.

Women around the world face the imperative to bear and rear children and to take primary responsibility for the home. Cultures value us as reproducers, homemakers and consumers but rarely as workers and producers. This "invisibility" is absurd, considering that women's participation worldwide in the agricultural labor force is between 50 and 90 percent.[3] Women produce 60 percent of the world's food; prepare, process and store food; and are integral to local distribution systems. Wherever water must be carried, young girls and women do it. In many cultures, women also have important roles as traders of foodstuffs.

REPRODUCTION: WOMAN/COMMUNITY-CONTROLLED REPRODUCTIVE RIGHTS

Control of our bodies is a core feminist issue. Whether it is forced sterilization in Puerto Rico or denial of sterilization in France, "family planning" centers in India or restricted availability of abortion in the United States, wife battering, sexual slavery, "crimes of passion"—the result is the same: Women are not free to control our own bodies. Patriarchal domination begins here. In the words of an Indian woman:

We are brought up to view our bodies with suspicion and contempt, and this gives us a poor self-image. We are taught to consider our very existence as women as a misfortune; we never understood the way our bodies functioned and always feared or were ashamed of natural happenings like menstruation, pregnancy, childbirth.

A healthy attitude towards our bodies would help us develop our self-respect, and such self-awareness is the first step towards playing an active role in our communities, to change the unjust structures of which we are a part.[4]

When we say women must have reproductive freedom, we mean the possibility of controlling for ourselves, in a real and practical way—that is, free from economic, social or legal coercion—whether and under what conditions we will have children.[5]

Women all over the world increasingly see reproductive-rights issues as central to self-determination. Because the forces manipulating women's reproduction are many and powerful—governments, multinational corporations, the population control establishment, churches, the medical establishment and antiabortion organizations—we need international networks to counteract them effectively.

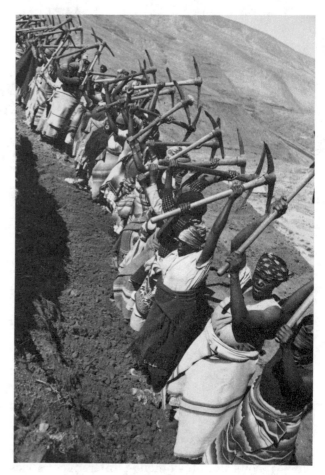

Women building a cross-country road in Lesotho.

United Nations/Muldoon

Birth control and population control (see Population Control Has Not Gone Away, p. 723) are *not* the same. We must ask many questions about birth control programs overseas: Who controls the program being offered? Who funds it, and what strings are attached? Who distributes the contraceptives and what kind? What kind of information and instructions are offered? Most important, how much and what kinds of birth control do people really want?

Contraception and sterilization can never substitute for safe, legal abortion services, either, despite antiabortion groups' claims. An estimated 500,000 to 1,000,000 women die in developing countries annually from illegal abortions and other preventable pregnancy-related causes.* More than half of these pregnancies are unwanted. Even where abortions are legal, as in India and Italy, we know from women's groups that the situation can still be dangerous and unfair. In India,

---

*Estimates vary because of secrecy and falsification. The World Health Organization's 1988 maternal mortality estimate of more than 500,000 deaths has changed little since 1983.

few women are aware that an abortion is legal, fewer still have access, and those who do get to a facility often receive deplorable treatment. In Italy and Greece many doctors refuse to perform abortions in hospitals on grounds of conscience but manage to overcome their scruples if a woman pays a large sum as a private patient. In the United States Medicaid cuts for abortion mean that many minority and poor women must end up being sterilized when that isn't what they really want.

The international public health establishment has begun a new focus on maternal mortality in many developing countries, but it is grass-roots women's groups worldwide who have made a public issue of maternal mortality in the context of reproductive rights. Coordinated by the Women's Global Network on Reproductive Rights (see Resources), groups everywhere have organized as never before, demanding safe abortion services, legalization of abortion, an end to sterilization abuse and safer, higher-quality birth control methods and services. Groups are in touch with one another, recognizing that they confront similar opposition and sharing strategies in a common commitment to stop the unnecessary deaths of women.

EXPORTING MISGUIDED PRIORITIES

Development

The word *development* usually means modernization. Here we talk about development as the conscious exportation of the process of modernization according to a Western model. Development theory is based on the history of Western industrialization and assumes that Third World countries could and would choose to follow the same path of economic growth. "Development experts," mostly Western males, study poverty, low productivity and unemployment as "problems of underdevelopment." They conceptualize programs to alleviate these "problems" after talking only with male spokesmen in the countries involved. They then try to get individual governments or international/multinational agencies like the United Nations or the World Bank (to which they

---

AFRICAN WOMEN STRUGGLE FOR REPRODUCTIVE HEALTH

African women are speaking out in their own way about reproductive rights and health, often with different priorities from women in other world regions. Because they produce up to 80 percent of all food and bear almost all the responsibility to care for and educate their children (who belong to fathers in most cases), their daily lives are often much harder than women's elsewhere. Being unmarried is always undesirable and even unacceptable in many places; producing (many) children is usually central to women's status and power in patriarchal, tribal groups, whose diversity is much greater than in other developing regions. Many African traditions of family and sexuality are nearly destroyed by colonial systems of exploitation, but contemporary replacement by traditions in extremist religions from the West or the East have done little to improve women's lot. Instead, this combination of imported and traditional beliefs has contributed to the ignorance and repression that fuels the rise of AIDS and spreads the practice of female circumcision in the mistaken belief that devoutness requires it.

Against these obstacles, African women have decided to fight against female circumcision in the context of other harmful traditional practices and with support from Western women rather than interference. They have also begun to tackle the AIDS epidemic, realizing that neither outsiders nor the governments can give the same quality of commitment as women themselves are able to bring to families and individuals. As they begin to acknowledge both AIDS and the steep rise in teenage pregnancy, some African women also are beginning to demand more accountability and responsibility from African men for men's sexual behavior. The "blame the victim" mentality in women's health is slowly becoming increasingly unacceptable. In recent years, networking with women in other African countries and other developing and Western countries, African women have begun to exchange ideas and build campaigns to improve maternal mortality, fighting for access to birth control and abortion in some places and fighting against coercive population control programs elsewhere. African women's extraordinary strength and determination is a model for all of us; as they continue to define their needs we will need to continue to offer them support and solidarity.

often belong) to fund these programs either with low-interest loans or free assistance. The end products of such aid are often extremely high levels of debt for developing nations and dependency on foreign goods and money.

Women worldwide criticize this kind of development policy, which largely ignores both their traditional role as major food producer and the devastating effects of the policy itself on women and children. Because the Western model assumes that only men work in agriculture, these programs usually give land titles only to men, thus denying women access to their traditional family-subsistence plots.

In Africa, for instance, women have the main responsibility to feed their children (i.e., grow, harvest and cook the food), pay school fees and purchase clothes and supplies. How can they accomplish these things when their land is taken away from them? The health of the community also declines, because subsistence crops (women's domain) are the stuff people eat, while cash crops (men's domain) are grown to be sold. Men control the money made from cash crops and are not as likely as women to spend it on food or on the family.

Also, development programs usually offer extension programs and training only to men, thereby denying women opportunities for learning new skills. When women are included, their workload is often increased, as for example in the high-yield grains that require more hours of weeding and harvesting. Planners find it hard to grasp that women need paid work. An Indian woman writes:

There is a prevailing myth that women live like parasites off the earnings of their husbands, but we found the reverse to be true. The women who came to Saheli [a women's resource center in Delhi, India] were women who had worked before and after marriage—they earned their own living and had often built assets (i.e., dowry) for their new homes—yet when the marriage broke up, they usually lost all these assets.[6]

Western and Third World academic and development experts of the women and development school push Western-style development in the name of women's liberation. However, development theory will never adequately benefit women if it does not address the question of patriarchy.

Society's acceptance of male-domination pervades development work. Though much lip-service is paid to the equal participation of women in the male-dominated development circles, there is little thought or real effort toward genuine power sharing with women.[7]

We need a new theory of development that both acknowledges women's central role in production and challenges the economic and political systems that oppress women. More women in every country must be involved in designing and implementing flexible programs to meet women's needs and to reflect their productive roles both inside and outside the home.

Multinational Corporations

The multinational corporations (MNCs) we are discussing here are those that have branches in different countries but retain concentration of capital and authority in the industrialized West. Even though they are often women's only source of paid employment, they have a primarily negative effect on Third World women's lives.

The MNCs force women to compete with one another. For example, women in the United States buy products produced by the toil of Third World women under sweatshop conditions. Whenever women (in South Korea, for example) begin to organize for better wages and working conditions, industries pick up and move to another community. U.S. women face unemployment because U.S. industries relocate to the Third World.

Textiles, electronics and agribusiness are three

Oxfam, America

industries that locate in developing countries because of tax incentives and the promise of cheap and docile labor. Women perform 80 to 90 percent of low-skilled assembly jobs. The MNCs pay low wages for long hours in unhealthy working conditions and then claim they are "liberating" women by giving them work.

In the Philippines . . . starting wages in U.S.-owned electronics plants are between $36–$46 a month, compared to a cost of living of $37 a month; in Indonesia the starting wages are actually about $7 a month less than the cost of living. "Living" is interpreted minimally: a diet of rice, dried fish, and water (a Coke might cost a half-day's wages), lodging in a room occupied by four or more people.[8]

Female workers worldwide earn 30 to 60 percent less than their male counterparts. Single women enlist for these new jobs often at the insistence of their families, who desperately need their earnings. Their move to urban areas means an upheaval—they lose their kin and community networks and in return receive no wage protection, work benefits, priority or seniority. They are the most exploited section of the formal labor force.

Health hazards abound in MNC workplaces. In the electronics industry, one of the safest and cleanest of the exporting industries, toxic chemicals and solvents sit in open containers filling the air with powerful fumes. An AFSC (American Friends Service Committee) worker in Northern Mexico heard about cases where ten or twelve women passed out at once. The newspapers reported this as "mass hysteria." In Malaysia, mass hysteria has become a form of resistance. One young woman sees a *hantu* or *jin* (hideous varieties of ghosts) and falls screaming to the floor in convulsions, and within minutes the hysteria spreads up and down the assembly line. Sometimes the plant has to close for a week or more to exorcise the spirits. Malaysian academics point out that the attacks are likely to be preceded by a speedup or a tightening of plant discipline.[9]

The stress of peering through a microscope at tiny wires for seven to nine hours at a time, straining to meet quotas at a pay rate of two dollars per day, could make anyone hysterical. Electronics workers often lose the 20/20 vision required for the job. One study in South Korea found severe eye problems in electronics assembly workers; after only one year of employment, 88 percent had chronic conjunctivitis, 44 percent had become nearsighted and 19 percent had developed astigmatism. In one stage of the electronics assembly process, workers have to dip the circuits into open vats of acid. In Penang, Malaysia, women wear gloves and boots to do dipping, but when these

leak, burns are common, and the workers sometimes lose fingers in painful accidents.[10]

Textile and garment industry conditions rival those of any nineteenth- or twentieth-century Western sweatshop. Workers are packed into poorly lit rooms where summer temperatures rise above 100 degrees Fahrenheit; textile dust, which can cause permanent lung damage, fills the air; rush orders require forced overtime of as much as forty-eight hours at a stretch, with the management supplying pep pills and amphetamine injections as needed. In her diary, published in a magazine now banned by the government, a thirty-year-old South Korean sewing-machine operator describes conditions in the garment factory where she works from seven A.M. to eleven-thirty P.M.

When apprentice workers shake the waste threads from the clothes, the whole room fills with dust, and it is hard to breathe. Since we've been working in such dusty air, there have been increasing numbers of people getting tuberculosis, bronchitis, and eye diseases. . . .

It seems to me that no one knows our blood dissolves into the threads and seams, with sighs and sorrow.[11]

Stress is probably the most invidious health hazard. Visits to the bathroom are a privilege; in some cases, workers must raise their hands for permission and wait up to half an hour. Working days one week and then nights the next wreaks havoc with sleeping patterns. Stomachaches and nervous problems reflect internalized anxieties and pressures of meeting production quotas. Management actually encourages a high turnover rate in many industries; because wages rise with seniority, it is cheaper to train a new batch of teenagers than to pay for an experienced "older" (i.e., twenty-three- or twenty-four-year-old) woman.

The MNCs say they are contributing to development, but they come into a country for one thing—cheap labor—and when the labor stops being so cheap, they move on. What kind of development is it that depends on people staying poor? Saralee Hamilton, an AFSC staff person working on the issue of women and global corporations, says:

The multinational corporations have deliberately targeted women for exploitation. If feminism is going to mean anything to women all over the world, it's going to have to find new ways to resist corporate power internationally.[12]

Infant Formula

After the postwar baby boom (when birth rates declined in the West), infant formula companies looked to the relatively untouched Third World markets. Convinced by aggressive and often unethical advertising practices that a bottle-fed baby will be healthier and more likely to survive than a breastfed baby,* millions of Third World mothers stopped breastfeeding but were unable to maintain the sanitary conditions for mixing and storing the formula and often couldn't afford to purchase it in sufficient quantities. The result was 10 million cases of severe malnutrition each year and approximately 3 million infant deaths.[13]

At times, the infant formula industry has promoted sexism, convincing women who have borne healthy babies that their bodies cannot keep the babies healthy and that they need an expert, often a male doctor, to tell them what to do.

Citizens around the world organized a major campaign to stop these unethical practices. During the 1970s and 1980s the Infant Formula Action Coalition (INFACT) and International Baby Food Action Network (IBFAN) began a boycott against Nestlé, a Swiss company, which is the world's largest multinational food corporation and generated almost half of all infant formula sales in the developing world.[14] This, the largest U.S. non-union boycott in history, involved over 300 national groups and forty-one countries. The demands: an end to direct consumer advertising, an end to promotion through and to members of the health care professions, an end to company "milk nurses" and an end to free samples.

The boycott had an economic impact.† In 1978 the Norwegian Dairy Sales Association canceled its exclusive contract with Nestlé for the distribution of Jarlsberg cheese; when Notre Dame in the United States became a "Nestlé-free campus," the food service stopped using $40,000 per week of Nestlé products. The greatest success of the boycott has been the consumer education impact, which has brought the whole issue to the international governmental-agency level for serious debate and action. As a result, the World Health Organization (WHO) developed an International Infant Formula Code of Marketing Behavior for the industry. When the World Health Assembly voted on the code in May 1980, every country voted in favor of it except the United States, whose representatives stated that it infringed upon the free enterprise system.

It's not enough just to get rid of infant formula. Breastfeeding is not always easy or possible, because many women have to work full-time outside the home and many have tremendous family responsibilities. Women's fight is not only against a technological culture that says it's better to bottle-feed, but also for alternatives—increased maternity leave with pay, workplaces where breastfeeding is part of the schedule and acceptance of the fact that women have a right to make choices in these matters. As a Senegalese woman puts it:

It's not enough to talk about the natural superiority of breast milk and the advantages to both the mother and infant. We have to create the conditions to make it possible for women to do this. Yes to breastfeeding, but . . . how?[15]

Drugs—Not Merely a Local Matter: The Impact of the U.S. Drug Industry on Third World Women

Dominated by some of the most powerful and profitable MNCs in the world, the pharmaceutical industry continues to exploit Third World health systems. By 1980 in the United States, patents for most of the 200 largest-selling drugs had expired. Having exploited the domestic market thoroughly, U.S. firms are now looking more aggressively to developing countries for new consumers—most especially women.* The U.S. government is eager to encourage export of drugs as a means of improving the balance of international payments. Weak restrictions in underdeveloped countries mean that these companies can promote their products with impunity. This is not good news for Third World women. Furthermore, in the past efforts to find safe drugs for women in the United States often involved testing on poor and Third World women. The high-dose birth control pill was first tested on women (usually poor and illiterate) in Puerto Rico and later in El Salvador, sometimes without their knowledge and with severe consequences to their health.

Pharmaceutical companies develop drugs for "rich country" diseases, like heart complaints, depression, insomnia and cancer but don't do much research into the tropical diseases affecting approximately a billion people in the Third World.[16] They dump drugs that regulations or consumer

---

*Infant formula manufacturers use a large repertoire of promotion tactics, including billboards and posters showing healthy children next to company products. They send sales personnel dressed in nurses' uniforms to offer mothers advice on infant feeding and give them free samples. Taking advantage of the medicalization of childbirth, they vigorously promote their products to and through health-care providers, especially in hospitals.

†The Nestlé boycott ended in early 1984, but the work of investigating other corporations involved in marketing breast-milk substitutes and commercial products for children in developing countries continues. U.S. corporations, in particular, will be under pressure to conform to the terms agreed on by Nestlé, and monitoring of all corporations' compliance will be important.

---

*Third World women are increasingly the targets for psychoactive drugs in particular.

complaints make unmarketable in the United States. Sending a multitude of representatives to the Third World, they sometimes spend more on promotion and advertising than Third World countries spend on health budgets. They promote many drugs that are ineffective and others for the wrong diseases, in which case their use may be hazardous. They provide minimal information on negative effects and contraindications, even to the professionals who will dispense the drugs.

Women health activists and consumer coalition groups have been working against these abuses. Health Action International (HAI) was established in Geneva in May 1981 to coordinate activities and share ideas and resources internationally among consumers and development and public interest groups, as well as provide the framework for international campaigns. HAI has set up an international clearinghouse for information on the drug industry's structure, ownership and marketing practices and has established an international consumer product warning network, the Consumer Interpol. They must be doing something right, because they have the pharmaceuticals worried. The July 17, 1981, *Food and Drug Letter* (Washington Business Information, Inc.) talked about a "group of activists—fresh from their work against infant formula industry marketing practices—[which] has set its sights on [the issue of] selling drugs to consumers in the Third World Nations."[17] The *Letter* was worried that HAI would conduct a media campaign against multinational drug firms along the lines of the Nestlé boycott. But most worrisome for the industry is the possibility that HAI may influence WHO to adopt a regulatory drug code similar to the one on infant formula marketing. The International Federation of Pharmaceutical Manufacturers' Associations (IFPMA) has developed a provisional, voluntary Code of Pharmaceutical Marketing Practice in an effort to head off the mounting criticism and avoid regulation. The IFPMA code is vague, incomplete and difficult to interpret or monitor. It makes no references to gifts or samples, the content of advertising, methods of production or product liability. Also, the requirements are so broad it is safe to assume nothing is likely to change.

Western Medicine Versus Indigenous Systems

We export Western medicine all over the world under the guise of sharing "expertise" (the so-called transfer of technology). A tragic result is the devaluation and persecution of indigenous health systems. For example, U.S.-assisted health care planning in newly independent India (in 1948) assumed a need for increased Western medical science and technology, in spite of the histor-

Women preparing enriched porridge in Chad.
International Federation of Red Cross and Red Crescent Societies

ical existence and availability of the traditional Indian system of Ayurveda (use of herbs) and yoga. Ayurvedic medicine, through its holistic approach, provides effective prevention for a range of health problems untouched by Western medicine. Ayurveda, like many traditional systems, is decentralized, giving individuals more control over their own health, a crucial factor in a country like India where 85 percent of the people live in rural areas.[18] Rural people are most often in need of simple, preventive services. Infectious diseases are still prevalent; public health measures like clean water, sanitation and a proper diet could prevent much more ill health than new machines, drugs and factories ever will.

Women all over the world suffer when governments accept physicians' monopoly over the direction of health policy. Two centuries ago, the medical establishment in the Western world began to ostracize and persecute women healers, the midwives and abortionists who had always served poor and rural women. Development often means a similar shift in the Third World. Because most women live in rural areas, most countries

SISTERHOOD IS POWERFUL; INTERNATIONAL SISTERHOOD IS EVEN MORE POWERFUL

The past few decades have witnessed the development of many new women's organizations. Here are just a *few* examples of what women have been doing to link internationally.

1974
ISIS, an international women's information and communication service, began as a resource and documentation center in the international women's movement. It makes materials from local women's groups available to women all over the world and publishes a quarterly bulletin and several guides.

1975
Designated by the United Nations as International Women's Year. The official conference took place in Mexico; there was an unofficial parallel conference, called the Tribunal, to which NGOs (nongovernmental organizations) and women's groups sent delegates.

1976 to 1985
U.N. International Women's Decade. Countries were instructed to look at their national priorities in development and to include women.

1976
International Tribunal of Crimes Against Women, Brussels. Out of this conference the International Feminist Network (IFN) was established. The IFN, coordinated by ISIS, is a communication channel through which women in one country can ask those in others for help—for instance, in the form of telegrams and letters expressing solidarity with an action they are taking.

1977
First International Women and Health Meeting, Rome.

1977
As part of International Women's Decade, there was a National Women's Conference in Houston, Texas, which 20,000 women attended. A delegation from the International Wages for Housework Campaign was present. Wilmette Brown, of Black Women for Wages for Housework (U.S.), stated, "Our fight for money of our own is not so we can join the *man* sitting on top of the world. Our victory is an open invitation to share the wealth."

1979
Feminist Conference, Bangkok. Third World women participants decided to embrace the term *feminism*, despite its distorted media image. They recognized an *indigenous feminism*, which was comprised in part of Third World women questioning the whole concept of "development" and asking whether women *wanted* integration into this process, no matter how equally. These women defined feminism in terms of two long-term goals: first, the achievement of women's equality, dignity and freedom of choice through power to control our bodies and lives, inside and outside the home; second, the removal of all forms of inequity and oppression through the creation of

Striking domestic workers of Poona.   Navrose Contractor

720

a more just social and economic order, nationally and internationally.

1980

Mid-Decade U.N. Conference on Women, Copenhagen. There was also an NGO Forum, a parallel conference that 8,000 women attended. The theme was Development, Equality, and Peace.

1980

Second International Women and Health Meeting, Hanover, Germany.

1981

Third International Women and Health Meeting, Geneva, organized by ISIS and Dispensaire des Femmes. Five hundred women, working in self-help in thirty-five countries, convened to exchange knowledge, experiences and ideas.

1981

First Latin American/Caribbean Feminist Meeting, Bogotá, Colombia.

1982

National New Zealand Women's Health Conference.

1984

Women's International Tribunal and Meeting on Women's Reproductive Rights, Amsterdam.

1985

Women's NGO Forum, Nairobi, Kenya, at time of End-of-Decade U.N. Conference on Women.

The International Women's Decade has served primarily to make all of us more deeply aware of the vast extent of women's *exclusion* from the political process on every continent. A challenge for the next decades is to maintain this new awareness of the need for change and full involvement for women, as well as to push for the implementation of the gains we have so painstakingly won.

1987

Fifth International Women and Health Meeting, San José, Costa Rica. This was a gathering of over 600 women from five continents (the first time this international feminist meeting was held outside Europe).

1990

Sixth International Women and Health Meeting, Manila, the Philippines. Over 400 women from sixty countries in attendance.

need to keep health in the hands of community health providers, traditional healers and village health workers and to use doctors as auxiliaries or consultants, the role they should have in any case, based on their narrow, highly technical training.

Tourism

Tourism is an increasingly important source of income in the Third World, in some cases the third or fourth largest source of foreign currency. A strong incentive for tourism is the availability of women in these countries either explicitly as prostitutes or disguised as hospitality girls, massage and bath attendants, performers in sex shows, hostesses and waitresses in clubs. Closely related to the sex-tourism industry is the "rest and relaxation" (R-and-R) business that has grown up around many permanent U.S. military bases in Asia. The sex-tourism and R-and-R industries exploit the vast majority of their employees both sexually and economically. Women enter this type of employment out of economic necessity and because there are often no alternatives for them.

In Thailand, the gap in incomes and opportunities between the city and countryside is enormous, setting the way for rural–urban migration. For women from poor rural backgrounds, migration provides an earning power which is simply astounding compared to normal rural budgets. Two or three years' working as a masseuse/prostitute enables a [woman's] family to build a house of size and quality few people in the countryside could hope to achieve with the earnings of a lifetime. Many families, indeed entire villages, have raised their standard of living through the bodies of their daughters.[19]

Most of the money generated by sex tourism goes to tourist agencies, hotels, club owners, tour operators, pimps and other organizers of the business. Tourist agencies and airlines in industrialized countries reap huge profits. Because they see it as an important source of income, some governments condone or encourage sex tourism outright: Some officials even exhort their women to prostitution as a form of great patriotism! The most blatant examples are in the Philippines, South Korea and Thailand. Some 700,000 women work in Bangkok's massage parlors, teahouses, nightclubs, brothels and disco-restaurants. From a Dutch travel agency's promotional material:

. . . Thailand is a world full of extremes and possibilities are unlimited. Anything goes in this exotic country, especially when it comes to girls. . . . However, it may be a problem for visitors to Thailand to find the right places where they can indulge in

unknown pleasures. It is frustrating to have to ask the hotel receptionist in broken English where you can pick up pretty girls. Rosie has done something about this. For the first time, you can book a trip to Thailand with erotic pleasures included in the price....[20]

Dutch men board charter flights from Amsterdam to Bangkok where they can buy a woman for twenty-five guilders a night (twelve and a half dollars), a hundred guilders a week. The "girls," on the other hand, earn about eighty guilders a month when they can find work. The fact that 70 percent of the women suffer from sexually transmitted diseases does not serve as a deterrent, and the airplane home was nicknamed the "gonorrhea express."[21]

Japanese businessmen often fly on one-night *Kisaeng* (i.e., sex) tours to South Korea. The following appeared in a Japanese magazine:

There are only two types of people who don't sleep with South Korean women: those with no money and those with something wrong with a certain part of their body.

A young Japanese male asked this magazine:

"I've heard that you can do absolutely anything you want with South Korean women. Is this true? If I travel, I'd like to taste women to the full, so I'd like to know a little more about South Korean "service."

The magazine answered:

No, it is not an exaggeration to say that South Korea fully deserves its reputation as a "Male Paradise." These special tours cost a little more, but you can still buy a woman for only 75 dollars. In addition, these Korean girls are young, between 18 and 25, and very ripe. If you want our advice, get going to the "Male Paradise," South Korea.[22]

Prostitution in the Philippines has always flourished where there is a heavy concentration of foreigners, for example, in the row of "clubs" adjacent to the U.S. military bases in Angeles City (Clark Air Force Base, effectively closed in 1991) and Olongapo (Subic Bay Naval Base, scheduled to close in the mid-1990s). About 6,500 American military and civilian personnel used to go to Olongapo every day for R and R. Average monthly earnings for an Olangapo hostess is between 500 and 600 pesos (seventy to eighty-four dollars). Some girls start work at age thirteen or fourteen through arrangement with club owners and managers, and women work until their late forties or fifties or as long as the owners will allow it. Upon retirement, most have no savings or Social Security benefits and end up as poor and exploitable as when they

began. Analysts have predicted that wherever the U.S. military bases remain (the Subic and Clark operations are moving elsewhere), the profitable and powerful existing R-and-R trade will thrive.[23]

Women's and church groups in Asia have protested these activities, many seeking international solidarity. Responding to appeals by South Korean, Thai and Philippine women, women's groups in Japan and elsewhere have organized information campaigns and actions against the tourist agencies involved.

South Korean women organized a demonstration at the airport where the *Kisaeng* airplanes land. They carried placards in Japanese saying: "We will throw you beyond the sea, Japanese sex monsters!"[24]

"TO TALK FEMINISM IS NEVER TO TALK NONSENSE"*

International women's organizations, such as ISIS and the Women's Global Network for Reproductive Rights, along with the hundreds of local groups in every region on every continent, point to feminist efforts in organizing a strong women's international presence. We must nurture and expand these groups so that women may truly learn about the lives of their sisters by exchanging information, experiences and hopes. The numerous feminist magazines further these goals. *Broadsheet* (New Zealand), *Manushi* (India), *Spare Rib* (England), *Courage* (Germany), *FemPress* (Mexico) and *Off Our Backs* (United States) are just a few of our important "spokeswomen." This kind of exchange can help diminish some of the barriers of region, race, class and fear that now divide us, and can strengthen the similarities we share. As the Korean garment worker quoted on p. 717 wrote in her diary, "We all have the same hard life. We are bound together by one string."[25] And, from a woman in India:

We will be able to derive strength for all our efforts if all women stand united, convinced of our worth, and angry at our oppression.[26]

*Donna Awatere, a Maori woman, New Zealand.

POPULATION CONTROL HAS NOT GONE AWAY

After almost twenty years of feminist and progressive opposition, population control remains a dominant element in development strategy and a primary goal of international family planning programs. At the World Bank, the United Nations, the U.S. Agency for International Development (USAID) and a host of other public and private agencies, the old population establishment is alive and well. While it often incorporates the language of women's rights into its goals, for example, by calling for the education of women, it rarely calls for critical structural changes such as land reform, the redistribution of economic and political power and the repudiation of international debt. By focusing primarily on the narrow issue of population, it often obscures the main causes of poverty, environmental degradation and the economic and political dislocations of the new world order.

Like any ideology, population control has evolved and changed over time. In response to the failure of past family planning efforts, a reformist wing has emerged that calls for higher-quality care and the expansion of programs to address other aspects of women's reproductive health. Although this is welcome, it has little impact on the dominant view. More important, it fails to challenge the fundamental assumption of population control policy: that rapid population growth is one of the main causes of underdevelopment in the Third World.

Over the years this assumption has been tailored to the times and rapid population growth blamed for a variety of serious problems: in the 1970s for hunger and poverty, in the 1980s for unemployment and economic crisis and now in the 1990s for environmental degradation. Today the poor are not only held responsible for their own misery, but for the destruction of the entire planet.

Today in the United States, mainstream environmental organizations, such as the Sierra Club, National Wildlife Federation and Audubon Society, have formed a political alliance with population agencies around the dangers of high birth rates and the need for massive increases in U.S. population assistance. "Because of its pervasive and detrimental impact on global ecological systems, population growth threatens to overwhelm any possible gains made in improving living conditions," reads a "Priority Statement on Population" circulated within the population and environment community. The document calls for massive increases in family planning aid.

These groups seriously downplay the principal causes of the environmental crisis: dominant economic systems that squander natural and human resources in the drive for short-term profits; the displacement of peasant farmers and indigenous peoples by agribusiness, timber, mining and energy firms; the policies of international lending institutions; war and arms production; and the wasteful consumption patterns of industrialized countries and wealthy elites in the world.

While women in many countries could benefit from expanded access to birth control and abortion, how the population problem is defined, however, profoundly affects the nature of birth control methods developed and the programs that distribute these methods. For example, the World Bank and other agencies often promote intensive family planning programs as a condition of aid and at the expense of other equally important health care services.

Today, the international aid community is concentrating its population control efforts in sub-Saharan Africa, where according to the World Bank, family planning should be the "cornerstone" of health and development policy. USAID's Office of Population, for example, has dramatically increased its aid for Africa, so that the continent now accounts for more than a third of family-planning service delivery funds and half the expenditure of the policy division.

One controversial aspect of family planning programs in some countries is the use of incentives. According to a Bank working paper, "Ethical Approaches to Family Planning in Africa," incentives and disincentives "may have a place in family planning programs, but they should never have discriminatory or coercive effects." Then in a dazzling display of contorted logic, the authors state, "By their nature, incentives and disincentives are aimed primarily at the poor, since it is mainly the poor who will be susceptible to them."

In many cases, policymakers have also advocated an extremely "casual" approach toward medical screening and follow-up for certainly highly effective and somewhat riskier contraceptives. For example, a letter from

continued

continued

USAID's Office of Population to the International Planned Parenthood Federation states:

All too often, in our view, family planning programs impose numerous medical barriers to service which we are convinced hinder program effectiveness and impact, especially for hormonal contraception. A common example of what we mean by medical barriers includes conservative medical thinking (e.g. taking a woman off the pill for a while if she develops a headache just to play it "safe" . . .) . . . we prefer not even to use the term . . . contraindications . . . which may have very negative connotations. . . .

The concrete dangers of such a cavalier approach to contraceptive safety are illustrated by the case of Norplant in Indonesia. Developed by the Population Council in New York, Norplant is a progestin implant system inserted under the skin of a woman's arm, which prevents pregnancy for at least five years (see p. 288). Both insertion and removal require local anesthesia and medical skill. Ethical use of the drug depends on adequate medical screening and follow-up, and, most important, on access to removal on demand.

An internal Population Council report provides chilling evidence of how Norplant has been misused in the Indonesian population program. Nearly a half million women had Norplant inserted, often without counseling on the side effects or on alternative contraceptive options, pregnancy screening and sterilization of equipment. Many were not told that the implant must be removed after five years.

Moreoever, removal on demand was not guaranteed, not only because of lack of trained personnel, but, more important, to serve the Indonesian government's demographic objectives. As one Indonesian population official put it, "People are told it has to last five years, they give their word . . . and rural people don't go back on their word. If they request removal, they are reminded that they gave their word."

At the same time women confront overly zealous population control programs, they must also struggle against a well-funded antiabortion, anticontraception movement that would deny women access to basic birth control and abortion services. Between the two extremes, mainstream population control may appear reasonable to many. But its narrow focus on human *numbers* obscures the human *systems* of exploitation—exploitation of women by men, poor by rich, dark-skinned by light-skinned—that have created those high numbers in the first place. Population control will never be a substitute for social justice.

This is an updated and expanded version of a plenary address, "Population Policies and Programs: A Feminist Assessment," by Betsy Hartmann, delivered at the Sixth International Women and Health Meeting, Manila, Philippines, November 5, 1990. Hartmann is the author of *Reproductive Rights and Wrongs: The Global Politics of Population Control and Contraceptive Choice*, New York: Harper & Row, 1987.

THE POCKETBOOK AND THE PILL: REFLECTIONS ON GREEN CONSUMERISM AND POPULATION CONTROL

by H. Patricia Hynes, Institute on Women and Technology, North Amherst, MA 01059. Abridged from *Issues in Reproductive Genetic Engineering*, Vol. 4, No. 1 (1991), pp. 47–52.

Environmental pollution is intimately linked to the technology of the West. The specific technologies developed for our basic needs of energy, transportation, waste removal and treatment, food, health, and consumer products are themselves the major sources of hazardous waste and the pollution of local air, water, and soil, the sea, and the global atmosphere. Also, technologies and products are marketed within a culture that baptizes the new as progressive and desirable, a culture that turns desires into needs and reduces citizens to consumers. This culture of consumption cohabitates with a culture of production within the western view of the world as an economic arena in which a country's "degree of civilization . . . [is] measured by the level of its production."[27] The consequences of this world-view are that we produce in a style and to a degree that is destroying our environment; we exercise dominance in the world by endless economic penetration; and we export the concept of the world as an economic arena in our view of development and underdevelopment. (I say "we" when I mean they, because women did not invent western development schemes and institutions nor this view of the world as an economic arena. In industrial countries, however, 90 percent of consumer advertising is directed toward women, and 80 percent of consumer buying is done by women.)

Western environmentalists have endeavored to wrest some control over industrial production and marketing of new products, by launching a green consumer movement. "Consumers have the power to change the market" was the upbeat salvo sounding forth from Earth Day 1990 events. Green consumerism urges shoppers to "buy green," that is, to replace products which pollute or whose manufacture causes pollution by buying new products which cause, or claim to cause, less pollution. And there has been some success: demand for organic produce doubled from 1988 to 1989 in the United States and business in recycled paper products and nontoxic household cleaners is brisk and growing. However, the message that buying power can change the world is simplistic, shallow, and incomplete; a movement based on it will fare no better. Let women be wary of green consumerism.

First, green buying reduces people to consumers and nature to market commodities. In this brand of economics, the value of a mountain is calculated by polling people on how much they would pay to hike it.

Second, green consumerism rarely addresses rigorously the reality that our enormous per capita consumption in the west steals natural resources from third world countries, depends on the labor of their children, and contributes excessively to global climate change. Buying with environmental consciousness should be, first, buying less, and then, buying differently. Green companies, consultants and catalogues do not prompt us to ask ourselves if we truly need something or simply want it. The power of absence—consuming less—diminishes the dominant role of economics, while the power of a different presence—buying green—does not.

Third, major corporate polluters who see a new marketing opportunity in green products are rapidly overtaking the green consumer movement. The steps in pollution prevention that some corporations are taking—waste reduction and minimization, energy efficiency, recyclable packaging—are necessary but long overdue. Few, if any, are changing *the products* they manufacture to eliminate toxicity; where there are beneficial changes in product ingredient, which happens more because of consumer pressure than because of industry initiative, industry often tries to take the credit. Some industries engage in deception by: marketing plastic as degradable when there are no standard definitions or tests for degradability in plastic; labeling plastic as recyclable when the industrial capacity for recycling plastic hovers around 1 percent of "post-consumer" plastic; and promoting genetically engineered plants and bacteria as organic, natural, and ecological. Without an analysis of corporate interests and power, the green consumer movement will be outmaneuvered by corporate marketing and will fail to reform industry.

continued

continued

Fourth, green consumerism contains little critical vision of development and little analysis of the effects of international trade on local industrial and agricultural self-reliance. We need to move away from the idea of one global economic village to the goal of a "globe of villages" that "allows us to produce most of what we need from our own local human, natural and capital resources on a sustainable basis."[28]

Fifth, the classic rule upon which green consuming is based—supply follows demand—does not bear out even in efficient, market-based economies. Organic agriculture in the United States supplies less than 4 percent of commercial food; yet, if demand did drive supply, commercial organic food supply would easily be five to ten times as much. What are the impediments to supply? A shortage of public and private funds for the multidisciplinary research needed, federal grading standards based on the cosmetic appearance of fruits and vegetables, and a system of government price supports and land management requirements that favors chemical-intensive agriculture. Government policy, then, binds farmers to agriculture with high inputs of artificial fertilizer, pesticides, and antibiotics and obstructs the transition to sustainable agriculture.

Sixth, green consumerism lacks an analysis of sexual politics. If a cosmetic is made with natural ingredients but is advertised with pictures that objectify women and promote the message that aging in women is unattractive, is that product a "green" product? In *The Green Consumer* (Penguin, 1987), a bestselling British guide to purchasing "environmentally friendly" products, authors John Elkington and Julia Hailes recommend Playboy deodorant because it does not contain ozone-deplet-ing chlorofluorocarbons. Already accused of being little more than "green capitalism," this brand of consumer movement will advance nothing if pornographic images and sexist messages stay intact in "green" products.

The issue of population growth and control is one in which the shallow, apolitical, and incomplete thinking that characterizes consumer environmentalists is framing the debate. "Population" recently has moved up the chain of causes to become a major cause of environmental degradation, according to many environmental organizations and journals. Quick-fix solutions are being proposed which short-circuit women's complex path to autonomy, integrity, and dignity. The call for population control principally through greater use of the pill and longer lasting hormonal implants and injectables is rapidly sealing off the deeper questions of why women have children, why men are not expected to take responsibility for contraception, and how women can gain gender justice.

Ironically, this push for greater use of long-acting contraception comes during an era when sexually transmitted diseases, including AIDS, are epidemic, when, instead, we should be placing greater emphasis upon barrier methods of contraception, like the male condom, female condom, cervical cap, and diaphragm. Also, in many cases, it is not the lack of birth control methods or poverty but male-dominated cultural, legal, and religious pressures that force women into unwanted pregnancies. Long-acting methods do not free women from pressures to have male children, from assumptions that they are less than whole without a child, and from forced sex by husbands and others.

Is the best remedy for the environment one of population control or consumption control?

NOTES

1. T. K. Sundari. "Women's Camp," July 30–August 3, 1981, p. 35. Available from Rural Women's Social Education Centre and Rural Development Society, 15/1. Periya Melamaiyur, Chingleput 603 002, Tamil-nadu, S. India.

2. *ISIS International Bulletin* 3 (April 1977), p. 3.

3. Anita Anand. "Rethinking Women and Development: The Case for Feminism," in *Women and Development Resource Guide.* Philadelphia: New Society Publishers, 1983.

4. T. K. Sundari. "Women's Camp," p. 33.

5. *International Women and Health Resource Guide.* Boston: BWHBC and ISIS, 1980, p. 51. No longer in print.

6. *Saheli.* Indian Women's Resource Center, Unit Above Shop, 105–108 Shopping Center, Defense Colony Bridge (South Side), New Delhi 110024 India.

7. Anita Anand. "Rethinking Women and Development," in *Women and Development Resource Guide.*

8. Barbara Ehrenreich and Annette Fuentes. "Life on the Global Assembly Line," *Ms.* (January 1981), p. 55.

9. Barbara Ehrenreich and Annette Fuentes. "Life on the Global Assembly Line," p. 55.

10. Barbara Ehrenreich and Annette Fuentes. "Life on the Global Assembly Line," p. 56.

A small segment of the world's population in the industrial countries uses far more energy and more natural resources—10- to 100-fold in some cases—than the populous developing countries. Industrial countries generate most of the world's waste, including the majority of airborne chemicals and gases that deplete the ozone layer and contribute to global warming. In other words, a family of eight in Rwanda or Nicaragua neither depletes nor pollutes the Earth anywhere near the amount that does a family of four in Great Britain or the United States. The average Indian uses only 4 percent of the energy consumed by the average U.S. citizen.

Rich nations have borrowed from the Earth's commonly held ecological system, such as clean air, and left in its place the "junk" of acid rain and greenhouse gases. The industrial nations have incurred an environmental debt in order to finance their economic development and wealth. The best remedy for what ails the Earth is consumption control in industrial countries coupled with a rapid shift to technologies for agriculture, transportation, and energy that deplete and pollute the environment as little as it is technically possible.

As for the question of population, what really matters is *reproductive self-determination* for all women. This approach advocates improvements in the status of women in society, improvements in living standards through equitable social and economic development, and the provision of safe and effective birth control services as part of the larger system of primary health care. It does not subordinate women's health and well-being to the population goals of husbands, family, community or government.

11. Barbara Ehrenreich and Annette Fuentes. "Life on the Global Assembly Line," p. 57.

12. Barbara Ehrenreich and Annette Fuentes. "Life on the Global Assembly Line," p. 60. See also the monthly newsletter of the Pacific Studies Center for the Global Electronics Information Project, 222B View Street, Mountain View, CA 94101.

13. Fred Clarkson. "Growing Nestlé Boycott Haunts Infant Formula Makers," *WIN Magazine* (March 1, 1981), p. 12.

14. Sally Austen Tom. "Hazards of Infant Formula," *Heresies*, Vol. 4, No. 1, Issue 13 (1981), p. 74.

15. Marie-Angelique Savané. "Yes to Breastfeeding, But . . . How?" *Assignment Children*, UNICEF Vol. 49/50 (Spring 1980), p. 82.

16. "Women and Health," Part 1, *ISIS International Bulletin* 7 (Spring 1978), p. 5.

17. *The Food and Drug Letter*, an independent bi-weekly from Washington Business Information, 235 National Press Building, Washington, DC 20045, July 17, 1981, p. 1.

18. J. Bandyopadhyay and V. Shiva. "Alternatives for India, Western or Indigenous Science," *Science for the People*, Vol. 13, No. 2 (March/April 1981), pp. 22–28.

19. Pasuk Phongpaichit. "Bangkok Masseuses: Holding Up the Family Sky," in "Tourism: Selling Southeast Asia," *Southeast Asia Chronicle*, Issue 78 (April 1981), p. 23.

20. "Tourism and Prostitution," *ISIS International Bulletin* 13 (November 1979), p. 9.

21. "Tourism and Prostitution," p. 9.

22. "Tourism and Prostitution," p. 22.

23. "Tourism and Prostitution," p. 20.

24. "Tourism and Prostitution," p. 8.

25. Barbara Ehrenreich and Annette Fuentes. "Life on the Global Assembly Line," p. 60.

26. T. K. Sundari. "Women's Camp," p. 36.

27. Wolfgang Sachs. "On the Archaeology of the Development Idea," *The Ecologist* (March/April 1990), pp. 42–43.

28. David Morris. "Free Trade: The Great Destroyer," *The Ecologist* (September/October 1990), pp. 190–95.

RESOURCES

Books

Asian and Pacific Women's Resource Collection Network. *Health*. 1990. Available from Asian and Pacific Development Centre, Kuala Lumpur, Malaysia.

Barry, Kathleen. *Female Sexual Slavery*. New York: Avon Books, 1981.

Bhagat, Mukurram. *Aspects of the Drug Industry in India*. February 1982. Available from Centre for Education and Documentation, 3, Suleman Chambers, 4 Battery Street, Bombay 400 039 India.

Boston Women's Health Book Collective. *Our Bodies, Ourselves*. List of over fourteen foreign-language editions available from BWHBC, P.O. Box 192, West Somerville, MA 02144.

Bunch, Charlotte and Roxanna Carillo. *Gender Violence: A Development and Human Rights Issue*. $5.00. Available from the Center for Women's Global Leadership, Rutgers University, 27 Clifton Avenue, New Brunswick, NJ 08903, 1991.

Center for Women's Global Leadership. *Report of the First Women's Leadership Institute*. $5.00. Available from the Center for Women's Global Leadership, 27 Clifton Avenue, New Brunswick, NJ 08903. Summarizes the discussion and findings of a two-week institute where women from twenty-three countries met to share strategies around violence against women.

El Saadawi, Nawal. *The Hidden Face of Eve*. Boston: Beacon Press, 1980.

Hardon, Anita, Sjaak van der Geest, Hanna Geerling and Amanda le Grand. *The Provision and Use of Drugs in Developing Countries*. Amsterdam: University of Amsterdam and Health Action International Europe, 1991.

Hartmann, Betsy. *Reproductive Rights and Wrongs*. New York: Harper & Row, 1987.

Hosken, Fran P. *The Childbirth Picture Book*. Available from WIN News, 187 Grant Street, Lexington, MA 02173. Available in Hindi, Gujarati, Tegulu and Bengali.

———. *The Hosken Report: Genital Mutilation and Sexual Mutilation of Females*. 1983. Available from WIN News, 187 Grant Street, Lexington, MA 02173.

———. *The Universal Childbirth Picture Book*. Available from WIN News, 187 Grant Street, Lexington, MA 02173. Available in Arabic, English, French and Spanish.

ISIS International. *Violence Against Women in Latin America and the Caribbean: A Bibliographic Catalogue*. Santiago, Chile: ISIS International, 1990.

Jacobson, Jodi. *Global Politics of Abortion*, Worldwatch Paper 97. Washington, DC: Worldwatch Institute, 1990.

Koblinsky, Marge, Judith Timyan and Jill Gay, eds. *Women's Health: A Global Perspective*. Boulder, CO: Westview Press, 1993. This book is a detailed exploration based on the 1991 Conference on Women's Health sponsored by the National Council on International Health in Washington, DC.

Matsui, Yayori. *Women's Asia*. London: Zed Books, 1987.

McClain, Carol, ed. *Women as Healers: Cross-Cultural Perspectives*. New Brunswick, NJ: Rutgers University Press, 1989.

McDonnell, Kathleen, ed. *Adverse Effects: Women and the Pharmaceutical Industry*. Toronto: Educational Press, 1986.

Newland, Kathleen. *Infant Mortality and the Health of Societies*, Worldwatch Paper 47. Washington, DC: Worldwatch Institute, 1981.

Pan American Health Organization and the American Association of Retired Persons. *Mid-Life and Older Women in Latin America and the Caribbean*. Washington, DC: 1989.

Panos Institute. *Triple Jeopardy: Women and AIDS*. 1990. Available from Panos Publications, Ltd., 9 White Lion Street, London N1 9PD, England.

Parker, Richard. *Bodies, Pleasure and Passions: Sexual Culture in Contemporary Brazil*. Boston: Beacon Press, 1991.

Petchesky, Rosalind, and Jennifer Weiner. *Global Feminist Perspectives on Reproductive Rights and Reproductive Health*. New York: Reproductive Rights Education Project, Hunter College, 1990. Selected proceedings from the IV International Congress on Women.

Rogers, Barbara. *The Domestication of Women: Discrimination in Developing Societies*. London/New York: Tavistock, 1980.

Sai, F., et al. "The Role of the World Bank in Shaping Third World Population Policy," in Godfrey Roberts, ed. *Population Policy: Contemporary Issues*. New York: Praeger, 1990.

Schuler, Margaret. *Freedom from Violence: Women's Strategies Around the World*. New York: UNIFEM, 1992. This book tells the stories of women organizing to combat gender violence in eleven developing countries and the United States.

Silverman, Lee, et al. *Prescriptions for Death: Drugging the Third World*. Berkeley: University of California Press, 1982.

Taylor, Jill, and Sheelagh Stewart. *Sexual and Domestic Violence: Help, Recovery and Action in Zimbabwe*. Harare, Zimbabwe: Women and Law in Southern Africa, 1991. Available from P.O. Box UA 171, Union Avenue, Harare, Zimbabwe. This is a practical hands-on manual for doing work in an African context.

Toubia, Nahid, ed. *Women of the Arab World: The Coming Challenge (Papers of the Arab Women's Solidarity Conference)*. London: Zed Books, 1988.

Toubia, Nahid, and Virginia Kallianes. *Information and Methodological References for Research on Unwanted Pregnancy and Abortion*. New York: The Population Council, 1991.

Turshen, Meredith. *The Politics of Public Health*. New Brunswick, NJ: Rutgers University Press, 1989.

United Nations. *Violence Against Women in the Family*. New York: United Nations, 1989. Sales No. E89.IV.5. This report synthesizes the findings of the Expert Group Meeting on Violence Against Women in the Family, held in Vienna, Austria, December 1989.

United Nations Development Programme. *Human Development Report 1990*. Oxford: Oxford University Press, 1990.

Van Esterik, Penny. *Beyond the Breast/Bottle Controversy*. New Brunswick, NJ: Rutgers University Press, 1989.

Vukani Makhosikazi Collective. *South African Women Speak*. Birmingham, England: Third World Publishers, 1985.

Werner, David. *Donde No Hay Doctor (Where There Is No Doctor)*. 1982. Available from from the Hesperian Foundation, Box 1692, Palo Alto, CA 94302. Available in Spanish, English, Portuguese, Swahili and Hindi.

Women's Global Network on Reproductive Rights: Uganda Chapter. *Report on First African Regional Meeting of Women and Health, 23–27 October, 1989*, Kampala, Uganda, 1990.

World Health Organization Regional Office for Europe. *Having a Baby in Europe, Report on a Study, Public Health in Europe 26*. Copenhagen: World Health Organization, 1985.

Wright, Martha, Zena Stein and Jean Scanlyn, eds. *Women's Health and Apartheid: The Health of Women and Children and the Future of Progressive Health Care in Southern Africa*. New York: Columbia University, Committee on Health in Southern Africa, 1988.

Articles

Bruce, Judith. "Users' Perspectives on Contraceptive Technology and Delivery Systems: Some Feminist Issues," *Technology and Society*, Vol. 9 (1987).

Bunch, Charlotte. "Women's Rights as Human Rights: Toward a Revision of Women's Rights," *Women's Health Journal*, No. 19 (July–September 1990). The *Journal* is published by ISIS in Santiago, Chile.

"Reproductive Health: A Strategy for the 1990's," a program paper of the Ford Foundation. New York: Ford Foundation, 1991.

Gay, Jill, and Tamara Underwood. "Women in Danger: A Call for Action," background paper for the 1991 National Council for International Health Conference. Available from the National Council for International Health, 2121 Virginia Avenue, Suite 303, Washington, DC 20037.

Grant, James M. "The State of the World's Children—1991." Available from the U.S. Committee for UNICEF, 331 East 38th Street, New York, NY 10016.

Hartmann, Betsy. "Population Control as Foreign Policy," *Covert Action*, No. 39 (Winter 1991–92).

Heise, Lori. "The Global War Against Women," *Washington Post* (April 9, 1989).

———. "Violence Against Women: The Missing Agenda," in *Women's Health: A Global Perspective.* Marge Koblinsky, Judith Timyan and Jill Gay, eds. Boulder, CO: Westview Press, 1992. This article outlines the dimensions of gender violence throughout the world and explores its health consequences. It outlines a five-point rationale explaining why violence against women should be taken up as an international women's health issue.

Karkal, Malini. "Abortion Laws and the Abortion Situation in India," *Issues in Reproductive and Genetic Engineering.* Vol. 4, No. 3 (1991).

———. "The Invisibility of the Girl Child in India," *The Indian Journal of Social Work*, Special Edition on the Girl Child, Vol. 52, No. 1 (January 1991).

Standing, Hilary, and Mere Kisekka. "Sexual Behavior in Sub-Saharan Africa," annotated bibliography prepared for the Overseas Development Administration, Eland House, Stag Place, London, England SW1E 5DH, April 1989.

World Health Organization. "Women's Health: Across Age and Frontier." Geneva, Switzerland: WHO, 1992. Document prepared for the 1992 World Health Assembly on women's health.

Audiovisual Materials

Abortion Stories from North and South, a 55-minute video by the National Film Board of Canada. Documentary examines abortion cross-culturally in Ireland, Japan, Thailand, Peru, Colombia and Canada. Available from the Cinema Guild, 1697 Broadway, Suite 802, New York, NY 10019.

The Double Day (Doble Jornada), a 56-minute 1975 film. The efforts of Latin American working women to achieve equality in the home and workplace—a "double day." Classic. Available from the Cinema Guild, 1697 Broadway, Suite 802, New York, NY 10019.

Global Assembly Line, a 60-minute, 16-mm film. Produced by Lorraine Gray, Anne Bohlen and Patricia Fernandez. A documentary about the impact of twin plant production on working women and their families in the United States and free trade zones of developing countries. Available from New Day Films, 121 West 27th Street, Suite 902, New York, NY 10001.

La Operación, a 40-minute 16-mm film. A powerful documentary about female sterilization abuse and economic development in Puerto Rico. In English and Spanish with subtitles. Available from the Cinema Guild, 1697 Broadway, Suite 802, New York, NY 10019.

Still Killing Us Softly: Advertising's Image of Women, a 30-minute, 16-mm 1987 film. An examination of the advertising industry's manipulation of sex roles to sell products. Available from Cambridge Documentary Films, Inc., Box 385, Cambridge, MA 02139.

The Ultimate Test Animal, a 40-minute video available in all formats. This documentary examines the history and controversy around the use of the birth control injection Depo-Provera, primarily in the United States. Available from the Cinema Guild, 1697 Broadway, Suite 802, New York, NY 10019.

Periodicals

Broadsheet
P.O. Box 56147
Auckland, New Zealand
Excellent in-depth coverage of women's health issues in New Zealand.

Healthsharing
Women Healthsharing
14 Skey Lane
Toronto, Ontario M6J 3S4 Canada
An excellent quarterly newsletter covering a wide range of women's health concerns.

Links: Health and Development Report
P.O. Box 202
New York, NY 10276
Quarterly published by the National Central American Health Rights Network (NCAHRN). Frequently covers women and health.

Manushi
C/1202 Lajpat Nagar 1
New Delhi 110024 India
A feminist magazine (*manushi* means "woman") that encourages women to write in and tell their stories as well as analyze their situations and move toward a shared understanding. Lively, interesting and sometimes very grim, as it reflects the Indian woman's often harsh reality. Published in English and Hindi, it deserves wider circulation.

Radical America
38 Union Square
Somerville, MA 02143
An excellent monthly socialist journal covering a variety of topics not exclusive to women but with a feminist perspective when women are discussed.

Sauti Ya Siti (Tanzania women's magazine)
Tanzania Media Women's Association
P.O. Box 6143
Dar es Salaam, Tanzania

SPEAK (Magazine for Women)
Office 7
Conlyn House, 17th Floor
156 Pleasant Street
Johannesburg 2001 South Africa

WIN News
Women's International Network News
187 Grant Street
Lexington, MA 02173
A quarterly covering a wide range of topics of concern, including statistical data and reports on conferences.

Organizations

(Many publish periodicals and other materials)
AAWORD
B.P. 11007
CD Annexe
Dakar, Senegal

Acción para la Liberación de la Mujer Peruana (ALI-MUPER)
A.A. 2211
Lima, Peru
An autonomous socialist–feminist group that sees women as a socially oppressed sector needing to develop their own line of action.

Asian Women's Association, English Newsletter Section
Shibuya Coop 211, 14-10, Sakaragoaka
Shibuya-ku, Tokyo, Japan 150
One of the major groups involved in campaigns against sex tourism. In their newsletter, Asian Women's Liberation, they continually bring the issue up and report on actions taking place.

Boston Women's Health Book Collective
P.O. Box 192
West Somerville, MA 02144
The Women's Health Information Center, open to the public, includes many foreign-language books, periodicals and documents, as well as English-language materials on women's international issues. Send for literature lists.

CHETNA (Centre for Health Education, Training and Nutrition Awareness)
Drive-in Cinema Building, 2nd Floor
Thaltej Road
Ahmedabad-380 053, Gujarat, India

Coletivo Feminista Sexualidade e Saude
Rua Fradique Coutinho, 316, Apt. 3112
São Paulo, SP 5416 Brazil

Committee on Women in Asian Studies (CWAS)
Asian Studies Program
University of Pittsburgh
Pittsburgh, PA 15260
Since 1971, the organization has supported research and dissemination of knowledge concerning gender in Asia and among Asians living outside of Asia. Newsletter published three times a year.

Comunicación, Intercambio y Desarrollo Humano en America Latina (CIDHAL)
Apartado 579
Cuernavaca, Morelos, Mexico
A documentation center for Latin American women, CIDHAL holds classes, publishes pamphlets on health and education for women and organizes meetings and study groups. They have also started a clinic and offer holistic approaches.

DAWN (Development Alternatives for Women in the New Era)
c/o WAND
Women's Studies
UWI Pinelands
St. Michael, Barbados

FFGZ (Feminist Women's Health Center)
Bambergerstrasse 51
1000 Berlin 30, Germany

FINRRAGE (Feminist International Network of Resistance to Reproductive and Genetic Engineering)
P.O. Box 583
London NW3 1RQ England

GELEDES Instituto de Mulher Negra
Rua Jorge Utsumi 40
Villa Sonia
São Paulo, 00519 6190 Brazil

Health Action International (HAI)
c/o International Organisation of Consumers' Unions (IOCU)
P.O. Box 1045
10830, Penang, Malaysia
An international network of consumer and professional groups whose main concern is to resist ill treatment of consumers by multinational drug companies. It produces a bimonthly newsletter.

Healthsharing Women
318 Little Bourke Street, 5th Floor
Melbourne, Australia 3000

Inter-African Committee on Traditional Health Practices Affecting Women
c/o Economic Commission for Africa, ATRCW
P.O. Box 3001
Addis Ababa, Ethiopia
or:
c/o Inter-African Committee
147, rue de Lausanne
CH-1202 Geneva, Switzerland

Interfaith Center on Corporate Responsibility (ICCR)
475 Riverside Drive
New York, NY 10027
ICCR tries to make corporations responsible for their policies. They bring stockholder resolutions to try to change policies they don't agree with. They have developed an information/action packet on the whole issue of pharmaceutical marketing in the Third World.

International Network Against Violence Against Women
878 Peachtree Street NE, Room 508
Atlanta, GA 30309

International Women's Health Coalition
24 East 21st Street, 5th Floor
New York, NY 10010
Produces in-depth analyses of women's reproductive health issues. Works with selected groups in particular Southern countries.

International Women's Rights Action Watch
Women, Public Policy and Development Project
Humphrey Institute of Public Affairs
University of Minnesota
   301 19th Avenue South
   Minneapolis, MN 55455
Publishes a regular newsletter, *The Women's Watch*.

ISIS Internacional
   Ricardo Lyon 1735
   Casilla 2067
   Cor. Central Santiago, Chile
or
ISIS International
   85-A East Maya Street
   Philamlife Homes
   Quezon City, Philippines
ISIS is an international women's information and communication service with a resource and documentation center. They provide original and in-depth feminist analyses of a wide variety of topics. Their *Women's Health Journal* is a must for feminist health activists (available in Spanish and English).

ISIS-WICCE
   3 Chemin des Campanules
   1219 Aire
   Geneva, Switzerland

Latin American and Caribbean Black Women's Network
Joselina da Silva, information coordinator
   366 Rua do Catete
   Copacabana
   Duque de Caxias, RJ 2500 Brazil

MADRE
   121 West 27th Street, Room 301
   New York, NY 10001
Peace and justice focusing on women and children in the United States and abroad; includes health.

MATCH International Centre
   200 Elgin Street, Suite 1102
   Ottawa, Ontario K2P 1L5 Canada

National Women's Health Network
   1325 G Street NW
   Washington, DC 20005
The only national membership organization devoted exclusively to women and women's health, NWHN is the "umbrella" of the U.S. women's health movement. NWHN documents international dimensions of selected women's health issues.

The Northern Israel Women's Project
   Isha L'Isha-Haifa Feminist Center
   Arlosoroff 88
   Haifa 33276 Israel
The project works to involve both Jewish and Arab women in the northern region of Israel.

Rural Women's Social Education Center
c/o Centre for Development Studies
   Aakulan Road
   Ullor Trivandrum
   Kerala 695011 India
A group of rural Indian women who meet regularly and plan literacy programs and health education programs for their respective villages.

Saheli
   Unit Above Shop
   105–108 Shopping Center
   Defense Colony Bridge (South Side)
   New Delhi 110024 India
A group of feminists working to build awareness of women's issues and rights in India. It began by organizing against dowry burnings and tortures and now covers a broad range of women's issues, including health and reproduction.

SNDT
Research Centre for Women's Studies
   Juhu Campus
   Bombay 400049 India
The unit publishes a newsletter covering feminist activities around Bombay and distributes studies they have done.

Sos Corpo
   Rua do Hospicio
   859- 4o andar, Boa Vista
   Recife, PE 50050 Brazil

Taller Salud
   Apartado 2172
   Hato Rey, PR 00919
A self-help, advocacy and activist collective that produces publications and carries out community-based health education projects.

TATA Institute of Social Sciences
Women's Studies Unit
   P.O. Box 8313
   Donear
   Bombay 400088 India

WAND
Women's Studies
   UWI Pinelands
   St. Michael, Barbados

Womanhealth Philippines
   125B Gonzales Street
   Loyola Heights
   Quezon City 1108 Philippines
One of the organizers of the 6th International Women and Health Meeting held in Manila in 1991.

Women Living Under Muslim Law
   B.P. 23
   Grabels 34790 France

Women's Action Group
   P.O. Box 135
   Harare, Zimbabwe

Women's Development Programme
   Asian and Pacific Development Center
   P.O. Box 12224
   50770 Kuala Lumpur, Malaysia
Creating a women and health documentation center as well as other women's health programs.

Women's Global Network for Reproductive Rights (WGNRR)
   NZ Voorburgwal 32
   1012RZ Amsterdam, The Netherlands

Their newsletter and annual maternal mortality campaign and reports are indispensable women's health activist resources.

Women's Global Network for Reproductive Rights
    Uganda Chapter
    Plot I 2/4, City-House
    William Street
    Kampala, Uganda

Women's Health Action Foundation (formerly Women and Pharmaceuticals Project)
    PB 4263
    1009 AG Amsterdam, The Netherlands

Publishes excellent materials on fertility regulation technologies and seeks to improve women's health services and to increase the role of women in developing health policies and programs.

Women's Health Information Resource Collective, Inc.
    P.O. Box 187
    North Carlton
    Victoria, Australia 3054
Produces excellent pamphlets and brochures on many issues. Send for a list.

INDEX